Biotechnology in Medicine and Agriculture
Principles and Practices

Biotechnology in Medicine and Agriculture

Principles and Practices

Editors

Anil Kumar

Professor and Head

Coordinator Pantnagar Biotechnology Programme

Department of Molecular Biology and Genetic Engineering

College of Basic Science and Humanities

G. B. Pant University of Agriculture and Technology, Pant Nagar

Ashwani Pareek

Associate Professor

School of Life Sciences

Jawaharlal Nehru University, New Delhi

Sanjay Mohan Gupta

Scientist

Molecular Biology and Genetic Engineering Laboratory

Defence Institute of Bio-Energy Research (DIBER), DRDO, Haldwani

I.K. International Publishing House Pvt. Ltd.

NEW DELHI • BANGALORE

Published by

I.K. International Publishing House Pvt. Ltd.
S-25, Green Park Extension
Uphaar Cinema Market
New Delhi–110 016 (India)
E-mail : info@ikinternational.com
Website: www.ikbooks.com

ISBN: 978-93-81141-40-3

Published by Krishan Makhijani for I.K. International Publishing House Pvt. Ltd., S-25, Green Park Extension, Uphaar Cinema Market, New Delhi–110 016 and Printed by Rekha Printers Pvt. Ltd., Okhla Industrial Area, Phase II, New Delhi–110 020.

Dedicated
to
our revered parents
and esteemed teachers
To
Mani-Riddhi-Siddhi
for
Mani-Riddhi-Siddhi

" सर्वमंगल मांगल्ये शिवे सर्वार्थसाधिके "

FOREWORD

Discoveries in biology, more than ever before, are today dependent on the Techniques, Tools and Technology driven by modern and sophisticated instrumentation. One can attempt to answer most difficult questions with proper methodology and powered by computational analysis and supported by the best equipment. It is therefore extremely essential that the student of modern biology is exposed to the available technologies. This not only will help to use these in their research programmes but would also help them to understand the scientific papers that are published at an exemplary pace.

I am, therefore, very happy that authors have attempted to write the book entitled "Biotechnology in Medicine and Agriculture: Principles and Practices" covering latest emerging concepts in recent-past technologies under biotechnology. Globally, biotechnology is expanding in a very big way and developing countries are also catching up in the utilization of potential of biotechnology for the socio-economic developments. In the last thirty years, a revolution has taken place that has put molecular biology and biotechnology at the heart of all the biological sciences with extensive and innovative applications in agriculture, health, industry and environment. Biotechnologists today are confronted with myriads of diagnostic, therapeutic, debatable and emerging issues. Needless to mention, all of them find an appropriate and state-of-the-art presentation in this book. Majority of biotechnology books describe the concept of molecular biology and the role of other interdisciplinary branches of the life science rather than focusing on technologies and their potential applications in medical, agriculture and industry which is the hallmark of this book. This book covers basic scientific concepts, multistaged biotechnological applications and impact of biotechnology on society. The present book covers various disciplines of biotechnology including general, plant and animal biotechnologies.

I convey my appreciation to all the contributors and to the editors in compiling this book which will be useful not only for students but also for scientists and teachers. I give my compliments to Dr. Anil Kumar and his team for compiling this valuable book and I sincerely hope that all readers will find it extremely useful.

Sudhir K. Sopory

PREFACE

Biotechnology is most exciting, challenging and promising field in the 21st century and considered to revolutionize the every walk of life. The tremendous impetus received for biotechnological research and education has been due to its direct impact on human and animal health, agricultural productivity and environmental issues. Due to increasing acceptance of genetically modified foods and agricultural produce, big pharmaceutical and agribusiness companies are investing huge funds in the biotechnology R&D sector. It is felt that the second green-blue-white revolution can be achieved only through sustained improvement in the genetic upliftment of native crops and livestock. In the last thirty years, a revolution has taken place that has put molecular biology and biotechnology at the heart of all the biological sciences with extensive applications in agriculture, health, industry and environment. However, the major problems of developing biotechnology in the developing countries are lack of skilled, trained quality human resources and availability of resource materials for quality teaching.

This textbook is an attempt to compile information about some of the biotechnological processes for their easy access at a single platform which at present, is lacking. The aim of this book is not only to bring together the various fields of biotechnology, but also to present the basic principle (in a relatively understandable form) behind each of the potential biotechnologies emerging in recent-past. Our main objective has been to present a complete view of biotechnology to students, especially those who have just ventured into this field and need a head start. In order to keep high academic standards and quality teaching, it is now mandatory to have basic and applied paradigms about the molecular biology and biotechnology amongst the graduate, postgraduate students and research scholars which will also enable them to understand the tools and techniques used for the exploration of living system.

The book has been edited and compiled to include five sections having a total of 35 chapters covering diverse technologies with their basic principles and practices so that students can develop interest and appreciate the role of biotechnology for future research and advancement of agriculture, veterinary, biomedical, industrial development and environmental protection for the welfare of mankind in particular and society, in general. Information is provided in textbook style with good illustrations which makes this book a more suitable reading material for the beginners in the area. At the same time, we also provide the updated references for further clarification and detailed information about specific topics. The flow in each chapter is uniform and logical to help the students in providing sufficient background knowledge for each technology. Each chapter begin with a set of clearly defined objectives of the technology followed by its concept with historical perspectives, details of the experimental methods, medical, veterinary, agricultural and industrial applications and finally concluding with future prospective of the technology. Many technological concepts have been made clearer with suitable illustrations and the latest information using models to help the students visualize and interpret difficult concepts. For those students who wish to pursue particular topics, a reference section at the back of the text provides chapter-by-chapter listing of review articles and articles in the original literature. The present book has been designed with an intention of covering all the potential technologies and their applications in both medicine as well as agriculture. It describes the processes and methods used to manipulate living organisms or the substances and products from these organisms for medical, agricultural, and industrial purposes. It is hoped that this textbook will serve a sort of "essential reading" for all the students of biotechnology, biochemistry, biosciences and applied microbiology, and for researchers in biotechnology industries.

At present, in India the number of companies involved in R&D or product development or production related to biotechnology and life sciences products has grown close to 350. Sustenance of these efforts, biotechnology R&D as well as education sector needs highly skilled human resources, good infrastructure and quality teaching material in the form of textbook to explain basic paradigms for inventing and creating value-added products through intervention of biotechnology. Additionally, in view of the fast expanding scope of Molecular Biology and Biotechnology, several new postgraduate programmes, non-existent a few decades ago have now been conceptualized in hundreds of public and private universities and institutes and are being opted by thousands of students. Twenty-seven agricultural universities now offer Biotechnology teaching programmes either at graduate and/or postgraduate level, some of which offer both Animal Biotechnology and Plant/Agricultural Biotechnology & Molecular Biology Programmes. In addition, various Bioinformatics programme are also being offered in few institutions. Department of Biotechnology, Ministry of Science & Technology supports PG Biotechnology programmes at 67 places out of which ten are agricultural universities. Keeping these developments in view, there is an absolute need of good quality textbooks for both UG and PG programmes in 'Molecular Biology and Biotechnology'. The contents of the book cover syllabus for many of the courses being offered in different programmes in Molecular Biology & Biotechnology at national and international level. In India, the curricula of the programmes have been revised by Department of Biotechnology and Indian Council of Agricultural Research, Govt. of India, New Delhi keeping in view the advances in the respective subject area. Accordingly, contents of the present book have been modified to make them contemporary.

The Editors are thankful to Hon'ble Vice Chancellors Professor B. S. Bisht (GBPUAT) and Professor Sudhir K. Sopory (JNU), for their consistent support and guidance to work in directional manner. Dr. B. R. K. Gupta, Dean, College of Basic Sciences & Humanities, has been the main source of inspiration for bringing this book in the present shape. It would have been impossible together all the information and data required for this book without the valuable assistance of our colleagues and our friends from other institute. We are highly indebted to them for their kind cooperation and help at each step. We are thankful to several of our Master's and Doctoral's students who have helped us to put thoughts together in this book. We especially express thanks to our students Mr. Rajhans Tyagi, Mr. Alok Kumar Gupta, Mr. Manoj Singh, Mr. Netrapal Sharma, Ms. Sanveen Kaur, Ms. Sadhna Singh, Dr. Vikram S. Gaur, Dr. Arti Gupta, Dr. Dinesh Pandey, Dr. Gohar Taj, Dr. Supriya Gupta, Dr. Sumita Kumari, Dr. Brijesh Gupta, Mr. Kamlesh K. Nutan, Preeti Teotia, Amit Tripathy, Ajit Ghosh and Jyoti Mallik for their contribution. The efforts put by one of student Atul Kumar Gupta who really worked day and nights for bringing this book in the present form are highly appreciative. We also express heartfelt thanks to our families who always stood by us for providing every kind of support and not expressing their suffering for the cause of student's community. Last but not the least, contributions of Dr. Sneh L. Singla-Pareek (ICGEB) during the stage of proofreading is highly appreciated.

Finally, the authors solicit suggestions for further improvement of this book from the instructors, student and any other person who may be interested in promoting this discipline.

Anil Kumar
Ashwani Pareek
Sanjay Mohan Gupta

ABBREVIATIONS

AA	Acrylic acid
ABS	Alkyl benzyl sulfonate
ADA	Adenosine deaminase
AFLP	Amplified fragment length polymorphism
AFM	Atomic Force Microscopy
AHL	Acryl homoserine lactone
AIV	Avian influenza virus
AK	Aspartokinase
AM	Acrylamide
AMD	Age related Macular Degeneration
Amp–B	Amphotericin–B
AmpR	Ampicillin resistance
ANF	Atrial natriuretic factor
APC	Adenomatous polyposis coli
APCI	Atmospheric pressure chemical ionization
APPI	Atmospheric pressure photoionization
APS	Adenosine phosphosulfate
ARMS	Amplification refractory mutation system
ASO	Allele specific oligonucleotide
asRNA	Antisense RNA
ATPase	Adenosine triphosphatase
AVR	Acute vascular rejection
BAC	Bacterial Artificial Chromosome
BCG	Bacillus Calmette Guerin
bFGF	Basic fibroblast growth factor
BGTC	Bis (guanidinium)-tren-cholesterol
BILs	Backcross Inbred Lines
BLB	Bacterial leaf blight
BMA	Butyl methacrylate

BMPs	Bone morphogenetic proteins
BNF	Biological Nitrogen Fixation
BOD	Biological oxygen demand
Bp	Base pairs
BSA	Bovine serum albumin
BSE	Bovine spongiformis encephalopathy
BST	Bovine somatotrophin
BVDV	Bovine viral diarrhea virus
BYDV	Barley yellow dwarf virus
cad	Cinnamyl aldehyde dehydrogenase
CAEV	Caprine arthritis-encephalitis virus
CaMV	Cauliflower mosaic virus
CAPS	Cleaved Amplified Polymorphic Sequences
CBESC	Cord blood-derived embryonic like stem cells
CCD	Charge-coupled device
ccr	Cinnamoyl CoA reductase
CD	Circular Dichroism
cDNA	Complementary DNA
CDV	Canine distemper virus
CEA	Carcinoembryonic antigen
CEC	Corneal endothelial cells
CF	Cystic fibrosis
CFTR	Cystic fibrosis transmembrane regulator
CGA	Colletotrichum gloeosporioides f. sp. aeschynomene
CGH	Comparative Genomic Hybridization
CHI	Chalcone isomerases
ChIP	Chromatin Immunoprecipitation
CHS	Chalcone synthase
CHV	Canine herpesvirus
CI	Chemical ionization
CIM	Composite interval mapping
CIRB	Central Institute for Research on Buffalo
CL	Corpora lutea
CLEA	Cross linked enzyme aggregates
CLEG	Cross linked enzyme crystals
CLSD	Cross linked spray dried enzyme
cM	Centimorgans
Cm^R	Chloramphenicol resistance
CMR	Continuous flow membrane reactor
CNS	Central nervous system
CNTs	Carbon nanotubes
Con A	Concanavalin A
COPD	Chronic Obstructive Pulmonary Disease
COS	Conserved orthologous set

CpDNA	Chloroplast DNA
CPV	Canine parvovirus
CRR	Centromeric retrotransposons
CsA	Cyclosporine A
CSC	Cancer stem cells
CSF	Cerebrospinal fluid
CSSLs	Chomosomal Segment Substitution Lines
CSTR	Continuous flow stirred tank reactor
CSTRs	Continuous stirred tank reactor
CTB	Cholera toxin B subunit
CYP	Cytochrome P450
2,3-DPG	2,3-Diphosphoglycerate
3D	Three dimensional
DAB	Diaminobutane
DART	Direct analysis in real time
DARTT	DNA Amplification-restricted Transcription Translation
DCA	3, 4-dichloroaniline
DDT	1,1,1- Trichloro-2,2-bis[4-chlorophenyl]ethane
DEAE	Di ethyl amino ethyl
DESI	Desorption electrospray ionization
DFMs	Direct functional markers
DFR	Dihydroflavonol 4-reductase
DGGE	Denaturing gradient gel electrophoresis
DHDPS	Dihydrodipicolinic acid synthase
dHFR	Dihydrofolate reductase
DHPLC	Denaturing high-performance liquid chromatography
DIMS	Direct infusion mass spectrometry
DMAEMA	Dimethylaminoethyl methacrylate
DMS	Dimethyl sulfate
DMSO	Dimethyl sulphoxide
DNA	Deoxyribo nucleic acid
dNTPs	Deoxynucleoside triphosphates
DOPE	Dioleoylphosphatidylethanolamine
DOPG	Direct oxidation pathway of glucose
DOTMA	Dioleoyl-propyl-trimethylammonium
DOXP	Deoxyxylulose-5-phosphate
dPAGE	Discontinuous polyacrylamide gel electrophoresis
DR	Direct repeat
DRRV	Dog-related rabies virus
dRT-PCR	Duplex reverse transcription-polymerase chain reaction
DUS	Distinctness, uniformity, and stability
eCG	Equine chorionic gonadotropin
ECM	Extracellular matrix
EDC	Endocrine Disrupting Chemicals

EESI	Extractive Electro-spray Ionization
EGCs	Embryonic germ cells
EGDMA	Ethyleneglycol bismethacrylate
EI	Electron ionization
ELISA	Enzyme-linked immunosorbent assay
EMBL	European Molecular Biology Laboratory
EMS	Ethyl methane sulfonate
EMSA	Electrophoretic Mobility Shift Assay
ENFET	Enzyme Field Effect Transistor
ePCR	Electronic PCR
EPR	Enhanced Permeability and Retention
EPSPS	Enzyme 5-enol pyruvyl shikimate-3-phosphate synthase
ES	Embryonic stem
ESCs	Embryonic stem cells
ESI	Electrospray ionization
ESTs	Expressed Sequence Tags"
ET	Embryo transfer
ETEC	Enterotoxigenic *E. coli*
ETT	Embryo transfer technology
f5h	Ferulate 5-hydroxylase
FACS	Fluorescence assisted cell sorter
FAV	Fowl adenovirus
FBR	Fluidised bed reactor
FGF	Fibroblast growth factor
FIA	Flow-injection analysis
FISH	Fluorescent *in situ* hybridization
FMDV	Foot-and-mouth disease virus
FMs	Functional markers
FN3	Fibronectin type III domain
FSH	Follicle stimulating hormone
FT-ICR	Fourier transform ion cyclotron resonance
FTIR	Fourier Transform Infrared
FUE	Fertilizer Use Efficiency
GA	Gluconic acid
GADH	Gluconate dehydrogenase
GAG	Glycosaminoglycans
GALT	Gut associated lymphoid tissue
GC	Gas chromatography
GC-MS	Gas chromatography-mass spectrophotometry
GDH	Glucose dehydrogenase
GEO	Gene Expression Omnibus
GGDP	Geranyl geranyl diphosphate
GISH	Genomic *in situ* Hybridization
GMMs	Genic Molecular Markers

GMOs	Genetically Modified Organisms
GnRH	Gonadotrophin releasing hormone
GO	Gene ontology
GPCR PD	G-Protein Coupled Receptor Proteome Database
GTMs	Gene-targeted markers
GV	Gemini virus
GWS	Genome-wide selection
HA	Hemagglutination assay
HAR	Hyperacute rejection
HBED	N,N'-bis[2-hydroxybenzyl]-ethylene-diamine-N,N'-diacetic
HbsAg	Hepatitis B surface antigen
HBV	Hepatitis B virus
HCEC	Human donor-derived corneal endothelial cells
HCPro	Helper-component proteinase
HCV	Hepatitis C virus
HFCS	High-fructose corn syrup
HGP	Human Genome Project
HGPRT	Hypoxanthine-quinine phosphoribosy1 transferase
Hib	Haemophilus influenzae type b
HILIC	Hydrophilic interaction chromatography
HIV	Human immune deficiency virus
HIV-1	Human immunodeficiency virus type 1
hMADS	Human multipotent adipose derived stem cells
HN	Haemagglutinin-neuraminidase
HPLC	High performance liquid chromatography
HPRT	Hypoxanthine Phosphorisyl Transferase
HPSD	Human Proteome Survey Database
HPT	Hygromycin B phosphotransferase
HR	Hypersensitive response
HSF	Heat-shock transcription factor
HSV	Herpes simplex virus hour post-infection (HPI)
HUGO	Human Genome Organization
HuMAbs	Human monoclonal antibodies
HVRs	Hypervariable regions
IBD	Infectious bursal disease
IBDV	Infectious bursal disease viruses
IBV	Infectious bronchitis virus
ICAT	Isotope-coded affinity tag
ICM	Integrated Crop Management
IETS	International Embryo Transfer Society
IFMs	Indirect functional markers
iGEM	International Genetically Engineered Machines
IGF-II	Insulin like growth factor II
ILT	Infections laryngotracheitis

Indels	Insertion-deletion
IPF	Idiopathic Pulmonary Fibrosis
IPG	Immobilized pH gradient
IPR	Intellectual Property Right
iPS	Induced Pluripotent stem
ISH	*In situ* hybridization
ISS	Immune Stimulatory Sequences
IST	Induced systemic tolerance
IUPAC	International Union of Pure and Applied Chemistry
IVF	*In vitro* fertilization
IVM/IVF	*In vitro* maturation/ *in vitro* fertilization
IVRI	Indian Veterinary Research Institute
JEV	Japanese Encephalitis Virus
KA	Potassium acrylate
K_A	Affinity constant
KGA	ketogluconic acids
KLH	Keyhole Limpet Haemocyanin
KOs	Knockouts
LA	Linear array
LBA	Line blot assay
LC	Liquid chromatograpy
LD	Linkage Disequilibrium
LDLs	Low-Density Lipoproteins
LDTD	Laser diode thermal desorption
LEA	Late embryogenesis abundant
LGC-1	Low Glutelin Content-1
LH	Luteinizing hormone
LILA	Liposome immune lyses assay
LiPA	Line probe assay
LKR/SDH	Lysine-ketoglutarate reductase/saccharophine
LMOs	Living Modified Organisms
LMPCR	Ligation mediated Polymerase chain reaction
LOPU	Laparoscopic aided ovum pick-up
LOX	Lactate oxidase
LRR	Leucine Rich Repeat
LT	Labile toxin
LTRs	Long terminal repeats
LUV	Large unilamellar vesicle
MAB	Marker-assisted-breeding
MABC	Marker-assisted backcrossing
MAC	Mycobacterium avium complex
MALDI-TOF	Matrix-assisted laser desorption/ionization time-of-flight
MAML	Microarray Markup Language
MAP	Modified atmosphere packaging

MARS	Marker assisted recurrent selection
MAS	Marker assisted selection
MCMC	Markov Chain Monte Carlo
MCS	Multiple Cloning Site
MD	Muscular Dystrophy
MDV	Marek's disease viruses
MFA	Metabolite/metabolic flux analysis
MGED	Microarray Gene Expression Database
MGMT	O-6-methylguanine-DNA methyltransferase
MIM	Multiple interval mapping
MLPA	Multiplex ligation-dependent probe amplification
MLST	Multilocus sequence typing
MLV	Multilamellar vesicle
MoAbs	Monoclonal antibodies
MPB	Methane-producing bacteria
MPC	Multipotent progenitor cell
mPCR	Multiplex PCR
MRP	Moroccan Rock Phosphate
MS	Mass spectrometry
MSAD	Microgravity Science and Applications Division
MSCs	Mesenchymal stem cells
MSW	Municipal solid waste
MVA	Modified Vaccinia Ankara
MVV	Multivesicular vesicle
NAAT	Nicotianamine aminotransferase
NAGase	N-acetylglucosaminidase
NASA	National Aeronautics and Space Administration
nat-si	Natural antisense siRNAs
NBS	Nucleotide Binding Site
NDDB	National Dairy Development Board
NDRI	National Dairy Research Institute
NDV	Newcastle disease virus
NEB	New England Biolabs
NIF	Nitrogen fixing genes
NIH	National institute of health
NII	National Institute of Immunology
NILs	Near isogenic lines
NIR	Near Infrared
NMR	Nuclear magnetic resonance
nPCR	Nested PCR
NPDES	National Pollutant Discharge Elimination System
NPK	Nitrogen, phosphorous and potassium
nt	Nucleotides
NT	Nuclear transfer

OAS	O-acyl serine sulphydrase
ODAP	N-oxalyl, L-diamino propionic acid
ODNs	Oligodeoxynucleotides
omt	O-methyltransferase
ori	Origin of replication
P	Phosphoprotein
PAA	Poly (acrylic acid)
PAAC	Polyacrylamide-chitosan
PAAK	Potassium poly acrylate
PAC	P1 derived Artificial Chromosome
PAM	Polyacrylamide
PAN	Poly (N-isopropylacrylamide)-chitosan polyacrylonitrile
PBR	Packed bed reactor
PC	Phytochelatin
PCBs	Polychlorinated biphenyls
PCL	Polycaprolactone
PCMC	Protein coated micro crystals
PCR	Polymerase chain reaction
PD	Parkinson's disease
PDEAAm	Poly (N,N-diethylacrylamide)
PDEAEM	Poly (N,N, 9 -diethylaminoethyl methacrylate)
PDV	phocine distemper virus
PEBBLE	Probes Encapsulated by Biologically Localized Embedding
PEO	Poly (ethylene oxide)
PEPC	Phosphoenol pyruvate carboxylase
PERVs	Porcine endogenous retroviruses
PFC	Perfluorocarbons
PFR	Plug -flow reactor
PG	Polygalacturonase
PGA	Polyglycolic acid
PGPR	Plant Growth Promoting Rhizobacteria
PGRS	Polymorphic GC rich repeat sequence
PGS	Poly (glycerol–sebacate)
PHAs	Polyhydroxyalkanoates
PHB	Polyhydroxybutyrate
pHEMA	Poly(2-hydroxyethyl methacrylate)
PIC	Polymorphic information content
PKU	Phenylketonuria
PLGA	Poly (lactic-co-glycolic acid)
PLLA	Polylactic acid
PM/MM	Perfect Match/Mismatch
PMO	Phosphorodiamidate morpholino oligomers
PMT	Photo-multiplicator tube
PNA	Peptide nucleic acid

PNIPAAm	Poly (N-isopropylacrylamide)
PPi	Inorganic pyrophosphate
PPO	Poly(propylene oxide)
PPR	Peste des petitsruminants
PRSV	Papaya ring spot virus
PTAC	Polyvinyl alcohol–tetraethylorthosilicate–alginate–calcium oxide
PTGS	Post-transcriptional gene silencing
PTMCLA	Poly (trimethylene carbonate–co-lactide)
PUFA	polyunsaturated fatty acids
QCM	Quartz crystal microbalance
QDs	Quantum dots
QPM	Quality protein maize
QPSO	Quantum behaved particle swarm optimization
QTLs	Quantitative Trait Loci
QTMFs	Quantitative trait modifying factors
RACE	Rapid Amplification of cDNA Ends
RAMP	Randomly Amplified Microsatellite Polymorphism
RAPD	Random Amplified Polymorphic DNA
RCA	Rolling circle amplification
RCRA	Resource Conservation Recovery Act
RDMs	Random DNA Markers
RES	Reticuloendothelial system
RF	Radio frequency
RFLPs	Restriction Fragment Length Polymorphisms
RGHP	Resistance Gene Homologue Polymorphism
rhEPO	Human recombinant erythropoietin
RI	Refractive index
RIA	Radioimmunoassay
rif^R	Rifampicin resistance
RISC	RNA-induced silencing complex
RLB	Reverse line blot hybridization
RLC	Risc loading complex
RLS	Resonance Light Scattering
RN	Rendment Napole
RNAi	RNA Interference
RNB	Reverse northern blotting
ROS	Reactive oxygen species
RP	Rinderpest
rRNA	Ribosomal RNA
RSC	Respiratory syncytial virus
RSV	Rous sarcoma virus
RT	Reverse Transcribed
RT-PCR	Reverse transcription-polymerase chain reaction
SAGE	Serial analysis of gene expression

SAHH	S-adenosyl homocysteine hydrolase
SAM	Self Assembled Monolayer
SAPs	Superabsorbent polymers
SBH	Sequencing by hybridization
SCAR	Sequence characterized amplified region
SCNT	Somatic Cell Nuclear Transfer
SCP	Single Cell Protein
SCS	Stem cell science
SDA	Strand displacement amplification
SDS	Sodium dodecyl sulphate
SEGE	Serial Expression of Gene Expression
SELDI	Surface enhanced laser desorption ionization
SELEX	Systematic Evolution of Ligands by Exponential
SEM	Scanning electron microscopy
SEPTIC	Sensing of Phage-Treggered Ion Cascade
SF-ANOVA	Single factor analysis of variance
SH	Subtractive hybridization
SIM	Simple interval mapping
SIP	Selective infective phage
siRNA	Small interfering RNA
SLE	Systematic Lupas Erythematosus
SMBL	Systems Biology Modeling Language
SNP	Single Nucleotide Polymorphism
SOD	Superoxide dismutase
SPM	Scanning Probe Microscope
SPR	Surface Plasmon Resonance
SPS	Sucrose phosphate synthase
SRAP	Sequence-Related Amplified Polymorphism
SSB	Single Strand DNA Binding proteins
SSCP	Single-strand Conformation Polymorphism
ssDNA	Single-stranded DNA
SSLP	Simple Sequence Length Polymorphism
SSRs	Simple Sequence Repeats
ST	Stable toxin
STEM	Scanning Tunnel Electron Microscopy
STMS	Sequence tagged microsatellite site
STR	Short tandem repeat
STR	Stirred tank batch reactor
STS	Sequence Tagged Sites
STS	Silver thiosulfate
SUV	Small unilamellar vesicle
SV40	Simian virus 40
SVDV	Swine vesicular disease virus
TAD	Tissue Array Database

TAM	Tamoxifen
TASP	Template-assembled synthetic proteins
TCAB	3, 3' 4, 4'-tetrachloroazobenzene
TCPs	Tissue culture polystyrene dishes
TCS	Transmembrane Carrier System
TEL	Telomere sequences
TEM	Transmission electron microscopy
TEMED	N,N'-tetramethyl ethylene diamine
TGEV	Transmissible gastroenteritis virus
TGF-â1	Transforming growth factor beta
TILLING	Targetting Induced Local Lesions In Genomes
TK	Thymidine kinase
TLRs	Toll-like receptors
TMA	Transcription-mediated amplification
TMP	Trimethoprime
TMV	Tobacco mosaic virus
tPA	Tissue plasminogen activator
TPH	Tissue print hybridization
TRAP	Target Region Amplification Polymorphism
T-RFLP	Terminal-Restriction Fragment Length
TRP-2	Tyrosine-related protein-2
TTHA	Triethylenetetraamine hexaacetic acid
UC	Umbilical cord
UCB	Umbilical cord blood
USSC	Unrestricted somatic stem cells
UTRs	Un-translated regions
VAM	Vesicular Arbuscular Mycorrhiza
VEGF	Vascular Endothelial Growth Factor
VH	Heavy-chain variable region
VIGS	Viral Induced Gene Silencing
VIP	Vasoactive intestinal peptide
VL	Light-chain variable region
VLP	Virus-like particles
VNTR	Variable number of tandem repeat
VPBA	Vinyl phenyl boronic acid
VSV	Vesicular Stomatitis virus
WCIMV	White colour mosaic virus
Y2H	Yeast two-hybrid
YAC	Yeast Artificial Chromosomes

CONTRIBUTORS

Alok Kumar Gupta	Department of Molecular Biology & Genetic Engineering, C.B.S.H, G. B. Pant University of Agriculture & Technology, Pantnagar-263145
Ambika Gupta	25, Mahendra Puri Colony, Near Girl's Polytechnic, Gwalior Road, Jhansi
Anil Kumar	Department of Molecular Biology & Genetic Engineering, C.B.S.H, G. B. Pant University of Agriculture & Technology, Pantnagar-263145
Annapurna, K.	Division of Microbiology, Indian Agricultural Research Institute, New Delhi-110012
Ashok Kumar	Department of Biological Sciences and Bioengineering, Indian Institute of Technology, Kanpur-208016
Ashwani Pareek	Stress Physiology and Molecular Biology Laboratory, School of Life Sciences, Jawaharlal Nehru University, New Delhi-110067
Atul Kumar Gupta	Department of Molecular Biology & Genetic Engineering, C.B.S.H, G. B. Pant University of Agriculture & Technology, Pantnagar-263145
B. M. Prasanna	CIMMYT (International Maize and Wheat Improvement Center), ICRAF House, United Nations Avenue, Gigiri, Nairobi, Kenya
Chanchal Acharya	Department of Microbiology, C.B.S.H, G. B. Pant University of Agriculture & Technology, Pantnagar-263145
Deepa Bisht	Department of Biochemistry, National JALMA Institute for Leprosy & Other Mycobacterial Diseases, Agra-282001
Dhiraj Kumar Ray	H.C.S.T., Rarah, Mathura, (UP)
Dinesh Pandey	Department of Molecular Biology & Genetic Engineering, C.B.S.H, G. B. Pant University of Agriculture & Technology, Pantnagar-263145
Gita Satpathy	Ocular Microbiology, Dr R. P. Centre for Ophthalmic Sciences, All India Institute of Medical Sciences, Ansari Nagar, New Delhi-110029
Gohar Taj	Department of Molecular Biology & Genetic Engineering, C.B.S.H, G. B. Pant University of Agriculture & Technology, Pantnagar-263145

Hemant R. Kushwaha	Center for Computational Biology and Bioinformatics, School of Information Technology, Jawaharlal Nehru University, New Delhi-110067
Indira Ghosh	Stress Physiology and Molecular Biology Laboratory, School of Life Sciences, Jawaharlal Nehru University, New Delhi-110067
Indu Shekhar Thakur	School of Environment Sciences, Jawaharlal Nehru University, New Delhi-110067
J. P. Jaiswal	Department of Genetics & Plant Breeding College of Agriculture, G. B. Pant University of Agriculture & Technology, Pantnagar-263145
K. Premalatha	Department of Microbiology, C.B.S.H, G. B. Pant University of Agriculture & Technology, Pantnagar-263145
K. N. Singh	Department of Plant Molecular Biology and Genetic Engineering, Narendra Dev University of Agriculture and Technology, Kumarganj, Faizabad-224229, (UP)
Meenal Rathore	Plant Biotechnology, Directorate of Weed Science Research, Adhartal, Jabalpur-482004, Madhya Pradesh
Manoj Prasad	National Institute for Plant Genome Research (NIPGR); Aruna Asaf Ali Marg, New Delhi-110067
Manoj Singh	Department of Molecular Biology & Genetic Engineering, C.B.S.H, G. B. Pant University of Agriculture & Technology, Pantnagar-263145
Mumtesh Kumar Saxena	Animal Biotechnology Section, College of Veterinary and Animal Sciences, G. B. Pant University of Agriculture & Technology, Pantnagar-263145
N. K. Singh	Department of Genetics & Plant Breeding College of Agriculture, G. B. Pant University of Agriculture & Technology, Pantnagar-263145
Neeti Sanan-Mishra	Plant Molecular Biology, International Center for Genetic Engineering and Biotechnology, Aruna Asaf Ali Marg, New Delhi-110067
Neha R. Tomar	Department of Molecular Biology & Genetic Engineering, C.B.S.H, G. B. Pant University of Agriculture & Technology, Pantnagar-263145
Pallavi Shah	Department of Molecular Biology & Genetic Engineering, C.B.S.H, G. B. Pant University of Agriculture & Technology, Pantnagar-263145
Partha Roy	Department of Biotechnology, Indian Institute of Technology, Roorkee-247667
Pradipto Mukhopadhyay	Plant Molecular Biology, International Centre for Genetic Engineering and Biotechnology, Aruna Asif Ali Marg, New Delhi-110067
Rohit Joshi	Stress Physiology and Molecular Biology Laboratory, School of Life Sciences, Jawaharlal Nehru University, New Delhi-110067
Rajiv Kumar	Animal Biotechnology Section, C.S.W.R.I., Avikanagar, Rajasthan
Rashmi Singh	Department of Veterinary Microbiology, College of Veterinary and Animal Sciences, G. B. Pant University of Agriculture & Technology, Pantnagar-263145
Ratna Karan	Stress Physiology and Molecular Biology Laboratory, School of Life Sciences, Jawaharlal Nehru University, New Delhi-110067
Ravindra Soni	Department of Microbiology, C.B.S.H, G. B. Pant University of

	Agriculture & Technology, Pantnagar-263145
Reeta Goel	Department of Microbiology, C.B.S.H, G. B. Pant University of Agriculture & Technology, Pantnagar-263145
R. S. Sangwan	Department of Metabolic and Structural Biology, Central Institute of Medicinal and Aromatic Plants, P.O.-CIMAP, Near Kukrail Picnic Spot, Lucknow-226015,
S. K. Khare	Department of Chemistry and Biochemistry, Indian Institute of Technology, New Delhi
S. K. Sopory	Plant Molecular Biology, International Centre for Genetic Engineering and Biotechnology, Aruna Asif Ali Marg, New Delhi-110067
Sameer Shrivastava	Division of Animal Biotechnology Indian Veterinary Research Institute, Izatnagar-243122
Shaili Srivastava	School of Environment Sciences, Jawaharlal Nehru University, New Delhi-110067
Shiv Prasad	Animal Reproduction, Gynaecology & Obstetrics, College of Veterinary and Animal Sciences, G. B. Pant University of Agriculture & Technology, Pantnagar-263145
Smita Rastogi	Department of Biotechnology, Integral University, Kursi Road, Lucknow-226026
Sanjay Gupta	Department of Biotechnology, SBS PG Institute of Biomedical Sciences, Balawala, Dehradun
Sanjay Mohan Gupta	Molecular Biology and Genetic Engineering Laboratory, Defence Institute of Bio-Energy Research (DIBER), DRDO, Haldwani-263139
Sarika Gupta	National Institute for Plant Genome Research (NIPGR); Aruna Asaf Ali Marg, New Delhi-110067
Satish Kumar	Division of Animal Biotechnology Indian Veterinary Research Institute, Izatnagar-243122
Satyanarayana, T.	Department of Microbiology, University of Delhi, South Campus, New Delhi-110021
Sneh L. Singla-Pareek	Plant Molecular Biology, International Centre for Genetic Engineering and Biotechnology, Aruna Asif Ali Marg, New Delhi-110067
Senthil Kumar, M.	Radiation Application Research Division, Advanced Radiation Technology Institute, Korean Atomic Energy Research Institute, Sinjeong, Jeongeup, 580-185, Republic of Korea
Soma S. Marla	Division of National Genomic Resource Centre, National Bureau of Plant Genetic Resources, Indian Council of Plant Genetic Resources, New Delhi-110012
Sonal	Division of Animal Biotechnology Indian Veterinary Research Institute, Izatnagar-243122
Sumona Karjee	Plant Molecular Biology, International Center for Genetic Engineering and Biotechnology, Aruna Asaf Ali Marg, New Delhi-110067
Sunil K. Mukherjee	Plant Molecular Biology, International Center for Genetic Engineering and Biotechnology, Aruna Asaf Ali Marg, New Delhi-110067
Supriya Gupta	Department of Molecular Biology & Genetic Engineering, C.B.S.H,

	G. B. Pant University of Agriculture & Technology, Pantnagar-263145
Sumrita Bhat	Department of Biological Sciences and Bioengineering, Indian Institute of Technology, Kanpur-208016
Swati Srivastava	Department of Biotechnology, Indian Institute of Technology, Roorkee-247667
Tapas Kumar Ghose	Department of Botany, Bose Institute, 93/1, A. P. C. Road, Kolkata-700009
U. N. Dwivedi	Department of Biochemistry, University of Lucknow, Lucknow-226007
V. Suresh	Division of National Genomic Resource Centre, National Bureau of Plant Genetic Resources, Indian Council of Plant Genetic Resources, New Delhi-110012
Vikram S. Gaur	Department of Molecular Biology & Genetic Engineering, C.B.S.H, G. B. Pant University of Agriculture & Technology, Pantnagar-263145
Vikrant Gupta	Genetic Resources and Biotechnology Division, Central Institute of Medicinal and Aromatic Plants, Lucknow-226015
Vineeta Singh	Department of Molecular Biology & Genetic Engineering, C.B.S.H, G. B. Pant University of Agriculture & Technology, Pantnagar-263145

CONTENTS

SECTION B: BIOTECHNOLOGY FOR CROP APPLICATIONS

SECTION D: BIOTECHNOLOGY FOR INDUSTRIAL APPLICATIONS

EDITORS

Anil Kumar is presently working as Professor & Head since 2006 and was also Incharge since 2004 in the Department of Molecular Biology & Genetic Engineering and actively involved in teaching and research since last 25 years. Based on his meritorious services for the cause of teaching and research he has been given the responsibility of Coordinator, Human Resource Development in Agricultural Biotechnology, Coordinator, Sub-DIC in Bioinformatics and Co-coordinator in Programme Mode Support in Agricultural Biotechnology funded by Department of Biotechnology, Govt. of India., New Delhi. He has published more than 80 research papers in reputed national and international journals, around 50 popular articles and book chapters and seven books to his credit. He was involved in teaching since last more than 20 years as demonstrator, JRO and Lecturer in Medical Institutions till 1993. Further, he joined back to his alma mater in Plant Biotechnology research group at Pantnagar and was involved in signal transduction research in relation to host-pathogen interaction taking Karnal bunt-wheat and *Alternaria* blight-*Brassica* as a model system. He is engaged on three aspects of molecular plant pathology i.e., plant disease surveillance through molecular diagnostics, pathogen indexing programme through molecular pathotyping and characterization of disease resistance and pathogenesis through molecular signalling investigating the role of MAP kinases and Cystatin gene families as candidate genes. He visited the University of Jerusalem, Rehovot as FAO Fellow during 2000-2001. Anil has also visited USA under World Bank-NATP programme during 2004-05 and worked on molecular characterization and cloning of transcription factors for investigating its role in carbon and nitrogen metabolism. Currently, he is involved in the identification of potential candidate and/or master regulator genes associated with carbon and nitrogen metabolism as well as calcium accumulation in finger millet with the intention to explore the seed biology for development of nutraceuticals. Based on his long experience, Anil is developing animal cell culture facilities for production of hybridoma and cell culture based assays which can be used for screening pharmaceutically important molecules for re-inventing the old principles of Auyrvedic biology into newer perspectives. Anil has also been awarded the 'Shiksha Rattan', 'Scientist of Excellence Award' and Member of National Academy of Sciences India for his meritorious services to the cause of biotechnology education and research.

Ashwani Pareek was born in New Delhi, India, in 1969. Currently, he is an Associate Professor of Life Sciences at the Jawaharlal Nehru University (JNU), New Delhi. He obtained his B.Sc. (Botany) and M.Sc. (Plant Molecular Biology) in 1990 and 1992, respectively, from the University of Delhi, India. He was introduced to the exciting field of *Stress Physiology* and *Molecular Biology* of plants during his Master's thesis and his Ph.D. research work under the guidance of Professor Anil Grover at the Department of Plant Molecular Biology, University of Delhi South Campus (UDSC), New Delhi. His research work during Ph.D. focused on the analysis of heat shock proteins (HSPs, especially HSP90) and salt stress proteins (SSPs) in rice. After completing his Ph.D. in 1997, he worked at the laboratory of Professor Ralph S. Quatrano, at the University of North Carolina, Chapel Hill, NC, USA to learn "advanced plant molecular biology." In 1998, he joined the laboratory of Professor Deepak Pental as a Research Scientist at Delhi University to work on herbicide tolerant *Brassica juncea*. Soon thereafter, he was appointed as a Lecturer at the newly established GGS Indraprastha University, New Delhi, India, where he played a key role in establishing the School of Biotechnology. After serving this university for four years, he was appointed, in 2003, on the faculty of the School of Life Sciences (SLS) at JNU. The main focus of his research has been towards an understanding of the signaling machinery in plants operative under osmotic stresses such as salinity and drought. He uses the tools of functional genomics, transgenics, bioinformatics and metabolomics to dissect out the cascades of events leading to these stresses in plants, especially the steps involved in "osmosensing". During this period of research, he has highly benefited from collaborations with laboratories of Professor Hans Bohnert (at the University of Illinois at Urbana-Champaign, Illinois, USA), and Professor Roger A. Leigh (University of Cambridge, UK). Ashwani's honors include: the Indian National Science Academy (INSA)-ROYAL SOCIETY (UK) exchange visitor's fellowship 2005 (to work at University of Cambridge, UK); the BOYSCAST Fellowship by Ministry of Science and Technology, Government of India (2001); award of "The Rockefeller Foundation" Post-doctoral fellowship in the area of advanced 'Plant Molecular Biology' as a part of the 'Rice Biotechnology Program' to work in the laboratory of Professor Ralph S. Quatrano. He has been awarded Associateship from National Academy of Agricultural Sciences (NAAS) and he is also nominated a member of National Academy of Sciences, India (NASI).

Sanjay Mohan Gupta did his Masters in Biotechnology from School of Biotechnology, Devi Ahilya University, Indore in 1999 and was ranked second in the university. In his Master's dissertation, he worked on enzyme immobilization technology and developed an indigenous bed-reactor using brick dust immobilized CM-Cellulase enzyme isolated from Cowpea (*Vigna sinensis* L.). He did his Ph.D. degree in Biochemistry in 2007 from University of Lucknow, Lucknow and worked on genetic manipulation of banana fruit ripening. He has isolated and characterized ethylene regulated and ripening related 27 novel genes from banana pulp tissue by differential-display (DDRT-PCR) method and also studied ethylene biosynthesis, respiratory climacteric and activities of the various ripening related enzymes during ripening in banana. In his professional career, he has been working as senior scientist at Defence Institute of Bio-energy Research (DIBER) since 2004. He is involved in research project funded by DRDO and investigating the isolation and characterization of cold tolerant genes from the high altitude indigenous cold tolerant Seabuckthorn (*Hippophae salicifolia* L.) plant for genetic transformation of the vegetable crops. He has published 20 research papers, semi scientific papers in leading national and international journals. He is a coauthor of two books in the field biotechnology. He is also a member of the Indian Science Congress, professional society and other various scientific committees.

CHAPTER 1

Biotechnology: An Introduction

Biotechnology is not a recent development. In prehistoric times, ethanol was probably the first organic substance of alcoholic fermentation. Microorganisms have been used to produce beer, vinegar, yoghurt, and cheese for over 8 millennia. Biotechnology covers a wealth of specialized disciplines, which include not only the new genetic engineering techniques but also "old fermentation", which our ancestors practised thousands of years ago. Its origins go back to the dawn of civilization, when women first began to domesticate animals and plants gradually changing their characteristics. Selection for certain characteristics may have occurred on purpose, as well as unwittingly. Discoveries of fermentation, use of fungi for taste development and preservation led to culture selection and improvement of microorganisms for food preparation. All this is known as old biotechnology. Though the term was coined by Karl Ereky as late as 1919, biotechnology is as old as today's man.

In the second half of the 19th century, the pioneering work of Pasteur and a number of other microbiologists and chemists showed that in microorganism, many important physiological, metabolic reactions take place, which could be considered for technical utilization. Following this realization, manufacturing processes for a whole series of primary metabolic products were rapidly developed. The major products of old biotechnology industry are food and flavour ingredients, industrial alcohol, antibiotics and citric acid, which amount about hundreds of billion dollars annually on world-wide basis. The first period of historical development of biotechnology continues to influence one present trends and is currently still being extended in parallel to other, more modern, areas of biotechnology. In the past few decades, dramatic new developments in the ability to select and manipulate genetic material have sparked unprecedented interest in the medical uses of living organisms. As farmers and industry became more interdependent and as the biotech industries developed, plants and microbes were modified to suit industrial needs. In recent years, many exciting developments have taken place, and especially in the eyes of the public, the field has gained greatly its importance.

OLD BIOTECHNOLOGY VS NEW BIOTECHNOLOGY

The origin of biotechnology can be traced back to prehistoric times, when microorganisms were used for processes like fermentation. Although a molecular biologist may consider cloning of DNA to be the most important event in the history of biotechnology, the latter has actually been rediscovered in 1970s for the third time during the present century. In 1920s, *Clostridium acetobutylicum* was used by Chaim Weizmann for converting starch into butanol and acetone; the latter was an essential component of explosives during World War I. This raised hopes for commercial production of useful chemicals through biological processes, and may be considered the first rediscovery of biotechnology in the present century. Similarly, during World War II (in 1940s), the production of penicillin (as an antibiotic discovered by Alexander Fleming in 1929) on a large scale from cultures of *Penicillium notatum*, marked the second rediscovery of biotechnology. This was the beginning of an era of antibiotic research. The third rediscovery of biotechnology is its recent reincarnation in the form of recombinant-DNA technology, which led to the development of a variety of gene technologies and is thus considered to be the greatest scientific evolution of this century. Thus, even though biotechnology had its origin in the past, it has assumed special significance only in 1970s and 1980s. The field of modern biotechnology is thought to have largely begun on June 16, 1980, when the United States Supreme Court ruled that a genetically modified microorganism could be patented in the case of Diamond v. Chakrabarty. Indian-born Ananda Chakrabarty, working for General Electric, had developed a bacterium (derived from the *Pseudomonas* genus) capable of breaking down crude oil, which he proposed to use in treating oil spills.

Biotechnology, as the word indicates, is the product of interaction between the science of biology and technology. This relationship between science and technology has been observed to be complex, so that not only the science has influenced technology, but the technology has also influenced science. Because of this complex relationship and its major impact on human welfare, it is believed that biotechnology in future may become a major force for human existence. Already, the products of biotechnology (including diagnosis, prevention and cure of diseases; new and cheaper chemical products, e.g., pharmaceutical drugs and the new food sources; devices for environment protection and energy conservation, etc.) are playing a very important role in employment, productivity, trade, economies and the quality of human life throughout the world. It has been recognized that a complete definition of biotechnology is difficult due to such a wide range of its usage. Fermentation, by some microorganisms, formation of yoghurt (curd) and cheese from milk and that of vinegar from molasses, production of antibiotics like penicillin from certain fungi and the processes of baking and brewing are often included in describing what is called old biotechnology. The other examples of reaction (PCR), cell culture and fusion and bio-processing which became possible only through the researches in molecular biology have been described as new biotechnology (according to OTA, i.e., Office of Technology Assessment).

WHAT IS BIOTECHNOLOGY?

At its simplest, biotechnology is the commercial and large scale exploitation of living organisms or their components, e.g., enzymes for the welfare of mankind through molecular genetics. The major foundation of biotechnology arose out of empirical developments in the field of molecular genetics. Understanding the molecular basis of life processes and life will help in the development of molecular biology and in turn biotechnology.

Year	Historical Events in Biotechnology
1750 BC	The Sumerians brew beer.
500	The Chinese use moldy soybean curds as an antibiotic to treat boils.
250	The Greeks use moldy crop rotation to maximize soil fertility.
100	Powdered Chrysanthemum is used in China as an insecticide.
1590 AD	The first compound microscope is invented by Zacharias Jansen.
1663	Cells are first described by Hooke.
1675	Leeuwenhoek discovers protozoa and bacteria.
1797	Jenner inoculates a child with a viral vaccine to protect him from smallpox.
1833	The cell nucleus is discovered. The first enzymes are isolated.
1855	The *Escherichia coli* bacterium is discovered as production tool for biotechnology.
1863	Mendel, in his study of peas, discovers that traits were transmitted from parents to progeny by discrete, independent units, later called genes.
1869	F. Miescher discovers Nuclein (now known as DNA) from pus cells.
1877	A technique for staining and identifying bacteria is developed by Koch.
1879	Flemming discovers chromatin, the rod-like structures inside the cell nucleus.
1883	The first rabies vaccine is developed.
1907	The first *in vivo* culture of animal cells is reported.
1909	Genes are linked with hereditary disorders.
1911	The first cancer-causing virus is discovered by Rous.
1915	Phages, or bacterial viruses are discovered.
1919	The word "biotechnology" is first used by a Hungarian agricultural engineer.
1927	Muller discovers that X-rays cause mutation.
1928	Fleming discovers penicillin, the first antibiotic.
1941	The term "genetic engineering" is first used by a Danish microbiologist.
1942	The electron microscope is used to identify and characterize a bacteriophage- a virus that infects bacteria.
1943	Oswald T. Avery demonstrates that DNA is the "transforming factor" and is the material of genes.
1951	McClintock discovers transposable elements, or "jumping genes," in corn.
1953	Watson and Crick reveal the three-dimensional structure of DNA.
1954	Cell-culturing techniques are developed.
1956	Kornberg discovers the enzyme DNA polymerase I, leading to an understanding of how DNA is replicated.
1960	Exploiting base pairing, hybrid DNA-RNA molecules are created. Messenger RNA is discovered.
1961	The genetic code is understood for the first time.
1967	The first automatic protein sequencer is perfected.
1969	An enzyme is synthesized *in vitro* for the first time.
1970	Specific restriction nucleases are identified, opening the way for gene cloning reverse transcriptase (RT) is discovered independently in murine and avian retroviruses.
1971	RT is shown to have ribonuclease H (Rnase H) activity.
1972	Purified RT is first used to synthesize cDNA from purified mRNA *in vitro*.
1973	Cohen and Boyer perform the first successful recombinant DNA experiment, using bacterial genes.
1974	The NIH forms a Recombinant DNA Advisory Committee to oversee recombinant genetic research.
1975	Colony hybridization and Southern blotting are developed for detecting specific DNA sequences. The first monoclonal antibodies are produced.
1976	The tools of recombinant DNA are first applied to a human inherited disorder.
1977	Genetically engineered bacteria are used to synthesize human growth protein.

Contd.

1978	Hutchinson and Edgell show that it is possible to introduce specific mutations at specific sites in a DNA molecule.
1979	The first monoclonal antibodies are produced.
1780	The U.S. Supreme Court, in a landmark case Diamond v. Chakrabarty, approves the patenting of genetically engineered life forms. The U.S. patent for gene cloning is awarded to Cohen and Boyer.
1981	The first 'gene-synthesizing' machines are developed. The first genetically engineered plant is reported.
1982	Humulin, Genentech's human insulin drug produced by genetically engineered bacteria for the treatment of diabetes, is the first biotech drug to be approved by the Food and Drug Administration.
1983	The Polymerase Chain Reaction (PCR) technique is conceived. The first genetic transformation of plant cells by Ti plasmids is performed. The first artificial chromosome is synthesized.
1984	The DNA fingerprinting technique is developed. The first genetically engineered vaccine is developed. Chiron clones and sequences the entire genome of the HIV virus.
1985	Fully active murine RT is cloned and over-expressed in *E. coli*.
1986	The first biotech-derived interferon drugs for the treatment of cancer, Biogen's Intron A and Genentech's Roferon A, are approved by the FDA. The first genetically engineered human vaccine, Chiron's Recombivax HB, is approved for the prevention of hepatitis B.
1987	Advanced Genetic Sciences's Frostban, a genetically altered bacterium that inhibits frost formation on crop plants, is field tested on strawberry and potato plants in California, the first authorized outdoor tests of an engineered bacterium. Reverse transcription and PCR are combined to amplify mRNA sequences.
1988	Congress funds the Human Genome Project, a massive effort to map and sequence the human genetic code as well as the genomes of other species.
1989	Microorganisms are used to clean up the Exxon Valdez oil spill.
1990	The first federally approved gene therapy treatment is performed successfully on a 4-year old girl suffering from an immune disorder.
1991	Amgen develops Neupogen, the first of a new class of drugs called colony stimulating factors, for the treatment of low white blood cells in chemotherapy patients. Immunex's Leukine, used to replenish white blood counts after bone marrow transplants, is approved.
1992	The three-dimensional structure of HIV RT is elucidated. Recombinate, developed by Genetics Institute and used in the treatment of hemophilia A, becomes the first genetically engineered blood clotting factor approved. Chiron's Proleukin is approved for the treatment of renal cell cancer.
1993	The FDA declares that genetically engineered foods are "not inherently dangerous" and do not require special regulation.
1994	Calgene's Flavr Savr tomato, engineered to resist rotting, is approved for sale.
1995	The first full gene sequence of a living organism other than a virus is completed for the bacterium *"Haemophilus" influenzae*.
1996	Biogen's Avonex is approved for the treatment of multiple sclerosis. The company builds a $50 million plant in Research Triangle Park, N.C., to manufacture the recombinant interferon drug.
1997	Scottish scientists report cloning a sheep (Dolly), using DNA from adult sheep cells. A new DNA technique combines PCR, DNA chips, and a computer program, providing a new tool in the search for disease-causing genes.
1998	Human skin is produced *in vitro*. Embryonic stem cells are used to regenerate tissue and create disorders mimicking diseases. The first complete animal genome for the elegans worm is sequenced.
1999	The complete genetic code of the human chromosome is first deciphered. The rising tide of public opinion in Europe brings biotech food into the spotlight.
2000	"Golden Rice," modified to make vitamin A, promises to help third-world countries alleviate night blindness.

Contd.

2001	The sequence of the human genome is published in Science and Nature, making it possible for researchers all over the world to begin developing treatments.
2002	Kurt Wüthrich developed nuclear magnetic resonance spectroscopy for determining the three-dimensional structure of biological macromolecules in solution.
2003	Dolly, the cloned sheep that made headlines in 1997, is euthanized after developing progressive lung disease. Dolly was the first successful clone of a mammal.
2004	Approval of Xolair (omalizumab, for use in asthma); Raptiva (efalizumab, for use in psoriasis); Avastin (bevacizumab, for the treatment of cancer).
2005	A first draft of the chimpanzee genome is published.
2006	Discovery of RNA interference-gene silencing by double-stranded RNA.
2007	Discovery of principles for introducing specific gene modifications in mice by the use of embryonic stem cells.
2008	Paolo Macchiarini carries out the world's first tissue-engineered whole organ transplant, replacing a Colombian woman's windipipe made with the patient's own stem cells.
2009	Discovery of how chromosomes are protected by telomeres and the enzyme telomerase.
2010	Dr. Craig Venter and his team of geneticists at the J. Craig Venter Institute (JCVI) create a synthetic life form by using chemically-created chromosomes in empty cells, causing those cells to multiply.
2011	Discovery and development in nanoparticles based products.
2012	Development of genetically engineered stem cells to seek out and kill HIV in mice.

Definitions

Biotechnology, broadly defined, includes any technique that uses living organisms (or parts of organism) to make or modify products, to improve plants or animals, or to develop microorganisms for specific uses. However, other definitions are also given below:

- Biotechnology is the application of biological organisms, system or process to manufacturing and service industries.
- Biotechnology is the integrated use of biochemistry, microbiology, and engineering sciences in order to achieve technological (industrial) application of the capabilities of microorganisms, cultured tissue cells and parts thereof.
- Biotechnology is a technology using biological phenomena for copying and manufacturing various kinds of useful substances.
- Biotechnology is the controlled use of biological agents, such as microorganisms or cellular components, for beneficial use.
- Any technological application that uses biological systems, living organisms, or derivatives thereof, to make or modify products or processes for specific use.

Developments in Biotechnology

Biotechnology is the use of microbiology, biochemistry, genetics and engineering in an integrated fashion with the goal of using microorganisms and cell and tissue cultures (or their parts) to manufacture useful products. Biotechnology is developing by close interweaving between these areas and can develop further only by means of an interdisciplinary cooperation between them. Basic research has produced a large number of results in the field of microbiology, biochemistry, enzyme research, molecular biology, genetic engineering and, chemical engineering, which are being practically used in biotechnological applications. Biotechnology is therefore an application oriented science of microbiology and biochemistry that is closely connected with technical chemistry and chemical engineering. The field of operation of biotechnology consists of three large areas of life science (a) microbiology, including microbial genetics, (b) biochemistry including physical chemistry and organic chemistry, and (c) process engineering and apparatus constructions.

With the discovery of restriction enzymes in 1970, biotechnology was given a boost that opened the avenue of genetic engineering. The freedom to play around with DNA molecules resulted in dramatic use of gene cloning and gene transfer technology (Modern Biotechnology). Modern biotechnology is only 50 years old, and in the last decades it has been witnessing tremendous developments. With the development of new approaches and modern techniques, traditional biotechnology industries are also acquiring new horizons enabling them to improve the quality of their products and increase the productivity of their systems. In the past few decades, dramatic new developments in the ability to select and manipulate genetic material have sparked unprecedented interest in the uses of living organisms.

In the 1980s, biotechnology became a major growth area. Many products can be manufactured only biotechnologically. This applies particularly to most of the secondary metabolic products e.g., antibiotics, etc. Since last thousands of years, biological processes have central importance in food industry, but it is only in the last 100 years that they have been applied more intensively in chemical technology. At present, modern biotechnology is capable of becoming a part of not only medical industry but also other industrial developments of increasing importance like agro-industries. It is predicted that modern biotechnology will account for a much larger fraction of the total biotechnology industry in years to come.

Biotechnology has applications in four major industrial areas, including health care (medical), crop production and agriculture, non-food (industrial) uses of crops and other products (e.g. biodegradable plastics, vegetable oil, biofuels), and environmental uses. For example, one application of biotechnology is the directed use of organisms for the manufacture of organic products (examples include beer and milk products). Another example is using naturally present bacteria by the mining industry in bioleaching. Biotechnology is also used to recycle, treat waste, clean up sites contaminated by industrial activities (bioremediation), and also to produce biological weapons.

A series of derived terms have been coined to identify several branches of biotechnology, for example:

- **Bioinformatics** is an interdisciplinary field which addresses biological problems using computational techniques, and makes the rapid organization and analysis of biological data possible. The field may also be referred to as *computational biology*, and can be defined as, "conceptualizing biology in terms of molecules and then applying informatics techniques to understand and organize the information associated with these molecules, on a large scale." Bioinformatics plays a key role in various areas, such as functional genomics, structural genomics, and proteomics, and forms a key component in the biotechnology and pharmaceutical sector.

- **Blue biotechnology** is a term that has been used to describe the marine and aquatic applications of biotechnology, but its use is relatively rare.

- **Green biotechnology** is biotechnology applied to agricultural processes. An example would be the selection and domestication of plants via micropropagation. Another example is the designing of transgenic plants to grow under specific environments in the presence (or absence) of chemicals. One hope is that green biotechnology might produce more environment-friendly solutions than traditional industrial agriculture. An example of this is the engineering of a plant to express a pesticide, thereby ending the need of external application of pesticides. An example of this would be Bt corn. Whether or not green biotechnology products such as this are ultimately more environment friendly is a topic of considerable debate.
- **Red biotechnology** is applied to medical processes. Some examples are the designing of organisms to produce antibiotics, and the engineering of genetic cures through genetic manipulation.
- **White biotechnology,** also known as industrial biotechnology, is biotechnology applied to industrial processes. An example is the designing of an organism to produce a useful chemical. Another example is the using of enzymes as industrial catalysts to either produce valuable chemicals or destroy hazardous/polluting chemicals. White biotechnology tends to consume less in resources than traditional processes used to produce industrial goods. The investment and economic output of all of these types of applied biotechnologies is termed as bio-economy.

COMPONENTS OF BIOTECHNOLOGY

To keep pace with the ever expanding knowledge in the field of molecular genetics and molecular biology it necessitates harnessing this knowledge for the development of potential technologies and products for the welfare of mankind. In order to facilitate the development of biotechnology, we have to look upon three major components: objective, tools and methodology or techniques. Thus, in biotechnology, objective is the product of gene or metabolism; the tools are microorganisms (bacteria, fungi and viruses) and cultured cells of higher organisms; and the techniques employed are those used for development of commercially important biotechnologies.

Biological Organisms as Tools

Biotechnology always deals with reactions which, in principle, are of biological nature. These reactions are performed either by living microbial cells or plant and animal cells and their tissues or by enzymes from cells or parts of cells. The microorganisms, such as bacteria, actinomycetes, cyanobacteria, and yeasts and other fungi, viruses and mycoplasmas widely occur in nature. They function in industry as synthesizers of several useful products of fermentation and bioconversion. They have been the major tools in the study of molecular genetics and molecular biology which, in turn biotechnology. The production of biomass from the organisms or parts of organisms mentioned is also an area of biotechnology. In 1960s, considerable excitement was generated by the prospect of using microbial cells (or biomass) as a source of protein, the so-called single cell protein (SCP). However, introduction of SCP has not been a success.

Microorganisms figure principally as tools in biotechnology, especially for genetic engineering and gene cloning studies.

Biotechnology Processes

Microorganisms are the deciding factor of a biotechnological process. Basically, most biotechnological processes can be reduced to a simple equation:

$$\text{Substrate} + \text{Microbial cells} \xrightarrow{\text{Process Engineering}} \text{Product}$$

Process engineering consists of the manufacturing process proper and the subsequent recovery procedure (isolation of the product or the cells).

The product may be cell biomass, a metabolic product of the cells, or a transformation product of a given starting material, which is formed by the living microorganism or enzymes. Furthermore, an initially complex substrate can be replaced by a definite chemical compound, which is converted into a product in one or a few steps. Then the equation runs, for example:

$$\text{Substrate} + \text{Enzyme} \xrightarrow{\text{Process Engineering}} \text{Product}$$

These reactions are already simplified biotechnological processes. In general, however, biotechnological processes are altogether more complex and employ various technologies.

The Technologies

The novel methodology and techniques used in biotechnology are extremely powerful because they allow a large amount of control over biological system. Biotechnology as practised today is much more than recombinant DNA technology. It includes various technologies (as discussed below). However, if these are performers, gene manipulation is the star of show. The ability to splice genes has revolutionized the industry and is leading to the development of countless new products and improved methods for well established processes, which have wide applications in agriculture and medicine. However, besides recombinant DNA technology, some other potential biotechnologies have wide applications in agricultural and medical sciences and are briefly described below. (Principles and practices of these potential biotechnologies in agriculture and medicine are covered in the form of full chapters subsequently in this book).

Recombinant DNA technology

Recombinant DNA technology is a set of molecular techniques for locating, isolating, altering, and studying DNA segments. The term *recombinant* is used because frequently the goal is to combine DNA from two distinct sources. Genes from two different bacteria might be joined, for example, or a human gene might be inserted into a viral chromosome. Commonly called genetic engineering, recombinant DNA technology now encompasses an array of molecular techniques that can be used to analyze, alter, and recombine virtually any DNA sequences. In addition to providing valuable new information about the nature and function of genes, recombinant DNA technology has many applications. These applications include the production of pharmaceuticals and other chemicals, specialized bacteria, agriculturally important plants, and genetically engineered farm animals. The technology is also used extensively in medical testing and, in a few cases, is even being used to correct human genetic defects. Hundreds of firms now specialize in developing products through genetic engineering, and many large multinational corporations have invested enormous sums of money in recombinant DNA research. These techniques are also used in many other fields, including biochemistry, microbiology, developmental biology, neurobiology, evolution, and ecology. Recombinant DNA technology is also used to create a number of commercial products, including drugs, hormones, enzymes, and crops. An entirely new industry—biotechnology—has grown up around the use of these techniques to develop new products. In medicine, recombinant DNA techniques are used to probe the nature of cancer, diagnose genetic and infectious diseases, produce drugs, and treat hereditary disorders.

Nucleic acid probes technology

Nucleic acid probes technology has been developed that relies on the use of DNA or RNA probes to detect particular gene sequences. The application of the technique includes the diagnosis of genetic and infectious diseases. Through intensive research efforts in both chemical synthesis and bioassay development, molecular probes scientists have developed rapid and exceptionally sensitive fluorescence-based assays for quantitation of nucleic acids (DNA, RNA) and protein samples. The double-helical structure of nucleic acids, in which one strand binds specifically to its exact complement, is a fortuitous design for the study of biology. The ease of constructing assays based on this feature is responsible for the incredibly fast pace that has characterized molecular biology research since its inception. With the incorporation of fluorescence technologies, the ability to design multiplexed and high-throughput assays has increased the pace still further to the point in which sophisticated bioinformatics is required to analyze the huge outpouring of data. Experiments in which labeled sample nucleic acids are hybridized to nucleic acids on solid supports, most notably Southern and Northern blots, have been core technologies in the field of molecular biology. Conventionally, samples were labeled with radioisotopes, hybridized to nucleic acids on the membrane and imaged for long periods with X-ray film. Although some users still employ radioactive labeling for microarray experiments, fluorescent labeling and detection now dominate the field. Fluorescence provides an important advantage because the majority of microarray experiments rely on comparison of hybridization signals between two or more samples, and fluorescence detection allows the analysis of multiple samples on the same array, minimizing artifact variation in signals.

Polymerase chain reaction technology

The polymerase chain reaction (PCR) is a biochemistry and molecular biology technique originally conceived by Kary Mullis for exponentially amplifying DNA via enzymatic replication without using a living organism (such as *E. coli* or yeast). As PCR is an *in vitro* technique, it can be performed without restrictions on the form of DNA, and it can be extensively modified to perform a wide array of genetic manipulations. PCR is commonly used in medical and biological research labs for a variety of tasks, such as the detection of hereditary diseases, the identification of genetic fingerprints, the diagnosis of infectious diseases, the cloning of genes, paternity testing, and DNA computing. PCR was invented by Kary Mullis. At the time he thought up PCR in 1983, Mullis was working in Emeryville, California for Cetus Corporation, one of the first biotechnology companies. There, he was charged with making short chains of DNA for other scientists. Mullis has written that he conceived of PCR while cruising along the Pacific Coast Highway one night in his car. He was playing in his mind with a new way of analyzing changes (mutations) in DNA when he realized that he had instead invented a method of amplifying any DNA region. Mullis has said that before his trip was over, he was already savoring the prospects of a Nobel Prize. He shared the Nobel Prize in Chemistry with Michael Smith in 1993. PCR technology has wide application such as genetic fingerprinting, paternity testing, detection of hereditary diseases, cloning genes, mutagenesis, analysis of ancient DNA, genotyping of specific mutations, comparison of gene expression and many more.

DNA-protein interaction technology

DNA–protein interactions are fundamental to the existence of life forms, providing the key to the genetic plan as well as mechanisms for its maintenance and evolution. The specific binding of a protein to a nucleic acid is a first step in several central processes in a living cell. Sequence-specific protein–DNA interactions are crucial for the functional read-out of genetic information. The study of these interactions is therefore fundamental to our understanding of growth, development, differentiation, evolution, and disease. The manipulation of DNA-protein interactions is also becoming increasingly important to the biotechnology industry, permitting among other things the reprogramming of gene expression. DNA-protein complexes may be studied at three distinct levels—at the level of the DNA, of the protein, and of the complex. At the level of the DNA, the DNA binding site may be delimited and exact base sequence requirements defined. The DNA conformation can be studied and the exact bases contacted by the protein identified. At the protein level, the protein species binding a given DNA sequence can be identified. The amino acids contacting DNA and the protein surface facing the DNA may be defined and the amino acids essential to the recognition process can be identified. Furthermore, the protein's tertiary structure and its conformational changes on complex formation can be studied. Finally, global parameters of a DNA-protein complex such as stoichiometry, the kinetics of its formation and dissociation, its stability, and the energy of interaction can be measured. Filter binding, electrophoretic mobility shift assay (EMSA/gel shift), DNaseI footprinting, and Southwestern blotting have been the most commonly used techniques to identify potentially interesting DNA target sites and to define the proteins that bind them. DNA-protein crosslinking has in recent years become a very important approach to investigate the relative positions of proteins in multicomponent protein-DNA complexes such as the transcription initiation complex. When combined these methods are capable of providing a picture of the protein-DNA complex with a great deal of molecular detail, surpassed only by the more demanding methods of crystallography and nuclear magnetic resonance (NMR).

Genomics technology

Genomics is the study of the genomes of organisms. The field includes intensive efforts to determine the entire DNA sequence of organisms and fine-scale genetic mapping efforts. The field also includes studies of intragenomic phenomena such as heterosis, epistasis, pleiotropy and other interactions between loci and alleles within the genome. In contrast, the investigation of single genes, their functions and roles, something very common in today's medical and biological research, and a primary focus of molecular biology, does not fall into the definition of genomics unless the aim of this genetic pathway, and functional information analysis is to elucidate its effect on, place in, and response to the entire genome's networks. For the United States Environmental Protection Agency, "the term "genomics" encompasses a broader scope of scientific inquiry associated technologies than when genomics was initially considered. A genome is the sum total of all an individual organism's genes. Thus, genomics is the study of all the genes of a cell, or tissue, at the DNA (genotype), mRNA (transcriptome), or protein (proteome) levels. A major branch of genomics is still concerned with sequencing the genomes of various organisms, but the knowledge of full genomes has created the possibility for the field of functional genomics, mainly concerned with patterns of gene expression during various conditions.

Proteomics technology

Proteomics technology is an interdisciplinary science that includes biology and protein chemistry. A broader definition of proteomics includes systematic experimental and computational attempts at determining protein-protein interaction maps for an entire organism. This information is crucial to an understanding of how genes work in concert to generate a working cell. Functional proteomics constitutes an emerging research area in the proteomic field whose approaches are addressed towards two major targets: the elucidation of the biological function of unknown proteins and the definition of cellular mechanisms at the molecular level. The identification of interacting proteins in stable complexes *in vivo* is essentially achieved by affinity-based procedures. The basic idea is to express the protein of interest with a suitable tag to be used as a bait to fish its specific partners out from a cellular extract. Individual components within the multi-protein complex can then be identified by mass spectrometric methodologies. The association of an unknown protein with partners belonging to a specific protein complex involved in a particular mechanism is strongly suggestive of the biological function of the protein. Furthermore, a detailed description of the cellular signaling pathways might greatly benefit from the elucidation of protein–protein interactions *in vivo*. Since proteomics is a young and rapidly evolving field, the best approach is to gain a general understanding of the questions and technologies involved and then pursue the primary literature for detailed information on the latest developments.

Signalomics technology

The goal of signalomics technology is to track down faulty cellular signal proteins and to develop custom-made therapeutics, theranostics and diagnostics for complex illnesses that result from errors in cellular signal transduction. The ability to specifically influence cellular signals will make it possible to create individualized medications which are custom-designed for the patient. This is the revolutionary strategy that signalomics is pursuing. In its study of intracellular processes, signalomics makes use of functional proteomics, nano-biotechnology, computational biology and bioanalysis using fluorescent dyes. Signalomics makes it possible to observe dynamic molecular processes and interactions even in living cells. Furthermore, it is also possible to detect a variety of binding partners simultaneously.

Metabolomics technology

Metabolomics is the "systematic study of the unique chemical fingerprints that specific cellular processes leave behind"—specifically, the study of their small-molecule metabolite profiles. The metabolome represents the collection of all metabolites in a biological organism, which are the end products of its gene expression. Thus, while mRNA gene expression data and proteomic analyses do not tell the whole story of what might be happening in a cell, metabolic profiling can give an instantaneous 'snapshot' of the physiology of that cell. One of the challenges of systems biology is to integrate proteomics, transcriptomics, and metabolomics information to give a more complete picture of living organisms. Metabolomics was conceived in 1970 by Arthur Robinson, an assistant professor in the Department of Chemistry at the University of California, San Diego. Metabolomics can be an excellent tool for determining the phenotype caused by a genetic manipulation, such as gene deletion or insertion. Metabolic profiling (especially of urine or blood plasma samples) can also be used to detect the physiological changes caused by toxic insult of a chemical (or mixture of chemicals).

Bioinformatics and in silico technology

Bioinformatics and *in silico* technology occupies a unique niche amongst the sciences, lying at the intersection of biology, genetics, biochemistry, computer science, mathematics, statistics, and numerous other allied fields. The inherent strength of the field of bioinformatics comes from the relationships between investigators in these allied fields. Collaborations between these individuals has led to the development of novel methods and approaches, furthering advances in each of these areas. Such collaborations also set the stage for the piloting of experiments on computers, followed by the verification of the computational results in the laboratory. DNA sequences generated by the human genome project, protein structures, gene expression patterns, etc. carry with them an enormous amount of valuable information. To uncover all the information, however, will still take many more years of research. Bioinformatics, as we have seen, is set to become an indispensable tool. This is not to say that wet-bench work is not required; on the contrary, bioinformatics will give researchers the tools necessary to guide their bench work and handle computers as easily as they do the microscope. *In silico* technologies in drug target identification and validation addresses the challenge of testing a growing number of new potential targets and reviews currently available *in silico* approaches for identifying and validating these targets and determine the biological functionality of potential targets more effectively.

System biology technology

Systems biology aims at understanding biological systems at system level. Systems biology, just like all other emerging scientific disciplines, is built on multiple efforts that share the vision. Systems biology clearly includes both experimental and computational or analytical studies. However, systems biology is not a mere combination of molecular biology and computing science to reverse engineer gene networks. Of course, it is one of the topics included, but system-level understanding requires more than understanding structures. Understanding of (1) system structures, (2) dynamics, (3) control methods, and (4) design methods are major four milestones of systems biology research. To understand biology at the system level, we must examine the structure and dynamics of cellular and organismal function, rather than the characteristics of isolated parts of a cell or organism. However, many breakthroughs in experimental devices, advanced software, and analytical methods are required before the achievements of systems biology can live up to their much-touted potential. Systems biology works towards understanding the intricacies of cellular life through the collaborative efforts of biologists, chemists, mathematicians and computer scientists and recently, a number of laboratories around the world have embarked upon such research agendas. Systems biology will bring about a revolution in the practice of medicine. Knowledge of specific genetic traits, coupled with multi-parameter diagnostics, will generate routine procedures for assessing health and disease status. Knowledge of disease-perturbed networks will facilitate drug discovery, and pharmacological intervention will focus on preventing disease-mediated transitions. This predictive and preventative medicine will lead naturally to a personalized medicine, in which therapeutic strategies will be tailored to individual needs. In this sense, systems biology will fundamentally transform society.

Microarray technology

Microarray is an advanced and high throughput method based on DNA chips, which consists of very high density arrays of short oligonucleotides synthesized on a silicon wafer by a combination of conventional oligonucleotide synthesis chemistry and photolithography. There are two parallel methods to monitor the genes, which are differentially expressed in a particular sample, oligonucleotide microarrays and cDNA microarrays. Both of these methods offer tremendous advantages in speed of analysis, allowing thousands of cDNA sequences to be surveyed in a single set of experiments. This method has been applied for profiling of differentially expressed genes from various plant samples and recently there are also some reports for their usefulness in profiling of ripening related genes. This technology has wide applications, such as in quantitative gene expression; mutation detection; disease profiling (diagnostics); patient monitoring (prognostics) and many more.

Antisense technology

Antisense technologies are a suite of techniques that, together, form a very powerful weapon for studying gene function (functional genomics) and discovering new and more specific treatments of diseases in humans, animals, and plants (antisense therapeutics). A conventional definition of antisense refers to the laboratory manipulation and/or modification of DNA or RNA so that its components (nucleotides) form a complementary copy of normal, or "senses", messenger RNA (mRNA). The binding, or hybridization of antisense nucleic acid sequences to a specific mRNA target will, through a number of different mechanisms, interrupt normal cellular processing of the genetic message of a gene. This interruption, sometimes referred to as "knock-down" or "knock-out" depending upon whether or not the message is either partially or completely eliminated, allows researchers to determine the function of that gene. The impact of biotechnology on antisense technology is expected to increase dramatically as the links between genetics, protein production and disease are better understood. Currently, antisense technology is used to design therapeutic compounds, which target specific mRNA sequences to obstruct the production of certain disease-causing proteins. Traditional drug therapies focus on a drug's interaction with the disease-causing proteins. However, antisense drug therapies inhibit the production of the disease-causing proteins altogether. Applications of antisense technology in therapeutics are expected to increase substantially as the link between diseases and genes are made.

RNA interference technology

RNA interference (RNAi) technology has become one of the key methods used in functional genomics. RNAi is used to block the expression of genes and create phenotypes that can potentially yield clues about the function of these genes. It was discovered unexpectedly during attempts to experimentally manipulate the expression of specific genes. This naturally occurring phenomenon was first described for the nematode worm *Caenorhabditis elegans*. RNAi is believed to be an ancient cellular defense against certain viruses and mobile genetic elements in both plants and animals. RNAi is initiated by long double-stranded RNA molecules, which are processed into 21-23 nucleotides long RNAs by the dicer enzyme. These small interfering RNAs (siRNAs) are then incorporated into the RNA-induced silencing complex (RISC), a protein AERNA complex, and guide a nuclease, which degrades the target RNA. RNA interference has been used for applications in biotechnology, particularly in the engineering of food plants that produce lower levels of natural plant toxins. Recently, this technology has been applied for manipulation of ripening related gene expression to improve the post-harvest life of fruits.

Hybridoma technology

Hybridoma technology for production of monoclonal antibodies was discovered in 1975 by two scientists, Georges Kohler of West Germany and Cesar Milstein of Argentina (now working in U.K.), who jointly with Niels Jerne of Denmark (now working in Germany) were awarded the 1984 Nobel Prize for Physiology and Medicine. A hybridoma, which can be considered a hybrid cell, is produced by the injection of a specific antigen into a mouse, procuring the antibody-producing cell from the mouse's spleen and the subsequent fusion of this cell with a cancerous immune cell called myeloma cell. Monoclonal antibodies (Mabs) can be produced from these hybrid cells (hybridoma cells) through a technique now popularly known as hybridoma technology. Mabs can potentially be used for many purposes including the diagnosis and treatment of diseases and the purification of proteins. The fused hybrid cells (called hybridomas), being cancer cells, will multiply rapidly and indefinitely and will produce large amounts of the desired antibodies. They have to be selected and subsequently cloned by limiting dilution. Supplemental media containing Interleukin-6 (such as briclone) are essential for this step.

Molecular diagnostics technology

Molecular technology that has been implemented into diagnostic testing is called molecular diagnostic technology. The molecular diagnostics involves the molecules-molecules interaction based on their complementarities and affinity. These include broadly ligand-binder such as the DNA-DNA, DNA-RNA, DNA-protein, protein-protein and more specifically the antigen-antibody interaction that makes the basis of development of immuno-technologies for diagnostic and analytical purposes in medical, veterinary and even in agricultural sciences. Recently, several programs that educate clinical laboratory professionals have had to incorporate molecular-based diagnostic testing into their curricula just as rapidly despite the lack of formal resources. This technology has wide applications such as detection and identification of microorganisms, DNA polymorphisms and *human identification*, molecular detection of inherited diseases, gene mutations, resolution and detection of nucleic acids, nucleic acid amplification, analysis and characterization of nucleic acids and proteins, chromosomal structure and chromosomal mutations, quality assurance and quality control in the molecular laboratory, DNA-based tissue typing, molecular oncology and many more. Molecular and cytogenetic analyses are a critical component of diagnostic testing, especially for diseases that arise from known genetic events. The identification of a molecular or chromosomal abnormality is a direct observation of the source of some diseases. Genetic lesions in single-gene disorders are detected by a variety of hybridization/amplification methods and nucleotide sequencing.

Biosensor technology

Biosensor technology deals with the use of an analytical device that converts a biological response into an electrical signal. The term 'biosensor' is often used to cover sensor devices used in order to determine the concentration of substances and other parameters of biological interest even where they do not utilize a biological system directly. Enzymes are the biologically responsive material, but it should be recognized that other biological systems may be utilized by biosensors, for example, whole cell metabolism, ligand binding and the antibody-antigen reaction. Research and development in biosensor is wide and multidisciplinary, spanning biochemistry, bioreactor science, physical chemistry, electrochemistry, electronics and software engineering. Most of this current endeavor concerns potentiometric and amperometric biosensors and colorimetric paper enzyme strips. However, all the main transducer types are likely to be thoroughly examined for use in biosensors over the next few years. A successful biosensor must be highly specific for the purpose of the analyses; stable under normal storage conditions and show good stability over a large number of assays; tiny and biocompatible; having no toxic or antigenic effects; the response should be accurate, precise, reproducible and linear over the useful analytical range; free from electrical noise; should not be prone to fouling or proteolysis and should be cheap, portable and capable of being used by semi-skilled operators.

Protein engineering

Protein engineering is the process of developing useful or valuable proteins. It is a young discipline, with much research currently taking place into the understanding of protein folding and protein recognition for protein design principles. There are two general strategies for protein engineering. The first is known as *rational design*, in which the scientist uses detailed knowledge of the structure and function of the protein to make the desired changes. This has the advantage of being generally inexpensive and easy, since site-directed mutagenesis techniques are well developed. Computational protein design algorithms seek to identify amino acid sequences that have low energies for target structures. While the sequence-conformation space that needs to be searched is large, the most challenging requirement for computational protein design is a fast, yet accurate, energy function that can distinguish optimal sequences from similar suboptimal ones. The second strategy is known as directed evolution. This is where random mutagenesis is applied to a protein, and a selection regime is used to pick out variants that have the desired qualities. Further rounds of mutation and selection are then applied. This method mimics natural evolution and generally produces superior results to rational design. An additional technique known as DNA shuffling mixes and matches pieces of successful variants in order to produce better results. This process mimics recombination that occurs naturally during sexual reproduction. Rational design and directed evolution techniques are not mutually exclusive; good researchers will often apply both. In the future, more detailed knowledge of protein structure and function, as well as advancements in high-throughput technology, will greatly expand the capabilities of protein engineering.

Nano-biotechnology

Nano-biotechnology is one of the most future-oriented technologies of the 21st century. Nano-biotechnology is becoming established in the interdisciplinary area, supported by a dynamic boom in innovations and will promote close cooperation between the life sciences, physical and chemical sciences as well as engineering. It is bridging the gap between inanimate and animate nature and aims at understanding the basic principles of biological functional units as well as creating extremely small components at "nano-scale" in a controlled way with technical materials. In April 2000, the BMBF established the "Nano-biotechnology" funding measure in order to develop this new research area in Germany and to make it internationally competitive. The convergence of nanotechnology and biomedical sciences opens a wide variety of biological research topics and medical uses at the molecular and cellular level. The long-term goal of nano-biotechnology is to contribute to the information transfer and to the explosive growth of this important research area. Nano-biotechnology used in biotechnology is definitely a life-saving innovation that has come as a boon to mankind. The real applications can turn around the life cycle of human beings in the years to come.

Molecular marker technology

Molecular marker technology has opened exciting new windows to view the natural biological world. DNA-based molecular markers have acted as versatile tools and have found their own position in various fields like taxonomy, physiology, embryology, genetic engineering, behavioral ecology, organism evolution, genetics, ecology, phylogeny, etc. DNA markers offer several advantages over traditional phenotypic markers, as they provide data that can be analyzed objectively. Molecular marker is any kind of molecule indicating the existence of a chemical or physical process. Molecular markers are used in molecular biology and biotechnology experiments to identify a particular sequence of DNA. As the DNA sequences are highly specific, they can be identified with the help of the known molecular markers, which can find out a particular sequence of DNA from a group of unknown. Molecular markers have been used to monitor DNA sequence variation in and among the species and create new sources of genetic variation by introducing new and favorable traits from landraces and related species. In recent years, different marker systems such as Restriction Fragment Length Polymorphisms (RFLPs), Random Amplified Polymorphic DNAs (RAPDs), Sequence Tagged Sites (STSs), Amplified Fragment Length Polymorphisms (AFLPs), Simple Sequence Repeats (SSRs) or microsatellites, Single Nucleotide Polymorphisms (SNPs) and others have been developed and applied to plants and animals. Improvements in marker detection systems and the techniques used to identify markers linked to useful traits has enabled great advances to be made in recent years.

Marker-assisted selection technology

Marker assisted selection is a complementary technology for use in conjunction with more established conventional methods of genetic selection for plant and animal improvement. Marker assisted selection (MAS) involves establishing the linkage between the inheritance of a particular trait, which might be desirable as in the case of milk yield, or undesirable, as in the susceptibility to a disease, with the segregation of particular genetic markers. Thus, even if the gene that controls the trait is unknown, its presence can be inferred from the presence of the marker that segregates with it. MAS is an established plant breeding technology widely used by plant breeding programs around the world to supplement and enhance field-based phenotypic selection programs. Based on copious genetic and chromosome mapping research published in recent years, usable molecular markers that are associated with economic traits of interest are now available for public use. This technology is user-friendly and can be utilized at a relatively low cost by programs with limited technological capabilities. MAS can be used in an applied breeding program with two basic strategies. The first strategy recognizes that the superior genetic background identified by long term selection and evaluation is the most important aspect of an elite cultivar. Lines exhibiting statistically improved grain yield potential are rarely identified and highly valued when found since they likely represent a unique new combination of genes. Commonly during selection, lines possessing a superior combination of the key traits of grain yield, adaptation, and quality are identified, which lack other simply inherited traits that would enhance or protect their performance. Thus, this strategy attempts to improve and enhance genetic backgrounds documented to have superior yield performance by correcting deficiencies and/or enhancing the levels of secondary, simply inherited genetic traits that can be improved relatively easily using marker assisted selection. A second strategy for MAS is to cross two elite parents, one of which carries economically important genes that can be identified by appropriate molecular markers. Progeny are screened during generation advancement for molecular markers and progeny carrying markers associated with traits of value are retained. Selection for yield and other traits of importance is imposed secondary to selection for the gene being followed by MAS. Both types of MAS are valuable and necessary in an applied program for cultivar development.

Integrating MAS into breeding strategies could become increasingly important in the coming years to realize genetic gains with greater speed and precision. The promise of MAS for improving polygenic traits in a quick time-frame and a cost-effective manner is still elusive. There is a wider appreciation that simply demonstrating that a complex trait can be dissected into QTLs and mapped to approximate genomic locations using DNA markers would not serve the ultimate goal of trait improvement. In facing the challenge of improving several lines for quantitative traits, MAS strategies use DNA markers in one key selection step to maximize their impact.

Plant transgenic technology

Transgenic technology has provided important tools for sustainable development of agriculture and forestry and can be of significant help in meeting the food needs of a growing and increasing urbanized population. The genetic engineering of plants by inserting a foreign DNA segment into the plant genome is called transgenesis and the developed plant a transgenic plant. All genetically engineered plants are GMOs (Genetically Modified Organisms), also known as LMOs (Living Modified Organisms). Common LMOs include agricultural crops genetically modified for agronomic traits. The advantage or potential benefit of transgenic plants is the applications for which they are being developed, the new traits being introduced. In brief, a GM plant allows expression of a trait not found inherently, regulated temporal and spatial expression of desired trait. With depleting natural resources and changing global climate, conventional agricultural practices alone are unable to sustain the quality and quantity of the produce. With the advent of modern biotechnology, newer tools permitting gene transfer across the species: transgenics, opened an avenue for solving the age old problem. Genetically modified crops can be produced by several ways, be it a physical or chemical delivery method of inserting gene of choice. The aims of gene transfer are – breeding crops with improved traits – as well as molecular farming, the production of pharmaceuticals, therapeutic molecules or specialty chemicals for industry. Transgenics have potential to reduce usage of insecticides, herbicides and weedicides, improve tolerance to stress, and function as edible vaccine and biosensors.

Bioinoculant technology

Bioinoculant technology deals with the prospect of improving agriculture by inoculation with biofertilizers, which is of great importance for less intensive, ecofriendly, restore natural soil fertility and low-input agricultural system existing in many developing countries. Agricultural fields that are deficient in a nutrient and are devoid of native populations of microorganisms capable of supplying the deficient nutrients are the appropriate locations for using biofertilizers for inoculations. The need for the use of biofertilizers has arisen primarily due to two reasons. First, because increase in the use of biofertilizers leads to increased crop productivity, and second because increased usage of chemical fertilizer leads to damage in soil texture and raises other environmental problems. Broadly, bioinoculants include biofertilizers, biopesticides and organic decomposers. Biofertilizers are live cells of beneficial microbial isolates that provide necessary nutrients (nitrogen, phosphorous, etc.), excrete growth promoting compounds and provide resistance to a variety of diseases that culminates to enhanced yield and production. While biopesticides are live microbial isolates or their metabolic products that eradicate/kill known insects/pests of crops. The third component of bioinoculants is the organic decomposers that include certain fungal species, bacterial genera and actinomycetes that hasten decomposition of organic compounds and make available nutrients held as organic matter. The main types of bioinoculants, which are present in market include:

(1) soil inoculants: to improve soil biological activity;

(2) plant inoculants: to improve plant nutrient uptake and disease resistance; and

(3) residue inoculants: to improve the breakdown of crop and litter residues.

Before using a bioinoculant product you need to be sure of the purpose that you want to add it for. Is it for soil or plant biology? You then need to match the product to your specific need.

Bioinoculant technology includes selection of appropriate bacterial strains, large scale production of their biomass, development of formulations (liquid, powder or granules), and their applications methods in the field. Reliable commercial use of bioinoculants on a large scale depends on formulations that are simple, economical, unaffected by long storage, and easy to transport and apply. It also depends on application technology that facilitates timely, easy, and precise delivery in the field. The study of a formulation process is generally undertaken when the choice of an efficient strain has already been made. However, the development of an economically viable production processes is a significant hurdle in the commercialization of bioinoculants. A primary method of achieving this goal is through strain engineering. Evolutionary engineering has been practiced for decades in the form of classic strain improvement. The process of genetic diversification and functional screening has now become a powerful means of improving the function of diverse biological systems from genes and enzymes to whole genomes. Gene shuffling is a method for effecting genetic diversification in evolutionary engineering programs that incorporate recombination into the evolutionary algorithm. This approach dramatically accelerates the process of directed evolution and is arguably the most robust method for the purposeful manipulation of biological structure and function. In addition, the optimization of formulation is largely independent of the strain, since strains within one genus or species share many cultural properties. A process developed for one strain of a genus may also be generally applicable to the other strains of the same genus, requiring only a few adaptations or modifications.

Embryo transfer technology

Embryo transfer technology is a technique by which embryos are collected from a donor female and transferred to recipient females, which serve as surrogate mothers for the remainder of pregnancy. Embryo transfer techniques have been applied to nearly every inter-generic and intra-specific species of domestic animals and too many species of wildlife and exotic animals, including humans and non-human primates. Within the past decade, the degree of sophistication of embryo transfer procedures has evolved to permit complete utilization of non-surgical procedures in the cow, long term embryo culture and storage with cryopreservation, and, more recently, micromanipulation and many techniques associated with genetic engineering. This is a rapidly developing science with a very short lag-time between discovery and application. The potential applications continue to increase with the development of new technology. This technology achieves a surprisingly rapid rate of multiplication of animals of the selected superior genotype. In natural course, a single female will produce a single progeny in about one year. But using super-ovulation and embryo transfer technology, it is possible to collect around 36 embryos from one female in one year. Assuming an average success rate of 50% in the embryo transfer, an average of 18 progeny can be derived from one superior female in one year. Although the embryo transfer procedure has, fundamentally, remained unchanged, modifications in the technique to improve the efficiency, the donor and recipient safety, and the success rate, as well as the advent of embryo freezing, embryo micromanipulation and embryo sexing have kept the industry dynamic and extremely challenging.

Stem cell technology

Stem cells are characterized by the ability to renew themselves through mitotic cell division and differentiating into a diverse range of specialized cell types. Although most cells of the body, such as heart cells or skin cells, are committed to conduct a specific function, a stem cell is uncommitted and remains uncommitted, until it receives a signal to develop into a specialized cell. Research in the stem cell field grew out of findings by Canadian scientists Ernest A. McCulloch and James E. Till in the 1960s. The two broad types of mammalian stem cells are embryonic stem cells that are isolated from the inner cell mass of blastocysts, and adult stem cells that are found in adult tissues. Highly plastic adult stem cells from a variety of sources, including umbilical cord blood and bone marrow, are routinely used in medical therapies. Embryonic cell lines and autologous embryonic stem cells generated through therapeutic cloning have also been proposed as promising candidates for future therapies. Stem cells may hold the key to replacing cells lost in many devastating diseases like Parkinson's disease, diabetes, chronic heart disease, end-stage kidney disease, liver failure, and cancer are just a few for which stem cells have therapeutic potential. Today, science has brought us to a point where the immune response can be subdued, so that organs from one person can be used to replace the diseased organs and tissues of another. Scientists in academic and industrial research are vigorously pursuing all possible avenues of research, including ways to direct the specialization of adult and embryonic stem cells to become pancreatic islet-like cells that produce insulin and can be used to control blood glucose levels. Researchers have recently shown that human embryonic stem cells be directly differentiated into cells that produce insulin. Predicting the future of stem cell applications is impossible, particularly given the very early stage of the science of stem cell biology. To date, it is impossible to predict which stem cells those derived from the embryo, the fetus, or the adult or which methods for manipulating the cells, will best meet the needs of basic research and clinical applications. The answers clearly lie in conducting more research.

Animal transgenic technology

Animal transgenic technology deals with the production of transgenic animals that depends upon the success of a series of several complex technical experimental manipulations. Even under the best of circumstances, the success of these manipulations can be somewhat variable, depending upon the genetic background of the host or the recipient cells as well as upon the biological consequences of gene or DNA-sequence modification. Nevertheless, the construction of transgenic animals is available as a resource in most research settings, thus allowing for the systematic *in vivo* evaluation of the consequences of deleting, altering, or over-expressing a single gene or DNA sequence of interest. While both transgenic rats and mice useful for toxicological studies have been generated, thus far most efforts have focused on the generation of transgenic mouse model systems. Indeed, these systems provide excellent experimental models for the evaluation of gene-specific interactions in the studies of metabolism, pharmacology, and carcinogenesis.

Potentially, specifically modified transgenic animals will be generated that allow for a limited response to a toxic agent, thereby better defining the role of a specific gene product in the cellular or organism response pathway. In addition to the development of new and more elaborate transgenic models, one can expect to see an increasing number of applications of molecular biology in studies of toxicology in the future.

Liposome technology

Liposomes are amphipathic in nature, i.e., one part of their structure is water-soluble (hydrophilic or water-loving) and the other part is oil-like (hydrophobic or water-fearing or fat-soluble). They are well-recognized delivery vehicles that have been developed to enhance the therapeutic activity of several drugs. Liposomes are the smallest artificial vesicles of spherical shape that can be used as drug carriers and loaded with a great variety of molecules, such as vaccines, proteins, genes, enzymes and even plasmids to the body. Liposomes are extremely versatile and due to the variability of their composition they can be used for a large number of applications such as gene therapy, cancer therapy, clinical pathogenesis, enzyme replacement theory, chelation therapy, immunomodulation, thermal transitions of phospholipids, neurobiological applications, leukocyte phagocytosis, botanical research, drug interactions with membranes, bacterial cell wall synthesis, lectin receptor interactions, microvillus formation in cells and many more. These are only a few of the applications for which liposomes have been used. Reports of new types of liposomes and as well as new uses for liposomes appear almost daily.

Vaccine technology

Vaccines are suspensions of live, killed, or attenuated microorganisms such as bacteria or viruses or their components. They are designed for human or veterinary use to prime the immune system to produce antibodies or cellular responses that ward off future diseases by pathogenic organisms or their toxins. Research into vaccine technology continues on many fronts to provide safe, efficacious, and affordable vaccine products. One approach to improve coverage that is being adopted by many vaccine manufacturers is to combine antigens into single preparation so that immunity to two or more diseases can be achieved with a single injection. Time release polymeric preparations are also being explored even for monovalent preparations to achieve repeated antigenic stimulation of the immune system without the need for multiple injections. Other research initiatives seek to eliminate the need for needles for delivery of vaccines through the use of oral vaccines, aerosolizers for inhalation, or needleless devices that use compressed gases at high pressure to deliver transdermal doses of vaccine preparations. The tremendous amount of research in the past few years has led to the development of vaccines against disease targets associated with bacterial, viral, and parasitic infections and provides hope for combating autoimmune and inflammatory diseases as well as cancer.

Synthetic biologicals technology

There is no agreed definition of synthetic biology, but it is best understood as the deliberate design of biological systems and living organisms using engineering principles. Synthetic biology is the design and construction of new biological entities, such as enzymes, genetic circuits, and cells, or the redesign of existing biological systems. The goal of synthetic biology, which builds on advances in molecular, cellular, and systems biology, is to transform biology in the same way that synthesis transformed chemistry and integrated circuit design transformed computing. The aims of synthetic biology include:

(1) the production of minimal living genomes;
(2) the design of interchangeable parts that can be assembled into pathways for the fabrication of novel components;
(3) the construction of entirely artificial cells; and
(4) the creation of synthetic biomolecules.

Research within synthetic biology can be explored through one of the two approaches: top-down, or bottom-up. The top-down approach attempts to eliminate the problem of natural complexity by removing it, e.g., by stripping a genome of all genetic material that is not absolutely essential for replication and functionality. The bottom-up approach uses naturally occurring organisms that appear to have little complexity and adds the required functions by engineering them into the existing genome. There are a number of major areas of research that constitute the field of synthetic biology such as making minimal genomes; designing modular components; pathway engineering; expanding the genetic pool; production of artificial cells; and creation of synthetic biomolecules. Just as engineers now design integrated circuits based on the known physical properties of materials and then fabricate functioning circuits and entire processors (with relatively high reliability), synthetic biologists will soon design and build engineered biological systems.

Bioengineering

Bioengineering (also known as Biological Engineering) is the application of engineering principles to address challenges in the fields of biology and medicine. Bioengineering integrates physical, chemical, biochemical and mathematical competencies and expertise with engineering approaches for applications in the field of biology, medicine, health and food industry. It applies engineering principles to the full spectrum of living systems. This is achieved by utilizing the existing methodologies in such fields as molecular biology, biochemistry, microbiology, pharmacology, cytology, immunology and neuroscience and applies them to the design of medical devices, diagnostic equipment, biocompatible materials, and other important medical needs. Bioengineering is not limited to the medical field. Bioengineers have the ability to exploit new opportunities and solve problems within the domain of complex systems. They have a great understanding of living systems as complex systems, which can be applied to many fields including entrepreneurship. Much as other engineering disciplines also address human health (e.g., prosthetics in mechanical engineering), bioengineers can apply their expertise to other applications of engineering and biotechnology, including genetic modification of plants and microorganisms, bioprocess engineering, and biocatalysis. However, the main fields of bioengineering may be categorized as: Biomedical Engineering, Biomedical technology, Biomedical Diagnosis, Biomedical Therapy, Biomechanics, Biomaterials, Genetic Engineering, Cell Engineering and Tissue Culture Engineering. "Bioengineering" is also used to describe the use of vegetation in civil engineering constructions. The term bioengineering may also be applied to environmental modifications such as surface soil protection, slope stabilization, watercourse and shoreline protection, windbreaks, vegetation barriers including noise barriers and visual screens, and the ecological enhancement of an area.

Immobilized biocatalyst technology

Immobilized biocatalyst technology can be defined as "enzymes physically confined or localized in a certain defined region of space with retention of their catalytic activities, and which can be used repeatedly and continuously". Accordingly, enzymes modified to a water-insoluble form by suitable techniques satisfy this definition of immobilized enzymes. This is known as immobilization and may be achieved by fixing the enzyme to, or within, some other material. It provides stability and easy separation of the enzyme from the products of the catalyzed reaction that minimizing downstream processing costs and possible effluent handling problems, particularly if the enzyme is noticeably toxic or antigenic. It also allows continuous processes to be practicable, with a considerable saving in enzyme, labor and overhead costs. During the last three decades, immobilization of enzymes, cells, and organelles has found vast analytical, technological, and medical applications. Biological materials have a great variety of properties, and for each particular application, the proper choice of support and immobilization method may not always be easy to accomplish. Immobilized biocatalyst technology is presently going through a phase of maturation and evolution. The evolution is shown by the ever broadening range of enzymic applications. Immobilized enzymes will clearly be more widely used in the future and this will be reflected in the number of enzymes available on an industrial (and research) scale, the variety of reactions catalyzed and the range of environmental conditions under which they will operate. Established immobilized enzymes will be put to new uses and novel enzymes, discovered within their biological niches or produced by design using enzyme engineering, will be used to catalyze hitherto unexploited reactions. This is just the start of the immobilized biocatalyst technology era.

Bioprocess engineering

Bioprocess engineering is the sub-discipline within biotechnology that is responsible for translating the discoveries of life science into practical products, processes, or systems that can serve the needs of society. Bioprocess engineers work at the frontiers of biological and engineering sciences to "Bring engineering to life" through the conversion of biological materials into other forms needed by mankind. Application areas commonly associated with bioprocess engineering include the production of biofuels, ethanol, amino acids and other organic acids, antibiotics, design and operation of fermentation systems, development of food processing systems, application and testing of product separation technologies, design of instrumentation to monitor and control biological processes, and many more. Like other engineering disciplines, bioprocess engineers are trained in the application of engineering sciences and problem solving techniques. What separates them from other engineers is their understanding of how every engineering field relates to living materials. With the rapid growth of biologically based technologies, bioprocess engineers are uniquely qualified to solve the problems of today and tomorrow. The demand for bioprocess engineers continues to grow. They provide a bridge between the research lab and the economic, large-scale implementation of biotechnologies and food production systems.

Metagenomics technology

Metagenome technology (metagenomics) uses a culture-independent approach to collect, sort, categorize and identify sequences of microbes retrieved from environmental samples such as soil or water. The emerging field of metagenomics provides a new way of viewing the microbial world that will not only transform modern microbiology, but also may revolutionize understanding of the entire living world. Through metagenomics, scientists can apply the power of genomic analysis to entire communities of microbes, bypassing the need to isolate and culture individual community members. Metagenomics involves studying the genetic makeup of many microbes in an environment simultaneously, and makes accessible the many types of microbes that cannot be grown in the laboratory and therefore cannot be studied using the central tool of classical microbiology. Metagenomics has been applied to many environments, including the oceans, soils, thermal vents, hot springs, and the human mouth and gastrointestinal tract. Areas in which metagenomics offers particular value include: medicine, alternative energy, environmental remediation, biotechnology, agriculture, biodefense, and forensics. Increased understanding of microbes will lead to new concepts of genomes, species, evolution, and ecosystem robustness that will have effects beyond the specific field of microbiology. Metagenomics can help scientists address questions such as "How do microbes evolve?" "What is the role of microbes in maintaining the health of their hosts?" and "How diverse is life?".

Bioremediation technology

Bioremediation is a process which relies on microorganisms to break down and detoxify organic chemicals such as hydrocarbons and some organochlorines. Carbon dioxide and water are the final degradation products for hydrocarbon wastes using this process. Bioremediation has a number of applications within the mining industry, including the treatment of the various types of wastes. Bioremediation has proven to be a non-disruptive, non-toxic, non-pathogenic cost-effective and highly efficient method of safely breaking down many environmentally persistent toxic chemicals. Bioremediation is gaining attention as it is fast, economical, and does not require heavy machinery or skilled labor, according to the analyst of this research service. These technologies are also efficient in the biodegradation of contaminants to create end products that are not hazardous to the environment. Bioremediation technologies in various companies generally vary from one site to another depending on the kind of contaminants, the hydrogeology, and the accessibility of the contaminants.

BIOTECHNOLOGY REGULATIONS

The National Institute of Health (NIH) was the first federal agency to assume regulatory responsibility in the United States. The Recombinant DNA Advisory Committee of the NIH published guidelines for working with recombinant DNA and recombinant organisms in the laboratory. Agencies responsible for the biotechnology regulations are: US Department of Agriculture (USDA) regulates plant pests and medical preparation from living organisms, Environment Protection Agency (EPA) regulates pesticides and herbicides, and the Food and Drug Administration (FDA) ensures that the food and drug products are safe and effective.

The Regulatory framework in India: To ensure the compliance of safeguards on various levels, drafting of guidelines and their implementation is indispensable. The activities and use of GE organism and products thereof are regulated under the "Rules for the manufacture, use/import/ export and storage of hazardous organisms/GE organism or cells notified under the Environment Protection Act, 1986, commonly referred as Rules, 1989. These rules and regulations are implemented by the Ministry of Environment and Forest (MOEF) & Department of Biotechnology (DBT) and state governments. Six competent authorities and their composition have been p rovided for in the Rules to handle various aspects (http://www.dbtbiosafety,nic,in-stepwise procedure) are as follows:

- Recombinant DNA Advisory Committee (RDAC)
- Review Committee on Genetic Manipulation (RCGM)
- Genetic Engineering Approval Committee (GEAC)
- Institutional Bio-safety Committee (IBSC)
- State Border Coordination Committee (SBCC)
- District Level Committees (DLCs)

While RDAC is advisory in function, the IBSC, RCGM & GEAC are for regulatory functions, SBCC & DLC are for monitoring purpose. In addition to the above, a monitoring-cum-evaluation committee (MEC) has been set up by RCGM to monitor the field performance of GM crops. DBT has issued certain guidelines for applicants seeking approval for environmental release of GE plants in India under Rules, 1989. Specifically these protocols address key elements of the safety assessment of foods and/or livestock feeds that may be derived from GM crops. The results are submitted to appropriate regulatory bodies, i.e., RCGM and GEAC as required. DBT reviewed these guidelines in 2008 and made them available as draft guidelines on its website. DBT has prepared five protocols each based on best international practices including guidance and peer reviewed from the codex Alimenatrius Commission, FAO, WHO and Organization for Economic Cooperation and Development and the ILSI (http://www/dbtbiosafety.nic.in-protocols). These include:

- Acute oral safety limit study in rats or mice
- Sub-chronic feeding study rodents
- Protein thermal stability
- Pepsin digestibility assay
- Livestock feeding assay

For additional guidance, the ICMR guidelines for the safety assessment of foods derived from genetically engineered plants that provide a comprehensive summary of information and data required must be provided to regulatory authorities of demostrate the GE plants, may also be reviewed (http://www/dbtbiosafety.nic.in-protocols). With the increase in Indian biotechnology sector, significant implementation in area of regulation is expected. The 2004 Report of Task Force on Application of Agricultural Biotechnology (The Swaminanthan Report) and the 2005 report of

Task Force of Recombinant Pharma (The Mashelkar report) both have recommended the establishment of a national biotechnology regulatory authority (NBRA). The NBRA will be an autonomous, statutory agency established by GOI with a mandate to safeguard the health of the people of India and to protect the environment by identifying risks posed by, or as a result of, modern biotechnology, and deployment of biotechnology products and processes. In order to empower NBRA, DBT has defined a new legislation namely the Biotechnology Regulatory Bill in April 2008 (www/agbios.com/sabp – June 2008).

FURTHER READINGS

1. Anne S.U. (2002) Biophysical aspects of using liposomes as delivery vehicles. *Journal of Bioscience Reports* **(22):** 129-149.
2. Avise (1994) ed., *Molecular Markers, Natural History and Evolution,* Chapman and Hall, New York, pp. 1-5.
3. Babu R., Nair S.K., Prasanna B.M. and Gupta H.S. (2004) Integrating marker-assisted selection in crop breeding-Prospects and challenges. *Current Sci.* 87 **(5):** 607-619.
4. Becker A.J., McCulloch E.A. and Till J.E. (1963) Cytological demonstration of the clonal nature of spleen colonies derived from transplanted mouse marrow cells. *Nature*. **(197):** 452-454.
5. Betteridge K.J. (1981) A historical look at embryo transfer. *J. Reprod Fert.* **(62):** 1-13.
6. Bradford, G.E. and Kennedy, B.W. (1980) Genetic aspects of embryo transfer. *Theriogenology.* **(13):** 13-26.
7. Canton B., Labno A. and Endy D. (2008) Refinement and standardization of synthetic biological parts and devices. *Nat. Biotechnol.* **(26):** 771-774.
8. Cercós M., Soler G., Iglesias D.J., Gadea J., Forment J. and Talón M. (2006) Global analysis of gene expression during development and ripening of citrus fruit flesh. A proposed mechanism for citric Acid utilization. *Plant Mol. Biol.* **(62):** 513-527.
9. Chawla H.S. (2002) Transgenics in crop improvement In: Introduction to plant Biotechnology, 2nd edt. Oxford and IBH Publishing Co. Pvt. Ltd., New Delhi, pp. 396-427.
10. Cheetham, P.S.J. (1987) Screening for novel biocatalysts. *Enzyme and Microbial Technology* **(9):** 194-213.
11. Chotai K. and Payne S.J. (1998) A rapid, PCR-based test for differential molecular diagnosis of Prader-Willi and Angelman syndromes. *Journal of Medical Genetics.* **(35):** 472-475.
12. Choudhary K., Choudhary O.P. and Shekhawat N.S. (2008) Marker Assisted Selection: A Novel Approach for Crop Improvement. *American-Eurasian Journal of Agronomy.* 1 **(2):** 26-30.
13. Chrispeels, M.J. and Sadava, D.E. (1994) Plant biotechnology: An overview. *In: C Plants, Genes and Agriculture*. Jones and Barlett Publishers, Boston, London. pp. 58-81.
14. Collins, F.S., Green, E.D., Guttmacher, A.E., and Guyer, M.S. (2003) A vision for the future of genomics research. *Nature.* **(422)** 835-847.
15. Conrad S., Renninger M., Hennenlotter J., *et al.* (2008) Generation of pluripotent stem cells from adult human testis. *Nature.* 456 **(7220):** 344-349.
16. Dahm, R. (2005) "Friedrich Miescher and the discovery of DNA". *Developmental biology.* 278 **(2):** 274–88.
17. Dekkers J.C.M. (2004) Commercial application of marker-and gene-assisted selection in livestock:strategies and lessons. *J. Animal Sci.* **(82):** 313-328.
18. Edwards S.W. and Preston R.J. (2008), Systems biology and mode of action based risk assessment. *Toxicol. Sci.* **(106):** 312-318.
19. Entani, E., S. Ohmori, H. Masai, and K. Suzuki. (1985) *Acetobacter polyoxogenes* sp. nov., a new species of an acetic acid bacterium useful for producing vinegar with high acidity. *J. Gen. Appl. Microbiol.* **(31):** 475-490.

20. Fire A., S.Q. Xu, M.K. Montgomery, S.A. Kostas, S.E. Driver and C.C. Mello (1998) Potent and specific genetic interference by double stranded RNA in Caenorhabditis elegans. *Nature.* **(391):** 806-811.
21. Franklin, W.A., Shpall, E.J., Archer, P., Johnston, C.S., Garza-Williams, S., Hami, L., Bitter M.A., Bast R.C. and Jones R.B. (1996) Immunocytochemical detection of breast cancer cells in marrow and peripheral blood of patients undergoing high dose chemotherapy with autologous stem cell support. *Breast Cancer Res. Treat.* 41 **(1):** 1-13.
22. Ghosh, A.K., Spriggs, A.I., Taylor-papadimitriou, J. and Mason, D.Y. (1983) Immunocytochemical staining of cells in pleural and peritoneal effusions with a panel of monoclonal antibodies. *J. Clin. Pathol.* **(36):** 1154-1164.
23. Glick, Bernard and Jack Pasternak (1998) *Molecular Biotechnology: Principles and Applications of Recombinant DNA,* 2nd ed. Washington, DC: ASM Press.
24. Guisan Jose M. *et al.* (2007) Improvement of enzyme activity, selectivity and stability via immobilization techniques". *Enzyme and Microbial Technology.* 40 **(6):** 1451-1463.
25. Hall, E.A.H. (1986) The developing biosensor arena. *Enzyme and Microbial Technology.* **(8):** 651-657.
26. Handelsman J. (2005) How to find new antibiotics: metagenomics could be the way to mine the soil beneath our feet. *The Scientist.* 19 **(19):** e20.
27. Hiroaki Kitano (2002) Systems Biology: A Brief *Overview Science* 1, 295. **(5560):** 1662-1664.
28. Igor Kovalchuk and Kovalchuk (2008) Transgenic plants as sensor of environmental pollution genotoxicity. *Sensor.* **(8):** 1539-1588.
29. Jean M.M., Gary R.M., Lynn E.S. and Carl R.A. (1999) Oil in water liposomal emulsions: Characterization and potential use in vaccine delivery. *Journal of Pharmaceutical Sciences.* 88 **(2):** 1332-1339.
30. Johansson J.F., Paul L.R. and Finlay R.D. (2004) Microbial interactions in the mycorrhizosphere and their significance for sustainable agriculture. *FEMS Microbiol. Ecol.* **48:** 1-13.
31. Kennedy, J.F. and Cabral, J.M.S. (1987) Enzyme immobilisation. In Biotechnology, vol. 7a, Enzyme Technology, ed. J.F. Kennedy, pp. 347-404. Weinheim: VCH Verlagsgesellschaft mbH.
32. Kumar Anil; Jaiswal, J.P., Hota, M. and Garg, G.K. (2007) LMOs! !GMOs!! Are they safe? Frequently asked questions on Biotechnology and Biosafety. pp. 4.
33. Kurreck J. (2003) Antisense technologies: Improvement through novel chemical modifications. European *Journal of Biochemistry.* **(270):** 1628 1644.
34. Lehmann, M., Loch, C., Middendorf, A., *et al.* (2002) The consensus concept for thermostability engineering of proteins: further proof of concept. *Protein Eng.* **(15):** 403-411.
35. Li L., Nie Y., Zhu R., Shi S., Luo K., He B., Yang Y., Yang J. and Gu Z. (2008) Preparation and gene delivery of alkaline amino acids-based cationic liposomes. *Arch. Pharm. Res.* 31 **(7):** 924-931.
36. Lumelsky, Anna (2005) "Diamond v. Chakrabarty: Gauging Congress's response to dynamic statutory interpretation by the Supreme Court". *University of San Francisco Low Review*. 39 **(3):** 641.
37. Lowe, C.R. (1984) Biosensors. *Trends in Biotechnology.* **(2):** 59-64.
38. Maria Monti, Stefania Orru', Daniela Pagnozzi and Piero Pucci (2005) Functional proteomics. *Clinica Chimica Acta*. **(357):** 140-150.
39. Mullis K.B. (1990) The unusual origin of the polymerase chain reaction. *Sci Am*. 262 **(4):** 56-61 & 64-65.
40. Mullis, Kary (1998) *Dancing Naked in the Mind Field.* New York: Pantheon Books.
41. Nanba A., Kimura K., and Nagai S. (1985) Vinegar Production by Acetobacter rancens cells fixed on a hollow fiber module. *J. Ferment. Technol.* 63 **(2):** 175-179.
42. Patterson S.D. and Aebersold R.H. (2003) Proteomics: the first decade and beyond. *Nat. Genet.* **(33):** 311-323.
43. Pauling L., Robinson A.B., Teranishi R. and Cary P. (1971) Quantitative analysis of urine vapour and breath by gas-liquid partition chromatography. *PNAS, USA.* **(68):** 2374-2376.
44. Pavlov A.R., Pavlova N.V., Kozyavkin S.A. and Slesarev A.I. (2004) Recent developments in the optimization of thermostable DNA polymerases for efficient applications. *Trends Biotechnol.* **(22):** 253-260.

45. Rabie G.H. and Almadini A.M. (2005) Role of bioinoculants in development of salt-tolerance of *Vicia faba* plants under salinity stress. *African Journal of Biotechnology.* 4 **(3):** 210-222.
46. Ramos S., Hernandez M., Roces A., *et al.* (1998) Molecular diagnosis of alkaptonuria mutation by analysis of homogentisate 1,2 dioxygenase mRNA from urine and blood. *American Journal of Medical Genetics*. **(78):** 192-194.
47. Roos, D. (2001) Bioinformatics: Trying to swim in a sea of data." *Science*. 291 **(5507):** 1260-1266.
48. Sanger F., Air G.M., Barrell B.G., Brown N.L., Coulson A.R., Fiddes C.A., Hutchison C.A., Slocombe P.M. and Smith M. (1977) Nucleotide sequence of bacteriophage phi X174 DNA. *Nature.* 265 **(5596):** 687-695.
49. Schena M., Shalon D., Davis R.W. and Brown P.O. (1995) Quantitative monitoring of gene expression patterns with a complimentary DNA microarray. *Science.* **(270):** 467-470.
50. Scherer L.J. and Rossi J.J. (2003) Approaches for the sequence specific knockdown of mRNA. *Nat. Biotech.* **(21):** 1457-1463.
51. Sreenan, J.M. (1983) Embryo transfer procedure and its use as a research technique. *Vet. Rec.* **(112):** 494-500.
52. Tingey, S. V., Rafalski, J. A. and Williams, J. G. K. (1993) *Application of RAPD Technology to Plant Breeding* (ed. Neff, M.), ASHS Publishers, Minnesota, pp. 3-8.
53. Tiwari S., Goyal A.K., Khatri K., Mishra N. and Vyas S.P. (2008) Gel core liposomes: An advanced carrier for improved vaccine delivery. *J. Microencapsul*. **(25):** 1-8.
54. Toudjarska I., Kilpatrick M.W., Lembessis P., *et al.* (2001) Novel approach to the molecular diagnosis of Marfan syndrome: Application to sporadic cases and in prenatal diagnosis. *American Journal of Medical Genetics.* **(99):** 294-302.
55. Trabulo S., Mano M., Faneca H., Cardoso A.L., Duarte S., Henriques A., Paiva A., Gomes P., Simões S. and de Lima M.C. (2008) S4 (13)-PV cell penetrating peptide and cationic liposomes act synergistically to mediate intracellular delivery of plasmid DNA. *J. Gene Med.* 10 **(11):** 1210-1222.
56. Tuch B.E. (2006) Stem cells—a clinical update. *Australian Family Physician*. 35 **(9):** 719-21.
57. Turner, A.P.F., Karube, I. and Wilson, G.S. eds. (1987) *Biosensors: Fundamentals and Applications.* Oxford, U.K: Oxford University Press.
58. Wan Q., Zhang X.G. and Song M. (2007) Fruit-specific RNAi-mediated restraining expression of Lcy gene to enhance lycopene content in tomatoes. *Chinese Journal of Biotechnology*. **(23):** 29-43.
59. Warwick, B.L. and Berry, R.O. (1949) Inter-generic and intra-specific embryo transfers. *J. Hered.* **(40):** 297-303.
60. Weising, K., Nybom, H., Wolff, K. and Meyer, W. (1995) *DNA Fingerprinting in Plants and Fungi* (ed. Arbor, A.) CRC Press, Boca Raton, pp. 1-3.
61. Whitesides G.M. (2003) The right size in nanobiotechnology. *Nat. Biotechol.* **(21):** 161-165.
62. Xiong A.S., Yao Q.H., Peng R.H., Li X., Han P.L. and Fan H.Q. (2005) Different effects on ACC oxidase gene silencing triggered by RNA interference in transgenic tomato. *Plant Cell Rep.* **(23):** 639-646.
63. Young N.D. (1999) A cautiously optimistic vision for marker-assisted breeding. *Molecular Breeding.* **(5):** 505-510.

SECTION A

Biotechnology for Wider Applications

CHAPTER

2

Recombinant DNA Technology

Recombinant DNA technology is recombining of DNA molecules from two different species inserted into a host organism to produce new genetic combinations that are of value to science, medicine, agriculture, or industry. This chapter deals with the basic principles and practical applications of recombinant DNA technology that can be used to study mutations and their biological effects, gene therapy, reverse genetics, diagnostics, genomics, and protein manufacture.

Keywords: Recombinant DNA technology; genetic engineering; gene cloning; genetic transformation.

INTRODUCTION

Recombinant DNA is a form of artificial DNA that is engineered through the combination or insertion of one or more DNA strands, thereby combining DNA sequences that would not normally occur together. In terms of genetic modification, recombinant DNA is produced through the addition of relevant DNA into an existing organismal genome, such as the plasmid of bacteria, to code for or alter different traits for a specific purpose. It differs from genetic recombination in that it does not occur through processes within the cell or ribosome, but is exclusively engineered. Recombinant DNA technology utilizes techniques for cleaving DNA and splicing it into a carrier molecule (vector) that make it possible to transfer genetic information from one organism to an unrelated organism, where it may be expressed. The host cells will then synthesize the foreign protein from the recombinant DNA. When the cells are grown in vast quantities, the foreign or recombinant protein can be isolated and purified in large amounts. Recombinant DNA technology is also called Hybridization and Genetic Engineering *in vivo* and *in vitro* respectively.

The recombinant DNA technique was engineered by Stanley Norman Cohen and Herbert Boyer in 1973. They published their findings in a 1974 paper entitled "Construction of Biologically Functional Bacterial Plasmids *in vitro*", which described a technique to isolate and amplify genes or DNA segments and insert them into another cell with precision, creating a transgenic bacterium. Recombinant DNA technology was made possible by the discovery of restriction endonucleases by Werner Arber, Daniel Nathans, and Hamilton Smith, for which they received the 1978 Nobel Prize in Medicine.

Recombinant DNA technology is not only an important tool in scientific research, but it has also impacted the diagnosis and treatment of diseases and genetic disorders in many areas of medicine. It has enabled many advances, including isolation of large quantities of pure protein; identification of mutations; diagnosis of affected and carrier states for hereditary diseases; and transferring of genes from one organism to another. Because of the importance of DNA in the replication of new structures and characteristics of living organisms, it has widespread importance in recapitulating via viral or non-viral vectors, both desirable and undesirable characteristics of a species to achieve characteristic change or to counteract effects caused by genetic or imposed disorders that have effects upon cellular or organismal processes. Through the use of recombinant DNA, genes that are identified as important can be amplified and isolated for use in other species or applications, where there may be some form of genetic illness or discrepancy, and provides a different approach to solve complex biological problem. Applying these techniques has already brought significant changes in industry and medicine. Future applications of recombinant DNA technology will transform our lives.

CONCEPTS

The history of recombinant DNA technology follows a classic pattern for scientific discoveries. At first there was a phase of slow development as a few unconnected theories were formed about fundamental biological processes. Then, quite suddenly, many of these different lines of work converged. There followed a rapid expansion as these theories led to techniques, and the techniques found valuable practical uses.

The foundation for recombinant DNA technology can be traced to Thompson's discovery of the electron in 1887 that laid the foundation for biochemistry, Miescher's isolation of DNA, Avery's demonstration of DNA as genetic material in 1944, Watson and Crick's proposal of DNA's double helix structure in 1953, plasmidology by Cohen *et al.* in 1973. The development of recombinant DNA tools and techniques in the early 1970s led to much concern about developing genetically modified organisms with unanticipated and potentially dangerous properties. This concern led to a proposal for a voluntary moratorium on recombinant DNA research in 1974, and to a meeting in 1975 at the Asilomar Conference Center in California. Participants at the Asilomar Conference agreed to a set of safety standards for recombinant DNA work, including the use of disabled bacteria that were unable to survive outside the laboratory. This conference helped to satisfy the public about the safety of recombinant DNA research, and led to a rapid expansion of the use of these powerful new technologies. Using recombinant DNA technology, first fungal gene was cloned and expressed in *E. coli* in 1976, followed by a hormone, Somatostatin, responsible for the growth, Dihydrofolate reductase and Proinsulin in 1978 and Hepatitis B genes in 1979. The list went on and continues to expand even today. Genetic engineering has now become integral part of our lives. Scientific views on DNA and genes are challenging the fundamental concepts of the nature of the life, society and humanities. The ethical and social aspects of genetic engineering are being debated intensely today. The concept of using recombinant molecules is mainly for two purposes: first, for the basic study of gene structure (e.g., discovery of the split gene in eukaryotes), and secondly to endow (or assurance) the host with the capability of producing substances, which it normally is unable to do (e.g., biosynthesis of insulin, growth hormone, interferon, etc.).

PRINCIPLES

The basic principles of recombinant DNA technology involve digesting a vehicle e.g., plasmids or viral DNA with a restriction enzyme, which is the molecular scissors that cuts DNA at specific sites. A DNA molecule from the organism of interest is also digested in a separate tube with the same restriction enzyme. The two DNAs are then mixed together and joined, this time using an enzyme called DNA ligase, to make an intact double-stranded DNA molecule. So the vehicle containing the foreign DNA is then introduced into the recipient organism by transformation or transfection. It is important to make sure that the vehicle has a replication origin, which is recognized by the DNA synthesis machinery of the host. After this the foreign DNA is multiplied manifold in the new host (Figure 2.1). It is also essential to ensure that the signals involved in the

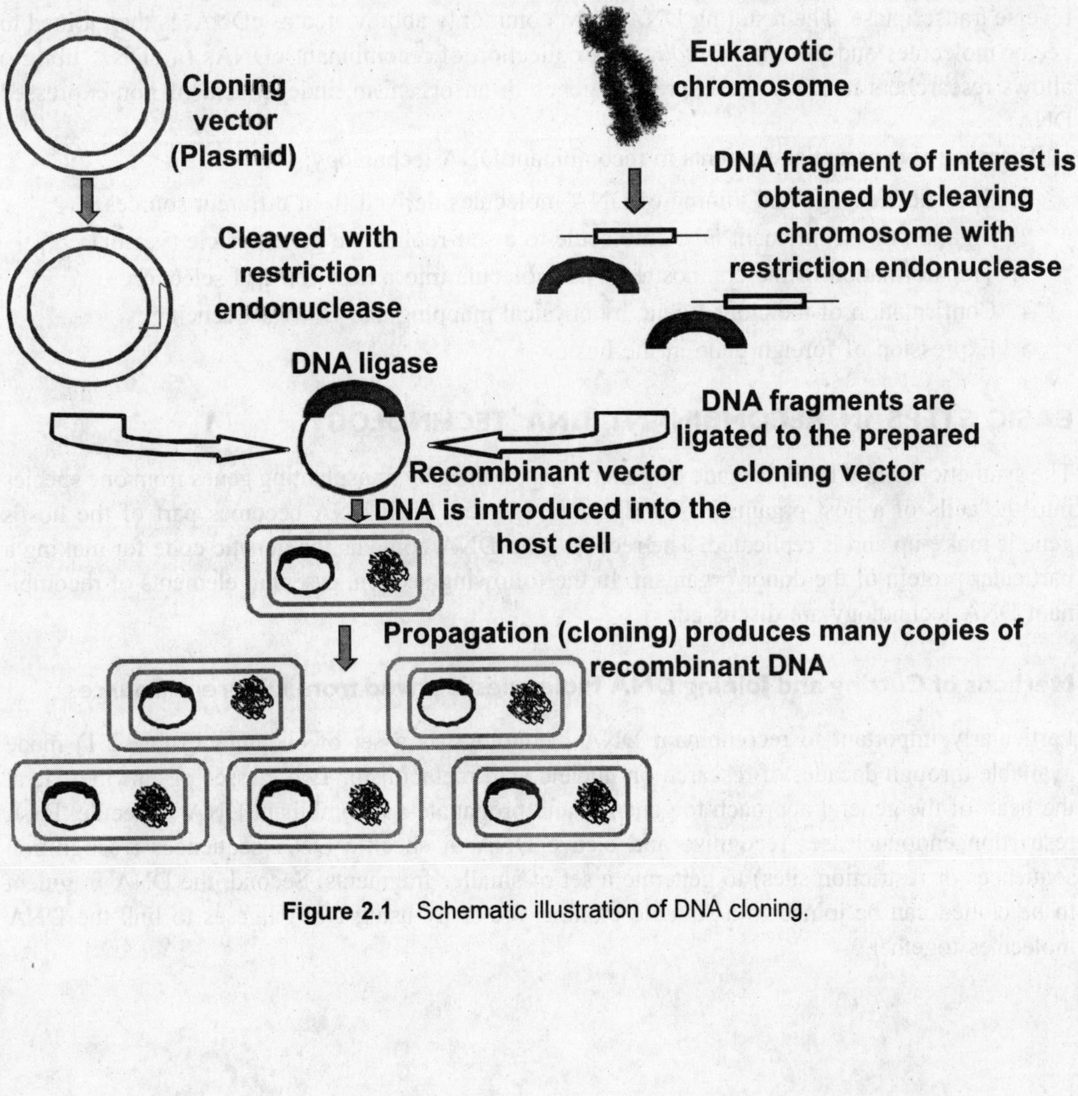

Figure 2.1 Schematic illustration of DNA cloning.

expression (transcription and translation) of the new gene are compatible with the expression machinery of the host. This novel DNA molecule is then isolated from the host cells and analyzed to make sure that the correct construct was produced. This DNA can then be sequenced, used to generate protein from *E. coli* or another host, or for many other purposes. There are many variations of this basic method of producing recombinant DNA molecules. For example, sometimes researchers are interested in isolating a whole collection of DNAs from an organism. In this case, they digest the whole genome with restriction enzyme, join many DNA fragments into many different vector molecules, and then transform those molecules into *E. coli*. The different *E. coli* cells that contain different DNA molecules are then pooled, resulting in a "library" of *E. coli* cells that contain, collectively, all of the genes present in the original organism. Another variation is to make a library of all expressed genes (genes that are used to make proteins) from an organism or tissue. In this case, RNA is isolated. The isolated RNA is converted to DNA using the enzyme called reverse transcriptase. The resulting DNA copy, commonly abbreviated as cDNA, is then joined to vector molecules and put into *E. coli*. This collection of recombinant cDNAs (a cDNA library) allows researchers to study the expressed genes in an organism, independent of non-expressed DNA.

There are five essential elements in recombinant DNA technology:

1. Specific cleavage and joining of DNA molecules derived from different sources.
2. Ligation of recombinant DNA molecule to a self-replicative gene vehicle (vector).
3. Transformation of the composite DNA molecule into a host cell and selection.
4. Confirmation of the cloned gene by physical mapping and DNA sequencing.
5. Expression of foreign gene in the host.

BASIC STEPS IN RECOMBINANT DNA TECHNOLOGY

The synthetic form of DNA is made by genetic engineering by transplanting genes from one species into the cells of a host organism of a different species. Such DNA becomes part of the host's genetic make-up and is replicated. The recombinant DNA contains the genetic code for making a particular protein of the donor organism. In the following section, essential elements of recombinant DNA technology are discussed.

Methods of Cutting and Joining DNA Molecules Derived from Different Sources

Particularly important to recombinant DNA technology is a set of enzymes (Table 2.1) made available through decades of research on nucleic acid metabolism. Two classes of enzymes lie at the heart of the general approach to generate and propagate a recombinant DNA molecule. First, restriction endonucleases recognize and cleave DNA at specific DNA sequences (recognition sequences or restriction sites) to generate a set of smaller fragments. Second, the DNA fragment to be cloned can be joined to a suitable cloning vector by using DNA ligases to link the DNA molecules together.

Table 2.1 Some enzymes used in recombinant DNA technology.

Enzyme	*Function*
Restriction endonucleases (type II)	Cleave DNAs at specific base sequence
DNA Ligase	Joins the two DNA molecules
DNA Polymerase I	Additions of nucleotides at 3′ ends of duplex DNA molecule for filling gaps
Reverse transcriptase	Makes a DNA copy of an RNA molecule
Polynucleotide kinase	Adds a phosphate to 5′-OH end of a polynucleotide
Terminal transferase	Adds homopolymer tails to the 3′-OH ends of a linear duplex
Exonuclease III	Removes nucleotide from the 3′ ends of a DNA molecule
Bacteriophage I exonuclease	Removes nucleotide from the 5′ ends of a duplex to expose single-stranded 3′ ends
Alkaline phosphatase	Removes terminal phosphate from either the 5′ or 3′ end (or both)

The recombinant vector is then introduced into a host cell, which amplifies the fragment in the course of many generations of cell division. Restriction endonucleases are found in a wide range of bacterial species. Werner Arber discovered in the early 1960s that their biological function is to recognize and cleave foreign DNA (the DNA of an infecting virus). Such a DNA is said to be restricted. In the host cell's DNA, the sequence that would be recognized by its own restriction endonuclease is protected from digestion by methylation of the DNA, catalyzed by a specific DNA methylase. The restriction endonuclease and the corresponding methylase are sometimes referred to as a restriction-modification system. There are three types of restriction endonucleases, designated I, II, and III. Types I and III are generally large, multisubunit complexes containing both the endonuclease and methylase activities. Type I restriction endonucleases cleave DNA at random sites that can be more than 1,000 base pairs (bp) from the recognition sequence. Type III restriction endonucleases cleave the DNA about 25 bp from the recognition sequence. Both types move along the DNA in a reaction that requires the energy of ATP. Type II restriction endonucleases, first isolated by Smith and Wilox in 1970, are simpler, require no ATP, and cleave the DNA within the recognition sequence itself. The extraordinary utility of this group of restriction endonucleases was demonstrated by Daniel Nathans, who first used them to develop novel methods for mapping and analyzing genes and genomes. Thousands of restriction endonucleases have been discovered in different bacterial species, and more than 100 different DNA sequences are recognized by one or more of these enzymes. The recognition sequences are usually 4 to 6 bp long and palindromic. Table 2.2 lists sequences recognized by a few type II restriction endonucleases. Some restriction endonucleases make staggered cuts on the two DNA strands, leaving two to four nucleotides of one strand unpaired at each resulting end. These unpaired strands are referred to as sticky ends, because they can base-pair with each other or with complementary sticky ends of other DNA fragments. Other restriction endonucleases cleave both strands of DNA at the opposing phosphodiester bonds, leaving no unpaired bases on the ends, often called blunt ends (Figure 2.2).

The average size of the DNA fragments produced by cleaving genomic DNA with restriction endonucleases depends on the frequency with which a particular restriction site occurs in the DNA molecule. In a DNA molecule with a random sequence in which all four nucleotides were equally abundant, a 6 bp sequence recognized by a restriction endonuclease such as BamHI would occur on an average once every 4^6 (4,096) bp, assuming the DNA had a 50% G-C content. Enzymes that

Table 2.2 Recognition sequences for some type II restriction endonucleases.

Enzyme	Recognition sequence	Enzyme	Recognition sequence
BamHI	(5') G GATCC (3') CCTAGG	*HindIII*	(5') AAGCTT (3') TTCGAA
ClaI	(5') ATCGAT (3') TAGCTA	*NotI*	(5') GCGGCCGC (3') CGCCGGCG
EcoRI	(5') GAATTC (3') CTTAAG	*PstIII*	(5') CTGCAG (3') GACGTC
EcoRV	(5') GATATC (3') CTATAG	*PvuIII*	(5') CAGCTG (3') GTCGAC
HaeIII	(5') GGCC (3') CCGG	*Tth111*	(5') GACNNNGTC (3') CTGNNNCA

Arrows indicate the phosphodiester bonds cleaved by each restriction endonuclease. Asterisks indicate bases that are methylated by the corresponding methylase (where known). N denotes any base. Note that the name of each enzyme consists of a three-letter abbreviation (in italics) of the bacterial species from which it is derived, sometimes followed by a strain designation and Roman numerals to distinguish different restriction endonucleases isolated from the same bacterial species. Thus BamHI is the first (I) restriction endonuclease characterized from *Bacillus amyloliquefaciens*, strain H.

recognize a 4 bp sequence would produce smaller DNA fragments from a random-sequence DNA molecule; a recognition sequence of this size would be expected to occur about once every 4^4 (256) bp. In natural DNA molecules, particular recognition sequences tend to occur less frequently than this because nucleotide sequences in DNA are not random and the four nucleotides are not equally abundant. In laboratory experiments, the average size of the fragments produced by restriction endonucleases cleavage of a large DNA can be increased by simply terminating the reaction before completion; the result is called a partial digest. Fragment size can also be increased by using a special class of endonucleases called homing endonucleases. These recognize and cleave much longer DNA sequences (14 to 20 bp). Once a DNA molecule has been cleaved into fragments, a particular fragment of known size can be enriched by agarose or acrylamide gel electrophoresis or by HPLC. After the target DNA fragment is isolated, DNA ligase can be used to join it to a similarly digested cloning vector, i.e., a vector digested by the same restriction endonuclease. A fragment generated by *EcoRI*, for example, generally will not link to a fragment generated by *BamHI*. DNA ligase catalyzes the formation of new phosphodiester bonds in a reaction that uses ATP or a similar cofactor. The base-pairing of complementary sticky ends greatly facilitates the ligation reaction. Blunt ends can also be ligated, albeit less efficiently. Researchers can create new DNA sequences by inserting synthetic DNA fragments (called linkers) between the ends that are being ligated. Inserted DNA fragments with multiple recognition sequences for restriction endonucleases (often useful later as points for inserting additional DNA by cleavage and ligation) are called polylinkers. The effectiveness of sticky ends in selectively joining two DNA fragments was apparent in the earliest recombinant DNA experiments. Before restriction endonucleases were widely available, some workers found they could generate sticky ends by the combined action of the bacteriophage l, exonuclease and terminal transferase. The fragments to be joined were given complementary homopolymeric tails. Lobban and Kaiser used this method in 1973 in the first experiments to join naturally occurring DNA fragments. Similar methods were used soon after in the laboratory of Paul Berg to join DNA segments from simian virus 40 (SV40) to DNA derived from bacteriophage l, thereby creating the first recombinant DNA molecule with DNA segments from different species.

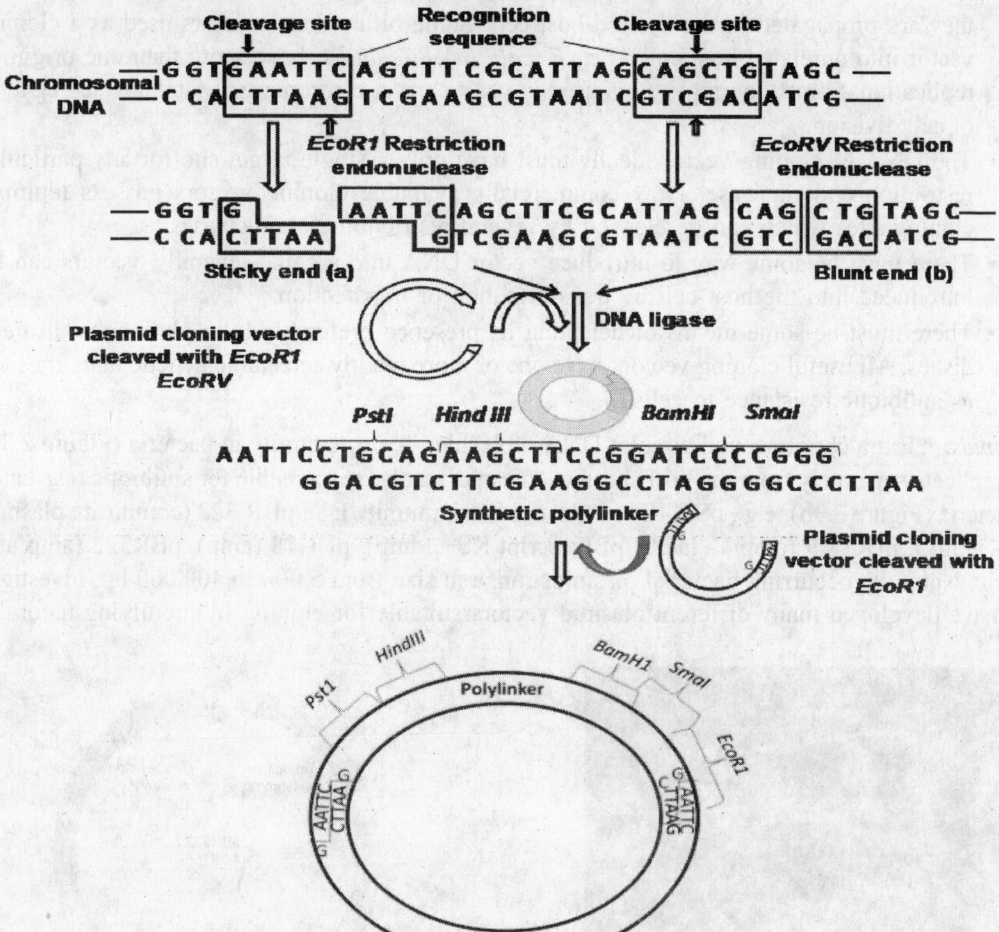

Figure 2.2 A synthetic DNA fragment (polylinker) with recognition sequences for several restriction endonucleases can be inserted into a plasmid that has been cleaved by a restriction endonuclease.

Cloning Vectors Allow Amplification of Inserted DNA Segments

Most segments of DNA do not have an inherent capacity for self-replication, and in order to reproduce themselves in a biological system, they need to integrate into DNA molecules that can replicate in the particular system (gene cloning) and for maintaining through generations. Even a

DNA segment that can replicate in its original host was not likely to have specific genetic sequences (signals) required to replicate in different hosts, so if a foreign DNA has to be propagated in bacteria, a suitable vehicle or carrier is required. They are also called vectors or cloning vehicles or carrier molecule, e.g., plasmids, cosmids, bacteriophages, M-13 vectors, shuttle vector, etc. Hundreds of different cloning vectors have been described and constructed for special purposes. However, cloning vehicles should have the following features:

- It must be able to replicate, i.e., possession of an origin of replication, which ensures that they are propagated in the desired host cell. Some bifunctional vectors used as a cloning vector into unrelated host cells, i.e., *E. coli* and *B. subtilis*, have more than one origin of replication. Some cloning vectors used in yeast carry a centromere to facilitate segregation of cell division.
- The DNA of cloning vector ideally must have only a single target site for any particular restriction endonuclease. Now commercially available cloning vectors possess multiple cloning sites which can be cleaved by several restriction endonucleases.
- There must be some way to introduce vector DNA into a cell. Generally, vectors can be introduced into the host cell by transformation or transfection.
- There must be some means of detecting its presence preferably by a plating test in Petri dishes. All useful cloning vectors have one or more readily selectable genetic markers such as antibiotic resistance to cells.

Plasmids: Extra chromosomal circular DNA molecules occur naturally in bacteria (Figure 2.3a) that replicate separately from the host chromosome and are also responsible for antibiotic resistance in bacteria (Figure 2.3b), e.g., pSC 101 (tetR), col E1 (immunity E1), pBR 322 (composite plasmid tet^R - amp^R), pUC 8/9 (amp< - lacZ), pBluescript KS+ (amp), pUC18 (amp), pBR322 (amp and tet) etc. Naturally occurring bacterial plasmids range in size from 5,000 to 400,000 bp. Investigators have developed many different plasmid vectors suitable for cloning by modifying naturally

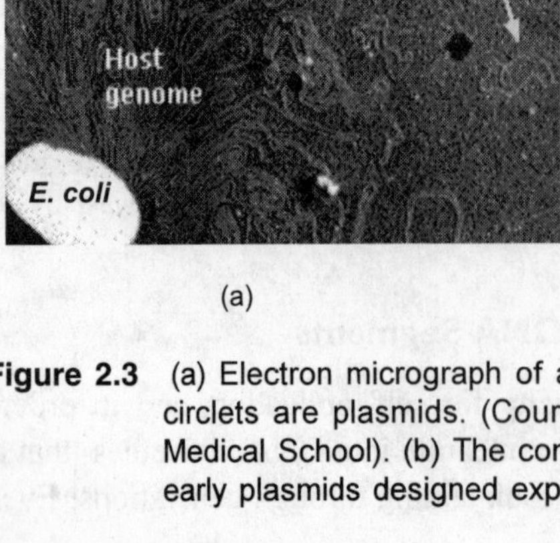

(a)

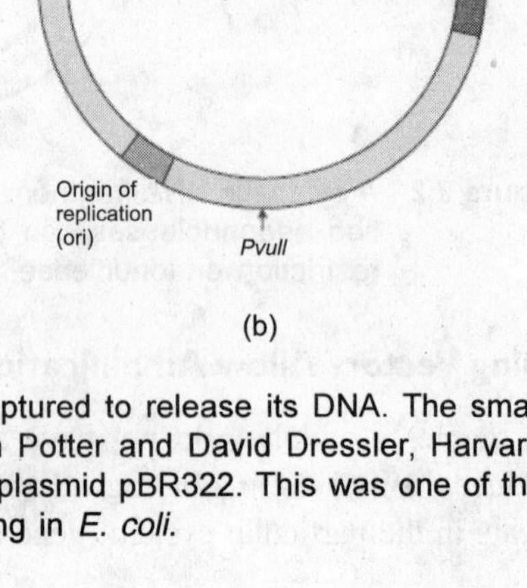

(b)

Figure 2.3 (a) Electron micrograph of an *E. coli* cell ruptured to release its DNA. The small circlets are plasmids. (Courtesy: Huntington Potter and David Dressler, Harvard Medical School). (b) The constructed *E. coli* plasmid pBR322. This was one of the early plasmids designed expressing for cloning in *E. coli*.

occurring plasmids. Transformation of typical bacterial cells with purified DNA (never a very efficient process) becomes less successful as plasmid size increases, and it is difficult to clone DNA segments longer than about 15,000 bp when plasmids are used as the vector.

Viral vectors: Bacterial viruses were though of as the most likely vehicles for genetic manipulation, however, it was the plasmid that first served as a vehicle for introducing foreign genes into a bacterium and that provided a mechanism for replication and selection of foreign DNA. Both viruses and plasmids are suitable vehicles and have been successfully used. SV40 has been the most commonly used vector for introducing foreign genes into animal cells. Virus infects animal's cells and has a covalently closed circular DNA of about 5200 bp that can be divided into "early" and "late" regions. Between the early and late regions there is a DNA sequence containing the origin of viral DNA replication. The early region is expressed throughout the lytic cycle, whereas expression of the late genes occurs only after viral DNA replication has begun.

Phage vectors: Bacteriophage λ has a very efficient mechanism for delivering its 48,502 bp of DNA into a bacterium, and it can be used as a vector to clone somewhat larger DNA segments. Two key features contribute to its utility: firstly, about one-third of the λ genome is nonessential and can be replaced with foreign DNA, and secondly DNA is packaged into infectious phage particles only if it is between 40 to 53 kb long, a constraint that can be used to ensure packaging of recombinant DNA only. Researchers have developed bacteriophage λ vectors that can be readily cleaved into three pieces, two of which contain essential genes but which together are only about 30 kb long. The third piece, "filler" DNA, is discarded when the vector is to be used for cloning, and additional DNA is inserted between the two essential segments to generate ligated DNA molecules long enough to produce viable phage particles. In effect, the packaging mechanism selects for recombinant viral DNAs. Bacteriophage λ vectors permit the cloning of DNA fragments of up to 23 kb (Table 2.3). Once the bacteriophage λ fragments are ligated to foreign DNA fragments of suitable size, the resulting recombinant DNAs can be packaged into phage particles by adding them to crude bacterial cell extracts that contain all the proteins needed to assemble a complete phage. This is called *in vitro* packaging. All viable phage particles will contain a foreign DNA fragment. The subsequent transmission of the recombinant DNA into *E. coli* cells is highly efficient.

Cosmids: (Phage cos-site carrying plasmids) These are novel vectors that combine the features of a plasmid and phage to increase the probability of selecting a recombinant plasmid carrying foreign DNA. A typical cosmid is circular col E1 plasmid carrying both the gene for resistance to the drug rifampicin (rif^R) and the cos-site of phage. The cosmid has two cleavage sites for the *Hind III* restriction enzyme, which separate the *rif* gene from the cos site and the col E1 region. Cloning the eukaryotic genome in phage limits the size of the eukaryotic segment that can be cloned to about 15 kilobases (kb), i.e., smaller genes. However, for cloning larger gene of 35 to 40 kb, phage is not suitable. Therefore, cosmids are generally used for this purpose (Table 2.3). A technique for cloning much larger eukaryotic fragments in *E. coli* is known as "cosmid cloning". The cos sites are necessary for packaging DNA into phage heads. The cos sites of phage have been cloned into ampicillin resistance gene of pBR322, leaving the tetracycline gene intact.

Bacterial artificial chromosomes (BACs): Bacterial artificial chromosomes are simply plasmids designed for the cloning of very long segments (typically 100,000 to 300,000 bp) of DNA (Table

2.3). They generally include selectable markers such as those having resistance to the antibiotic chloramphenicol (Cm^R), as well as a very stable origin of replication (ori) that maintains the plasmid at one or two copies per cell. DNA fragments of several hundred thousand base pairs are cloned into the BAC vector. The large circular DNAs are then introduced into the host bacteria by electroporation. These procedures use host bacteria with mutations that compromise the structure of their cell wall, permitting the uptake of the large DNA molecules.

Yeast artificial chromosomes (YACs): *E. coli* cells are by no means the only hosts for genetic engineering. Yeasts are particularly convenient eukaryotic organisms for this work. The genome of the most commonly used yeast, *Saccharomyces cerevisiae*, contains only 14×10^6 bp (less than four times the size of the *E. coli* chromosome), and its entire sequence is known. Yeast is also very easy to maintain and grow on a large scale in the laboratory. Plasmid vectors have been constructed for yeast, employing the same principles that govern the use of *E. coli* vectors described above. Convenient methods are now available for moving DNA into and out of yeast cells, facilitating the study of many aspects of eukaryotic cell biochemistry. Research work with large genomes and the associated need for high-capacity cloning vectors led to the development of yeast artificial chromosomes (YAC). YAC vectors contain all the elements needed to maintain a eukaryotic chromosome in the yeast nucleus: a yeast origin of replication, two selectable markers, and specialized sequences needed for stability and proper segregation of the chromosomes at cell division. Before being used in cloning, the vector is propagated as a circular bacterial plasmid. Cleavage with a restriction endonuclease *(BamHI)* removes a length of DNA between two telomere sequences (TEL), leaving the telomeres at the ends of the linearized DNA. Cleavage at another internal site *(EcoRI)* divides the vector into two DNA segments, referred to as vector arms, each with a different selectable marker.

Table 2.3 Cloning capacity of commonly used vectors.

Vector	***Insert size range (Kb)***
Plasmid	≤ 10
λ Phage	≥ 23
Cosmid	30-45
P1 artificial chromosome (PAC)	130-150
Bacterial artificial chromosome (BAC)	≤ 300
Yeast artificial chromosome (YAC)	200-2000

Shuttle vectors: A shuttle vector is a vector that can replicate in different organisms. The first shuttle vector, which contained *E. coli* and yeast components, was used to clone yeast genes. If a yeast gene were cloned into an *E. coli* plasmid and then *E. coli* cells were transformed by the recombinant plasmid, in general the yeast gene would not be expressed for usual reasons–lack of recognition of yeast promoters in *E. coli* and incorrect processing. Shuttle vectors, which contain sequences from *E. coli* plasmid and a particular region of yeast genome, were designed to avoid this problem. Essential features of this shuttle vector are two replication origins (one active in yeast and one in *E. coli*), two selective markers (trp, detectable in yeast, and amp, detectable in *E. coli*), and restriction sites next to a yeast promoter. A problem with these vectors is that they are not particularly stable in yeast because they lack a centromere (the portion of chromosome by which the chromosome is attached to the mitotic spindle), thus replicas are not efficiently segregated into daughter cells.

Expression vectors: An expression vector, otherwise known as an expression construct, is generally a plasmid that is used to introduce and express a specific gene into a target cell. Once the expression vector is inside the cell, the protein that is encoded by the gene is produced by the cellular transcription and translation machinery. The plasmid is engineered such that it contains a highly active promoter, which causes the production of large amounts of mRNA. Some important expression vectors used now-a-days are pBI121, pCAMBIA, pgD–DHFR, etc.

Different Cloning Strategies

DNA technique for placing and maintaining a new gene in bacteria is called cloning i.e., isolation of a specific new DNA sequence from one organism and placing this gene into another organism with the help of a vehicle that proliferates to form a population of identical descendants clone. Three approaches were generally used for cloning—shotgun, cDNA cloning and synthetic gene cloning. A comparison has been made between these cloning strategies in Table 2.4.

Shotgun: Theoretically it is possible to clone any desired gene in one organism from another organism by the technique known as shotgunning. In this case, we take the entire genome of the first organism and digest it with a restriction endonuclease to produce a random mixture of fragments. The vehicle is also cleaved off by the same restriction endonucleases, and hence we get sticky ends of foreign DNA and vehicle that can be ligated and the recombinant plasmids transformed into the desired host cell. Since each recombinant plasmid will contain a different fragment of foreign DNA, it is a major task to select those transformed cells that carry the cloned gene of interest.

cDNA cloning: The next approach is that the desired gene is present somewhere on the DNA of the eukaryotic cell. The eukaryotic DNA is divided into exons and introns and the information is broken. In prokaryotes, genes have a very simple structure and all the genetic information between the initiation and stop codon is translated into protein. In eukaryotes, genes containing exons are transcribed into mRNA in the usual manner, but the corresponding intron sequences are spliced out. As bacteria cannot splice out introns, they cannot be used directly to express many genes from mammals or other eukaryotes. One solution to the problem of introns is to clone the gene of interest in yeast, which can mediate splicing. Unfortunately, cloning directly into yeast is much less efficient than cloning into bacterium such as *E. coli* and this technique is not favored. A better approach is to start by isolating mRNA than the DNA from the original organism, e.g., isolation of mRNA from the human pancreatic cells in case of insulin, as these are rich in insulin specific m-RNA from which introns have already been spliced out. So if we have a mixture of mRNA, prepare cDNA from it and then integrate into cloning vector. Isolate the positive clones on a medium having a particular drug for which the cloning vector is carrying resistance. From these clones, isolate DNA, denature them, and add the mixture of mRNA that was earlier used to form cDNA. Keep the temperature to hybridizing temperature and then transfer it to a medium containing all translation machinery and radioactive labeled amino acids. At last, add antibody attached to beads. If the clone contains the right gene, all the mRNA complementary to it will be involved in hybridization and hence there will not be the synthesis of that particular protein. When we add antibodies, it will not find its correct protein to bind and remains as such, whereas in all other fractions, in which the gene of interest is absent and hence no hybridization of its mRNA and hence synthesis of that protein that will be bound by antibodies, proves that it is not a gene of our interest. Using the enzyme reverse transcriptase it is possible to convert this m-RNA into a DNA copy. This copy DNA (cDNA) that carries uninterrupted genetic information for insulin production can then be cloned. This is cDNA, has blunt ends instead of sticky ends but it still can be inserted into plasmid vector using blunt ends ligation.

Synthetic gene cloning: An alternative way of avoiding the problem of introns is to synthesize an artificial gene in the test tube starting with deoxy ribonucleotides. If we know the amino acid composition of the protein, we can predict its mRNA and hence DNA. In practice various oligonucleotides are synthesized and ligated together before insertion into vehicle. But this approach is applicable only for small proteins (up to 500 amino acids long). For larger proteins it is difficult to synthesize long synthetic DNA in test tube. For making eukaryotic protein in bacterial cells, i.e., eukaryotic to prokaryotic transfer, a fragment of animal DNA that encodes the protein is inserted into a plasmid, a small, circular piece of bacterial DNA, which in turn serves as the vehicle for introducing the DNA into the bacterium.

Table 2.4 Advantages and disadvantages of different cloning strategies.

Cloning method	*Advantages*	*Disadvantages*
Shotgun method	Easy to do	(1) Many different clones are isolated, so a good selection method is needed to isolate the desired clone. (2) Genes with introns will not be correctly expressed in *E. coli,* the usual shotgun cloning host. (3) Expression dependent on recognition of foreign promoters by *E. coli.*
c-DNA cloning	(1) If desired mRNA is in abundance in the mRNA preparation used, desired clone should be easily detected. (2) Introns are not a problem as mRNA will contain spliced molecules	(1) Desired mRNA not always abundant so selection may be necessary. (2) Technically more difficult than shotgun cloning. (3) Cloned gene needs to be placed downstream from a promoter, since normal promoter eliminated by starting with mRNA. (4) Codon choice may not be optimal for *E. coli.*
Gene synthesis	(1) No selection needed after cloning (2) Sequence of promoters, ribosome binding sites etc. can be optimized. (3) Codon choice can be optimized for preferred host cell.	(1) Need to know protein sequence before synthetic gene can be designed.

A Means of Transferring Recombinant DNA into Functional Cells

Manipulating the sequence of gene in a test tube is not sufficient for discovering its functions. It is necessary to study the functioning of the gene in a living cell, and this requires persuading a cell to take up the gene. Fortunately many bacterial and yeast species can be directly transformed with DNA. The efficiency of the transformation has been improved by first treating bacteria with salts such as calcium chloride, adding plasmid DNA, and then exposing the cells to a brief heat shock, e.g., 42°C for 90 sec. Another effective approach for gene transfer is electroporation, in which cells are placed in a solution containing DNA and subjected to a brief electrical pulse that causes holes to open transiently in their membranes. DNA enters through the holes directly into the cytoplasm and then passes to the nucleus. There are a wide variety of methods used to transfer DNA directly in the cells. Perhaps the simplest to understand, although quite challenging to do, is microinjection, in which DNA is injected directly into the nucleus of cells through fine glass needles. When first developed, microinjection was a time-consuming process and only a few cells could be injected in a single experiment. Once again, computers have revolutionized techniques. In this case, computer-controlled, automated injection means that hundreds of the cells can be injected. The first method used for introducing DNA into animal cells en masse was to incubate the DNA with an inert carbohydrate polymer (dextran) to which a negatively charged chemical group (DEAE [diethyl-aminoethyl]) has been coupled. The DNA sticks to the DEAE-dextran via its negatively charged phosphate groups. These large DNA-containing particles in turn stick to the surface of the cells, which are though to take them in by a process known as endocytosis—a normal feature of membrane turnover. DNA can also be incorporated into artificial lipid vesicles called liposomes, which fuse with the cell membrane, delivering their contents directly to the cytoplasm.

A plant cell presents a special challenge to DNA transfer—they are encased in a thick cell wall made up of cellulose that poses a formidable barrier to efficient gene transfer. One approach is to remove this wall using fungal cellulase enzymes. The resulting protoplast is enclosed only by a plasma membrane and is much more amenable to experimental manipulations including transfection and electroporation. Protoplasts will take up macromolecules like DNA, and they are capable of regenerating whole plants, as are nearly all plant cells. In a stunningly direct approach, DNA can be absorbed on the surfaces of tungstun or gold microprojectiles, 1 μm in diameter, which is fired into intact cells as through pellets from a shotgun. Although first developed for plants, gene guns are also used to introduce DNA directly into animal cells in tissues. However, a number of nonlytic viruses drawn from the retrovirus, adenovirues, and adeno-associated virus groups have been modified to transfer genes to animal cells. Retroviruses after infecting cells use reverse transcriptase to convert their RNA genome to DNA. This viral DNA is efficiently integrated into the host genome as a "provirus", where it permanently resides, replicating along with the host DNA at each cell division. The most popular method for DNA transfer into many types of plants uses *Agrobacterium tumefaciens*, a bacterium that infects plant cells and drives the infected cells to multiply wildly, thus producing the plant tumors known as crown galls. The tumor-inducing agents in Agrobacterium are a plasmid, called Ti that integrates some of its DNA (T-DNA) into the chromosomes of its host plant cells. Ti plasmids are (200 kb large) double-stranded circular DNA that replicate independently in host cells. The process of transfer from the bacterial cells to the plant cells is mechanistically similar to the process of bacterial conjugation.

Methods of Selecting Recombinants Containing Right Gene

The task of isolating a desired recombinant from a population of transformed bacteria depends very much on the cloning strategy that has been adopted. For instance, if a synthetic gene has been cloned, no selection is necessary because every transformed cell will contain the correct sequence. When a cDNA derived from a purified or abundant mRNA is to be cloned, the task is relatively simple: only a small number of clones need to be screened. Isolating a particular single-copy gene sequence from a complete mammalian genomic library requires techniques in which hundreds of thousands of recombinants can be screened. A number of different methods have been devised to facilitate screening of recombinants. These include genetic, immunochemical and nucleic acid hybridization methods.

Genetic method: The simplest example of a genetic method is the complementations of nutritional defects, e.g., suppose a bacterial strain is available, which has a mutation in a gene encoding an enzyme involved in the biosynthesis of the amino acid histidine. Such a mutant strain, will grow

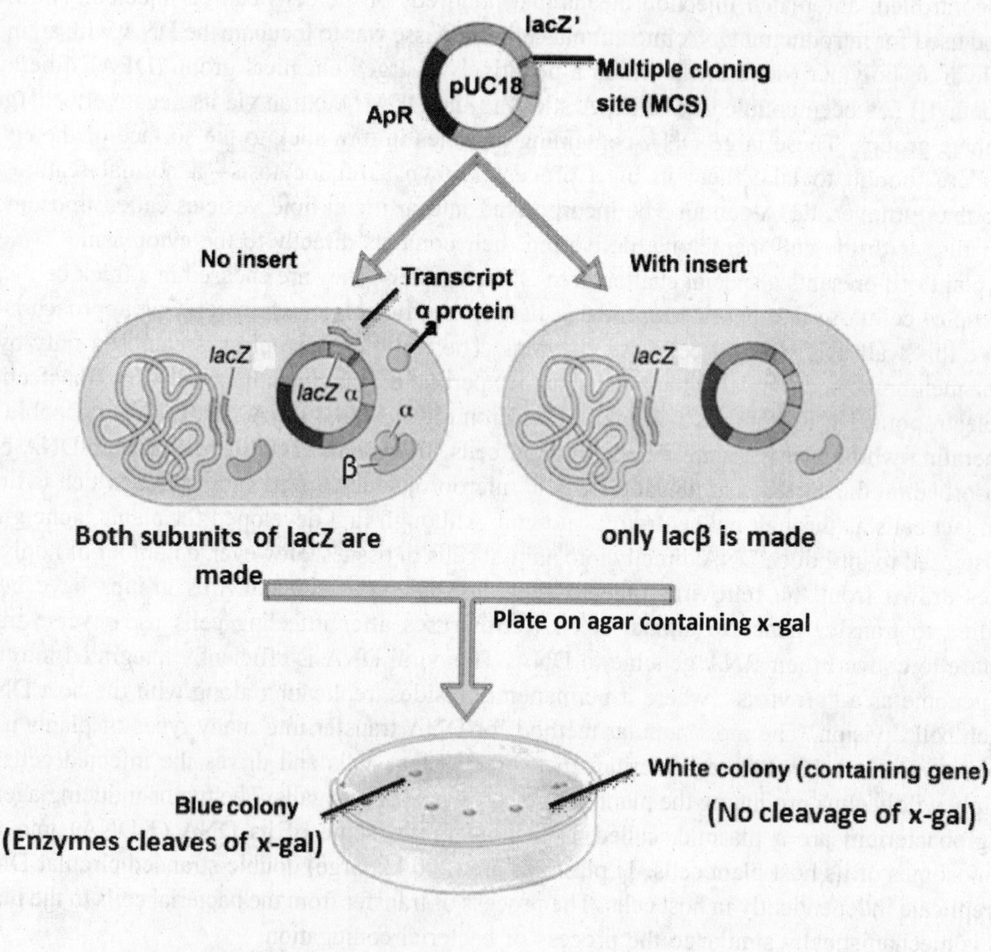

Figure 2.4 Blue/white screening to recognize vector containing inserts.

only in a medium supplemented with histidine. By cloning DNA from a normal strain, i.e., one that can synthesize its own histidine, in the mutant strain and selecting those transformants, which grow in the absence of histidine, it is possible to isolate the gene of interest. Even yeast and mammalian genes can be selected in this way. In another approach, marker genes were used in the plasmid having resistance towards antibiotic, so that the cells which have been transferred with the plasmid can be easily selected due to the death of the other unlabelled cells. Cells transformed with plasmid DNA reproduced themselves normally and produced a clone of bacteria, since each cell in the clone contained a DNA species having the same genetic and molecular properties as the plasmid DNA molecule that was taken up by a single bacterial cell. The procedure made possible the cloning of individual molecules even if they were originally present in a heterogeneous population of plasmids. In addition, blue/white screening can also be used to determine whether recombinant vector is present at high frequency in the library and picking white colonies or plaques excludes those containing empty vectors. This method relies on the β-galactosidase gene from the *lac* opern. The enzyme β-galactosidase hydrolyses the chemical X-gal to produce an insoluble blue dye. The cloning site of many vectors is within a copy of the β-galactosidase gene, so that the insertion of

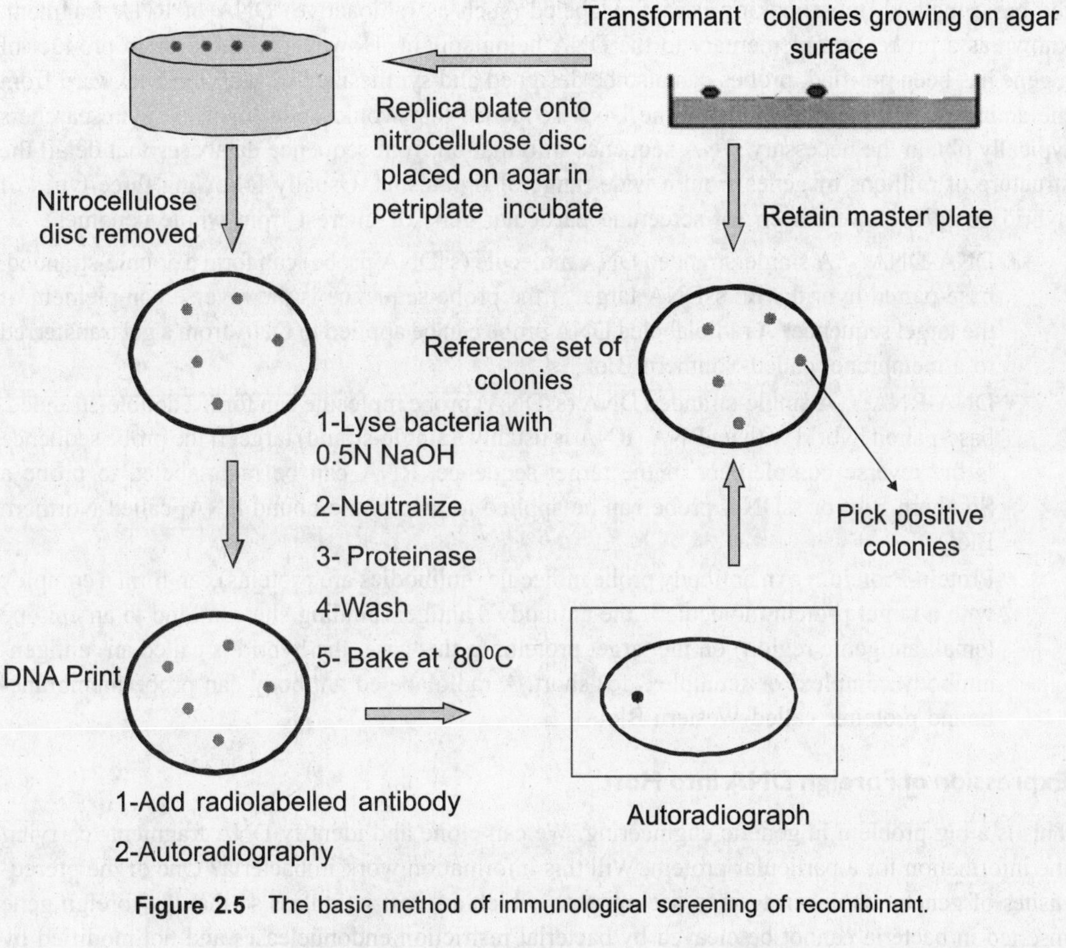

Figure 2.5 The basic method of immunological screening of recombinant.

the DNA disrupts the gene and bacterial colonies or phage plaques remain colorless (white) if X-gal is included in the culture medium. In contrast, colonies or plaques containing vectors without DNA inserts turn blue (Figure 2.4).

Immunological method: These are widely used to select particular recombinant clones, but demand the availability of a specific antibody against the desired protein product. When such antibody is available, the method works well as nucleic acid hybridization method. Transferred cells are grown on agar in a conventional Petri dish and a duplicate set of colonies prepared in a second Petri dish. Both duplicate sets of colonies are lysed by exposure to chloroform vapour and the released proteins blotted onto an absorbent matrix are then exposed to antibody, which has been radioactively labeled *in vitro* (Figure 2.5). Positively reacting lysates are detected by washing surplus radiolabelled material off the matrix and making an autoradiographic image. Many different variations of this technique have been adopted as radioactive antibody test for insulin producing colony and immunoprecipitation test for other protein producing colony.

Nucleic acid hybridization method: DNA hybridization is the most common sequence-based process for detecting a particular gene or a segment of nucleic acid. There are many variations of the basic method, most making use of a labeled (such as radioactive) DNA or RNA fragment, known as a probe, complementary to the DNA being sought. However, if the protein product of a gene has been purified, probes can also be designed and synthesized by working backward from the amino acid sequence, deducing the DNA sequence that would code for it. Now, researchers typically obtain the necessary DNA sequence information from sequence databases that detail the structure of millions of genes from a wide range of organisms. Usually following three types of hybrid complexes were seen for screening particular gene of interest from whole genome.

- DNA-DNA: A single-stranded DNA molecule (ssDNA probe) can form a double-stranded, base-paired hybrid with ssDNA target if the probe sequence is the reverse complement of the target sequence. A radiolabeled DNA probe can be applied to DNA from a gel transferred to a membrane, called-Southern Blot.
- DNA-RNA: A single-stranded DNA (ssDNA) probe molecule can form a double-stranded, base-paired hybrid with an RNA (RNA is usually a single-strand) target if the probe sequence is the reverse complement of the target sequence. RNA can be radiolabeled to probe a Southern Blot or ssDNA probe can be applied to membrane-bound RNA, called-Northern Blot.
- Protein-Protein: An antibody probe molecule (antibodies are proteins) can form a complex with a target protein molecule if the antibody's antigen-binding site can bind to an epitope (small antigenic region) on the target protein. In this case, the hybrid is called an 'antigen-antibody complex' or 'complex' for short. A radiolabeled antibody can probe membrane-bound proteins, called-Western Blot.

Expression of Foreign DNA into Host

This is a big problem in genetic engineering. We can clone and identify DNA fragments carrying the information for a particular protein. Will this information work in bacteria? One of the prerequisites of genetic engineering is to use mutants, which are restrictionless so that the foreign gene inserted in bacteria cannot be cleaved by bacterial restriction endonucleases and not modified by modification enzymes present in the bacteria. Regulatory signals, "where to start" and "where to stop" should be provided to the bacteria. For the expression of foreign DNA, all genes have two stop and two start signals—one for transcription and one for translation. A simple way to make the new protein sequences is to cut open the bacterial gene by restriction endonucleases and insert the new DNA there. So a hybrid protein will be formed. This has been done successfully in case of Somatostatin, a growth hormone. The DNA for those 14 amino acids and a stop signal was inserted. The bacterium made the hybrid protein that was cleaved off and purified to get a functional growth hormone. For getting maximum gene expression of a mammalian gene in a microorganism for facilitating commercial production of the corresponding gene product, some important factors are required:

(1) The number of copies of the plasmid vector per unit cell (copy number)
(2) The strength of the promoter
(3) The sequence of the ribosome binding site (rbs) and flanking DNA
(4) Codon choice in the cloned gene
(5) Genetic stability of the recombinant
(6) Proteolysis

The limiting factor in expression is the initiation of protein synthesis. Increasing the number of plasmids per cell increases the number of mRNA molecules transcribed from the cloned gene, and this results in increased protein synthesis. Similarly, the stronger the promoter, the more mRNA molecules are synthesized. The nucleotide base sequence of ribosome binding sites and the length and sequence of the DNA between the ribosome binding sites and the initiating AUG codon are so important that a single base change, addition or deletion can affect the level of translation up to 1000-fold. Another important factor is related to the redundancy of the genetic code. There are several trinucleotide codons for most amino acids, and different organisms favor different codons in their genes. If genes inserted into cells of another species utilized codons are in the host cell, the host's biosynthetic machinery may be starved of charged t-RNAs. This could result in premature protein chain termination or a high error frequency in the amino acid sequence of the protein. Heavy secretor of cells i.e. excess protein synthesizing cells have tendency to convert into non-secretor by spontaneous changes in gene sequence e.g. deletions and gene rearrangements. Thus it is advised to minimize recombinant gene expression by using controllable copy number. Example of controllable promoter is *E. coli* lactose operon, no transcription occurs unless lactose is added. Runaway plasmids are examples of vectors with controllable copy number. At low temperature, e.g., below 30°C, the copy number may be as low as 10 plasmids per cell, but when temperature is raised to 37°C, the copy number increases to several hundreds, or even several thousands. The enzymatic breakdown of protein (proteolysis) does not affect transcription and translation but influences the apparent rate of gene expression. Although proteolysis can be reduced, it is difficult to eliminate completely. One approach used widely is to 'protect' the desired protein by fusing it to a normal cellular protein, from which it must subsequently be released.

APPLICATIONS OF RECOMBINANT DNA TECHNOLOGY

There are many things that can be done more effectively with the help of cloning techniques. These include gene mapping, controlled mutagenesis and production of specific gene products. However, the major revolution occurred in eukaryotic biology with the development of DNA cloning that allows defining segments of any DNA to be isolated and characterized. Some applications of this technology in medical, veterinary, agricultural sciences and industrial applications that have possibly or greatly facilitated by DNA cloning are discussed.

Medical and Veterinary Applications

Diagnosis of genetic disease: One of the major medical applications of gene cloning is to safely predict or diagnose the genetic diseases in fetuses, which are untreatable by available therapeutic strategies, so that abortion can be offered to prevent the birth of incurably sick children. Several genetic diseases that can currently be diagnosed prenatally are various enzyumopathies that include inborn error of metabolism e.g., Tay Sachs disease, Gaucher's disease, Hurler's Syndrome, Galactosemia, hypercholesterolemia, Lesch-Nyhan Syndrome, Xerodema pigmentosum, emphysema, cystic fibrosis, muscular dystrophy, hemoglobinpathies such as sickle cell anaemia and β-thalassemias etc. The basic approach to fetal diagnosis is to obtain fetal cells—either fibroblasts or blood cells taken by amniocentesis (Figure 2.6)—and to test them for biochemical defects. Currently the tests are made for the gene products such as proteins or enzymes suspected of being defective rather than mutated gene themselves. It is also possible now to detect lethal recessive mutations directly on genome itself.

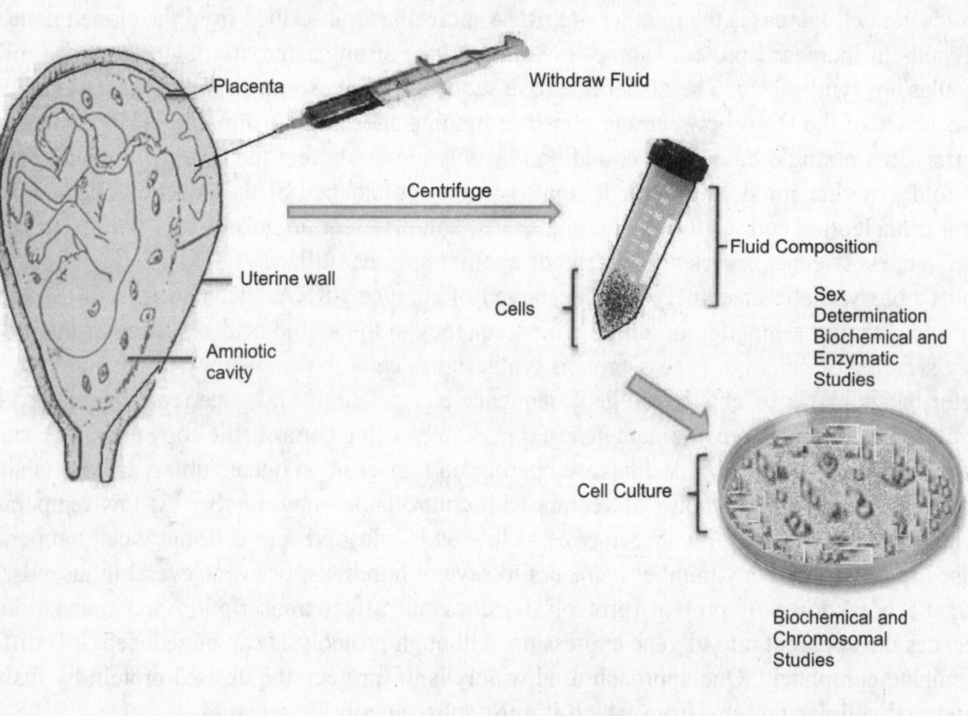

Figure 2.6 Amniocentesis. A sample of amniotic fluid is taken by inserting a needle into the amniotic cavity during or around the 16th week of gestation for diagnosis of the genetic diseases.

Gene therapy: It is the correction of an inborn error of metabolism by the insertion of a normal gene of either somatic or germ cells into the afflicted organism. In somatic therapy, healthy copy of a gene is inserted into somatic cells that are not involved in reproduction, and such an alteration is not carried to future generation. In contrast, germ-line therapy treats cells that make eggs and sperm, therefore affecting all future offspring. In gene therapy, cells need to be extracted from the body, grown in culture, genetically manipulated and then re-implanted into the patient from whom original tissue was taken. The first human experiment was carried out at NIH in 1990. The patient was born with virtually no natural protection against disease because her immune system lacked a critical gene. After inserting critical gene by gene therapy, the patient's body began generating a normal immune response. A second human experiment used altered genes to attack advanced melanoma, a disease that is always fatal. In this case, doctors removed from patients a type of cell called tumor infiltrating lymphocytes or TIL, which the body uses to attack cancers. A gene that manufactures a potent cancer fighter called tumor necrosis factor was inserted into the TIL cells. These cells were reproduced in millions and infected into the patients. Researchers hope that TIL cells will migrate naturally to the tumors and cure cancer. In 1993, Carly Todd had a single gene disease called adenosine deaminase (ADA) deficiency, in which her body could not produce working copies of the enzyme ADA because of a fault in the gene sequence. This defect has been cured successfully by implanting in her a genetically altered ADA gene containing bone marrow cells. Researchers at the National Institutes of Health reported that their work with laboratory rats showed that the flawed gene that causes cystic fibrosis can possibly be corrected in the lungs. The problem is that lung cells cannot be removed from the body, genetically altered and then returned. Somehow, the correct genes have to be inserted into the lung cell while they remain in place. The NIH team showed that this can be done in mice by placing the correct gene into the genetic make-up of cloned virus, which is then sprayed into the lungs. The virus is altered so that it does not cause infection, but is able to attack the cells in the lung. When this happens, the virus deposits the new gene into the DNA of the lung cells. With the new gene, the lung cells secrete a protein that prevents the deadly mucous from building up. In addition, Ohio University researchers have shown that gene can be inserted into fertilized mouse eggs, which will cause the rodents to be born with a genetic protection against a leukaemia virus by secreting a protein that keeps it from reproducing. Researchers caution that it will take decades before gene therapy can be used against most of the 4,000 genetic-related disorders. From birth defects in newborns to cancer in the elderly, several diseases can be cured by gene therapy, e.g., hemophilia, Lesch-Nyhan disease, Immuno-deficiency and combined immunodeficiency disease which are due to deficiency of factor VIII, Hypoxanthine-guanine phosphoribosy1 transferase (HGPRT), Pyramiding nucleoside phosphory-lase and adenosine deaminase.

Production of transgenic organisms: Recombinant DNA technology has made it possible to create transgenic organisms to produce human proteins, e.g., insulin, hemoglobin, etc. The aim of transgenesis is to produce organism with a hereditable change in their genotype such that the benefits of gene manipulation can be passed to their offspring. With mammals, the technique used is the microinjection of DNA into fertilized eggs followed by implantation of the manipulated ova in a foster mother. Scientists have introduced hemoglobin genes into pigs and made them produce human hemoglobin. In this method, the sows were first hormonally treated to produce a large numbers of eggs, which were then cultured *in vitro* with vectors carrying hemoglobin genes were then implanted into other sows specially prepared by hormones to receive their eggs. The blood of offspring of transgenic pigs had 15-20% of human Hb. Similarly, genetic engineers have successfully introduced the two human hemoglobin genes into Brewers yeast "*Saccharomyces cerevisiae*" and have got them to produce large amounts of human hemoglobin. *E. coli* is also presently being made to produce separately the two peptide chains of hemoglobin, which are then linked up with the iron containing heme to make up the complete hemoglobin. This technique has been used to place gene that codes for alpha-1 antitrypsin into a sheep embryo. As a result, this transgenic sheep produces milk that contains the protein that is used to treat patients with a particular type of inherited lung disease, congenital emphysema. In addition, it has also been used to manufacture bovine somatotrophin (BST), a hormone that increases by 10 to 15 % the amount of milk that cow can produce.

Agricultural Applications

Recombinant DNA technology is being applied to increase yields of plants, resistance to disease or pollution and to create new crops that can utilize previously wasted resources. New gene can be inserted to a section of a bacterium's DNA to transfer the genes to the plant cells.

Improving yields: There are different ways of increasing yields. You could either aim for a faster rate of growth, more efficient use of nutrients, or an increase in the quantity of the food produced by plants. In the case of cereal crops like wheat or rice, much attention has been given to increasing the number of the grains that grow in each head, whilst causing the plant to grow with a shorter stem, thus wasting less energy on this inedible part of the plant. In the past such development was carried out in prolonged breeding programmes, but now the rate of development can be accelerated. A major area of the research is dedicated to finding ways of moving nitrogen fixing genes (NIF genes) into agricultural crops. Nitrates are vital nutrients for most plants, and some bacteria are particularly good at creating them by biochemically reducing nitrogen. The gene, which produces the necessary NIF enzymes has been isolated, sequenced and cloned in *E. coli*. Now scientists are looking for ways of placing them into cells in crops such as wheat or rice. This would enable these crops to fertilize themselves effectively, saving much money and increasing yields. Placing the gene in crops grown in developing countries would have enormous impact on their ability to grow food, as currently they cannot afford the nitrogenous fertilizers used in more affluent countries.

Resistance to disease, pest or herbicides: Many crops are particularly vulnerable to attack from specific organisms, e.g., tomatoes are attacked by aphids, potatoes by viruses, and wheat by fungi. Farmers fight back by spraying their crops with chemicals that destroy the invading organisms. Now recombinant DNA technology is allowing plant breeders to introduce genes into crops, causing them to produce their own pesticides. For examples, a tomato plant had a gene placed in it that produces a protein, which kills tomato fruit worms. When modified tomato plants and normal plants were grown together in a laboratory and deliberately infected with fruit worms and pin worms, the normal plants were stripped of their leaves, but the modified plants were unaffected. In a similar way, crops can be adapted to make them resistant to herbicides. Most herbicides operate by blocking an enzyme that is vital for the plant's survival. The idea is to equip plants with a gene, which produces an enzyme that can destroy the herbicide. When the field is spread with the specific herbicide, the genetically modified plant will be unscathed, whilst all other plants will be killed. The first transgenic plant licensed for agricultural use in Europe (1994) was a tobacco plant that has built-in resistance to the herbicide, bromoxylnil.

Novel crops: One of the problems of the modern agriculture is that a crop is frequently grown many hundreds or thousand of miles from the customer. It can be difficult to get it to shops before it rots. Fruit and vegetables are often harvested before they ripe and then ripened artificially just before they are sold. This leads to a loss of flavour. In the case of tomatoes, the problem may now have been solved—researchers have now produced a tomato that is resistant to becoming soft and rotting once it has ripened. Fruit normally softens because it produces an enzyme called polygalacturonase (PG). This enzyme breaks down pectin in cell walls and so the fruit becomes soft. By inserting a gene, which has a sequence that is exactly the opposite of the gene coding for PG (an antisense gene), the cells produce an antisense strand of mRNA as well as a sense strand from the normal gene. These two mRNA strands are so perfectly matched that they stick together, thus rendering the sense strand useless. Without the mRNA, no enzyme forms, and without the enzyme the fruit stays firm.

Industrial Applications

Production of drugs: Perhaps the most glamorous aspect of recombinant DNA technology is its use to construct microorganisms, which synthesize human proteins with therapeutic potential as listed in Table 2.5. Several antibiotics can be overproduced by this technique, thereby reducing production costs. Another examples are human insulin, human growth hormone (Somatostatin) and an antiviral agent, interferon, which are being marketed. Many more are undergoing clinical trial. The interferon reduces the duration of viral infection, is effective against herpes virus infection of eye, reduces the incidence of attacks of multiple sclerosis, suppresses atherosclerosis in rats on high cholesterol diets, and is being examined for its antitumor activity. In 1985, tumor necrosis factor, a powerful anticancer substance in rats was cloned and animal studies began shortly afterwards. Interleukin-2, a substance that stimulates multiplication of certain cells in immune system, has also been cloned. It is being tested on patients with AIDS and other viral diseases and shows promise in shrinking cancers in humans.

Table 2.5 Some recombinant DNA products in medicine.

Product	*Examples/uses*
Anticoagulants	Tissue plasminogen activator (TPA); activates plasmin, an enzyme involved in dissolving clots; effective in treating heart attack patients.
Blood factors	Factor VIII; promotes clotting; it is deficient in hemophiliacs; treatment with factor VIII produced by recombinant DNA technology eliminates infection risks associated with blood transfusions.
Colorry-stimulating factors	Immune system growth factors that stimulate leukocyte production; treatmetnt of immune deficiencies and infections,
Erythropoietin	Stimulates erythrocyte production treatment of anemia in patients with kidney disease.

Contd.

Growth factors	Stimulate differentiation and growth of various cell types; promote wound healing.
Human growth homone	Treatment of dwarfism.
Human insulin	Treatment of diabetes.
Interferons	Interfere with viral reproduction; used to treat some cancers.
Interteukins	Activate and stimulate different classes of leukocytes; possible uses in treatment of wounds, HIV Infection, cancer, and immune deficiencies.
Monoclonal antibodies	Extraordinary binding specificity is used in: tumors as a cancer therapy; many other applications.
Superoxide dismutase	Prevents tissue damage from reactive oxygen species when tissues briefly deprived of O_2 during surgery suddenly have blood flow restored.
Vaccines	Proteins derived from viral coats are as effective in "priming" an immune system as is the killed virus more traditionally used for vaccines, and are safer; first developed was the vaccine for hepatitis B.

Production of synthetic vaccines: A major breakthrough in disease prevention has been the development of synthetic vaccines. Attempts have also been made to use genetic engineering to facilitate vaccine production. Production of certain vaccines such as anti-hepatitis B has been difficult because of extreme hazards of working with large quantities of the virus. The danger would be avoided if viral antigen could be cloned and purified in *E. coli* or yeast, because the pure antigen could be given as a vaccine, which has received regulatory approval from the U.S. food and drug administration. Now genes for the major subunits of a number of viruses e.g., foot and mouth disease virus, have been cloned in *E. coli*, but the results have been disappointing because peptides thus produced have been either poorly immunogenic or thermally instable. However, the use of vaccinia virus (the anti-smallpox agent) as a carrier has been fruitful. The procedure makes use of the fact that viral antigens are on surface of virus particles and some of these antigens can be engineered into the coat of vaccinia. By 1985, vaccinia hybrids (containing vaccinia DNA and viral antigen, which are produced by genetic recombination of normal vaccinia DNA and plasmid DNA containing viral-antigen gene in animal cell lines) with surface antigens of hepatitis B, influenza virus and vesicular stomatitis virus have been prepared and shown to be useful vaccines in animal tests. A surface antigen of *Plasmodium falciparum* (causative agent of malaria) has also been placed in the vaccine coat, which may lead to an antimalarial vaccine.

Food industries: We have already seen how recombinant DNA technology is affecting food production in standard agricultural situations. Now we turn to the other areas of the food industry that are making use of this technique. For example, bacteria can be designed to grow on virtually any energy-rich molecules. Some have been adapted to use methane gas as a nutrient and others grow successfully on paper pulp. This is already providing a new source of protein to the food industry. The growing bacteria can be harvested and their proteins are purified. These proteins may be of particular value as the numbers of people eating a vegetarian diet increase. This has two benefits: firstly, growing farm animals to supply us with protein is a very inefficient use of energy as it can take between 10 to 20 kg of protein in feeds to produce 1 kg of meat. However, bacteria are much more efficient. Secondly, waste materials such as pulped newspapers could form the basic nutrient supply for new bacteria. In addition, industrial cheese production uses a lot of enzyme called chymosin (commonly called rennin) to coagulate the protein casein, found in milk. Traditionally, this enzyme is obtained from the content of the abomasums (fourth stomach) of calf.

Bacteria are modified by transforming them with the inclusion of a gene that causes chymosin production for making the vegetarian cheese.

Other Biotechnological Applications

DNA sequence analysis: A great deal of information can be gained about a gene's operation once the sequence of bases is known. This was made possible because, like so many aspects of recombinant DNA technology, the process leads itself to automation. It requires homogeneous duplex segments that are produced by cloning because sequencing by Maxam-Gilbert or Sanger's methods requires microgram quantities (Figure 2.7).

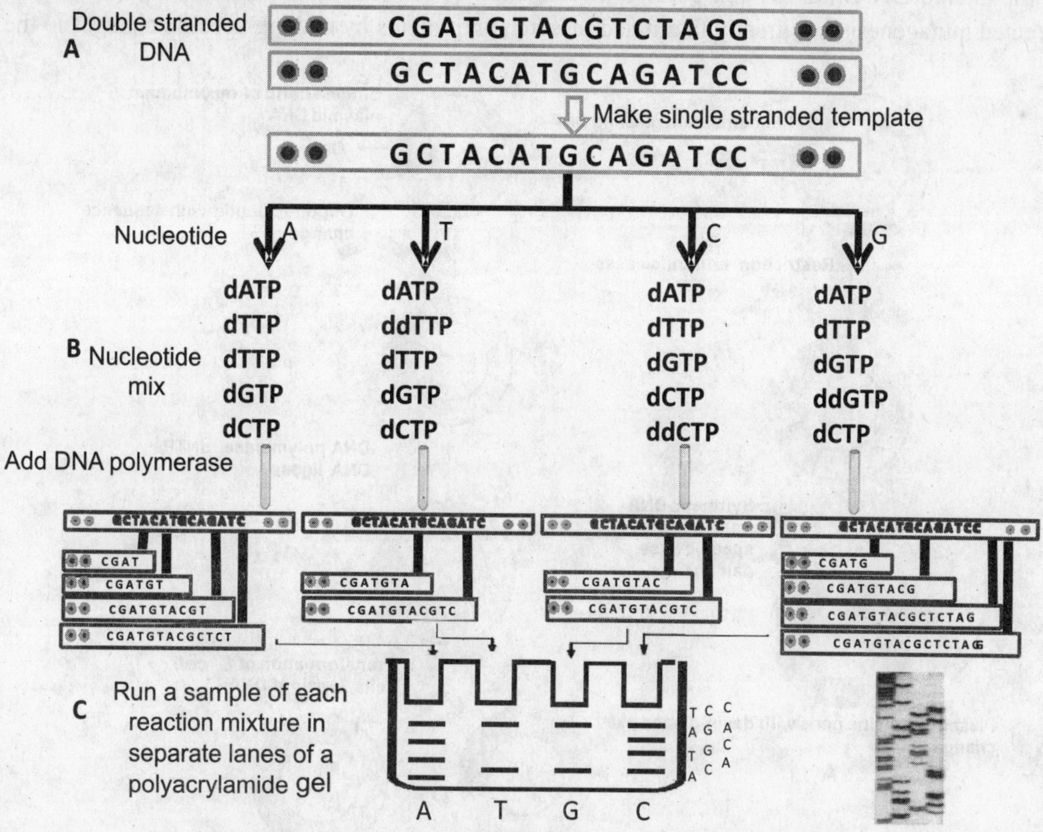

Figure 2.7 The Sanger dideoxy DNA sequencing procedure.

Site directed mutagenesis: Small regions of DNA can be specifically modified and reintroduced into the organism. This process is known as site-directed mutagenesis. After modification, the altered DNA can be amplified in bacteria and effect of the alterations can be studied either *in vitro* or *in vivo.* Specific amino acids may be replaced individually by site-directed mutagenesis. This powerful approach to study protein structure and function changes the amino acid sequence of a protein by altering the DNA sequence of the cloned gene (Figure 2.8). A short synthetic DNA strand with a specific base change is annealed to a single-stranded copy of the cloned gene within a suitable vector. The mismatch of a single base pair in 15 to 20 bp does not prevent annealing if it is done at an appropriate temperature. The annealed strand serves as a primer for the synthesis of a strand complementary to the plasmid vector. This slightly mismatched duplex recombinant plasmid is then used to transform bacteria, where the mismatch is repaired by cellular DNA repair enzymes. About half of the repair events will remove and replace the altered base and restore the gene to its original sequence; the other half will remove and replace the normal base, retaining the desired mutation. Transformants are screened until a bacterial colony containing a plasmid with the altered sequence is found. Parts of two different genes can also be ligated to create new combinations. The product of such a fused gene is called a fusion protein. Researchers have now developed ingenious methods to bring about virtually any genetic alteration *in vitro*. Reintroduction of the altered DNA into the cell permits investigation of the consequences of the alteration. Site directed mutagenesis has greatly facilitated research on proteins by making specific changes in the

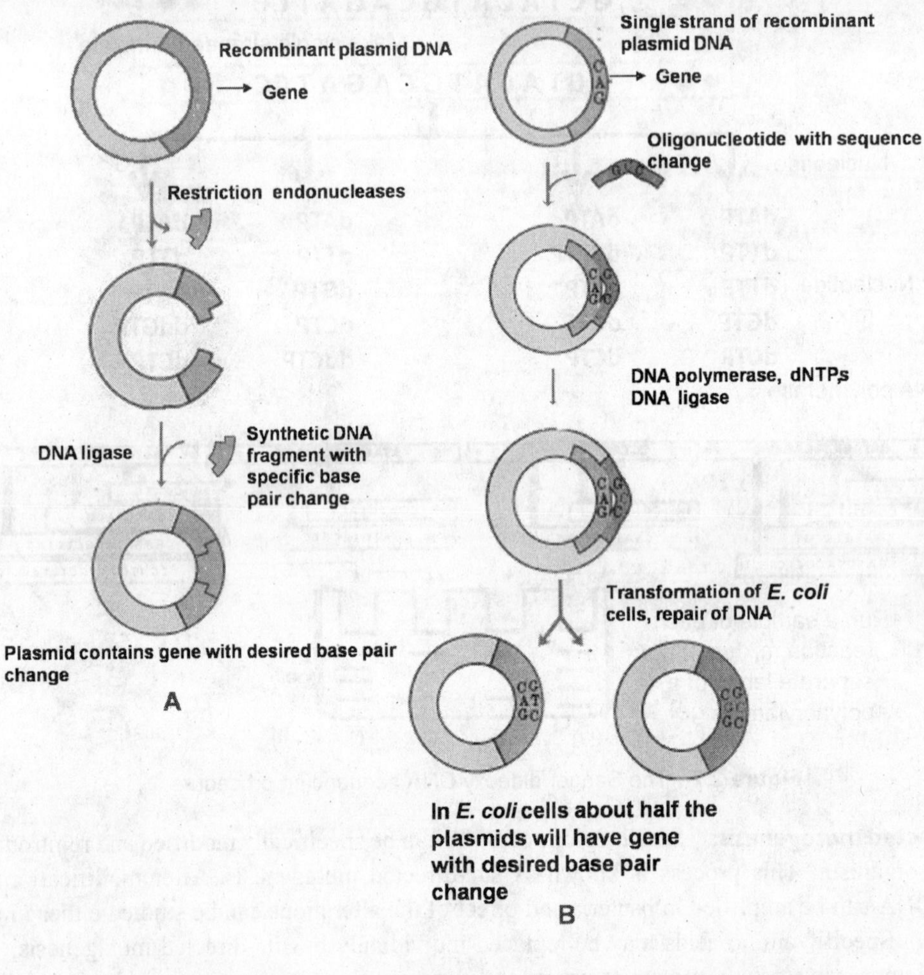

Figure 2.8 Two approaches for site-directed mutagenesis. (a) A synthetic DNA segment replaces a DNA fragment that has been removed by cleavage with a restriction endonuclease. (b) A synthetic oligonucleotide with a desired sequence change at one position is hybridized to a single-stranded copy of the gene to be altered.

primary structure of a protein and to examine the effects of these changes on the folding, three-dimensional structure, and activity of the protein.

Gene mapping: Studies using cloned DNA, e.g., *Saccharomyces cerevisiae* even in host were homologous between plasmid and host DNA not occur. One important approach involves the development of the technique known as Chromosome Walking. This is a process in which a set of cloned DNAs, is isolated so that a contiguous region of the genome is represented in the population of the clones. Chromosome walking is very useful for investigating the organization of genes in complex Eukaryotes, for which detailed genetic maps are almost impossible to obtain by other means. For example, Human Genome Organization (HUGO) project aims to produce a map of the entire genome on the 46 human chromosomes. The genome has been divided into a number of different regions, and some 250 individual laboratories around the world are working on sequencing each part. The potential benefit for medical is immense, as it will accelerate the rate at which genes can be located. Once the genes are located, genetic screening for many more conditions will be possible. In addition, it will increase our understanding of the codes that surround genes and control their activity.

Forensic science: When investigating a criminal offence, such as a burglary, serious sexual assault or murder, the police try to find evidence that will indicate who the criminals are. Recombinant DNA technology has now been used in a number of different ways. The best known example is DNA fingerprinting, which is based on two assumptions: firstly, each of a person's cells carries an identical set of DNA, and secondly, the DNA code for every individual person is unique. The sequences that code for genes are very similar throughout the population. However, sequence of DNA contain short sequences (15-100 bp) that repeat over and over again. The number of repeats in these areas of DNA are very different between individual people. Oligonucleotide probes, which code for one of the repeating sequences are used, each person's DNA producing a unique pattern. This means that if a few drops of blood or a few hair follicle cells attached to pieces of hair are left at the scene of crime, the DNA can be extracted, multiplied and then analyzed. The results can then be matched to those of a similar analysis carried out on samples taken from a suspect. If they match, this indicates that the suspect was at the crime site.

FUTURE PROSPECTS OF RECOMBINANT DNA TECHNOLOGY

The advent and development of recombinant DNA has been portrayed as very much a mixed blessing for mankind. A whole proponent have hailed it as a source of technology that will some day solve many of the problems of environmental pollution, food and energy shortages and human diseases. Gene manipulation opens the prospects of constructing bacterial cells, which can grow easily and inexpensively, and synthesize a variety of biological products like antibodies, hormones, enzymes, etc. In contrary, its opponents have bitterly criticized research in this area because of possibilities for accidental development and release of highly virulent forms of infective agents that may lead to epidemic diseases of unknown properties. Possibility exists that potentially biohazardous consequences might result from widespread injuditicious use of constructing novel organisms containing combinations of toxin producing capabilities and showing antibiotic resistance. Experiment involved in the introduction of DNA from tumor viruses into bacteria and infection of these bacteria to human beings will increase the incidence of cancer. Newly developed cloning methods offer the prospect of dealing with a wide variety of scientific and medical problems as well as other problems that trouble society.

CONCLUSION

The importance of recombinant DNA technology can be judged by the diversity of application and high market potential. There are more than 726 companies in the USA dealing with the products emanating from the application of genetic engineering. The Human Genome Project has relied on the recombinant DNA technology to generate libraries of genomic DNA molecules. Proteins for the treatment or diagnosis of disease have been produced using recombinant DNA techniques. Till date, over eighty products that are currently used for treatment of diseases or vaccination have been produced using recombinant DNA techniques. At least 350 additional recombinant-based drugs are currently being tested for safety and efficacy. Recombinant DNA technology has also been used to produce genetically modified foods with improved nutritional qualities. It is likely that this relatively new area of genetics will continue to play an increasingly important part in biological research into the foreseeable future. The basic information emerging out of this technology involves organization of the chromosomes, genetic switches in development and differentiation leading to amplification of genes which will have profound significance.

FURTHER READINGS

1. Adams, M.D., Kelley, J.M., Gocayne, J.D., Dubnick, M., Polymeropoulos, M.H., Xiao, H., Merril, C.R., Wu, A., Olde, B. and Moreno, R.F. (1991) Complementary DNA sequencing: expressed sequence tags and Human Genome Project. *Science.* **(252):** 1651-1656.
2. Alberts B., Johnson A., Lewis J., Raff M., Roberts K. and Walter P. (2002) *Molecular Biology of Cell.* Garland, New York (ISBN 0-8153-4072-9).
3. Alwine J.C., Kemp D. J. and Stark G.R. (1977) Method for detection of specific RNAs in agarose gels by transfer to diazobenzylomethyl-paper and hybridization with DNA probes. *Proc. Natl. Acad. Sci.* **(74):** 5463-5354.
4. Arat S., Rzucidlo S.J., Gibbons J., Miyoshi K. and Stice S.L. (2001) Production of transgenic bovine embryos by transfer of transfected granulosa cells into enucleated oocytes. *Mol. Reprod. Dev.* 60 **(1):** 20-26.
5. Archer J., Pinney J.W., Fan J., Simon-Loriere E., Arts E.J., Negroni M. and Robertson D.L. (2008) Identifying the Important HIV-1 Recombination Breakpoints. *PLoS Comput. Biol.* 4 **(9):** 100-117.
6. Avery O.T., MacLeod C.M. and McCarty M. (1944) Studies on the chemical nature of the substance inducing transformation of pneumococcal types. *J. Exp. Med.* **(79):** 137-158.
7. Bamshad, M. and Wooding, S.P. (2003) Signatures of natural selection in the human genome. *Nat. Rev. Genet.* **(4):** 99-111.
8. Brenner, S. (2004) Genes to genomics. *Annu. Rev. Genet.* **(38):** 20-25.
9. Brummell D.A. and Harpster M.H. (2001) Cell wall metabolism in fruit softening and quality and its manipulation in transgenic plants. *Plant Mol. Biol.* **(47):** 311-340.
10. Capecchi M.R. (1980) High efficiency transformation by direct microinjection of DNA into cultured mammalian cells. *Cell.* **(22):** 479-488.

11. Capper J.L., Castañeda-Gutiérrez E., Cady R.A. and Bauman D.E. (2008) The environmental impact of recombinant bovine somatotropin (rbST) use in dairy production. *Proc. Natl. Acad. Sci. USA.* 105 **(28):** 9668-9673.
12. Carbonaro D.A., Jin X., Cotoi D., Mi T., Yu X.J., Skelton D.C., Dorey F., Kellems R.E., Blackburn M.R. and Kohn D.B. (2008) Neonatal bone marrow transplantation of ADA-deficient SCID mice results in immunologic reconstitution despite low levels of engraftment and an absence of selective donor T lymphoid expansion. *Blood.* 111 **(12):** 5745-5754.
13. Cavazzana-Calvo M., Thrasher A. and Mavilio F. (2004) The future of gene therapy. *Nature.* 427 **(6977):** 779-781.
14. Clark, M.S. (1999) Comparative genomics: the key to understanding the human genome project. *Bioassays.* **(21):** 121-130.
15. Cohen S., Chang A., Boyer H. and Helgfing R. (1973) Construction of biologically functional bacterial plasmids *in vitro. Proc. Natl. Acad. Sci.* **(70):** 3240-3244.
16. Collins, F.S., Green, E.D., Guttmacher, A.E., and Guyer, M.S (2003) A vision for the future of genomics research. *Nature.* **(422):** 835-847.
17. Colowick, S. P. and Kapian, ON (1980) *Methods in Enzymology* - Volume 68; *Recombinant DNA.* Academic Press, ISBN 012181968X.
18. Cooper, Geoffrey (1997) *The Cell: A Molecular Approach.* Washington, DC: ASM Press.
19. David L. Nelson and Michael M. Cox (2001) Lehninger Principles of Biochemistry Fourth Edition University of Wisconsin–Madison) California, San Diego.
20. Felgner, P.L. T.R. Gadek, M. Holm, R. Roman, H.W. Chan, M. Wenz, J.P. Northrop, G.M. Ringold and M. Danielsen (1987) Lipofection: A highly efficient, lipid-mediated DNA-transfection procedure. *Proc. Nat. Acad. Sci.* **(84):** 7413-7417.
21. Garret, R.H. and Grisham, C.M. (2000) *Recombinant DNA Technology is also known as Transgenic Biochemistry,* Saunders College Publishers, (ISBN 0030758173).
22. Glick, Bernard and Jack Pasternak. (1998) *Molecular Biotechnology: Principles and Applications of Recombinant DNA,* 2nd ed. Washington, DC: ASM Press.
23. Grunstein M. and Hogness D.S. (1975) Colony hybridization: a method for the isolation of cloned DNAs that contain a specific gene. *Proc. Natl. Acad. Sci.* **(72):** 3961-3965.
24. Gunther M., Wagner E. and Ogris M. (2005) Specific targets in tumor tissue for the delivery of therapeutic genes. *Curr. Med. Chem. Anti. Canc. Agents.* 5 **(2):** 157-171.
25. Hansen, G. and Wright M.S. (1999) Recent advances in the transformation of plants. *Trends Plant Sci.* **(4):** 226-231.
26. Heyman Y., Zhou Q., Lebourhis D., Chavatte-Palmer P., Renard J.P. and Vignon X. (2002) Novel approaches and hurdles to somatic cloning in cattle. *Cloning Stem Cells.* 4 **(1):** 47-55.
27. Hohn B. and Murray K. (1977) Packaging recombinant DNA molecules into bacteriophage particles *in vitro. Proc. Natl. Acad. Sci.* **(74):** 3259-3263.
28. Houdebine L.M. (2003) *Animal Transgenesis and Cloning.* John Wiley & Sons, Inc. Hoboken, NJ, USA, pp. 34-73.
29. Jackson, D.A., Symons, R.H and Berg, P (1972) Biochemical method for inserting new genetic information into DNA of simian virus 40: circular SV40 DNA molecules containing lambda phage genes and the galactose operon of *Escherichia coli. Proc. Natl. Acad. Sci. USA.* **(69):** 2904-2909.
30. James D.W., Richard M.M., Amy A.C. and Jan A.W. (2007) *Recombinant DNA: Genes and Genomes–A Short Course.* Cold Spring Harbor Laboratory Press, New York.
31. Jeremy M. Berg, John L. Tymoczko and Lubert Stryer (1992) *Biochemistry.* San Francisco: W. H. Freeman., 2 Rev. edition (ISBN 0-7167-8724-5).
32. Kikkert J.R., Vidal J.R. and Reisch B.I. (2005) Stable transformation of plant cells by particle bombardment biolistics. *Methods Mol Biol.* **(286):** 61-78.

33. Klein T.M., Wolf E.D., Wu R. and Sanford J.C. (1987) Hugh-velocity microprojectiles for delivering nucleic acids into living cells. *Nature.* **(327):** 70-73.
34. Kreuzer, Helen, and Adrianne Massey (2000) *Recombinant DNA and Biotechnology,* 2nd ed. Washington, DC: ASM Press.
35. Kunkel T.A. (1985) Rapid and efficient site-specific mutagenesis without phenotypic selection. *Proc. Natl Acad. Sci. U S A.* 82 **(2):** 488-492.
36. Lai C.M., Lai Y.K. and Rakoczy P.E. (2002) Adenovirus and adeno-associated virus vectors. *DNA Cell Biol.* 21 **(12):** 895-913.
37. Lander, E.S., Linton, L.M., Birren, B., Nusbaum, C., Zody, M.C., Baldwin, J., Devon, K., Dewar, K., Doyle, M., FitzHugh, W., *et al.* (2001) Initial sequencing and analysis of the human genome. *Nature.* **(409):** 860-921.
38. Lanza R.P., Dresser B.L. and Damiani P. (2002) *Cloning Noah's ark, in Understanding Cloning.* Scientific American, Inc. and Byron Press Visual Publications, Inc, 24-35.
39. Lobban P and Kaiser AD (1973) Enzymatic end-to-end joining of DNA molecules. *J. Mol. Biol.* **(78):** 453-471.
40. Lodish H., Berk A., Zipursky S.L., Matsudaira P., Baltimore D. and Darnell J. (2003) *Molecular Cell Biology.* W.H. Freeman, New York.
41. Lorence A. and Verpoorte R. (2004) Gene transfer and expression in plants. *Methods Mol. Biol.* **(267):** 329-50.
42. Lynch S.V. and Wiener-Kronish J.P. (2008) Novel strategies to combat bacterial virulence. *Curr. Opin. Crit. Care.* 14 **(5):** 593-599.
43. Ma H. (2004a) Technique of animal clone. *Nature and Science.* 2 **(1):** 29-35.
44. Mahowald, M.B., Verp, M.S. and Anderson R.R. (1998) Genetic counselling: clinical and ethical challenges. *Annu. Rev. Genet.* **(32):** 547-559.
45. Maxam A.M. and Gilbert W. (1977) A new method of sequencing DNA. *Proc. Natl. Acad. Sci.* (74) 560-564.
46. McCutchan J.H. and Pagano J.S. (1968) Enhancement of the infectivity of simian virus 40 deoxyribonucleic acid with diethylaminoethyl-dextran. *J. Natl. Cancer. Inst.* 41 **(2):** 351-357.
47. Meselson M. and Yuan R. (1968) DNA restriction enzyme from *E. coli. Nature.* **(217):** 1110-114.
48. Nathan P. Kaplan, Nathan P. Colowick and Ray Wu (1980) *Recombinant DNA,* Vol. 68: *Recombinant D* Part F (*Methods in Enzymology*). Academic Press (ISBN 0-1218-1968-X).
49. Ohlstein, E.H., Ruffolo, R.R., Jr. and Elliott JD (2000) Drug discovery in the next millennium. *Annu. Rev. Pharmacol. Toxicol.* **(40):** 177-191.
50. Old, R.W., and S.B. Primrose (1994) *Principles of Gene Manipulation,* 5th ed. London: Blackwell Scientific Publications.
51. Pagano J.S. and Vaheri A. (1965) Enhancement of infectivity of poliovirus RNA with diethylaminoethyl-dextran (DEAE-D). *Arch Gesamte Virusforsch.* 17 **(3):** 456-464.
52. Palmiter, R.D., Brinster, R.L., Hammer, R.E., Trumbauer, M.E., Rosenfeld, M.G, Birnberg, N.C., and Evans, R.M. (1982) Dramatic growth of mice that develop from eggs microinjected with metallothionein-growth hormone fusion genes. *Nature.* **(300):** 611-615.
53. Peppin L., McEwing R., Carvalho G.R. and Ogden R.A. (2008) *DNA-Based Approach for the Forensic Identification of Asiatic Black Bear* (Ursus thibetanus) in a Traditional Asian Medicine [In press].
54. Peter Moore (1994) Recombinant DNA technology. The Biochemical Society, 59 Portland Place, London WIN 3AJ (ISBN 0-90449-8302).
55. Pfeifer, A. and Verma, I.M. (2001) Gene therapy: promises and problems. *Annu. Rev. Genomics Hum. Genet.* **(2):** 177-211.

56. Pinto G.A., Giordano R.L. and Giordano R.C. (2008) Remote engineering for a cheese whey biorefinery: an Internet-based application for process design, economic analysis, monitoring, and control of multiple plant sites. *Bioprocess Biosyst. Eng.* [In press].
57. Sambrook, J., Fritsch, E.F. and Maniatis, T. (1989) *Molecular Cloning: A Laboratory Manual*, 2nd edn, Cold Spring Harbor Laboratory Press, Cold Spring Harbor, NY.
58. Sanger F., Nicklen S. and Coulson A.R. (1977) A rapid method for determining sequencing with chain terminating inhibitors. *Proc. Natl. Acad. Sci.* **(74):** 5463-5467.
59. Shimizu M., Goto M., Hanai M., Shimizu T., Izawa N., Kanamoto H., Tomizawa K., Yokota A. and Kobayashi H. (2008) Selectable tolerance to herbicides by mutated acetolactate synthase genes integrated into the chloroplast genome of tobacco. *Plant Physiol.* 147 **(4):** 1976-1983. [In press].
60. Smith C.J.S., Watson C.P., MOlTis P.C., Bird C.R., Seymour G.B., Gray J.E., Arnold C., Tucker G.A., Schuch W., Harding S. and Grierson D. (1990) Inheritance and effect on ripening of antisense polygalacturonase genes in transgenic tomatoes. *Plant Mol. Biol.* **(14):** 369-379.
61. Smith H.O. and Wilox K.W. (1970) A restriction enzyme from *Hemophilus influenza*, I. Purification and general properties. *J. Mol. Biol.* **(51):** 373-391.
62. Southern E.M. (1975) Detection of specific sequences among DNA fragments separated by gel electrophoresis. *J. Mol. Biol.* **(98):** 503-517.
63. Tetteh K.K. and Polley S.D. (2007) Progress and challenges towards the development of malaria vaccines. *BioDrugs.* 21 **(6):** 357-373.
64. Umemoto Y., Sasaki S., Kojima Y., Kubota H., Kaneko T., Hayashi Y. and Kohri K. (2005) Gene transfer to mouse testes by electroporation and its influence on spermatogenesis. *J. Androl.* 26 **(2):** 264-271.
65. Uzogara S.G. (2000) The impact of genetic modification of human foods in the 21st century: a review. *Biotechnol Adv.* 18 **(3):** 179-206.
66. Wadhwa, P.D., Zielske, S.P., Roth, J.C., Ballas, C.B., Bowman, J.E. and Gerson, S.L. (2002) Cancer gene therapy: scientific basis. *Annu. Rev. Med.* **(53):** 437-452.
67. Wakabayashi H., Su Y.C., Ahmad S.S., Walsh P.N. and Fay P.J. (2005) A Glu113Ala mutation within a factor VIII Ca2+-binding site enhances cofactor interactions in factor Xase. *Biochemistry.* **(44):** 10298-10304.
68. Warden D. and Thorne H.V. (1968) The infectivity of polyoma virus DNA for mouse embryo cells in the presence of diethylaminoethyl-dextran. *J. Gen. Virol.* 3 **(3):** 371-377.
69. Watson J.D. and Crick F.H.C. (1953) Molecular structure of nucleic acids: a structure for deoxyribose nucleic acid. *Nature.* **(171):** 737-738.
70. Yan Y., Yang J., Dou Y., Chen M., Ping S., Peng J., Lu W., Zhang W., Yao Z., Li H., Liu W., He S., Geng L., Zhang X., Yang F., Yu H., Zhan Y., Li D., Lin Z., Wang Y., Elmerich C., Lin M. and Jin Q. (2008) Nitrogen fixation island and rhizosphere competence traits in the genome of root-associated Pseudomonas stutzeri A1501: *Proc. Natl. Acad. Sci. U S A.* 105 **(21):** 7564-7569.
71. Zambryski, P., Tempe J. and Schell J. (1989) Transfer and function of T-DNA genes from agrobacterium Ti and Ri plasmids in plants. *Cell.* **(56):** 193-201.
72. Zhu, H., Bilgin, M. and Snyder, M. (2003) Proteomics. *Annu. Rev. Biochem.* **(72):** 783-812.

CHAPTER

3

Nucleic Acid Probe Technology

Nucleic acid probe technology has been developed that relies on the use of DNA or RNA probes to detect particular gene sequences. The application of the techniques includes the diagnosis of genetic and infectious diseases. Through intensive research efforts in both chemical synthesis and bioassay development, molecular probes scientists have developed rapid and exceptionally sensitive fluorescence-based assays for quantitation of nucleic acids (DNA, RNA) and protein samples. In this chapter we present the basic concepts and practical applications of nucleic acid probe technology in agricultural, medical, veterinary and industrial applications that will have a marked influence on the development of new diagnostic strategies in the next future.

Keywords: Nucleic acid probe technology; hybridization techniques; probe labelling.

INTRODUCTION

Nucleic acid, i.e., DNA—the genetic code of all living organisms lying in the nucleus and extra-nuclear bodies—determines each individual's hereditary characteristics. Each person's genotype is different and is found in each living cell, so a hair, blood, skin or any part of the body can be used to identify and distinguish an individual from all other people. DNA probe technology has been used at many instances to prove the guilt or innocence of convict's involvement in a crime scene. DNA probe technology is routinely used in medical, clinical and microbiological research. It helps in the identification of new isolates of microbes in the culture and samples. This helps in drug discovery. Scientists looking for a disease gene typically used to study DNA samples from members of "disease families" and relatives, over several generations for disease history. It used to be extremely time taking and painful to find a gene marker linked to the disease under study. In the case of Huntington's disease, it took 10 years to advance from linked markers to the gene. Advances in nucleic acid probe technology have directly led to the development of widespread application of molecular hybridization techniques in diagnostic and molecular biology laboratories. A wide variety of microbial infections as well as genetic disorders are now diagnosed using hybridization techniques. In molecular hybridization, a specific nucleic acid probe is used to hybridize to complementary nucleic acid of a specific pathogen species directly in specimens or to analytes immobilized on solid phases. For genotype analysis, cloned genomic sequences are used to detect restriction fragment length polymorphisms in Southern blot hybridization protocols. Probes are labeled with either radionucleotide or biotin in order to permit the detection of specific hybrids. Hybridization is particularly useful in the diagnosis of microbial infections where the pathogen cannot be identified using conventional or classical diagnostic procedures. Some pathogens cannot be propagated in laboratory bioassays. Some viral pathogens may be present in latent states or integrated into host genomes. In such circumstances, transcriptional and translational processes are typically minimal and infectious agents may not be recoverable.

Two techniques are now widely used to diagnose infections by directly identifying the pathogen in clinical specimens: antigen detection using immunological techniques and nucleic acid detection using hybridization. Although both methods have proven to be sensitive and reliable for providing diagnostic results, molecular hybridization does permit diagnosis of certain infections and conditions where antigen detection cannot. For example, integrated or extra chromosomal nucleic acid of pathogens can be detected by hybridization, permitting diagnosis in the absence of gene expression.

The nucleic acid probe technology is increasingly being used in basic research in veterinary microbiology and in the diagnosis of infectious diseases of veterinary importance. Advances in molecular cloning techniques that made possible the preparation of gene-specific probes led to the use of hybridization techniques for the detection of bacterial and viral pathogens in clinical samples. Nucleic acid hybridization can provide a confirmation of diagnosis before the results of culture and biochemical tests are available. One key advantage of hybridization techniques is detection sensitivity of fraction of a picogram (one millionth of a microgram) and possibly femtogram of viral or bacterial nucleic acids without the loss of specificity. No other viral or bacterial detection method

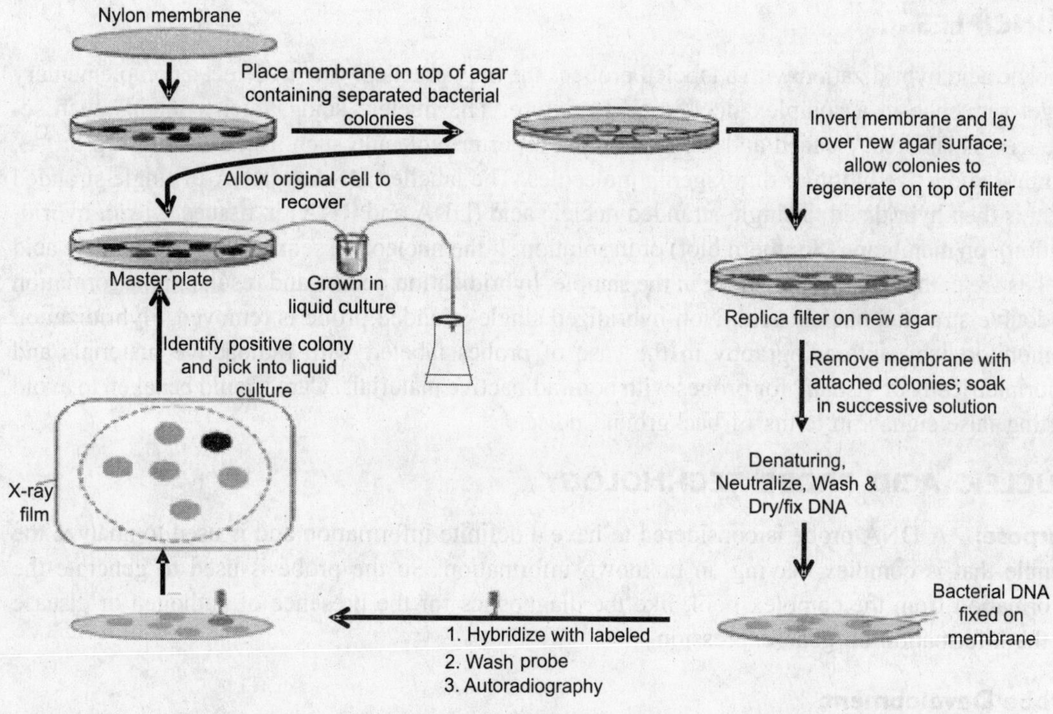

Figure 3.1 Colony hybridization involves replicating colonies on to a durable membrane prior to hybridization with a labeled nucleic acid probe. This method is popularly used to identify colonies containing recombinant DNA, should a suitable labeled probe be available.

has this degree of sensitivity (Figure 3.1). Probe technology has helped in the detection of virtually any organism in food, clinical samples or environment. It is now possible to detect a wide variety of viral, bacterial and protozoan pathogens in urine, stools, tissues and sputum using radiolabeled or non-radiolabeled assay systems. This technology is also useful in agricultural research for varietal identification and settlement of disputes arising due to the use of germplasm for varietal and hybrid development and biopiracy.

CONCEPTS

The detection of specific DNA sequences has always been an important issue in the biomedical field due to its application in DNA sequencing and diagnostics. Thirty years ago, the method by excellence to identify DNA was "sequencing by digestion", which was laborious and time-consuming. Soon thereafter, membrane-supported methods appeared based on "sequencing by hybridization" (SBH), which were simpler. However, the most important advance did not appear until the last decade, with the advent of DNA sensors and arrays. These two approaches overcame the problems of the previous technologies, such as low hybridization efficiency, low sequence discrimination, long analysis time and laborious procedures. Additionally, DNA arrays allow simultaneous multi-site detection, which further reduces the analysis time and facilitates genetic analysis. Miniaturized arrays allow small sample volumes and can be mass-produced.

PRINCIPLES

Nucleic acid hybridization with a labeled probe is the only practical way to detect a complementary target sequence in a complex nucleic acid mixture. The nucleic acid, which contains such sequences, is isolated, cleaned and labelled with a reporter molecule such as radioactive ^{32}p or ^{35}S, or non-radioactive biotin or digoxigenin molecules. The labelled DNA or RNA in single-stranded form is then hybridized to single-stranded nucleic acid (DNA and RNA) in tissues (*in situ* hybridization), on membrane (Southern blot) or in solution. If the nucleotide sequences in the nucleic acid probes are complementary to those in the sample, hybridization occurs and results in the formation of double-stranded nucleic acid. Non-hybridized single-stranded probe is removed. Hybridization is monitored by autoradiography in the case of probes labeled with radioactive materials and colorimetrically or visually for probes with non-radioactive materials. Care should be taken to avoid getting false signals in terms of background noise.

NUCLEIC ACID PROBE TECHNOLOGY

Purpose: A DNA probe is considered to have a definite information and is used to analyze the sample that is complex, having an unknown information. So the probe is used to generate the information from the complex pool, like the diagnostics for the presence of pathogen or disease or the information on gene expression.

Probe Development

For diagnosis, three major types of probe constructs are commonly used. First, genomic sequences or complementary DNA (cDNA) of RNA species of the organism of interest may be cloned into a vector system. Second, from the microbes, nucleic acid can be directly extracted and labelled for use as a probe. Third, if the sequence of the analyte is known, a complementary probe can be synthesized. Steps involved in the production of a probe are as follows:

1. Isolation of the desired nucleic acid sequences.
2. Cloning the sequences into an appropriate vector system by recombinant DNA technology.
3. Amplification of the sequences in a host vector system.
4. Recovery and labeling of the sequences.
5. Demonstration of the efficacy of the probe.

Choice of Probe

In order to interpret a hybridization experiment, hybrids must be distinguishable from nucleic acids that remain single stranded. This is accomplished by labelling one of the reacting nucleic acids, the probe, with a reporter molecule. After hybridization, the probe that has not reacted is washed away and the hybrids are recognized by virtue of the reporter molecule. In principle, any nucleic acid—double-stranded DNA, single-stranded DNA, oligonucleotides, mRNA and RNA—can act as a probe. The choice is determined by the purpose of the experiment and the materials available (Figure 3.2).

a. ***DNA probes:*** Double-stranded DNA probes are very commonly used and consist of double-stranded DNAs that have been denatured and added quickly to the hybridization mix before they have time to reassociate. Single-stranded DNA probes are usually derived by reverse transcription of RNA. If the template is mRNA, the cDNA will consist of many different sequences and the complexity of the DNA will be high.

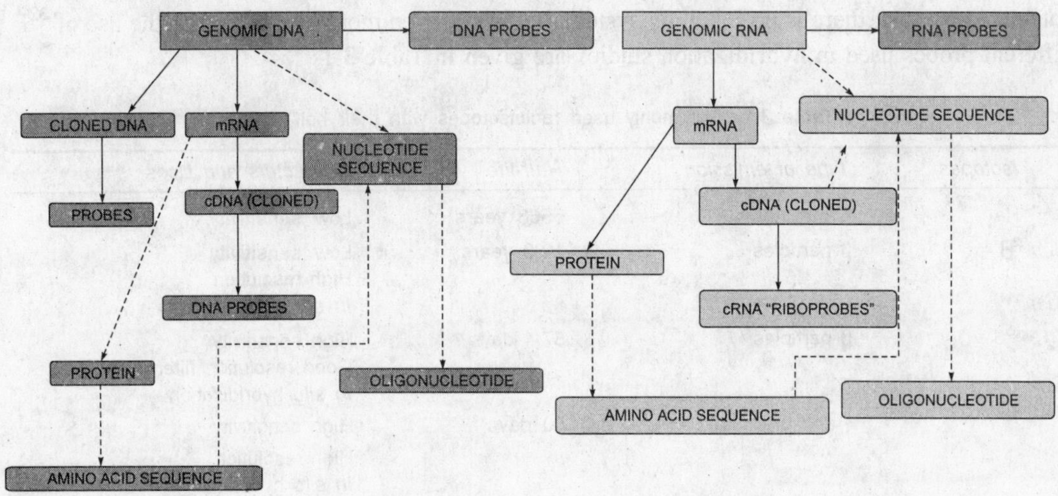

Figure 3.2 Sources of DNA (left) and RNA (right) probes. Heavy solid lines = primary means of obtaining probes; light lines = minor sources of probes; dotted lines = transmission of sequence data to synthesize oligonucleotide probes.

b. ***RNA probes:*** Single-stranded probes may be prepared by labelling isolated RNA, but it is more common to transcribe cloned sequences from recombinant plasmids in which the cloned sequences are flanked by promoters for bacteriophage RNA polymerases. The advantages of RNA probes are that they are relatively easy to prepare and RNA: DNA and RNA: RNA hybrids are more stable than the corresponding DNA: DNA hybrids. However, their main disadvantage is that they are more difficult to handle than DNA probes because of the widespread presence of ribonucleases.

c. ***Oligonucleotide probes:*** Oligonucleotide probes are short (typically 17-50 nt in length) and are usually chemically synthesized. In theory, they may be oligodeoxyribonucleotides (more commonly used), oligoribonucleotides or molecules with a modified backbone such as peptide nucleic acids. One of the most useful properties of oligonucleotide probes is that they can discriminate between target sequences that differ by as little as a single nucleotide. The main disadvantage in their use is that hybrids containing oligonucleotides are much less stable than hybrids containing longer nucleic acids.

Commonly used Isotopic and Non-isotopic Chemicals for Labelling of Probe

The most commonly used tag for the probe is phosphorus 32 (^{32}P) which is incorporated into the probe by enzymatic polymerization of nucleoside phosphates. This is an excellent tag for most research applications where short half-life and the hazards of radioactive materials are not the major concerns. ^{32}P has the highest specific activity and emits α-particles of high energy. This gives maximum sensitivity in the shortest time in autoradiography. Limitations are short half-life of ^{32}P-Iabelled probe, cost, inconvenience of radioactivity disposals, and the hazards of working with the isotope. At present, there is no labelling system that has proven more sensitive than the use of ^{32}P. Different probes used in hybridization studies are given in Table 3.1.

Table 3.1 Commonly used radioisotopes with their half-life.

Isotopes	*Type of emission*	*Half-life*	*Characters and Uses*
He	β particles	5568 years	Low sensitivity
^{3}H	β particles	12.6 years	Low sensitivity High resolution *In situ* hybridization
^{35}S	β particles	87.4 days	High sensitivity Good resolution filter *In situ* hybridization
$^{125}1$	γ and β	60 days	High sensitivity High resolution *In situ* hybridization
$^{131}1$	γ and β	8.6 days	High radiation Rarely used
^{32}p	β	14.2 days	High sensitivity Filter hybridization
^{33}p	β	24.5 days	Filter hybridization

Recently a new radioisotope, ^{33}P, has been developed. This has a half-life of 24.5°C days and emits radiation with E_{max} of 0.249. The ^{33}P with its radiation characteristics in between those of ^{32}P and ^{35}S strikes a reasonable balance between the sensitivity of ^{32}P and the resolution of ^{35}S. The maximum energy of ^{33}P is 1.5 times that of ^{35}S, but is 5 times weaker than ^{32}P. The specific activity of ^{33}P is in the same range as that of ^{32}P, but at the same time the resolution is at par with ^{35}S. ^{33}P is less sticky compared to ^{35}S and hence reduces the non-specific background *in situ* hybridization. The relatively longer half-life of ^{33}P as compared to ^{32}P leads to increased shelf life of the labeled probe and hence they can be reused over longer periods of time.

Recently, non-isotopic reporter systems have been used for detection of microbes using biotin or digoxigenin probes. These techniques retain the exquisite sensitivity and specificity of nucleic acid hybridization without the drawbacks associated with radioisotopes. After hybridization, the reaction is detected immunologically by enzyme immunoassay or immunofluorescence. Advantages of the non-isotopic detection system include the following:

(1) Biotinylated probes are stable for a year or more at 4°C.
(2) Picogram levels of nucleic acid can be detected.
(3) Hybridization can be detected rapidly within a matter of hours.
(4) Radioisotopes are not used, precluding problems with licensing, hazard and disposal problems.
(5) Hybridization tests are readily conducted in clinical or field situations.

Probe Labelling Techniques

For detection and quantitation of a test gene by hybridization of a nucleic acid probe, it is essential that the probe should be labelled. Labelling of the probe is done by either *in vivo* or *in vitro* methods. Previously, probes with radioactive label were prepared from bacteria grown in the presence of radioisotopes. Recently, methods of labelling probes *in vitro* have been devised. Labelling is generally accomplished by the incorporation of labelled precursor molecules such as adenosine triphosphate in the probe. The two methods are: (1) radioisotopic labelling and (2) non-isotopic labeling.

Radioisotopic probe labelling

The radioisotopes like ^{32}P, ^{33}P, ^{35}S, ^{3}H are the usual labels for probes used in blotting techniques, while ^{3}H (tritium), which has a shorter track length in photographic emulsions and therefore, allows more precise localization at the histological level, is preferred for *in situ* hybridization studies in tissue sections. For *in vitro* radioisotopic labelling, generally four types of methods, *viz.*, nick translation, random primer, end labeling, and *in vitro* transcription are being used.

(i) **Nick translation method:** DNA can be uniformly labelled by nick translation (Figure 3.3). This procedure depends on the concerted action of two enzymes, DNase I and *E. coli* DNA polymerase I. DNase I introduces single-stranded nicks into a double-stranded DNA template at a frequency that depends on the amount of enzyme present. Starting at a nick, the 5' to 3' exonuclease activity of *E. coli* DNA polymerase I excises nucleotides from the newly created 5' end. At the same time, the 5' to 3' polymerase activity adds template-specific nucleotides at the 3' end. The net result is that the nick is moved (translated) in the 5' to 3' direction as new nucleotides are added in the same direction. If one of the added nucleoside triphosphates is labelled, a uniformly labelled product is generated. The proportion of bases replaced by DNA polymerase I and hence the specific activity of the product depends on the number of nicks introduced into the DNA. The advantage of random priming is that it tends to give higher specific activity of probes than nick translation, but nick translation gives better control of the length of the probe.

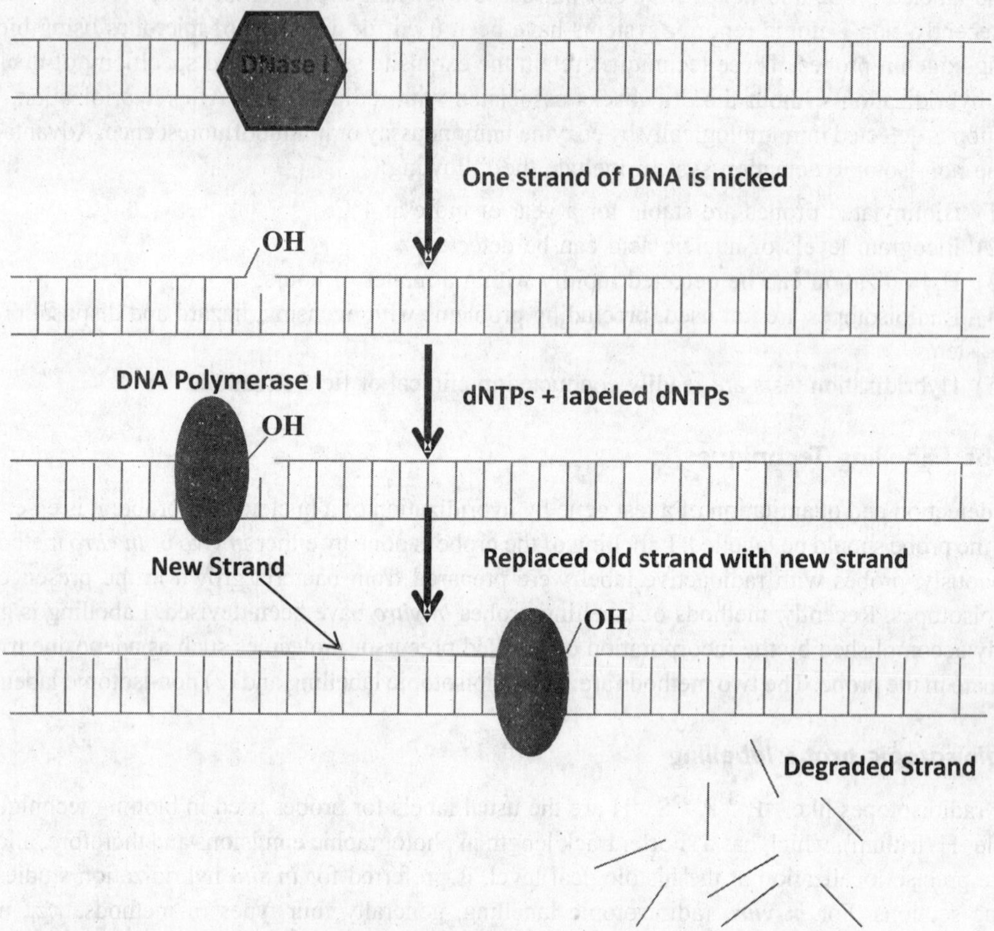

Figure 3.3 DNA labelling by nick translation.

(ii) Random priming method: The most common method for uniform labelling of DNA is random priming (Figure 3.4). DNA is denatured and incubated with short primers or random sequences, which anneal to the DNA. The primers are extended by the Klenow fragment of DNA polymerase I in the presence of labelled dNTPs to create labeled products. This is a good method by which DNA probes can be produced. These probes have ten times higher specific activity than those prepared by nick translation.

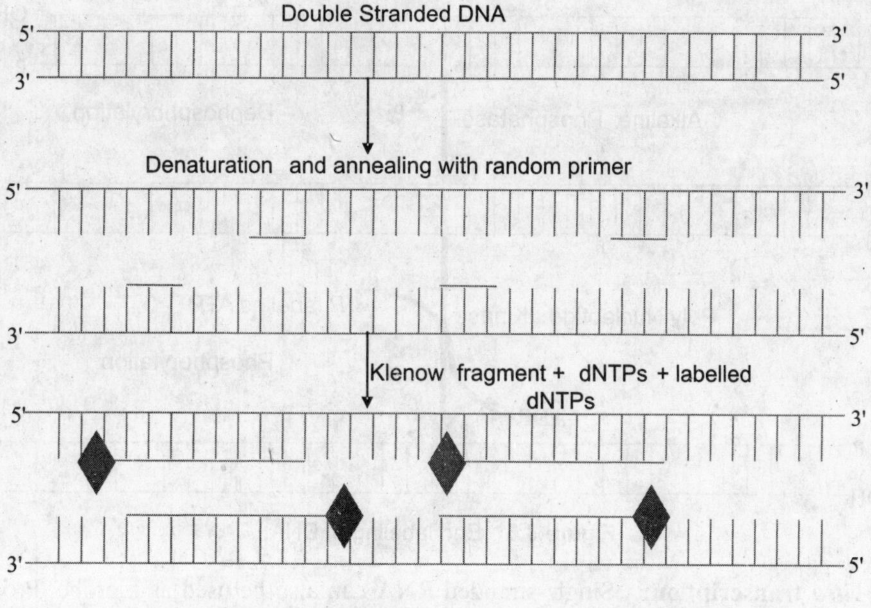

Figure 3.4 DNA labelling by random primer method.

(iii) End labelling: DNA, RNA or oligonucleotides can be radiolabelled at the 5' ends by T4 polynucleotide kinase, which catalyses the transfer of the γ-phosphate from [^{32}P] ATP to a free 5' hydroxyl group (Figure 3.5). Chemically synthesized oligo nucleotides have a free 5' hydroxyl group, and radioactive phosphate can be attached directly with no pretreatment of the oligonucleotide. The reaction is very efficient and high specific activities of ~109 cpm mg^{-1} oligonucleotide are readily achieved. DNA fragments derived by restriction enzyme digestion usually carry 5' phosphates, which must be removed with phosphatase to generate free 5' hydroxyl groups. The phosphatase must then be completely inactivated or removed, otherwise the [^{32}P] phosphate attached by the kinase will be removed by residual phosphatase activity. Calf intestinal alkaline phosphatase is used in preference to calf thymus phosphatase because it is easier to inactivate. The specific activity of these probes is less, as the molecules are labeled at the end. In the same way the double-stranded DNA can be labeled with the PNK. Enzyme like Klenow fragment can be used for labelling double-stranded DNA in the restricted end by filling-in.

Labelling DNA or oligonucleotides at the 3' end depends on the ability of the enzyme terminal transferase to add nucleotides to the free 3' hydroxyl in a template-independent manner. Short, labelled, homopolymer tails can be added by incubating the enzyme and DNA with a labelled reporter-dNTP (usually dATP). This is called DNA tailing. A useful feature of tailing is that it provides several reporter molecules per DNA or oligonucleotide molecule. This makes detection more sensitive than when a single reporter molecule is present.

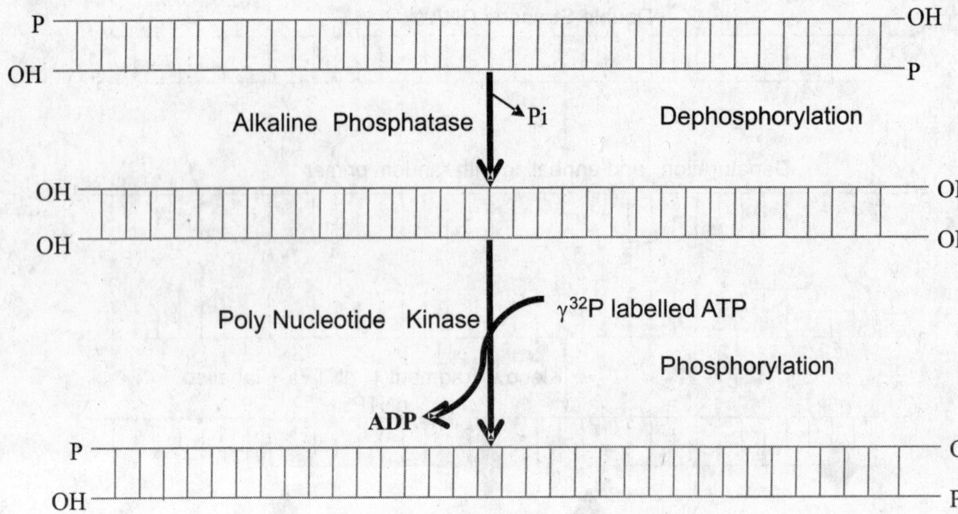

Figure 3.5 End labeling of DNA.

(iv) ***In vitro*** **transcription:** Single-stranded RNA can also be used as a probe. Probes composed of mRNA can be prepared readily by *in vitro* transcription from cloned complementary DNA in the presence of RNA polymerase and suitably labelled precursor molecules. These are most sensitive probes for any diagnostic procedure based on hybridization because the rate and stability of hybridization is far greater in RNA-DNA hybrid than in DNA-

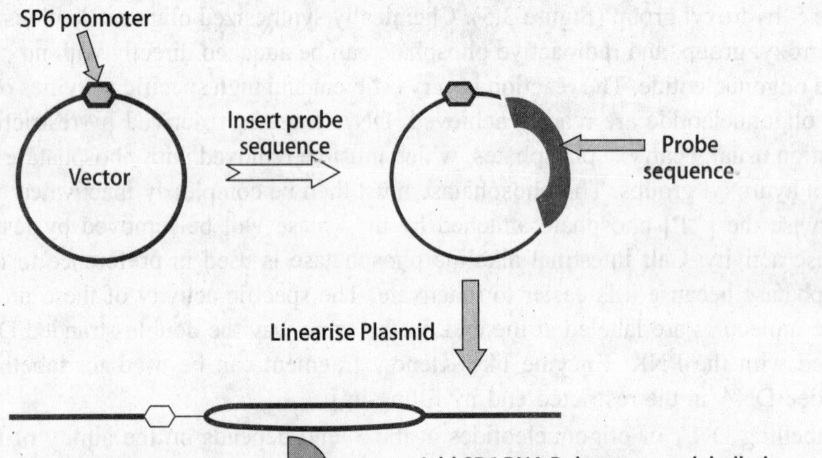

Figure 3.6 The SP6 system for preparing labelled RNA.

DNA hybrid. Most of the present-day cloning vectors have the promoter sites of T7, T3 and SP6 on the either side of the multiple cloning site (MCS) (Figure 3.6). If the probe that needs to be labelled is cloned, it can be labelled by transcription from any of these promoters and option is available for the strand to be labelled. The plasmid is linearized with a suitable restriction enzyme and then incubated with RNA polymerase and the four NTPs. If one of the NTP is radioactively labelled, the incubation mix will contain labelled RNA, which can be added directly to the hybridization mixture. Instead of cloning in the vector, the promoter sequence can be added to the primer sequences and *in vitro* transcription can be done on the PCR amplified product.

Non-radioactive labelling

Probes required for the detection of DNA or RNA sequences that are present only in small numbers (e.g., one or two copies per cell) must be highly radioactive and unfortunately pose serious health and disposal problems, which prevents their widespread use in routine tests. These radiolabelled probes are also not found suitable because of shorter shelf life and unavailability of quality control in diagnostic laboratory. The shelf life of probes can be extended by using radioactively labelled thionucleotides.

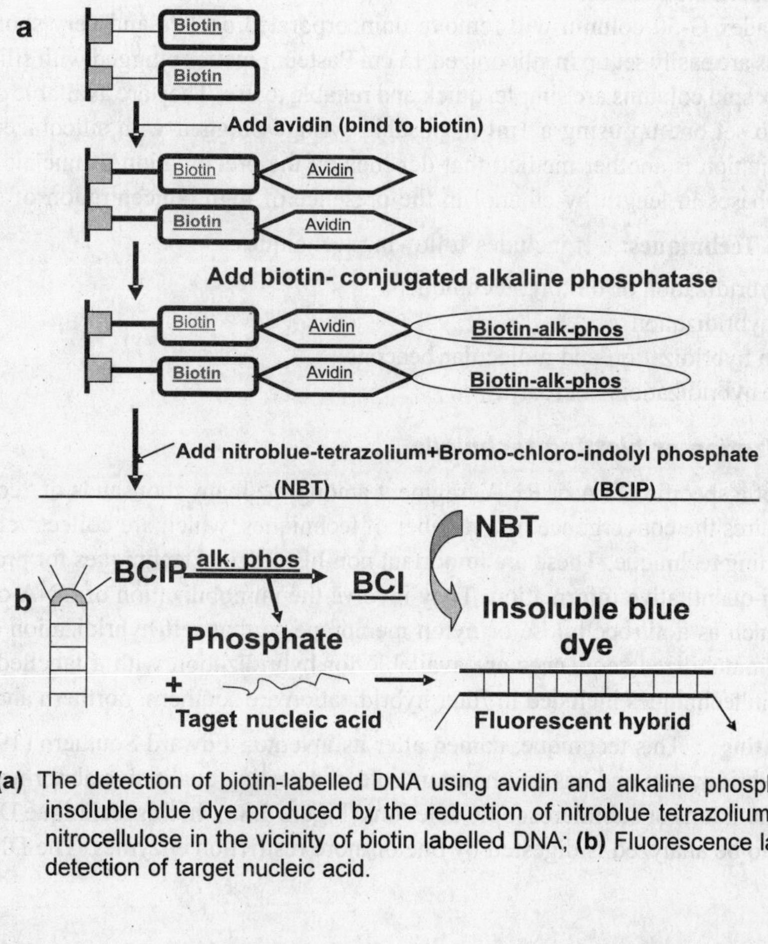

Figure 3.7 (a) The detection of biotin-labelled DNA using avidin and alkaline phosphatase. The insoluble blue dye produced by the reduction of nitroblue tetrazolium 'stains' the nitrocellulose in the vicinity of biotin labelled DNA; **(b)** Fluorescence labelling and detection of target nucleic acid.

An alternative approach is to use the nucleotides modified with reporter molecules, which does not affect its ability to be recognized by the enzymes and thus added to the probe. There are two types in non-radioactive labeling—labelling with direct detection of the molecule with reporter like flourescein or indirect detection with enzyme conjugates for the reporter like biotin and digoxigenin (Figure 3.7a and b). Enzyme conjugate detection could be done either by colorimetric or chemiluminescence, wherein the labeled nucleotides are incorporated into the probe and the probe is localized by affinity conjugates like avidin or streptavidin for the biotin, and anti-dig antibody for the digoxigenin. Probes for filter hybridization are most commonly labelled with biotin, digoxygenin, fluorescein or enhanced chemiluminescence method. The enzymes alkaline phosphatase and horseradish peroxidase are fairly common reporter molecules.

Removal of Unincorporated Nucleotides

After the probe has been labelled, it is usual to remove unincorporated radioactive label because during hybridization free labelled nucleotides may bind non-specifically to the filter causing high backgrounds. However, removal of radioactive label may not be necessary if more than about 70% has been incorporated into the probe. Non-radioactive labelled nucleotides tend to have very low affinity for the commonly used types or filter and so unincorporated label is seldom removed. There are several standard methods for removing unincorporated nucleotides. Size exclusion chromatography on Sephadex G-50 column will remove unincorporated dNTPs and very short oligonucleotides. Columns are easily set up in siliconized 15 cm Pasteur pipettes plugged with siliconized glass wool. Sephadex spin columns are simple, quick and reliable to use. They are available commercially, but it is easy to set one up using a 1ml disposable syringe plugged with siliconized glass wool. Ethanol precipitation is another method that depends on the precipitation of nucleic acids greater than about 20 bases in length by ethanol in the presence of high concentration of salt.

Hybridization Techniques: It includes following techniques:

1. Filter hybridization or blotting technique
2. *In situ* hybridization
3. Solution hybridization and molecular beacons
4. Reverse hybridization/Microarray

Filter hybridization or blotting technique

Visualization of a specific DNA or RNA fragment among the many thousands of "contaminating" molecules requires the convergence of a number of techniques, which are collectively termed blot transfer or blotting technique. These are important non-histological techniques for providing qualitative and semi-quantitative information. They involve the immobilization of DNA or RNA on an inert support such as a nitrocellulose or nylon membrane so that self-hybridization does not take place but the immobilized sequences are available for hybridization with a labelled nucleic acid probe. The main techniques included in filter hybridization are southern, northern and dot blotting.

Southern Blotting: This technique, named after its inventor, Edward Southern (1975), involves DNA: DNA hybridization and has an important role in detecting qualitative abnormalities in DNA such as point mutations or submicroscopic deletions (Figure 3.8a). In this technique DNA extracted from the cells to be analyzed is digested by one or more restriction enzymes. The DNA fragments so produced are separated on the basis of size by gel electrophoresis. The fragments are then denatured into single strands and "blotted" onto nitrocellulose membranes. A radiolabelled DNA probe is then applied to the nitrocellulose paper. If any DNA fragment contains a sequence complementary to that of the probe, hybridization occurs. Since the probe is radioactive, the hybridizing band can be revealed by autoradiography.

Northern Blotting: It involves mRNA: DNA hybridization. This procedure is utilized to detect whether a given gene is being expressed (Figure 3.8a). Total cellular mRNA is extracted and subjected to agarose gel electrophoresis that separates mRNA species on the basis of size. Subsequent steps are same as described with Southern blotting. By this procedure, the presence or absence of a given mRNA as well as the size of the transcript can be determined. 'Northern' is a parody on the use of Southern's name. The joke has been extended with the term 'Western' blotting, which refers to the sizing of polypeptides by gel electrophoresis, blotting and detection of the relevant bands with labelled antibody.

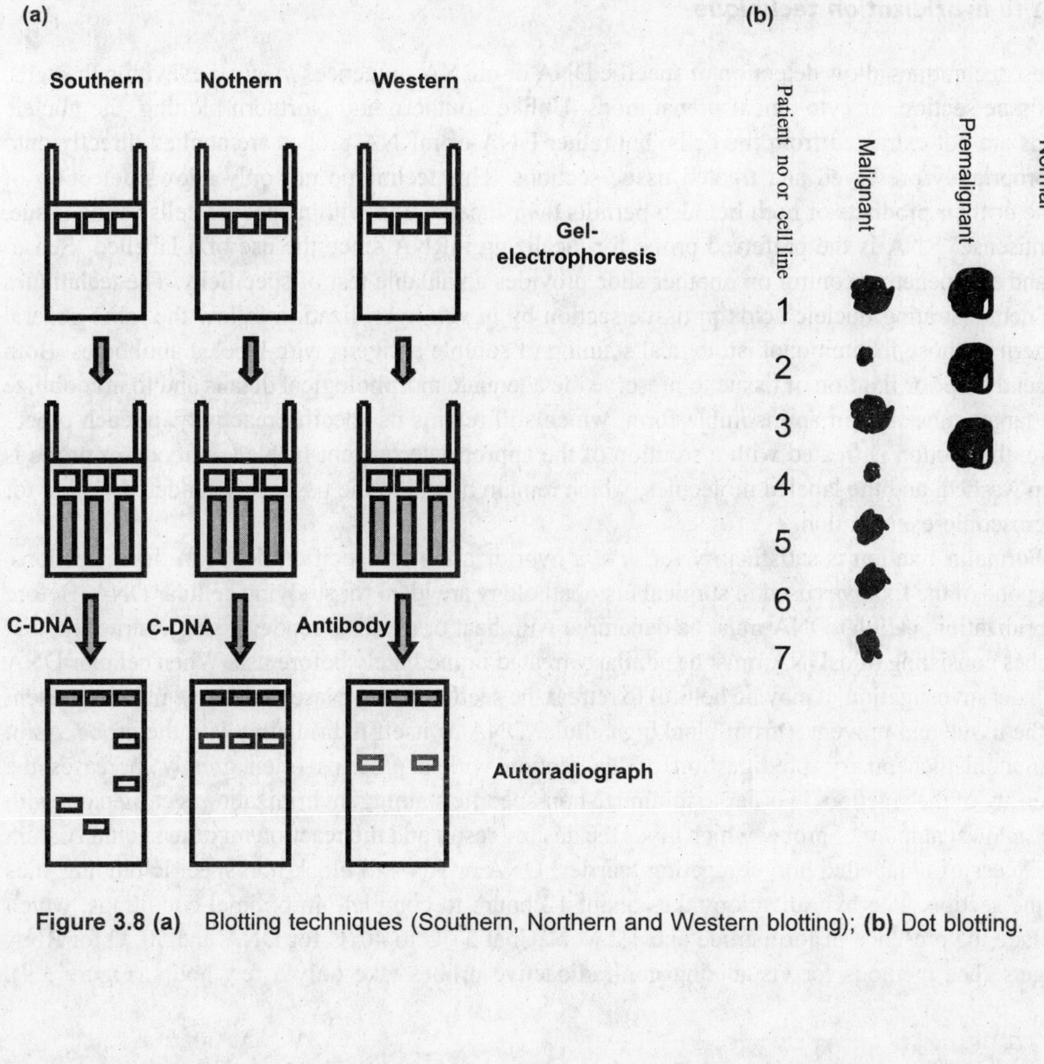

Figure 3.8 (a) Blotting techniques (Southern, Northern and Western blotting); **(b)** Dot blotting.

Dot Blotting: It differs from Southern and Northern blotting in that it does not involve restriction digestion or size fractionation (Figure 3.8b). In the simplest form of hybridization, measured amount of DNA or RNA is extracted from cells such as tumor. The RNA or DNA to be tested is applied onto a moistened nitrocellulose membrane as 4 mm diameter 'Dots', denatured (e.g., with alkali) and immobilized by baking at 80°C for two hrs. A labelled-single stranded probe is then applied in a solution containing salt, formamide and to block non specific uptake of probe by the membrane, an excess of carrier DNA or RNA. After overnight hybridization at 42°C the membrane is washed to remove unreacted probe. The duration, temperature and salt content of the wash determines the stringency of the reaction. The intensity of labelling of each dot is proportional to the concentration of specific sequences it contains, and the results can be calibrated by comparison with 'dots' prepared from standard. In this way, assay of specific sequences in DNA can detect gene amplification in pathological tissue such as duplication of a particular oncogene, while measurement of the corresponding mRNA can indicate to what extent the gene is being transcribed.

In situ hybridization technique

These techniques allow detection of specific DNA or mRNA sequences *in situ*, i.e., within the cells, in tissue section, or cytological preparations. Unlike Southern and Northern blotting, the nucleic acids are not extracted from the cells, but rather DNA or mRNA probes are applied directly onto appropriately preserved and treated tissue sections. This technique not only allows detection of gene or their products or both but also permits their localization within specific cells of the tissue. 'Antisense' RNA is the preferred probe for localizing mRNA since the use of a labelled 'Sense' strand as a negative control on another slide provides a valuable test of specificity. The techniques for demonstrating nucleic acids in tissue section by *in situ* hybridization follow the same general pattern as those for immunohistological staining of soluble antigens with labeled antibodies. Both depend on prior fixation of tissue to preserve the adequate morphological details and to immobilize the target substance in an insoluble form, which still retains its specific reactivity. In each procedure, the section is treated with a solution of the appropriate reagent-labeled antibody or probe is then washed, and the labeled molecules, which remain bound to the tissue, are rendered visible for microscopic examination.

Formalin fixation is satisfactory for *in situ* hybridization of specific mRNA in tissue sections, but none of the fixatives used in surgical histopathology are ideal for studying cellular DNA. Before hybridization, cellular DNA must be denatured with heat or alkali to render it single-stranded, and probes consisting of dsDNA must be similarly treated immediately before use. When cellular DNA is under investigation, it may be helpful to retreat the section with RNase to destroy mRNA present in the tissue and prevent it from blocking cellular DNA or itself hybridizing with the probe. As in immunohistochemistry, predigestion of the section with a proteins often greatly increases the intensity of the reaction. In order to minimize non-specific staining, hybridization is carried out with the smallest amount of probe, which gives the desired result and the reaction mixture should contain an excess of unlabelled non-competing 'carrier' DNA or RNA to block non-specific binding sites in the section. The hybridization takes about 12 hours to complete in optimal conditions, which include the presence of formamide and 1.2 M NaCl at 37°C to 40° C for DNA and 50° C for RNA targets. The methods for visualizing non-radioactive probes take only a few hours (Figure 3.9).

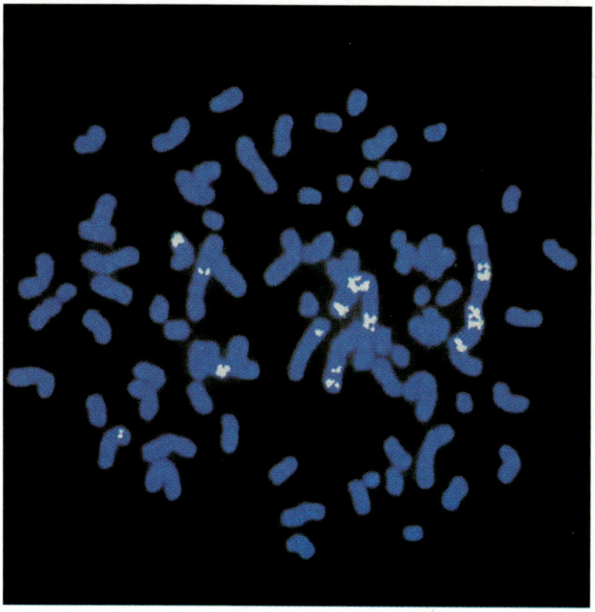

Figure 3.9 Chromogenic *in situ* hybridization (CISH) using DNA probe for the HER2 gene for the detection of breast cancer (Source: Saez *et al.*, 2006).

Solution hybridization and molecular beacons

Nucleotide acid probes can be used to detect molecules in solution by hybridization. Since the elimination of unhybridized probe is not possible in the solution, the detection of hybridization depends on the structural change in the probe upon hybridization with target molecule. Solution hybridization is mostly used to detect the target molecule in real time. Recent development of fluorescent reporters lead to the development of single-stranded hybridization probes, which are called molecular beacons. The probes can form the stem-loop structures with the target region in the loop. When hybridization occurs with the target molecule, the stem-loop structures are opened up or lost. Molecular beacons use a flourophore in one arm of stem and a non-emitting quencher in the other arm of the stem, so that when excited with light, the fluorescence from fluorophore is quenched by the quencher and no emission takes place. Upon hybridization, the stem-loop opens and the distance between the fluorophore and the quencher is increased so that flourecence is not quenched, which can be detected. Solution hybridization is routinely followed in the hybridization kinetic studies and preparative techniques like normalization, subtraction, etc. where the hybridized and unhybridized molecules are separated by affinity in carboxyapatite column, which has differential affinity for single and double-stranded DNA or in avidin affinity column where the probe is labelled with biotin.

Detection of proteins by molecular beacon aptamers: The concept of molecular beacons is even extended with development of nucleic acid aptamer, which has affinity for proteins or any molecule. Aptamers are nucleic acids that have high affinity and selectivity with the target molecule. The aptamers can be developed for the target molecules by a process called SELEX (Systematic

Evolution of Ligands by Exponential Enrichment). The process involves the isolation of high affinity oligos from the random oligonucleotide pool. The *oligos* with the affinity to target molecule are purified by affinity chromatography or gel shift assay and extraction. The affinity purification is repeated for many rounds of selection. The molecular aptamers are also used similarly to molecular beacons wherein the structural change in the aptamer upon binding of the target molecule can be visualized by the change in fluorescent properties. The nucleotide aptamers can also be used in an array for the detection of protein molecules similar to the microarray for detection DNA.

Reverse hybridization/microarray

In reverse hybridization, the probe is immobilized on the membrane or on glass slide and the sample to be analyzed is labelled and hybridized with probe. Usually many probes are spotted on the array or synthesized *in situ* on the slide. Analysis can be carried out in parallel for many probes simultaneously. Arrays are used for global gene expression analysis of many genes simultaneously or for diagnosis of many pathogens from single hybridization.

APPLICATIONS OF NUCLEIC ACID PROBE TECHNOLOGY

Nucleic acid probe technology has got several implications in clinical, medical, agricultural, veterinary and industrial fields. Some of the important applications are discussed below.

Medical and Veterinary Applications

Detection of pathogens in clinical samples

Nucleic acid probes provide a sensitive method for the detection of infectious agents. These probes have been used to detect bacteria, viruses and parasites in clinical samples. The DNA fragments that encode for heat-stable toxin (ST) and heat-labile toxin (LT) were radiolabelled and used as probes for detection of enterotoxic *E. coli*. ^{32}P-labelled DNA probes are used for the detection of leptospires in blood, urine and liver specimens. Specific ^{125}I labelled single-stranded DNA probes complementary to rRNAs of the target organisms were used for rapid identification of *Mycobacterium avium*, *M. intracellulare* and *M. tuberculosis*. This method was also used to differentiate *M. paratuberculosis* from *M. avium*, which are indistinguishable by cultural and biochemical tests. Allison *et al.* (2005) described a set of rRNA-based oligonucleotide probes that specifically detected either *M. intracellulare*, the two *M. avium* subspecies associated with human disease, or all members of the *Mycobacterium avium* complex (MAC). The most important application of nucleic acid probes is the detection of fastidious organisms. Many organisms such as *Mycoplasma* and *Mycobacterium* spp. cannot be cultured easily, or require 3 weeks to 3 months to culture. Nucleic acid probes have been developed and are being successfully used for their detection either directly in clinical specimens or following short culture periods. A dot blot hybridization method was used for the detection of *Campylobacter* spp. in stools using ^{32}P-labelled probes. *Mycoplasma hyorhinis*, which causes chronic arthritis in swine, was differentiated from other mycoplasma organisms using DNA probes in Southern blot hybridization. *Mycoplasma haemosuis* DNA was detected in experimentally infected splenectomized pigs by *in situ* hybridization (ISH) with a non-radioactive digoxigenin-labeled DNA probe. An 839-base-pair DNA probe targeting a 16S rRNA gene was generated by the polymerase chain reaction. The ISH method developed in this study was useful for the detection of *M. haemosuis* DNA in formalin fixed, paraffin wax-embedded tissues and may be valuable for studying the pathogenesis of *M. haemosuis infection.*

Detection of *Haemophilus parasuis* in naturally infected pigs was studied by *in situ* hybridization with a non-radioactive digoxigenin-labelled DNA probe. Twenty pigs were selected on the basis of bacterial isolation and histopathological lesions. An 821-base-pair DNA probe from the 16S small subunit ribosomal RNA (rRNA) was generated by the polymerase chain reaction. Hybridization signals were detected in formalin-fixed, paraffin-wax-embedded tissues (lung, heart, spleen and liver). It was concluded that *in situ* hybridization was a valuable tool for the diagnosis of *H. parasuis* infection. Specific DNA probes are also available for the detection of other bacteria like *Yersinia, Salmonella, Usteria* and *Clostridium* spp. Among viral infections, ^{32}P-labelled probes prepared with polymerase sequences of FMD virus detected the virus in oesophageal and pharyngeal fluids using dot blot hybridization. A 3-kb DNA fragment of porcine parvovirus was cloned and used as probe for detection of parvovirus. Direct filter hybridization was used for the detection of pseudorabies virus in nasal and tonsillar cells. Bluetongue virus serogroup-specific and serotype-specific single-stranded DNA probes labelled with ^{35}S-CTP was used to identify bluetongue virus in infected cell lines. DNA probes have been produced for RNA viruses such as rotavirus and influenza A virus by synthesis of complementary DNA (cDNA) from the viral RNA using the enzyme reverse transcriptase. After synthesizing the homologous strand, cDNA can be inserted into a bacterial plasmid or phage and molecularly cloned to produce recombinant DNA probes. Specific DNA probes have been used for detection of other viruses like herpesvirus, canine parvovirus, infectious laryngotracheitis virus and adenovirus from clinical samples.

Two non-radioactive probes using digoxigenin or biotin were developed for detecting canine herpesvirus (CHV) and compared for their sensitivities by *in situ* hybridization (ISH) in formalin-fixed, paraffin-embedded sections, which has been used routinely in veterinary fields. The best result was obtained by the optimized ISH protocol using digoxigenin-labelled probe for detection of CHV DNA. The optimized ISH assay, which developed in this study, may be a valid tool for the study of pathogenesis and diagnosis of CHV infection. A digoxigenin-labelled probe was produced from the Pasteur virus strain for the detection of the rabies virus N gene. The probe hybridization was performed from amplified N gene obtained by reverse transcription polymerase chain reaction, and the results from RT- PCR and hybridization showed 100% agreement. The hybridization, when carried out in products amplified by RT-PCR, increased the sensitivity of this technique even more and conferred specificity to the diagnosis. The technique described in this work would be useful in rabies diagnosis laboratories.

An improved method for the diagnosis of canine parvovirus using *in situ* hybridization in standard formalin-fixed, paraffin-embedded tissue sections was developed by Nho *et al.* (1997). A digoxigenin-labeled probe complementary to DNA sequences that coded for the entire sequence of the capsid protein VP-1 and the middle part of the sequence of the capsid protein VP-2 was designed. Specific histologic localization of canine parvovirus-infected cells was demonstrated in the small intestine, tonsil, lymph node, thymus, spleen, heart, liver, and kidney from dogs diagnosed at necropsy with canine parvovirus infection. The *in situ* hybridization accurately pinpointed the specific sites of viral infection. The detection of canine parvovirus in liver, kidney, and heart tissues together in the same pups could represent an enhanced virulence of this strain of canine parvovirus, and suggests a broadened tissue tropism not seen before in Korean strains of canine parvovirus.

Mondal and Cardona (2003) used slot blot hybridization of the hypervariable regions of the Sl subunit of spike peplomer gene to identify and characterize infectious bronchitis virus (IBV) strains. Template DNA was created from six reference IBV strains of different serotypes and immobilized on a nitrocellulose membrane. Digoxigenin-labelled probes were synthesized from reference and unknown field viruses and hybridized to template DNA. All reference strains could be distinguished and isolates identified by serotype if they were at least 95% identical to a reference strain. This slot blot hybridization procedure was specific and reproducible, and strain typing was consistent with the S1 sequencing of the IBV genome. This study thus provides a simple and rapid method for typing of IBV. Among parasitic infections, DNA probes had been developed for diagnosis of anaplasmosis, babesiosis, cowdriosis and trypanosomiasis. The DIG-labelled probe specific to *Babesia bigemina* generated from monomorphic RAPD fragment of approximately 873 bp size amplified by a 10 mer CGGTGGCGAA, detected up to 100 ng of template DNA. This non-radioactive probe also detected *B. Bigemina* in preparations of larval tick DNA from two of the five samples on dot blot hybridization.

A reverse line blot hybridization (RLB) one-stage nested PCR (nPCR) for *Anaplasma centrale* and a nested PCR for *Anaplasma marginale* were used to detect infected cattle grazing within an endemic region in Israel. A novel set of PCR primers and oligonucleotide probes based on a 16S ribosomal RNA gene was designed for RLB detection of both Anaplasma species, and the performance of the molecular assays compared. The RLB and the nested PCR procedures showed bacteraemia with sensitivity of 50 infected erythrocytes per millilitre.

Epidemiological studies

The development of specific probes for organisms, groups of organisms or specific serotypes provide a valuable tool for epidemiological studies. Such tests can be developed in a few reference laboratories and distributed to diagnostic laboratories to determine prevalence and incidence of specific organisms. Probes will be especially useful for determining the epidemiology of microorganisms, which are difficult to culture or type. Antero *et al.* (2005) have used DNA probe technology for epidemiological studies of tegumentary leishmaniasis in Mato Grosso State.

Study of Mechanisms of Pathogenesis

Nucleic acid probes are excellent tools for the determination of molecular mechanisms of pathogenesis. Mechanism of latency induction by herpesvirus has been studied by *in situ* hybridization. Only selected regions of the viral genome were transcribed in neurons of latently infected rabbits, whereas all regions of the genome were transcribed in lytically infected cells. These studies indicate that transcription of BHV-1 is restricted to the latent phase of infection and suggest that transcription of specific genes may be important in the establishment and maintenance of latency.

Microarrays for Diagnosis

Baxi *et al.* (2006) developed a microarray-based test that used a FMD DNA chip containing 155 oligonucleotide probes, 35-45 base pairs (bp) long, and serotype-specific, designed from the VP3, VPl-2A region of the genome. A set of two forward primers and one reverse primer was also designed to allow amplification of approximately 1100 bp of target sequences from this region. The amplified target was labelled with Alexa-Fluor 546 dye and applied to the FMD DNA chip. A total of 23 different FMDV strains representing all seven serotypes were detected and typed by the FMD DNA chip. Microarray technology offers a unique capability to identify multiple pathogens in a single chip.

Sachse *et al.* (2005) developed a microarray assay for detection and differentiation of all currently defined chlamydial species belonging to the genera Chlamydia and Chlamydophila using the Array Tube system, which they found to be particularly user-friendly and economical. The test included PCR amplification of a 23S rDNA target region with concurrent biotinylation and subsequent hybridization in the ArrayTube, a micro-reaction tube carrying the microarray chip on the bottom. In addition to high specificity, the assay was shown to allow detection and genetic characterization of single PCR-amplifiable target DNA copies.

A DNA microarray targeting O-serotype-specific genes was developed to detect 15 serotypes of *Shigella* and *E. coli*, including *Shigella sonnei*; *Shigella flexneri* type 2a; *Shigella boydii* types 7, 9, 13, 16, and 18; *Shigella dysenteriae* types 4,8, and 10; and *E. coli* O55, O111, O114, O128, arid 0157. The microarray was tested against 186 representative strains of all *Shigella* and *E. coli* O serotypes, 38 clinical isolates, and 9 strains of other bacterial species that are commonly present in stool samples and was shown to be specific and reproducible. The detection sensitivity was 50 ng genomic DNA or 10^4 cfu per m1 in mock stool specimens. This is the first report of a microarray for serotyping *Shigella* and pathogenic *E. coli*. The method has a number of advantages over traditional bacterial culture and antiserum agglutination methods, and is promising for applications in basic microbiological research, clinical diagnosis, food safety, and epidemiological surveillance.

Wang *et al.* (2007) described a rapid(<4 h) high-throughput detection and identification system that used polymerase chain reaction (PCR) primers to amplify a variable region of bacterial16S rRNA gene, followed by reverse hybridization of the products to species-specific oligonucleotide probes on a chip. This procedure was successful in discriminating 204 strains of bacteria from pure culture belonging to 13 genera of bacteria. When this method was applied directly to 115 strains of bacteria isolated from foods, 112/115 (97.4%) were correctly identified; two strains were indistinguishable due to weak signal, while one failed to produce a PCR product. The array was used to detect and successfully identify two strains of bacteria from food poisoning outbreak samples, giving results through hybridization that were identical to those obtained by traditional methods. The sensitivity of the microarray assay was 10^2 cfu of bacteria. Thus, the oligonucleotide microarray is a powerful tool for the detection and identification of pathogens from food.

Hybridization in Diagnosis

Nucleic acid probes and hybridization provide an alternate technique for the diagnosis of microbial infections and genetic disorders. Selected applications of this technique have been described to illustrate the potential and unique capabilities and the nature of complexcities of these techniques. Takahashi *et al.* (1999) developed a sensitive probe using a repetitive sequence of *Leptospira interrogans* serovar icterohaemorrhagiae strain Ictero No.1 for demonstration of *Leptospira interrogans* strains. Hybridization experiments showed positive reactions with the strains of *L. interrogans* and *L. kirschneri*, but not with any strains of *L. borgpetersenii*, *L. weilli* and *L. meyeri* or *L. biflexa*. O'Brien *et al.* (1996) developed a cloned probe from the region of the *Mycobacterium bovis* genome, pUCD, which generated a clear, highly polymorphic banding pattern when used as an RFLP probe on AluI restriction-digested *M. bovis* genomic DNA. When used to type 60 Irish *M. bovis* isolates, pUCD exhibited greater discriminatory power than the commonly used mycobacterial RFLP probes IS611O, PGRS (highly repetitive polymorphic GC rich repeat sequence) and DR (Direct repeat) and detected an equivalent number of strain types to a combination of these three probes.

Zhang and Kitching (2000) developed an *in situ* hybridization method/protocol using biotin-labeled oligodeoxynucleotides and tyramide signal amplification for sensitive detection of foot-and-mouth disease virus in infected cells. The tyramide signal amplification detection enhances by at least l00-fold compared to the sensitivity of *in situ* hybridization. The genome segments of infectious bursal disease viruses (IBDV) in the bursa of Fabricius from experimentally infected chicken or field samples were detected by tissue print hybridization (TPH) with subsequent reverse Transcriptase-PCR. Bursae were imprinted onto nylon membrane and then hybridized with a cloned digoxygenin-labeled cDNA probe. Tissue prints ón nylon membrane were readily distinguished from control prints by colour development and differences in signal intensity. *In situ* hybridization was used in a pathogenesis study of three vaccine pathotypes (Delaware variant A, D78 and Bursa Vac) of IBDV. With an antisense VP2 gene probe, viral nucleic acid was detected in bursa from both D78 and Bursa Vac-infected chicken at 24,48,72 and 120 hour post-infection (HPI). However, viral RNA was detected only in the Delaware variant A-infected birds at 72 HPI.

BHV-l is an important disease of bovines that can cause a variety of disease syndromes including infectious bovine rhinotracheitis, conjunctivitis, encephalitis, vulvovaginitis/ balanoposthitis and abortion. Latent infection often follows viral infection. Biotinylated nucleic acid hybridization probes have been developed to detect BHV-l nucleic acid in cells by *in situ* hybridization and in tissue homogenate and nasal exudates by blot hybridization. A series of HBV-l probes have been prepared by *Hind* III digestion of BHV-I DNA and fragments cloned into pBR 322. One probe, pCB-31, proved to be the most sensitive and specific for *in situ* hybridization. Another probe, a pCB 2 probe (9.6 kb *Hind* III fragment), proved to be the most sensitive for blot hybridization.

Enterotoxigenic *E. coli* (ETEC) is a major cause of diarrhoeal illness in humans and animals throughout the world. Diagnosis of ETEC diarrhoea has been complicated by the difficulty in differentiating enterotoxigenic strains from normal flora. ETEC produce both heat labile (LT) and heat stable (ST I and ST II) toxins. Recently, genes coding for these toxins have been cloned, labeled with ^{32}P and used to detect toxic genes coding for A (1.3 kb) and B (0.85 kb) subunits of porcine LT, porcine ST (PST, 157 bp) and human ST (HST, 510 bp) and were used to genotype 20 strains of *E. coli*. Probes were labelled with Bio-11-dUTP or ^{32}P, by nick translation or random priming. ^{32}P-labelled hybrids were detected by autoradiography; biotinylated probes were detected by streptavidin/biotin-conjugated polyalkaline phosphatase/ NBT-BCIP system. About 160 pg of target DNA was detected with biotin system; however, the ^{32}P-labelled probes were approximately eightfold more sensitive.

Pre-Natal Detection of Inherited Defect

Amniocentesis is a technique whereby a syringe is carefully inserted through the abdomen of a pregnant woman and a sample of the amniotic fluid is withdrawn, which surrounds the fetus. This amniotic fluid contains some cells (amniocytes) derived from the developing child and, if desired, these can be cultured *in vitro* to increase their number. These amniotic cells are an accurate reflection of the genetic composition of the fetus. Using cloned gene probes, it is possible to determine whether the fetus is carrying a particular inherited metabolic disorder e.g., sickle cell anaemia β-thalassemia, cystic fibrosis, and subsequently arrangements can be made for abortion, if so desired.

Prenatal diagnosis of many of these genetic disorders is not possible with the analysis of foetal DNA being isolated from cells in amniotic fluid. Linkage analysis of DNA polymorphism has been used to identify foetuses at risk of sickle cell anaemia and thalassemias. For example, a variant *Hpa*I restriction site is frequently associated with the sickle gene in the genome of Black Americans. Greater specificity can be introduced into the diagnosis of sickle cell anaemia by the use of specific restriction enzymes that recognize the DNA sequences involved in the sickle mutation, CCTGAGG to CCTGTGG. For example, the restriction enzyme *"Dde I"*, which recognizes CTNAG (where N is any nucleotide), has been used to detect sickle mutation. A culture of amniotic fluid is necessary to obtain sufficient DNA for analysis. An alternate enzyme *Mst* II has an additional two-base specificity (CCTBAGG), which results in larger cleavage products. Thus, its use increases the sensitivity of the assay and precludes the need for culture of amniotic cells.

Tumor Pathology

A major application of DNA probes has been the study of mutational events in somatic cells (such as colonic epithelium, osteocytes etc.), which give rise to clones of genetically abnormal neoplastic cells with increased capacity for growth. In the normal genome of man and other species there are at least two categories of genes, which have fundamental roles in carcinogenesis when their functions are altered. They are proto-oncogenes (contribute to tumor formation in active form) and anti-oncogenes (exert antitumor effects). Despite their potential value in tumor classification and prognosis, the cellular proto-oncogenes and anti-onocogenes have not yet found a place in routine tumor diagnosis. Viral oncogene is also responsible for tumor formation. By testing with cDNA probes prepared against V-oncs, a set of structurally similar (but not identical) genes have been discovered in normal human DNA and their chromosomal locations have been determined by *in situ* hybridization on karyotypic preparations.

Forensic Pathology

DNA fingerprints can be applied forensically. DNA can be isolated from stains such as blood or/ and semen even of several years old. Particularly in rape cases, sperm nuclei can be separated from the vaginal cellular debris present in semen contaminated vaginal swabs. Southern blots on human

DNA of such specimens with a probe for one set of such sequences show up to 50 polymorphic bands, which provide evidences about the culprit. These are also used to provide unequivocal evidence of parent-child relationship in case of disputed paternity.

Veterinary Microbiology

Nucleic acid probe technology is increasingly being used in veterinary microbiology and in diagnosis of infectious diseases of veterinary importance. The major applications of nucleic acid probes include detection of pathogens in clinical samples, especially those organisms which are fastidious and difficult to cultivate, differentiation of virulent from avirulent organisms and vaccine strains from wild type isolates, typing of microorganisms, mapping genes, screening libraries of cloned DNA for specific genes, detection of latently infected or carrier animals, study of mechanisms of pathogenesis, epidemiological studies and food safety.

Agricultural Applications

Food safety: There is increasingly more emphasis on the rapid detection and identification of microorganisms in food. In the past, this has been generally accomplished by the isolation and identification of bacteria using conventional methods that are time-consuming and require the presence of viable microorganisms. Nucleic acid probes provide a more rapid method for the identification of microorganisms in food. Nucleic acid probes have been developed and are commercially available for the detection of microorganisms of public health importance like toxigenic *E. coli*, *Listeria* spp., *Salmonella* spp. and *Yersinia enterocolitica*.

Other Biotechnological Applications

Differentiation of virulent from avirulent organisms

The differentiation of virulent from avirulent organisms and vaccine strains from wild type isolated is extremely important in diagnostic medicine and epidemiological studies. This can be accomplished immunologically by monoclonal antibodies and genetically by restriction endonuclease analysis, sequence analysis and via probes. *Treponema hyodysenteriae*, causative agent of swine dysentery, cannot be easily distinguished from a non-pathogenic treponema, *Treponema innocens*, which is commonly present in normal swine. A nucleic acid probe prepared from a plasmid associated with *T. hyodysenteriae* was successfully used to differentiate pathogenic from non-pathogenic treponemas.

Typing of microorganisms

Typing of microorganisms has usually been based on biological and antigenic characteristics. These classical procedures have been found to be unsatisfactory in many cases. Genetic tools like hybridization methods with specific probes have been used for typing microbes. Nucleic acid probes have been used to type pilus and enterotoxigenic gene types to differentiate *Campylobacter* spp. *E. coli*, *Leptospira* spp., *Mycobacterium* spp., and rotavirus group, subgroup and serotypes. Ramadass *et al.* (1992) used DNA homology studies with serovar-specific nucleic acid probes, and classified 40 *L. biflexa* serovars into six homology groups and 65 *L. interrogans* serovars into six homology groups.

Mapping genes

The isolation of a specific gene from an entire genome requires a technique that will discriminate one part in a million. DNA hybridization technique is used to localize specific genes to distinct chromosomes and thus to define a map of the human genome. This is already yielding useful information in the definition of human disease. For this purpose, a simple and more direct procedure is used which is known as *in situ* hybridization. A radioactive probe is added to a metaphase spread of chromosome on a glass slide. The exact area of hybridization is localized by layering photographic emulsion over the slide and, after exposure, lining up the grains with some histologic identification of the chromosome. This often places the gene at a location on a given band or region on the chromosome. More than 100 genes of human genome have been mapped. Some of the human genes localized using this technique are listed in Table 3.2.

Table 3.2 Localization of human genes.

Gene	*Chromosome**	*Disease associated with deficient or abnormal production of the gene products.*
Insulin	11 p 15	
Prolaction	6 p 23 q 12	
Growth hormone	17 q 21 – qter	Growth hormone deficiency
α – globin	16 p 12 – pter	α – Thalassemia
β-globin	11 p 12	β–Thalassemia, sickle cell
Adenosine deaminase	20 q 13 – qter	Adenosine deaminase deficiency
Phenylalanine hydroxylase	12 q 24	Phenylketonuria
Hypoxanthine guanine Phosphoribosyl transferase	X q 26 q 27	Lesch-Nyhan syndrome
Ribosyl transferase DNA segment G B	4 p	Huntington's Chorea

*The chromosome involved is indicated by the first (underlined) number or letter. The other numbers and letters refer to precise localization.

Gene expression analysis

Any given cell expresses only a limited number of its encoded genes. The number of genes expressed and the level of expression varies according to factors such as cell type, stage of development and response to external stimuli. Understanding gene expression and how it is regulated depends on analyzing many transcripts simultaneously. Hybridization with labelled RNAs to targets on chips allows quantitative and qualitative measurement of transcripts to be made with a sensitivity of one to five transcripts per cell. Transcripts from two different cell types can be labelled with different fluorescent dyes. The probes are mixed and hybridized simultaneously to chip bound targets. The two-colour fluorescence of hybrids allows differential gene expression to be monitored.

Detection of mutations and polymorphisms

Arrays can be prepared to include oligonucleotides that cover known mutations within a gene. An improved method is to include in the array oligonucleotide sequences that have the other three bases at the sites of known mutations. The alternative bases are the centre of the oligonucleotides where mismatching has the most disruptive effect on the stability of hybrids. On hybridization, the mutant gene should hybridize to one of these mutant sequences. Test arrays of 100,000 oligonucleotides of 20 mers have been used to screen for mutations in exon 11 of the human *BRCAI* gene. This exon codes for about 60% of the protein. Sequences covered the normal sequence as well as oligonucleotides covering insertions, deletions and substitutions. All known mutations were detected with no false positives. Diagnostic arrays are likely to be of increasing importance and arrays of HIV oligonucleotides are already available. In several conditions, such as the thalassemias and haemoglobinopathies, mutations in several different positions within the gene can give rise to disease. Overlapping oligonucleotide arrays are potentially well-suited to screening rapidly for the absence of mutations (Figure 3.10). Arrays of overlapping oligonucleotides of the gene to be screened are hybridized to DNA probes from normal and patient samples. By labelling the probes from each source with a different fluor, hybridization can be carried out with both probes at once.

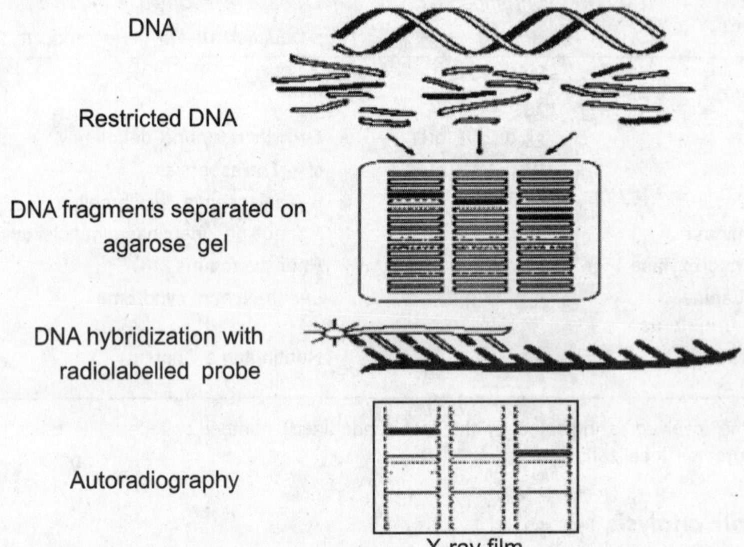

Figure 3.10 Radiolabelled DNA probe used to find a target gene mutation in a sample of DNA that matches part of the gene. The single-stranded probe seeks and binds to the gene. Radioactive signals from the probe are then visualized on x-ray film, showing the spots where the probe and gene matches.

DNA sequencing by hybridization

An array may contain all possible oligonucleotides of a chosen length. Hybridizing a probe to such an array provides information on all the constituent sequences of length in the probe. Sufficient information can be generated to allow assembly into a reconstructed sequence of the probe. This approach is known as sequencing by hybridization. When the probe is hybridized to the array, some oligonucleotides will hybridize and some will not. The sequence of those oligonucleotides that have hybridized can be aligned by overlapping their sequences to reconstruct the complete sequence. Each non-terminal n-mer will overlap the next by n-1 nucleotides. This method of sequencing is useful in terms of speed, cost, ease of automation and quality of data. However, there are two main problems with the technique. First, it is a major operation to align overlapping sequences correctly. Second, the technique runs into difficulties if the probe contains repeated sequences because the overlaps will not be unique. The reconstruction stops at a repeated sequence. Confirmation of the sequence of the entire human mitochondrial genome has been obtained using oligonucleotide arrays.

DNA fingerprinting for genotype analysis

Most of the genetic analyses are based on changes in DNA sequences that introduce or destroy restriction enzyme cleavage sites or cause restriction fragment length polymorphisms (RFLPs). These changes in the size of restriction fragments have been related to major genetic diseases. In a family, if one pattern is produced from the DNA of diseased individuals, but not from normal individuals, then this pattern or polymorphism serves as a marker for the disease gene. A 7.5-kb deletion within the human growth hormone gene results in dwarfism. Homozygous β-thalassemia (hydrops fetalis) is characterized by the absence of an *EcoRI* fragment, which is approximately 14 kb in size and is present in the normal individuals' globin gene.

Analysis of restriction fragment length polymorphisms (RFLPs) is widely used in genetic studies, linkage studies of inherited disorders and in forensic medicine. DNA fingerprinting is produced upon RFLPs associated with hypervariable minisatellite or variable number of tandem repeat (VNTR) regions present in the human genome. DNA fingerprints can be obtained from ml quantities of blood or semen and from specimens dried for up to 4 years. The probability that fingerprints of individuals will be identical is less than 10-20, and the DNA fingerprints are stably inherited. The presence of highly polymorphic patterns with DNA of equine, murine and canine origin was also reported. DNA fingerprinting is proving to be a significant tool with applications in paternity testing, forensic medicine and the more conventional genetic analysis. The potential for application of this technique for genotyping and pedigree analysis of animal species would seem to be enormous.

CONCLUSION

The use of DNA probes technology by microbiologists is growing at a significant rate to detect and identify pathogens, with the increasing use of hybridization technology by microbiology community for incorporating DNA probe tests into their laboratories. The usefulness of this technology needs to be assayed in the area of diagnostic microbiology that reduces the time required for the identification of fastidious pathogens. Probes can be used both for the direct identification of organisms in clinical specimens and for confirming the identity of organisms grown in culture. The availability of a variety of commercially produced DNA probe kits is indeed making the realization of each of these functions of DNA probes in clinical laboratories possible. One of the major concerns among clinical microbiologists with respect to the use of DNA probes is the sensitivity of the assays, particularly in complex clinical samples like stool and sputa. Additional concerns of microbiologists regarding probes include their cost-effectiveness, impact on workflow, the use of radio-isotopic detection systems, the biohazards associated with sonicating, and the short shelf life of kits.

It therefore appears that several frontiers remain to be mastered before molecular probe technology is used on a large-scale, routine basis: replacement of radioisotopes with more sensitive non-isotopic detection techniques; reduction of labor investment, with parallel decrease in turnaround time; increased demonstration of clinical significance for probe results; development of quality-assurance programs; and assessment of cost/benefit ratio for these tests. Automation can be expected to solve some of these problems (i.e., sample handling, analysis and signal detection, reliability, and reproducibility), but the remaining ones will need to be addressed by the clinical laboratory. Training and subsequent involvement of knowledgeable laboratory personnel will also be of paramount importance to the increased utilization of this exciting technology.

FURTHER READINGS

1. Abbott M.A., Poiesz B.J., Byrne B.C., Kwok 5, Sninsky J.J. and Ehrlich G.D. (1988) Enzymatic gene amplification: qualitative and quantitative methods for detecting proviral DNA amplified *in vitro*. *J. Infect Dis.* **(158)**: 1158-1169.
2. Aibretson C., Haukanes B-I., Aasland R. and Kleppe K. (1988) Optimal conditions for hybridization with oligonucleotides: a study with myc-oncogene DNA probes. *Anal Biochem.* **(170)**: 193-202.
3. Allison L. St. Amand, Daniel N. Frank, Mary Ann De Groote, and Norman R. Pace (2005) Use of specific rRNA oligonucleotide probes for microscopic detection of *Mycobacterium avium* complex organisms in Tissue. *Journal of Clinical Microbiology.* 43 **(4)**: 1505-1514.
4. Andrade, A.S.R., Fernandes, O., Heub, M., Carvalho, M.L.R., Fontes C.J. and Melo, M.N. (2005) The use of radionuclide DNA probe technology for epidemiological studies of tegumentary leishmaniasis in Mato Grosso State. *Brazilian Archives of Biology and Technology.* **(48)**: 201-204.
5. Andrade, A.S.R., Gomes, R.F., Fernandes, O. and Melo, M.N. (2001) Use of DNA-based diagnostic methods for human leishmaniasis in Minas Gerais. *Brazil. Acta Trop.* **(78)**: 261-267.
6. Antero Silva Ribeiro de Andrade, Octávio Fernandes, Marcia Heub, Maria de Lourdes Ribeiro Carvalho, Cor Jesus Fontes and Maria Norma de Melo (2005) The use of radionucleotide DNA probe technology for epidemiological studies of tegumentary leishmaniasis in Mato Grosso State. *Broz. Arch. Biol. Technol.* **(48)**: 201-204.
7. Baxi Mohit K., Baxi Shailja, Alfonso Clavijo, Kimberly M. Burton and Dirk Deregt (2006) Microarray-based detection and typing of foot-and-mouth disease virus. *The Veterinary Journal.* 172 **(3)**: 473-481.
8. Beaucage, S.L. (2001) Strategies in the preparation of DNA oligonucleotide arrays for diagnostic applications. *Curr. Med. Chem.* **(8)**: 1213-1244.
9. Campbell A. K. (1988) *Chemiluminescence: Principles and Applications in Biology and Medicine*. New York: VCH Publishers. pp. 469-472.
10. Cardullo H.A., Agarwal S., Flores C., Zamechik P.C. and Wolf D.E. (1988) Detection of nucleic acid hybridization by non-radioative fluorescence resonance transfer. *Proc. Natl. Aced. Sd. USA.* **(85)**: 8790-8794.
11. Carnieli Jr P., Brandão E.P., Castilho J.G., Bueno C.R., Carrieri M.L., Macedo C.I., Oliveira R.N., Zanetti C.R. and Kotait I. (2005) Phylogeny of a rabies virus identified in a cat closely related to vampire-bat rabies base don the nucleoprotein gene. *Virus Reviews and Research.* **(10)**: 38-44.

12. Chee, M. *et al.* (1996) Accessing genetic information with high-density DNA arrays. *Science* **(274):** 610-614.

13. Chu B.C.F. and Orgel L. (1985) Detection of specific DNA sequences with short biotin-labeled probes. *DNA.* **(4):** 327-331.

14. Collins M.L. and Hunsaker W.R. (1985) Improved hybridization assays employing tailed oligonucleotide probes: a direct comparison with 5'-end-labeled oligonucleotide probes and nick-translated oligonucleotide probes and nick-translated plasmid probes. *Anal Biochem.* **(151):** 211-224.

15. Dattagupta N., Rabin D., Michaud G. and Rae P.M.M. (1987) A simple method for generation of high specific activity oligonucleotide probes. *Biotechniques.* **(5):** 38-43.

16. Degrave, W., Fernandes, O., Campbell, D. Bozza, M. and Lopes, U (1994) Use of molecular probes and PCR for detection and typing of *Leishmania* – a minireview. *Mem. Inst. Oswaldo Cruz.* **(89):** 463-469.

17. Feinberg A.P. and Vogelstein B. (1985) A technique of radiolabeling DNA restriction endonuclease fragments to high specific activity. *Anal Biochem.* **(137):** 266-268.

18. Feldman G.L., Williamson R., Beaudet A.L. and O'Brien W.E. (1988) Prenatal diagnosis of cystic fibrosis by DNA amplification for detection of KM-19 polymorphism. *Lancet.* **(2):** 109.

19. Fodor S.P., Read J.L., Pirrung M.C., Stryer L., Lu A.T. and Solas D. (1991) Light-directed, spatially addressable parallel chemical synthesis. *Science.* 251 **(4995):** 767-773.

20. Gasparini P., Savoia A., Pignatti P.F., Dallapiccola B. and Novelli G. (1988) Amplification of DNA from epithelial cells in urine. *N. Engl. J. Med.* **(320):** 809.

21. Gebhart C.J., Fennell C.L., Murtaugh M.P. and Stamm W.E. (1989) *Campylobactor* cinaedi is normal intestinal flora in hamsters. *J. Clin. Microbiol.* **(27):** 1692-1694.

22. Ha S.K., Jung K., Choi C., Ha Y., Song H.C., Lim J.H., Kim S.H. and Chae (2005) Development of *In-situ* Hybridization for the Detection of *Mycoplasma haemosuis* (*Eperythrozoon suis*) in Formalin-fixed, Paraffin Wax-embedded Tissues from Experimentally Infected Splenectomized Pigs. *Journal of Comparative Pathology.* 133 **(4):** 294-297.

23. Hill, W.E., W.L. Payne, and C.C.G. Aulisio (1983) Detection and enumeration of virulent *Yersinia enterocolitica* in food by DNA colony hybridization. *Appl. Environ. Microbiol.* **(46):** 636-641.

24. Hughes M.R., Malloy P.J., Kieback D.O. *et al.* (1988) Point mutations in the human vitamin D receptor gene associated with hypocalcemic rickets. *Science.* **(242):** 1702-1705.

25. Jablonski E., Moomaw E.W., Tullis R.H. and Ruth J.L. (1986) Preparation of oligodeoxynucleotide-alkaline phosphatase conjugates and their use as hybridization probes. *Nucleic Acids Res.* **(14):** 6115-6128.

26. Jeffreys A.J. (1987) Highly variable *minisatellites* and DNA fingerprints. *Biochem. Soc. Trans.* **(15):** 309-315.

27. Jung K. and Chae C. (2004) *In-situ* Hybridization for the Detection of *Haemophilus parasuis* in naturally infected pigs. *Journal of Comparative Pathology.* 130 **(4):** 294-298.

28. Kotani H. and McGarrity G.J. (1986) Ureaplasma infection of cell cultures. *Infect Immun.* 52 **(2):** 437-444.

29. Krell P.J., Salas T. and Johnson R.P. (1988) Mapping of porcine parvovirus DNA and development of a diagnostic DNA probe. *Veterinary Microbiology.* 17 **(1):** 29-43.

30. Landry ML and Fong CKY (1986) Nucleic acid hybridization in the diagnosis of viral infections. *Clin. Lab. Med.* **(5):** 513-529.

31. Langer P.R., Waldrop A.A. and Ward D.C. (1981) Enzymatic synthesis of biotin-labeled polynucleotides: novel nucleic acid affinity probes. *Proc. Natl. Acad. Sci. USA.* **(78):** 6633-6637.

32. Lathe R. (1985) Synthetic oligonucleotide probes deduced from amino acid sequence data. Theoretical and practical considerations. *J. Mol. Biol.* **(183):** 1-12.

33. Li H., Gyliensten U.B., CuiX, Saiki R.K., Erlich H.A. and Arnheim N. (1988) Amplification and analysis of DNA sequences in single human sperm and diploid cells. *Nature* (London). **(335):** 414-417.

34. Li, F. and Stormo, G.D. (2001) Selection of optimal DNA oligos for gene expression arrays. *Bioinformatics.* **(17):** 1067-1076.

35. Linne T., Berg M., Bergvall A.C., Hjertner B. and Moreno-Lopez J. (1992) The molecular biology of the porcine paramyxovirus LPMV. *Vet. Microbiol.* **(33):** 263-273.
36. Lo Y.M.D., Mehal W.Z. and Fleming K.A. (1988) Rapid production of vector-free biotinylated probes using the polymerase chain reaction. *Nucleic Acids Res.* **(16):** 871-879.
37. Lowe J.B. (1986) Clinical applications of gene probes in human genetic disease, malignancy, and infectious disease [Review]. *Clin Chim Acts.* **(157):** 1-32.
38. Malouin, F., Bryan, L.E., Shewciw, P., Douglas, J., Li, D., Van den Elzen, H., and Lapointe, J.R. (1988) DNA probe technology for rapid detection of *Haemophilus influenzae* in clinical specimens. *J. Clin. Microbiol.* 26 **(10):** 2132-2138.
39. Mathews J.A., Bathi A., Hynds C. and Kricka L.I. (1985) Enhanced chemiluminescent method for the detection of DNA dot-hybridization assays. *Anal Biochem.* **(151):** 205-209.
40. Mei, R. *et al.* (2003) Probe selection for high-density oligonucleotide arrays. *Proc. Natl. Acad. Sci.* U. S. A. **(100):** 11237-11242.
41. Melton D.A., Krieg P.A., Rebagliati M.R. Maniatis T., Zinn K. and Green M.R. (1984) Efficient *in vitro* synthesis of biologically active RNA and RNA hybridization probes from plasinids containing a bacteriophage SP6 promoter. *Nucleic Acids Res.* **(12):** 7035-7056.
42. Moaley S.L., Huq M.I., Alim A.R.M.A., Samadpour-Motalebi M. and Falkow S. (1980) Detection of *E. coli* by DNA colony hybridization. *J. Infect Dis.* **(142):** 892-897.
43. Molad T., Mazuz M.L., Fleiderovitz L. *et al.* (2006) Molecular and serological detection of A. central and A. marginale infected cattle grazing within an endemic area. *Vet. Microbiol.* **(113):** 55-62.
44. Mondal Shankar P. and Cardona Carol J. (2003) Characterization of Infectious Bronchitis Virus Isolates by Slot Blot Hybridization. *Avian Diseases.* 47 **(3):** 725-730.
45. Muffin T.E., Bowden J., Lovell M.A. *et al.* (1987) Comparison of radioactive (^{32}P and ^{35}S) and biotinylated probes for detection of cytomegalovirus DNA. *Chin Biochem.* **(20):** 231-235.
46. Nakamura Y., Leppart M., O'Connel P. *et al.* (1987) Variable number of tandem repeat (VNTR) markers for human gene mapping. *Science.* **(235):** 1616-1622.
47. Nho W.G., Sur J.H., Doster A.R. and Kim S.B. (1997) Detection of canine parvovirus in naturally infected dogs with enteritis and myocarditis by *in situ* hybridization. *Journal of Veterinary Diagnostic Investigation.* 9 **(3):** 255-260.
48. O'Brien, K.L., Dietz, H.C., Romagnoli, M and Eiden, J. (1996) Evaluation of inhA gene and catalase-peroxidase gene among isoniazid-sensitive and resistant *Mycobacterium tuberculosis* isolates. *Mol. Cell Probes.* **(10):** 1-6.
49. Orkin S. H., Markham A.F. and Kazazian H. H., Jr. (1983) Direct detection of the common Mediterranean beta-thalassemia gene with synthetic DNA probes. An alternative approach for prenatal diagnosis. *J. Clin. Invest.* 71 **(3):** 775-779.
50. Ou, C.Y., Kwok, S., Mitchell, S.W., Mack, D.H., Sninsky, J.J., Krebs, J.W., Feorino, P., Warfield, D. and Sehoehetman, G. (2005) DNA amplification for direct detection of HIV-1 in DNA of peripheral blood mononuclear cells. *Science.* **(239):** 295-297.
51. Pease W., Vandenberg J. and Hooper K. (1991) Comparing alternative approaches to establishing regulatory levels for reproductive toxicants: DBCP as a case study. *Environmental Health Perspectives.* **(91):** 141-155.
52. Peterson, A.W. *et al.* (2002) Hybridization of mismatched or partially matched DNA at surfaces. *J. Am. Chem. Soc.* **(124):** 14601-14607.
53. Ramadass, P., Jarvis, B.D.W., Corner R.J., Penny D. and Marshall, R.B. (1992) Genetic characterization of pathogenic *Leptospira species* by DNA hybridization. *Int. J. Syst. Bacteriol.* **(42):** 215-219.
54. Ravindran, R., Mishra, A.K. and Rao, J.R. (2007) Development of a *Babesia bigemina* Specific Probe from Monomorphic Fragment of RAPD-PCR. *Journal of Applied Animal Research.* 31 **(2):** 54-57.

55. Rigby P.W.J., Dieckmann M., Rhodes C. and Berg P. (1977) Labeling deoxyribonucleic acid to high specific activity *in vitro* by nick translation. *J. Mol. Biol.* **(113):** 237-251.
56. Riley L.K., Marshall M.E. and Coleman M.S. (1986) A method for biotinylating oligonucleotide probes for use in molecular hybridizations. *DNA.* **(5):** 333-337.
57. Rossi M.S., Sadir A.M., Schudel A.A. and Palma E.L. (1988) Detection of foot-and-mouth disease virus with DNA probes in bovine esophageal-pharyngeal fluids. *Arch Virol.* **(99):** 67-74.
58. Rouillard, J.M. *et al.* (2002) Oligo-Array: Genome-scale oligonucleotide design for microarrays. *Bioinformatics.* **(18):** 486-487.
59. Sachse Konrad, Hotzel Helmut, Slickers Peter, Ellinger Thomas and Ehrich Ralf (2005) DNA microarray-based detection and identification of *Chlamydia* and *Chlamydophila* spp. *Molecular and Cellular Probes.* 19 **(1):** 41-50.
60. Saez A., Andreu F.J., Segui M.A., Bare M.L., Fernandez S., Dinares C. and Rey M. (2006) HER-2 give amplification by chromogenic *in situ* hybridization (CISH) compared with fluorescence *in situ* hybridization (FISH) in breast cancer-A study of two hundred cases. *Breast.* 15 **(4):** 519-527.
61. Saiki R.K., Chang C.A., Levenson C.H., *et al.* (1988) Diagnosis of sickle cell *anemia* and beta-thalassemia with enzymatically amplified DNA and non-radioactive allele-specific probes. *N. Engl. J. Med.* **(319):** 537-541.
62. Saiki R.K., Scharf S., Faloona F., *et al.* (1985) Enzymatic amplification of a-globin genomic sequences and restriction site analysis for diagnosis of sickle cell anemia. *Science.* **(230):** 1350-1354.
63. Schena, M. *et al.* (1998) Microarrays: Biotechnology's discovery platform for functional genomics. *Trends Biotechnol.* **(16):** 301-306.
64. Sellers H.S., Villegas P.N., *et al.* (2001) Detection of infectious Bursal disease virus in experimentally infected chickens by *in situ* hybridization. *Avian Diseases.* **(45):** 26-33.
65. Seriwatana, J., Eeheverria, P., Taylor, D.N., Sakuldaipeora, T., Changchawalit, S. and Chivoratanond, O. (1987) Identification of enterotoxigenic *Escherichia coli* with synthetic alkaline phosphatase-conjugated oligonucleotide probes. *Journal of Clinical Microbiology.* **(25):** 1438-1441.
66. Sheldon E.L., Kellogg D.E., Watson H., Levenson C.H. and Erlich H.A. (1986) Use of nonisotopic M13 probes for genetic analysis: applications to HLA class II loci. *Proc. Natl. Aced. Sci. USA.* **(83):** 9085-9089.
67. Southern, E.M. (1975) Detection of specific sequences among DNA fragments separated by gel electrophoresis. *J. Mol. Biol.* **(98):** 503-517.
68. Takahashi, Y., Kishida, M., Yamamoto, S. and Fukunaga, M. (1999) Repetitive sequence of *Leptospira* interrogans serovar icterohaemorrhagiae strain Ictero No.1: A sensitive probe for demonstration of Leptospira interrogans strains. *Microbiol. Immunol.* **(43):** 669-678.
69. Tenover F.C. (1988) Diagnostic deoxyribonucleic acid probes for infectious diseases [Review]. *Clin. Microbiol Rev.* **(1):** 82-101.
70. Tenover, F.C. (1988) Diagnostic deoxyribonucleic acid probes for infectious diseases. *Clinical Microbiology Reviews.* **(1):** 82-101.
71. Theodore E. MIfflIn (1989) Use and applications of nucleic acid probes in the clinical laboratory. *Clin. Chem.* 35 **(9):** 1819-1825.
72. Urdea M.S., Running J.A., Horn T., Clyne J., Ku L. and Warner B.O. (1988) A novel method for the rapid detection of specific nucleotide sequences in crude biological samples without blotting or radioactivity, applications to the analysis of hepatitis B virus in human serum. *Gene.* **(6):** 253-264.
73. Walker J. and Dougan G. (2008) DNA probes: A new role in diagnostic microbiology. *Journal of Applied Microbiology.* 67 **(3):** 229-238.
74. Wallace S.J., Mandelzweig V.B., Schneider D.M. and Van Orden J.W. (1981) Multiple scattering theory and local field effects. *Phys. Rev.* **(24):** 799-801.

75. Wang Qiong, Garrity George M., Tiedje James M. and James R. Cole (2007) Naïve Bayesian classifier for rapid assignment of rRNA sequences into the new bacterial taxonomy. *Applied and Environmental Microbiology.* 73 **(16)**: 5261-5267.
76. Wetmur, J.G (1991) DNA probes: Applications of the principles of nucleic acid hybridization. Crit. Rev. *Biochem. Mol. Biol.* **(26)**: 227-259.
77. Wolfe H.J. (1988) DNA probes in diagnostic pathology. *Am J Clin. Pathol.* **(90)**: 340-344.
78. Xu C., He, P. and Fang, Y. (2000) Electrochemical labeled DNA probe for the detection of sequence-specific DNA. *Analytica Chimica Acta.* 411 **(1-2)**: 31-36.
79. Zhang Zhidong and Kitching Paul (2000) A sensitive method for the detection of foot and mouth disease virus by *in situ* hybridisation using biotin-labelled oligodeoxynucleotides and tyramide signal amplification. *Journal of Virological Methods.* 88 **(2)**: 187-192.

CHAPTER 4

PCR Technology

Polymerase chain reaction (PCR) has been developed for exponentially amplifying DNA, via enzymatic replication, without using a living organism. PCR is commonly used in medical and biological research labs for a variety of tasks, such as detection of hereditary diseases, identification of genetic fingerprints, diagnosis of infectious diseases, cloning and expression of genes, mutagenesis, paternity testing, and DNA computing and many more. In this chapter we present the basic concepts and practical applications of PCR technology in agricultural, medical, veterinary and biotechnological applications that will have a marked influence on the development of new diagnostic strategies in the future.

Keywords: Polymerase chain reaction; *in vitro* DNA amplification, RT-PCR, Q-PCR, Touch down PCR.

INTRODUCTION

The polymerase chain reaction (PCR) is an *in vitro* technique, which allows the amplification of a specific deoxyribonucleic acid (DNA) region that lies between two regions of known DNA sequences. This technique was invented by Kary Mullis in 1983 while working for Cetus Corporation in California. In 1993, the Nobel Prize for Chemistry was awarded to Dr. Mullis for having invented PCR. The PCR amplification of DNA is achieved by using oligonucleotide primers, also known as amplimers. These are short, single-stranded DNA molecules that are complementary to a defined sequence of DNA template. The primers are used for extensions of a denatured single-stranded DNA (template) by a DNA polymerase in the presence of deoxynucleoside triphosphates (dNTPs) under suitable reaction conditions. This results in the synthesis of new DNA strands complementary to the template strands. These strands exist at this stage as double-stranded DNA molecules. Strand synthesis can be repeated by heat denaturation of the dsDNA, annealing of primers by cooling the mixture and primer extension by DNA polymerase at a temperature suitable for the enzyme reaction. Each repetition of strand synthesis comprises a cycle of amplification. Each new DNA strand synthesized becomes template for any further cycle of amplification and so the amplified target DNA sequence is selectively amplified, cycle after cycle. The first extension products result from DNA synthesis on the original template, and these do not have a distinct length as the DNA polymerase will continue to synthesis new DNA until it either stops or is interrupted by the start of the next cycle. The second cycle extension products are also of intermediate length. In the 3rd cycle, fragments of "target" sequence are synthesized that are of defined length corresponding to the position of the primers on the original template. From the 4th cycle onwards, the target sequence is amplified exponentially. After each cycle, the number of templates doubles.

This number can be calculated by applying the formula: $M_f = M_i \times 2^n$, where M_i is the initial number of molecule, M_f is the final number of DNA molecule produced by the PCR and n is the number of cycles performed. Potentially after 20 cycles of PCR, there will be 220-fold amplification, assuming 100% efficiency during each cycle. However, in practice, only 20-30% efficiency is achieved in PCR methods.

Nucleic acid amplification techniques are most useful for the detection and characterization of viruses for which cell culture and serological methods are difficult, expensive or unavailable. Especially, the very high level of sensitivity provided by DNA amplification makes PCR the method of choice to detect viral DNA directly in clinical samples. The most obvious advantage of PCR for virus diagnosis is the selective amplification of extremely small number of viral DNA or RNA molecules in clinical samples to amounts sufficient for detection by simple methods. The high sensitivity of PCR makes this technique especially appropriate for diagnosis of various viral infections. This is particularly true for latent virus infections including herpesvirus, retrovirus or papilloma virus infections. The polymerase chain reaction is such a powerful technique, that for majority of laboratory experiments, it has now largely replaced the gene cloning undertaken with the help of vectors. The basic principles and the methodology involved in PCR (including its various modified forms) and its various applications are discussed in this chapter.

CONCEPTS

The techniques of recombinant DNA and gene cloning, permit us to obtain an unlimited supply of identical copies of a gene sequence or DNA segment, which is cloned in a prokaryotic or a eukaryotic cell with the help of a vector. This technique, discovered around 1975, proved extremely useful in all experiments of molecular biology and genetic engineering and thus became an essential tool in all molecular biology laboratories. In 1985, yet another remarkable tool in molecular biology was discovered, which is known as polymerase chain reaction (PCR), later nick named as 'people's choice reaction'. The methodology is so important that the prestigious journal *Science* published from USA considered PCR the major scientific development of the year 1989, and had chosen Taq DNA polymerase, the enzyme used in PCR, as the molecule of the year 1989. Kary Mullis, who discovered this reaction in 1985, described in his article published in April 1990 issue of *Scientific American*, how he got the basic idea of this reaction while driving through the red wood mountains of California, USA. In view of the significance that PCR and its varied applications achieved within a few years after its discovery, the 1993 Nobel Prize in Chemistry was shared by Karry Mullis for his discovery of PCR, with Michael Smith, for his discovery of site directed mutagenesis.

PRINCIPLES

Any process used to obtain large quantities of DNA is based on the basic structure of the DNA molecule. DNA normally exists as double strands bind around one another. The base pairing is the key to DNA's role as molecule for storing and copying hereditary information. Each strand contains all the information needed to build its opposite strand. Moreover, for every sequence of DNA there can be complementary sequences, which will bind to it. This same complementarity is what makes DNA work as a unique genetic information carrier. It also forms the basis of DNA replication and polymerase chain reaction.

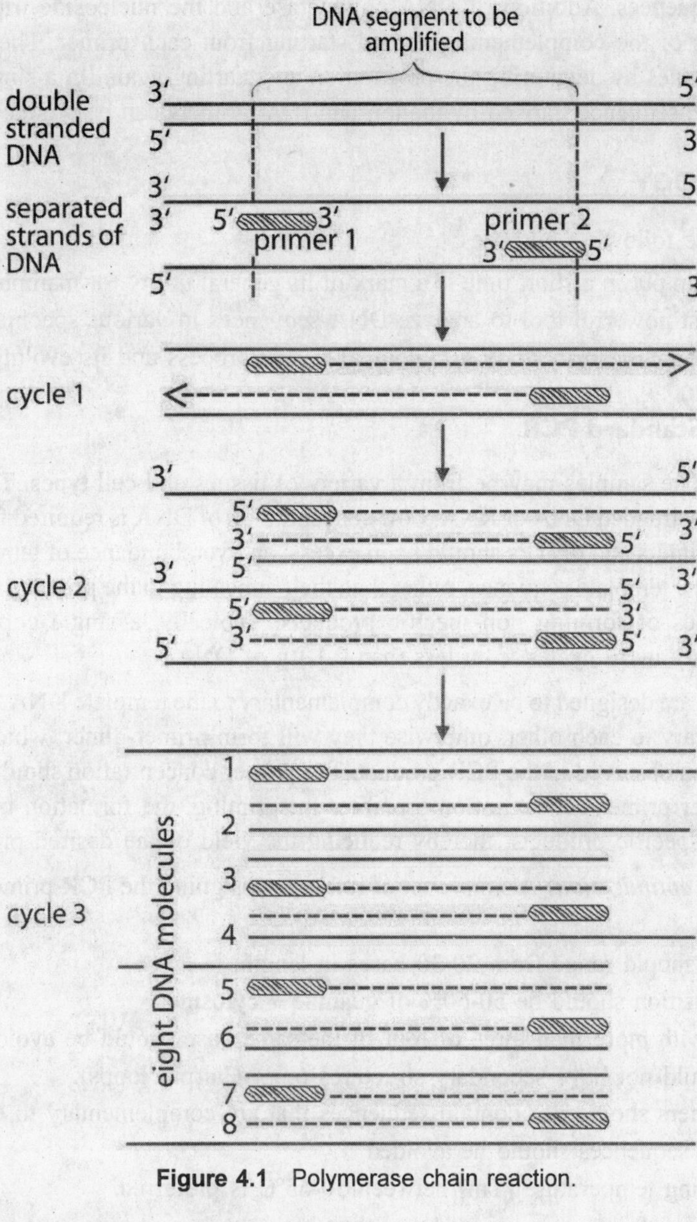

Figure 4.1 Polymerase chain reaction.

In normal cells dsDNA is replicated by DNA polymerase to produce two daughter strands. Besides the template, this enzyme requires a primer to carry out the polymerization of nucleotides and produce complementary strands. In PCR, as in the normal cells, essentially identical reactions take place but in a tube. When dsDNA are denatured by heating at 95°C, the two strands separate by breaking the bonds between bases, which normally hold them together. Two primers, one recognizing each strand and bordering the sequence to be amplified, are mixed and the whole mix is cooled to 40 to 60°C. This process is called renaturation and allows the primers to bind complementary sequences. Addition of DNA polymerase and the nucleoside triphosphates will allow the synthesis of the complementary strand starting from each primer. The entire cycle is repeated 20 to 30 times by denaturing the preparation and starting again. In a single afternoon, a billion copies of the sequence flanked by the left and right primers can be produced (Figure 4.1).

PCR TECHNOLOGY

Purpose: It has the following purposes:

1. PCR has been put in a short time is a mark of its general utility for manipulation of DNA.
2. It is the most powerful tool to analyze DNA sequences in various specimens.
3. It is a novel approach to study a biological system/process and its evolutionary aspects.

Components of Standard PCR

Template DNA: The samples may be from a variety of tissues and cell types. The sample may be single- or double-stranded DNA or RNA. Low concentration of DNA is required for optimal PCR because both the primers and dNTPs should be in excess; an overabundance of template DNA will form annealing of the template sequence, rather than their annealing to the primer pair and will also increase the chances of forming non-specific products. Typically, a single copy gene can be amplified sufficiently in 30 cycles from less than 0.1 μg of DNA.

Primers: Primers are designed to be exactly complementary to the template DNA. Primers should not be complementary to each other, otherwise they will form primer-dimer, which is the amplification artifact often observed in the PCR product. The primer concentration should not be greater than 10 μM. Higher primer concentration promotes mispriming, the formation of primer or the generation of non-specific products, thereby reducing the yield of the desired product.

Primer design and optimization: A simple set of rules for designing the PCR primers includes the following:

1. Primer size should range from 20-30 bases in length.
2. Base composition should be 50-60% of guanine + cytosine.
3. Long runs with more than three or four of the same base should be avoided.
4. Primers should not have secondary structures (e.g., Hairpin loops).
5. Ideally, primers should not contain sequences that are complementary to each other.
6. Palindromic sequences should be avoided.
7. Primer melting temperature (Tm) between 50-65°C is preferred.

The melting temperature (Tm) for a particular primer can be calculated using the following formula:

$$Tm = [(\text{no. of } A + T) \times 2°C + (\text{no. of } G + C) \times 4°C].$$

Deoxynucleotide triphosphates (dNTPs): PCR is normally performed with dNTP concentration around 50 μM to 200 μM. However, the PCR optimally performed with dNTPs depends on (a) the $MgCl_2$ concentration, (b) the reaction stringency, (c) the primer concentration, (d) the length of the amplified product and (e) the number of cycles of PCR. Higher concentration encourages misincorporation by the DNA polymerase. Final concentration of 50 μM and 200 μM of each dNTP in PCR reaction is sufficient to synthesize 6.5 μg and 25 μg of DNA, respectively.

PCR Buffers and $MgCl_2$: There are several buffers available for PCR and the most commonly used buffer has the following components in a 10 times concentration and must be diluted 1:10 (v/v) prior to use. The 10 × buffer contains 500 mM KCl, 100 mM Tris.HCl (PH 8.3), 15 mM $MgCl_2$ and 0.1% (w/v) gelatin. The appropriate concentration of magnesium ions in the reaction buffer is also important for maximal Taq polymerase activity, and since the dNTPs bind magnesium ions, the reaction mixture must contain excess magnesium ions. As a rule of thumb, the magnesium concentration in the reaction mixture is generally 0.5 to 2.5 mM greater than the concentration of dNTPs. The concentration of magnesium ions also influences the efficiency of primer to template annealing. As a result, it is possible to modify the magnesium concentration rather than the annealing temperature to regulate primer specificity. Generally, insufficient Mg^{2+} leads to low yields and excess Mg^{2+} results in the accumulation of non-specific products. The $MgCl_2$ concentration in the final reaction mixture can be varied usually within the range of 1.0 to 1.5 mM. Salts like KCl and NaCl may help to facilitate primer annealing, but concentration of 50 mM will inhibit Taq polymerase activity. Detergents such as Tween 20, Triton X-100 or Nonidet P-40 and/or extra protein (e.g., gelatin or bovine serum albumin) may also be added to the reaction buffer. The addition of these reagents helps to prevent precipitation of the hydrophobic Taq polymerase in aqueous solutions.

PCR enzymes: The most commonly used DNA polymerase is Taq DNA polymerase, which is isolated from a bacterium *Thermus aquaticus* found in hot springs. This works optimally at 72°C and over the pH range of 7.5 to 8.0, adding 100 nucleotides/sec to the primer under these conditions. One drawback of Taq polymerase is its lack of 3′ to 5′ exonuclease (proof reading) activity, which can lead to the misincorporation of nucleotides (~1 in 9000 bases). Table 4.1 lists some of the polymerases commonly in use in PCR.

Table 4.1 Thermostable DNA polymerases and their sources.

DNA polymerase	*Natural/recombinant*	*Source*
Taq	Natural	*Thermus aquaticus*
AmplitaqR	Recombinant	*T. aquaticus*
Hot TubTM	Natural	*Thermus flavus*
VentTM	Recombinant	*Thermococcus litoralis*
Tth	Recombinant	*Thermus thermophilus*
Pfu	Natural	*Pyrococcus furiosus*
UlTmaTM	Recombinant	*Thermotoga maritima*

DNA polymerases are enzymes that catalyse the synthesis of long polynucleotide chains from monomer deoxynucleoside triphosphate using one of the original parental strands as template for the synthesis of a new complementary strand. DNA synthesis always proceeds in a 5′ to 3′ direction, since polymerization is always from the 5′ phosphate to 3′ terminal hydroxyl group of the growing DNA strand.

Inhibitors and enhancers of PCR: Many different types of biological specimens are used for PCR, including animal tissues and body fluids, bacterial samples, forensic and archaeological materials and plant tissues. Human DNA is typically obtained from peripheral blood cells, urine, faecal samples, cells, smears, hair roots, semen, cerebrospinal fluid, biopsy material, amniotic fluid, placenta and chorionic villus. In addition to these sources, DNA from animals and birds can be extracted from tail sections and feather roots, respectively. Many of these crude preparations contain inhibitory substances, which have not been identified. Heparin, a commonly used anticoagulant, should not be used for collection of blood if PCR is to be performed on the extracted DNA, since heparin is a potent PCR inhibitor. Other substances in the blood, probably porphyrin compounds that are also strong inhibitors of PCR, can be eliminated from the DNA preparation by lysis of the red blood cells and centrifugation to pellet the white cells. Extraction of DNA from different sources routinely use detergents for cell lysis and denaturation. Often non-ionic detergents (e.g., Triton X-100, Tween-20, Nonidet P40) are used and these generally do not inhibit PCR at concentrations of up to 5%. On the other hand, ionic detergents such as sodium dodecyl sulphate (SDS) can only be tolerated at extremely low concentration and therefore should be removed by phenol extraction and used at the level of 1-2% (v/v) and SDS inhibits Taq DNA polymerase at concentration higher than 0.01% (w/v). The inhibitory effects of low concentration of SDS (e.g., 0.01%) can be removed by certain non-toxic detergents (e.g., 0.5% Tween-20 and Nonidet P40). In addition, Taq DNA polymerase is susceptible to protease digestion and so proteinase K must be removed or inactivated. Many researches have reported substances that can be added to PCR to increase the efficiency or specificity. Formamide at a concentration of 5%, dimethyl sulphoxide (DMSO) at a concentration of 10%, polyethylene glycol 6000 at a concentration of 50-15%, glycerol at a concentration of 10-15% and tween-20 at 0.25% are found to enhance PCR amplification.

Steps involved in PCR: The components of PCR are mixed in reaction tubes and placed in a thermal cycler-PCR machine. The thermal block is controlled by a microprocessor in order to increase and decrease the temperature rapidly in accordance with a preselected programme. PCR commences with an extended initial denaturation step (usually 5 minutes at 94°C), which ensures that there is complete strand separation of the template DNA. The reaction mixture is then cycled usually between 30-35 times. A typical temperature programme would be: denaturation at 94°C for 20–30 seconds; primer annealing at ~50–60°C (depends on primer sequence) for 30–60 seconds; extension at 72°C for 30–60 seconds (one min/kb). Cycling concludes with a final extension step at 72°C, usually for 5 minutes, assuming that all templates DNA are in double-stranded conformation.

Comparison Between PCR and Conventional Cloning

Before the discovery of the PCR in 1983, the standard method used for getting enough DNA was gene cloning by which bacteria are transformed into tiny cloning factories. Isolating analyzable amounts of a single gene by using the bacterial cloning technique is an enormously intricate task. The entire process can take days, weeks or even months. Thus, there is no hesitation to say that the PCR will ultimately replace gene cloning to a large extent because it can do this in a few hours (Table 4.2).

Table 4.2 Comparison between PCR and conventional cloning.

S. No.	*Parameter*	*PCR*	*Gene cloning*
1.	Concentration of starting material	Nanogram	Microgram
2.	Biological reagents required	DNA polymerase	Restriction enzymes, ligase, vector, bacterial cell
3.	Selectivity of the specific segment from complex DNA	First step	Last step
4.	Manipulation	*In vitro*	*In vitro* & *in vivo*
5.	Cost	Less	More
6.	Labour intensive	No	Yes
7.	User skill	Not required	Required
8.	Time for a typical experiment	4 hours	24 hours
9.	Final result	Selective amplification of specific sequences	Selective amplification of specific sequences with vector sequences
10.	Error probability	Less	More
11.	Automation	Yes	No
12.	Applications	More	Less

Different Schemes/Variants of PCR

In the previous section, we discussed the basic outline of PCR technique, outlining how billions of copies of a DNA sequence can be obtained within a few hours, without the use of a vector and a host as done in gene cloning. However, there are several variations to this basic PCR technique, which allow varied applications.

Inverse PCR: In this technique, the amplification of those DNA sequences takes place, which are away from the primers, and not those, which are flanked by the primers. For instance, if the border sequences of a DNA segment are not known and those of a vector are known, then the sequence to be amplified may be cloned in the vector and border sequences of vector may be used as primers in such a way that the polymerization proceeds in inverse direction i.e., away from the vector sequence flanked by the primers and towards the DNA sequence of inserted segment. Similarly, if the gene sequence is known, one can use its border sequences as primers for an inverse PCR (Figure 4.2) reaction, to amplify the sequences flanking this gene such as, the regulatory sequences.

Anchored PCR: In the basic PCR technique and the inverse PCR, one has to use two primers representing the sequences lying at the ends of sequences to be amplified. But sometimes, we may have knowledge about sequence at only one of the two ends of the DNA sequence to be amplified. In such cases, anchored PCR (Figure 4.3) may be used, which will utilize only one primer instead of two. In this technique, due to the use of one primer, only one strand will be copied first, after which a poly-G tail will be attached at the end of the newly synthesized strand. This newly synthesized strand with poly G tail at its 3' end will then become template for the daughter strand synthesise utilizing an anchor primer with which a poly-C sequence is linked to complement with poly-G of the template. In the next cycle, both the original primer and anchored primer will be used for gene amplification.

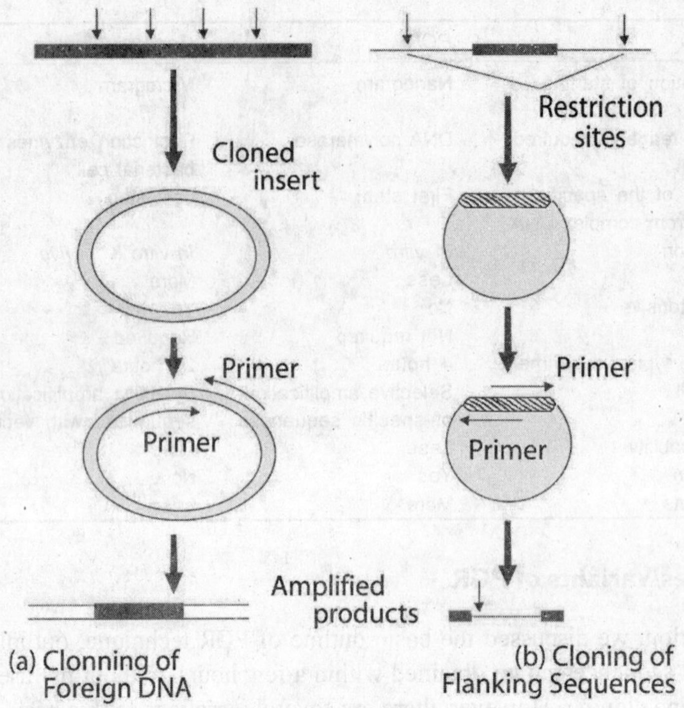

Figure 4.2 Inverse PCR.

Nested PCR: The sensitivity and specificity of PCR can be increased by using nested PCR (nPCR). In nPCR, two separate amplifications are used. The first uses a set of primers that yields a longer product, which is then used as a template for the second amplification. The second set of primers anneal to sequence within the initial product producing a second smaller product. The primers for the second round of amplification are either both different from the first set or both located within the amplified DNA region. If only one of the second round primers is located within the amplified region and is used together with one of the first round primers, it is termed seminested PCR. Nested PCR increases the specificity of the reaction because the formation of the final product depends upon the binding of two separate sets of primers, which may preclude the need for verification of the PCR product by blotting, restriction digestion or sequencing. The second set of primers also serves to verify the specificity of the first product. Nested PCR primers are one that are internal to the first primer pair. The longer fragment produced by the first round of PCR is used as the template for the second PCR. Nested PCR can also be performed with one of the first primer pair and a single nested primer. Using the nested PCR method can dramatically increase the sensitivity and specificity of both DNA and RNA amplification. The specificity is particularly enhanced because this technique almost always eliminates any spurious non-specific amplification products. This is because after the first round of PCR, the non-specific products are unlikely to be sufficiently complementary to the nested primers to be able to serve as template for further

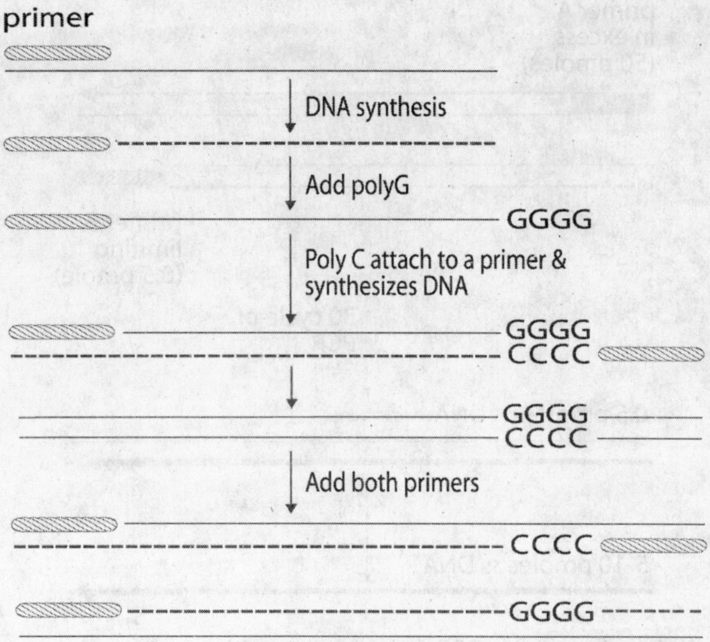

Figure 4.3 Anchored PCR.

amplification. Thus, the desired target sequence is preferentially amplified. However, the increased risk of contamination is a drawback of this extreme sensitivity.

Asymmetric PCR: In this method, the addition of one primer in vast excess over the other during the PCR results in the generation of an excess of one amplified strand relative to the other, i.e., an asymmetric amplification (Figure 4.4). The single-stranded product is usually used for dideoxy sequencing. Asymmetric PCR can be performed directly on any given template, although reproducible high yields of single-stranded products are often difficult to obtain. Alternatively, it is more common to isolate a double-stranded PCR product by conventional symmetrical methods and re-amplify this by asymmetric PCR, using only one primer for approximately 20 cycles. The single-stranded product increases arithmetically with each cycle. Dideoxy DNA sequencing of asymmetric PCR products can be performed either with the original PCR primer or by using a complementary sequence internal to the asymmetric PCR product. Asymmetric PCR sequencing is particularly useful for a particular region where the asymmetric PCR conditions can be standardized.

Multiplex PCR: In multiplex PCR (mPCR), two or more primer pairs specific for different targets are included in the same amplification reaction. The major advantages of mPCR are conservation of reagents and template and reduction in preparation and analysis time required to identify multiple target sites in one assay, as opposed to running separate analysis for each target. However, the system requires careful optimization of the PCR conditions to ensure that one PCR reaction is not dominant over the other. Futhermore, the products obtained in each reaction should

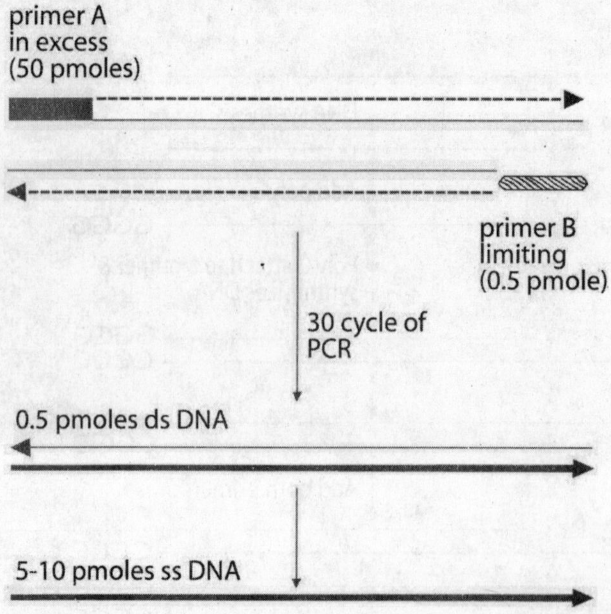

Figure 4.4 Asymmetric PCR for generating ssDNA for DNA sequencing.

also be of different sizes to enable their visualization on agarose gel. The co-amplification of two or more products in a single reaction is dependent on the compatibility of the PCR primers used in the reaction. All the primers in the reaction must have similar melting temperature, so they anneal to and dissociate from complementary DNA sequences at approximately the same temperature, allowing each amplification to proceed at the selected temperature. Each amplification proceeds independently of the other and each specific amplification product is synthesized in an unencumbered way.

Arbitrarily primed PCR: This method is also called random amplified polymorphic DNA fingerprinting and is based on the amplification of genomic DNA with a single primer selected from an arbitrary nucleotide sequence. We use a short oligonucleotide primer to produce random but reproducible sets of amplified DNA fragments. The multiple products resulting from RAPD analysis are then separated according to size by conventional agarose gel electrophoresis and the DNA binding patterns of different isolates can then be compared. This technique has proven to be very useful for subtyping diverse bacterial species.

RT (Reverse Transcribed)-PCR: In a number of situations, when mRNA transcript needs to be examined, reverse transcription is first used to obtain cDNA, which is then used as a template for PCR reaction. Often the synthesis of cDNA is initiated by primers that are either complementary to poly (A) tail or to specific sequences known to be present on one or more specific subsets of RNA species. Adapters of known sequences may also be ligated to mRNA to facilitate designing of primers. cDNA synthesized thus by RT-PCR (Figure 4.5), is then used as a template for PCR using Taq polymerase and specific primers. One of the important uses of RT-PCR is the identifica-

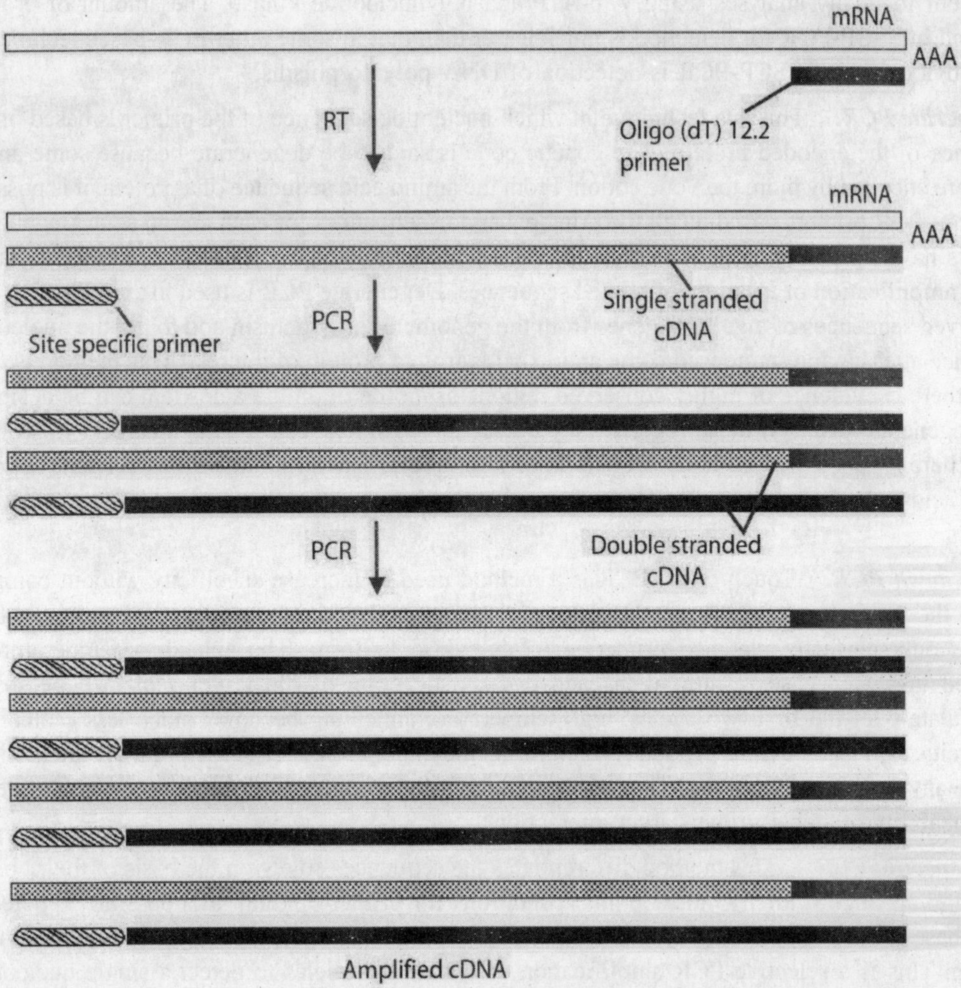

Figure 4.5 Different steps involved in RT-PCR.

tion of differences in two mRNA samples using the technique of differential display, leading to isolation of specific genes.

Quantitative PCR: Quantitative PCR involves co-amplification of two templates: a constant amount of a preparation containing the desired target sequence and serial dilutions of a reference template that is added in known amounts to a series of amplification reactions. The concentration of the target sequence is determined by simple interpolation into a standard curve.

Single-strand conformation polymorphism PCR (SSCP-PCR): In SSCP-PCR, the target sequence is first labelled and amplified simultaneously by the PCR of the genomic DNA and cDNA using labelled substrates. The PCR product is then denatured and resolved by PAGE and mutations are detected as altered mobility of separated single strands in the autoradiogram. Thus, the overall procedure is rapid and simple. Primers or deoxynucleotides are also labelled efficiently in a batch sufficient for many analyses using γ^{32}p-ATP and polynucleotide kinase. The amount of product required in SSCP-PCR for detection is much lesser than that in some other PCR-based techniques. One obvious use of SSCP-PCR is detection of DNA polymorphisms.

Degenerate PCR: This is a technique in which nucleotide sequence of the primer is based on the sequence of the encoded protein. The genetic code is said to be degenerate because some amino acids are encoded by more than one codon. From the amino acid sequence of a protein, it is possible to design PCR primers based on all the principal codon sequences for each amino acid. Degenerate primers have a number of options at several positions in the sequences so as to allow annealing to and amplification of a variety of related sequences. Degenerate PCR is used to amplify (fish out) conserved sequences of a gene or genes from the genome of an organism and to get the nucleotide sequence after having sequenced some amino acids from a protein of interest. This method is used when there is evidence of highly conserved regions or motifs of amino acids that can be designed into degenerate primers; these regions may be conserved interspecies. This method is also used when there is successful isolation of gene family members. The terminals of this protein (or some amino acids) are then sequenced. The amino acid sequence can then be used to design degenerate primers.

Touch down PCR: Touch down PCR is a method used to increase specificity without compromising the yield. The principle is to initiate synthesis at a very high annealing temperature, which permits only perfectly matched primer template-hybrid to form. The annealing temperature is dropped in a step-wise fashion with each cycle. One copy of the target sequence begins to accumulate over the first two cycles, high temperature annealing becomes much less critical for specificity, as it is a previous product, which forms the major template. These products are unlikely to have any sites for mispriming. The benefit of decreasing the annealing temperature is to increase the probability of stable primer-target interaction.

Allele-specific PCR: This method differentiates the sequences solely on the basis of their ability to bind to an oligo primer. Under optimal conditions for primer binding, it is possible to detect a single base mismatch because only the precise primer-targets complementarity will support amplification. This is a selective PCR amplification of one of the alleles to detect a single nucleotide polymorphism (SNP). Selective amplification is usually achieved by designing a primer such that the primers will match/mismatch one of the alleles at the 3′ end of the primer.

Major Advantages of PCR Technology

Because of its simplicity, PCR is a popular technique with a wide range of applications, which depend on three major advantages of the method.

Speed and ease of use: DNA cloning by PCR can be performed in a few hours using relatively unsophisticated equipment. This compares favorably with the time required for cell-based DNA cloning, which may take weeks. Clearly, some time it is also required for designing and synthesizing oligonucleotide primers, but this has been simplified by the availability of computer software for primer design and rapid commercial synthesis of custom oligonucleotides. Once the conditions for a reaction have been tested, the reaction can be repeated simply.

Sensitivity: PCR is capable of amplifying sequences from minute amounts of target DNA, even the DNA from a single cell. Such exquisite sensitivity has afforded new methods of studying molecular pathogenesis and has found numerous applications in forensic science, diagnosis, genetic linkage analysis using single-sperm typing and in molecular palaentology studies, where samples may contain minute numbers of cells.

Robustness: PCR can permit amplification of specific sequences from material in which the DNA is badly degraded or embedded in a medium from which conventional DNA isolation is problematic. As a result, it is again very suitable for molecular anthropological and palaentological studies, for example, the analysis of DNA recovered from archaeological remains. It has also been used successfully to amplify DNA from formalin-fixed tissue samples, which has important applications in molecular pathology and, in some cases, genetic linkage studies.

Problem in PCR Technology

Theoretically, the number of copies of target sequence grows exponentially i.e. doubles with each cycle. In practice, it doubles with each cycle until reaching a plateau at which more primer-template accumulates than the enzyme can extend during the cycle, and then the increase in target DNA becomes linear.

APPLICATIONS OF PCR TECHNOLOGY

Polymerase chain reaction technique has proven a powerful tool because it is very simple to perform with the help of automatic machines, extremely specific, extremely efficient, and even extremely cost efficient. It is now used in a very wide number of practical applications in the areas of molecular biology, medicine and biotechnology. Some of the important applications of PCR technology are discussed below.

Medical Applications

PCR as diagnostics tools

PCR technology is very much useful in clinical diagnosis. The most profound technological impact of PCR is being felt in the field of diagnostic assays for the detection of infectious or genetic diseases. Considering the popularity of PCR in diagnostic applications, it is no surprise that PCR kits are already available, and commercial diagnostic systems employing PCR technology are expected to reach the market in less than two years.

Detection of AIDS: PCR provides much more direct evidence of infection by spotting and amplifying minute quantities of the AIDS (HIV) virus genes. Existing tests detect the virus by measuring antibodies produced to fight it. But antibodies may not be produced for months or years after infection. Thus, this PCR based test is most sensitive for the AIDS virus. With this, it is also possible to test babies born to mothers infected with AIDS virus. Babies, even perfectly healthy ones, usually carry their mother's antibodies for the first year or so of their life. Thus, it will give positive result using antibody test. This renders standard test useless. However, PCR can distinguish healthy babies from infected ones.

Pre-natal detection of genetic diseases: The medical industry has already used PCR in pre-natal screening of various inherited diseases (called monogenic disorders) such as hemophilia- A, beta thalassemia, sickle cell anemia, phenylketonuria, cystic fibrosis (Duchene muscular dystrophy), Tay Sach's disease, congenital isolated thyrotrophic (TSH) deficiency and several other disorders. These diseases can be detected within hours of taking the biological samples. Indeed the PCR was first used to detect sickle cell anemia. These can be diagnosed by obtaining samples of fetal cells and analyzing the genetic material with radioactive DNA probes that specifically pick up the gene mutations causing these diseases. But before this, cells have to be grown in culture for a week or so to obtain sufficient DNA to carry out the test. But with PCR, a single cell is sufficient for amplification making the culture step unnecessary. PCR plays an important role in the early diagnosis of inherited diseases screened at the level of embryo with the possibility of safer and less traumatic abortions. It is a speedy procedure for detecting defective genes in conventionally conceived embryos or embryos obtained by *in vitro* fertilization. Couples going for *in vitro* fertilization could choose to have those embryos for implantation that do not carry the defective gene in question. Prenatal diagnosis of sickle cell anemia with enhanced sensitivity was perhaps the first application of PCR for diagnosis of a human disease. Using PCR, this is done in less than one day in contrast to several days/weeks needed, when southern blots are used for hybridization with a probe. The test has also been used for diagnosis of phenylketonuria (PKU), β-thalassemia, hemophilia, etc. The PCR product in all these cases is examined using a labelled probe, to suggest whether or not mutant sequence causing the disease is found. Sometimes, RFLP pattern of PCR products in healthy and defective feti (singular = fetus) differ, thus enabling prenatal diagnosis. In still other cases, PCR product may be sequenced to reveal the difference (for sequencing with PCR, consult).

Sex determination: This approach can be used for selective breeding of one sex over the other or to avoid a girl if the parents are at a risk for alpha-linked disorders in their offspring. However, this technique should not be used to abort a perfectly healthy female fetus in this male dominated society. One could determine the sex of the *in vitro* fertilized egg using PCR. The presence of the Y- chromosome can be detected at the 6-10 cells cleavage embryo without affecting the life of embryo. Since DNA sequences in single cells can be studied using PCR, sex of human or livestock embryos fertilized *in vitro* can be determined before implantation. For this purpose, PCR primers and probes specific for sex chromosomes (e.g., ZFY or ZFX sequences) can be used. Y-specific primers and probes in humans are available for this purpose. This technique can also be used to detect sex-linked disorders in the fertilized embryos.

PCR in histopathology

PCR analysis has been performed on DNA extracted from formalin fixed paraffin embedded tissues, and promises to play an important role in bridging the gap between histopathology and molecular genetics. It has already been used successfully to detect papilloma virus in histological specimens.

PCR in forensic science

PCR technology is used in forensic DNA fingerprinting for identification of criminals and disputed parentage. Some well-characterized sequences of microsatellites are being used for designing primers, so that DNA fingerprinting may be achieved through PCR. PCR has found a niche in forensic medicines too. DNA samples found at the scene of crime such as small pieces of tissue, semen, blood, and even a single hair or one sperm lingering after a rape are often of poor quantity and quality therefore cannot be analyzed by other forensic techniques. PCR can do needful by amplifying these DNA samples, which can then be compared with the samples from the suspects to pin point the identity of the criminals and to convict or exonerate them in rape and murder cases.

Veterinary Applications

In detecting pathogens: PCR is used to detect a wide range of organisms, whether they are present in foodstuff, environment or biological or histological materials. The detection of pathogens is therefore an essential application of PCR with relevance to the food industry, environmental monitoring, medical, veterinary and botanical sciences. Meyer *et al.* (1991) used PCR for detection of foot-and-mouth disease virus in infected bovine and porcine tissues. Silva (1992) used PCR for differentiation of pathogenic and non-pathogenic serotypes of Marek's disease viruses (MDV). PCR method has been used for the detection of sites of latency of infections laryngotracheitis (ILT) virus in chicken. It was used to detect a DNA sequence from the ILT thymidine kinase gene. PCR was compared with virus isolation (VI) and hemagglutination assay (HA) for the detection of canine parvovirus (CPV) in faecal specimen. Pratelli *et al.* (2000) reported that the nPCR was more sensitive than regular PCR for the detection of canine coronavirus from faecal samples of pups. An improved PCR assay was used for the detection of canine parvovirus from faecal samples. Similarly, it was used for detection of *Mycoplasma pneumoniae* in throat swab samples. A 88-bp amplified product was obtained, which was specific for *M. pneumoniae*. PCR method has been used for the detection of carrier cattle by detection of *Theileria annaulata* from blood samples. PCR was also used for detection of leptospires from clinical samples like urine, hserum, mastitis milk and cerebrospinal fluids from dogs and cattle. Berg *et al.* (2006) compared microscopy, culture and PCR for the diagnosis of anthrax in blood samples from sheep and cattle. Recently, PCR assay was evaluated for the detection of *Brucella canis* in canine semen, and the results were compared with that of bacterial isolation, serological tests and PCR assay of blood.

A strain-specific RT-PCR and RFLP analysis was used for differentiating dog-related (DRRV) and rabies viruses (RV) in Brazil. Amude *et al.* (2006) evaluated RT-PCR for antemortem CDV detection in hospitalized dogs with neurological disturbances without typical findings of distemper. Antognoli *et al.*(2001) used one tube nPCR for detection of *Mycobacterium bovis* in milk samples. Handberg *et al.* (1999) developed RT-PCR technique using common and strain-specific primers for infectious bronchitis virus in allantoic fluid and tracheal tissue preparations. Ramadass *et al.* (2003) used RT-PCR method for detection of infectious bursal disease virus from bursal sample collected from suspected flocks for amplification of 474-bp product from variable region of the VP2 gene. *In situ* RT-PCR method was used for early detection of IBDV in chicken experimentally infected. Similarly, a duplex reverse transcription-polymerase chain reaction (dRT-PCR) assay was developed for the simultaneous, rapid and specific detection/discrimination of avian influenza virus (AIV) and Newcastle disease virus (NDV).

A multiplex PCR (mPCR) assay was found to be specific, sensitive and cost effective for simultaneous detection of four avian mycoplasma. Wang and Khan (1999) developed an mPCR for simultaneous detection of Massachusetts and Arkansas serotypes of infectious bronchitis virus. Similarly, Sato *et al.* (2005) investigated the usefulness of multiplex reverse transcription-polymerase chain reaction (RT-PCR) for determining the origin of 54 rabies virus (RV) isolates from various host species in Brazil. A nested mPCR assay was developed for genotyping of bovine viral diarrhea viruses, BVDV1 and BVDV2 using cattle blood samples. In addition, mPCR assay has been used for detection of *Campylobacter coli* and *C. jejuni, Clostridium perfringens* toxins, enterohaemorrhagic *E. coli* 0157:H7 toxic genes, *Brucell abortus* and *Mycobacterium bovis* in cattle, *Staphylococcus aureus* enterotoxins and canine parvovirus infection and leptospirosis in dogs. Recently, mPCR assay was developed for the rapid detection of *Brucella ovis, Actinobacillus seminis* and *Histophilus somni* in fresh ram semen samples.

A nested and real-time PCR was used for detection of *B. anthracis* spores in soil. Real-time PCR and culture methods were compared for detection of *Mycobacterium avium* subsp. paratuberculosis in dairy cattle and bovine semen. *Mycoplama gallisepticum* was rapidly detected from chicken tracheal swabs by real-time PCR by Light Cycler system. A real-time fluorogenic RT-PCR assay was developed for the specific detection of all seven serotypes of foot and mouth disease virus in epithelial suspensions and cell culture virus preparations. A rapid, sensitive and reproducible real-time PCR assay for detecting and quantifying canine parvovirus type 2 (CPV-2) DNA in the faeces of dogs with diarrhoea was described. A real-time RT-PCR assay was developed for detection and quantitation of canine distemper virus.

Agricultural Applications

The agricultural biotechnology industry applies polymerase chain reaction (PCR) technology at numerous points in product development. Commodity and food companies as well as third-party diagnostic testing companies also rely on PCR technology for a number of purposes. The primary use of the technology is to verify the presence or absence of genetically modified (GM) material in a product or to quantify the amount of GM material present in a product. PCR techniques have the potential to revolutionize plant pathology diagnostics. They offer in theory, an increase in specificity and sensitivity of some orders of magnitude over existing methods such as ELISA. The novel agricultural applications of the PCR are discussed below.

Applications in food authenticity and legislation

PCR is now an accepted analytical tool in the food industry. Its principal role has been one of assisting the legislative authorities, major manufacturers and retailers to confirm the authenticity of foods. The most obvious role is the detection and quantification of GMOs, but real-time PCR makes a significant contribution in many other areas of the food industry, including food safety and other specialty analyses such as the detection of common wheat adulteration in pasta and the detection of allergenic species. The role of quantitative real-time PCR in determining the actual amount of these materials, which are subject to considerable regulation, is discussed together with a consideration of the uncertainty of the methods.

Genetically modified material testing: Entering the second decade of commercialization of biotech crops, the global area cultivated with transgenic plants constantly expands and national legislations in many countries, particularly in the European Union, require identification and labeling of genetically modified material in food and feed. Here we discuss the characterization of transgenic material of unknown origin present in conventional seed lots using a genome walking strategy for isolation and characterization of the junction between the inserted transgene construct and the host plant genomic DNA. The procedure was applied to transgenic cotton detected as adventitious or technically unavoidable presence in a conventional commercial cultivar. The structure of the isolated region revealed that the transgenic material derived from Monsanto's event 1445 transgenic cotton. Due to the random incorporation of the transgene into the host plant's genome, the sequence of the junction region obtained using the genome walking strategy, provided the means to develop an event-specific identification method without prior knowledge for the nature of the transformation event.

Diagnosis of recalcitrant disease: The mounting prevalence of invasive and recalcitrant disease is exacerbated by PCR-based amplification approaches that have been developed to address this problem because conventional methods for pathogen identification lack sensitivity, specificity and speed, and some infectious organisms are difficult to culture. PCR amplification of ribosomal genes and their internal transcribed spacer regions coupled with sequence-specific detection probes are the most reliable approaches for disease identification.

Gene tagging

PCR has also been utilized for developing molecular markers closely linked to specific genes of economic importance. For instance, in tomato, 144 random primers were used to produce 625 PCR products from a set of near isogenic lines (NILs which differ only for the presence and absence of a specific gene) for *Pseudomonas* resistance. At least three of these PCR products were present in one and not in the other of a pair of NILs showing linkage with *Pseudomonas* resistance gene (Pto). These PCR products could be mapped close to Pto. Such tagging of genes through PCR will be used in future for marker-aided selection (MAS) in plant breeding (selection of desirable plants in segregating populations) and also for isolation of genes.

Other Biotechnological Applications

Study of DNA polymorphism using PCR

DNA polymorphism can be studied at a loci with known DNA sequence (using primers based on known sequences) or at random sites (using primers having unknown to random DNA sequences, called random primers). A restriction fragment length polymorphism (RFLP) is a variation in the DNA sequence of a genome that can be detected by breaking the DNA into pieces with restriction enzymes and analyzing the size of the resulting fragments by gel electrophoresis. It is the sequence that makes DNA different from different sources and RFLP analysis is a technique that can identify some differences in sequence (that occur in a restriction site). Analysis of RFLP variation was an important tool in genome mapping, localization of genetic disease genes, determination of risk for a disease, genetic fingerprinting, and paternity testing.

Randomly amplified polymorphic DNA (RAPD) markers are decamers (10 nucleotide length) DNA fragments from PCR amplification of random segments of genomic DNA with single primer of arbitrary nucleotide sequence and which are able to differentiate between genetically distinct individuals. If a mutation has occurred in the template DNA at the site that was previously complementary to the primer, a PCR product will not be produced, resulting in a different pattern of amplified DNA segments on the gel. In recent years, RAPD has been used to characterize and trace the phylogeny of diverse plant and animal species. Based on a 10 mer primer, an RAPD method for typing *Campylobacter coli* isolated from pits was developed. Tcherneva *et al.* (2000) used RAPD method to differentiate different species of Brucella. Faggi *et al.* (2001) used PCR fingerprinting for the identification of species and varieties of common dermatophytes using a single primer (GACA). Butler *et al.* (2001) used AP-PCR method to investigate *Mycoplasma bovis* outbreaks and they characterized different isolates using this method.

A short tandem repeat (STR) in DNA occurs when a pattern of two or more nucleotides repeated and the repeated sequences are directly adjacent to each other. By identifying repeats of specific sequences, it is possible to create a genetic profile of an individual. A Variable Number Tandem Repeats (VNTR) is a location in a genome where a short nucleotide sequence is organized as a tandem repeat. VNTRs were an important source of RFLP genetic markers used in linkage analysis (mapping) of genomes. Now that many genomes have been sequenced, VNTRs have become essential in forensic crime investigations, via DNA fingerprinting and the CODIS database. VNTR analysis is also being used to study genetic diversity and breeding patterns in populations of wild or domesticated animals. There are two principal families of VNTRs: microsatellites and minisatellites. The former are repeats of sequences less than about 5 base pairs in length (an arbitrary cutoff), while the latter involve longer blocks. Confusing this distinction is the recent use of the terms Short Tandem Repeat (STR) and Simple Sequence Repeat (SSR), which are more descriptive, but whose definitions are similar to that of microsatellites.

Amplified fragment length polymorphism (AFLP) is a PCR-based tool used in genetic research, DNA fingerprinting, and in the practice of genetic engineering. AFLP uses restriction enzymes to cut genomic DNA, followed by ligation of adaptors to the sticky ends of the restriction fragments. A subset of the restriction fragments are then amplified using primers complementary to the adaptor and part of the restriction site fragments. The amplified fragments are visualized on denaturing polyacrylamide gels either through autoradiography or fluorescence methodologies. AFLP-PCR is a highly sensitive method for detecting polymorphisms in DNA. A variation of AFLP is cDNA-AFLP, which is used to quantify differences in gene expression levels. Another variation of AFLP is TE Display used to detect transposable element mobility. There are many advantages of AFLP when compared to other marker technologies including RFLP, RAPD and microsatellites. AFLP not only has higher reproducibility, resolution, and sensitivity at the whole genome level compared to other techniques, but it also has the capability to amplify between 50 and 100 fragments at one time and detect various polymorphisms in different genomic region simultaneously. In addition, no prior sequence information is needed for amplification. As a result, AFLP has become extremely beneficial in the study of taxa including bacteria, fungi, and plants, where much is still unknown about the genomic makeup of various organisms.

Cloning, expression and sequencing of the PCR product

The amplified PCR product can be cloned if restriction sites for specific enzymes are introduced at the 5' end of each primer. These restriction sites do not interfere with amplification and can be used for cloning with a variety of vectors in the usual manner. Similarly, incorporation of a T7 promoter at the 5' end of one primer will allow the use of RNA polymerase enzyme to get RNA copies of PCR product. PCR amplified products can also be cloned without using modified primers in PCR reactions. For this purpose the amplified product is purified using QIA quick PCR purification kit (QIAGEN, USA) and ligated to Promega's pGEM-T or pGEM-T Easy vector (Holton and Graham, 1991). The chimeric vector is transformed in *E. coli* cells and the insert (PCR product) is sequenced using universal M13 primers.

PCR for site directed mutagenesis

PCR technique is used for introducing mutations at the desired place in a DNA sequence by altering the sequences of primers (Figure 4.6). Since mutations are introduced only through primers, mutations are limited to the ends of the gene sequence. A variation of this technique allows mutations to be introduced at any place of interest in the gene.

In two separate PCR reactions, a particular gene is amplified into two separate segments. In each of the two reactions, there is one primer at the end of the gene and the other (with desired alteration for mutation) internal to the sequence. The internal modified primers in two reactions are complementary to one another, so that the amplified products will have their ends internal to the original sequence. These internal ends of products in two reactions will overlap, so that if the two PCR products are mixed and used again for PCR, their internal ends function as primers. Extension of these primers by Taq polymerase results in the formation of a complete gene with mutations incorporated at internal sites.

Isolation of differentially expressed genes by DDRT-PCR

This method was developed by Liang and Pardee (1992) in which PCR was used to amplify and display many cDNAs derived from the mRNAs of a given cell or tissue type. The method relies on two different types of synthetic oligonucleotides: anchored antisense primers and arbitrary sense primers. A typical anchored primer is complementary to approx. 13 nucleotides of the poly(A) tail of mRNA and the adjacent two nucleotides of the transcribed sequence. Anchored primers therefore anneal to the junction between the poly(A) tail and the 3′-untranslated region of mRNA templates, from where they can prime the synthesis of first-strand cDNA (A second primer, an arbitrary sequence of approx 10 nucleotides, is then added to the reaction mixture, and double-stranded cDNAs are produced by conventional PCR, carried out at low stringency). The products of the amplification reaction are separated by electrophoresis through a denaturing polyacrylamide

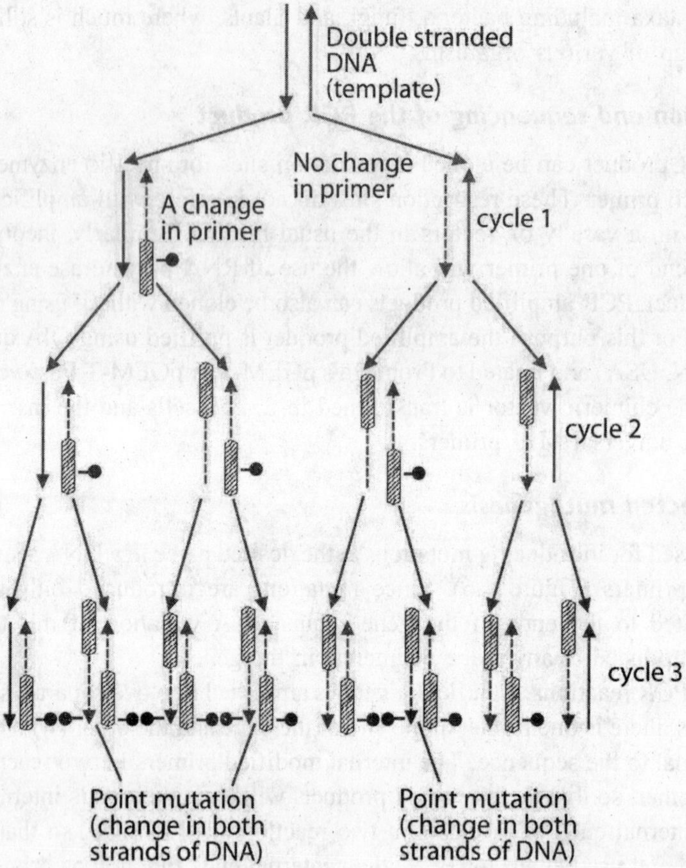

Figure 4.6 Site directed mutagenesis using PCR.

gel and visualized by autoradiography. By comparing the banding patterns of cDNA products derived from two different cell types, or from the same cell type grown under different conditions, it is sometimes possible to identify the products of differentially expressed genes (Figure 4.7). The bands of interest can then be recovered from the gel, amplified further, cloned and/or used as probes to screen northern blots, cDNA libraries, etc.

Rapid amplification of cDNA ends (RACE)

This method is used to extend partial cDNA clones by amplifying 5′ and 3′ end sequences of the corresponding mRNAs. The technique requires knowledge of a small region of sequence within the partial cDNA clone. During PCR, the thermostable DNA polymerase is directed to the appropriate target RNA by a single primer derived from the region of known sequence; the second primer required for PCR is complementary to a general feature of the target in the case of 5′RACE, to a

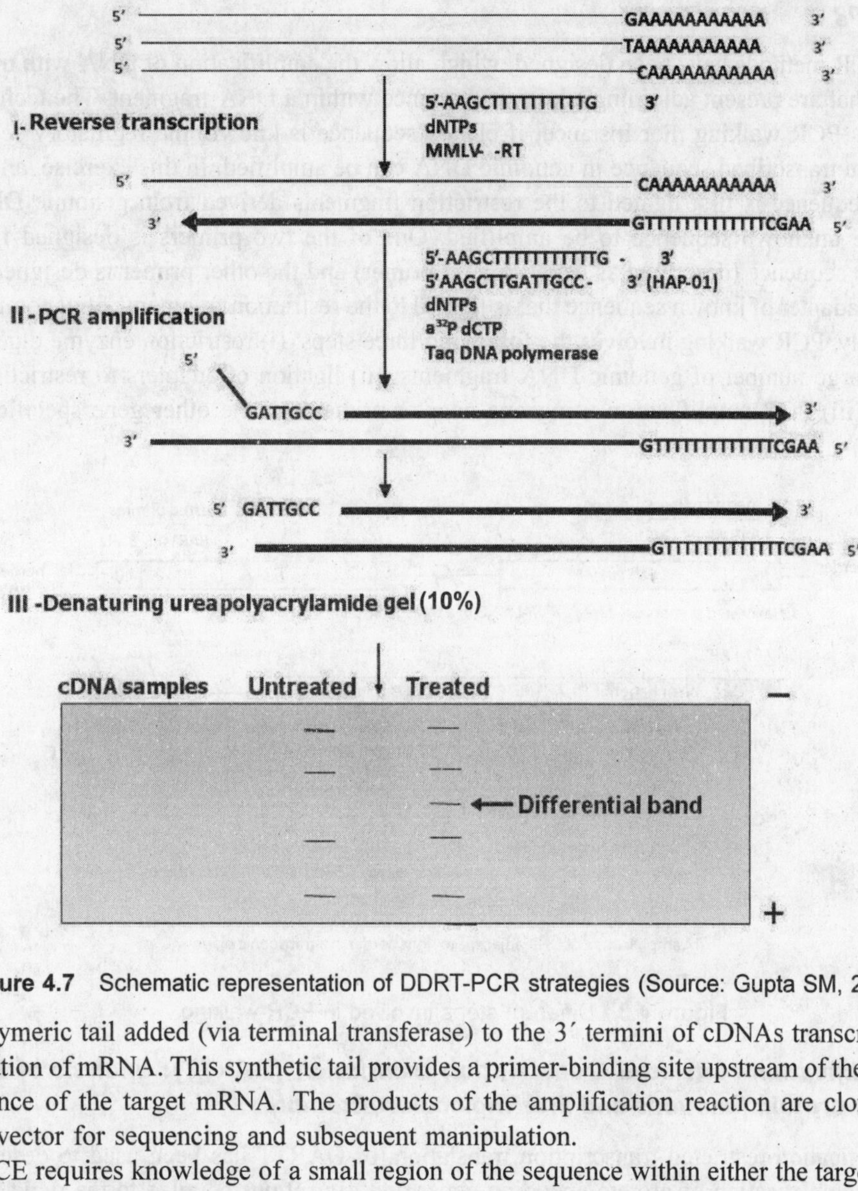

Figure 4.7 Schematic representation of DDRT-PCR strategies (Source: Gupta SM, 2007).

homopolymeric tail added (via terminal transferase) to the 3′ termini of cDNAs transcribed from a preparation of mRNA. This synthetic tail provides a primer-binding site upstream of the unknown 5′ sequence of the target mRNA. The products of the amplification reaction are cloned into a plasmid vector for sequencing and subsequent manipulation.

3′RACE requires knowledge of a small region of the sequence within either the target RNA or a partial clone of cDNA. A population of mRNAs is transcribed into cDNA with an adaptor-primer consisting at its 3′ end of a poly (T) tract and at its 5′ end of an arbitrary sequence of 30-40 nucleotides. Reverse transcription is usually followed by two successive PCRs. The first is primed by a gene-specific sense oligonucleotide and an antisense primer complementary to the arbitrary sequence in the (dT) adaptor-primer. If necessary, the products of the first PCR can be used as templates for a second nested PCR, which is primed by a gene-specific sense oligonucleotide internal to the first, and a second antisense oligonucleotide complementary to the central region of the (dT) adaptor-primer. The products amplified in the second PCR are isolated from an agarose gel, cloned, and characterized.

PCR walking

Recently PCR methods have been designed, which allow the amplification of DNA with unknown sequences that are present adjoining a known sequence within a DNA fragment. The technique is described as PCR walking. For instance, if cDNA sequence is known, the regulatory sequences adjoining the transcribed sequence in genomic DNA can be amplified. In this exercise, an adapter of known sequence is first ligated to the restriction fragments derived from genomic DNA that contains the unknown sequence to be amplified. One of the two primers is designed from the known gene sequence (described as gene specific primer) and the other primer is designed on the basis of the adapter of known sequence that is ligated to the restriction fragments of genomic DNA. Consequently, PCR walking involves the following three steps: (i) restriction enzyme digestion to produce a large number of genomic DNA fragments; (ii) ligation of adapters to restriction fragments and (iii) PCR amplification using one adapter primer and the other gene specific primer (Figure 4.8).

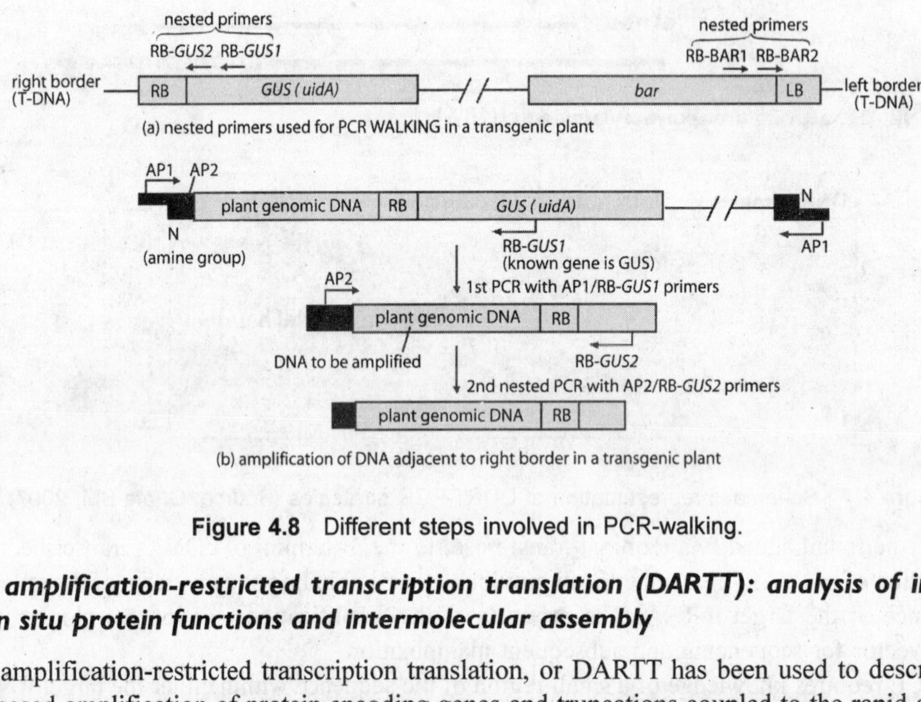

Figure 4.8 Different steps involved in PCR-walking.

DNA amplification-restricted transcription translation (DARTT): analysis of in vitro and in situ protein functions and intermolecular assembly

DNA amplification-restricted transcription translation, or DARTT has been used to describe the PCR-based amplification of protein encoding genes and truncations coupled to the rapid analysis of protein functions following transcription and translation of the encoded protein. Transcriptional initiation signals are added to genes during amplification, and runoff RNA transcripts are synthesized. PCR-generated RNAs are used to prime *in vitro* translation reactions with or without PCR-added, ATG translational initiation signals. DARTT has been used to define functionally active portions of polypeptides truncated at the amino and carboxy termini. Initially DARTT was used to define the minimum polypeptides required to recognize neutralizing monoclonal antibodies (Figure 4.9). Subsequently, it has been used to define the amino acids necessary for oligomerization

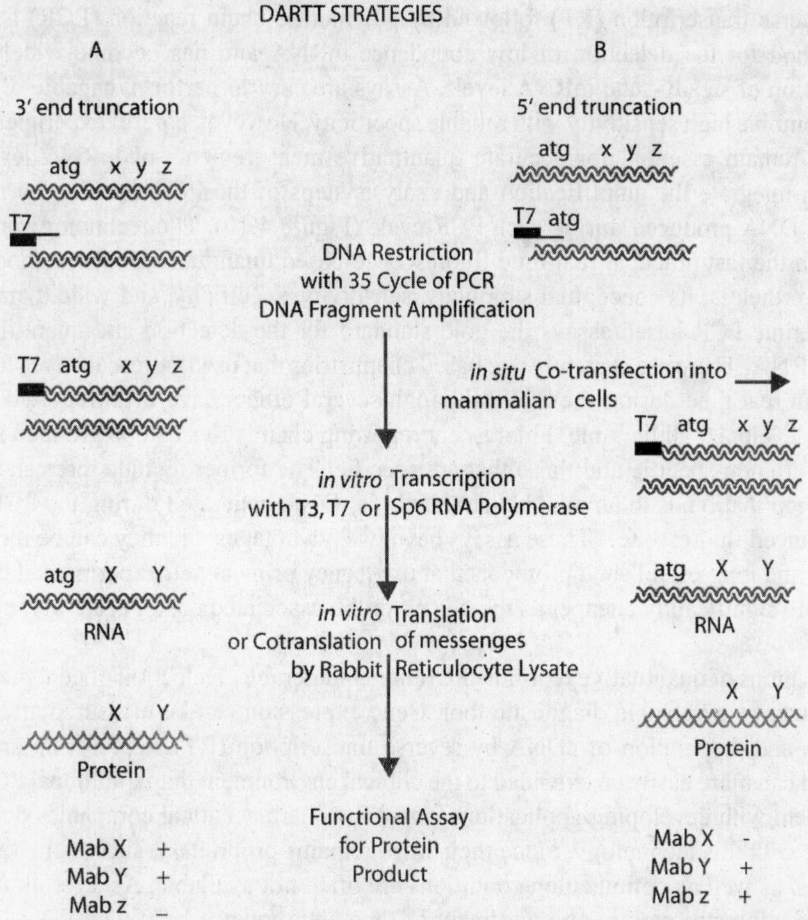

Figure 4.9 DARTT strategies for protein-function analysis.

of protein subunits and for the assembly of viral particles. More recently, DARTT has been extended to generating truncated polypeptides in transfected tissue culture cells by providing the sturdy cloned T7 RNA polymerase in trans. This extended use of DARTT should allow the rapid definition of protein processing and assembly signals within the cell as well as the identification of cell regulatory or enzymatically active polypeptides. A brief synopsis of the tissue culture adaptation of DARTT follows *in vitro* protocol. The ability to rapidly generate truncated polypeptide products via PCR in either an *in situ* or *in vitro* system is the advantage of the DARTT system for defining functionally active peptide fragments.

Meaningful quantification of mRNA using real-time PCR

Its conceptual and practical simplicity, capacity for high throughput, and combination of high sensitivity with specificity has made the fluorescence-based real-time reverse transcription polymerase chain reaction (qRT-PCR or RT-PCR) today's method of choice for the quantification of RNA. Reverse transcription (RT) followed by polymerase chain reaction (PCR) is the most sensitive method for the detection of low abundance mRNA and has become widely used for the quantification of steady-state mRNA levels. Assays are easy to perform, capable of high throughput, can combine high sensitivity with reliable specificity. However, careful experimental design and validation remain essential for accurate quantitative measurements of mRNA levels. Real-time techniques integrate the amplification and analysis steps of the PCR reaction by monitoring the amount of DNA produced during each PCR cycle (Figure 4.10). The technology is still relatively novel, with the fast practical real-time fluorescence-based quantitative PCR method developed in 1996. Nevertheless, its conceptual simplicity, sensitivity, specificity, and wide dynamic range has made real time PCR-based assays the gold standard for the detection and quantification of both DNA and RNA. There are currently dye based chemistries that use fluorescent dyes to monitor PCR reactions in real time during the PCR, although several others have been reported and new ones are being developed all the time. Fluorescent reporting chemistries can be grouped into two types: those that are non-specific and those that are specific. The former include intercalating dyes, e.g., SYBR-Green that binds to any double-stranded (ds) DNA generated during the PCR reaction and emits enhanced fluorescence. These assays have two advantages: (1) they can be incorporated into optimized and long-established protocols that use legacy primers and experimental conditions, and (2) They are significantly cheaper as there is no probe-associated cost. Furthermore, they can yield *quasi.*

The applications of quantitative real-time PCR are innumerable. Detection of genomic or viral DNA in tissues can be a valuable diagnostic tool. Gene expression can be measured after extraction of total RNA and preparation of cDNA by reverse transcription (RT) step. Set-up and analysis are simple and can more easily be extended to the clinical environment than traditional PCR techniques. One problem with developing applications is that the pharmaceutical companies do most research conducted with this technology. Since their work remains proprietary, successful TaqMan primers and probes, as well as optimization conditions are often not available. As a result, *de novo* design and optimization still require an investment of time and money.

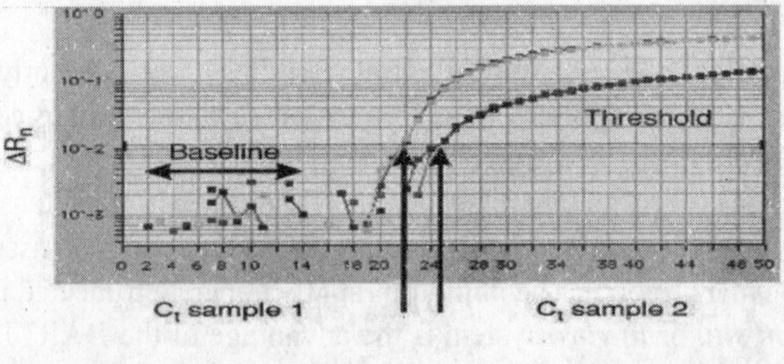

Figure 4.10 Typical amplification plots obtained using a real-time PCR assay. An amplification plot is the plot of fluorescence signal vs. cycle number. An increase in fluorescence above the baseline indicates the detection of accumulated PCR product, and the threshold cycle (Ct) is defined as the cycle number at which the fluorescence passes that threshold.

Molecular haplotyping by PCR

Molecular real-time PCR methods can determine whether two or more mutations are on the same or different chromosomes. This ability to haplotype without family studies is useful for research and clinical purposes and can give an advantage over genotyping. Haplotyping by real-time PCR with hybridization probes has been demonstrated for adjacent repeats and single base alterations, with a probe that covers both the sites. However, base alterations may be separated by distances greater than a traditional hybridization probe will cover. We described a probe design that covers both (or all) sites, but does not include the entire sequence between the sites. When hybridized with the template, the template is forced to form a loop. This "loop-out" probe will dissociate from the template as a unit, therefore allowing haplotyping of base alterations separated by over 80 bp. Examples of haplotyping by traditional probes for adjacent sequence variants, as well as examples of "loop-out" probes are presented.

Generation of single-chain antibody fragments by PCR

The ability to generate monoclonal antibodies revolutionized the use of antibodies for scientific analysis, immunodiagnostics, and immunotherapeutics. Monoclonal antibodies have traditionally been generated via hybridoma technology which is expensive, time-consuming, and small number of clones producing antibodies of the desired specificity. Recently, the production of monoclonal antibodies generated through recombinant DNA technology (recombinant antibodies) has been demonstrated in bacteria. This recombinant antibody technology is easier and less time-consuming than mammalian cell culture techniques. Recombinant antibody fragments assembled as fusion proteins on the surface of bacteriophages can be directly selected for antigen binding ability, circumventing the need for extensive screening procedures. The cloned antibody fragments can also be easily manipulated to improve their binding affinity through a number of techniques, including *in vitro* mutagenesis—a step that could not be carried out using the traditional hybridoma technology. For these reasons, the recombinant antibody technology should soon replace traditional hybridoma techniques for creating antibody molecules for diagnostic and therapeutic use.

Pyrosequencing technology

The ability to determine nucleic acid sequences is important for the detailed study of biological systems. Pyrosequencing is an alternative to the traditional Sanger method for *de novo* DNA sequencing. The pyrosequencing technology is especially suited for short-read sequencing, although the method has recently been improved to allow sequencing of up to hundred bases. It is broadly applicable for analysis of single nucleotide polymorphism (SNPs) and for identification of short DNA sequences used in bacterial, fungal (unpublished data), and viral typing. In addition, the methodological performance of the pyrosequencing technology has been used to determine difficult secondary structures, mutations, and for tag sequencing of a selected cDNA library. Pyrosequencing employs coupled enzymatic reactions in order to monitor the inorganic pyrophosphate (PPi) released during nucleotide incorporation (Figure 4.11). A sequencing primer is hybridized to a single-stranded DNA template and mixed with the enzymes, DNA polymerase, ATP sulfurylase, luciferase, and apyrase, as well as the substrates, adenosine phosphosulfate (APS) and luciferin. Then the rest of four deoxynucleotide triphosphates (dNTP) are added to the reaction. DNA polymerse catalyzes the incorporation of the deoxynucleotide into the DNA strand only if it is complementary to the base in the template strand. Each incorporation event is accompanied by the release of PPi in a quantity equimolar to the amount of incorporated nucleotide. ATP sulfurylase quantitatively converts PPi to ATP in the presence of APS.

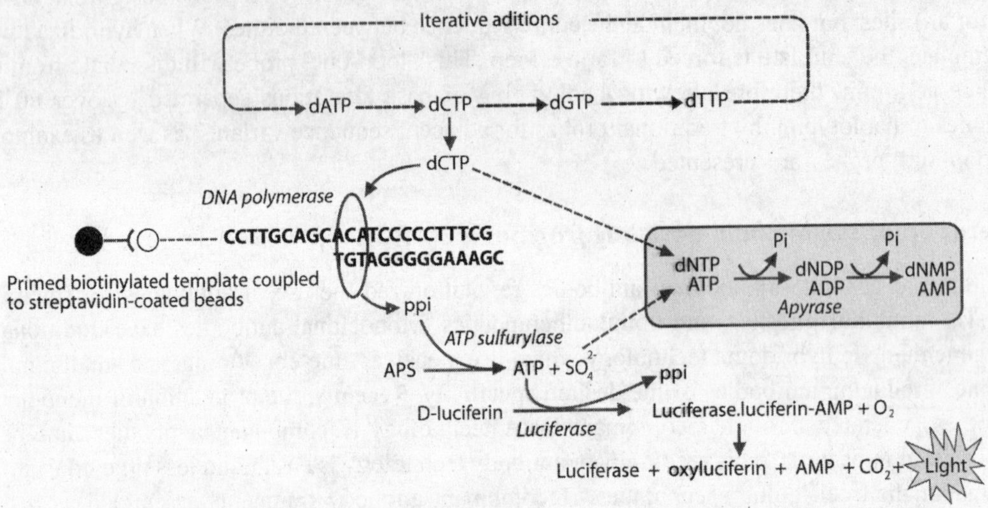

Figure 4.11 A schematic representation of the pyrosequencing reaction.

The produced ATP drives the luciferase-mediated conversion of luciferin to oxyluciferin that generates visible light in amounts that are proportional to the amount of ATP. The light produced in the luciferase-catalyzed reaction is detected by a charge-coupled device (CCD) camera and seen as a peak in a Pyrogram. Each light signal is proportional to the number of nucleotides incorporated. Apyrase, a nucleotide-degrading enzyme, continuously degrades ATP and unincorporated dNTPs. When degradation is complete, another dNTP is added. Addition of dNTPs is performed one at a time. As the process continues, the complementary DNA strand is built up and the nucleotide sequence is determined from the signal peaks in the Pyrogram. Pyrosequencing has the advantages of accuracy, flexibility, simple automation, and parallel processing.

Biodefense

With the public's reawakened concern regarding use of biological agents as weapons, the rapid detection, discrimination, and identification of pathogenic organisms and toxins has become a priority for state and federal government agencies. High confidence, cost effective, and near real-time diagnostic methods are essential to protect national health security whether the target is public health, agriculture, commodities, or water supply infrastructures. While culture-based methods have been, and will likely remain, the gold standard for microbiological diagnostics, PCR-based tests offer significant advantages in sensitivity, specificity, speed and data richness that make them invaluable to diagnostic laboratories.

Recent Advancement in PCR Technology

Electronic-PCR (ePCR)

In the post-genomic era, massive data on DNA sequences are now available in different databases. The approach of data mining using bioinformatics tools is employed for making good use of data. This data can also be utilized for conducting PCR on the computer. For instance, primers for a specific conserved DNA sequence can be designed and used on the computer to find out the expected length of the amplified product. This approach has been successfully utilized for conducting electronic PCR (ePCR) without the use of PCR machine or PCR reaction mixtures.

Future Prospects of the PCR Technology

Currently, nucleic acid amplification techniques are still labor intensive and expensive to perform, which limit their use to large commercial laboratories or research oriented diagnostic laboratories at universities. The ability to automate PCR procedures is therefore considered a key factor in determining how large the role of PCR will be in the future for the average laboratory. For a variety of human pathogens including viruses, commercially available PCR kits have been introduced. The present technology for doing PCR, about the size of a microwave oven and costing several thousand dollars seems destined for further radial improvement. Extraordinary miniaturization of the hardware is also underway, as experimenters squeeze the PCR onto chip-sized devices. Criss-crossed with the tiniest of troughs to hold the reagents and the DNA, the chips are heated electrically and cooled down much faster than the present generation of machines, so amplification is even speedier than today's swift process. Already researchers have reported using a handheld battery-powdered gadget to copy pieces of DNA that contained eight different cystic fibrosis mutation sites. While such experimental chip-based devices are not yet ready for prime time, they are hastening the day when scientists can take them on the road, and patients will be able to get on the spot readouts of their DNA. It may soon be quite routine to diagnose an infectious or genetic disorder, or even detect an inherited predisposition to cancer or heart disease right in the doctor's office.

CONCLUSION

PCR has, no doubt, established itself as one of the most commonly used techniques in the life sciences. But the numbers of papers per year mentioning PCR now remain at a constant level or are even slightly decreasing. It is interesting to compare this trend with that in a somewhat older key technology of the life sciences, monoclonal antibodies. For both, there was a rapid increase in the number of published papers in the past decade after their introduction (1974 to 1986 for monoclonals, 1985 to 1995 for PCR). Thereafter, the output slowed down. At least for PCR, all major improvements in the technology so far were made during the last 10 years. An interesting exception is the real-time PCR, a relatively young invention. Still, PCR remains the most popular technology in the life sciences, and for the moment there is no serious contender in sight. Isothermal amplification methods can be performed on simpler instruments. However, this advantage is offset by their need for more complex reaction mixtures, resulting in higher reagent costs and decreased robustness. This makes these methods less attractive for high throughput and quantitative applications. Thus, the unique strength of PCR remains its versatility, e.g., the same instruments and related expertise can be used for a large variety of demands. These will remain high for some time since the genome sequences of several key organisms have just recently been completed. Polymorphism and expression data obtained with the aid of these sequences are expected to yield a wealth of clinical and commercially important data, and PCR is at the forefront of the genomics revolution. It will be interesting to see whether this will lead not only to further specialization, but also major developments in the technique. The amazing number of uses to which the PCR has been put in short time is a mark of its general utility for manipulation of DNA, but also clearly a mark of its simplicity and robustness. Never in the history of biotechnology has such enthusiasm and unreserved welcome been accorded to an analytical technique as like for polymerase chain reaction.

FURTHER READINGS

1. Ahmed J.S., Shayan P., Hugel F.U., Biermann R., Ewald Ch., Schein E. and Gerdes J. (1997) Acroschizonts of *Theileria annulata* as vaccine and diagnostic tools. *Tropical Animal Health and Production.* 29 **(4):** 128S-132S.
2. Amude A.M., Alfieri A.A. and Alfieri A.F. (2006) Antemortem Diagnosis of CDV Infection by RT-PCR in Distemper dogs with neurological deficits without the typical clinical presentation. *Archives of Virology.* 30 **(6):** 679-687.
3. Antognoli M.C., Salman M.D., Triantis J., Herna´ndez J. and Keefe T. (2001) A one-tube nested polymerase chain reaction for the detection of *Mycobacterium bovis* in spiked milk samples: an evaluation of concentration and lytic techniques. *J. Vet. Diagn. Invest.* **(13):** 111-116.
4. Berg T., Suddes H., Morrice G. *et al.* (2006) Comparison of PCR, culture and microscopy of blood smears for the diagnosis of anthrax in sheep and cattle. *Lett. Appl. Microbiol.* **(43):** 181-186.
5. Bespalova I.N., Adkins S. and Burmeister M. (1998) 3′-RACE: Skewed ratio of specific to general PCR primers improves yield and specificity. *BioTechniques* **(24):** 575-577.
6. Bögli-Stuber K., Kohler C., Seitert G., Glanemann B., Antognoli M.C., Salman M.D., Wittenbrink M.M., Wittwer M., Wassenaar T., Jemmi T. and Bissig-Choisat B. (2005) Detection of *Mycobacterium avium* subspecies paratuberculosis in Swiss dairy cattle by real-time PCR and culture: a comparison of the two assays. *Journal of Applied Microbiology.* 99 **(3):** 587-597.
7. Bordignon J., Brasil-dos-Anjos G., Bueno C.R., Salvatiera-Oporto J., Dávila A.M.R., Grisard E.C. and Zanetti C.R. (2005) Detection and characterization of rabies virus in Southern Brazil by PCR amplification and sequencing of the nucleoprotein gene. *Archives of Virology.* 150 **(4):** 695-708.
8. Budowle B., Chakraborty R., Giusti A.M., Eisenberg A.J. and Allen R.C. (1991) Analysis of the VNTR locus DIS80 by the PCR followed by high-resolution PAGE. *Am. J. Hum. Genet.* **(48):** 137.
9. Butler J.A., Pinnow C.C., Thomson J.U., Levisohn S. and Rosenbusch R.F. (2001) Use of arbitrarily primed polymerase chain reaction to investigate *Mycoplasma bovis* outbreaks. *Veterinary Microbiology.* 78 **(2):** 175-181.
10. Clapp L.L. and Patton J.T. (1991) Rotavirus morphogenesis: domains in the major inner capsid protein essential for binding to single-shelled particles and for trimerization. *Virology.* 180 **(2):** 697-708.
11. Decaro N., Elia G., Martella V., Desario C., Campolo M., Di trani L., Tarsitano E., Tempesta M. and Buonavoglia C. (2005) A real-time PCR assay for rapid detection and quantitation of canine parvovirus type 2 DNA in the feces of dogs. *Vet. Microbiol.* **(105):** 19-28.
12. Eckert K.A. and and Kunkel T.A. (1990) High fidelity DNA synthesis by the *Thermus aquaticus* DNA polymerase. *Nucleic Acids Res.* **(18):** 3739-3744.

13. Elia G., Decaro N., Martella V., Cirone F., Stella M.L., Lorusso E., Livia D.T. and Canio B. (2006) Detection of canine distemper virus in dogs by real-time RT-PCR. *Journal of Virological Methods.* 136 **(1-2):** 171-176.
14. Faggi E., Pini G., Campisi E., Bertellini C., Difonzo E. and Mancianti F. (2001) Application of PCR to distinguish common species of dermatophytes. *J. Clin. Microbiol.* **(39):** 3382-3385.
15. Farkas T., Antal M., Sámi L., Germán P., Kecskeméti S., Kardos G., Belák S. and Kiss I. (2007) Rapid and simultaneous detection of avian influenza and newcastle disease viruses by duplex polymerase chain reaction assay. *Zoonoses and Public Health.* 54 **(1):** 38-43.
16. Ferre F. (1992) Quantitative or semi-quantitative PCR: Reality versus myth. *PCR Methods Appl.* **(2):** 1-9.
17. Figueroa J.V., Chieves L.P., Johnson G.S. and Buening G. M. (1992) Detection of *Babesia bigemina*-infected carriers by polymerase chain reaction amplification. *J. Clin. Microbiol.* 30 **(10):** 2576-2582.
18. Foley K.P., Leonard M.W. and Engel J.D. (1993) Quantitation of RNA using the polymerase chain reaction. *Trends Genet.* **(9):** 380-385.
19. Fratamico P.M., Sackitey S.K., Wiedmann M. and Deng M.Y. (1995) Detection of *Escherichia coli* O157:H7 by multiplex PCR. *Journal of Clinical Microbiology.* 33 **(8):** 2188-2191.
20. Freeman W.M., Walker S.J. and Vrana K.E. (1999) Quantitative RT-PCR: Pitfalls and potential. *BioTechniques.* **(26):** 112-125.
21. Frohman M.A., Dush M.K. and Martin G.R. (1988) Rapid production of full-length cDNAs from rare transcripts: Amplification using a single gene-specific oligonucleotide primer. *Proc. Natl. Acad. Sci.* **(85):** 8998-9002.
22. Gelfand D.H. and White T.J. (1990) Thermostable DNA polymerases. *In: PCR Protocols: A Guide to Methods and Applications* (ed. Innis MA, Gelfand DH, Sninsky JJ and White TJ), Academic Press, San Diego, pp. 129-141.
23. Gharizadeh B. *et al.* (2001) Long-read Pyrosequencing using pure 2 deoxyadenosine-5-O-(1-thiotriphosphate) Sp-isomer. *Anal. Biochem.* **(301):** 82.
24. Gilbert S.A., Burton K.M., Prins S.E. and Deregt D. (1999) Typing of bovine viral diarrhea viruses directly from blood of persistently infected cattle by multiplex PCR. *Journal of Clinical Microbiology.* 37 **(6):** 2020-2023.
25. Gussow D. and Clackson T. (1989) Direct clone characterization from plaques and colonies by the polymerase chain reaction. *Nucleic Acids Res.* **(17):** 4000.
26. Halford W.P. (1999) The essential prerequisites for quantitative PCR. *Nat. Biotechnol.* **(17):** 835.
27. Handberg K.J., Nielsen O.L., Pedersen M.W. and Jorgensen P.H. (1999) Detection and strain differentiation of infectious bronchitis virus in tracheal tissues from experimentally infected chickens by reverse transcription polymerase chain reaction. Comparison with an immunohistochemical technique. *Avian Pathol.* **(28):** 327-335.
28. Harmon K.M., Ransom G.M. and Wesley IV. (1997) Differentiation of *Campylobacter jejuni* and *Campylobacter coli* by polymerase chain reaction. *Mol Cell Probes.* **(11):** 195-200.
29. Hartl D.L. and Ochman H. (1993) Inverse polymerase chain reaction. Methods Mol. Biol. **(58):** 293-301.
30. Herthnek1 D., Englund S., Willemsen P.T.J. and Bo¨ lske G. (2006) Sensitive detection of *Mycobacterium avium* subsp. paratuberculosis in bovine semen by real-time PCR. *Journal of Applied Microbiology.* **(100):** 1095-1102.
31. Holton T.A. and Graham M.W. (1991) A simple and efficient method for direct cloning of PCR products using DDT-tailed vectors. *Nucleic Acids Res.* **(19):** 1154.
32. Innis M.A. and Gelfand D.H. (1990) *Optimization of PCRs. In PCR protocols: A Guide to Methods and Applications* (ed. Innis MA, Gelfand DH, Sninsky JJ and White TJ), Academic Press, San Diego, pp. 3-12.
33. Jones M.D. (1993) Reverse transcription of mRNA by *Thermus aquaticus* DNA polymerase followed by polymerase chain reaction amplification. *Methods Enzymol.* **(218):** 413-419.

34. Kai M., Kamiya S., Yabe H., Takakura I., Shiozawa K. and Ozawa A. (1993) Rapid detection of *Mycoplasma pneumoniae* in clinical samples by the polymerase chain reaction. *J. Med. Microbiol.* **(38):** 166-170.
35. Kasai K., Nakamura Y. and White R. (1990) Amplification of a variable number of tandem repeats (VNTR) locus (pMCT118) by the polymerase chain reaction (PCR) and its application to forensic science. *J. Forensic Sciences.* **(35):** 1196.
36. Kaufman D.L. and Evans G.A. (1990) Restriction endonuclease cleavage at the termini of PCR products. *BioTechniques.* **(9):** 304-306.
37. Kawasaki E.S. and Wang A.M. (1989) Detection of gene expression. *In: PCR Technology: Principles and Applications for DNA Amplification* (ed. Erlich HA), Stockton Press, New York, pp. 89-97.
38. Keid L., Soares R., Vasconcellos S., Chiebao D., Megid J., Salgado V. and Richtzenhain L. (2007) A polymerase chain reaction for the detection of *Brucella canis* in semen of naturally infected dogs. *Theriogenology.* 67 **(7):** 1203-1210.
39. Latha D. and Ramadass P. (2002) Improved PCR assay for the detection of canine parvovirus from faecal samples. *Ind. J. Vet. Med.* **(26):** 335-338.
40. Latha D., Geetha M., Ramadass P. and Narayanan R.B. (2007) Development of recombinant nucleocapsid protein based IgM-ELISA for the early detection of distemper infection in dogs. *Vet Immunol Immunopathol.* **(119):** 278-286.
41. Leung D.W., Chen E. and Goeddel D.V. (1989) A method for random mutagenesis of a defined DNA segment using a modified polymerase chain reaction. *Technique.* **(1):** 11-15.
42. Liang P. and Pardee A.B. (1992) Differential display of eukaryotic messenger RNA by means of the polymerase chain reaction. *Science.* **(257):** 967-971.
43. Liang P. and Pardee A.B. (1997) Differential display. A general protocol. Methods Mol. Biol. **(85):** 3-11.
44. Mackow E.R., Yamanaka M.Y., Dang M.N. and Greenberg H.B. (1990) DNA amplification-restricted transcription-translation: rapid analysis of rhesus rotavirus neutralization sites. *Proc. Natl. Acad. Sci. U S A.* 87 **(2):** 518-522.
45. Madden R.H., Moran L. and Scates P. (1996) Sub-typing of animal and human *Campylobacter* spp. using RAPD. *Lett. Appl. Microbiol.* **(23):** 167-170.
46. Marchuk D., Drumm M., Saulino A. and Collins F.S. (1991) Construction of T-vectors, a rapid and general system for direct cloning of unmodified PCR products. *Nucleic Acids Res.* **(19):** 1156.
47. Meer R. and Songer G. (1997) Multiplex polymerase chain reaction assay for genotyping *Clostridium perfringens*. *Am. J. Vet. Res.* **(58):** 702-705.
48. Mehrotra M., Wang G. and Johnson (2000) Multiplex PCR for detection of genes for *Staphylococcus aureus* enterotoxin, exfoliative toxin, toxic shock syndrome toxin 1 and methicilin resistance. *J. Clin. Microbiol.* **(38):** 1032-1035.
49. Mekkes D.R. and Feberwee A. (2005) Real-Time PCR for the qualitative and quantitative detection of *Mycoplasma gallisepticum*. *Avian Pathology.* **(34):** 348-354.
50. Meudt H.M. and Clarke A.C. (2007) Almost forgotten or latest practice? AFLP applications, analyses and advances. *Trends Plant Sci.* 12 **(3):** 106-117.
51. Meyer R.F., Brown C.C., House C., House J.A. and Molitor T.W. (1991) Rapid and sensitive detection of foot-and-mouth disease virus in tissues by enzymatic RNA amplification of the polymerase gene. *J. Virol. Methods.* **(34):** 161-172.
52. Mueller U.G. and Wolfenbarger L.L. (1999) AFLP genotyping and fingerprinting. *Trends Ecol. Evol.* (Amst.) 14 **(10):** 389-394.
53. Nelson R.M. and Long G.L. (1989) A general method of site-specific mutagenesis using a modification of the *Thermus aquaticus* polymerase chain reaction. *Anal. Biochem.* **(180):** 147-151.
54. Nyrén P. (2001) Method of sequencing DNA based on the detection of the release of pyrophosphate and enzymatic nucleotide degradation, United States Patent, US 6, 258, 568 B1.

55. Ochman H., Ayala F.J. and Hartl D.L. (1993) Use of polymerase chain reaction to amplify segments outside boundaries of known sequences. *Methods Enzymol.* **(218):** 309-321.
56. Orita M.Y., Suzuki Y., Sekiya T. and Hayashi K. (1989b) Rapid and sensitive detection of point mutations and DNA polymorphisms using the polymerase chain reaction. *Genomics.* **(5):** 874-879.
57. Pratelli A., Buonavoglia D., Martella V., Tempesta M., Lavazza A. and Buonavoglia C. (2000) Diagnosis of canine coronavirus infection using nested-PCR. *J Virol. Methods.* **(84):** 91-94.
58. Preston G.M. (1993) Use of degenerate oligonucleotide primers and polymerase chain reaction to clone gene family members. *Methods Mol. Biol.* **(15):** 317-337.
59. Ramadass P. and Latha D. (2005) Multiplex PCR assay for diagnosis of canine parvovirus infection and leptospirosis. *Indian Veterinary Journal.* 82 **(4):** 365-367.
60. Ramadass P., Thiagarajan V., Parthiban M., Senthil Kumar T.M.A., Latha D., Anbalagan A., Krishnakumar M. and Nachimuthu K. (2003) Sequence analysis of infectious bursal disease virus isolates from India: phylogenetic relationships. *Acta Virol.* **(4):** 131-135.
61. Reid S.M., Ferris N.P., Hutchings G.H., Zhang Z., Belsham G.J. and Alexandersen S. (2002) Detection of all seven serotypes of foot-and-mouth disease virus by real-time, fluorogenic reverse transcription polymerase chain reaction assay. *J. Virol. Methods.* **(105):** 67-80.
62. Ronaghi M. *et al.* (1998) A sequencing method based on real-time pyrophosphate. Science. ***(281):*** 363.
63. Saiki R.K. (1989) The design and optimization of the PCR. *In: PCR Technology Principles and Applications* [or DNA amplilfication (ed. H. A. Erlich)], Stockton Press, New York, pp. 7-16.
64. Saiki R.K., Gelfand D.H., Stoffel S., Scharf S.J., Higuchi R., Horn G.T., Mullis K.B. and Erlich H.A. (1988) Primer-directed enzymatic amplification of DNA with a thermostable DNA polymerase. *Science.* **(239):** 487-491.
65. Sambrook J., Fritsch E.F. and Maniatis T. (1989) *In: Molecular Cloning: A Laboratory Manual* 2nd ed. (ed. C. Nolan), Cold Spring Harbor Laboratory, Cold Spring Harbor, New York, pp. 7.19-7.22.
66. Sanger F. *et al.* (1977) DNA sequencing with chain-terminating inhibitors. *Proc. Natl. Acad. Sci. U S A.* **(74):** 5463.
67. Saravanan M., Parthiban M. and Ramadass P. (2006) Genotyping of rotavirus of neonatal calves by nested-multiplex PCR in India. *Veterinarski Arhiv.* 76 **(6):** 497-505.
68. Sarkar G. and Sommer S.S. (1989) Access to a messenger RNA sequence or its protein product is not limited by tissue or species specificity. *Science.* **(244):** 331-334.
69. Sato G., Tanabe H., Shoji Y., Itou T., Ito F.H., Sato T. and Sakai T. (2005) Rapid discrimination of rabies viruses isolated from various host species in Brazil by multiplex reverse transcription-polymerase chain reaction. *J. Clin Virol.* **(33):** 267-273.
70. Saunders V.F., Reddacliff L.A., Berg T. and Hornitzky M. (2007) Multiplex PCR for the detection of *Brucella ovis, Actinobacillus seminis* and *Histophilus somni* in ram semen. *Australian Veterinary Journal.* 85 **(1-2):** 72-77.
71. Schaefer B.C. (1995) Revolutions in rapid amplification of cDNA ends: New strategies for polymerase chain reaction cloning of full-length cDNA ends. *Anal. Biochem.* **(227):** 255-273.
72. Scharf S.J., Horn G.T. and Erlich H.A. (1986) Direct cloning and sequence analysis of enzymatically amplified genomic sequences. *Science.* **(233):** 1076-1078.
73. Schowalter D.B. and Sommer S.S. (1989) The generation of radiolabeled DNA and RNA probes with polymerase chain reaction. *Anal. Biochem.* **(177):** 90-94.
74. Senthilkumar T.M.A., Murugan S. and Pachaikani R. (2008) Latex agglutination test for the detection of canine leptospiral antibodies using recombinant OmpL1 antigen. *Veterinarski Arhiv.* 78 **(5):** 393-399.
75. Sheffield V.C., Beck 1.S., Kwitek A.E., Sandstrom D.W. and Stone E.M. (1993) The sensitivity of single-strand conformation polymorphism analysis for the detection of single base substitutions. *Genomics.* **(16):** 325-332.

76. Silva R.F. (1992) Differentiation of pathogenic and non-pathogenic serotype 1 Marek's disease viruses (MDVs) by the polymerase chain reaction amplification of the tandem direct repeats within the MDV genome. *Avian Dis.* 36 **(3):** 521-528.
77. Skottman T., Piiparinen H., Hyytiäinen H., Myllys V., Skurnik M. and Nikkari S. (2007) Simultaneous real-time PCR detection of *Bacillus anthracis* , *Francisella tularensis* and *Yersinia pestis. European Journal of Clinical Microbiology & Infectious Diseases.* 26 **(3):** 207-211.
78. Spinardi L., Mazars R. and Theillet C. (1991) Protocols for an improved detection of points mutations by SSCP. *Nucleic Acids Res.* **19:** 4009.
79. Sreevatsan S., Bookout J.B., Ringpis F., Perumaalla V.S., Ficht T.A., Adams L.G., Hagius S.D., Elzer P.H., Bricker B.J., Kumar G.K., Rajasekhar M., Isloor S. and Barathur R.R. (2000) A multiplex approach to molecular detection of *Brucella abortus* and/or *Mycobacterium bovis* infection in cattle. *J. Clin. Microbiol.* **(38):** 2602-2610.
80. Studier F.W. and Moffatt B.A. (1986) Use of bacteriophage T7 RNA polymerase to direct selective high-level expression of cloned genes. *J. Mol Biol.* **(189):** 113-130.
81. Tcherneva E., Rijpens N., Jersek B. and Herman L.M. (2000) Differentiation of Brucella species by random amplified polymorphic DNA analysis. *J. Appl. Microbiol.* **(88):** 69-80.
82. Triglia T., Peterson M.G. and Kemp D.J. (1988) A procedure for *in vitro* amplification of DNA segments that lie outside the boundaries of known sequences. *Nucleic Acids Res.* **(16):** 81-86.
83. Vos P., Hogers R., Bleeker M. *et al.* (1995) AFLP: a new technique for DNA fingerprinting. *Nucleic Acids Res.* 23 **(21):** 4407-4414.
84. Vrioni G., Gartzonika C., Kostoula A., Boboyianni C., Papadopoulou C. and Levidiotou S. (2004) Application of a polymerase chain reaction enzyme immunoassay in peripheral whole blood and serum specimens for diagnosis of acute human brucellosis. *Eur. J. Clin. Microbiol Infect Dis.* 23 **(3):** 194-199.
85. Walsh P.S., Erlich H.A. and Higuchi R. (1992) Preferential PCR amplification of alleles; Mechanisms and solutions. *PCR Meth. Appl.* **(1):** 241.
86. Wang H., Fadl A.A. and Khan M.I. (1997) Multiplex PCR for avian pathogenic mycoplasmas. *Mol. Cell. Probes.* **(11):** 211-216.
87. Wang X. and Khan M.I. (1999) A multiplex PCR for Massachusetts and Arkansas serotypes of infectious bronchitis virus. *Molecular and Cellular Probes.* 13 **(1):** 1-7.
88. Washington D.C., Persson M.A.A., Caothien R.H. and Burton D.R. (1991) Generation of diverse high-affinity human monoclonal antibodies by repetoire cloning. *Proc. Natl. Acad. Sci. U S A.* **(88):** 2432-2436.
89. Welsh J. and McClelland M. (1993) The characterization of pathogenic microorganisms by genomic fingerprinting using arbitrarily primed polymerase chain reaction (AP-PCR). In: *Diagnostic Molecular Microbiology* (eds. Persing D H, Smith TF, Tenover FC and White TJ), ASM Press, pp. 595-602.
90. Welsh J., Chada K., Dalal S.S., Cheng R., Ralph D. and McClelland M. (1992) Arbitrarily primed PCR fingerprinting of RNA. *Nucleic Acids Res.* **(20):** 4965-4970.
91. Williams J.G., Hanafey M.K., Rafalski J.A. and Tingey S.V. (1993) Genetic analysis using random amplified polymorphic DNA markers. *Methods Enzymol.* **(218):** 704-740.
92. Williams R.A., Bennet M., Bradbury J.M., Gaskell R.M., Jones R.C. and Jordan F.T.W. (1992) Demonstration of sites of latency of infectious laryngotracheitis virus using the polymerase chain reaction. *Journal General Virology.* 73 **(9):** 2415-2430.
93. Woodward S.R., Sudweeks J. and Teuscher C. (1993) Random sequence oligonucleotide primers detect polymorphic DNA products, which segregate in inbred strains of mice. Mature. *Genome.* **(3):** 73-78.
94. Wu D.Y., Ugozzoli L., Pal B.K., Qian I. and Wallace R.B. (1991) The effect of temperature and oligonucleotide primer length on the specificity and efficiency of amplification by the polymerase chain reaction. *DNA Cell Biol.* **(10):** 233-238.
95. Zabeau M. and Vos P. (1993) Selective restriction fragment amplification: a general method for DNA fingerprinting. European Patent Office, publication 0534 858 A1, bulletin 93/13.
96. Zhang Y. and Frohman M.A. (1997) using rapid amplification of cDNA ends (RACE) to obtain full-length cDNAs. *Methods Mol. Biol.* **(69):** 61-87.

CHAPTER 5

DNA-Protein Interaction Technology

Gene expression, DNA replication and repair are three core bio-molecular mechanisms which are exclusively required for any living organism to continue its existence in this world. A detailed knowledge about these phenomena is required to develop strategies to combat lethal diseases and abnormalities and to provide advance qualities of crops and bio-products for human sustenance. As all the three aforementioned biological phenomena are dependent on DNA-protein interactions, gaining a clear insight about them becomes an automatic choice. In this chapter, the most commonly applied strategies for the study of DNA-protein interaction has been described briefly with examples of case studies from different classes of organisms.

Keywords: DNA footprinting; electrophoretic mobility shift assay; southwestern blotting.

INTRODUCTION

The function of DNA is governed by the interacting proteins. The DNA-protein interaction in any organism plays the central role in all the important cellular functions-replication, repair and transcription. Disruption of any DNA-protein interaction will alter the cellular homeostasis. These DNA-protein interactions are broadly of two types—DNA sequence specific and sequence non-specific. The transcription factors are best examples of sequence-specific interactions while the non-specific DNA-protein interaction could be typified by histone-DNA interactions. The DNA-protein interactions are quite strong and are mediated by hydrogen bonding (direct or via water molecules), ionic interaction between protein side chains and DNA backbone and others like van der Waals forces and hydrophobic interactions. In this chapter, we present a brief discussion on the most common methodologies available to study the DNA-protein interactions.

GENETIC ANALYSIS

Genetic analysis of DNA-protein interactions originally concerned isolation and analysis of mutants having mutation in the protein binding sites within the DNA such as isolation of operator-constitutive mutant in repressor binding sites. This kind of mutant analysis could really be of great help in understanding the functional significance of a DNA-protein interaction, but it is tough to isolate such mutants specifically in case of higher eukaryotes. In such cases, mutants of the protein interaction regions in the DNA are made to map the exact protein interaction sites and to determine the functional significance of such interaction. The regulation of promoters will be discussed here in this context.

For promoter study, regions estimated to be the promoter is amplified using PCR and various deletions and site directed mutations are generated within the isolated fragment. The isolated promoter region and its induced mutant counterparts are then tagged to a reporter in a suitable vector which is used to transform desired cells. Assay for reporter gene expression is done either for transient expression or after stable integration leading to a comprehensive genetic analysis. Depending on the expression of the reporter, the region of protein interaction in the promoter DNA sequence is determined. Figures 5.1, 5.2 and 5.3 indicate the strategies for generating different deletions and mutations of the promoter fragment. This method has been implicated in the study of numerous promoters in various organisms.

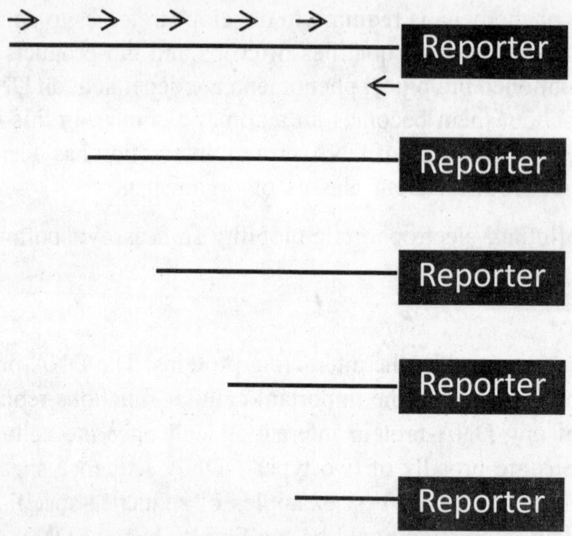

Figure 5.1 A schematic representation showing 5′ seriel deletion of the promoter using PCR. The arrows indicate the different primers that can be used to make the serial deletion. Different fragments are tagged to a reporter and are used for promoter: reporter assays.

ADH (Alcohol Dehydrogenenase) from *Arabidopsis* is induced by cold, drought and hypoxia. Using 5' deletion and site-directed mutagenesis, different elements responsive to different stress conditions were identified. Another example is the discovery of UP1 elements in the genes expressed in cells of axillary bud after main stem capitation of *Arabidopsis*. Transcriptome of axillary bud was analysed after main stem decapitation. The region upstream of these genes was analyzed *in silico* to find the common enriched sequences. The found sequences were mutagenized using site-directed mutagenesis and were subjected to promoter:reporter assays which indicate UP1 is an important transcription factor binding site needed to express the mentioned genes. Site-directed mutagenesis has been applied for the study of osmotically regulated *proU* promoter in *Salmonella typhimurium*.

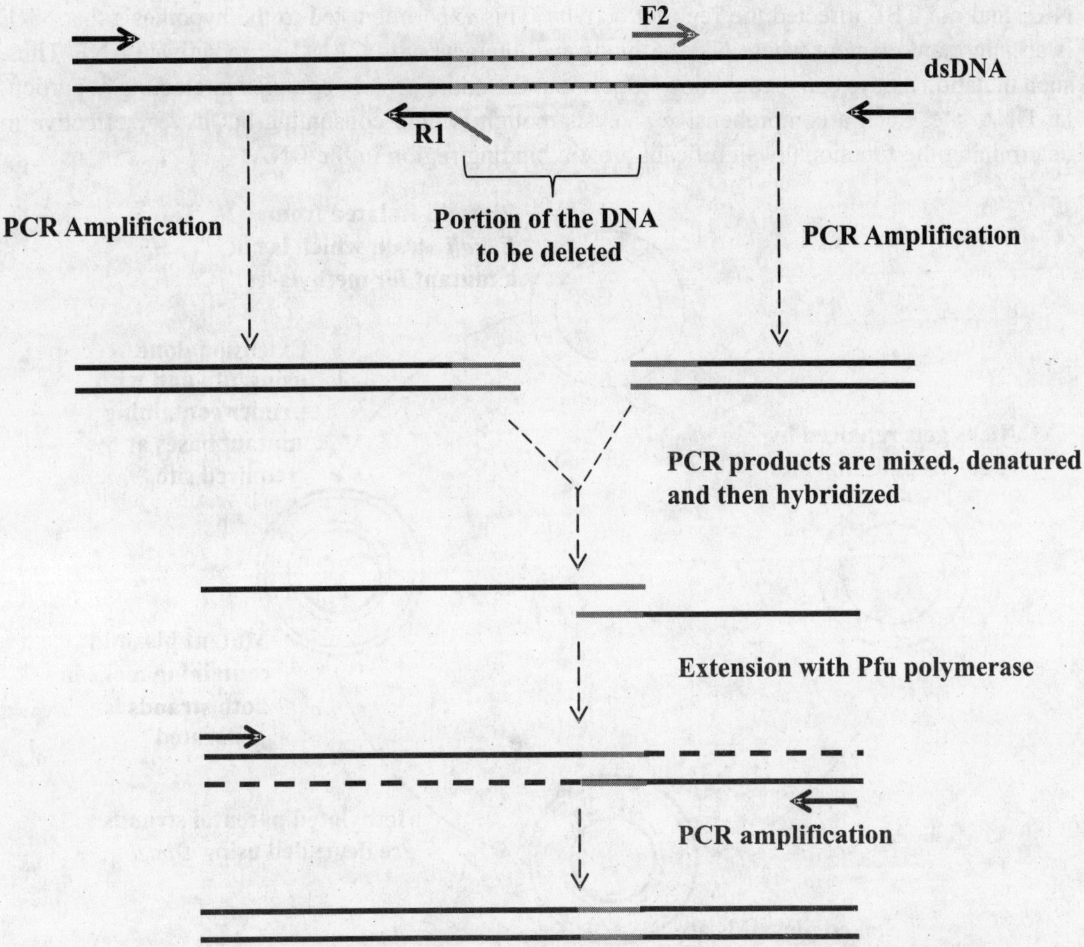

Figure 5.2 A schematic representation showing a strategy for deletion of a central region in the promoter. The arrows indicate the different primers that are used at various steps of PCR amplification. The Primer R1 carries an extra DNA tag, the sequence of which is complementary to the binding region of Primer F2.

Atrial natriuretic factor (ANF) gene is a cardiac-specific marker of hypertrophic signaling. A cDNA expression screen by expressing pool of clones from various cDNA expression libraries in COS cells and assaying for activation of a luciferase reporter controlled by the ANF promoter led to the discovery of CAMTA2 as a strong activator of ANF. Serial deletion of the promoter from -624 bp to -97 bp relative to the transcription initiation site did not impair activation of the promoter by CAMTA2 in transfected COS cells but deletion to -74 bp resulted in a precipitous decline in responsiveness to CAMTA2. Deletion of central portion between the -74 and -30 (position of TATA box) from the -97 bp promoter fragment did not affect the reporter activity significantly indicating the region between -97 and -74 bp is important for ANF activation. An *in silico* analysis revealed the presence of Nkx2.5 and Tbx binding elements (NKE and TBE) in this region. Mutation in only

NKE and not TBE affected the reporter activity. This experiment led to the hypothesis that NKE is an important element where Nkx2.5 binds and interacts with CAMTA2 to activate ANF. Thus, such mutation assays can reveal knowledge about the entire protein complex interacting at particular DNA site. Such a comprehensive analysis though is time consuming but is very effective in determining the functionally significant protein binding region in the DNA.

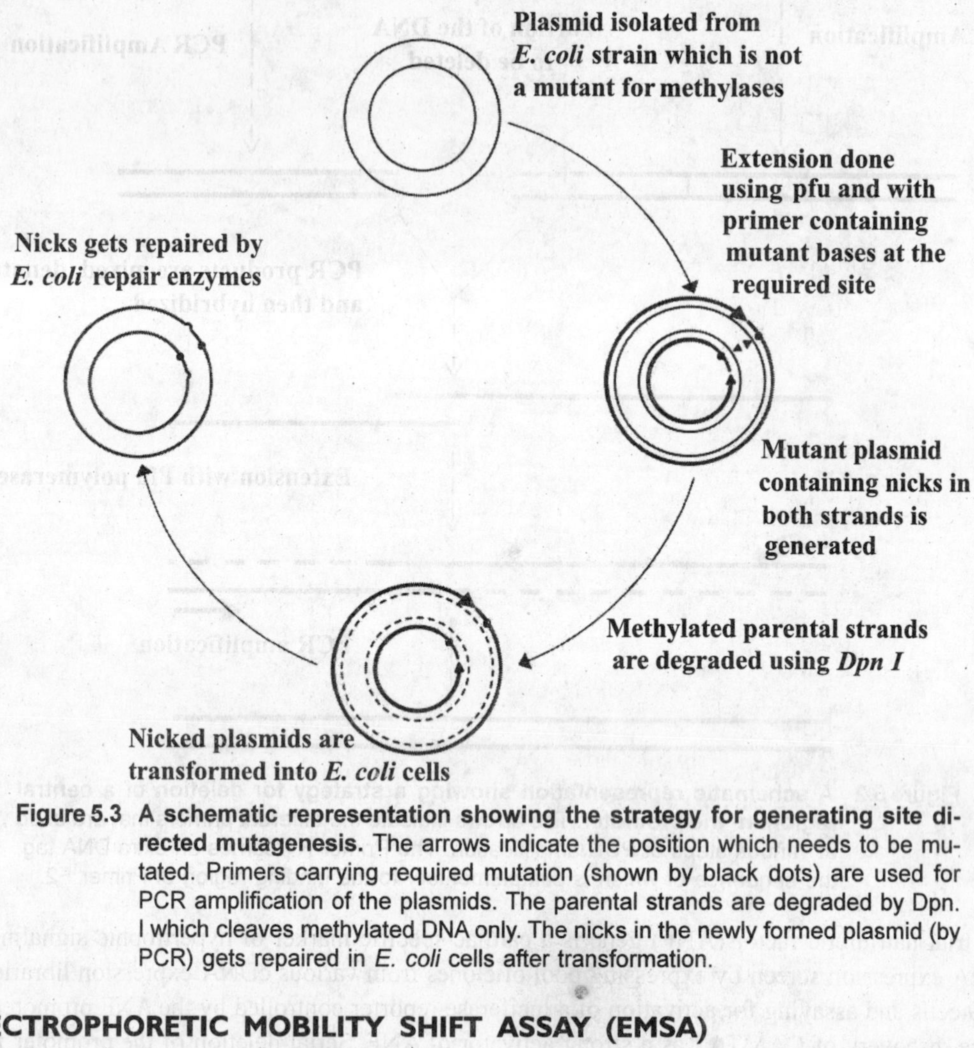

Figure 5.3 A schematic representation showing the strategy for generating site directed mutagenesis. The arrows indicate the position which needs to be mutated. Primers carrying required mutation (shown by black dots) are used for PCR amplification of the plasmids. The parental strands are degraded by Dpn. I which cleaves methylated DNA only. The nicks in the newly formed plasmid (by PCR) gets repaired in *E. coli* cells after transformation.

ELECTROPHORETIC MOBILITY SHIFT ASSAY (EMSA)

The EMSA or gel shift assay experiment includes incubating a ^{32}P-end labelled DNA with a protein or protein mixture in an incubation buffer wherein the DNA binding protein binds to the DNA. Upon electrophoresing, the incubated sample mixture on a non-denaturing polyacrylamide or agarose gel, the mobility of protein bound DNA is retarded and is detected as a separate higher order band in the autoradiogram (Figure 5.4). The size of the probe varies from few to hundreds of nucleotides. Sometimes short oligonucleotides of 20-25 bp might fail to form stable DNA-protein complex as the specific protein may require longer stretch of DNA for stable binding. The protein used in this experiment could be purified recombinant protein or nuclear extracts or total protein extracts. The assay could be used to find the binding sequence of a specified protein and the specificity of the protein binding to a particular sequence. ^{32}P-end labelling of DNA for EMSA could be achieved by using T4 polynucleotide kinase and γ-^{32}P ATP or by polymerization at 5' overhang using Klenow enzyme and α-^{32}P dNTP. Using the latter one for end labelling is more advantageous for doing EMSA for dsDNA binding proteins as only the annealed double stranded oligo will be labelled. If EMSA is being done with extracts from cells, the extracts should be prepared carefully. The lysis of the cells should be done with non-ionic detergents like NP-40 or Triton X-100. While preparing nuclear extracts the nuclear lysis is usually achieved by using NaCl or KCl containing high salt buffers. The proteins are generally concentrated using ammonium sulfate precipitation as very dilute protein preparation may fail to show DNA binding in EMSA.

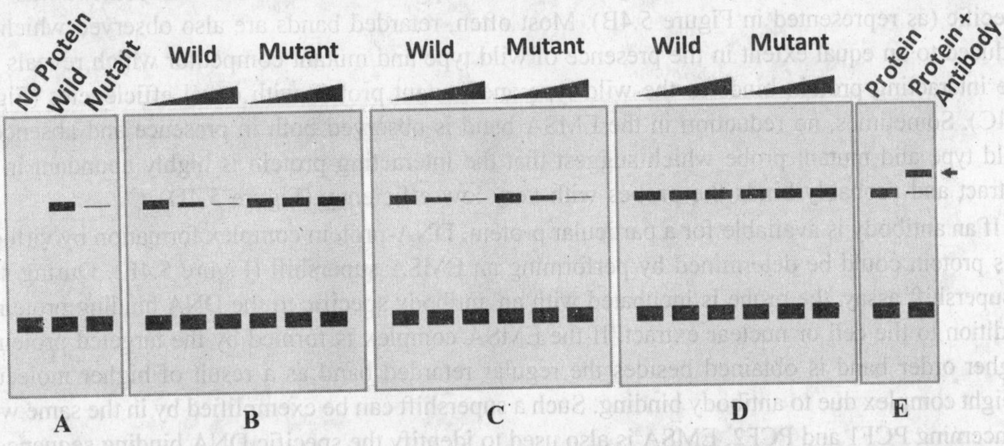

Figure 5.4 A schematic representation showing different kinds of bands that can appear in an EMSA experiment. (A) shows EMSA with wild type and with mutant probe. (B) – (D) shows the different kinds of results that can be obtained from competition assay with wild type and mutant DNA. (E) shows EMSA supershift experiment.

Concentration of DNA binding protein can also be increased by fractionating the extract through a heparin agarose or sepharose column under 0.1 M NaCl or KCl conditions and eluting the DNA binding proteins with 0.4M NaCl or KCl. Failure of nuclear extracts to generate gel shift band should be followed by repeating the EMSA with whole cell extracts or cytoplasmic extracts as many nuclear proteins leak into cytoplasmic fraction during the preparation of the extracts. Inclusion of a non-specific competitor (like poly dI-dC) in an EMSA experiment is usually recommended (from 0.1-10 μg) especially while working with total, cytoplasmic or nuclear extracts to reduce the chances of non-specific DNA binding. Different non-specific competitors can be added to detect a specific DNA-protein complex. In case some of the non-specific DNA binding proteins bind to one of the non-specific competitor DNA with low affinity and form non-specific complex with the analysed DNA with relatively higher affinity. To increase specificity and protein binding, varying salt concentration and sometimes including non-ionic detergents in the buffer are also recommended.

To further confirm the specificity of binding and to estimate the functional relevance of the protein binding, EMSA is generally done in the presence of unlabelled cold wild-type DNA and mutated DNA. An example of such an assay with recombinant PCF1 and PCF2 from rice is described here. From genetic analysis and yeast one-hybrid system, it was estimated that PCF1 and PCF2 binds to Site IIa and Site IIb elements. An EMSA done with oligo containing the binding sites of these proteins and an oligo containing a substitution mutation in the core sequence revealed that purified recombinant proteins do not bind to the mutated oligo, thus increasing the confidence that these proteins specifically bind to Site II elements (as represented in Figure 5.4A). An EMSA was done with nuclear extracts and Site IIa elements revealed a thick gel shift band. When unlabelled oligo containing Site IIa or Site IIb elements were added in excess to the above reaction, the retarded band vanished slowly. No reduction in the retarded band was observed when unlabelled mutated DNA was added, indicating that the DNA-protein interaction in the context was very specific (as represented in Figure 5.4B). Most often, retarded bands are also observed which are reduced to an equal extent in the presence of wild type and mutant competitor which reveals that the interacting protein binds to the wild type and mutant probes with equal efficiencies (Figure 5.4C). Sometimes, no reduction in the EMSA band is observed both in presence and absence of wild type and mutant probe which suggest that the interacting protein is highly abundant in the extract and probably binds the probes with very low efficiency (Figure 5.4D).

If an antibody is available for a particular protein, DNA-protein complex formation by virtue of this protein could be determined by performing an EMSA supershift (Figure 5.4E). During such a supershift assay, the probe is incubated with an antibody specific to the DNA binding protein in addition to the cell or nuclear extract. If the EMSA complex is formed by the targeted protein, a higher order band is obtained besides the regular retarded band as a result of higher molecular weight complex due to antibody binding. Such a supershift can be exemplified by in the same work concerning PCF1 and PCF2. EMSA is also used to identify the specific DNA binding sequence of a recombinant DNA binding protein through a method commonly known as oligo selection procedure. An outline of this procedure is shown in Figure 5.5. A mix of single stranded oligo having central (~20 bp) variable region with known flanking sequence is chemically synthesized. This single stranded DNA is made double stranded and radiolabelled by primer extension using α-^{32}P dNTP. An EMSA is then performed with this probe and the retarded band of DNA-protein complex is excised out of the gel (by superimposing the autoradiogram and the gel) and the DNA is isolated. The DNA is then PCR amplified using primers designed from the flanking known sequences of the probe and thereafter cloned in *E. coli* and sequenced to know the binding sequence. The procedure is repeated with the known sequences for better confirmation. This technique has been used to contain the specific binding sequences of many DNA binding proteins. We exemplify it here by the study done with rep68 and rep78 of adeno associated virus. These rep proteins were earlier shown to regulate AAV viral transcription, replication and integration. It was also known that these proteins bind to GAGC repeats. By oligo selection procedure, it became apparent that rep68 and rep78 can also form stable but low affinity complex with a single GAGC motif, if it is flanked by a string of G-residues. In *Arabidopsis*, the binding site of *Arabidopsis* AtSR1 to its cis-element (CGCG-Box) was determined by oligo selection procedure.

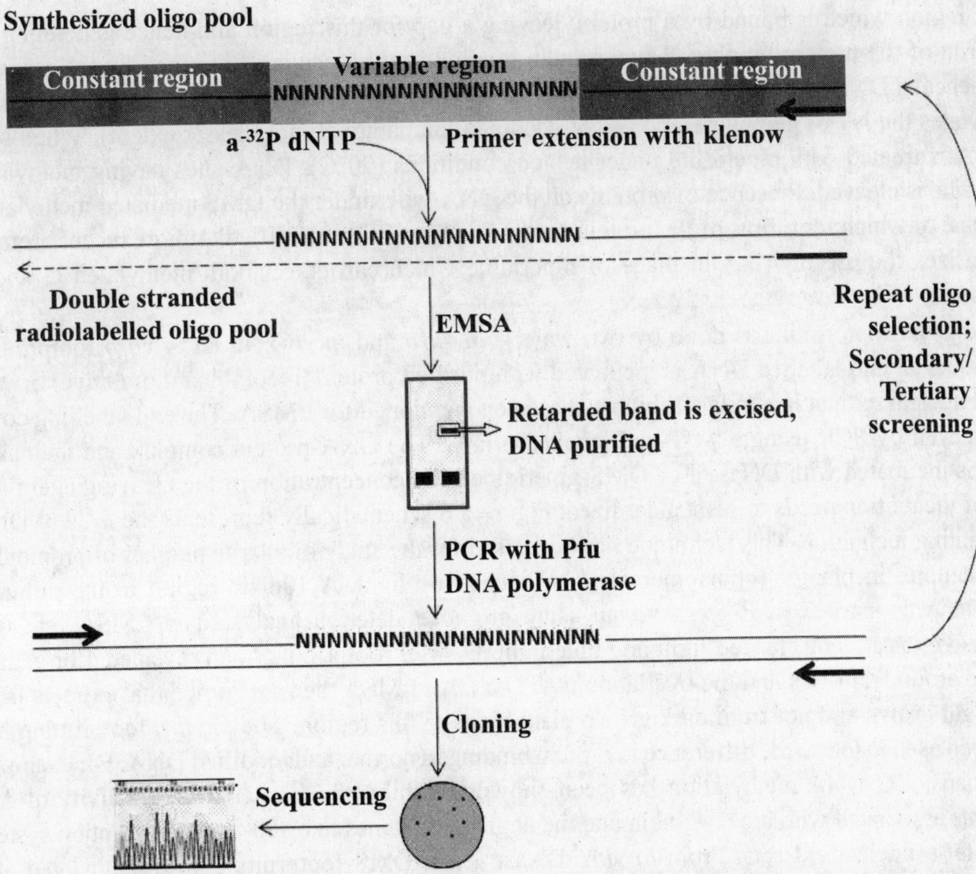

Figure 5.5 A schematic representation of oligo selection procedure. The two constant regions are two different known sequences. The bold arrows indicate the primers used for primer extension or PCR.

DNA FOOTPRINTING

This biochemical technique has been used to identify exact region in DNA which interacts with the protein binding factors. In this method, DNA is treated with DNA cleaving or nicking agent and then is electrophoresed on a denaturing urea-PAGE gel. If a protein is bound at a specific position in the DNA, the cleaving agent will fail to cut the DNA at that region. Hence, no band will be detected for the region of protein binding sequence which could be observed for a corresponding naked DNA. The protein will thus form a footprint showing the sequence of DNA with which it interacts. A marker is run alongside the DNA fragment to know the size of the bands (generally made by manual sequencing of the same clone fragment for which footprinting is being done).

Two of the most common agents used for DNA footprinting are DNase I and Dimethyl sulfate (in combination with piperidine; methylation interference). DNase I is a sequence non-specific DNA cleaving enzyme which interacts with the DNA in the minor groove. DNase I will not cleave the

DNA region which is bound by a protein, leaving a gap for this region and hence generating the footprint of the protein binding. Thus, protein binding in this case is determined by the presence or absence of DNA hypersensitive sites. Dimethyl sulfate (DMS) is a DNA methylating agent which methylates the N7 of guanidine and N3 of adenine (comparatively to a lesser extent). When such a DNA is treated with piperidine under heated conditions (90°C), DNA sites having methylated guanidine is cleaved. Presence of proteins on the DNA will hinder the DMS mediated methylation by virtue of which footprints of the protein on the DNA could be identified. A more recent protocol emphasizes the use of AlkA in place of piperidine which can detect both methylated G and A residues.

The DNA footprinting is done by two ways – *in vitro* and *in vivo.* In an *in vitro* footprinting technique, an end labelled DNA is incubated with purified protein (recombinant or native) or with cell or nuclear extract in similar fashion as has been mentioned for EMSA. The end labelling could be achieved by PCR using a γ-^{32}P end labelled primer. The DNA-protein complex and the naked DNA is incubated with DNase I or DMS-piperidine. The concentration of the cleaving agent and time of incubation needs to be standardized. Figure 5.6 schematically represents the *in vitro* DNA footprinting technique. This technique has been used for the study of a large number of promoters. For example, in plants, Topoisomerase 2 is induced by light. A 106 bp region in the minimal promoter was marked in *Pisum sativum* using promoter deletion analysis and EMSA that was responsive to red light, far red light and blue light. DNaseI footprinting then revealed 6 bp region centred around an I-box and the overlapping ATl box. An EMSA then confirmed that extracts from only light grown and not from dark grown plant binds to this region. The *in vitro* footprinting has also been used to locate the difference in protein binding in normal and modified DNA. For example, in humans, CG DNA methylation has been shown to inhibit the transcriptional activity of Alu elements associated with the α_1-globin and the angiogenin genes in a cell-free transcription system from HeLa nuclear extracts. From *in vitro* DNase I and DMS footprinting with methylated and unmethylated B control region (that exists in the Alu elements), it became evident that the specific nuclear proteins can interact with the unmethylated but not with methylated B control region.

The *in vivo* footprinting technique involves the detection of DNA regions interacting with specific proteins from within the cells and is also known as genomic footprinting. In such a case, the DNA cleaving or modifying agent is made to enter the cell or the isolated nucleus where it cleaves or modifies the genomic DNA in an *in vivo* condition leaving the protein binding site undisturbed. As a control, isolated genomic DNA is treated with the same agent under *in vitro* conditions. This technique is considered better than the *in vitro* footprinting because of its less chance of generating artifacts which could form due to external incubation of DNA and protein under a defined set of conditions during the *in vitro* footprinting. The major challenge while performing the *in vivo* footprinting is to identify the specific DNA fragments among the total genomic pool of DNA which is achieved by ligation mediated PCR (LMPCR). LMPCR is a powerful technique to detect any specific site of DNA cleavage within the genomic DNA. An outline of this technique is shown in Figure 5.7. The technique involves a primer extension step with primers designed from a known site that will generate a blunt end at the site of cleavage. To the blunt end, a double stranded oligo is ligated and 18-25 cycle PCR is done with one primer being designed from the interior to the first primer and the top strand of the double stranded oligo being used as the second primer. A primer extension is then done with radiolabelled primer to generate the final DNA fragments. For this method, the annealing temperature of the DNA and the $MgSO_4$ concentration should be empirically determined and all operations are performed with Vent or pfu DNA polymerase. A simple work flow of the *in vivo* foot printing is shown in Figure 5.8.

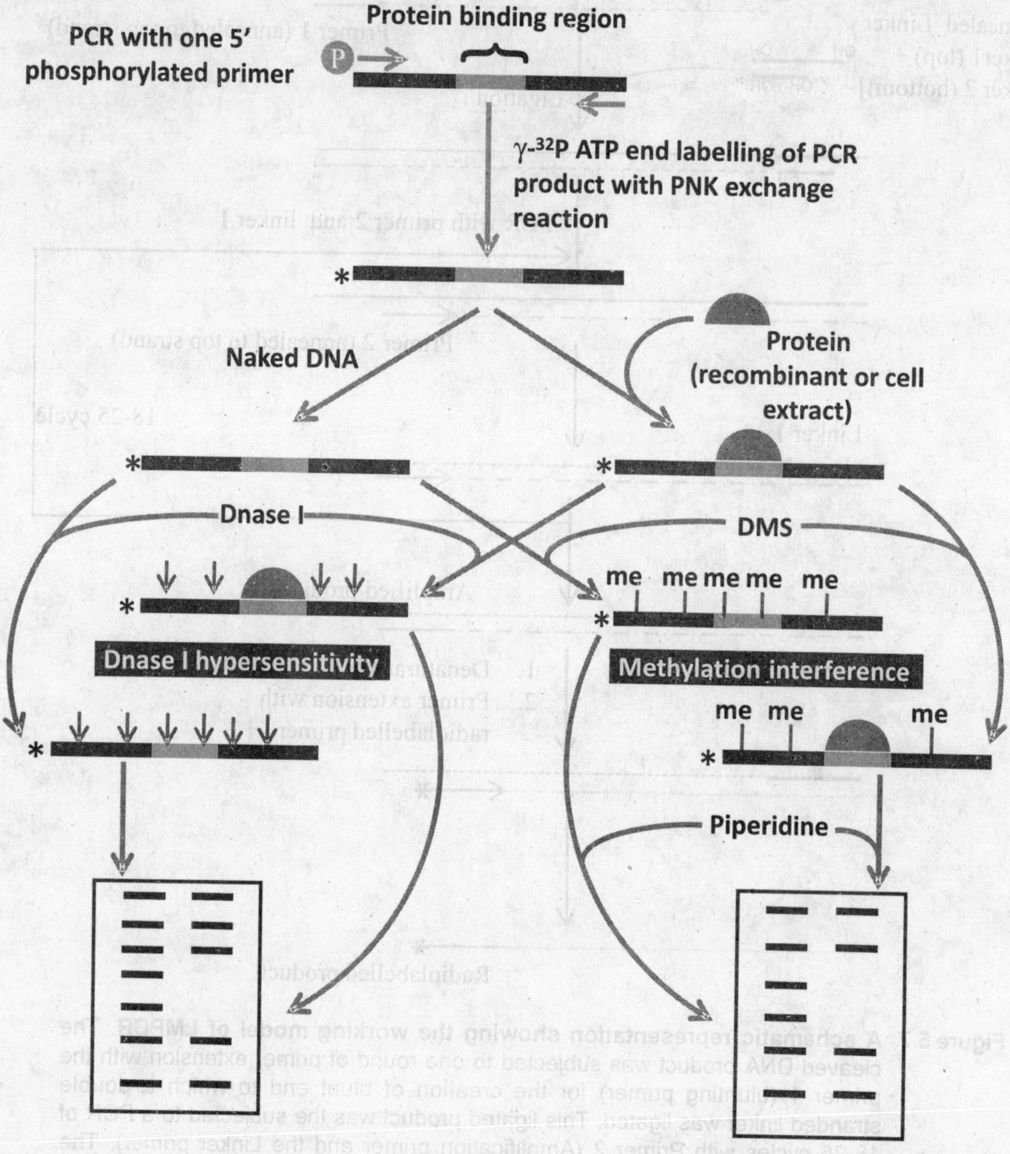

Figure 5.6 A schematic representation showing *in vitro* footprinting using Dnase I and DMS. *indicates end labelled DNA. PNK indicates Polynucleotide kinase. Ⓟ indicates 5′ phosphorylation.

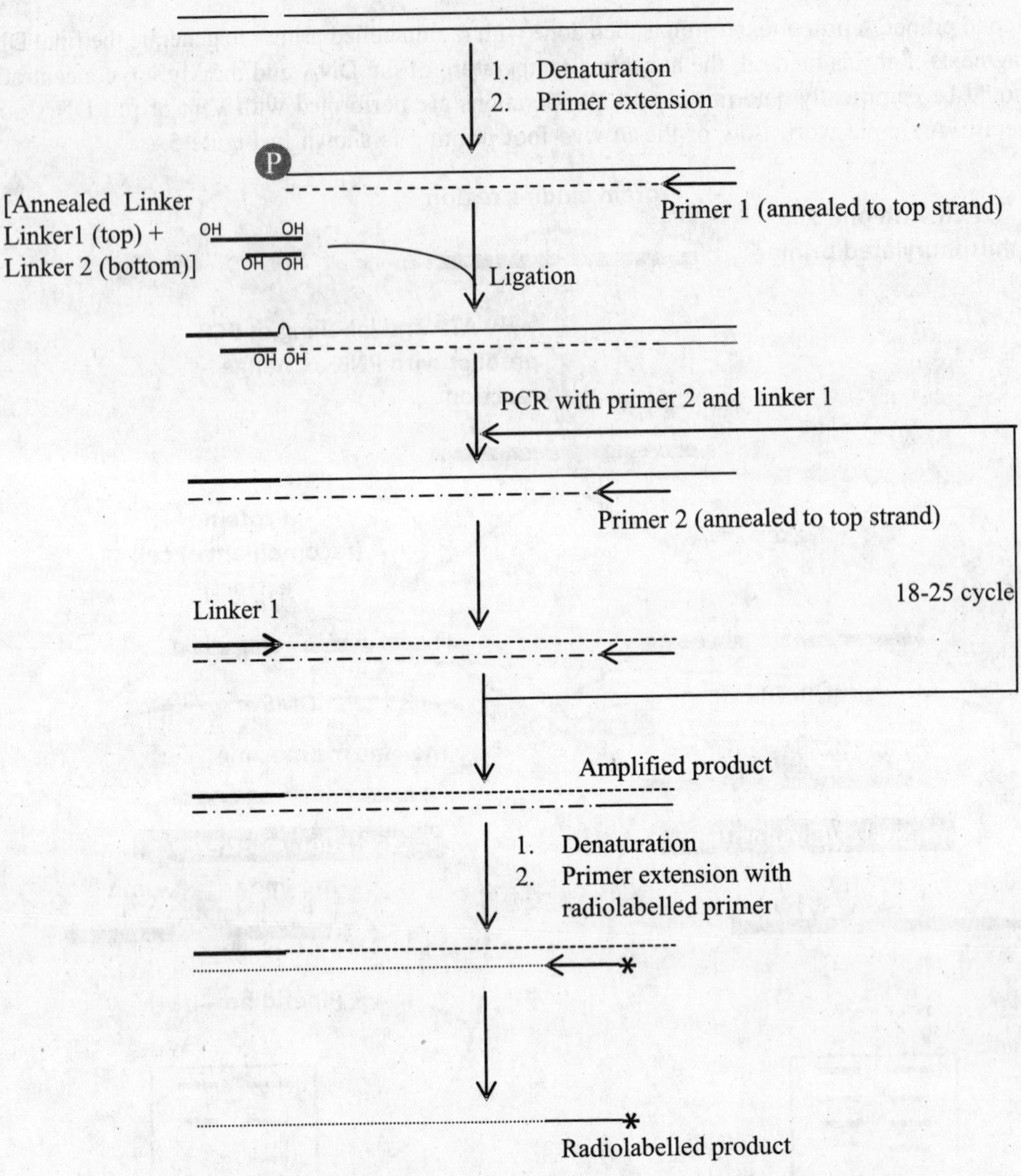

Figure 5.7 A schematic representation showing the working model of LMPCR. The cleaved DNA product was subjected to one round of primer extension with the primer 1 (blunting primer) for the creation of blunt end to which a double stranded linker was ligated. This ligated product was the subjected to a PCR of 18-25 cycles with Primer 2 (Amplification primer and the Linker primer). The amplified products were then subjected to radiolabelling via primer extension with ^{32}P end labelled Primer 3 (labelling primer).

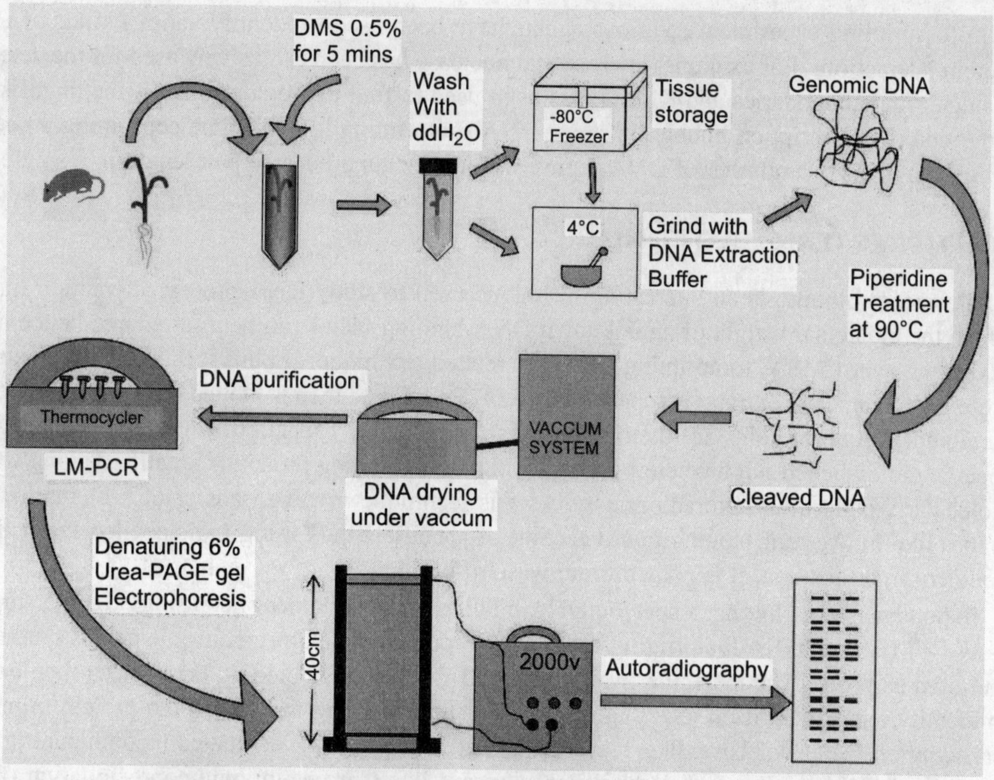

Figure 5.8 A schematic representation showing the work flow of *in vivo* footprinting using DMS. After DMS treatment the samples can be directly processed for DNA isolation or can be stored at -80°C. The DMS concentration and the time of incubation has to be experimentally determined after piperidine cleavage by running alkaline denaturing gel. The condition that gives major band size of around 500 bp (average) should be considered.

Like the *in vitro* DNA footprinting, the *in vivo* footprinting has been used in a number of cases. In humans, 11α-Hydroxysteroid dehydrogenase type 2 is selectively expressed in aldosterone target tissues. Using DMS-LMPCR *in vivo* footprinting, two GC-rich sequences were observed in the first exon and two upstream elements were observed where the occupancy of the proteins correlated with transcriptional state of the gene. In plants, the phaseolin gene is expressed only during seed embryogenesis and does not express in leaf tissue. A detailed DNase I and DMS *in vivo* footprinting indicated that in leaf tissue, the promoter is associated with a nucleosome which is rotationally present over the three TATA-boxes. Under active condition in seed, the region is free of the nucleosome and the TATA-box was found to form nucleo-protein complexes. *In vivo* footprinting could many times help in detecting DNA regions associated with the formation of nucleo-protein complexes which cannot be detected by *in vitro* footprinting. For example, during the analysis of Carcinoembryonic antigen (CEA) promoter in the colon carcinoma lines III -29 and SW403 before and after IFN-γ, three footprint regions were discovered by *in vitro* footprinting while *in vivo* footprinting detected a fourth printing region also.

In footprinting experiments, various agents have been used to identify various kinds of DNA-protein interactions. For example, micrococcal nuclease has been exclusively used for the detection of nucleosome boundaries and $KMnO_4$ has been used to find the region of DNA melting, like the formation of transcription bubble. In short, DNA footprinting is a less time consuming procedure which can identify a number of DNA region within few hundred base pair length in a single trial.

SOUTHWESTERN BLOTTING

Southwestern blotting is an interesting technique used to study DNA-protein interaction through which the molecular weight of an unknown DNA binding factor can be inferred and hence has an advantage over EMSA, footprinting and other related techniques. In this technique, the mixture of proteins (like nuclear extract) is separated by SDS-PAGE and then is blotted onto a membrane. The membrane bound proteins are then renatured *in situ* (using TNED buffer) and is probed with a specific radiolabelled oligo where by the specific DNA binding protein is identified along with its molecular weight after autoradiography. As this technique involve transfer of proteins to membranes like in Western blotting and detection of specific bands using radiolabelled DNA like in Southern hybridization, it is named Southwestern blotting.

In Southwestern blotting, a specific DNA binding element is identified using promoter-reporter assays, EMSA and DNA footprinting. Oligos corresponding to DNA binding element is synthesized and used as probe. The molecular weight inferred for the DNA binding protein can then be used to identify the protein itself (See Figure 5.9). For this, keeping the size of the protein in mind, a transcription factor database, like TransFac is searched and if the estimated recombinant proteins and/or antibodies against them are available, assays like Chromatin immunoprecipitation (ChIP), EMSA and EMSA supershift can be carried out for the confirmation of specific DNA binding to these proteins. Using such an approach, the interaction of NF1 transcription factor with hLHX3b promoter was established. In humans, two different proximal promoter regions encode two different transcripts (LHX3a and LHX3b) from LHX3 gene. The promoter encoding LHX3b lies within the genomic region corresponding to intron 1a of LHX3a ORF. The promoter-reporter assays and EMSA identified a region, -1444 to -1414, which is necessary for LHX3b expression. A Southwestern blot with a double stranded oligo with the sequence of the aforesaid region and pituitary cell extracts identified a protein with molecular weight of 60-65 kDa. An *in silico* analysis identified a NF1 binding site within the mentioned region and NF1 has a similar molecular weight as was identified by Southwestern blotting. EMSA and ChIP experiments then confirmed the binding of NF1 to its binding region in the promoter.

A more direct approach to identify DNA binding proteins is to perform the Southwestern blots by separating the proteins on a 2D-gel whereby the identified spot in the blot can be excised out from a duplicate Coomassie blue stained gel. The isolated protein is then subjected to trypsin digestion followed by mass spectrometry like MALDI-TOF or LC-MS. DNA triple helix binding proteins were isolated from Hela cell extracts using this methodology. For this, Hela cell extracts were separated by 2D gel electrophoresis and were electroblotted onto PVDF membranes. After renaturation of proteins, blots was subjected to Southwestern blotting with a panel of DNA probes adopting intramolecular triple helices and varying in their sequence and structure. A few spots were detected on the blots that showed good reproducibility. The same spots were then excised out of a preparative gel and were subjected to trypsin digestion. Following MALDI-TOF fingerprinting analysis, five proteins showing homology to hnRNPs were identified. Thus, Southwestern blotting is a useful tool which can be used in combination with other technologies to find a specific DNA binding protein.

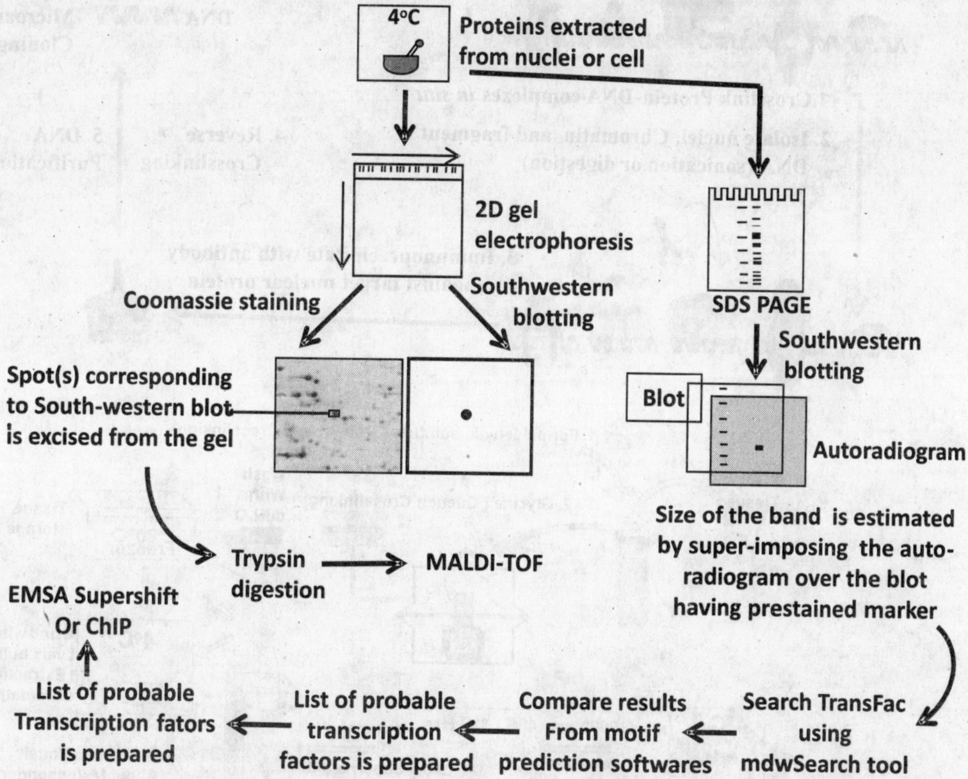

Figure 5.9 A schematic representation showing the application of Southewestern blotting in identifying a DNA binding protein. To get the protein identity, the obtained protein band can be analysed using MALDI-TOF or by *in silico* tools followed by EMSA.

CHROMATIN IMMUNOPRECIPITATION (CHIP)

Chromatin Immunoprecipitation (ChIP) is a powerful tool to identify the *in vivo* interaction of a specific protein at particular region in the chromatin (Figure 5.10). It involves crosslinking of the proteins and DNA within the cell by the application of formaldehyde (generally 1%). The crosslinked chromatin is then subjected to sonication for fragmenting the chromatin to about 500 bp size. The sonicated chromatin is precleared for a short duration with Protein A or Protein G sepharose or agarose and then is incubated with a specific antibody. Upon incubation with Protein A or Protein G sepharose or agarose, the specific nucleoproteic-complexes are precipitated. After decrosslinking the immunoprecipitated chromatin [heating at 65°C, DNA is then purified and subjected to various applications depending on the need like PCR (ChIP-PCR), cloning (ChIP-cloning) and microarray (ChIP on Chip)]. The ChIP technique mentioned above is known as X-ChIP (involves formaldehyde crosslinking). A method of doing ChIP without formaldehyde crosslinking (Native or N-ChIP) has also been implied in many cases.

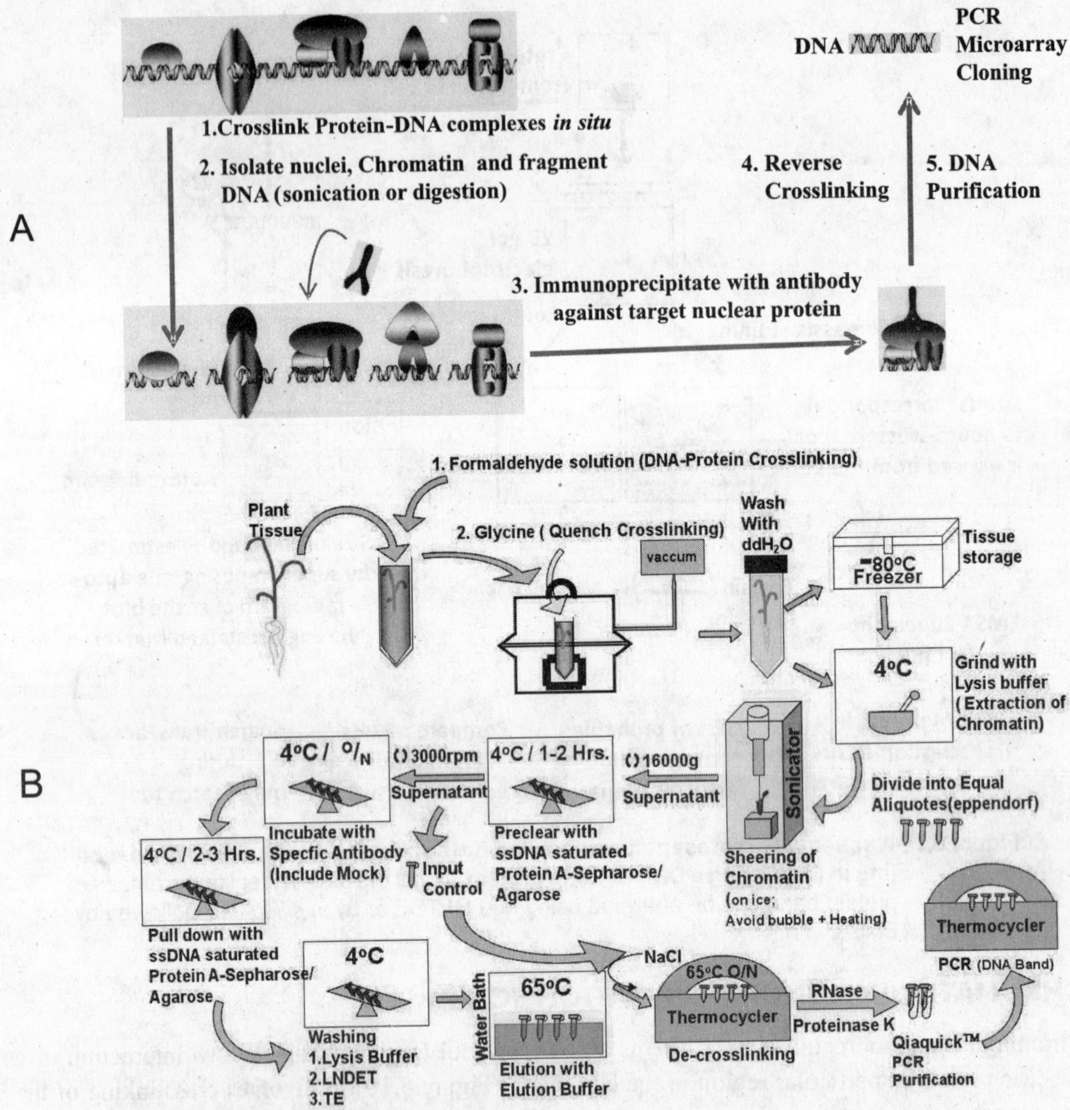

Figure 5.10 A schematic representation of ChIP assay. (A) Shows the principle of X-Chip **(B)** Shows the work flow of X-ChIP.

Sonication is the most critical step in the X-ChIP experiment. Condition for sonication should be so adjusted that frothing and heating does not occur. It is considered better to do sonication at low amplitude and in shorter pulses. Less sonication will cause less amount of chromatin yield and generation of false signals during PCR. A protocol using a combination of *Mnase* and sonication to shear the chromatin in order to obtain consistent amount of chromatin yield is described at the websites of New England Biolabs (NEB). Formaldehyde is the reagent of choice for crosslinking step in ChIP because the crossslinked chromatin can be decrosslinked very easily. The time of crosslinking is also an important factor as reduced time will cause improper crosslinking and more time will cause over crosslinking that could be detrimental for proper sonication, chromatin yield and antibody binding. The quality of antibody is critical to the success of ChIP experiment. Antibody should not crossreact with other proteins. Hence, it is better to raise antibody from a peptide rather than the whole protein. Monoclonal antibodies are best suited for ChIP experiment but then it will result in less amount of immunoprecipitated chromatin. The chances of success of using a particular antibody are first determined by immunoprecipitating the protein from cell lysates and by performing EMSA supershift.

The ChIP-PCR technique is the most widely used ChIP application. The presence of a huge array of post-translational modifications of N-terminal tail of histones at different chromatin locus in a large number of organisms and cell lines has been studied in relation to different contexts using ChIP-PCR. The N-terminal tails of the histones and its associated modification are highly conserved and the best quality antibodies against them are commercially available. That is why such studies have been implicated to a large range of eukaryotes. For animal system, a large range of ChIP quality antibodies against various proteins are available. For systems like plants, where very few specific antibodies are available, developing ChIP quality antibody is a tedious job. One alternative is to make constructs with the target protein tagged to a known peptide (Like FLAG or HA) and then perform ChIP in cells transformed with such chimeric constructs using antibodies against the tag. The binding of TCP-20 to ribosomal protein promoters in *Arabidopsis* fast cycling cells was observed by ChIP-PCR using antibody against HA-tag TCP20 that was used to transform these cell lines.

In humans, RUNX1 is an important transcription factor and is also a tumour suppressor and developmental determinant. RUNX1 has been shown to bind to protein kinase Cβ by ChIP-PCR in U397 cells transfected with FLAG tagged RUNX1 and using anti-Flag antibody. While performing ChIP certain controls need to be considered. A small aliquot of the chromatin is taken out before immunoprecipitation step (input control). A PCR with the input control should always amplify a specific DNA region and provides us the information about the relative amount of chromatin that has been used for the ChIP experiment. To one sample no antibody (mock control) or a negative antibody (negative control) is added and theoretically should not give any PCR product or if it does, the amount should be significantly lower than the signals from the immunoprecipitated samples. A PCR for a region of the DNA where the specific sequence is known to bind should also be performed to be used as the internal control. A detailed methodology for quantitative analysis and data normalization for ChIP-PCR is also available.

For a genome wide analysis of the targets of particular transcription factor, ChIP cloning or ChIP-on-Chip is done. For ChIP-cloning and ChIP-microarray, the first step is to generate blunt ends (as sonication results in overhanging ends) by end filling with T4 DNA polymerase. The ChIP-on Chip is done with genomic tilling microarray (microarray prepared from intergenic portions of the genome). One of the successful methods involve amplification of the ChIP DNA, before performing microarray, using LMPCR. After blunting, a unidirectional double stranded linker is ligated to the blunt ends and then the DNA is amplified using PCR. The PCR products of immunoprecipitated DNA is then labelled with Cy5 and that of input sample is labelled with Cy3. The labelled DNA is then subjected to genomic tilling microarray to find the target regions of a specific protein within the genome. Such a protocol is described in detail at http://www.genomecenter.ucdavis.edu/farnham/protocols.html. The regulatory network of Rel/NFkappaB has been recently established using ChIP-on-Chip method. For ChIP-cloning, after blunting, the DNA is ligated to adapter having cleaved restriction enzyme sites and then cloned in suitable vectors or is subjected to A-tailing by Taq DNA polymerase and then cloned in a TA-cloning vector. The sequences are then aligned to find the common element. For example, in *Oryza,* the centromeres of rice have two conserved components centromeric retrotransposons (CRR) and a 155 bp satellite repeat (CentO). For few species, CentO was not reported. A ChIP cloning was carried out with antibodies against CenH3 (which interacts with CentO) and three CenO fragment were discovered in *Oryza rhizomatis* and *Oryza brachyantha;* (species where CentO was not reported earlier. All ChIP studies involving CenH3 in rice has been done using N-ChIP. In summary, ChIP is powereful technique, which if standardized properly, will directly locate the DNA regions in the genome which are involved in interaction of a specific protein.

YEAST ONE-HYBRID SYSTEM

Yeast one-hybrid system has been developed to trap specific DNA binding protein and is a modification of yeast two-hybrid system which is generally used to study the protein-protein interaction. Figure 5.11 describes the yeast one-hybrid system. For this, a cDNA library is made in fusion with GAL4 transcription factor activation domain. The specific DNA element for which the binding protein needs to be screened out is then cloned in another plasmid in multiple copies adjacent to a yeast minimal promoter which is tagged to a reporter gene. Each of these plasmids have their own selection markers. Upon co-transformation with these two plasmids, the clones of the cDNA library having the specific region to bind the DNA element in question will bind to the same element in the other plasmid. Upon binding, the GAL4 activation domain will activate the reporter gene. The colonies are then finally screened on a medium specific for the three markers (triple drop out). From the appeared colonies, the plasmid is isolated and sequenced to know the protein factor which is further needed to be confirmed by assays like EMSA and chromatin immunoprecipitation as the appearance of false positive is a common problem associated with yeast two-hybrid and yeast one-hybrid systems.

This assay has been used to identify transcription factors from various organisms. Very recently a jasmonic acid inducible novel *Tc*AP2 transcription factor from *Taxus cuspidata* has been cloned using yeast one-hybrid system. A modified yeast one-hybrid system has been developed to find different kinds of DNA binding proteins. A method has been developed to screen CG methylated DNA binding protein. In such a system, LexA fused M.SssI DNA methyltransferase is recruited to the LexA operator sequences adjacent to the bait DNA (target site). Using this system, methyl

DNA binding protein MBD1 and Kaiso were screened out. In another modification, mutation in the ligand binding domain of estrogen receptor was screened out. It was found that a fusion protein consisting of the GAL4 DNA-binding domain and the estrogen receptor can interact with a GAL4 upstream activating sequence and induce the expression of an integrated GALI-IacZ gene only in the presence of estradiol. Using this, mutations affecting the transactivational activity were screened. Thus, yeast one-hybrid system provides an *in vivo* system to screen DNA binding proteins and its modifications could be used for various other applications.

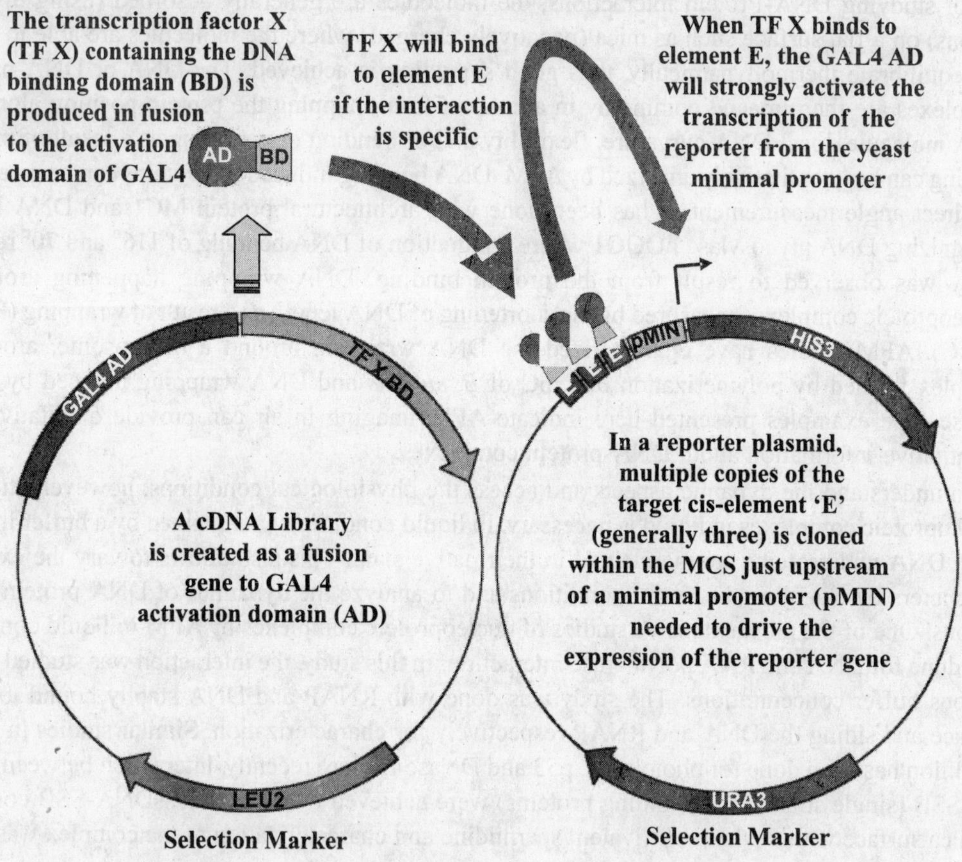

Figure 5.11 **A schematic representation showing the principle of yeast one-hybrid system.** The selection markers HIS3, LEU2 and URA3 codes for Histidine, Leucine and Uracil respectively.

ATOMIC FORCE MICROSCOPY (AFM) IMAGING

AFM imaging is a unique direct visualization technique that is used to characterize mechanism involved in DNA-protein recognition and DNA-protein complex formation in different conditions (air and liquid). A schematic representation of the cross-sectional view of a AFM is shown in Figure 5.12A. To obtain atomic scale resolution by AFM, a sharp stylus (tip) is attached to a cantilever which is used to scan an object (done by a piezoelectric tube) and contouring it while a constant small force is applied to the stylus (Figure 5.12B). A laser is reflected from the back of the cantilever onto a position-sensitive detector. AFM tips and cantilever are microfabricated from Si to Si_3N_4. The tip radius ranges from a few to tens of nanometer. The force between the tip and the sample is calculated indirectly by measuring the deflection of the lever and knowing the stiffness of the cantilever using the formula $F = -kz$ (Hooks law), where F is the force, k is the stiffness of the lever and z is the distance the lever is bent.

For studying DNA-Protein interactions, the molecules are generally adsorbed (using divalent cations) on a flat surface such as mica (negatively charged) where the molecules are able to move and equilibrate thermodynamically, thus good spreading is achieved. The DNA or DNA-protein complexes are then imaged commonly in air. Apart from mapping the protein position along the DNA molecule, local DNA curvature, flexibility and/or bending or wrapping as a result of protein binding can be quantitatively analyzed by AFM. DNA bending induced by proteins can be measured by direct angle measurement as has been done with architectural protein MC1 and DNA lesion recognizing DNA glycosylase hOGG1 where a induction of DNA bending of 116° and 70° respectively was observed to result from the protein binding. DNA wrapping happening around a nucleoproteic complex is measured by the shortening of DNA length as a result of wrapping (Figure 5.12 C). AFM studies have characterized the DNA wrapping around a nucleosome, around a complex formed by polymerization of LrpC of *B. subtilis* and DNA wrapping induced by DNA gyrase. The examples presented here indicate AFM imaging in air can provide qualitative and quantitative information about DNA-protein complexes.

To understand the dynamic aspects and access the physiological conditions, however, study of nucleoproteic complexes in liquid is necessary. In liquid conditions (maintained by a buffer in fluid cell), DNA and proteins are maintained in their native state. This also allows to vary the external parameters by changing the buffer conditions and to analyze the dynamics of DNA protein interactions. One of the most extensive studies of nucleoproteic complexes by AFM in liquid condition was done for DNA and RNA polymerase interaction. In this study, the interaction was studied under various buffer concentrations. The study was done with RNAP and DNA stabily bound to mica surface and siding the DNA and RNAP respectively for characterization. Similar studies in liquid condition has been done for photolyase, p53 and DNase I. More recently, interaction between DNA and SSB (single strand DNA binding proteins) were achieved by adsorbing ssDNA-SSB complex to mica surface with the help of trivalent spermidine and characterization of the complex was done at low and high ionic strength and for various monovalent salt concentration.

With the cantilever of AFM (spring constant near to 10pN/nm), piconewton range of forces of interaction between DNA and protein can be measured. "Force distance curve" (using Hooke's law) with piconewton range force resolution and sub-nanometer distance resolution is obtained when cantilever tip covalently attached with ligand is brought near to the surface where it interacts with its target to form a complex and then retracts from the sample. The complex is increasingly loaded upon retraction until ruptures. By repeating the same process, distribution of unbinding force probability is obtained from which the thermodynamic parameters related to the energy barriers involved in the interaction can be estimated. This methodology has been used to study the interaction between ExpG of *Sinorhizobium meliloti* and three domains of a promoter region. AFM,

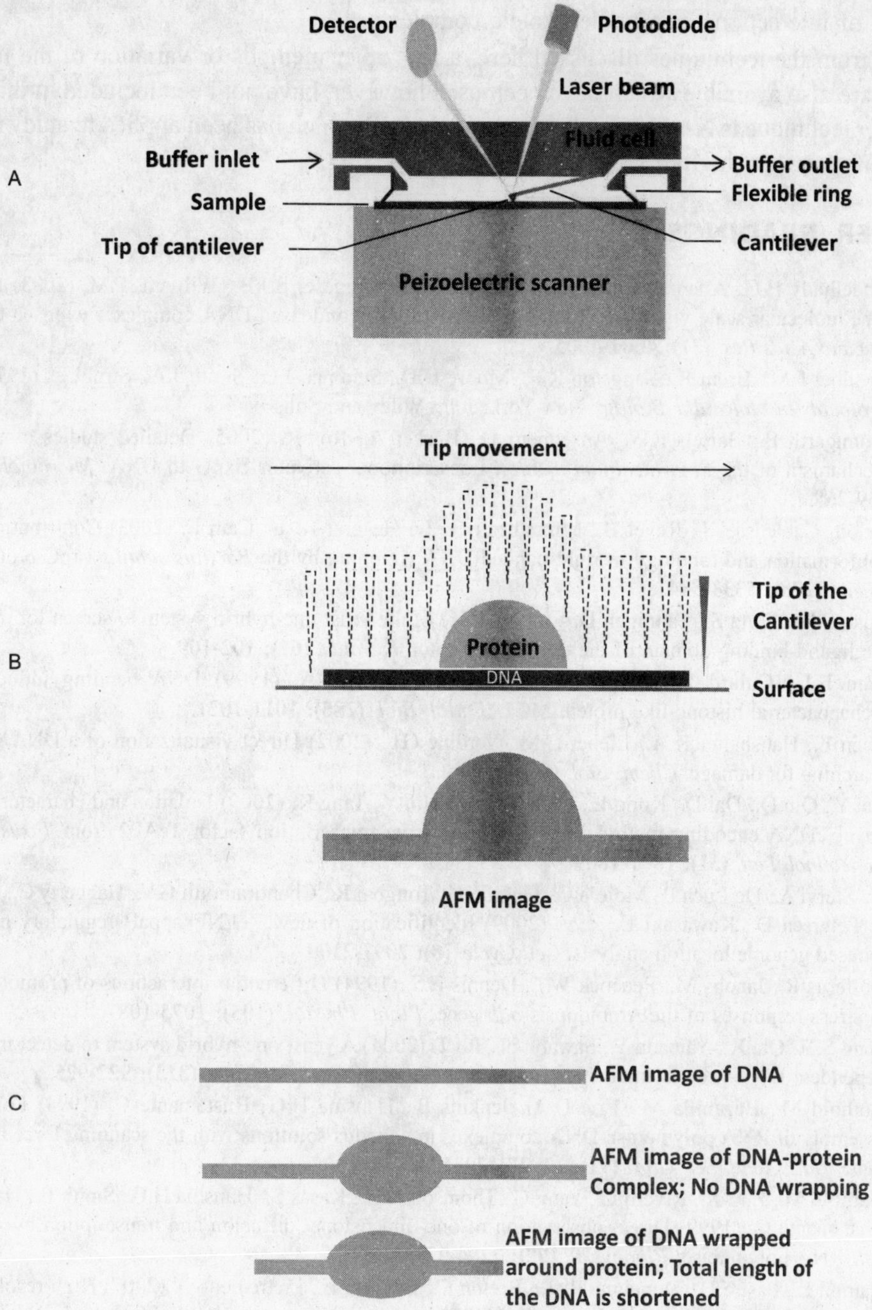

Figure 5.12 A schematic representation analysing DNA-protein interaction using AFM. **(A)** shows a transverse section of AFM instrument. **(B)** shows the principle of imaging a DNA protein complex by AFM. **(C)** Shows the principle of detecting DNA wrapping around a protein.

thus, provides a high resolution method to study the DNA protein interaction and also to measure the force of interaction for a nucleoproteic complex.

Apart from the techniques discussed here, a few other methods or variation of the mentioned methods are also available which have been used however, have not been included in this chapter. One major technique is X-ray crystallography and NMR which has been applied to study the DNA-protein interaction at highest resolution.

FURTHER READINGS

1. Abdelhady H.G., Allen S., Davies M.C., Roberts C.J., Tendler S.J.B., Williams P.M. (2003) Direct real-time molecular scale visualisation of the degradation of condensed DNA complexes exposed to DNase I. *Nucleic Acids Res.* **(31):** 4001-4005.
2. Ausubel F.M., Brent R., Kingston R.E., Moore D.D., Seidman J.G., Smith J.A., Struhl K. (1994) *Current Protocols in Molecular Biology* New York: John Wiley and Sons.
3. Baumgarth B., Bartels F.W., Anselmetti D., Becker A., Ros R. (2005) Detailed studies of the binding mechanism of the *Sinorhizobium meliloti* transcriptional activator ExpG to DNA. *Microbiology.* **(151):** 259-268.
4. Beloin C., Jeusset J., Revet B., Mirambeau G., Le Hegarat F., Le Cam E. (2003) Contribution of DNA conformation and topology in right-handed DNA wrapping by the *Bacillus subtilis* LrpC protein. *J. Biol Chem.* **(278):** 5333-5342.
5. Bush S.M., Folta S., Lannigan D.A. (1996) Use of the yeast one-hybrid system to screen for mutations in the ligand-binding domain of the estrogen receptor. *Steroids.* **(61):** 102-109.
6. Cam E.L., Culard F., Larquet E., Delain E., Cognet J.A. (1999) DNA bending induced by the archaebacterial histone-like protein MC1. *J. Mol. Biol.* **(285):** 1011-1021.
7. Chen L., Haushalter K.A., Lieber C.M., Verdine G.L. (2002) Direct visualization of a DNA glycosylase searching for damage. *Chem. Biol.* **(9):** 345-350.
8. Dai Y., Qin Q., Dai D., Kong L., Li W., Zha X., Jin Y., Tang K. (2009) Isolation and characterization of a novel cDNA encoding methyl jasmonate-responsive transcription factor TcAP2 from *Taxus cuspidata. Biotechnol. Lett.* **(31):** 1801-1809
9. De Siervi A., De Luca P., Moiola C., Gueron G., Tongbai R., Chandramouli G.V., Haggerty C., Dzekunova I., Petersen D., Kawasaki E. *et al.* (2009) Identification of new Rel/NFkappaB regulatory networks by focused genome location analysis. *Cell Cycle.* **(8):** 2093-2100.
10. Dolferus R., Jacobs M., Peacock W.J., Dennis E.S. (1994) Differential interactions of promoter elements in stress responses of the Arabidopsis *adh* gene. *Plant. Physiol.* **(105):** 1075-1087.
11. Feng S.Y., Ota K., Yamada Y., Sawabu N., Ito T. (2004) A yeast one-hybrid system to detect methylation-dependent DNA-protein interactions. *Biochem. Biophys. Res. Commun.* **(313):** 922-925.
12. Guthold M., Bezanilla M., Erie D.A., Jenkins B., Hansma H.G., Bustamante C. (1994) Following the assembly of RNA polymerase-DNA complexes in aqueous solutions with the scanning force microscope. *Proc. Natl. Acad. Sci. USA.* **(91):** 12927-12931.
13. Guthold M., Zhu X., Rivetti C., Yang G., Thomson N.H., Kasas S., Hansma H.G., Smith B., Hansma P.K., Bustamante C. (1999) Direct observation of one-dimensional diffusion and transcription by *Escherichia coli* RNA polymerase. *Biophys. J.* **(77):** 2284-2294.
14. Hamon L., Pastre D., Dupaigne P., Le Breton C., Le Cam E., Pietrement O. (2007) High-resolution AFM imaging of single-stranded DNA-binding (SSB) protein–DNA complexes. *Nucleic Acids Res.* **(35):** e58.
15. Haring M., Offermann S., Danker T., Horst I., Peterhansel C., Stam M. (2007) Chromatin immunoprecipitation: optimization, quantitative analysis and data normalization. *Plant Methods.* **(3):** 11.

16. Heddle J.G., Mitelheiser S., Maxwell A, Thomson N.H. (2004) Nucleotide binding to DNA gyrase causes loss of DNA wrap. *J. Mol. Biol.* **(337):** 597-610.
17. Hettiarachchi G.H., Yadav V., Reddy M.K., Chattopadhyay S., Sopory S.K. (2003) Light-mediated regulation defines a minimal promoter region of TOP2. *Nucleic. Acids. Res.* **(31):** 5256-5265.
18. Hug B.A., Ahmed N., Robbins J.A., Lazar M.A. (2004) A chromatin immunoprecipitation screen reveals protein kinase Cbeta as a direct RUNX1 target gene. *J. Biol. Chem.* **(279):** 825-830.
19. Jiao Y., Cherny D.I., Heim G., Jovin T.M., Schäffer T.E.. (2001). Dynamic interactions of p53 with DNA in solution by time-lapse atomic force microscopy. *J. Mol. Biol.* **(314):** 233-243.
20. Kochanek S., Renz D., Doerfler W. (1995) Transcriptional silencing of human Alu sequences and inhibition of protein binding in the box B regulatory elements by 5'-CG-3' methylation. *FEBS Lett* **(360):** 115-120.
21. Kosugi S., Ohashi Y. (1997) PCF1 and PCF2 specifically bind to cis elements in the rice proliferating cell nuclear antigen gene. *Plant Cell.* **(9):** 1607-1619.
22. Lee H.R., Zhang W., Langdon T., Jin W., Yan H., Cheng Z., Jiang J. (2005) Chromatin immunoprecipitation cloning reveals rapid evolutionary patterns of centromeric DNA in *Oryza* species. *Proc. Natl. Acad. Sci. USA.* **(102):** 11793-11798.
23. Li C., Potuschak T., Colón-Carmona A., Gutiérrez R.A., Doerner P. (2005) *Arabidopsis* TCP20 links regulation of growth and cell division control pathways. *Proc. Natl. Acad. Sci. USA.* **(102):** 12978-12983.
24. Szabo P.E., Pfeifer G.P., Miao F., O'Connor T.R., Mann J.R. (2000) Improved *in vivo* Dimethyl Sulfate Footprinting Using AlkA Protein: DNA-Protein Interactions at the Mouse H19 Gene Promoter in Primary Embryo Fibroblasts. *Anal. Biochem.* **(283):** 112-116.
25. Tatematsu K., Ward S., Leyser O., Kamiya Y., Nambara E. (2005) Identification of cis-Elements That Regulate Gene Expression during Initiation of Axillary Bud Outgrowth in *Arabidopsis*. *Plant Physiol.* **(138):** 757-766.
26. van Noort S.J., van der Werf K.O., Eker A.P., Wyman C., de Grooth B.G., van Hulst N.F., Greve J. (1998) Direct visualization of dynamic protein-DNA interactions with a dedicated atomic force microscope. *Biophys. J.* **(74):** 2840-2849.
27. Yaden B.C., Garcia M., 3rd, Smith T.P., Rhodes S.J. (2006) Two promoters mediate transcription from the human LHX3 gene: involvement of nuclear factor I and specificity protein 1. *Endocrinology.* **(147):** 324-337.
28. Yang T., Poovaiah B.W. (2002) A calmodulin-binding/CGCG box DNA-binding protein family involved in multiple signaling pathways in plants. *J. Biol. Chem.* **(277):** 45049-45058.
29. Zhang X., Fletcher S.A., Csonka L.N. (1996) Site-directed mutational analysis of the osmotically regulated proU promoter of *Salmonella typhimurium. J. Bacteriol.* **(178):** 3377-3379.

CHAPTER

6

Genomics Technology

Genomics is the study of the genomes of organisms. The field includes intensive efforts to determine the entire DNA sequence of organisms and fine-scale genetic mapping efforts. The field also includes studies of intragenomic phenomena such as heterosis, epistasis, pleiotropy and other interactions between loci and alleles within the genome. In contrast, the investigation of the roles and functions of single genes is a primary focus of molecular biology or genetics and is a common topic of modern medical and biological research. Research of single genes does not fall into the definition of genomics unless the aim of this genetic, pathway, and functional information analysis is to elucidate its effect on, place in, and response to the entire genome's networks. For the United States Environmental Protection Agency, the term "genomics" encompasses a broader scope of scientific inquiry associated technologies than when genomics was initially considered. A genome is the sum total of all individual organism's genes. Thus, genomics is the study of all the genes of a cell, or tissue, at the DNA (genotype), mRNA (transcriptome), or protein (proteome) levels".

Keywords: Genomics, genome, genotype.

INTRODUCTION

Genomics, the term coined by T.H. Roderick in 1987, refers to the study of genome which is an entire complement of chromosomal and extrachromosomal genes present in an organism. It mainly includes genetic mapping and complete sequencing of the genome with an objective to understand organization and function of complete genetic information contained in the organism, to study the interactions among genes and gene products, to perform comparative study of genomes and analyse the evolution of genomes. The determination of complete genome sequence of desired organism serves as raw material to perform above processes. The first DNA-based genome sequencing of bacteriophage Φ-X174 was performed by Frederick Sanger in 1977. Since 1995, when complete genome sequence was determined for the first free-living organism, *Haemophilus influenza*, a number of genomes have been sequenced for different organisms. By the end of 2007, the complete genomes of about 1879 viruses, 577 bacterial species and around 23 eukaryotes were sequenced. Most of the bacterial genomes that have been completely sequenced are disease-causing agents like *Haemophilus influenza*, *Plasmodium* and *Mycobacterium*. Of the other species, genomes of *Saccharomyces cerevisiae*, *Drosophila melanogaster*, *Caenorhabditis elegans*, *Mus musculus*, *Homo sapiens*, *Arabidopsis thaliana*, *Oryza sativa*, *Vitis vinifera*, *Populus* etc. have been completely sequenced. This huge biological sequence information obtained from sequencing projects is available online in the form of various databases. These data are extremely important for researchers in veterinary, agriculture and medicine to understand the functions of key genes and proteins involved in growth, development and resistance to numerous diseases and unfavorable conditions. However, there exists a wide gap between genotype and phenotype in manifestation of a trait. To fill this gap, research is conducted at different levels—whole plant, cellular, biochemical, gene and protein levels. All these areas of unparalleled scientific efforts further increase the amount of biological information. The need to handle, store and analyze this biological information has led to evolution of a new field of science known as "Bioinformatics", which performs this job through computer software and programs. Enhanced bioinformatic tools along with genome research have facilitated the identification of suitable candidate genes and gene products, which can be precisely manipulated in a biological system so as to produce a desirable product or phenotype. This has also triggered paradigm shift from single gene approach (i.e., gene by gene approach) in understanding the mechanism of biological phenomenon to working with several genes at a time. This shift has resulted from the observation that any biological response results from cross talk of many biomolecules, which act in interdependent manner. Many high throughput technologies under the field of genomics have potential to provide holistic view of molecules involved in the mechanism of some recalcitrant problems of agricultural and medicinal importance. Therefore, the development of superior designer crops resistant to various biotic and abiotic stresses, or design of effective medicines, vaccine and gene therapy has now become possible with the advent of genomics.

CONCEPTS

Genomics can broadly be divided into two main categories as "structural genomics" and "functional genomics". Structural genomics includes construction of high resolution genetic and physical map, determination of complete genome sequence and determination of structures of proteins encoded by the genes. Construction of physical or genetic map helps in assembly of genome sequences. One of the aims of structural genomics is to unravel the protein structure, which is a powerful means of discovering the gene's function through detection of homology between protein structures. Since the protein structures are evolutionally conserved, this method enables to detect homologies that otherwise are undetectable through simple gene sequence comparisons. For example, although horse hemoglobin and whale sperm myoglobin gene sequences are different, they were shown to be homologues and to have identical function by comparison of their protein structures.

The knowledge of complete genome sequences has led to the development of functional genomics, which studies gene expression pattern and gene functions. Functional genomics utilizes the holistic genome based experimental approaches to assess the gene functions by utilizing the data generated by structural genomics. Thus, it aims at shifting the biological investigation from studying single gene, its transcript and protein product to all genes, transcripts and proteins simultaneously and thus narrows down the gap between the sequence and its possible function. Functional genomics thus also includes transcriptomics, which is the study of whole transcripts encoded by the genome, and proteomics, which is the study of all the proteins encoded by the genome.

PRINCIPLES

The genes present in an organism are encoded by its genomic DNA, which is first copied into an intermediate, RNA, and the RNA molecules are used to make proteins that carry out the basic processes of life. In general, a gene is the stretch of DNA, including regulatory elements that specifies a RNA or protein. A key question regarding the behavior of biological system is to understand how the expression of different genes is regulated under different environmental conditions and how different proteins collaborate to perform a particular task. The first step toward answering these questions is determination of a genome's complete sequence. A prerequisite for any genome sequencing is to construct its genetic or physical map based on the molecular markers or the cloned DNA fragments aligned to the chromosomes. Mapping is done at different levels using various resources and techniques such as Restriction Fragment Length Polymorphism (RFLP), Amplified Fragment Length Polymorphism (AFLP), Random Amplified Polymorphic DNA (RAPD), Microsatellites like Simple Sequence Repeats (SSRs) and Simple Sequence Length Polymorphism (SSLP), Cleaved Amplified Polymorphic Sequences (CAPS), and Single Nucleotide Polymorphism (SNP). Complete physical and genetic maps of human, mouse, rice, tomato, potato, pepper and several microorganisms are available. A complete physical map consisting of ordered recombinant genomic clones spanning an entire genome is essential. A high resolution physical map at the level of DNA length directly provides DNA clones located at distinct positions of the genome for further study. Physical mapping with YAC/BAC/PAC-based large insert clones ensures to revolutionize genomics of large and complex genomes. BAC (Bacterial Artificial Chromosome) based physical maps of *Drosophila melanogaster*, human, *Arabidopsis* and rice were used as templates in sequence finishing. The cytogenetic maps could be intermediates between physical and genetic maps showing approximate locations of genes and molecular markers, heterochromatin bands and secondary constriction on any chromosome. Cytogenetic maps link together the information from linkage maps and the distribution of crossover-events and physical maps.

Once the genome has been mapped, it acts as a blueprint for sequencing. In the past recent years, development of several advanced techniques for DNA sequencing has enabled sequencing of large DNA fragments and even complete genomes. An important step towards the large-scale sequencing is the development of automated DNA sequencers based on Sanger technology and Pyrosequencing.

A 'completed' genome sequence is the one that is contiguous without any gaps in between and is a rarely possible situation. Even if each base of a genome has been determined, there are still likely to be errors present because of some limitations of the present sequencing technology. The proportion of a genome that codes for genes is usually very small. It is not possible to sequence only the coding regions present on a genome. Therefore, sequencing of entire transcriptome of an organism having a cumbersome genome would be a logical step. This can be well achieved by developing "Expressed Sequence Tags" (ESTs). ESTs are single pass sequences of cloned mRNAs (cDNA clone taken from a cDNA library). A large number of EST sequences from many animal and plant species are available in the databases. As enormous information regarding the role of noncoding DNA (often called junk DNA) is being generated, it is becoming more important to have a complete genome sequence as a background for understanding the genetics and biology of any given organism.

Genome sequences are used first to predict the set of possible proteins, which are compared with all known sequences in central databases. In many instances, for approximately half of the proteins, there is a reasonable match to a previously sequenced protein from another organism. Since the functions of many proteins have already been determined in some organisms, and similarity in sequence generally reflects similarity in function, these database comparisons can at least partially interpret a substantial fraction of the genome. But how are the functions of the many uncharacterized genes on a genomewide basis?

Screening of mutants induced by insertion element, followed by isolation of causative genes using these sequences as molecular tags (called gene tagging), is one of the most important methods for functional characterization of genes in plants. The insertion sequences that are commonly used for mutagenesis include transposable elements and T-DNA (transfer-DNA). Many of the important genes from plants such as phytochrome A *(phyA)*, zeaxanthin epoxidase (*OsABA1*) and *OsTATC* showing homology to bacterial Sec-independent translocase *TATC* have been cloned using gene tagging method. Another most widely used method for isolation and functional characterization of genes in plants is "map-based cloning". "Positional cloning" or "map-based cloning" is an indirect approach, which utilizes the genetic mapping of the allele or mutation by successively excluding all other parts of the genome. Once the interval is defined, the mutated gene is identified and isolated from YAC/BAC large insert libraries. By crossing the mutant and wild type plants, a segregating population is generated followed by the assignment of the approximate position to the mutation on the genetic map by identifying linked markers by segregant analysis. Finally, the mutation containing region is further narrowed down by process of fine-mapping. A number of agronomically important genes such as *pto*, receptor kinase-like protein gene *Xa21*, disease resistance genes like *Xa1*, *Xa5* and *Xa26*(t), stem rust resistance genes *Rpg1* and *Rpg4*, tospovirus resistance gene (*Sw-5*) from different plant species have been identified and characterized by positional or map-based cloning. Several other important genes such as pyridoxal kinase gene (*SOS4*) required for root hair development, *KNAT1* and *ERECTA* genes regulating inflorescence architecture, *PICKLE* gene responsible for embryonic to vegetative development and *COBRA* genes involved in cell expansion have also been identified by this approach.

With the discovery of double-stranded RNA-mediated gene silencing, targeted disruption of expression of individual genes has become possible. This newly discovered biological phenomenon called RNA interference (RNAi) has practical implications for functional genomics. RNA interference has been proved to be a rapid method to test gene functions in a high throughput fashion in the nematode *Caenorhabditis elegans*. Most of the genes on *C.elegans* chromosome I and III were tested for knockout phenotypes utilizing the RNAi phenomenon. Important insight into gene function is gained by expression profiling. For example, many genes are up-regulated or certain other genes are down-regulated by external signals. Many genes have developmental stage or cell-type-specific expression in multicellular organisms. Northern blotting, reverse northern blotting, nuclease protection assay, reverse transcriptase polymerase chain reaction and western blotting are traditional ways of gene expression analyses. These techniques give opportunity to study only one gene at a time. In the recent years, advancements in the technology have made possible to study the expression of thousands of genes simultaneously. Serial analysis of gene expression (SAGE) and microarrays are such powerful tools to study global gene expression. SAGE takes advantage of high throughput sequencing to obtain a quantitative profile of cellular gene expression. In SAGE, concatemers of short tags of cDNA are produced, cloned and sequenced, which ultimately determine the level of gene expression in an organism at a particular stage/environmental condition. Expression profiles of tens of thousands of genes can be monitored simultaneously in a single attempt using microarray technique. GeneChip (DNA microarray) has become a key tool in the area of functional genomics. DNA/cDNA or oligonucleotides derived from transcripts are arrayed individually on a solid matrix, which is subsequently probed with labeled cDNAs from total RNA pools representing control and sample tissues. After hybridization, the chips are scanned and analyzed for expression of spotted genes. DNA chips have been successfully used to study developmental responses, interactions of the pathways, transcript regulation in response to biotic and abiotic stresses and disease control.

GENOMICS TECHNOLOGY

Structural Genomics

A plethora of high throughput techniques and instrumentation are currently being utilized in the field of genomics. These techniques include:

(i) mapping the genome;
(ii) sequencing the genome; and
(iii) understanding the genome sequence.

Genome Mapping

The genome mapping is of two types: 1. Genetic mapping and 2. Physical mapping.

Genetic mapping

This includes the use of genetic techniques to show the position of various genetic markers including Restriction fragment length polymorphism (RFLP), Randomly amplified polymorphic DNA (RAPD), Simple sequence length polymorphism (SSLP's) and single nucleotide polymorphism (SNPs). Linkage analysis is the basis of genetic mapping. In this method, parents of known genotypes are crossed and their progenies are analyzed. The genotypes of the gametes resulting from meiosis are analyzed directly by typing the genetic markers by using PCR or restriction digestion. The frequency of recombination that occurs during crossing over stage in meiosis is calculated. A linkage map shows the order of the genetic markers and the distances between them in the form of recombination frequencies, which are expressed in the form of centimorgans (cM). 1 cM is that distance which corresponds to 1% recombination frequency between the markers.

Physical mapping

It utilizes various molecular biological techniques to show the exact location and distance between different markers in base pairs. The physical mapping techniques fall in three categories:

Construction of chromosome specific libraries

In order to facilitate genome mapping process, the library of genomic DNA fragments is constructed by selecting one chromosome at a time. For this, the single chromosome is isolated from the cell by using various techniques, some of which are listed below:

Pulsed field gel electrophoresis (PFGE)

Since chromosomes differ with respect to size and shape, they can be resolved and isolated by following the technique of PFGE.

Fluorescent activated chromosome sorting (FACS)

In this procedure, metaphase chromosomes are stained with a fluorescent dye. Cells are disrupted to release the whole chromosomes in liquid suspension which is diluted so that each droplet contains single chromosome. The droplets containing single chromosome are allowed to pass through a laser beam which excites the fluorescence. Each chromosome has a specific level of fluorescence depending upon which it is deflected in an electric field and collected separately.

Somatic cell hybrid technology

This has been utilized for selecting the specific human chromosome. A specific human chromosome can be selected by fusing the human cell with the rodent cell. The hybrid cell containing a particular chromosome can be selected by utilizing a marker gene on the chromosome that compliments a missing function on the rodent chromosomes.

DNA fragmentation

The genomic DNA obtained from the specific chromosome is fragment by digesting it with restriction endonucleases or a hydroshear can be used to fragment the genomic DNA.

Cloning of DNA fragments

The vectors that can carry large inserts, e.g., YACS, BACS, PACS, or cosmids are utilized to clone the DNA fragments.

Contig development

The cloned DNA fragments are characterized in some way to determine overlaps. On the basis of overlaps, a set of overlapping DNA fragments is determined which is known as contig. Various techniques are used to determine the order of fragments in a contig, which are described below:

Restriction mapping: It locates the relative positions of restriction sites for various restriction endonucleases on a DNA fragment. In this technique, a particular genomic DNA segment is digested with two different restriction endonucleases singly and in combination. Each digested sample is separated using gel electrophoresis, and the sizes of different DNA fragments are compared with each other. Since the size of individual DNA fragment depends upon the positions of restriction site, each restriction site can be mapped according to sizes of the fragments. The data about fragment sizes obtained from double digestion of restriction endonucleases are very crucial in mapping the restriction sites.

Fluorescent in situ hybridization (FISH): It enables the relative positions of different markers to be directly visualized on the chromosome. For this the particular DNA fragment is labeled with a fluorescent probe and is allowed to hybridize with denatured chromosomal preparation. The position at which the probe hybridizes to the chromosomal DNA is visualized by detecting the fluorescence signal emitted by the labeled DNA. The map created by this technique is known as cytogenetic map. FISH is a widely used accurate cytogenetic tool for mapping single copy sequences and repetitive DNA sequences on chromosomes. Various plants such as maize, tomato, wheat, rye and rice serve as model species for such cytogenetic studies.

Related to FISH (Fluorescence *in situ* Hybridization), there is a technique known as GISH (Genomic *in situ* Hybridization) where whole genomic DNA from one species is labeled and used as a probe to find out alien chromosomes in other species. GISH allows chromosomes from different parents or ancestors to be distinguished by means of differential hybridization of entire genomic probes. Using this technique it is possible to determine the genome origin of paired and unpaired chromosomes in hybrids at metaphase.

STS content mapping: STSs are sequence tagged sites that are short sequences detected by PCR using STS specific primers. ESTs (expressed sequence tags) are STSs from the transcribed region of the genome. The physical location of a particular STS can be determined on a large DNA fragment by FISH. A clone library contains different DNA fragments whose relative order and position on a given large DNA segment remains unknown. STS content mapping can be utilized to order the cloned DNA fragments on the underlying DNA segment and builds a physical map for ordered cloned DNA fragments. The procedure first determines which cloned DNA fragments contain which STS. This can be easily achieved by performing PCR using STS specific primers and the cloned DNA fragment as template. PCR will amplify the STS only if it is present in the DNA fragment. By running down this experiment for the pair of cloned DNA fragments, a data is generated that is used to order the DNA fragments present in the cloned library.

Genome Sequencing

The genome can be sequenced in two steps: first step is DNA fragmentation followed by their cloning and amplification under *in vitro* conditions and second step is use of a suitable method of sequencing.

Cloning and amplification of DNA fragments to be sequenced

The genomic DNA is fragmented with the help of a suitable restriction endonuclease enzyme, then cloned into a plasmid vector and introduced in to host bacterial cell such *E. coli*. The plasmid DNA is isolated from individual bacterial colony and sequencing is preformed by using a suitable method.

Methods for sequencing

Two different techniques exist for sequencing the genome: (1) The chain termination method by Sanger *et. al.* 1977 and (2) Maxam and Gilbert's chemical degradation method. However, the former method has been widely used for genome sequencing projects because of its ease and complete automation.

The chain termination method

In Sanger's chain termination method, the DNA strand is treated with a variety of nucleotides, a set of enzymes, and a specific primer to generate a collection of smaller DNA fragments. Four fluorescent tags, each specific for a given base, are part of the mixture. Each of the fragments differs in length by one base and is marked with a fluorescent tag that identifies the last base of the fragment. The fragments are then separated according to size and passed by a detector that reads the fluorescent tag. Then, a computer reconstructs the entire sequence of the long DNA

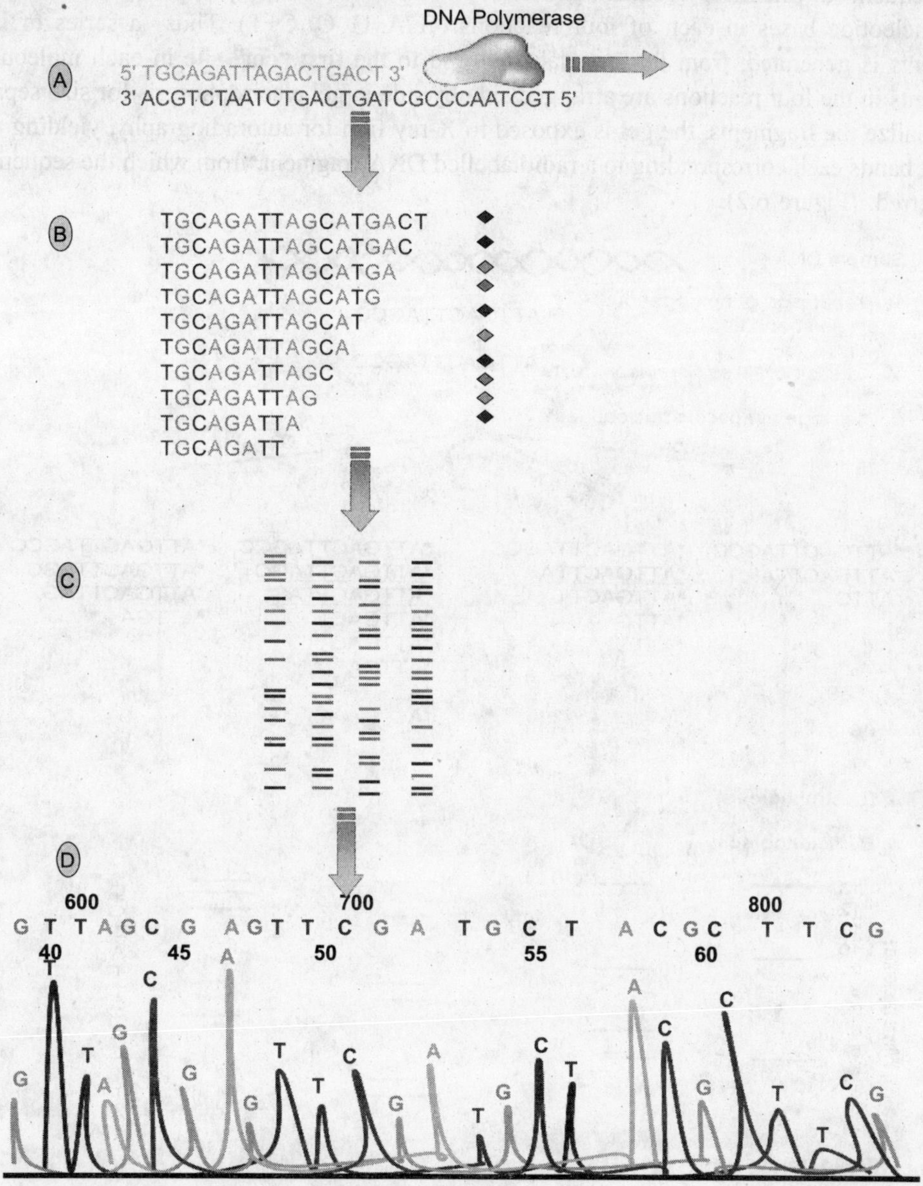

Figure 6.1 Chain termination method to sequence DNA.

strand by identifying the base at each position from the size of each fragment and the particular fluorescent signal at its end (Figure 6.1).

Maxam Gilbert's chemical degradation method

This was the first method developed in 1976-77 to determine the sequence of DNA molecule of upto 500bp. It is based on chemical modification of DNA and subsequent cleavage at specific bases. This process requires radioactive labelling at one end and purification of the DNA fragment to be sequenced. Chemical treatment generates breaks at a small proportion of one or two of the four nucleotide bases in each of four reactions (G, A+G, C, C+T). Thus a series of labelled fragments is generated, from the radiolabelled end to the first "cut" site in each molecule. The fragments in the four reactions are arranged side by side in gel electrophoresis for size separation. To visualize the fragments, the gel is exposed to X-ray film for autoradiography, yielding a series of dark bands each corresponding to a radiolabelled DNA fragment, from which the sequence may be inferred. (Figure 6.2)

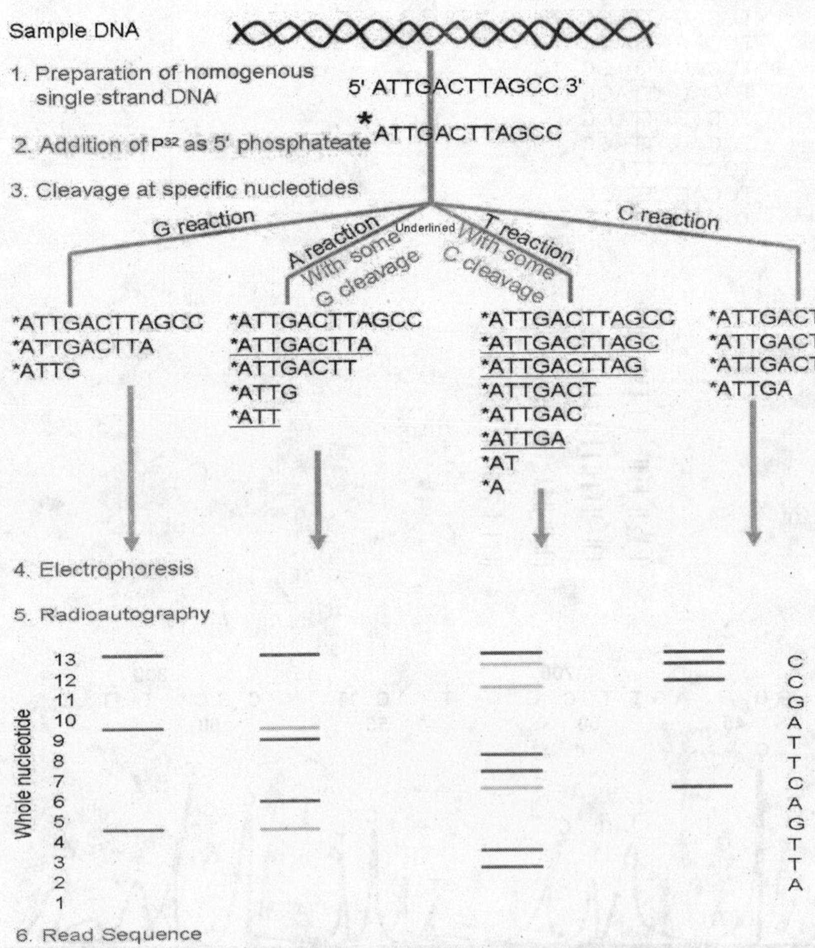

Figure 6.2 Maxam and Gilbert's chemical degradation method.

Automated DNA sequencing

Automated DNA sequencing utilizes fluorescent tracers instead of radioisotopes to label the DNA which is mainly used in conventional DNA sequencing techniques thereby reducing the use of radioactive materials in some research laboratories. Modern automated DNA sequencing instruments (DNA sequencers) can sequence up to 384 fluorescently labelled samples in a single batch (run) and perform as many as 24 runs a day. It can carry out only DNA size separation by capillary electrophoresis, detection and recording of dye fluorescence, and data output as fluorescent peak trace chromatograms. In dye-terminator sequencing, each of the four dideoxynucleotide chain terminators is labelled with a different fluorescent dye, each fluorescing at a different wavelength, resulting in unequal peak heights and shapes in the electronic DNA sequence trace chromatogram after capillary electrophoresis. It permits sequencing in a single reaction, rather than four reactions as in the labelled-primer method. The dye-terminator sequencing method, along with automated high-throughput DNA sequence analyzers, is now being used for the vast majority of sequencing projects.

Next generation DNA sequencing methods

The pace of data generation from traditional DNA sequencing methods was slow producing 1000 bp per day which led to the development of next generation sequencing platforms available today by which an entire genome can be sequenced in a few days. Following five next generation sequencing platforms are available:

454 Pyrosequencing: The 454 system was the first next generation sequencing platform which utilizes the principle of emulsion PCR and pyrosequencing.

Emulsion PCR: Individual DNA fragments to be sequenced are *in vitro* amplified by Emulsion PCR in which the first step is DNA fragmentation followed by ligation of common adaptors to the fragmented DNA. In the next step, the library of *in vitro* constructed adaptor flanked shotgun library is PCR amplified. For this, the primers specific for adaptor sequences are immobilized on micron scale beads and mixed with DNA fragments along with other PCR reaction components. This is taken in the compartment made up of oil water emulsion and PCR is allowed in that compartment only. The template and bead concentration is adjusted in such a way that each emulsion compartment contains only one template. Thus, this method results in amplification of a single DNA fragment on the surface of a bead within the emulsified compartment. The emulsion is broken to release the bead and pyrosequencing is performed to sequence the fragment on the surface of bead.

Pyrosequencing

This method is based on the detection of pyrophosphate, a byproduct of DNA synthesis, which is converted to adenosine triphosphate (ATP), which then stimulates luciferase activity, causing the emission of a chemiluminescent signal. The reaction includes adenosine 5' phosphosulfate (APS) and ATP sulfurylase, which convert APS into ATP in the presence of pyrophosphate. Also present is luciferin (the substrate of luciferase) and apirase, which continuously degrade unincorporated dNTPs and excess ATP. The dNTPs are added to the reaction one by one, and only complementary dNTP will extend the primer, releasing pyrophosphate in equimolar quantity, thus producing ATP, which generates a chemiluminescent signal (Figure 6.3).

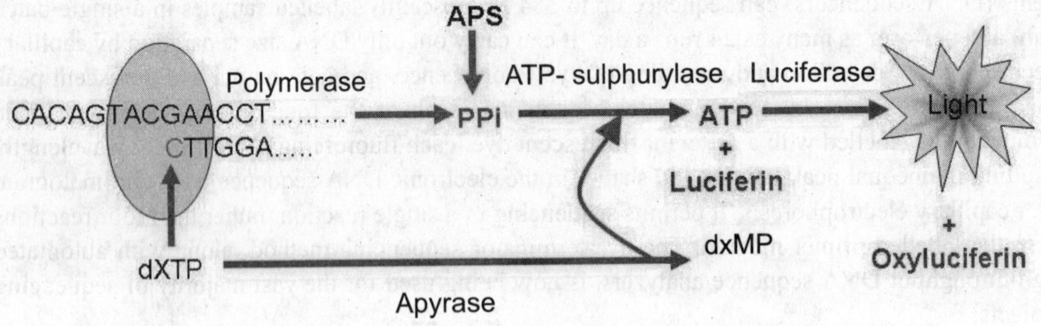

Figure 6.3 Pyrosequencing.

Illumina Genome analyzer

This is commonly referred to as "the Solexa" technology for sequencing. In this method DNA fragments are ligated with specific adaptor fragments and amplified *in vitro* by the method known as bridge PCR. In this approach, primers complementary to adaptors remain attached at their 5' ends on a solid substrate with the help of linkers. One end of DNA fragment becomes attached to the solid surface with the help of adaptor and the other end bends on the surface and pairs with complementary primer leading to formation of a bridge. Next, this bridge is amplified by PCR. In this way, different fragments are amplified on a specific physical location in a solid surface. In order to sequence different fragments, amplified fragments are denatured and a sequencing primer is annealed to the fragment. The sequencing is done by single base extension method carried out with the help of a modified DNA polymerase and a mixture of four modified nucleotides. The four nucleotides are labelled with four different fluorescent dyes and bear a chemical moiety at 3' hydroxyl moiety. This allows the single insertion of nucleotide in each cycle. The identity of incorporated nucleotide is known through detection of fluorescence by an imaging system. After each cycle, the chemical moiety is removed from 3' hydroxyl moiety from incorporated nucleotide and the cycle is repeated.

AB SoLid

This system has been adopted by Applied Biosystems to develop the sequencers. In this method, library of adaptor flanked DNA fragments is constructed by emulsion PCR. After breaking the emulsion, amplicons linked to paramagnetic beads are recovered and immobilized on a solid surface. Sequencing of amplified DNA fragments is done on the surface of beads with the help of a DNA ligase instead of DNA polymerase. In this method, a universal primer is first hybridized with the adaptor sequence and an octamer oligonucleotide is ligated with the primer by DNA ligase. The octamer is fluorscently labeled and structured in such a way that it has central 4th and 5th base available for complementary base pairing. The identity of 4th and 5th base is correlated with fluorescent signal which is obtained when the octamer is hybridized with the complementary fragment. Identity of bases at 4th and 5th position can be disclosed in all the fragments by using a specifically designed octamer. After ligation and imaging the labelled portion of octamer is removed leading to exposure of a free end to which new octamer can be ligated. Thus, the discontinuous sequence of bases in different fragments (i.e. 5th, 10th, 15th .... and so on) can be deciphered with the help of serial ligation of octamers. The system is reset by denaturing the extended primer and by annealing a different primer set back from the original position by one or several bases. Serial ligation of the same set of octamers then leads to interrogation of different set of discontinuous bases. Several such cycles with different primers and octamers lead to deciphering of complete sequence of all DNA fragments.

Polonator

This system is similar to AB SoLid system in that emulsion PCR is used for clonal amplification of DNA fragments and sequencing is done with the help of DNA ligase. However, in this method, nonamers are ligated with primer instead of octamers.

HeliScope

In this technology, the DNA fragments are sequenced without clonal amplification. Poly A tail is added to DNA fragments generated by random DNA fragmentation. Next, they are immobilized on a solid surface through hybridization between poly A tail and poly T oligomers linked with the surface. This generated a set of single copy primed DNA fragments which are to be sequenced. Now DNA polymerase in reaction mixture is added to the platform and incorporation of a fluorescent labelled nucleotide is detected through imaging system. All four fluorescently labelled nucleotides are added one by one in cyclical manner and their incorporation is simulatenously detected in different DNA fragments.

Sequencing Strategies

There is a dramatic difference in size and complexity between the genomes of different organisms. Eukaryotic genome is typically characterized by the presence of large repetitive sequences. Therefore, the strategies for sequencing different genomes have to be different. Several strategies and approaches that are involved in whole genome sequencing include "clone by clone" sequencing, sequence tag connector, random whole genome shotgun sequencing and transposon-mediated genome sequencing. There are two approaches:

Clone contig approach

The "clone-by-clone" strategy involves the construction of genomic DNA libraries in suitable vectors such as PAC (P1 derived Artificial Chromosome) and BAC (Bacterial Artificial Chromosome), which can clone up to 150 kb of DNA fragment. A genetic map would help screening the libraries for picking clones belonging to a particular marker region on a chromosome. A minimum tiling path is constructed covering the entire chromosome having least possible overlaps among the neighbor clones. The clones falling in the minimum tiling path are then picked one by one, and randomly sheared using a sonicator or hydroshear to generate inserts of 2 kb to 5 kb size. These small sheared fragments (derived from PAC or BAC clones) are then ligated with a suitable vector such as pUC or Bluescript to generate a sub-library of clones known as shotgun library. Around 2000-3000 white colonies having insert are then picked and stocked at -80°C. DNA (plasmid) from all the 2000-3000 sub-clones are isolated and sequenced randomly in a high through fashion from both the insert ends using universal vector-specific primers. Sequence reads thus generated are subjected to quality check using PHRED software and finally good quality reads are assembled into contigs using powerful software such as PHRAP or CAP3. Contigs are then oriented and ordered to get the contiguous sequence of the cloned DNA fragment. The gaps present between the contigs are filled by the complete sequencing of the bridge sub-clones (clones joining the two neighbor contigs) or by PCR amplification of the gap region followed by sequencing of the product. Finally, the complete sequence is checked for any error and edited for any discrepancy found.

Shotgun approach

Whole genome shotgun is another widely used strategy for genome sequencing (Figure 6.4). Total genomic DNA isolated from an organism is randomly sheared and sub-cloned in a suitable plasmid vector to construct a shotgun library. Randomly picked clones are stocked, DNA isolated and sequenced from both the ends using vector-specific primers. High throughput sequence data is generated and assembled using assembly software. In this case, minimum tiling path using a large

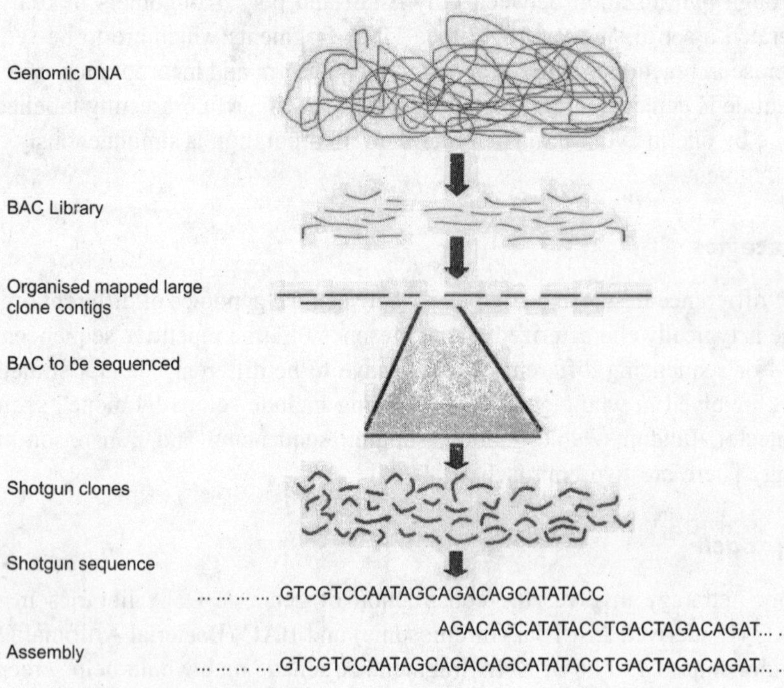

Figure 6.4 Hierarchical shotgun sequencing strategy.

insert library (PAC or BAC vector) for the organism is not prepared. Millions of sequence reads are assembled, which generate thousands of contigs. Now these contigs are anchored on the chromosomes with the help of marker sequences present in the assembled contigs. Most of the time, a large number of contigs remain unanchored and unoriented. As compared to the "clone-by-clone" approach, the gap filling or finishing process is a cumbersome job in "whole genome" shotgun approach. Presence of repeat regions within the genome raises difficulty in proper assembly of the sequence reads into contigs. Mis-assembled sequences are often found in many contigs, which are identified and subsequently re-sequenced using alternative approaches.

Assembly of the Sequence

Various computational methods and sophisticated algorithms are used to identify overlapping DNA sequences and reconstruct the genome by generating a set of scaffolds (Figure 6.5).

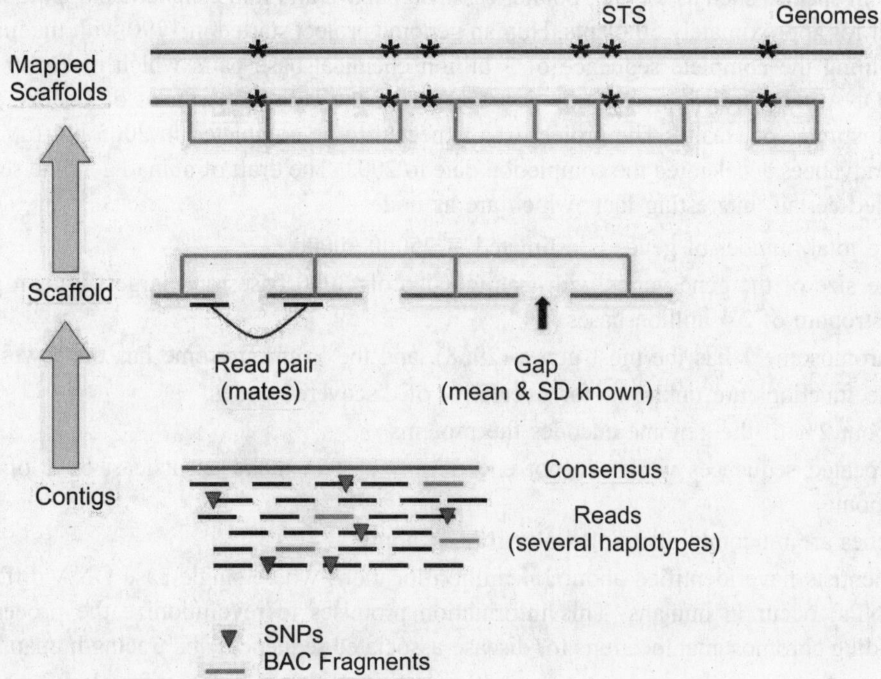

Figure 6.5 Whole genome assembly.

Genome Annotation

Generation of long contiguous sequence is of no use unless it is annotated for the presence of coding sequences or genes. Genome annotation is the process of integrating biological information to genomic sequences. It consists of two main steps: identifying elements on the genome, a process called Gene Finding, and tagging these elements with biological information. Structural annotation consists of identification of ORFs and their localization, gene structure, coding regions and location of regulatory motifs. Functional annotation assigns biological information to genomic sequences such as biochemical function, regulatory function, cell metabolism and signal transduction. FGENESH, GENSCAN, GLIMMER, GENEMARK. HMM and JIGSAW are some of the gene prediction tools commonly used for annotation. In any genome, there are usually regions that are difficult sequence (often regions with highly repetitive DNA).

Genome Projects

The main aim of genome project is to determine the complete genome sequence of an organism. So far, the genome projects for all the model organisms including *E. coli, Bacillus subtilis, Archaeoglobus fulgidus, Sacchoromyces cerevisae, Arabidopsis thaliana, C. elegans, Drosophila melangaster* have been completed. Complete genome sequences for eight crop species including arabidopsis, rice, soybean, maize, sorghum, grape, black cottonwood and *Medicago truncatula* have become available till date. Whole genome or gene space sequencing is being carried out for several plant species such as tomato, potato, cassava, papaya and lotus. Genetic mapping is being carried out for approximately 50 plants. Human genome project started in 1990 with the main aim of determining the complete sequence of 3 billion chemical base pairs which make up human genomic DNA. The project was jointly coordinated by the U.S. Department of Energy and the National Institutes of Health. The project was expected to be completed in 2005 but rapid technological advances accelerated the completion date to 2003. The draft of human genome sequence has revealed certain interesting facts which are as under :

1. The total number of genes is estimated at 25000-30000.
2. The size of the gene varies with average size of 3000 bases and largest known gene is dystrophin of 2.4 million bases.
3. Chromosome 1 has the most genes (2968), and the Y chromosome has the fewest (231)
4. The functions are unknown for over 50% of discovered genes.
5. About 2% of the genome encodes the proteins.
6. Repeated sequences which do not encode any protein make up at least 50% of human genome.
7. Genes are randomly distributed along the genome.
8. Scientists have identified about 1.4 million locations where single-base DNA differences (SNPs) occur in humans. This information promises to revolutionize the processes of finding chromosomal locations for disease-associated sequences and tracing human history.
9. The ratio of germline (sperm or egg cell) mutations is 2:1 in males vs females. Researchers point to several reasons for the higher mutation rate in the male germline, including the greater number of cell divisions required for sperm formation than for eggs.

Functional Genomics

Various techniques of transcriptomics and proteomics are utilized to study the gene function.

Transcriptome Analysis

The transcriptome may be analysed in a simultaneous and comprehensive manner by various high-throughput methods. These methods include:

- serial analysis of gene expression (SAGE); and
- microarray-based transcript analyse.

Serial analysis of gene expression (SAGE)

The SAGE technology is based on the principle that a 10-bp cDNA fragment, the tag, contains sufficient information to unambiguously identify a transcript, provided that the tag has been isolated from a defined position within the transcript. The original SAGE protocol is based on the construction of SAGE libraries, which contain concatenates of up to 50 short sequence tags, each representing a single mRNA. Initially, double-stranded cDNA is synthesised with a biotinylated oligo(dT) primer and bound to streptavidine-coated beads. The cDNA is cleaved with a restriction endonuclease, the anchoring enzyme, revealing specific fragments of the 3' ends of every single cDNA. Next, specific linker sequences, which contain a recognition site of a Type IIS restriction endonuclease, the tagging enzyme, are ligated to these fragments. Cleavage with this enzyme results in unique sequence tags of 10 bp or 11 bp, plus the 4-bp recognition site of the anchoring enzyme of every cDNA species. The tags are concatenated and ligated into a cloning vector to create a SAGE library. Each sequencing reaction of one of these cloned concatenates determines the tags of up to 50 mRNA species, accelerating the speed of EST sequencing up to fiftyfold. Sequencing appropriate numbers of clones from SAGE libraries yields hundreds of thousands of tags, and tag identification and counting have identified gene expression profiles of many different cell types and tissues.

Microarray based transcript analysis

The basic concept behind all microarrays is the precise positioning and immobilisation of a defined amount of gene-specific DNA fragments (probes) at high density on a solid support. These sequences are then queried by hybridisation with labelled copies of nucleic aciom biological samples (targets). The underlying theory is that the greater the expression of a gene, the greater the amount of labelled target and, hence, the greater the output signal. In principle, this approach is the reversion of a classical Northern blot with the advantage that in a single experiment, the expression level of as many genes as are arrayed on the solid support can be determined. Microarrays vary, according to, principally:

(a) the solid support used (e.g., filters or glass);
(b) the surface modifications with various substrates;
(c) the type of DNA fragments on the array (e.g., cDNA or oligonucleotides);
(d) whether the gene fragments are presynthesised and deposited or synthesised *in situ*; and
(e) the machinery used to place the fragments on the array (e.g., ink jet printing or spotting).

Combinations of these variables are used to generate three main types of microarray: 1) filter arrays, 2) spotted glass slide arrays and 3) oligonucleotide arrays synthesised *in situ*.

Filter arrays and spotted arrays can be produced in academic facilities or purchased from commercial sources, but high-density oligonucleotide arrays that are synthesised *in situ* can only be obtained from commercial sources. An example is the Affymetrix GeneChip® technology, which uses photolithography and combinatorial chemistry to synthesise probes on quartz wafer (Figure 6.6).

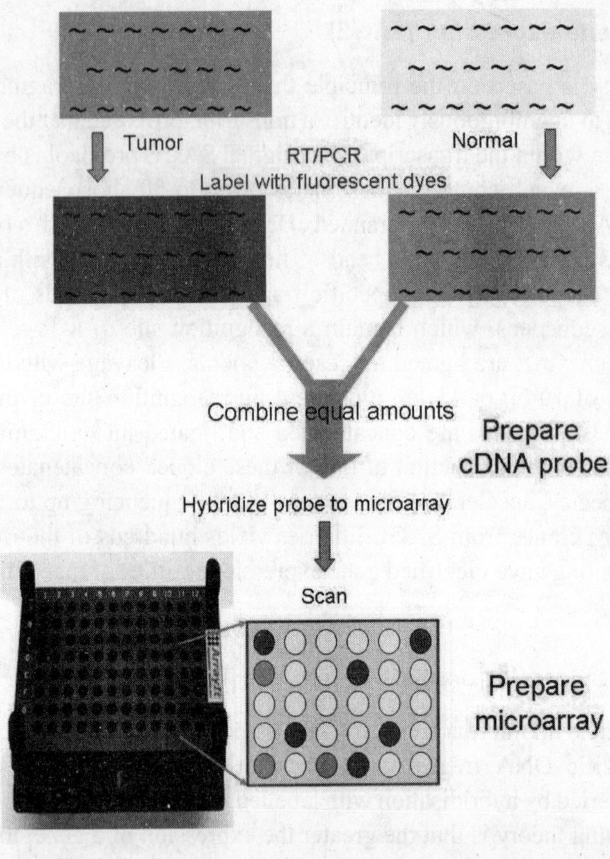

Figure 6.6 Schematic representation of detection of cancer critical genes by microarray.

APPLICATIONS OF GENOMICS TECHNOLOGY

Agricultural Applications

Complete genome sequence of *Arabidopsis thaliana* (first plant) and rice (first crop plant), and their analyses will always remain a scientific landmark. The increasing role of public databases of these model organisms and bioinformatics tools in data mining presents a new opportunity as well as a challenge to researchers to develop more focused molecular tools for gene discovery. Comparative genomics has shown that the organization of genes within plant genomes has remained more conserved during evolution than what was previously thought. The genome sequencing of a species is just the beginning of a new venture to unravel genetic information and to gain better insight into the genetics of other species. Insights from Arabidopsis and rice genome sequences, which have less repetitive DNA, are likely to boost developments in agricultural science. The biggest challenge today is to use this sequence information intelligently and to extend it to food, feed and fibre crops. Today, the search for a gene of interest starts with sequence information including EST, genomic DNA sequence and protein sequence. Various high-throughput sequencing projects have generated enormous information, which is publicly available for large scale analysis from GenBank at NCBI and European Molecular Biology Laboratory (EMBL). This genome related databases have already become an invaluable part of the scientific community. The model system databases could be mined by other but related crop specialists to design markers for marker-assisted selection and aided introgression methods. Hunting new genes that add value to agricultural crops and their products has immense value in agri-business. Molecular techniques have changed the way of plant breeding. Molecular markers allow transferring greater variety of genetic information in a more precise and controlled manner. Marker-assisted selection for important but complex traits will enhance the breeding in terms of better plant products and also save time and resources. Data mining utilizes the use of pattern recognition technologies and statistical techniques to examine large data sets. Generation of microsatellite markers through screening of SSR-enriched genomic libraries is highly time consuming and expensive. An alternative to this *de novo* approach is the screening of the public databases of related model species where abundant sequence data is already available. This *in silico* approach also offers the possibility of identifying rare microsatellite motifs, which would otherwise be uneconomical to identify *de novo*. Maps based on molecular markers of crops of the semi-arid tropics (such as chickpea, cowpea, groundnut and pigeonpea) are relatively less dense as compared to the other related crops like soybean. Data from other, related crop plants could be mined to develop maps and markers. Comparative gene mapping is based on the observation that closely linked genes in one species tend to be closely linked in other while loosely linked genes in one tend to be unlinked in other related species. The probabilities that linkage or synteny will be conserved or disrupted depend on the chromosomal rearrangements accumulated since divergence of the lineages leading to the two species being considered. Comparison of genes controlling qualitative and quantitative traits across species shows that quantitative traits (QTLs) and major genes are the same. If a gene responsible for a trait in one species has already been isolated, a candidate for the corresponding QTL is available for other plants. In agricultural crops, new alleles are constantly accumulated during selection. Understanding of these alleles at the molecular level has stimulated new genomic approaches to map quantitative trait loci (QTL). Large number of quantitative trait nucleotides responsible for QTL variation has been described. An increase in the rate of their discovery is expected with the adoption of linkage disequilibrium and candidate gene strategies for fine mapping and cloning of QTL. In the coming decades, the successful integration of data mining, gene discovery, marker development and gene deployment will become routine practice in crop improvement programs.

Medical Applications

Major impact of the availability of the human genome sequence information is the understanding of disease etiology. A catalog of diseases can now be easily completed through *in silico* investigations. The most challenging task today is to decipher the etiology of common diseases such as obesity, cardiovascular malfunctioning, allergic, auto-immune, degenerative disorders etc. Identification of causative genes of all inherited diseases is one of the most expected consequences of the completion of human or other mammalian genome. Most of the human ailments (diseases), other than the infectious ones and trauma, has some basis in our genes. Until today, doctors were able to consider genes or genetics only in cases of birth defects and a limited set of other diseases. There were conditions, such as sickle cell anaemia, which have very simple and predictable inheritance patterns. Each is caused by a heritable change in a single gene. In the post-genomic era, scientists and clinicians have now much more powerful tools to study the role that genetic factors play in complex diseases like cancer, diabetes, and cardiovascular diseases. Medical research based on genomic sequence is enabling scientists to develop more effective diagnostic tools to better understand the health needs of people based on their individual genetic make-ups, and to design new treatments for diseases. It often takes considerable time, effort, and money to bring discoveries from the scientific laboratory to the medical clinic and finally to the society. Essentially, the new drugs developed by genome-based approach are estimated to be at least 10-15 years away from the society. It usually takes more than a decade for a drug company to conduct the kinds of clinical studies needed to receive approval from the Food and Drug Administration. A rapid progress is anticipated in the emerging field of pharmacogenomics, which involves using information about a patient's genetic make-up to better tailor drug therapy to their individual needs.

Genome-based therapy comprises pharmacogenetics dealing with individual differences in reactivity to drugs. It also includes pharmacogenomics in which high throughput screening of molecules is performed looking for specific genomic targets and, Pharmacoproteomics where proteins themselves are used as drugs. Various pharmaceutical companies are using these novel approaches massively. The emerging and promising stem cell therapy (also known as regenerative medicine) will benefit from basic scientific progress and knowledge in cell biology deriving from genome deciphering. Still, a deeper understanding of genetics will shed light on more than just hereditary risks by revealing the basic components of cells and, ultimately, explaining how all the elements work together to affect the human body in both health and disease.

Industrial Applications

Human population is increasing faster than the increase in crop productivity. In developing countries, several million people are undernourished and suffer from various diseases due to malnutrition. In the same way, there is acute shortage of drinking water of good quality and safety problems arise because the raw materials, ingredients and finished foods are not tested using the accurate and sensitive techniques required to ensure the quality of these products. Knowledge of human genome has increased our understanding of the functioning of human cells and subsequently the functioning of the human body. This information combined with high-throughput screening capabilities and information technology will drive the cultivation of plants and development of fermentation processes. It will enable the agro food industry to transform into a high-technology/high-value business. Epidemiological and intervention studies have shown that certain dietary components have beneficial effects on human health. These components comprise not only the vitamins and minerals, which are needed for human development, but also include components like antioxidants, unsaturated fatty acids, probiotics etc. Functional foods will be particularly required for the rapidly growing number of elderly people for improving the quality of their life style. Genomics has already provided new insights into aging and human disease. Now it has been very well established that many cognitive functions, some of which are genetically determined, that are impaired in the elderly people are related to gene products that can be influenced by components present in the food they consume. Many food items sometimes contain components that have a negative effect on human health and should be inactivated or removed such as proteins causing an allergic response. The finished human genome sequence and various databases of single nucleotide polymorphisms tell that although humans are 99.9% same at the genomic DNA level, still 0.1% difference is there. It clearly means that variants of our ~30,000 genes are present, of which some may be neutral, and others may, sooner or later, cause severe health problems. Substantial screening of metabolites from plants and microorganisms will identify a broad range of components beneficial to human health. Food industry has to follow the same route to find these functional components as followed by pharmaceutical industry. It will involve the high-throughput screening of components in cell cultures, tissues, model organisms and finally in human feeding studies. Genomics can help to design elaborative and effective experiments which will provide new insights into how cells respond to these components. Genetic engineering has the potential to increase crop yields and develop plants that are more resistant to pathogens and can grow under non-favourable conditions. Recombinant DNA technology or genetic engineering has successfully created 'Golden Rice', genetically modified rice for its provitamin A content. A thorough knowledge of plant genomes would provide sufficient information to the scientists to successfully use recombinant DNA techniques.

Pharmaceutical industry has been aware of the impact of genomic information, which is accumulating at a very fast rate. Unlike any other single discipline except informatics, genomic technologies promise to impact all facets of the drug discovery and development, i.e., from idea generation to marketed products. Vaccine industry has been benefited the most by complete sequencing of bacterial genomes. A critical examination of genetic content as well as transcription and expression profiles, a detailed understanding of bacterial pathogenesis can be obtained. Moreover, a whole-genome perspective would provide significant contribution to vaccine development, particularly to target those pathogens for which the traditional approaches have failed. By tremendous increase in the number of complete genome sequences, it has become possible to compare and analyze closely related bacterial genomes. Particularly, genetic variability analysis between pathogenic and closely-related non-pathogenic microorganisms leads to the rapid identification of the complete set of genes potentially responsible for acquisition of virulence and has tremendous practical implications in vaccine discovery. Novel vaccine candidates can be rapidly identified *in silico* before being subjected to confirmatory *in vitro* studies. Transcriptome and proteome analysis offer a great opportunity to gain a better understanding of pathogen biology and also its interactions with the immune system of the host. The analysis of the entire proteome (the entire set of proteins expressed by a genome) becomes a valuable and useful tool for antigen discovery. Advancements in protein gel electrophoresis and mass spectrometry analysis has enabled separation of entire set of proteins of a given cell. Proteomics has been used to identify novel bacterial vaccine candidates against several human pathogens. Genomic mining coupled with proteomics has been successfully used to characterize the surface proteins of *C. pneumoniae* and discovery of antigens from *H. pylori*, *S. aureus*, *Streptococcus agalactiae*, *Plasmodium falciparum*, *Bacillus anthracis*, and *H. influenzae*. The development of large scale testing assays of vaccine candidates will have a crucial role in expanding the potential of this reverse vaccinology strategy.

CONCLUSION

A significant increase in genetic sequence information for a wide variety of species is seen in the genomic era. It opens a challenging new area of research for scientists and engineers to extract sense out of this enormous sequence information. Initial phase of the genomic era, i.e., the generation of genomic sequence information, has been made possible by the development of high-throughput DNA sequencing technologies. The genomic databases have necessitated a drift towards a holistic approach to biological research and the development of new analysis tools. Various computational methods are being generated and applied to interpret and link genes in these databases by comparing and identifying sequence homology, evolutionary pathways, gene expression, and proteome analysis. Genomics and proteomics data in combination with informatics tools will lead to improved descriptions of gene networks and their underlying regulation mechanisms.

FURTHER READINGS

1. Adams M.D., Celniker S.E., Holt R.A., *et al.* (2000) "The genome sequence of *Drosophila melanogaster*". *Science.* 287 **(5461):** 2185-95.
2. Collins F.S., Morgan M., Patrinos A. (2003) The human genome project: lessons from large-scale biology. *Science*. **(300):** 286-290.
3. Daniel Lang, Andreas D. Zimmer, Stefan A. Rensing, Ralf Reski (2008) Exploring plant biodiversity: the Physcomitrella genome and beyond. *Trends in Plant Science.* **(13):** 542-549.
4. Ewing B., Green P. (1998) Base-calling of automated sequencer traces using phred. II. Error probabilities. *Genome Res.* **(8):** 186-194.
5. Ewing B., Hillier L., Wendl M.C., Green P. (1998) Base-calling of automated sequencer traces using phred. I. Accuracy assessment. *Genome Res.* **(8):** 175-185.
6. Fiers W., Contreras R., Duerinck F., Haegeman G., Iserentant D., Merregaert J., Min Jou W., Molemans F., Raeymaekers A., Van den Berghe A., Volckaert G., Ysebaert M. (1976) "Complete nucleotide sequence of bacteriophage MS2 RNA: primary and secondary structure of the replicase gene". *Nature.* 260 **(5551):** 500-507.
7. Fiers W., Contreras R., Haegemann G., Rogiers R., Van de Voorde A., Van Heuverswyn H., Van Herreweghe J., Volckaert G., Ysebaert M. (1978) "Complete nucleotide sequence of SV40 DNA". *Nature.* 273 **(5658):** 113-120.
8. Fiers W., *et al.* (1976) "Complete nucleotide-sequence of bacteriophage MS2-RNA - primary and secondary structure of replicase gene". *Nature.* 260 **(5551):** 500-507.
9. Fleischmann R., Adams M., White O., Clayton R., Kirkness E., Kerlavage A., Bult C., Tomb J., Dougherty B., Merrick J. (1995) "Whole-genome random sequencing and assembly of Haemophilus influenzae Rd". *Science.* 269 **(5223):** 496-512.
10. Forster A.C., Church G.M. (2006) "Towards synthesis of a minimal cell". *Mol. Syst. Biol.* 2 **(45):** 45.
11. Frederick R.. Blattner, Guy Plunkett III, *et al.* (1997) "The Complete Genome Sequence of *Escherichia coli* K-12". *Science.* 277 **(5331):** 1453-1462.
12. Glass JI, Assad-Garcia N., Alperovich N., Yooseph S., Lewis M.R., Maruf M., Hutchison C.A. 3rd, Smith H.O., Venter J.C. (2006) "Essential genes of a minimal bacterium.". *Proc. Natl. Acad. Sci. USA.* 103 **(2):** 425-30.
13. Gregory, T.R. (2005) Animal Genome Size Database. http://www.genomesize.com". http://www.genomesize.com/statistics.php?stats=entire#stats_top.

14. Greilhuber, J., Borsch, T., Müller, K., Worberg, A., Porembski, S., and Barthlott, W. (2006) "Smallest angiosperm genomes found in Lentibulariaceae, with chromosomes of bacterial size". *Plant Biology.* 8 **(6):** 770-777.
15. Herrero A. and Flores E., ed (2008) *The Cyanobacteria: Molecular Biology, Genomics and Evolution* (1st ed.). Caister Academic Press.
16. Joshua Lederberg and Alexa T. McCray (2001) "'Ome sweet 'Omics — A. genealogical treasury of words". *The Scientist.* 15 **(7):** 8.
17. Madigan M., Martinko J. (eds.) (2006) *Brock Biology of Microorganisms* (11th ed.). Prentice Hall.
18. Margulies M., Egholm M., Altman W.E. *et al.* (2005) Genome sequencing in microfabricated high-density picolitre reactors. *Nature*. 437 **(7057):** 376-380.
19. McGrath S. and van Sinderen D., ed. (2007) *Bacteriophage: Genetics and Molecular Biology* (1st ed.). Caister Academic Press.
20. Min Jou W., Haegeman G, Ysebaert M., Fiers W. (1972) "Nucleotide sequence of the gene coding for the bacteriophage MS2 coat protein". *Nature.* 237 **(5350):** 82-88.
21. Nakabachi A., Yamashita A., Toh H., *et al.* (October 2006) "The 160-kilobase genome of the bacterial endosymbiont Carsonella". *Science.* 314 **(5797):** 267.
22. Parfrey, L.W.; Lahr, D.J.G.; Katz, L.A. (2008) "The dynamic nature of eukaryotic genomes". *Molecular Biology and Evolution.* 25 **(4):** 787.
23. Ridley, M. (2006) *Genome*. New York, NY: Harper Perennial. ISBN 0-06-019497-9.
24. Sanger F., Air G.M., Barrell B.G. *et al.* (1977) Nucleotide sequence of bacteriophage phiX174 DNA. *Nature*. **(265):** 687-695.
25. Sanger F., Air G.M., Barrell B.G., Brown N.L., Coulson A.R., Fiddes C.A., Hutchison C.A., Slocombe P.M., Smith M. (1977) "Nucleotide sequence of bacteriophage phi X174 DNA". *Nature.* 265 **(5596):** 687-695.

26. Sanger F., Air G.M., Barrell B.G., Brown N.L., Coulson A.R., Fiddes C.A., Hutchison C.A., Slocombe P.M., Smith M. (1977) "Nucleotide sequence of bacteriophage phi X174 DNA". *Nature.* 265 **(5596):** 687-695.

27. Shendure J., Mitra R.D., Varma C. *et al.* (2004) Advanced sequencing technologies: methods and goals. *Nat. Rev. Genet.* **(5):** 335-344.
28. Shendure J., Porreca G.J., Reppas N.B. *et al.* (2005) Accurate multiplex polony sequencing of an evolved bacterial genome. *Science*. **(309):** 1728-1732.
29. Wade, Nicholas (2007) "Genome of DNA pioneer is deciphered". *New York Times.*

CHAPTER

7

Proteomics Technology

Proteomics technology deals with the large-scale study of protein properties such as expression levels, post-translational modifications and interactions with other molecules to obtain a global view of cellular processes at the protein level. Proteomics approach has become possible in recent years due to rapid developments of techniques which allow study of thousands and millions of proteins in parallel. This approach has also made the approach of reverse genetics truly feasible, because from a study of proteins, one can deduce the function of the corresponding gene and then the trait which this gene controls.

Keywords: Proteomics, polyacrylamide gel electrophoresis (2-DE), liquid chromatography (LC) and isotope-coded affinity tag (ICAT) labeling, HPLC, LC-MS, GC-MS, MALDI.

INTRODUCTION

Although the genome of every cell is same, yet changes in pattern of gene expression bring about changes in cellular and developmental pathways of different cells of an organism. Different physiological processes under particular set of conditions result from changes in global gene expression or the proteome level while number of genes in the genome remains same. (Figure 7.1)

The complete set of proteins expressed by a cell is known as "proteome", and proteomics is the quantitative study of gene expression at protein level. The term "proteomics" or "proteome" was introduced in 1995 and was defined as large-scale characterization of entire complement of proteins from a cell line, tissue or organism. The major aim of proteomics is to make inventory

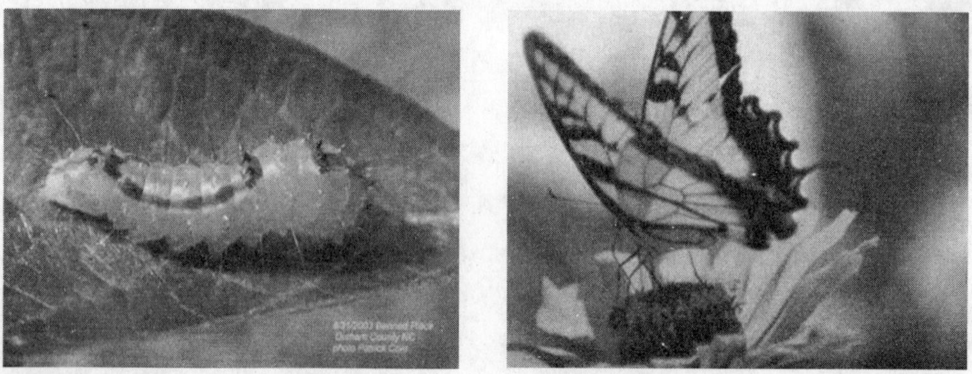

Figure 7.1 A butterfly (right side) and its larva caterpillar (left side) contain the same genome but different proteome.

of all proteins encoded in the genome of a given organism and analysis of interaction of these proteins. This new molecular biological approach for proteome analysis was rather enabled by the availability of complete sequences of genomes and high sensitivity mass spectrometry techniques and instruments for analyzing peptides and proteins. To understand proteomics, one must have to understand proteins first. A protein is a macromolecule that consists of a long chain of amino acids and is translated according to RNA sequence that has been transcribed from DNA and ultimately folds to one of the four 'levels' of protein structure. Studying proteins helps us to determine how proteins affect cell processes and vice-versa. Since proteins act as the molecular machinery of a cell, knowing exactly how proteins function and interact allows unprecedented insight into larger systems. It is now clear with the finishing of human genome sequencing project that the ratio of genes to proteins is not usually one to one as previously thought. For example, human genome contains about 30,000 genes, whereas there are 0.3 to 1 million proteins in human cell. In order to understand mechanisms that make this amazing flexibility possible, proteomics studies, which explain expression of proteins, their intra-cellular location and post translational modification etc. are required. The information generated will ultimately lead to development of new drugs, clinical applications and newer therapies for disease treatment. The studies also help in unraveling the complexity of plant's responses to various environmental and developmental stimuli. Hence, this approach also helps agriculture through the development of new superior crop plants, which have enhanced tolerance to biotic and abiotic stresses and more nutritional value. Thus, in the post-genomic era, proteomics is a rapidly growing field of scientific interest that is becoming important day by day.

CONCEPTS

Proteomics is often considered the next step in the study of biological systems after genomics. Scientists are inclined towards proteomics because it gives a much better understanding of an organism as compared to genomics. The proteins encoded by the organism cannot be studied by studying all the genes, as one gene does not encode one protein (Figure 7.2).

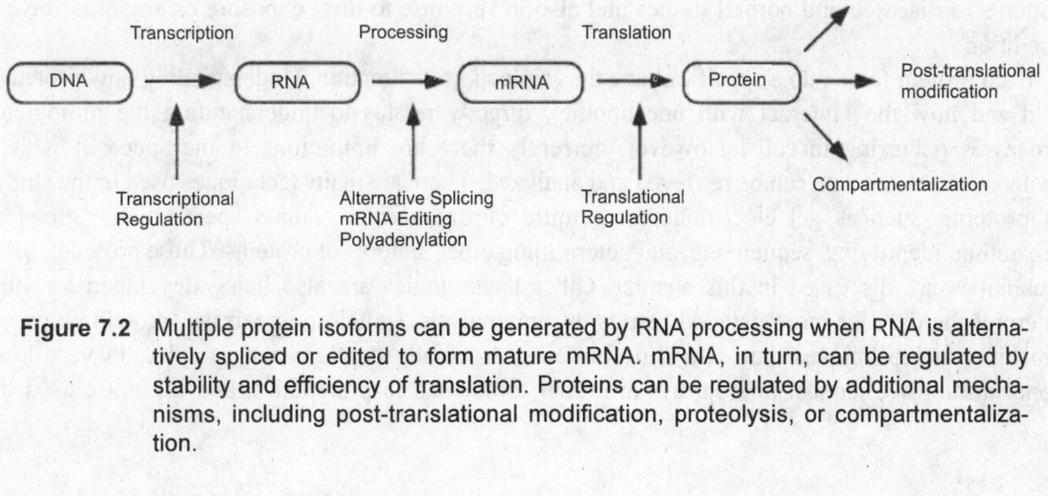

Figure 7.2 Multiple protein isoforms can be generated by RNA processing when RNA is alternatively spliced or edited to form mature mRNA. mRNA, in turn, can be regulated by stability and efficiency of translation. Proteins can be regulated by additional mechanisms, including post-translational modification, proteolysis, or compartmentalization.

An mRNA produced in abundance may be degraded or translated insufficiently, resulting in lesser amount of protein. Many proteins undergo post-translational modifications, which profoundly affect their activities. For example, many proteins like kinases become active and inactive through phosphorylation and dephosphorylation respectively. Many transcripts give rise to more than one protein through alternative splicing or alternative post-translational modifications. Finally, many proteins form complexes with other proteins or RNA molecules and function only in the presence of other molecules. Therefore the goal of proteomics is to obtain global and integrated view of biology by studying all the proteins of a cell at a given point of time rather than all the genes. It not only identifies the protein but also attempts to study protein-protein interaction, protein modification, protein structure, function and its localization within the cell. Considering this the proteomics can be divided into three main types:

- **Expression proteomics:** It refers to the study of the differential expression of proteins under two different experimental conditions. This helps in precisely pin-pointing the proteins expressed in a particular condition and thus helps in identifying the role of proteins in a particular condition.
- **Structural proteomics:** It identifies the proteins present in a protein complex, elucidates their structure and studies their location and protein-protein interaction. Recently the structure of nuclear pore complex was analyzed using structural proteomics.
- **Functional proteomics:** This is a broad term and includes purification of a selected group of proteins isolated from a specific cellular condition and complete characterization of function of the proteins. This provides important insight into protein signaling and protein-protein or protein-drug interactions.

PRINCIPLES

Proteomes, unlike the genome, are temporally and spatially dynamic, with each analytical pattern exhibiting a unique moment in time, and therefore analysis of proteomes is much more complicated and challenging. If all proteins a cell ever needed were always present, it would be easier to correlate genes with proteins. Variable protein expression allows us to see what is up and down regulated with a given set of circumstances. This is very useful in analyzing differences in protein expression patterns of diseased and normal tissues and also in response to drug exposure or any other given condition.

Each protein folds into a specific shape thus reflecting its function. Understanding how proteins fold and how they interact with one another, directly relates to understanding the biological processes occurring in cells. However, currently there are limitations to the speed at which proteomics-related data can be retrieved and analyzed. There are many techniques used in the study of proteins, such as gel electrophoresis, liquid chromatography, mass spectrometry, etc. for separating, identifying, sequencing, and determining other features of proteins. These protocols and techniques are discussed in this chapter. Other technologies are also being developed to help interpret the data for more detailed results during analysis. Protein microarrays (protein chips or biochips) are techniques that determine proteins, especially peptides and samples, in very low concentrations. Chemical microarrays are other tools used in proteomics, and these are used in peptide analysis as well as analysis of other small molecules. Nanotechnology seems to be a very promising field in proteomics, and some scientists are producing nanoparticles as labeling devices, such as SERRS tags.

One of the major problems in proteomics is the study of low abundance proteins. Since many proteins exist in very high concentrations, their presence can mask lower-concentration proteins. Methods with fairly high resolution have the problem of not being able to isolate a large number of different proteins, and need a great deal of sample preparation. Combining different techniques with complementary strengths shows a lot of promise in proteomics studies. Another problem with proteomics is the analysis of the data gathered in the study. Researchers are trying to analyze the data and simulate the different proteins folding through distributed computing. Distributed programming is essentially using many computers, interpreting their normal idle time, in contrast to a specific programming procedure so as to characterize and analyze data that a parent computer sent them. These and other types of improvements show great promise in nurturing the study of proteins. High throughput analysis and tools are being used to overcome these limitations in the data collection process. High throughput proteomics incorporates large scale purification methods like affinity tags. Some microscale productions are being used to examine protein profiles including protein chips and microfluid separations. High-throughput prescreening techniques are being developed as well to help assure sample quality and allow for quicker results from testing, like for cancer patients.

BASIC STEPS IN PROTEOMICS TECHNOLOGY

Significant technological advances have been made to study the proteome of the cell for the last two decades. However, there is still difficulty in conducting several types of proteomics due to limitations of advanced and robust technologies. Hence the quest for newer and improved technology is still going on to realize the full potential of proteomics.

Like any other area of research, attention must be imparted to proper experimental planning and designing in order to get meaningful results. The three commonly employed steps in proteomic studies are (a) sample preparation (b) protein separation and (c) identification of proteins.

Sample Preparation

Appropriate sample preparation is absolutely essential for good results. Sample preparation basically involves efficient and effective solubilization of proteins from biological samples. Since proteins are not a homogenous entity (having different chemical and biophysical properties), it is important that the solubilization process be optimized for each sample type. Ideally, the process will result in the complete solubilization, disaggregation, denaturation and reduction of the proteins in the sample. When developing a sample preparation strategy, it is important to have clear idea of what is desired in the final result. Reducing agents, detergents and chaotropic are generally used for sample preparations. Also to minimize non-desirable protein modifications different inhibitors (like protease, kinase and phosphatase) can be included in the extraction buffer used for sample preparation.

Protein Separation

The next step following sample preparation is separation of proteins. It mainly includes two-dimensional polyacrylamide gel electrophoresis (2-DE), liquid chromatography (LC) and isotope-coded affinity tag (ICAT) labeling.

Two-dimensional polyacrylamide gel electrophoresis

Despite landmark progress made in the development of alternative protein separation techniques, two-dimensional polyacrylamide gel electrophoresis (2-DE) of proteins is still the most powerful analytical technique for the study of protein expression patterns. 2-DE separates proteins based on two parameters, isoelectric point (pI) in the first dimension and molecular size in the second dimension (Figure 7.3).

In isoelectric focusing, the proteins migrate in the pH gradient to the pH at which they have no net charge. 2-DE using an immobilized pH gradient (IPG) strip in the first dimension has proven to be a boon for protein analysis as it is highly flexible. High resolution 2-DE can resolve up to 10,000 protein spots per gel. Stains such as Commassie blue, silver, SYPRO Ruby can be used to visualize the proteins. Using 2-DE based approach, several workers have made significant contributions to identification of proteins from various organisms. However, the technique has some inherent limitations like it is time consuming, labor intensive, low dynamic range and gel to gel variability. Also hydrophobic and alkaline proteins are often under-represented in 2-DE.

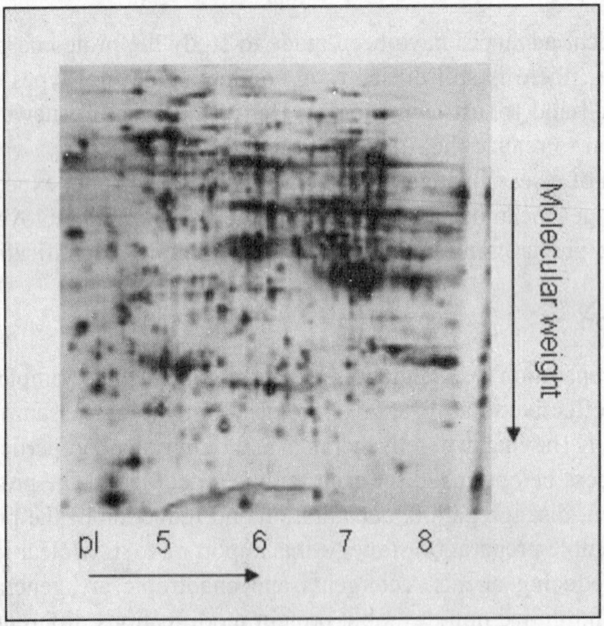

Figure 7.3 Two-dimensional gel electrogram of separated proteins.

Liquid Chromatography

Liquid chromatography (LC) is an analytical chromatographic technique used for separating molecules or ions dissolved in a solvent. If the sample solution is in contact with a second solid or liquid phase, different solutes will interact with the other phase to differing degrees due to differences in adsorption, ion-exchange, partitioning or size. These differences allow the mixture components to separate from each other. Conventional LC is mostly employed in preparative scale work to isolate and purify some components of a mixture. Analytical separations of solutions for detection or quantification typically use more sophisticated high-performance liquid chromatography (HPLC) instruments. HPLC instruments use a pump to force the mobile phase through and provide higher resolution and faster analysis time.

HPLC is a form of chromatography that separates compounds dissolved in solution. The instrument consists of a reservoir of mobile phase, a pump, an injector, a separation column and a detector. The different components in the mixture pass through the column at different rates due to differences in their partitioning behaviour between the mobile liquid and the stationary phase. The presence of analytes in the column is recorded by detecting a change in refractive index, UV-VIS absorption at a given wavelength, fluorescence after excitation with a suitable wavelength or electrochemical response. Mass spectrometers can also be interacted with LC to provide structural information and help identify the separated analytes.

There are increasing applications of LC in proteomics research due to its ability to analyze large and fragile molecules. With advancements in ionization methods and instrumentation, LC combined with MS has become a powerful technology for the characterization and identification of peptides and proteins. LC-MS approach to proteomics generally involves protease digestion followed by LC-MS with peptide mass fingerprinting or LC-MS/MS to get sequence of individual peptides. Multi-dimensional protein identification technology, which separates peptides in two-dimensional LC is another significant development. The separation can be interfaced directly with the ion source of a mass spectrometer.

Isotope-coded affinity tag labeling

There are several protocols for the use of stable isotopes in proteomics, out of which the isotope-coded affinity tags (ICAT) has received the greatest attention. This method relies on the labeling of protein samples from two different sources with two chemically identical reagents that differ only in mass as a result of isotope composition. Differential labeling of samples by mass allows the relative amount of protein between two samples to be quantitated in the mass spectrometer. Here two different samples are allowed to react with two different forms of the ICAT reagent, an isotopically light form (linker contains eight hydrogens) and other heavy form (linker contains eight deuterium atoms). The ICAT reagent reacts with cysteine residues via thiol-reactive group and contains a biotin moiety to facilitate purification. Peptides are recovered with the help of biotin tag by avidin affinity chromatography and are then analyzed by mass spectrometry (MS). Difference between the light and heavy peptide ions peak heights is directly correlated with the difference in protein abundance.

One of the major advantages of the ICAT labeling is the elimination of two-dimensional gel for protein quantitation and therefore increased amount of sample can be used to enrich low-abundant proteins. Further the labeling reaction is compatible with commonly used reagent of 2-DE. However, the technique has certain disadvantages as it requires cysteine containing proteins, provides only relative quantitation and peptides must contain appropriately spaced protease cleavage sites flanking the cysteine residues. Also ICAT label is large (approximately 500 kDa) and remains with peptide throughout the analysis, thus making database search more difficult especially for small peptides. A more recent ICAT is isobaric tags for relative and absolute quantitation (iTRAQ), where a set of isobaric reagents allows the identification and quantitation of four different samples simultaneously. The technique exhibits enhanced sensitivity and more extensive proteome coverage. Isobaric tags require that the quantitation occurs in MS/MS mode, thus simplifying the analysis. A good number of proteomics studies have used ICAT labeling strategy.

Protein Identification

Edman sequencing

One of the earliest methods used for protein identification was sequencing by Edman degradation to obtain N-terminal amino acid sequences. Though little has changed in Edman chemistry since its inception, advancements in the technology have increased the sensitivity and ease of sequencing. Although Edman sequencing is waning from the field of proteomics, it is still an important tool for few reasons. For example, it is used to get the N-terminal sequence of a protein (provided N-terminal not blocked) to determine its true start, and Edman sequencing of abundant protein is a viable alternative to MS.

The N-terminal sequencing of proteins was developed by Pehr Edman in 1949. Edman degradation relies on the specific reactivity of a protein's N-terminal amino acid (amino acid reacts with phenylisothiocyanate) and the selective removal of the derivatized amino acid from the protein, while leaving the rest of the molecule intact. The resulting PTH-amino acids are analyzed sequentially (by HPLC) to determine the amino acid sequence of the protein or peptide. This cyclic process provides the primary structure. Today, it is most often used to identify proteins after they are transferred to membranes. The development of membranes compatible with the chemicals allowed Edman sequencing to become more applicable method for the identification of proteins separated on gels. One of the biggest problems that has hampered the success of Edman sequencing is N-terminal modification of proteins. To overcome this problem, a novel approach called mixed-peptide sequencing has been developed. In this approach, a protein is converted into peptides by cleavage with cyanogen bromide (methionine) or skatole (tryptophan), and the peptides are sequenced in an Edman sequencer simultaneously.

Mass spectrometry

Protein analysis by mass spectrometry (MS) is used as a powerful platform in proteomics. MS provides protein structural information like peptide masses or amino acid sequences, which can be used to identify the protein by nucleotide and protein databases searching. A mass spectrometer separates proteins and other analytes according to their mass-to-charge (m/z) ratio. The molecule is ionized and the ion is propelled into a mass analyzer by an electric field that resolves each ion according to its m/z ratio and then the detector passes the information to the computer for analysis. The most common ionization methods used are electrospray ionization (ESI), matrix-assisted laser desorption ionization (MALDI) and surface enhanced laser desorption ionization (SELDI) as they cause almost no fragmentation, thus maintaining the sample integrity.

(a) **Electrospray ionization:** In ESI, liquid sample flows from a microcapillary tube into the orifice of the mass spectrometer, where a potential difference between the capillary and the inlet results in the generation of fine charged droplets. Solvent is removed from the droplet by heat or another form of energy like collision with a gas and multiple charged ions are formed. While decreasing in size, the droplets ultimately reach a point where they become unstable and explode into much finer droplets. Finally, electrostatic repulsion is sufficiently high to cause desorption of the ions, which are then passed to the mass spectrometer. Significant improvement in ESI technology occurred with the development of nanospray ionization. In nanospray ionization, the microcapillary tube has a spraying orifice of 1 to 2 μm and flow rates as low as 5 to 10 nl/min. A quadrupole analyzer is frequently used with ESI. Only ions of a certain m/z ratio will have the correct oscillation path that enables it to reach the detector in the presence of electric field. Electrospray sources have been connected in line with liquid chromatography systems that automatically purify and deliver the sample to mass spectrometer.

(b) **Matrix-assisted laser desorption ionization:** In MALDI, the sample is incorporated into matrix molecules (small, organic and UV-absorbing molecules) and then subjected to irradiation by a laser. Here laser promotes the formation of molecular ions. The crystal absorbs energy at the same wavelength of the laser that is used to ionize the protein. The laser energy strikes the matrix to cause rapid excitation of the matrix, and then the matrix and analyte ions are subsequently passed into gaseous phase. The principal ion detected for MALDI is ($M+H^+$), although signals for multiple charged ions and oligomeric forms of the analyte may be seen, especially for large proteins. The ionized protein is accelerated by an electrostatic field and expelled into a flight tube. As it exits the flight tube, the mass analyzer (time-of-flight) is encountered (Figure 7.4). This time-of-flight analyzer is based on the principle that when accelerated by applying constant voltage, the velocity with which an ion reaches the detector is determined by its mass. Information obtained from MALDI analysis can be automatically submitted to a database search for further examination.

MALDI is able to analyze proteins down to femtomole quantities and can detect biomolecules over 300,000 Da in size. As sample application can be performed by a robot, the entire process including data collection and analysis can be automated. Another advantage of MALDI is that samples can be used directly without any purification after in-gel digestion. MALDI is a very fast and sensitive technique, implemented on small, relatively inexpensive instruments that do not require extensive expertise in mass spectrometry. Such instruments are ideally suited for biological scientists that need molecular mass information more quickly and accurately than can be obtained by gel electrophoresis.

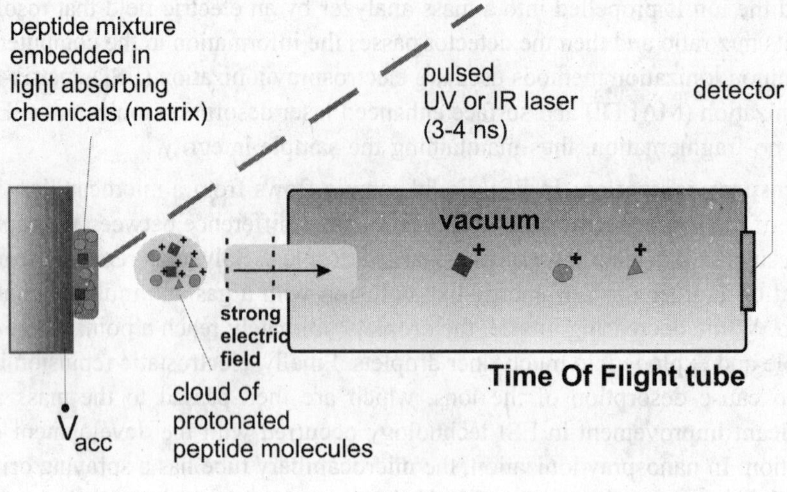

Figure 7.4 Principle of MALDI-TOF mass spectrometry.

(c) **Surface-enhanced laser desorption ionization:** SELDI mass spectrometry is an ultra high throughput screening system for protein purification, expression profiling or protein interaction profiling. SELDI is designed to perform mass spectrometric analysis of protein mixtures retained on chromatographic chip surfaces. In this method, different selective surfaces such as cation or anion exchange surfaces, hydrophobic surfaces, metal binding surfaces, antibodies for specific proteins or DNA can be used on protein chip array to capture proteins and study protein-protein interactions and protein-DNA interactions to identify proteins. In SELDI, the sample is applied on the selective surface of the protein chip so that a subset of proteins is bound to the protein chip. After the capture step, the array is washed to reduce nonspecific binding. An energy absorbing molecular assembly solution (like matrix in MALDI) is added on the top of each spot to facilitate desorption and ionization. Then it is subjected to short bursts of laser light, which leads to uncoupling from the array surface of the retained proteins and are analyzed by laser desorption/ionization TOF MS. The obtained data (protein spectrum of different molecular masses present in the chip) is transferred to a specialized software package to facilitate data collection and further analysis.

With one microliter of sample, a high resolution mass spectrum following a complete chromatographic separation can be obtained. It can detect the mass of compounds ranging from small molecules and peptides of less than 1 kDa to proteins of 500 kDa or more. The power of technology is the integration of on-chip selective capture, relative or absolute quantitation, and partial characterization of proteins and peptides from small molecules, which allows rapid protein discovery and differential expression analysis. Moreover many type of analysis can be carried out. However, a difficulty of SELDI is that proteins must often remain folded in the correct conformation during the preparation and incubation with the array for protein-protein interactions to occur.

Tandem Mass Spectrometry (MS/MS)

Tandem mass spectrometry is basically the connection of two MS in series. It provides amino acid sequence information on peptide fragments of the parent protein. In MS/MS, the first MS generates the PMF spectra; the peptide fragment of interest is selected and isolated by an ion gate voltage that excludes all other fragments but allows the passage of the selected peptide fragment of interest into the second MS where it is fragmented. Fragmentation may occur through metastable decay from the ion's own internal energy or induced by collisions with a gas. As amino acids are sequentially removed from the selected peptide, the decreasing mass of the fragment is used to determine the amino acid sequence. Peptide mass information obtained from MALDI-TOF along with peptide sequence information from MS/MS provides a strong basis for protein identification.

Phage Display

Phage display is another technique contributing to proteomics. It involves the creation of peptide or protein libraries on viral surfaces that are screened for activity as a group. Here peptides or proteins remain associated with their corresponding genes, thus helping in identification. Cloning of ligand targets is an alternative to phage display. It uses ligands, which are small peptide sequences that bind to larger domain units within proteins to identify new domains and ultimately new proteins. Phage display has been used mainly *in vitro* and in animal models to generate ligands so as to identify disease related targets. By applying phage display selection on myeloid cell lines, Geuijen *et al*. (2005) have reported a panel of myeloid cell binding single chain variable fragments followed by the identification of several antibody target molecules on malignant cells.

Bioinformatics

Bioinformatics is an integration of mathematical, statistical and computational methods to analyze biological, biochemical and biophysical data. Bioinformatic databases are used to elucidate protein or nucleic acid structure and function. The aim of database searching is to be able to quickly and accurately identify large number of proteins. The success of database searching depends on the quality of the data obtained in the mass spectrometer, quality of the database searched, and the method used to search the database. If the amino acid sequence of a protein is known or if peptide mapping has been performed, then it is possible to cross-reference the information against private and/or public databases. This is a fast and inexpensive method of obtaining information concerning the unknown protein's ultimate structure and function. For example, if the protein of interest is 95% identical to a known protein in the database, then there is a strong chance that it is in the same protein fam..y and its nature can then be hypothesized and tested. Generally used search websites for peptide mass fingerprinting are: http://www.Matrixscience.com (MASCOT), http:pospector.ucsf.edu/(ProteinProspector), http://prowl.rockefeller.edu/cgi-bin/Profound (ProFound), www.expasy.ch/tools/peptident.html (PeptIdent). Sophisticated bioinformatics tools are being developed to handle the vast quantity of data resulting from genomics and proteomics studies. Databases of computationally derived protein structures are available to aid in the design of molecules capable of interacting with the protein of interest. A wide range of research areas in molecular biology and medicinal chemistry require information about chemical structure of molecules, such as drug designing, ligand docking, metabolic network reconstruction and systems biology. Bioinformatic tools are important for converting raw data into knowledge and ultimately into meaningful applications. Development of methodology by Shen *et al.* (2007) for predicting protein-protein interactions based on sequence information can be a very good example.

APPLICATIONS OF PROTEOMICS TECHNOLOGY

Proteomics has unique and significant advantages as an important complement to genomics approach, and applications for this technology are readily apparent.

Medical Applications

Clinical proteomics is the application of proteomic techniques and strategies to the field of medicine.

Drug development

Drug development is generally based around the desire to up-regulate or down-regulate a specific activity implicated in disease pathogenesis or in treatment-associated side effects. Proteins are the functional molecules in cells and are the major targets for drug action. Proteomics plays an important role in the multi-step drug development process. The process includes target identification and validation, lead selection, small-molecular screening and optimization and toxicity testing. Changes observed in the proteome of an animal model of disease or a clinical subject can be utilized as a biomarker to detect disease, or used as the basis for the development of pharmacological targets for therapeutic interventions. Once the target is identified and the resultant changes in protein structure, function or expression are elucidated, a drug to counteract such aberrations can be rationally designed. An example is the development of an inhibitor of the BCR-ABL tyrosine kinase in chronic myeloid leukaemia. Similarly, identification of protein which is pivotal in a biological process has led to the designing of drugs to manipulate these properties. Use of neutralizing antibodies or inhibitors of the receptor tyrosine kinases to inhibit angiogenesis induced by vascular endothelial growth factor in tumours is one such example. An example of validation is the study showing the actions of the cholesterol-lowering agent, lovastatinin, affecting proteins involved with cholesterol metabolism. An excellent example of the use of proteomics in toxicity was the study of the toxic activity of cyclosporine A (CsA) in kidney. One of the downregulated protein spots with CsA treatment was identified as calbindin (involved in calcium binding and transport). This is an example where 2D gel analysis of kidney tissues gave new insights into side effects related to CsA.

Infectious diseases

The aim of such studies is to develop novel vaccines, drugs or diagnostics. *Mycobacterium tuberculosis*, causative agent of tuberculosis in humans is the most studied microorganism. Tuberculosis remains a major global health problem and is the most frequent cause of death from a single infectious agent. Attempts for primary prevention using BCG (Bacillus Calmette Guerin) and other vaccines prepared from integral mycobacteria have generally been disappointing. Culture filtrates of M. tuberculosis provide effective vaccination in animal models and several groups have been systematically characterizing the mycobacterial proteome, particularly the secreted proteins. After further screening for reactivity in humans, several of the antigens identified by these studies have now been incorporated into trial vaccines. Studies examining the humoral response in vivo have also identified relevant antigens, with several having diagnostic potential in early tuberculosis.

Heart disease

Heart failure is one of the leading causes of morbidity and mortality in more developed countries. Changes in protein expression in heart disease and heart failure using proteomics-based approach may provide some new insights into the cellular mechanisms involved in cardiac dysfunction, new diagnostic markers and therapeutic opportunities. Federated two-dimensional electrophoresis databases of human cardiac proteins have identified several hundred cardiac proteins (www.expasy.ch/ch2d/2d-index.html). Proteomic studies carried out on dilated cardiomyopathy have shown the differential expression of at least hundred cardiac proteins, most of which are less abundant in the diseased than in the normal heart. Studies carried out with animals like cattle and dogs have shown similarities with the proteomic analysis of human dilated cardiomyopathy. The affected proteins were mainly identified as cytoskeletal or associated with mitochondria and energy metabolism. In addition, several cardiac antigens that elicit specific antibody responses *in vivo* are being identified and their role in rejection after cardiac transplantation is being investigated.

Neurological disorders

Although still at very early stages of development, knowledge of specific protein abnormalities in neurological disorders may lead to the development of therapeutic approaches. A study on peptides designed to reverse the conformational changes seen in PrP showed a greatly reduced infectivity of prion infectious material in mice with experimental scrapie. Further immunochemical and electrophoretic analysis have shown that pathological tau differs from normal tau biochemically. Tau is the microtubule-associated major protein component of neurofibrillary tangles found in Alzheimer's disease. In view of the importance of protein-protein interactions and post-translational modifications in Alzheimer's disease and other neurological disorders, proteomic approach is likely to remain the principal approach in the future.

Cancer

Since proteins play a central role in the life of an organism, proteomics is instrumental in discovery of biomarkers, such as markers that indicate a particular disease. Most tumour markers in current use were identified from protein based studies, from the identification in 1800s of an abnormal urinary precipitate in myeloma (Bence-Jones protein) to the generation of tumour-specific antibodies against epithelial cancer cell lines. Proteomic analysis of kidney cells and cancerous kidney cells is producing promising leads for biomarkers for renal cell carcinoma and developing assays to test for this disease. In kidney related diseases, urine is a potential source for such biomarkers. Recently, it has been shown that the identification of urinary polypeptides as biomarkers of kidney related diseases allows to diagnose the severity of the disease several months before the appearance of the pathology. Studies in squamous-cell carcinoma of the bladder using proteomic approaches have also been reported. With two-dimensional electrophoresis six squamous-cell carcinomas were correctly identified from one hundred and fifty bladder tumours on the basis of characteristic protein-expression patterns. Proteomics-based studies of many tumour types are now underway, and they are likely to benefit from the use of complementary techniques such as laser capture microdissection to isolate malignant cells for electrophoretic analysis, thus facilitating the discovery of tumour-specific proteins.

Agricultural Applications

Proteomics has many applications in agriculture. In plant science, the number of proteome studies is expanding rapidly after the completion of the *Arabidopsis thaliana* genome sequence. The and proteome analysis of other crop plants are in progress or being initiated. Proteome analysis of plants is more challenging due to their rigid cell walls and complex variety of secondary metabolites.

Major disciplines gaining prominence in plant proteomics are environmental proteomics, symbiosome proteomics, phosphoproteomics and proteomics in genetic relationships. Environmental proteomics highlight the cataloguing of proteins induced or suppressed under specific stress conditions. It is remarkable that the abiotic stress responses have provided more insights into the protein changes. Recently proteomics approach has been used to understand the effect of O_3 and SO_2 (environmental gaseous pollutants) on rice. Symbiosome proteomics results in the identification of molecular events occurring in plant root symbiosis and associated processes. Symbiosome proteomics (Leguminoseae family) suggested that nodulins are not only involved in the symbiotic events, but also play a significant role in normal plant development, as evidenced from the identification of ENOD18 and a homologue of narbonin (two nodulins) in uninfected root tissues. Phosphoproteomics is the study of phosphorylated proteins. It has provided a good start towards the identification of phosphorylated proteins involved in signal perception and transduction pathways in plants, which will subsequently lead to the dissection of signaling network(s). Mutations in the FLS2 LRR-kinase in *Arabidopsis* render the plant insensitive to the bacterial elicitor, flagellin. Preliminary studies with *Arabidopsis* identified chloroplast thylakoid membrane phosphoproteins and their phosphorylation sites were identified using MALDI-TOF-MS and ESI-MS. Finally, in the late 1980s, it was shown that genetic relationship between species and genera could also be established based on the comparison of protein profiles. The significance of qualitative and quantitative variation of protein spots separated by two-dimensional electrophoresis for distinguishing closely related genotypes has been demonstrated. Comparative study of protein patterns among plants leads to the establishment of genetic relationship by proteomics. Further, proteomics also seems to be suitable for the evaluation of food safety in genetically modified plants. On comparing the protein profiles of transgenic tomato plant resistant to virus and its wild type by two-dimensional electrophoresis, no significant difference was detected suggesting that expression of major proteins was unaltered by genetic manipulation.

CONCLUSION

It is now clear that proteomics is not the study of individual proteins as has been done traditionally, but rather in an automated, large-scale manner which requires new technologies and considerable effort is currently being devoted to the development of novel tools. Proteomics is a powerful post-genomic paradigm that will contribute greatly to our understanding of gene function. Since it is often difficult to predict the function of a protein based on homology to other proteins or even their three-dimensional structure, determination of components of a protein complex or of a cellular structure is central in functional analysis and this aspect of proteomic studies is perhaps the area of greatest promise. After the revolution in molecular biology exemplified by the ease of cloning by DNA methods, proteomics will add to our understanding of the biochemistry of proteins, processes and pathways for years to come.

FURTHER READINGS

1. Aebersold R., Rist B. and Gygi S.P. (2000) Quantitative proteome analysis: methods and applications. *Ann. N. Y. Acad. Sci.* **(919):** 33-47.
2. Agrawal G.K., Rakwal R., Yonekura M., Kubo A. and Saji H. (2002) Proteome analysis of differentially displayed proteins as a tool for investigating ozone stress in rice (*Oryza sativa* L.) seedlings. *Proteomics.* **(2):** 947-959.
3. Agrawal G.K., Yonekura M., Iwahashi Y., Iwahashi H. and Rakwal R. (2005) System, trends and perspectives of proteomics in dicot plants Part III: Unraveling the proteomes influenced by the environment, and at the levels of function and genetic relationships. *Journal of Chromatography B.* **(815):** 137-145.
4. Aicher L., Wahl D., Arce A., Grenet O. and Steiner S. (1998) New insights into cyclosporine A nephrotoxicity by proteome analysis. *Electrophoresis.* **(19):** 1998-2003.
5. Alms G.R., Sanz P., Carlson M. and Haystead T.A. (1999) Reg1p targets protein phosphatase 1 to dephosphorylate hexokinase II in *Saccharomyces cerevisiae:* characterizing the effects of a phosphatase subunit on the yeast proteome. *EMBO J.* **(18):** 4157-4168.
6. Andersen P. (1994) Effective vaccination of mice against *Mycobacterium tuberculosis* infection with a soluble mixture of secreted mycobacterial proteins. *Infect. Immun.* **(62):** 2536-2544.
7. Andersen P., Andersen A.B., Sorensen A.L. and Nagai S. (1995) Recall of long-lived immunity to *Mycobacterium tuberculosis* infection in mice. *J. Immunol.* **(154):** 3359-3372.
8. Anderson N.L., Esquer-Blasco R., Hofmann J.P. and Anderson N.G. (1991) A two-dimensional gel database of rat liver proteins useful in gene regulation and drug effects studies. *Electrophoresis.* **(12):** 907-930.
9. Andersson T., Johansson M., Bolmsjö G. and James P. (2007) Automating MALDI sample plate loading. *J. Proteome Res.* **(6):** 894-896.
10. Banks R.E., Dunn M.J., Forbes M.A., Stanley A., Pappin D., Naven T. and Gough M. (1999) The potential use of laser capture microdissection to selectively obtain distinct populations of cells for proteomic analysis: preliminary findings. *Electrophoresis.* **(20):** 689-700.
11. Bisht D., Singhal N., Sharma P. and Venkatesan K. (2007) An improved sample preparation method for analyzing mycobacterial proteins in two-dimensional gels. *Biochemistry.* (Moscow) **(72):** 672-674.
12. Celis J.E., Celis P., Ostergaard M., Basse B., Lauridsen J.B., Ratz G., Rasmussen H.H., Orntoft T.F., Hein B., Wolf H. and Celis A. (1999) Proteomics and immunohistochemistry define some of the steps involved in the squamous differentiation of the bladder transitional epithelium: a novel strategy for identifying metaplastic lesions. *Cancer Res.* **(59):** 3003-3009.
13. Chen G., Pramanik B.N., Liu Y.H. and Mirza U.A. (2007) Applications of LC/MS in structure identifications of small molecules and proteins in drug discovery. *J. Mass Spectrom.* **(42):** 279-287.
14. Cho W.C. (2006) Research progress in SELDI-TOF MS and its clinical applications. *Chin. J. Biotech.* **(22):** 871-876.
15. Corbett J.M., Why H.J., Wheeler C.H., Richardson P.J., Archard L.C., Yacoub M.H. and Dunn M.J. (1998) Cardiac protein abnormalities in dilated cardiomyopathy detected by two-dimensional gel electrophoresis. *Electrophoresis.* **(19):** 2031-2042.

16. Corpillo D., Gardini G., Vaira A.M., Basso M., Aime S., Accotto G.P. and Fasano M. (2004) Proteomics as a tool to improve investigation of substantial equivalence in genetically modified organisms: the case of a virus-resistant tomato. *Proteomics.* **(4):** 193-200.
17. Damer C.K., Partridge J., Pearson W.R. and Haystead T.A. (1998) Rapid identification of protein phosphatase 1-binding proteins by mixed peptide sequencing and data base searching. Characterization of a novel holoenzymic form of protein phosphatase 1. *J. Biol. Chem.* **(273):** 24396-24405.
18. Dcan R.A. and Overall C.M. (2007) Proteomics discovery of metalloproteinase substrates in the cellular context by iTRAQ labeling reveals a diverse MMP-2 substrate degradome. *Mol. Cell. Proteomics.* **(6):** 611-623.
19. Druker B.J. and Lydon N.B. (2000) Lessons learned from the development of an Ab1 tyrosine kinase inhibitor for chronic myelogenous leukemia. *J. Clin. Invest.* **(105):** 3-7.
20. Duffes F., Jenoe P. and Boyaval P. (2000) Use of Two-dimensional electrophoresis to study differential protein expression in Divercin V41-resistant and wild-type strains of *Listeria monocytogenes*. *Applied & Environ. Microbiol.* **(66):** 4318-4324.
21. Edman P. (1949) A method for the determination of the amino acid sequence of peptides. *Arch. Biochem. Biophys.* **(22):** 475-483.
22. Emmert-Buck M.R., Bonner R.F., Smith P.D., Chuaqui R.F., Zhuang 1., Goldstein S.R., Weiss R.A. and Liotta L.A. (1996) Laser capture microdissection. *Science.* **(274):** 998-1001.
23. Evanko D. (2006) Systems biology for beginners. *Nat. Methods.* **(3):** 964-965.
24. Fenn J.B., Mann M., Meng C.K., Wong S.F. and Whitehouse C.M. (1989) Electrospray ionization for mass spectrometry of large biomolecules. *Science.* **(246):** 64-71.
25. Florens L. and Washburn M.P. (2006) Proteomic analysis by multidimensional protein identification technology. *Methods Mol. Biol.* **(328):** 159-175.
26. Geuijen C.A., Bijl N., Smit R.C., Cox F., Throsby M., Visser T.J., Jongeneelen M.A., Bakker A.B., Kruisbeek A.M., Goudsmit J. and de Kruif J. (2005) A proteomic approach to tumour target identification using phage display, affinity purification and mass spectrometry. *Eur. J. Cancer.* **(41):** 178-187.
27. Gomez-Gomez L. and Boller T. (2000) FLS2 An LRR receptor –like kinase involved in the perception of the bacterial elicitor flagellin in Arabidopsis. *Mol. Cell.* **(5):** 1003-1011.
28. Gorg A., Postel W., Baumer M. and Weiss W. (1992) Two-dimensional polyacrylamide gel electrophoresis, with immobilized pH gradients in the first dimension of barley seed proteins: discrimination of cultivars with different malting grades. *Electrophoresis.* **(13):** 192-203.
29. Gygi S.P., Rist B. and Aebersold R. (2000) Measuring gene expression by quantitative proteome analysis. *Current Opinion in Biotechnology.* **(11):** 396-401
30. Gygi S.P., Rist B., Gerber S.A., Turecek F., Gelb M.H. and Aebersold R. (1999) Quantitative analysis of complex protein mixtures using isotopecoded affinity tags. *Nature Biotechnology.* **(17):** 994-999.
31. Heinke M.Y., Wheeler C.H., Chang D., Einstein R., Drake-Holland A., Dunn M.J. and dos Remedios C.G (1998) Protein changes observed in pacing-induced heart failure using two-dimensional electrophoresis. *Electrophoresis.* **(19):** 2021-2030.
32. Humphery-Smith I., Cordwell S.J. and Blackstock W.P. (1997) Proteome research: complementarity and limitations with respect to the RNA and DNA worlds. *Electrophoresis.* **(18):** 1217-1242.
33. Hunt D.F., Henderson R.A., Shabanowitz J., Sakaguchi K., Michel H., Sevilir N., Cox A.L., Appella E. and Engelhard V.H. (1992) Characterization of peptides bound to the class I MHC molecule HLA-A2.1 by mass spectrometry. *Science.* **(255):** 1261-1263.
34. Hunter T. (1995) Protein kinases and phosphatases: the yin and yang of protein phosphorylation and signaling. *Cell.* **(80):** 225-236.
35. Jungblut P.R., Schaible U.E., Mollenkopf H.J., Zimny-Arndt U., Raupach B., Mattow J., Halada P., Lamer S., Hagens K. and Kaufmann S.H. (1999) Comparative proteome analysis of *Mycobacterium tuberculosis* and *Mycobacterium bovis* BCG strains: towards functional genomics of microbial pathogens. Mol. *Microbiol.* **(33):** 1103-1117.

36. Karas M. and Hillenkamp F. (1988) Laser desorption ionization of proteins with molecular masses exceeding 10,000 daltons. *Anal. Chem.* **(60):** 2299-2301.
37. Knecht M., Regitz-Zagrosek V., Pleissner K.P., Jungblut P., Steffen C., Hildebrandt A. and Fleck E. (1994) Characterization of myocardial protein composition in dilated cardiomyopathy by two-dimensional gel electrophoresis. Electrophoresis. *Eur. Heart J.* **(15):** 37-44.
38. Latif N., Rose M.L., Yacoub M.H. and Dunn M.J. (1995) Association of pretransplantation antiheart antibodies with clinical course after heart transplantation. *J. Heart Lung Transplant.* **(14):** 119-126.
39. Lauber W.M., Carroll J.A., Dufield D.R., Kiesel J.R., Radabaugh M.R. and Malone J.P. (2001) Mass spectrometery compatibility of two-dimensional gel protein stains. *Electrophoresis.* **(22):** 906-918.
40. MacDonald J.A., Borman M.A., Muranyi A., Somlyo A.V., Hartshorne D.J. and Haystead T.A. (2001) Identification of the endogenous smooth muscle myosin phosphatase-associated kinase. *Proc. Natl. Acad. Sci. USA.* **(98):** 2419-2424.
41. Mann M., Hendrickson R.C. and Pandey A. (2001) Analysis of proteins and proteomes by mass spectrometry. *Annu. Rev. Biochem.* **(70):** 437-473.
42. Nilsson C.L., Larsson T., Gustafsson E., Karlsson K.A. and Davidsson P. (2000) Identification of protein vaccine candidates from *Helicobacter pylori* using a preparative two-dimensional electrophoretic procedure and mass spectrometry. *Anal. Chem.* **(72):** 2148-2153.
43. Orme I.M. (1999) New vaccines against tuberculosis: the status of current research. *Infect. Dis. Clin. North Am.* **(13):** 169-185.
44. Ostergaard M., Rasmussen H.H., Nielsen H.V., Vorum H., Orntoft T.F., Wolf H. and Celis J.E. (1997) Proteome profiling of bladder squamous cell carcinomas: identification of markers that define their degree of differentiation. *Cancer Res.* **(57):** 4111-4117.
45. Pleissner K.P., Soding P., Sander S., Oswald H., Neuss M., Regitz-Zagrosek V. and Fleck E. (1997) Dilated cardiomyopathy-associated proteins and their presentation in a WWW-accessible two-dimensional gel protein database. *Electrophoresis.* **(18):** 802-808.
46. Qin J., Fenyo D., Zhao Y., Hall W.W., Chao D.M., Wilson C.J., Young R.A. and Chait B.T. (1997) A strategy for rapid high-confidence protein identification. *Anal. Chem.* **(69):** 3995-4001.
47. Quadroni M. and James P. (1999) Proteomics and automation. *Electrophoresis* **(20):** 664-677.
48. Rakwal R. and Agrawal G.K. (2003) Rice proteomics: Current status and future perspec-tives. *Electrophoresis.* **(24):** 3378-3389.
49. Roche P.W., Triccas J.A. and Winter N. (1995) BCG vaccination against tuberculosis: past disappointments and future hopes. *Trends Microbiol.* **(3):** 397-401.
50. Samanich K.M., Belisle J.T., Sonnenberg M.G., Keen M.A., Zolla-Pazner S. and Laal S. (1998) Delineation of human antibody responses to culture filtrate antigens of *Mycobacterium tuberculosis*. J. Infect. *Dis.* **(178):** 1534-1538.
51. Schlaeppi J.M. and Wood J.M. (2000) Targeting vascular endothelial growth factor (VEGF) for anti-tumor therapy, by anti VEGF neutralizing monoclonal antibodies or by VEGF receptor tyrosine-kinase inhibitors. *Cancer Metastasis Rev.* **(18):** 473-481.
52. Sell S. (1990) Cancer markers of the 1990s: comparison of the new generation of markers defined by monoclonal antibodies and oncogene probes to prototypic markers. *Clin. Lab. Med.* **(10):** 1-37.
53. Sethuraman M., Clavreul N., Huang H., McComb M.E., Costello C.E. and Cohen R.A. (2007) Quantification of oxidative posttranslational modifications of cysteine thiols of p21ras associated with redox modulation of activity using isotope-coded affinity tags and mass spectrometry. *Free Radic. Biol. Med.* **(42):** 823-829.
54. Shen J., Zhang J., Luo X., Zhu W., Yu K., Chen K., Li Y. and Jiang H. (2007) Predicting protein-protein interactions based only on sequences information. *Proc. Natl. Acad. Sci. USA.* **(104):** 4337-43341.

55. Soto C., Kascsak R.J., Saborio G.P., Aucouturier P., Wisniewski T., Prelli F., Kascsak R., Mendez E., Harris D.A., Ironside J., Tagliavini F., Carp R.I. and Frangione B. (2000) Reversion of prion protein conformational changes by synthetic b-sheet breaker peptides. *Lancet.* **(355):** 192-197.
56. Stratmann T. and Kang A.S. (2005) Cognate peptide-receptor ligand mapping by directed phage display. *Proteome Sci.* **(3):** 7.
57. Sullivan L. and Bennett G.N. (2006) Proteome analysis and comparison of *Clostridium acetobutylicum* ATCC 824 and Spo0A strain variants. *J. Ind. Microbiol. Biotechnol.* **(33):** 298-308.
58. Tolnay M. and Probst A. (1999) Review: tau protein pathology in Alzheimer's disease and related disorders. *Neuropathol. Appl. Neurobiol.* **(25):** 171-187.
59. Vener A.V., Harms A., Sussman M.R. and Vierstra R.D. (2001) *J. Biol. Chem.* **(276):** 6959-6966.
60. Wasinger V.C., Cordwell S.J., Cerpa-Poljak A., Yan J.X., Gooley A.A., Wilkins M.R., Duncan M.W., Harris R., Williams K.L. and Humphery-Smith I. (1995) Progress with gene-product mapping of the Mollicutes: *Mycoplasma genitalium. Electrophoresis.* **(16):** 1090-1094.
61. Weekes J., Wheeler C.H., Yan J.X., Weil J., Eschenhagen T., Scholtysik G. and Dunn M.J. (1999) Bovine dilated cardiomyopathy: proteomic analysis of an animal model of human dilated cardiomyopathy. *Electrophoresis.* **(20):** 898-906.
62. Weldingh K., Rosenkrands I., Jacobsen S., Rasmussen P.B., Elhay M.J. and Andersen P. (1998) Two-dimensional electrophoresis for analysis of *Mycobacterium tuberculosis* culture filtrate and purification and characterization of six novel proteins. *Infect. Immun.* **(66):** 3492-3500.
63. Wheeler C.H., Collins A., Dunn M.J., Crisp S.J., Yacoub M.H. and Rose M.L. (1995) Characterization of endothelial antigens associated with transplant-associated coronary artery disease. *J. Heart Lung Transplant.* **(14):** S188-197.
64. Wilkins M.R., Williams K.L., Appel R.D. and Hochstrasser D.F. (1997) *Proteome Research: New Frontiers in Functional Genomics,* Springer, Berlin.
65. Wilm M. and Mann M. (1996) Analytical properties of the nanoelectrospray ion source. *Analytical Chemistry.* **(68):** 1-8.
66. Wilm M., Shevchenko A., Houthaeve T., Breit S., Schweigerer L., Fotsis T. and Mann M. (1996) Femtomole sequencing of proteins from polyacrylamide gels by nano-electrospray mass spectrometry. *Nature.* **(379):** 466-469.
67. Yates J.R. III (1998) Mass spectrometry and the age of the proteome. *J. Mass Spectrom.* **(33):** 1-19.
68. Zhao S.Q., Cai Y.F. and Zhu Z.Y. (2005) Comparative proteomic analysis of B. *henselae* Houston and B. *henselae* Marseille by two-dimensional gel electrophoresis. *Biomed. Environ. Sci.,* **(18):** 341-344.
69. Zieske L.R. (2006) A perspective on the use of iTRAQ reagent technology for protein complex and profiling studies. *J. Exp. Bot.* **(57):** 1501-1508.
70. Zivy M., el Madidi S. and Thiellement H. (1995) Distance indices in a comparison between the A, D, I and R genomes of the Triticeae tribe. *Electrophoresis.* **(16):** 1295-1300.

CHAPTER

8

Signalomics Technology

A cell's final response to asset of signals depends upon interplay of many intercellular signaling proteins leading to expression and activation of various target proteins during signal transduction pathways. Signalomics is study of signalome which includes genome wide expression and activation of signaling proteins involved during a cell singaling response. Various techniques of transcriptomics such as serial analysis of gene expression (SAGE) or DNA chip microarray and proteomics such as 2D gel electrophoresis, liquid chromatography, mass spectroscopy can be utilized to study the signalome. The phosphorylation and dephosphorylation of intercellular signalling proteins and protein-protein interaction is crucial for activation of signalling proteins. Various techniques of proteomics which fall under the category of phosphoproteomics can be utilized to understand the phosphorylation status of signalling proteins. Various high throughput techniques like surface plasmon resonance, phage display, yeast two hybrid, fluorescence resonance energy transfer (FRET) technology are currently being utilized to study proteins and protein-protein interaction. With the advent of these techniques, it has become possible to dissect signalling pathways involved in various developmental processes in both plants and animals. This has opened new avenues for solving the problems of agriculture and medicine through recombinant DNA technology.

Keywords: Signalomics, signal transduction pathways, proteomics, phosphoproteomics.

INTRODUCTION

Cells in a multicellular organism constantly communicate with each other so as to co-operate and collaborate with each other in performing important functions like growth, cell division, differentiation, metabolism and other cellular activities. Cell to cell communication occurs through producing and receiving diverse kind of signaling molecules which trigger signal transduction pathways in the target cell leading to a response. Cells not only receive signals from their neigbouring cells but also from the environment which also regulates various cellular functions. Therefore, final response of a cell depends upon the number and nature of signaling molecules received by them. The ability of cells to perceive and correctly respond to their microenvironment is the basis of development, tissue repair, and immunity as well as normal tissue homeostasis in animals and plants. The errors in cell signal perception and transduction, therefore, leads to various malfunctions and diseases and various physiological disorders. Understanding the signaling pathways involved in mediating a particular response, therefore, is crucial in pinpointing the molecular basis of human disease, susceptibility of plants to various biotic and abiotic stresses, nutrient accumulation and utilization and in identification of drug targets. This knowledge can be utilized to restructure animal/ plant physiology by selective genetic manipulation through modern biotechnological interventions to solve some of the recalcitrant problems of agriculture, medicine and animal husbandry. Traditional studies on cell signal transduction have been focussed on studying the expression, activity and interaction of few signaling components. However, such studies fail to explain the complexity in signaling mechanisms which lead to complex biological responses. Signalomics is that branch of science which attempts to understand the change in whole complement of signaling molecules, known as signalome, during a cellular response to particular signal. It includes the functional genomics based high throughput techniques as a means to study the genome-wide expression, post-translational modification and interaction between the signaling components leading to dissection of signaling mechanisms involved in a particular cellular response. These studies are greatly facilitated due to the evolution of genomic information through whole genome sequencing projects and novel technologies which allow us to study change in signaling components simultaneously with accuracy. The objective of the present chapter is to discuss the basic principle of some of these techniques and their applications in the field of signalomics.

CONCEPTS

During cell signaling, the signaling molecule released from the signaling cell or surrounding environment is perceived by the extracellular or intracellular receptor proteins of target cell. Signal transduction begins when receptor proteins convert extracellular signal into an intracellular signal which affects a number of target proteins which determine the behaviour of the target cell. Thus cell signaling occurs in three stages:

1. Signal Reception: Most of the signaling molecules including amino acids, sugars, steroids, hormones, nucleotides, peptides, proteins, ions and even gases are synthesized inside the signaling cell and released outside the cell through the process of exocytosis or by membrane transport. Some of the signals are in form of environmental cues which include radiation, temperature, ozone, salinity and drought. Broadly, all signals can be categorized into two types. The first type includes the extracellular signaling molecules such as proteins, ions, peptides, nucleotides etc., which are hydrophillic or too large to cross the plasma membrane of target cell. Such signals are perceived by membrane bound receptor proteins which have an extracellular domain for specifically recognizing them. The second type belongs to small or hydrophobic kind of molecules such as steroid hormones and gases which cross the target cell membrane and bind the intracellular receptors which act either as gene regulatory proteins or enzymes (Figure 8.1). Upon signal reception, the extracellular receptors change their conformation or aggregate which initiates the process of signal transduction. The extracellular receptors are of three major types : G protein coupled receptors, enzyme linked receptors and ion-channel linked receptors. G protein coupled receptors are seven pass transmembrane proteins which remain associated with G protein which becomes active upon binding of GTP and activates an enzyme or ion channel which then generates an intracellular signal that initiates signal transduction. G protein coupled receptors play a dominant role in mediating diverse physiological functions in both plants and animals. Enzymes linked receptors aggregate upon signal binding and behave like enzyme or activate a downstream intracellular enzyme to trigger signal transduction. The predominant enzyme linked receptors in animals and plants are tyrosine kinase receptors and serine threonine kinase receptors respectively. Ion channel linked receptors allow the flow of ions through the receptor channel which changes the membrane potential and generates an electrical signal. Such receptors play important role in transmission of electrical signal by neurons in animals.

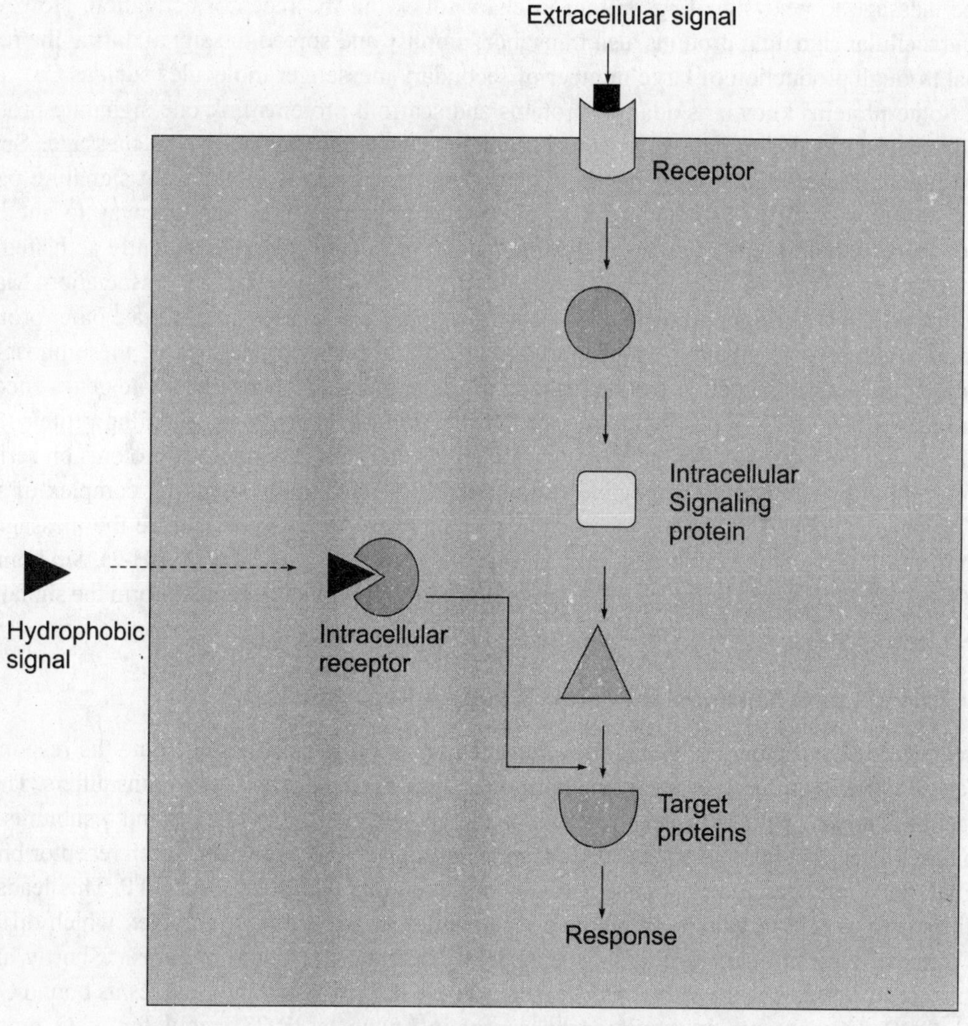

Figure 8.1 Signal transduction pathways activated by extracellular and intracellular (hydrophobic) molecules leading to celluler response.

2. Signal Transduction: The binding of signal to receptor changes its conformation leading to its activation. The activated receptor initiates the process of transduction by converting or transducing the signal into a form which can bring about a specific cellular response. Transduction sometimes occurs in a single step particulary in response to hydrophobic signals where receptor activation leads to activation of an intracellular signaling protein which directly brings about the response. However, most often transduction of extracellular hydrophillic signals is a multistep process which requires the activation of a number of intracellular signaling proteins in a series before a response is generated. This process by which a signal is converted into a cellular response through a series of steps is known as signal transduction pathway (Figure 8.1). Most of the intracellular signaling proteins of signal transduction pathway act as relay proteins which simply pass the message to next signaling protein in chain following the receptor activation. However, some intracellular signaling proteins also transduce, amplify and spread the signal during the relay of signal through production of large number of secondary messenger molecules such as Ca^{2+} and cAMP. Some proteins known as adaptor proteins and scaffold proteins link one signaling protein to another and hold the signaling proteins respectively without conveying the message. Some proteins function as integrator proteins which integrate the signals from different signaling pathways while others such as bifurcation proteins spread the signal from one pathway to another. Many of these signaling proteins function as molecular switches that are transiently activated by phosphorylation or GTP binding and inactivated by dephosphorylation or GTP dissociation. Many of the relay proteins in a signal-transduction pathway are protein kinases that activate other protein kinases in a sequence to create a "phosphorylation cascade." The importance of these phosphorylation cascades in cell signaling can be realized from the fact that 2% of vertebrate genes encode protein kinases. Two main types of kinases which function as intracellular signaling proteins are serine threonine kinases and tyrosine kinases which phosphorylate downstream proteins on serine/threonine and tyrosine residues respectively. Sometimes, the functional signaling complex of signaling proteins is formed by means of modular domains near to receptors before the message is relayed to cell interior. For example, various domains such as *Src* homology-2 (SH-2), *Src* homology-3 (SH-3) and Pleckstrin homology (PH) domains allow signaling proteins to form the signaling complex near to enzyme linked receptors which then triggers signal transduction.

Signal Transduction Through G Protein Coupled Receptors

G protein coupled receptors are seven pass transmembrane proteins which mediate the responses to variety of signaling molecules including hormones, local mediators and neurotransmitters. These receptors are coupled with G protein which is made up of three subunits α, β and γ subunits. In unstimulated state, α subunit is bound to GDP and G protein is idle. However, when receptor binds the signal, the stimulated receptor causes α subunit to lose its GDP and bind GTP. This leads to activation of G protein in which GTP bound α subunit detaches from βγ complex which diffuse in the plane of plasma membrane and independently activate the target proteins. Shortly after activation, α subunit is inactivated by its intrinsic GTPase activity which hydrolyzes its bound GTP back to GDP. This process is regulated by a protein known as RGS, regulator of G protein signaling. The loss of GTP inactivates α subunit which dissociates from its target protein and binds to βγ complex to form an inactive G protein. The G protein is now ready to couple with another receptor. G proteins are of two types : G_s protein stimulates the target protein and G_i protein inhbits the target protein. The target proteins for G protein subunits are either ion channels or membrane bound enzymes. The interaction of G protein with ion channel directly alters the membrane potential and hence immediately changes the cell behaviour. Their interactions with enzyme targets have complex consequences as it leads to producton of additional intracellular signaling molecules. Some G proteins activate the enzyme, adenyl cyclase which leads to production of cAMP as intracellular signaling molecules. In various cell types, cAMP has various effects. In most animal cells, cAMP production boosts up consumption of metabolic fuel. In skeletal muscle cell, for example, adrenalin acts through G protein mediated signaling pathway which leads to synthesis of cAMP that triggers glycogen breakdown. The above process makes more glucose available which is utilized for anticipated muscular activity. cAMP mediates these effects by activating an enzyme known as PKA (protein kinase A) which activates downstream intracellular target proteins through phosphorylation on their serine and threonine residues. Shortly after activation, this signal transduction pathway is shut off by phosphatases which deposphorylate the target proteins and by cAMP phosphodiesterase which degrades cAMP. In some cases, cAMP activated PKA activates gene regulatory protein through phosphorylation. The gene regulatory protein alters the pattern of gene expression which rgeulates the cell behaviour.

Some G protein coupled receptors exert their effects through G proteins which activate the enzyme, phospholipase which generate secondary messengers such as Inositol triphosphate (IP_3) and Diacylglycerol (DAG). IP_3 diffuses into the cytosol and binds the Ca^{2+} channels located on the membrane of endoplasmic reticulum resulting in an increase in the concentration of intracellular Ca^{2+}. Ca^{2+} along with DAG activate an enzyme known as protein Kinase C which phosphorylates various intracellular signaling proteins depending upon the cell type. Ca^{2+} also binds the Ca^{2+} sensitive proteins, most common of which are calmodulins. Ca^{2+} calmodulin complex activates certain kinases known as CaM kinases which phosphorylate down stream intracellular signaling proteins.

Signaling Through Enzyme Linked Receptors

Enzyme linked receptors have role in mediating responses to various growth factors which control the cellular processes such as growth, differentiation, division and survival etc. These receptors have extracellular domains which bind the signals whereas cytoplasmic domain functions as enzyme. The largest classes of enzyme linked receptors are those which have tyrosine kinase as a cytoplasmic domain and are known as tyrosine kinase linked receptors. The binding of signaling molecules to extracellular domain of tyrosine kinase receptors causes them to dimerize which brings the intracellular kinase domains close to each other. The contact between intracellular kinase domains activates them and allows them to phosphorylate each other on tyrosine residues. Each phosphorylated tyrosine residue acts as docking site for various intracellular signaling proteins having SH2 and SH3 which then relay the signal to cell interior. Various proliferative signals activate tyrosine kinase receptors which act as docking site for adaptor protein that recruits Ras activating protein. This protein in turn activates the protein Ras which then activates Mitogen activating protein (MAP kinase) signal transduction pathway leading to expression of genes of cell cycle machinery.

3. Response: Activation of signal transduction pathways eventually leads to regulation of activity of already existing proteins or enzymes or synthesis of new proteins. The nature of target proteins affected determines the type and rapidity of cellular response to a signal. Some signaling pathways alter the activity of metabolic enzymes or cytoskeletal proteins which lead to immediate or fast cellular response to the signal. Others affect the gene regulatory proteins which switch on the expression of some genes leading to delayed cellular response to the signals. However, the cellular response is affected by complexity in signal transduction pathways. A cell may be exposed to many signaling molecules present in the surrounding environment, but it responds to only those for which receptors are present on the target cell. The signal transduction pathways activated by a set of signals crosstalk with each other in such a way that the presence of one signal modifies the response of other. The basis for such crosstalk is convergence and divergence in signaling pathways due to presence of integrator and bifurcation proteins. Thus, one combination of signals may enable the cell to divide whereas another combination may cause it to divide. Further level of complexity is that a single stimulus can affect multiple cell functions because signaling pathways are interconnected. Therefore, the final cellular response is the sum of the effects of all signals which a cell recieves and on the intracellular signaling machinery through which signals propagate.

PRINCIPLES

Signalome includes the whole collection of such proteins and metabolites which express, become active, interact with other proteins or undergo post-translational modification such as phosphorylation in the presence of a signal molecule at a particular point of time and space. In those cases where signaling molecule triggers the expression of genes, signaling pathways eventually activate the transcription factors which regulate the gene expression. The activity of transcription factors, in turn, is regulated by several other regulatory proteins which bind them to form a transcription complex that affects the ability of RNA polymerase to bind promoter during gene expression. Hence signalome also includes regulome which refers to whole complement of regulatory components that control the expression of intracellular signaling proteins. High throughput technologies such as proteomics and transcriptomics allow the study of large number of proteins and metabolites which are the parts of regulome. An important component of regulomic is the study of post-translational modification such as phosphorylation of signaling proteins which regulates their activity within the signalome. Various techniques of proteomics which fall under the category of phosphoproteomics can be utilized to understand the phosphorylation status of signaling proteins. Signalome also includes interactome which is defined as the whole set of molecular interactions in the cell particularly protein-protein interaction network which operates during cell signal transduction. Various high throughput techniques like surface plasmon resonance, phage display, yeast two hybrid, fluorescence resonance energy transfer (FRET) technology are currently being utilized to study protein-protein interactions.

SIGNALOMICS TECHNOLOGY

The techniques used to study the genome-wide response to signals can be divided into three categories: techniques used to study (i) the global gene expression (ii) post-translational modification such as phosphorylation and (ii) protein-protein interaction.

Transcriptomics and Proteomics Approach to Study the Global Gene Expression

The techniques for studying the global gene expression help in initial identification of a group of genes which may be simultaneously regulated in response to a particular signal. As a first step towards this goal, one can check the global expression level of mRNA by using the techniques of transcriptomics such as serial analysis of gene expression (SAGE) or DNA chip microarrays. (Please refer to chapter on genomics in this book for detailed description of these techniques) However, transcriptome analysis is alone not sufficient to derive the information on the levels of proteins or proteome changed during signaling. This is based upon the fact that the mRNA abundance or expression does not necessarily correlate with the abundance of proteins. Furthermore, signal induced protein expression does not necessarily mean that signaling proteins will be functionally active. This is because the activity of signaling proteins depends upon the phosphorylation and dephosphorylation, a kind of post-translational modification. Therefore it is essential to follow those approaches which allow studying not only the level but also the post-translational modification of different proteins of cell signal transduction.

Proteomic techniques such as 2D gel electrophoresis, liquid chromatography, Mass spectroscopy etc. can be used to detect the change in the level of signaling proteins. (Please refer to the chapter on proteomics in this book for detailed description of these techniques) However, it requires further validation by other methods of protein biochemistry, cell biology to confirm that the changes occur due to the signal transduction pathway. In the technique of 2D gel electrophoresis, total protein is extracted from samples and resolved by utilizing the principle of isoelectric focussing and SDS- polyacrylamide gel electrophoresis. Comparison of protein profile from the sample exposed to the signal and from the sample, not exposed to any signal allows the changes in the protein expression to be detected in response to signal. The differentially expressed proteins can be identified by excising the proteins of interest from 2D gels and by analyzing them by mass spectrometry (MS) techniques coupled with database search. Matrix associated laser desorption/ionization time-of-flight MS (MALDI-TOF-MS) and surface-enhanced laser-desorption-ionization MS (SELDI-TOF-MS) are most commonly used MS techniques used for protein identification. However, it is difficult to detect changes in protein expression in large number of samples by 2D gel electrophoresis as it is labour intensive and time consuming. This method is also not suitable for identification of poorly expressed or low copy number proteins due to limitation of gel electrophoresis. In order to solve this problem, the techniques based upon liquid chromatography and MS have been developed. In these techniques, proteins are first converted into peptides which are then fractionated by liquid chromatography (LC) and finally peptides are identified by MS techniques. On the basis of this strategy, the techniques such as multi dimensional liquid chromatography, liquid chromatography coupled with MS (LC-MS) have been evolved. Another MS based technique which has been developed for detection of low abundance proteins is known as isotope code affinity tags (ICAT). This method relies on the labeling of protein samples from two different sources with two chemically identical reagents that differ only in mass as a result of isotope composition. Differential labeling of samples by mass allows the relative amount of protein between two samples to be quantitated in the mass spectrometer. Although these methods overcome the deficiency of gel electrophoresis methods yet they involve the analysis of each and every protein of proteome in order to check its role in signal transduction pathways. Many of the proteins analyzed may be irrelevant to a specific signal transduction pathway and their analysis unnecessarily increases investment of additional time and resources. Therefore, recent trend has been towards proteome mining to identify a subproteome which includes the proteins likely to be affected by the signal and excludes all other irrelevant proteins. An example of subproteome fractionation is isolation of proteins which act as kinases and therefore constitute kinome. In order to isolate kinome, affinity chromatography of protein samples is done by using α-^{32}P-linked ATP sepharose column which specifically binds protein kinases. The bound kinases can be later eluted from the column by using free ATP. This approach of subproteome isolation has two advantages. First, it enriches the proteins likely to be involved in signal transduction and thereby reduces the time in their analysis. Second, low abundance proteins can also be isolated and detected due to enrichment.

Phosphoproteomics Approach to Study Phosphorylation of Signaling Proteins

Most of the techniques of proteomics provide information about the protein expression in a sample in response to the signal which is not enough to dissect the signaling pathways. This is because, the signaling proteins are also modified by the reversible phosphorylation, the most common type of post-translational modification, which regulates their translocation, protein-protein interaction and activation-inactivation . Phosphoproteomics is that branch of proteomics which identifies and characterizes those proteins which are phosphorylated and thus, provides the information about the proteins which could be part of phosphorylation dependent signaling networks. Various methods have been developed to study phosphoproteome of the cell.

Detection of phosphoproteins by radiolabelling and 2 D gel electrophoresis

The most sensitive method of phosphoprotein detection is the labeling of proteins by radioactive $^{32}P_i$ or α-^{32}P-ATP. The proteins which carry radioactive phosphate groups can be detected by separation of protein sample by 2D gel electrophoresis followed by autoradiography. Proteins that undergo changes in phosphorylation are excised from the gel and identified by mass spectrometry techniques. Radiolabeling of phosphoproteins can be done either *in vivo* or *in vitro* conditions. Former method involves growing the cells in presence of ^{32}P inorganic phosphate so as to label all the phosphoproteins. The cells are then exposed to the signal and protein is extracted. The protein extract is subjected to ATP sepharose affinity column chromatography in order to isolate kinome which is then resolved by 2D gel electrophoresis. However, the exposure of living cells to radioactive reagents should be as low and as short as possible so as to prevent the possible cellular stress, DNA damage and apoptosis. During *in vitro* labeling, first the protein is extracted from the cell and then it is incubated with α-^{32}P-ATP. After appropriate incubation time, the protein sample is subjected to downstream phosphoprotein analysis. Major disadvantage of this method is unspecific phosphorylation which may occur due to unoptimized reagent concentration or reaction conditions.

Phosphostaining

Phosphoproteins can also directly be visualized in the gel by using commercially available phospho-specific stains. These stains have been designed to bind phosphorylated serine/threonine or tyrosine residues of proteins with the help of a metal chelator which remains conjugated with a fluorophore that has a particular excitation and emission maxima wavelength. An example of phosphostain is Phos-Tag developed by Perkin Elmer which binds phosphorylated serine/threonine and tyrosine residues. For phosphostaining, the protein sample is first run on either SDS-gel electrophoresis or 2D gel electrophoresis and then stained with phosphostain. The phosphoproteins are seen in the form of fluorescent bands when the gel is viewed under particular wavelength of light. Phosphostaining is a less sensitive method of phosphoprotein detection than the radioactive labeling but handling of phosphostains is more convenient than radioactive reagents.

Immunodetection of phosphoproteins by using phospho-specific antibodies

Phosphoantibodies are also being employed as an important tool to study the phosphorylation of signaling proteins by using various immunotechniques including western blotting, ELISA, flow cytometry and immunohistochemical analysis. These antibodies are developed by immunizing rabbits with synthetic phosphopeptides representing the amino acid sequence surrounding the phosphorylation site of the target protein. Various phosphoantibodies are commercially available which specifically recognize phosphorylated serine/threonine and tyrosine residues in phoshoproteins. However, the successful detection of phosphoproteins by utilizing phosphoantibodies depends upon the specificity and affinity of the antibody for the phosphoprotein of interest.

Enrichment of phosphoproteins

Since phosphoproteins comprise small fraction of total cellular proteins, many of them cannot be identified in the cell extract by using above techniques. Therefore, the following strategies have been developed to enrich the protein extract for phosphoproteins:

Immobilized metal affinity chromatography

Immobilized Metal Affinity Chromatography(IMAC) is based upon the electrostatic interaction of negatively charged phosphate group with a positively charged metal ion which is immobilized on the resin beads. In order to enrich the protein extract for phosphoproteins, the protein extract is passed through the column packed with beads having immobilized metal ion such as iron, zinc or gallium. Phosphoproteins or peptides bind to the beads whereas unphosphorylated proteins simply pass through the column. The bound phosphoproteins can be eluted by changing the pH or salt gradient of the elution buffer and can directly be identified by online mass spectrometer.The drawback of this technique is that many unphosphorylated acidic proteins or peptides also bind to the metal ion of resin beads via the carboxylate groups of aspartic and glutamic acids leading to their co-purification along with phosphoproteins.This problem has been overcome by prior esterification of carboxylate groups of acidic amino acids of the proteins. In this approach, the protein is first digested with a protease enzyme to produce peptide mixture which is then treated with HCl saturated dried methanol for esterification. Resulting mixture is subjected to IMAC for isolation of phosphoproteins which can be further separated by HPLC and eventually detected by MS. Another approach to decrease the copurification of acidic proteins or peptides is the use of TiO_2 column chromatography. Inorganic phosphates of phosphoproteins bind specifically with TiO_2 column matrix in acidic pH whereas all nonphosphorylated proteins do not bind. The bound phosphoproteins can be eluted from the column under alkaline pH.

Identification of phosphorylation sites in protein

In order to predict the role of a protein in signal transduction pathway, it is necessary to determine the phosphorylation sites in the protein. Currently following methods are used for this purpose:

1. Edman Degradation: In this method the phosphoprotein is radiolabelled with ^{32}P by *in vivo* or *in vitro* methods and then digested with protease to produce the peptides which are purified by HPLC. The isolated and purified peptides are linked to an inert membrane via their C termini. Each linked peptide is subjected to Edman degradation which releases the amino acid one by one from their N termini. After each round of Edman degradation, the radioactivity is measured in a scinJ.P. tillation counter which detects released ^{32}P. In this way, the phosphorylated amino acid is detected within the sequence of phosphopeptide. After this, the phosphorylated amino acids are placed in the amino acid sequence of whole phosphoprotein.

2. Mass Spectrometry: The phosphopeptides can also be analyzed by mass spectrometry to determine the phosphorylation sites. In this approach, proteins are first radiolabelled with ^{32}P by *in vivo* or *in vitro* methods and then individual phosphoprotein is fragmented to produce the mixture of peptides. The phosphopetides are identified from the mixture of petides by MALDI-MS using a method known as precursor ion scaning. In this method, MALDI-MS spectra are compared before and after treatment of phosphatase. If peptides are phosphorylated at serine and threonine residues then such peptides are heavier by 80 Da approximately before phosphatase treatment. The peptide is sequenced by MS/MS and location of phosphoserine or threonine is determined.

3. Bioinformatics approach: Some algorithms and bioinformatics programmes have been developed to predict the phosphorylation sites in the protein. An example of the programme is *Netphos* which analyzes the sequence around serine/threonine or tyrosine residues in a given protein. The sequence and structure around these amino acids is compared to verified phosphorylation sites available from the phosphobase database. Other programmes such as *Scansite* and *PROSITE* identify short protein sequence motifs that are recognized by modular signaling domains and phosphorylated by protein Ser/Thr- or Tyr-kinases.Various tools like *KinasePhos*, *Musite* and *PREDIKIN* have been developed to predict the phosphorylation sites present in the signaling proteins. A bioinformatics tool *PkaPs* is used specifically to predict the phosphorylation carried out by the enzyme protein kinase A.

Interactomics Approach to Study Protein-Protein Interaction

During signal transduction protein-protein interaction occurs to form signaling complex. For example signaling proteins containing SH2 domain binds to phosphorylated tyrosines on tyrosine kinase receptors. The interaction can occur briefly as in case of phosphorylation of a target protein by protein kinase. Therefore, knowledge about protein-protein interaction is important for dissection of signal transduction pathway. Plethora of techniques can be utilized for studying the protein-protein interaction; some of these are described below.

Fluorescene resonance energy transfer (FRET)

Forster or fluorescene resonance energy transfer (FRET) is a technique by which protein-protein interaction can be studied *in vivo*. Two fluoresecent molecules (donor and acceptor fluorophore) are used to label two suspected protein partners. The sample is excited at donor fluorophore's excitation wavelength and then fluorescence corresponding to emission wavelength of donor fluorophore is measured and compared with that of acceptor fluorophore. FRET occurs when an excited donor fluorophore transfers energy to an acceptor fluorophore, resulting in reduced donor fluorescence and enhanced acceptor fluorescence. This occurs only when the donor and the acceptor fuorophores are in close proximity (1-10 A) during interaction of two proteins. Another option to labeling proteins with fluorescent dyes is to express both partners as fusion proteins with different GFP (green fluorescent protein) tags. The most popular FRET pair for biological use is a cyan fluorescent protein (CFP)-yellow fluorescent protein (YFP) pair. Both are color variants of GFP (Figure 8.2). The genes for protein partners are cloned in suitable expression vectors and then introduced into the host cell. The cells are subjected to the light corresponding to excitation wavelength of donor.The FRET signal from the transformed cell can be detected by fluorescence microscopy or by fluorescence activated cell sorting.

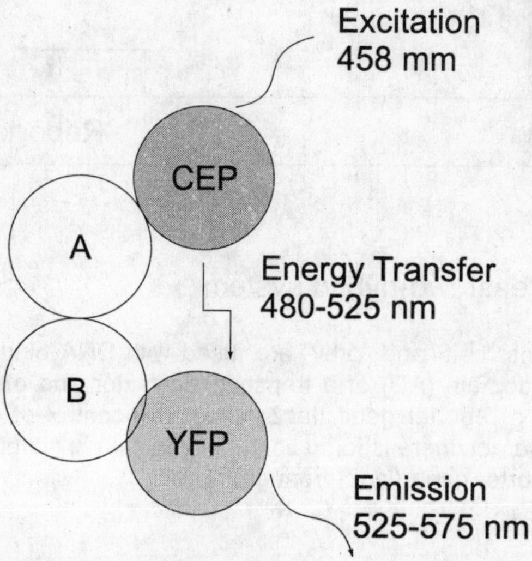

Figure 8.2. Fluorescence resonance energy transfer mechanism (FRET) Since proteins A and B labelled with CFP and YFP respectively interact, therefore CFP transfers the energy to YFP at its excitation wavelength of 458 nm and fluorescence is emitted coresponding to emission wavelength of 525-575 nm of YFP.

Yeast two-hybrid system

In yeast two-hybrid systems, the transcriptional activation of a reporter gene is used as a principle to screen the interacting proteins. The key to the two-hybrid screen is that in most eukaryotic transcription factors, the activating and binding domains are modular and can function in close proximity to each other without direct binding. In this technique, a protein known as "bait" is fused with DNA binding domain of transcription factor and another protein partner known as "prey" is fused with transcription activation domain of the same transcription factor. If the two proteins " bait" and "prey" interact with each other, there will be formation of functional transcription factor which will activate transcription of a reporter gene e.g. lac Z galactosidase (Figure 8.3). The genes for both "bait" and "prey" proteins are cloned into expression vectors which contain a selectable marker usually a gene for essential amino acid biosynthesis pathway. Both recombinant vectors are introduced into yeast cells which are grown in the medium that lacks the essential amino acids so that only the cells transformed with both plasmids will grow. The cells are then grown in the medium which contains the substrate for galactosidase such as X-gal. In such medium, only those cells will form blue colonies which will have interaction between both "bait" and "prey" proteins. The interacting proteins can be identified by sequencing the DNA isolated from these vectors from the yeast cells.

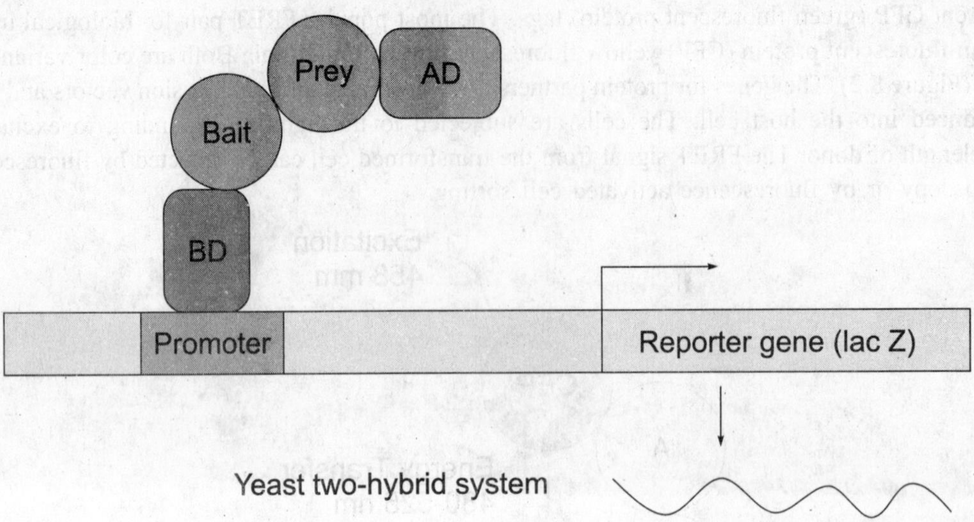

Figure 8.3 The proteins "bait" and "prey" are fused with DNA binding domain (BD) and activation domain (AD) of a transcription factor and expressed in yeast cell which has a reporter gene (lacZ) under the control of promoter. When both proteins interact, there is formation of functional transcription factor and expression of reporter gene (lacZ) from promoter.

Phage display method

Displaying the proteins or peptides on the surface of a filamentous phage such as M13, Ff etc. is known as "phage display" which has become a powerful technique to investigate the protein-protein interactions. The technique utilizes the principle that the polypeptides can be fused with coat protein of filamentous phage without losing their functions. In this technique, genes encoding different foreign polypeptides are fused with coat protein and cloned into the vector "phagemid" which is then introduced into host bacterial cells such as *E. coli*. This leads to preparation of a protein library in terms of virions or phage particles which express the protein on their surface. Next, this library is screened for the proteins which interact with a target protein by a method known as "panning". In order to perform "panning", the target protein is immobilized on a matrix and phage particles are allowed to interact with the target proteins. A phage that displays a protein that binds to target protein on its surface will remain bound to matrix while others are removed by washing. The phage particles which remain bound are eluted and amplified by reinfecting the bacterial host leading to a phage mixture which is enriched for relevant phages. The phagemids are isolated from these phage particles and relevant DNA sequences encoding the interacting proteins are identified.

Surface plasmon resonance

Surface plasmon resonance (SPR) is a phenomenon in which intensity of reflected light decreases when an incident light beam falls on metal surface (gold or silver) at a particular angle. At this angle of incidence, the photons of incidence light excite the metal surface plasmons resulting in plasmon resonance that decreases the intensity of reflected light. By monitoring the change in intensity of reflected light at different angles of incidence, one can detect an angle of incidence at which the loss in intensity of reflected light is maximum. This angle of incidence is known as resonance angle or SPR angle which is dependent on refractive index of media in contact with metal surface. If refractive index changes, then SPR angle also changes. This principle is utilized to detect protein protein interaction. In order to detect interaction, one protein known as ligand is immobilized on the metal surface and its suspected binding partner protein (analyte) is injected into a sample buffer that flows over the metal surface. If ligand binds to analyte protein on the metal surface then there is change in refractive index which can be monitored in real time by measuring the changes in SPR angle (Figure 8.4). The graph plotted between the shift in SPR angle and time is known as sensorgram. The association and dissociation constants between the ligand and analyte can be calculated through analysis of sensorgrams.

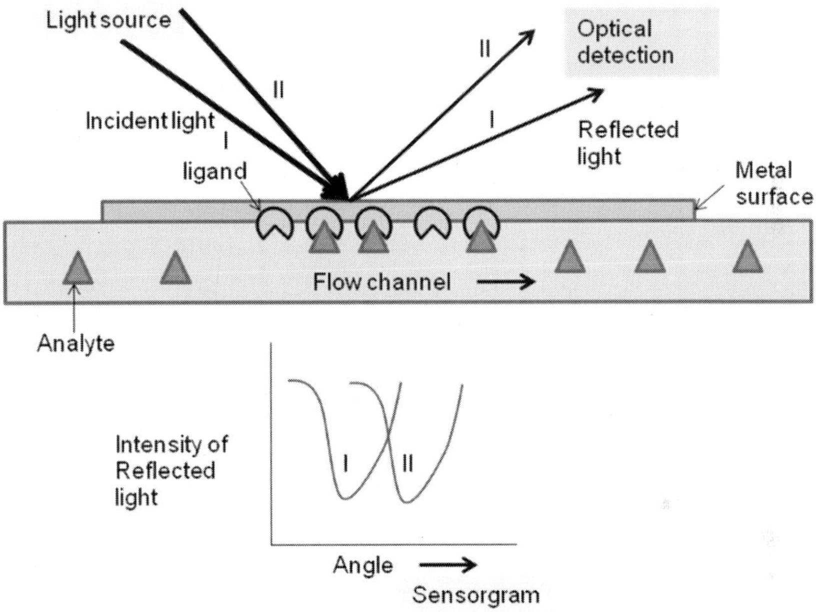

Figure 8.4 Diagram explaining the principle of SPR : SPR angle changes from I to II upon ligand and analyte interaction on the metal surface.

Computational methods for detection of protein protein interaction

Various computational methods based on comparative genomics have been developed to utilize genomic information so as to predict the protein-protein interaction.

Rosetta stone method or domain fusion method

This method utilizes the knowledge about the domains which interact with each other. If two domains A and B are fused with each other in a protein present in a genome then presence of these domains in two separate proteins in another genome indicates that the proteins might also interact with each other (Figure 8.5).

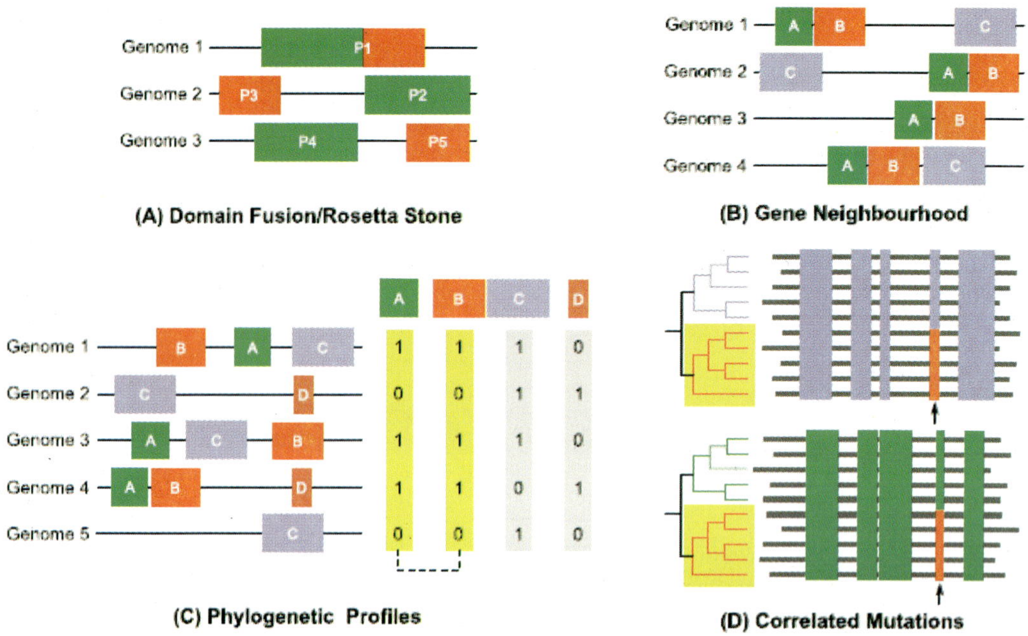

Figure 8.5 Prediction of functional linkages between proteins, based on different methods. (A) Method of domain fusion. The figure shows proteins predicted to interact by the Rosetta stone method (domain fusion). Each protein is shown schematically with boxes representing domains. Proteins P2 and P3 in Genomes 2 and 3 are predicted to interact because their homologues are fused in the first genome. (B) Gene neighbourhood. The figure shows four hypothetical genomes, containing one or more of the genes A, B and C. Since the genes A and B are co-localised in multiple genomes (1–4), they are likely to be functionally linked with one another. (C) Phylogenetic profiles. The figure shows five hypothetical genomes, each containing one or more of the proteins A, B, C and D. The presence or absence of each protein is indicated by 1 or 0, respectively, in the phylogenetic profiles given on the right. Identical profiles are highlighted — proteins A and B are functionally linked (dotted line), whereas proteins C and D, which have different phylogenetic profiles (shown in grey) are not likely to be functionally linked. (D) Correlated mutations. The alignments of two protein families are shown; conserved residues in either alignment are shown in the same colour (blue and green). Correlated mutations in either alignment (coloured red) are indicated by arrow marks. Common sub-trees of the phylogenetic trees are highlighted in yellow. The presence of correlated mutations in each family suggests that the corresponding sites may be involved in mediating interactions between the proteins from each family. (Raman, 2010)

Conserved neighbourhood method

If the genes that encode two proteins are neighbours on the chromosome in several genomes, the corresponding proteins are likely to be functionally linked. Therefore they are likely to interact with each other. This method is particularly useful in case of prokaryotes, where operons commonly exist, or in organisms where operon-like clusters are observed.

Phylogenetic profiling method

This method is based on the fact that if two proteins are functionally linked then they would interact and co-occur in many genomes. Phylogenetic profile of a particular protein can be indicated by scoring them for presence or absence in some genomes. If phylogenetic profiles of two proteins are exactly similar then it is likely that they are functionaly linked and interact with each other.

Methods based on coevolution

During evolution, one method of gene innovation is mutation which alters the proteins encoded by genome of a species. If two proteins interact then their pattern of evolution would be exactly similar. Therefore, in this method the protein families of two suspected protein partners are compared. If there is commonality of subtrees in their phylogenetic tree, it is indicative of their coevolution and hence their interaction.

Databases on protein-protein interaction

Use of above methods has resulted in accumulation of data about protein protein interaction in form of databases which are utilized as reference by scientists. Some databases which contain information about protein-protein interaction are as follows:

STRING

STRING (Search Tool for the Retrieval of Interacting Genes/Proteins; http://string.embl.de/) database contains data on protein protein interaction which are derived from various high-throughput experiments and computational methods described above.

HPRD

Human Protein Reference Database (HPRD; http://www.hprd.org/) houses information about proteins relevant to the human health and disease. The data are extracted from various published articles related to genome annotation.

DIP

The DIP (Database of Interacting Proteins; http://dip.doe-mbi.ucla.edu/) contains the information about protein-protein interaction which are derived from various wet lab experiments.

Predictome

This database contains the information about the links between the proteins of 44 genomes which are established by various methods such as by various computational methods and by wet lab experiments including yeast two hybrid screening, FRET, etc.

APPLICATIONS OF SIGNALOMICS TECHNOLOGY

The widest application of signalomics technology in agriculture has been in understanding the molecular biology of biotic and abiotic stress tolerance of agriculturally important plants. In order to understand host pathogen interaction at molecular level, proteomes of both host and pathogen are evaluated. The proteomics based approaches such as two dimensional electrophoresis and MS are being used to compare the proteome of a susceptible line of plant infected by a pathogen with that of mock inoculated line. This has led to identification of various pathogenicity and virulence factors and most of the host plant proteins which have defensive role.

FURTHER READINGS

1. Banning C., Votteler J., Hoffmann D., Koppensteiner H., Warmer M., *et al.* (2010) A flow cytometry-based FRET assay to identify and analyse protein-protein interactions in living cells. *PLoS ONE* 5 **(2):** 9344.
2. Graves P.R., Haystead T.A. (2002) Molecular biologist's guide to proteomics. *Microbiol. Mol. Biol. Rev.* **(66):** 39-63.
3. Hunter T. (1995) Protein kinases and phosphatases : the yin and yang of protein phosphorylation and signaling. *Cell.* **(80):** 225-36.
4. Lawrence David S. (2001) Functional proteomics: large-scale analysis of protein kinase activity. *Genome Biology.* 2 **(2):** 1-3
5. Raman Karthik. (2010) Construction and analysis of protein-protein interaction networks. *Automated Experimentation.* **(2):** 1-15
6. Schmelzle Katrin and White Forest M. (2006) Phosphoproteomic approaches to elucidate cellular signaling networks. *Current Opinion in Biotechnology.* **(17):** 406-414
7. Sergio de la Fuente van Bentem1 and Heribert Hirt. (2007) Using phosphoproteomics to reveal signalling dynamics in plants. *Trends in Plant Science.* 12 **(9):** 404-11

CHAPTER

9

Metabolomics Technology

Metabolites play vital roles in a biological system. They transport energy, facilitate cellular communication and control, and function as building blocks for other processes. Changes in metabolites provide valuable insight into underlying biochemistry and present a unique opportunity for phenotypic and dynamic profiling. They can serve as markers for disease and point to correlations between genes and functions. Metabolomics provides a useful avenue to the understanding of biological systems. It can be a powerful complement to genomic and proteomics analyses. Metabolomics, the comparative analysis of metabolites found in sets of similar biological samples, can identify potential biomarkers, identify effects of drugs or diseases on known biological pathways, or detect effects of drugs or diseases in unexpected biological pathways. The aim of this chapter is to provide an in-depth overview about metabolomics technology, explore how metabolomics networks can be connected to the underlying reaction pathway structure, and discuss the need to investigate integrative biochemical networks.

Keywords: Omics; metabolomics; liquid chromatography; gas chromatography; mass spectrophotometer; nuclear magnetic resonance; metabolite flux.

INTRODUCTION

Being the intermediates and end-products of biochemical reactions, metabolites play a very important role in connecting the different metabolic pathways and processes that operate within a living cell in particular and across the cells and tissues to realize a function or response for the state of molecular phenotype organism. Conventionally, the measurement of such metabolites was restricted to a few of them considered to be directly related to the process or pathway of study. The concept of systems biology emerged during the genomic era to emphasize the connectivity to be far and wide in the cell and the organism. Therefore, the post-genomic era has recognized the importance of assaying the status of full complement of transcripts (transcriptome), proteins (proteome) and metabolites (metabolome) and ions (ionome) for holistic understanding of the molecular physiology of the cell, tissue or organism under the normal or responsive (developmental, signaled or environmental) state to ensure the manifestation of a desired function system-wide. Accordingly, qualitative and quantitative measurement of the whole set of metabolites (pathway intermediates, end-products, signaling molecules, etc.) in the test sample(s) became imperative. The approach and associated technologies are collectively called the subject of 'metabolomics'. Despite technological challenges some which still exist, such as wide and high-throughput measurements with unprecedented sensitivity, metabolomics is now becoming a well-known approach for the study of all types of organisms, and is rapidly complementing the data obtained by the other 'omics' (genomics, transcriptomics, proteomics, ionomics). Its simple symbolic integration with the other 'omics' is represented in Figure 9.1. However, what is the critical mass/set (the number of metabolites) of measurements/profiles to qualify as 'metabolomics' and how does it relate to its other counterparts such as metabolic profiling, metabolic fingerprinting, or metabonomics are still the issues of diverse views?

Metabolite profiling measures the real outcome of potential changes suggested by genomics and proteomics.

Intricacy of complex and interconnected metabolic pathways

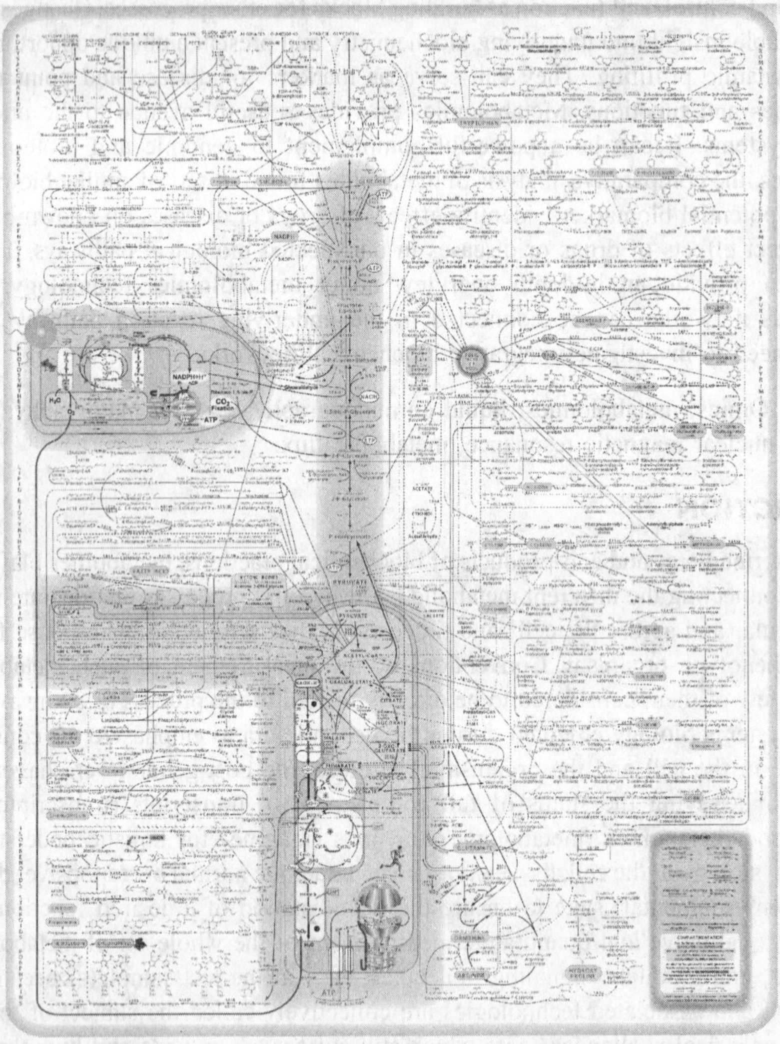

Metabolomics offers the opportunity to find patterns and changes in the entire metabolism, represented here by the metabolic pathways chart designed by Donald E. Nicholson, University of Leeds, England and Sigma-Aldrich.

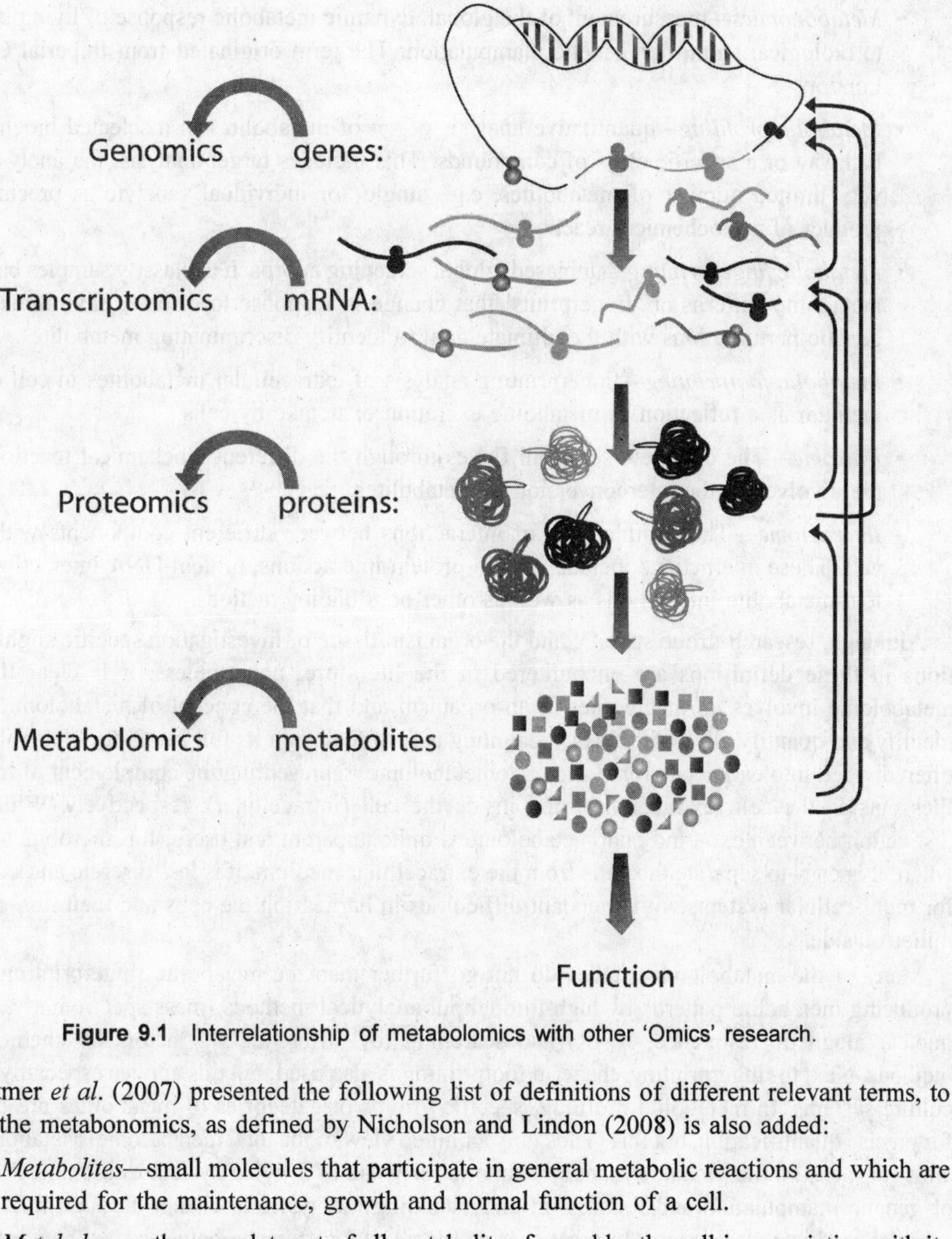

Figure 9.1 Interrelationship of metabolomics with other 'Omics' research.

Dettmer *et al*. (2007) presented the following list of definitions of different relevant terms, to which the metabonomics, as defined by Nicholson and Lindon (2008) is also added:

- *Metabolites*—small molecules that participate in general metabolic reactions and which are required for the maintenance, growth and normal function of a cell.
- *Metabolome*—the complete set of all metabolites formed by the cell in association with its metabolism.
- *Metabolomics*—identification and quantification of all metabolites in a biological system.

- *Metabonomics*—measurement of the global, dynamic metabolic response of living systems to biological stimuli or genetic manipulation. The term originated from Imperial College London.
- *Metabolic profiling*—quantitative analysis of set of metabolites in a selected biochemical pathway or a specific class of compounds. This includes target analysis, the analysis of a very limited number of metabolites, e.g., single "or individual" analyte as precursor or product of a biochemical reaction.
- *Metabolic fingerprinting*—unbiased, global screening approach to classify samples based on metabolite patterns or 'fingerprints' that change in response to disease, environmental or genetic perturbations with the ultimate goal to identify discriminating metabolites.
- *Metabolic footprinting*—fingerprinting analysis of extracellular metabolites in cell culture medium as a reflection of metabolite excretion or uptake by cells.
- *Fluxome*—The complete set of all fluxes through the different biochemical reactions that are involved in the interconversion of metabolites.
- *Interactome*—The complete set of interactions between different components within the cell. These interactions include protein-protein interactions, protein-DNA interaction, protein-metabolite interactions as well as other possible interactions.

Although, research-group specific and the organism/tissue of investigation specific slight variations in these definitions are encountered in the literature, nevertheless, it is clear that the metabolome involves all metabolites in an organism and that the concept of metabolomics is to identify and quantify all metabolites, a daunting task to realize in its full meaning. Metabolome is often divided into exometabolome and endometabolome, representing the complement of metabolites outside the cell (extracellular) and inside the cell (intracellular), respectively. Whilst this distinction between exo- and endometabolome is quite apparent and useful for microbial systems where it is easy to separate the cells from the extracellular medium, it is less discrete and complex for multi-cellular systems with attendant difficulties in harnessing the cells and their non-cellular milieu outside.

Many of the metabolomic studies do not go further than the metabolite fingerprinting stage: producing metabolite patterns by high-throughput analytical methods (mass spectrometry, MS or nuclear magnetic resonance, NMR) and searching for differentiating factors by chemometric methods. Next to fingerprinting, the term footprinting is also used, but this applies especially to cell culture systems. In metabolite profiling, specific groups or categories of metabolites are defined for precise quantification, but this yields only a limited view of the total metabolome. Metabonomics aims to measure the global, dynamic metabolic response of a living system to biological stimuli or genetic manipulation and focuses on understanding the systemic change through time in the complex multicellular system. In practice, there is no real difference between metabonomics and metabolomics, but the term metabonomics is traditionally more used in biomedical research to describe the fingerprinting of biochemical perturbations caused by disease, drugs, and toxins, often in biological fluids.

The difference between the two terms is hardly related to the choice of analytical platforms: although metabonomics is more associated with NMR spectroscopy and metabolomics with mass spectrometry-based techniques, truly it is the bias of choice of usage of the term by different research groups that have parallely popularized the two terms. While there is no absolute agreement, emerging consensus differentiates that 'metabolomics' implies as a comprehensive metabolite profiling emphatic approach, while 'metabonomics' as a description of multiple (but not necessarily comprehensive) metabolite changes as a consequence of biological perturbation(s). Hence, the highly significant commonality of analytical methodologies and instrumentation recruited in the analyses rationalizes their often synonymous usage in literature.

Although metabolite profiling has long been applied for medical and diagnostic purposes as well as for phenotypic characterization, the terminological transition to metabolomics emerged with the advent of high-throughput and sensitive hyphenated analytical technologies (mainly mass-spectrometric) enabling simultaneous analyses of enormously higher number of intracellular metabolites.

In this chapter, we discuss various historical and methodological aspects of metabolomic research including quenching of the metabolite, extraction of metabolites from living cells, sample collection, handling, storage, requirements for sample analysis, peak alignment, data interpretation using statistical approaches, metabolite identification and finally, recommendations for successful analysis of the data obtained.

HISTORY OF METABOLOMICS

Metabolomics was conceived in 1970 by Arthur Robinson, an Assistant Professor at that time in the Department of Chemistry at the University of California at San Diego. Robinson was investigating an idea of Linus Pauling's as to whether biological variability could be explained on the basis of far wider ranges of nutritional requirements than what was generally recognized. In analyzing the "messy" chromatographic patterns of urine from vitamin B_6-loaded subjects, Robinson realized that the patterns of hundreds or thousands of chemical constituents in urine contained much useful information. However, at that time, it was not known by the term, metabolomics.

In 1998, the term metabolome was introduced in a research paper on yeast genome by Oliver *et al.*, based on the analogy with the terms genome, proteome and transcriptome, which had been introduced already. From the year 2000, the term metabolomics came into use in publications, as can be seen from Figure 9.2 drawn from year-wise use of the term in research publications, as compiled by ISI Web of Science from Thomson Scientific. The term genome was the first one to be introduced, and from 1988, the term genomics came in use. Proteomics followed only in 1997 and transcriptomics in 1999 (Figure 9.2). It also appears that the term genomics only came into common use rather long after it had been introduced, but the number of papers rapidly increased since 1996 to about 2500–3000 per year over recent years. Proteomics research rapidly grew after 1998 and the number of papers surpassed the number of papers related to genomics since 2006, but like genomics, it seems to have reached its plateau with about 3000 papers a year. The number of papers about metabolomics and metabonomics showed a slower growth reaching to more than 600 in 2008. The slow growth might be due to the fact that metabolomics methods are complex, lack the level of automation and lack of availability of cheaper commercial services contrary to proteomics and genomics, (see below). Nevertheless, it seems probable that it would reach the same space in literature as that of proteomics and genomics.

When the term metabolomics was introduced, it was not a new process or a new concept, but it was more of a consequence of the development of the techniques that form the basis of metabolomics. In fact, the metabolite profiling which is the basis of metabolomics already had been performed since long. One can think of the TLC profiles of medicinal plant extracts, or the gas chromatography (GC) chromatograms of essential oils, fatty acid (as derivatized esters) and other normal or derivatized volaties. The increased resolution in NMR spectra by higher field magnets and the wider application of two-dimensional techniques has permitted the identification of metabolites in crude extracts or samples. Already from the mid-1980s, unmodified biological fluids were being studied by NMR, and in the early 1990s metabolic fingerprinting of plant materials came into use. Also, the development in chromatographic techniques, such as capillary columns for GC and small particle high performance liquid chromatography (HPLC) columns, permitted a wider application of these techniques. GC was successfully applied for the separation of relatively volatilizable underivatised substances. Derivatisation of the metabolites to their volatile form enabled GC based quantification of much higher range of compounds. Hyphenation of the separation technologies (GC, HPLC, capillary electrophoresis, etc.) with mass spectrometry (MS) led not only to direct identification of the compounds but also offered far better sensitivity of detection. This is heralded as the beginning of the instrumental opportunities for comprehensive profiling of samples. The next important analytical strength to the field of metabolomics came from the advances in chemometrics, that permitted the evaluation of large data sets and distilling out significant changes in relation to specific parameters.

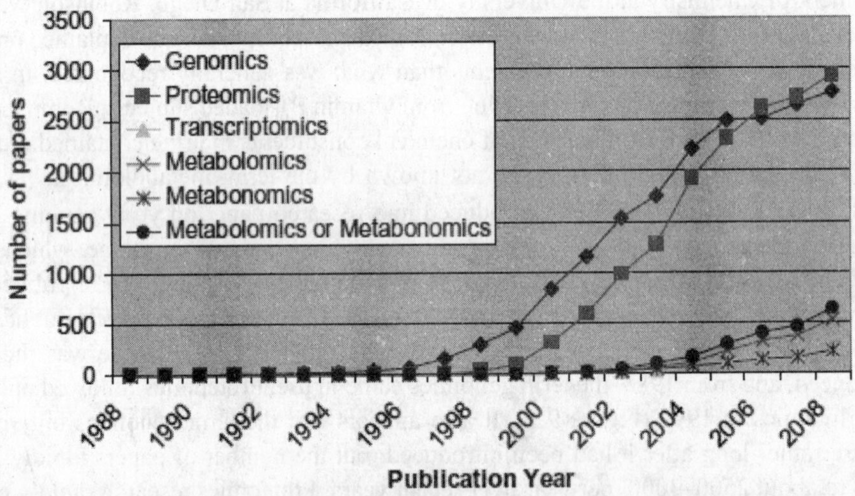

Figure 9.2 Number of papers appeared in different years related to the Science of 'Omics' as compiled by ISI Web of Science from Thomson Scientific (Jan Schripssma, 2009).

CONCEPTS

Metabolome analysis covers the identification and quantification of all intracellular and extracellular metabolites with molecular mass lower than 1000 daltons (Da) using different analytical techniques.

In common with the transcriptome and the proteome, the metabolome is context-dependent, and the levels of each metabolite depend on the physiological, developmental, environmental and pathological state of a cell, tissue or organism. However, an important difference is that, unlike mRNA and proteins, it is difficult or impossible to establish a direct link between genes and metabolites as they fall at the two ends of the relationship chain. Those compounds that are highly similar chemically though could be co-analyzed by the same high-throughput techniques but offer the obstacle of their discrete resolution from each other while those that are chemically quite dissimilar often fail to be extracted and/or analyzed with the same technique/methodology. Thus, the metabolome comprises a huge range of chemicals of varied structures, conjugation possessing diverse physico-chemical properties. These constituents of metabolome as chemical classes include ionic inorganic species to hydrophilic carbohydrates, volatile alcohols and ketones, protein amino acids and organic acids, hydrophobic lipids and complex natural products. This complexity makes it virtually impossible to simultaneously profile complete metabolome.

METABOLOMICS TECHNOLOGY

Purpose: The study of metabolomics is relevant to generate metabolic "signatures", monitor/measure metabolite flux, monitor enzyme/pathway kinetics, assess/identify phenotypes, monitor gene/environment interactions, track effects from toxins/drugs/surgery, monitor consequences from gene knockouts (KOs), identify functions of unknown genes, provide full-spectrum molecular phenotypes.

Intermediary Metabolism and Metabolomics

Understanding the chemical compositions and three-dimensional structures of biological molecules is not sufficient to understand how they are assembled to function together into organisms or how they function to sustain life or cohesively respond to changes in its environment. We must therefore examine the reactions by which the biological molecules are built, broken down or recombined to give rise to new chemical entities. We must also consider how free energy is consumed in building cellular materials and carrying out cellular work and how free energy is generated from organic or other sources. In other words, the metabolism of an organism (or of a cell) may be defined as 'the sum total of all the enzyme-catalysed reactions that occur in an organism (or in a cell)'. The large number of reactions in a cell are organized into relatively much small number of sets and subsets as defined sequence of reactions called metabolic pathways or routes. It is a highly coordinated and purposeful cell activity, in which multi-enzyme systems cooperate. This implies that the metabolism of even a simple unicellular organism is time-variant, i.e., all its aspects are not actually expressed at any given point. Metabolism, the overall process through which living systems acquire and use free energy to carry out their various functions, is traditionally divided into two parts and the terms catabolism and anabolism were coined by the physiologist Gasket in 1886:

- ***Catabolism:*** In which nutrients and cell constituents are broken down to salvage their components and/or to generate energy.
- ***Anabolism:*** In which bio-molecules are synthesized from simpler components.

The various activities powered by catabolism include mechanical movement, growth, reproduction, accumulation of foods, elimination of wastes, generation of electrical current or impulse, maintenance of temperature etc. The various anabolic activities may be exemplified by food manufacture etc.

Since, not only the metabolic reactions of a pathway are linked to each other, the pathways themselves are linked to each other in multifarious ways like sharing of the same precursor, intermediates of one serving as substrates for the committed step of another, intermediate or end-product of one modulating the catalytic activity of one or more of the enzymes of other pathways, two or more pathways conjointly leading to function or response, utility of one only in the presence or absence of other etc. Conventionally, while analysing a metabolic process or pathway, only the metabolites related to the specific biochemical reactions or at the most, all the metabolites of the pathway used to be assayed and interpreted. However, with the recent advent of the concept of systems biology (with respect to enzymes, genes and metabolites), a wholesome knowledge of the levels of intermediates of the directly and indirectly related metabolic pathways is intended for the realistic view of the metabolic and metabolite state that provide molecular phenotype to the cell, tissue, organ or the organism. Thus, metabolomics of pathway intermediates constitutes a key domain of understanding metabolism. At the highest order of differentiation, metabolism may be divided into two classes: primary metabolism and secondary (or specialized) metabolism. Accordingly, their metabolic intermediates and end-products are called primary metabolites and secondary metabolites, respectively. The precursors of secondary metabolism are either intermediates or end-products of primary metabolism. Thus, often metabolomic investigation of both is intended.

Primary and Secondary Metabolites

Bu'Lock borrowed the term "secondary metabolite" from plant physiology in 1961 and applied it to microbiology. While primary metabolites are essential for the normal developmental sustenance and progress of life and reproduction of cells and thereby primary metabolism operates and functions almost similarly in all microorganisms, the following is true for secondary metabolites and secondary metabolism:

- Every secondary metabolite is usually formed by only a few organisms.
- Secondary metabolites are seemingly not essential for growth and reproduction.
- Their formation is extremely dependent on environmental conditions.
- Some secondary metabolites are produced as a group of closely related structures; one strain of *streptomyces*, for example, produces 32 different anthracyclines.
- Some organisms form a variety of different classes of substances as secondary metabolites.
- The catalytic specificity of enzymes of secondary metabolism is quite flexible, as opposed to that of enzymes of primary metabolism.
- The regulation of the biosynthesis of secondary metabolites differs significantly from that of the primary metabolites.

There are several hypothesis about the role of secondary metabolites, of which Hans Zahner's illustrated in Figure 9.3, is the most elegant. Besides the five phases of the cell's own metabolism (intermediary metabolism, regulation, transport, differentiation and morphogenesis), secondary metabolism is considered a "playing field for the evolution of further biochemical development, which can proceed without damaging primary metabolism". Genetic changes leading to the modification of secondary metabolites would be expected not to have any major effect on normal cell function. If a genetic change leads to the formation of a compound that in some way is beneficial, then this genetic change would be fixed in the cell's genome, perhaps becoming essential. In this way with time the former secondary metabolites may be evolved into a primary metabolite. (Table 9.1).

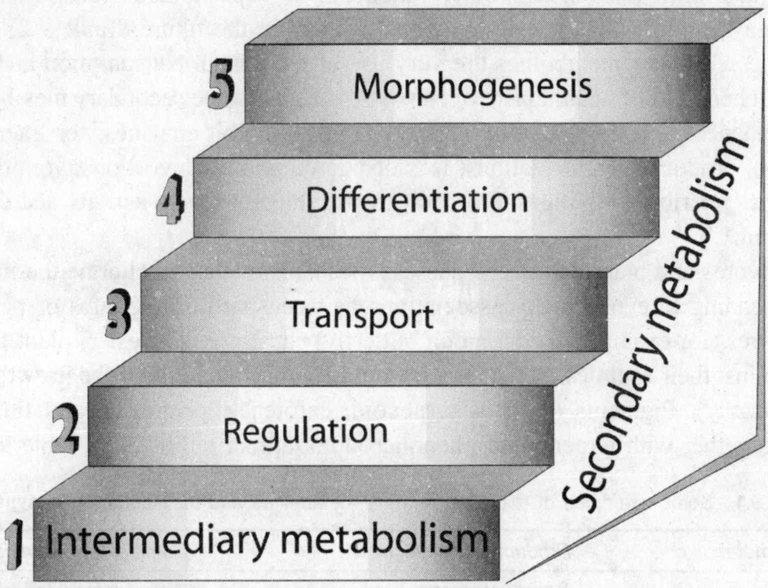

Figure 9.3 The five steps of primary metabolism with the "playing field" of secondary metabolism (Zahner, 1979).

Secondary metabolites are chemicals produced by plants (and microbes) for which no role has yet been found in growth, photosynthesis, reproduction, or other "primary" functions. These chemicals are extremely diverse; many thousands have been identified that are divisible into several major classes. Each plant family, genus and species produces a characteristic blend of these chemicals, and they can sometimes be used as taxonomic characters in classifying plants (chemotaxonomy). Humans use some of these compounds as medicines, flavorings, or recreational drugs. Secondary metabolites can be classified on the basis of chemical structure [for example, in terms of having rings, conjugation with sugars, polymeric state etc., composition (containing nitrogen or not), their solubility in various solvents, or the pathway by which they are synthesized (e.g. phenylpropanoid, which also leads to tannins), biogenetic origin (nature of committed precursor) etc]. A simple classification includes three main groups: the terpenes (made from mevalonic acid and/or deoxyxylulose-5-phosphate (DOXP), composed almost entirely of carbon hydrogen and oxygen), phenolics (originating from phenylalanine), and nitrogen-containing compounds (alkaloids-extremely diverse).

The apparent lack of primary function in the plant, combined with the observation that many secondary metabolites have specific adverse impacts on other organisms such as herbivores and pathogens, leads to the hypothesis that they have evolved because of their protective value or specialized function. Many secondary metabolites are toxic or repellant to herbivores and microbes and thus help defend plants producing them. Production of secondary metabolites often increases when a plant is attacked by herbivores or pathogens. Some compounds release volatiles into the air when plants are attacked by insects; these compounds attract parasites and predators that kill the herbivores. Recent research is identifying more and more primary roles for these chemicals in plants as signals, antioxidants, and other functions, so "specialized" rather than "secondary" metabolites may be more accurate designation for them in the future (Table 9.2).

While some secondary metabolites are very useful for human consumption and serve as non-nutrient phytochemicals of health, taste of flavor advantage, some secondary metabolites can have severe consequences. Alkaloids can block ion channels, inhibit enzymes, or interfere with neurotransmission, producing hallucinations, loss of coordination, convulsions, vomiting, and death. Some phenolics interfere with digestion, slow growth, block enzyme activity and cell division, or just taste awful.

Most herbivores and plant pathogens possess mechanisms that ameliorate the impacts of plant metabolites, leading to evolutionary associations between particular groups of pests and plants. Some herbivores (for example, the monarch butterfly) can store (sequester) plant toxins and gain protection against their enemies. Secondary metabolites may also inhibit the growth of competitor plants (allelopathy). Pigments (such as terpenoid, carotenes, phenolics, and flavonoids) color flowers and together with terpene and phenolic odors, attract pollinators (Table 9.3).

Table 9.1 Some examples of microbial primary metabolites and their commercial significance.

Primary metabolite	*Producing organism*	*Commercial significance*
Ethanol	*Saccharomyces cerevisieae*	'Active ingredient' in alcoholic beverages
Citric Acid	*Aspergillus niger*	Various uses in food industry
Glutamic acid	*Corynebacterium glutamicum*	Flavour enhancer
Lysine	*Corynebacterium glutamicum*	Feed additive
Polysaccharides	*Xanthomonas spp.*	Applications in food industry; enhanced oil recovery

Table 9.2 Some examples of microbial secondary metabolites and their commercial significance.

Secondary metabolite	*Commercial significance*
Penicillin	Antibiotic
Cephalosporin	Antibiotic
Streptomycin	Antibiotic
Griseofulvin	Antibiotic-antifungal
Pepstatin	Treatment of ulcers
Cyclosporin A	Immunosuppressant
Gibberellins	Plant growth regulator
Lovastatin	Cholesterol synthesis inhibitor

Table 9.3 Some example of plant secondary metabolites and their commercial significance.

Class	*Example Compounds*	*Example Sources*	*Some Effects and Uses*
NITROGEN-CONTAINING			
Alkaloids	Nicotine, cocaine, theobromine	Tobacco coca plant chocolate (cocao)	Interfere with neurotransmission, block enzyme action
NITROGEN-AND SULFUR-CONTAINING			
Glucosinolates	Sinigrin	cabbage, relatives	
TERPENOIDS			
Monoterpenes	Menthol, linalool	Mints,, many other plants	Interfere with neurotransmission, block ion transport, anesthetic
Sesquiterpenes	Parthenolide	Parthenium and relatives (*Asteraceae*)	contact dermatitis
Diterpenes	Gossypol	Cotton	Block phosphorylation; toxic
Triterpenes, cardiac glycosides	Digitogenin	Digitalis (foxglove)	stimulate heart muscle, alter ion transport
Tetraterpenoids	Carotene	many plants	Antioxidant; orange coloring
Terpene polymers	Rubber	Hevea (rubber) trees, dandelion	Gum up insects; airplane tires
Sterols	Spinasterol	Spinach	Interfere with animal hormone action
PHENOLICS			
Phenolic acids	caffeic, chlorogenic	all plants	Cause oxidative damage, browning in fruits and wine
Coumarins	Umbelliferone	carrots, parsnip	Cross-link DNA, block cell division
Lignans	podophyllin urushiol	mayapple poison ivy	Cathartic, vomiting, allergic dermatitis
Flavonoids	anthocyanin, catechin	almost all plants	Flower, leaf color; inhibit enzymes, anti- and pro-oxidants, estrogenic
Tannins	gallotannin,	oak, hemlock trees, birdsfoot trefoil, legumes	Bind to proteins, enzymes, block Digestion, antioxidants
Lignin	Lignin	all land plants	structure, toughness, fiber

Chemical and Physical Analysis of Metabolites

Biological systems are complex and their behaviour depends not only on the properties of the components but also the interactions between them as well as with the environment. Metabolome analysis presents one of the most exciting and also challenging investigations compared with the other cell product analyses, the "omes" such as the genome and transcriptome. This is because of the fact that each metabolite is characterized by its individual chemical structure, knowledge of the physical and chemical properties of the target compounds is useful for discerning the approach of their resolution and quantification. Therefore, each metabolite even from the same pathway can present very different chemistry requiring different methodology of sample preparation and analysis. The properties and chemistry of metabolites and their occurrence in the metabolism are governed by two major properties: the chemical and physical properties of metabolic compounds. These properties include molecular weight, molecular size, polarity, volatility, solubility, pKa and stability. It requires an assortment of procedures to enable accurate and comprehensive measurement of metabolites within a metabolomics approach.

Sample Preparation

Internal standards

Before extraction, samples are typically added with known amount of one or more internal standards to assess recovery during extraction and index chromatography and artefacts such as ion suppression etc. Standards can also be used as a normalization method and to help with chromatographic alignment if chromatography is used. For metabolic fingerprinting, internal standards may be used that represent all major classes of compounds (e.g. carbohydrates, organic acids, steroids, amines, etc.) under assay and for metabolic profiling, use of compounds that represent the metabolites of interest may be of advantage.

Metabolite extraction

The overall goal of extraction is to get the metabolites of interest solvated out of the cellular matrix after subjecting test sample to the quickest metabolic arrest so that the sample can be truly described in terms of its metabolome in a time, state, treatment or response context. Therefore, it involves choice of an appropriate sample processing that can inactivate enzymes and can catalyze the transformation of the metabolites or a solvent that can best solubilise the metabolites to facilitate their nearly complete recovery from the tissue or cells. Therefore, it is important that samples are collected in liquid nitrogen and be extracted soon after collection. The extracts may also be stored the same way at – 80°C to ensure their chemical and compositional stability. For metabolic fingerprinting, the goal is to develop a reproducible method to extract the most comprehensive set of metabolites possible while removing most of the macromolecules, particularly proteins. This can be challenging because of the physico-chemical diversity and range of abundances of cellular, tissue and bio-fluidic metabolites.

There are several techniques for metabolites identification and profiling that do not require extensive sample processing prior to detection as discussed ahead.

Direct infusion mass spectrometry (DIMS)

In this case, the analyte solution from a syringe flows to the ion source of the mass spectrometer using a syringe pump. Both atmospheric pressure chemical ionization (APCI) and electrospray ionization (ESI) are being used to detect metabolites in complex biological samples. This type of analysis can be helpful with metabolites that are challenging to measure by gas chromatography-mass spectrophotometry (GC-MS) and can increase the throughput of the analysis.

Derivatization

Derivatization is most commonly used for gas chromatography (GC) analysis so that the metabolites that are difficult to volatilize (hence difficult to detect and analyze by GC or GC-MS). Derivatization involves chemically modifying a compound to produce a new compound which is volatile and hence suitable for analysis using a GC. In some cases, metabolites are also derivatized for liquid chromatography (LC) for the ease of detection/resolution or advantage of enhanced sensitivity. Biological samples contain a variety of metabolites such as organic acids, sugars, sugar alcohols, amino acids and steroids many of which are not volatile. Derivatization reduces their polarity and leads to their increased volatility, stability and detectability enabling their separation by GC and followed by detection by MS. The most commonly used methods of derivatization for GC are presented in Table 9.4.

Table 9.4 Common derivatization methods.

Method	*Comment*	*Advantages*	*Disadvantages*
Silylation	Increases volatility and thermal stability	Compatible with a wide variety of compounds Large number of reagents available Easily prepared	Reagent are moisture sensitive Must use aprotic organic solvents TMS derivatives stable only for a short period of time thereafter re-derivatization is required
Acylation	Reduces the polarity of amino, hydroxyl, and thiol groups targets highly polar, multifunctional compounds (i.e., carbohydrate, amino acids)	Addition of halogenated carbons increased delectability by ECD Hydrolytically stable increases sensitivity by adding molecular weight can be used as a first step to activate carboxylic acids prior to alkylation	Derivatives can be difficult to prepare Reaction byproducts often need to be removed before analysis. Reagents are moisture sensitive Reagents are hazardous
Alkylation	Reduces polarity of compounds with acidic hydrogens (i.e., carboxylic acids, phenols)	Wide range of reagents available Wide range of reaction conditions are compatible Some reactions can be done in aqueous solutions Derivatives are generally stable	Limited to amines and acidic hydroxyls Reaction conditions are often severe Reagents are often toxic

Approaches used for Metabolome Analyses

Metabolome analyses usually involve two major approaches: discovery metabolomics and targeted metabolomics (Figure 9.4).

Discovery metabolomics typically includes:

toxic
- Profiling (also known as differential expression analysis), which involves finding the interesting metabolites with statistically significant variations in abundance within a set of experimental and control samples.
- Identification, which is the determination of the chemical structure of these metabolites after profiling.
- Interpretation, the last step in the workflow, which makes connections between the metabolites discovered and the biological processes or conditions.

Targeted metabolomics analyses focus on validation, which uses much larger numbers of samples to account for the effect of natural and biological variations to validate the previously identified metabolites. It is quantitative and requires analytical standards.

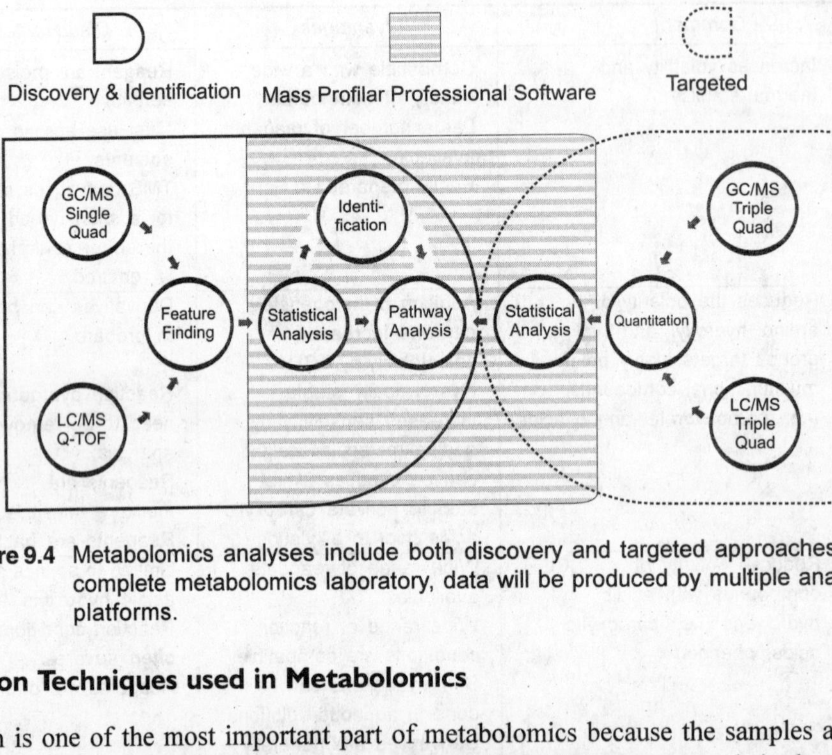

Figure 9.4 Metabolomics analyses include both discovery and targeted approaches. In a complete metabolomics laboratory, data will be produced by multiple analytical platforms.

Separation Techniques used in Metabolomics

Separation is one of the most important part of metabolomics because the samples are complex mixtures of several metabolites. Several chromatographic techniques are used singly or in combination to resolve the constituent chemical moieties of the mixture. The chromatographic information in the form of retention time or migration time of the separation is used to track and identify a metabolite undergoing analysis. This is necessary because MS alone cannot distinguish isobaric metabolites, whereas chromatography can be used to separate and identify isomers. The two most commonly used separation techniques are gas chromatography (GC) and liquid chromatography (LC). Each technique has its own strengths and weaknesses. GC requires analytes to be volatile which requires the use of chemically derived samples, if the targeted metabolites are not volatile *per se*. LC is highly versatile and can be used in several modes like reverse phase, normal phase etc. Although reverse phase is usually referred to as standard HPLC, it does not adequately address the separation of hydrophilic components of the metabolome. Capillary electrophoresis (CE) is very effective for hydrophilic metabolites, but the buffers used are not readily compatible with the ion source of the mass spectrometer. With the development of new column chemistries such as hydrophilic interaction chromatography (HILIC), they may be LC-MS alternative to CE-MS. The combination of separation and MS together make for a very sensitive and fast approach to examine samples containing hundreds to thousands of compounds. There is no other analytical technique so well suited to this task. The separation techniques most commonly used in metabolomic analyses are listed in Figure 9.5 and briefly described thereafter.

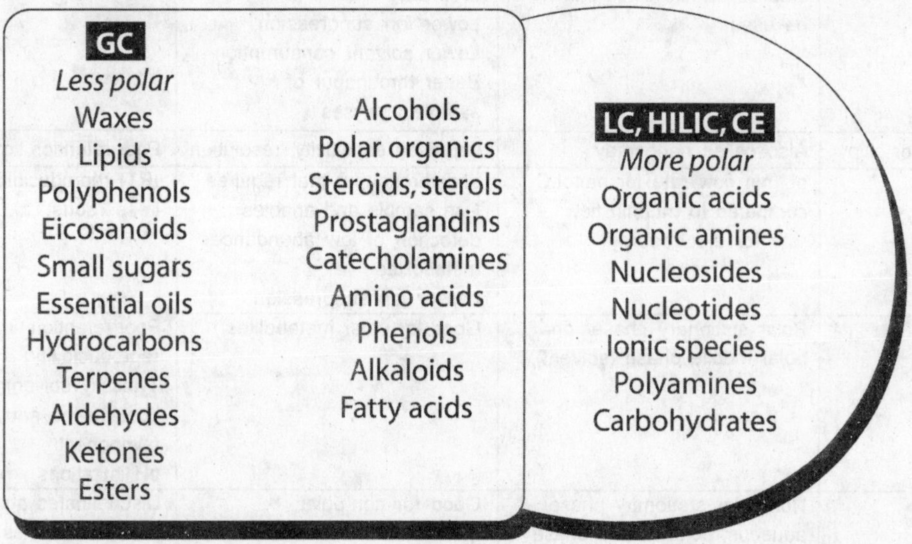

Figure 9.5 Most common types of chromatography and other methods of separation used in metabolomics.

Gas Chromatography (GC)

GC is the oldest form of automated separation. It uses a carrier gas as a mobile gas phase and a stationary liquid or polymer phase within a column. Nowadays, columns used in GC are capillary columns. The method requires the analyte to be volatile in order to migrate through the capillary. The analyte can be naturally volatile or be rendered volatile *via* chemical derivatization. The advantages of using GC include use of electron ionization (EI) that can ionize the molecules before they enter the mass spectrometer. Ionization of the analyte is a prerequisite for its measurement through mass-spectrometer (MS).

High Performance Liquid Chromatography (HPLC)

Liquid chromatography can reduce ion suppression by decreasing the number of competing analytes entering the mass spectrometer ion source at a given time. Liquid chromatography can separate metabolites that are nonvolatile, so a more diverse set of metabolites can be analyzed than toxicwith GC-MS. An overview of liquid chromatography (LC) columns with recommendations based on the known physical and chemical properties of the analyte(s) and the mode of analysis, is summarised in Table 9.5.

Table 9.5 Most common LC methods used in metabolomics.

LC Method	*Description*	*Advantages*	*Disadvantages*
U-HPLC (UPLC)	Higher pressure (up to 15,000 psi) than HPLC (6000 psi), columns with smaller particle sizes can be used	Increased resolution, throughput, peak capacity and sensitivity compared to HPLC Lower ion suppression Lower solvent consumption Better throughput of sample analyses	Increased pressure Faster deterioration of columns
Nano or chip Lc	Also called nanospray nL/min flow rate for nanoLC compared to mL/min flow rate for electrospray	Improved sensitivity, resolution and throughput that requires less sample and enables detection of low abundance metabolites Lesser ion suppression	Poor retention time (RT) reproducibility Less robust
NP	Polar stationary phase/non-polar mobile phase (solvent)	Good for polar metabolites	Poor retention-time reproducibility Typically solvent contains no aqueous component pH limitations
RP	Non-polar stationary phase/ aqueous, polar mobile phase (solvent)	Good for non-polar, hydrophobic metabolites	Discriminates against polar metabolites
HILIC	Polar stationary phase/ hydrophobic mobile phase	More reproducible retention time than NPGood for polar metabolites Enhanced sensitivity Lesser sample preparation time as mobile phase is 80% organic solvent Solvent system can include aqueous component	

Capillary Electrophoresis (CE)

In capillary electrophoresis, metabolites are separated based on charge and size. Advantages of CE include easily optimized resolution, much smaller dead volume and minimal sample effluent consumption. CE has been shown to work better for analysis of polar and low abundance compounds in complex mixtures. Some researchers have trouble in robustly coupling CE to MS.

Analyte Detection

Mass spectrometry

MS is a well-established detection method employed in many fields and is one of the essential instruments in an analytical laboratory. By measuring the m/z of elemental or molecular species, it allows the simultaneous detection of multiple analytes with high sensitivities. MS has been demonstrated as a potent platform for metabolomics because of its high sensitivity and thereby ability to detect metabolites present at very low levels (mM concentrations). Operationally, it involves ionization of the analytes. Atmospheric pressure ionisation includes common soft ionisation techniques that generally produce protonated molecules or deprotonated molecules. For metabolomic purposes and due to the fact that some metabolites can be observed exclusively in only one ionisation mode, acquisition should be performed in both positive and negative ion modes to maximise the metabolome coverage. The high mass accuracy of MS provides structural information about the analytes, as an exact molecular mass can be indicative of the molecular formula or fragments of the molecular structure. The vast majority of recent metabolomic studies have relied on this particular technique.

Ionization methods for mass spectrometry

In order to obtain a comprehensive LC-MS analysis for discovery metabolomics, positive and negative ion modes are used either by switching between the two modes in the same run or independent runs for the two modes.

Ionization methods that do not require sample preparation or upfront separation:

The methods described below are advantageous because they do not require sample preparation or separation before mass spectrometric analysis. Additionally, the methods are used at atmospheric pressure. Consequently they increase the throughput of metabolomic analyses. Limitations of these methods are related to the lack of upfront separation and therefore disadvantages of the technique include: (1) inability to distinguish chemical isomers (same mass), and (2) problems of signal suppression or its enhancement due to simultaneous introduction of all sample analytes leading to ion suppression.

Laser diode thermal desorption (LDTD)

The LDTD source contains an infrared diode laser with an X-Y moveable stage capable of holding one 96-well plate. Upon operation, the plunger powered by nitrogen inserts into a sample well, the programmable laser thermally desorbs the dried sample (2 μL spotted) by heating the back of the plate, and the desorbed neutral sample is passed by the carrier gas (air) along the transfer tube to the corona discharge needle to be ionized and then transmitted into the MS.

Desorption electrospray ionization (DESI)

DESI directs pneumatically assisted electrosprayed droplets onto a sample surface to produce ions. It is a gentle ionization method that produces electrospray-like spectra. This technique has been proved to work for polar and non-polar organic and biological compounds and enables *in situ* analysis of biological tissues.

Direct analysis in real time (DART)

This technique uses an atmospheric-pressure ion source that permits analysis of gases, liquids, solids, or materials on surfaces in open air at ground potential under ambient conditions. Samples are exposed to the DART gas stream which rapidly generates ions that are carried by the gas stream into the sampling orifice of the mass spectrometer atmospheric pressure interface. The gas stream can graze a solid sample surface or be reflected off the sample surface. Liquids can be sampled by dipping an object (such as a glass rod) into the liquid sample to be measured. Vapours are introduced directly into the DART gas stream.

Extractive electro-spray ionization (EESI)

EESI is a method for the ionization of analytes in complex matrices. EESI does not suffer from ion suppression effects which is common for traditional electrospray ionization (ESI). The technique was established for the direct analysis of vaporized samples such as breath for clinical diagnosis. Desorption of analytes from surfaces with a gentle gas stream allows the fast and efficient investigation of biological samples, or the detection of explosives from surfaces in real time. For EESI, a solvent is sprayed by electrospray while the sample is introduced as vapour. Charge is transferred from the electrospray plume to the analytes which leads to their ionization.

GC-MS Ionization Methods

Electron impact (EI)

The advantages of EI are that there are extensive spectral libraries that exist for metabolite identification; the technique has good sensitivity and unique fragmentation patterns. However, the molecular ion is commonly not detectable because the high energy fragmentation completely fragments the parent ion, which can make identification of unknown metabolites challenging. Also, the application of EI is restricted to thermally stable samples.

Chemical ionization (CI)

This method is less energetic than EI. Hence, it tends to produce more stable ions for easier determination of molecular weight of the metabolite. Quantification is almost impossible without internal standards.

LC-MS ionization methods

These methods are soft ionization, atmospheric pressure methods (unlike EI & CI) so that no fragmentation of the molecular ion occurs (Table 9.6). For more comprehensive coverage of metabolites, ionization should be performed in both positive and negative ion modes.

Electrospray ionization (ESI)/Nano-ESI

ESI is the most common ionization method used with LC-MS. This method is best used for analyzing polar and ionic metabolites. It provides excellent quantitative analysis and high sensitivity. Nano-ESI is performed at lower flow rates such as 200 nL/min which improves sensitivity and dynamic range.

Atmospheric pressure chemical ionization (APCI)

This technique is advantageous for analysis of nonpolar and neutral molecules that are thermally stable such as lipids and is tolerant to higher buffer concentrations. It can also be used with polar compounds so that a wide range of metabolites can be analyzed.

Atmospheric pressure photoionization (APPI)

APPI directly photoionizes metabolites and therefore can ionize compounds that cannot be ionized as effectively using other atmospheric pressure techniques such as less polar metabolites. This ion source uses low ionization energy, as a result it causes minimal fragmentation and relatively few adducts form, which makes it easier to identify the metabolite. This technique has a large linear dynamic range and minimal ionization of air and solvents.

Combination APCI/APPI

The PhotoMate combination APCI/APPI ion source allows for effective ionization of non-polar compounds. This unique ion source provides greater flexibility and the capability to analyze a larger range of compounds without changing hardware.

Table 9.6 Comparison of the most common analytical methods used for metabolomics.

Analytical method	*Advantages*	*Disadvantages*
NMR	Rapid analysis, in general, High resolution No derivatization required Non-destructive for sample More complete structural elucidation than MS	Relatively lower sensitivity than MS Difficult to interpret spectra>1 peak per metabolites High purity requirement of sample or peak in a hyphenated technique
GC-MS	Comprehensive EI spectral libraries for metabolite ID Sensitivity Robust Large linear range	Relatively slower method Derivatization required for non-volatiles Many analytes are too thermally labile for analysis
LC-MS	Typically no derivatization required More types of separation are compatible with LC Large sample capacity	Comprehensive spectral libraries do not exist

Contd.

CE-MS	Typically no derivatization required High resolution Smaller sample requirements Higher throughput analysis Analysis of neutrals & changed metabolites possible in a single run.	Limited spectral libraries do not exist.
Fourier Transform Infrared (FTIR) Spectroscopy	No derivatization required Rapid analysis High resolution of functional groups. Complete structural elucidation	Difficult to interpret spectra Challenging to identify metabolites >1 peak per metabolites Requires sample drying

Nuclear magnetic resonance (NMR)

NMR methods provide metabolite fingerprints with good chemical specificity for compounds containing elements with non-zero magnetic moments, such as ^{1}H, ^{13}C, ^{15}N and ^{32}P which are commonly found in most biological metabolites at different levels of low abundance. However, ^{1}H NMR spectra of plant extracts are inevitably crowded not only because there is a large number of contributing compounds, but also because of the low overall chemical shift dispersion (chemical shift is caused by the chemistry around the nucleus changing its resonance). Increased specificity and resolution can be achieved by using higher magnetic fields. Thus, NMR spectra of unpurified extracts of plants have the potential to provide a relatively unbiased fingerprint, containing overlapping signals of the majority of the metabolites present in the solvent extract.

The experimental operations and precautions in metabolomic analysis include quickest metabolic arrest of the target tissue by immersion in liquid nitrogen followed by storage at –80°C until analyzed. Although other methods of metabolic arrest like heating, organic solvent treatment or use of acid are also possible, they may lead to decomposition of metabolites and/or modifications of the metabolites. The nature of extraction solvent (from non-polar to highly polar) for the tissue would be governed by the types of metabolites targeted to be profiled. For programs that involve handling of a large number of samples at a time, even direct extraction with NMR solvents could be helpful, despite high cost involved therein as it not only reduces elaborate extraction procedures but also minimizes degradation or loss of metabolites. Typically, for direct extraction, the tissue can be extracted using MeOD (deuteriated methanol) and a buffer like KH_2PO_4 (pH 6.0 to 7.0). To reasonably compare the NMR data generated across the research groups, a large database is required (Table 9.6).

Fourier transform infrared spectroscopy (FT-IR)

Fourier transform infrared (FT-IR) spectroscopy primarily measures vibrations of functional groups and highly polar bonds. These (bio) chemical 'fingerprints' are made up of the vibrational features of all the sample's components. FT-IR spectrometers record the interaction of IR radiation with experimental samples, measuring the frequencies at which the sample absorbs the radiation and the intensities of the absorptions (Table 9.6). Determining these frequencies allows identification of the sample's chemical makeup since functional groups of the chemicals are known to absorb light at specific frequencies. However, there is a lack of differentiation between isomers, and the presence of fragment and adduct ions and problems of quantification caused by ion suppression make the use of powerful classification tools essential. The combination of FT-MS data with other chromatographic MS data is potentially powerful.

Number of Metabolites in Biological System

There have been many attempts to estimate the number of metabolites in a biological system. The size of the metabolome varies greatly, depending on the organism studied. The completion of whole genome sequences of many different species has enabled estimation of the number of metabolites, but owing to the lack of complete gene annotations in sequenced genomes, not all possible metabolic reactions can be predicted (Figure 9.6). For example, the well studied model of eukaryotic organism *Saccharomyces cerevisiae* contains more than 6000 genes of which only approximately 70% have been studied so far and hence there are almost 2000 genes whose function is unknown. Therefore, the number of metabolites estimated is uncertain and only represents a rough estimate. In general, it has been stated that the number of possible metabolites in a cell is lower than the number of all genes and proteins in a cell. However, the story seems otherway round. The number of genes is much lower than the number of metabolites as a single enzyme (gene) catalyzed reaction can deliver more than one product particularly as concerns secondary metabolism.

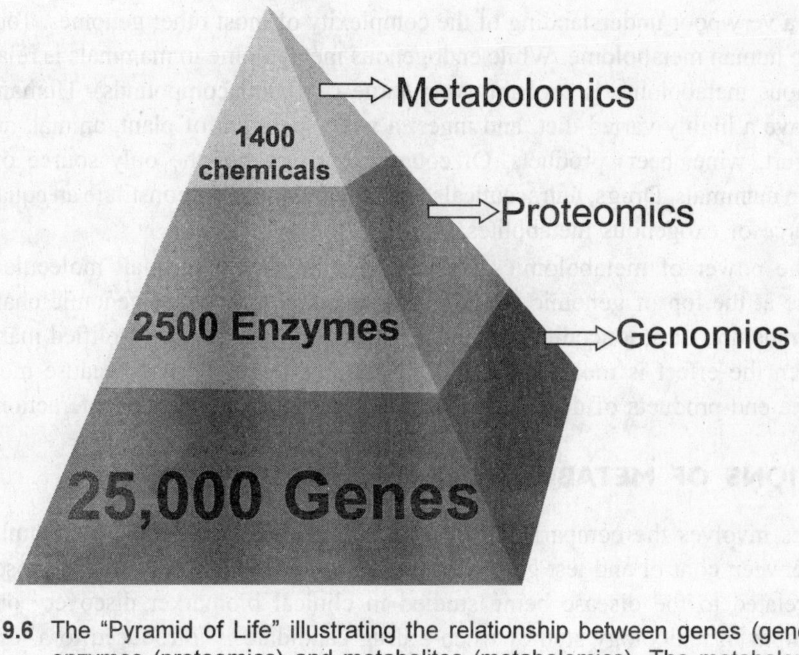

Figure 9.6 The "Pyramid of Life" illustrating the relationship between genes (genomics), enzymes (proteomics) and metabolites (metabolomics). The metabolomic estimate may be a serious underestimation.

In reality, it is extremely difficult to determine the number of metabolites and also other cell products, such as transcripts and proteins, at a given time in a given cell because of the lack of analytical techniques to measure all cellular components in a comprehensive manner. In many bacteria and also some eukaryotes such as baker's yeast, detailed genome-wide analyses have made great progress to get more information about the real complexity of these comparatively simpler cellular organisms. For example, in the well studied bacterium *E.coli,* there are about 4400 genes and it is estimated that only about 442 metabolic compounds are produced whereas for the eukaryote *S. cerevisieae*, which contains about 6200 genes, it has been estimated that it contains slightly more than 700 metabolites. While in higher organisms, the situation becomes much more complex. Additional dimensions, such as tissue specificity or organ structures, make correct estimations extremely difficult. For example, it has been estimated that the whole plant kingdom might be capable of producing between 200,000 and 400,000 primary and secondary metabolites and a similar number within the fungal kingdom. However, only about 5000 might be actually present in the well-studied plant model *Arabidopsis thaliana* at a given time point. This enormous difference in metabolic complexity can be rationalized by the fundamental differences in mobility between plants and animals (and microbes). Because mammals are able to run, walk, or fly, they require a much smaller arsenal of defensive chemical agents than plants, which must "stand and fight" when attacked by a predator or parasite.

Recall that 15 years ago no living organism had yet been fully sequenced, and the human genome project was only twinkling in a few scientists' eyes. In those early days, we had only widely incorrect estimates (150,000 vs. 23,000) of the number of genes that might be found in human genome and a very poor understanding of the complexity of most other genomes. Today the same is true for the human metabolome. While endogenous metabolome in mammals is relatively small, their exogenous metabolome is probably very large (>10,000 compounds). Humans, like most mammals, have a highly varied diet, and ingest a wide spectrum of plant, animal, and microbial (cheese, yogurt, wine, beer) products. Of course, food are not the only source of exogenous metabolites in mammals. Drugs, nutraceuticals and other xenobiotics constitute an equally large and complex source of exogenous metabolites.

Indeed, the power of metabolomics comes from the fact that small molecule metabolites effectively lie at the top of genomic pyramid. An imperceptibly small genomic change, such as single base transition or a noncoding polymorphism in a gene, can be amplified many thousands of times when the effect is measured at the metabolites level. This is because metabolites are essentially the end-products of dozens of interdependent macromolecular interactions.

APPLICATIONS OF METABOLOMICS TECHNOLOGY

Metabolomics involves the comparison of metabolomes (the full metabolite complement of an organism) between control and test groups to find differences in their profiles. Those differences may be correlated to the disease being studied in clinical biomarker discovery or changes in metabolic output in toxicology studies when a drug candidate is introduced to a test subject, as studied in pharmaceutical development. Environmental metabolomics is also growing in importance where studies are performed to assess chemical exposure to both the wildlife and the environment. In the agricultural/chemical industry, metabolomics may be used to develop herbicides and pesticides.

With increasing importance being placed on health and safety related aspects of our food, metabolomics can potentially be a valuable tool to monitor and improve the quality of what we eat; for example, in food processing and quality control, or in plant breeding for improved crop varieties and in the development of novel foodstuffs.

As the demand for energy increases along with the depletion of natural energy resources, alternative sources such as plant or microalgae biomass are sought. Metabolomics can be used to study the metabolism of these organisms under different environmental and genetic conditions to maximize production and types of hydrocarbons produced.

Unlike gene expression studies or proteomics analyses, which only reveal part of what might be happening in a cell, metabolomics profiling can give an instantaneous snapshot of the entire physiology of that cell. More importantly, if data from proteomics, transcriptomics and metabolomics studies can be integrated (a collective approach also known as systems biology), a more complete picture of a living organism's biology can be obtained.

Designing improved or new metabolic pathways for degradation of various chemicals, especially xenobiotics, examples include degradation of mixture of benzene, toluene, and xylene by *Pseudomonas putida* and degradation of polychlorinated biphenyls by *Pseudomonas* spp. could be facilitated by the metabolomics data.

Modification of cell properties that facilitate bioprocessing (fermentation and/or product recovery) requires *a priori* information about the metabolomics of the cell. Examples include better growth of *E.coli* and other microorganisms under microaerobic conditions, reduced acetate production in *E. coli*, uptake of glucose without consuming phosphoenolpyruvate in *E. coli*, and ammonia transport without ATP consumption in *Methylophilus methylotrophus*.

Metabolomic to Nutraceuticals and Functional Foods

Metabolomics is one of the newest 'omics' technologies in nutritional research. The metabolome in a time and state context reflects the outcome of the interaction of the genome with its environment. Nutritional metabolomics has the potential to provide insight into biochemical changes after dietary intervention and to impact food safety issues pertaining to genetically modified food. Metabolomic techniques such as NMR and MS combined with powerful bioinformatics platforms greatly enhance understanding of comprehensive dynamics of compositional metabolite in a nutrition perspectives and its metabolic origin. The first nutritional metabolomic approach to determine biochemical modifications following dietary intervention have shown that soy isoflavones induced changes in plasma components in healthy premenopausal women under controlled environmental conditions. The plasma biochemical profiles showed strong variability in each subject, indicating the complex interaction of factors such as genetics, age, health status, diet, and lifestyle. Despite the individual variability, there were clear diet intervention-related differences in the plasma lipoprotein, amino acid, and carbohydrate profile, suggesting a soy-induced alteration in energy metabolism. Metabolic responses to chamomile tea ingestion in human subjects have been evaluated by high resolution ^{1}H NMR spectroscopy coupled with chemometric methods, to reveal a clear differentiation in urinary excretion demonstrating an increased hippurate and glycine with decreased creatinine level after chamomile ingestion. This variation has been shown to be over and above the substantial variation among the subjects within the same experimental group. A similar study toxicevaluated the effects of black and green tea intake on human urinary metabolites. The study showed that green tea consumption resulted in a stronger increase in several citric acid cycle intermediates suggesting an effect of green tea flavanols on human oxidative energy metabolism.

Although metabolomics has contributed significantly to the 'omics' revolution, a global description of human metabolism is impossible at this point due to limitations in current technologies and diversity among individuals in terms of age, gender, diet, lifestyle, health status, and other internal and external factors. Currently, the extent to which food components in the human diet induce changes in nutritional metabolic profiles is poorly understood. However, with technological advances, the challenges of applying metabolomics in nutrition research can be overcome. Thus, it would provide the role of non-nutrient phytochemcials in body functions and health. Thus, metabolomics provides a stronger and more reliable platform for the potential nutraceuticals and their mechanisms of actions—a perspective of metabolomics from nutraceutical composition to its effect on human metabolism.

Metabolomics to Herbal and Pharmaceuticals

Currently, metabolomics research is being applied to myriad of different disciplines from plant sciences to medicine. In the plant science community, for instance, metabolomics research is utilized in studies relating to biomass accumulation, stress resistance/tolerance, secondary metabolite production, etc. Biomass accumulation and resistance to certain environmental stressors are important in plant science as they chiefly determine the productivity/utility of the plants for food, feed, forage and fuel. Breeding resistant or genetically modified plants can be a long and arduous task, and metabolite analyses using a metabolomic approach holds strong promise to provide early indication for increased utility of the targeted/developed plant biotype using metabolic biomarkers discerned through metabolomic approach.

Additionally, plants are an exceedingly rich source of nutrients and secondary metabolites useful in nutritional and medicinal research. Recently, there has been a resurgence in the interest for plant-based pharmaceutical compounds. A conservative estimate places the number of plant metabolic compounds at 200,000, which provides for an extensive searching ground for new and improved medicinal and nutritional products. On a related note, comparative metabolomics in humans may provide for enhanced diagnostic power and individualized treatment for illness and disease.

Metabolomics to the Environmental Sciences

Environmental metabolomics is to both recognize and highlight the growing number of metabolomics studies within the environmental sciences. Some may regard environmental metabolomics purely as the application of this technique to study organisms dwelling within the natural environment, with the goal to learn about the state or condition of the environment, including the application of metabolomics to areas such as ecophysiology—with a focus on understanding the underpinning biochemical responses of organisms to abiotic and biotic stressors in their environment; and to ecotoxicology and ecological risk assessment. Some of the pioneering work in environmental metabolomics includes characterising the responses of organisms to toxicity, stresses, temperature, etc. with the potential of discovering novel biomarkers for subsequent environmental diagnostics.

Taylor and colleagues described the first application of metabolomics to toxicity testing in *Daphnia magna*, a water flea that is used internationally for environmental risk assessment. They utilised direct infusion Fourier transform ion cyclotron resonance (FT-ICR) mass spectrometry to identify multiple metabolic responses to copper toxicity, and putatively identified more than a thousand low molecular weight polar metabolites in the tissue extracts. A time course study into the toxicity of the herbicide Prometryn on a unicellular green alga (*Scenedesmus vacuolatus*) has been reported by Kluender *et al.* (2009), Metabolic responses of *Eisenia fetida* to two pesticides, DDT and endosulfan, using both NMR and GC-MS based approaches. NMR and LC-MS based approaches has been reported to understand the molecular mechanisms associated with chronic stress in juvenile Atlantic salmon (*Salmo salar*), which is important both in context of ecology as well as aquaculture. The effects of environmental stress, specifically atmospheric temperature, on the metabolism of *Arabidopsis lyrata* ssp. Petraea has been analyzed by Davey *et al.* (2008). This investigation reported that plant populations sampled from different latitudes (and therefore varying minimal temperatures) exhibited differences in their metabolic phenotypes, suggesting differential adaptation to the local thermal environment. Similarly, biotic–biotic interactions have been the subject of the study by Jansen *et al.* (2009) to profile changes in the metabolomes of both the feral cabbage (*Brassica oleracea*) and small cabbage white caterpillar (*Pieris rapae*) in response to shoot and root induction. Further, metabolomics approach is useful for the faster discovery of bioactive compounds involved in ecological interactions.

Indeed, the environmental metabolomics applications go far beyond to cover ecotoxicology, chemical risk assessment and biomarker discovery, tools for assessing ecological and soil health, and assessment of the effects of other biotic and abiotic environmental stressors. The value of metabolomics to these fields is now being recognised by environmental scientists, both academics as well as "end-users" involved in regulation and monitoring.

Metabolic Engineering and Metabolomics

Metabolic engineering is the science that combines systematic analysis of metabolic and other pathways with molecular biological techniques to improve cellular properties by designing and implementing rational genetic modifications. Metabolic engineering involves modulation of a metabolic pathway in an organism by introduction of a new gene (transgene) or enhance or suppress/silent one of more of the native gene. Thus, how altered or new expression of one or more genes impacts the overall metabolic of the cell, tissue or organism is an important to understand intricate metabolic linkages of pathways and functions, metabolic fluxes and cell physiology.

E. coli is still the workhorse organism for the production of proteins as well as various metabolites. These include (a) a low copy number plasmid for stable expression of cloned genes, (b) the introduction of hairpins into the mRNA to modify its stability, (c) metabolic flux analysis and its application to evaluate the effect of new or modified pathway on cell growth and metabolism, and (d) a new *E. coli* strain that can achieve more precise control of gene expression by means of the phosphate starvation promoter because it is deficient in the ability to accumulate polyphosphate.

Plastics and other synthetic polymers, whose desirable properties include chemical and biological inertness, have become essential for a multitude of applications in modern technology as well as in common consumer products. However, increasing concerns about environmental pollution by these non-biodegradable polymers has created interest in the development of polymers that are completely biodegradable. Polyhydroxyalkanoates (PHAs) arc an important class of biodegradable polymers that can be produced by a number of microorganisms. However, the high production cost and some (but not all) of the poor material properties are preventing the use of PHAs in a wide range of applications.

The overproduction of metabolites is not a trivial matter, given the complex regulatory nature of cellular metabolism. Amino acid production is a representative example of the problems and issues encountered. The discovery by Japanese scientists of glutamate over excretion by *Corynebacterium* (Brevibacterium) was a great stimulus for research targeting the overproduction of other amino acids. Considering the enormous demand for amino acid production—one million tons is produced annually. Metabolic engineering for amino acid overproduction is an area of both fundamental and industrial significance. Regulatory retuning of productions in such heterologous systems itself involves a concerted interaction of metabolites, signals and receptors. Therefore, understanding their relative dynamics of determining levels of each other provides cues to strategise uninhibited overproduction of such targeted metabolites(s) of interest.

The excitement and potential of metabolic engineering to generate an enormous number of new organic molecules with antibiotic, anti-tumour, or antiviral properties is also immense. The basis of this approach (which arguably defines the classification proposed by Cameron and Tong), is based on three key traits of natural product biosynthesis, including the organization of the biosynthetic genes in clusters (regulons) and the mechanistic relationship among the synthetic pathways. The paradigm of this approach and potential is the biosynthesis of novel polyketides (polyketides include many well-known antibiotics) through "combinatorial biosynthesis." The combinatorial biosynthesis relies on the wide-substrate specificity of the enzymes, particularly those related to biosynthesis of secondary metabolites. These include methyltransferases, glycosyltransferases, terpene synthases, hydroxylases, epoxidases that can use a range of substrates. The transgenics for these genes, therefore, can generate a range of products depending upon the range of substrates available. Thus, an understanding of the resultant metabolomics in such single gene transgenics could provide a global glimpse of the substrate specificity when compared with the reference metabolomics of the organism.

The genetics and physiology of solventogenic clostridia is the basis for the emerging metabolic engineering of these anaerobic industrial organisms for the production of solvents and other oxychemicals. This class of organisms, which remain for now the paradigm of genetically reprogramming anaerobic metabolism, provided unexpected insights into the regulation and reprogramming primary metabolism. The almost complete sequence of the genome of the type strain (*Clostridium acetobutylicum* ATCC 824) offers enormous opportunities and challenges for the future, when global approaches based on master regulatory genes are promising to lead to superior industrial strains. Such strains will be beneficially deregulated for the expression of the genes that determine differentiation (sporulation) and product formation that depends on stage of growth, thus allowing solvent production throughout a continuous culture without the loss of cellular productivity associated with sporulation. The standard versus reprogrammed metabolomics of the organism is thus useful for the optimization of the productivity of the organism for these chemicals. Yeast used for the production of alcoholic beverages, fuel, ethanol, pharmaceutical proteins, enzymes etc. form another useful engineered system for metabolomic applications.

Metabolic Flux and Metabolite Flux Analysis (MFA)

Amplifying the activity of an enzyme or knocking out its competitors does not always result in increased flux through the desired metabolic pathway. This is because the control of the metabolic flux is frequently distributed among multiple enzymes. Thus, the concept of the "rate-limiting step," which states that one particular enzymatic reaction controls the rate of the entire pathway, is being increasingly indicated as both erroneous and potentially misleading. Since a number of controlling factors affect metabolic fluxes, it is difficult to predict the targets that must be modified to achieve the desired alteration of metabolic fluxes and their control by more research in cellular physiology with particular emphasis on quantitative aspects of pathway flux control. The determination of intracellular metabolic fluxes is of central and practical importance to successful metabolic engineering. A method now termed "metabolic flux (balance) analysis" has been developed and applied over the last 15 years or so. Metabolic flux analysis is based on stoichiometric balances of metabolic species and using the (pseudo) steady state assumption (hypothesis). This method requires information only on the stoichiometry of metabolic pathways and on metabolic demands. This is often useful because complete enzyme kinetic data seldom are available for most metabolic pathways, let alone the entire cellular metabolism.

Metabolite/metabolic flux analysis (MFA) represents a powerful tool for systems biology research on eukaryotic cells. Some of the recent advances, the challenges as well as applications of metabolic flux analysis comprising fungi, mammalian cells and plants are stated here in. While MFA is widely established and applied in microorganisms, it remains still a challenge to adapt these methods to eukaryotic cell systems having a higher complexity particularly concerning compartmentation or media composition. In fungi, MFA has been widely used to analyze a variety of conditions and factors and their effects on cellular metabolism. In mammalian cells, MFA has been applied mainly in cell culture technology and in medical and toxicological research. ^{13}C metabolic studies on native whole plants are additionally challenging by the fact that CO_2 is the only carbon source.

Metabolism is the "chemical engine" that drives the living process. The 25-30 year history of metabolic analysis has demonstrated the need to quantitatively describe the systemic aspects of cellular metabolism and develop mathematical models of linkages between pathways and pathway steps. There are significant incentives to study metabolomic dynamics. A quantitative description of metabolism and the ability to produce or "engineer" metabolic change not only is important to achieve specific bioprocessing or therapeutic goals but has general importance to our fundamental understanding of cell biology. Important applications of metabolic analysis include strain design for the production of therapeutics and metabolites, assessment of the metabolic consequences of genetic alteration, and synthesis of systematic methods to combat infectious disease and to design chemotherapies. Quantitative analysis of metabolism and its systemic properties is thus of fundamental and practical importance.

Detailed kinetics modelling of metabolism has been hampered by the requirement for extensive and explicit enzyme kinetics. In general, complete enzyme kinetics information is not available for the entire metabolism of a single cell. The human red blood cell is the only cell for which complete enzyme kinetics information is available and a full dynamic metabolic model is achievable. As often is the case in biology, this simple model system has proven very useful to develop methods and obtain deeper understanding of the issues associated with detailed kinetics models of metabolism. For instance, methods to simplify metabolic descriptions, such as modal analysis and metabolic pool representation, resulted from this activity. However, comprehensive enzyme kinetic information is not available for microbial cell, and metabolic modelling methods, especially approaches that rely on less detailed kinetic information, must be developed.

In recent years, an approach has been developed that is based on balancing metabolic fluxes. Based on the fundamental law of mass conservation, the flux balance method is able to provide insightful information about the systemic constraints placed on metabolic function. The analysis is performed under steady state conditions, and it requires information only about the stoichiometry of metabolic pathways and metabolic demands. Although different solution methods are used to obtain pathway flux distributions, no information on metabolite concentrations or transient behaviour results from this type of analysis.

A number of different objective functions have been used for metabolic analysis. These include the following:

1. Minimize ATP production: this objective is stated to determine conditions of optimal metabolic energy efficiency.
2. Minimize nutrient uptake: this objective function is used to determine the conditions under which the cell will perform its metabolic functions while consuming the minimum amount of available nutrients.
3. Minimize redox production: this objective function finds conditions where the cells operate to generate the minimum amount of redox potential.
4. Minimize the Euclidean norm: this objective has been applied to satisfy the strategy of a cell to minimize the sum of the flux values, or to channel the metabolites as efficiently as possible through the metabolic pathways.
5. Maximize metabolite production: this objective function has been used to determine the biochemical production capabilities of *Escherichia coli*. In this analysis the objective function was defined to maximise the production of a chosen metabolite (i.e., lysine or phenylalanine).
6. Maximize biomass and metabolite production: by weighing these two conflicting objectives appropriately, one can explore the trade-off between cell growth and forced metabolite production in a producing strain.

MFA in mammalian cells is still less established and more complicated compared to MFA in microorganisms or yeast owing to complex media composition and related unbalanced growth behaviour. Media consist usually of multiple substrates and the composition changes dramatically during cultivation resulting in metabolic shifts. The different flux estimation methods applied on mammalian cells are depicted and compared in Figure 9.7. Most of the flux calculations applied on mammalian cells were pure metabolite balancing and considered just a certain period, usually the exponential growth phase representing mean metabolic fluxes for the respective phase. However, metabolic steady state, which is a prerequisite for stationary MFA, or isotopic steady state, which is necessary for stationary ^{13}C MFA, is usually not reached during batch or fed-batch cultivation. Due to the complex and changing media composition, the metabolism is changing during the cultivation limiting the application of MFA. It seems generally possible to change the medium by targeted adaptation of substrate concentrations such that metabolic steady state is kept up for a longer period and isotopic steady state is asymptotically reached. However, if the metabolism in conventional, industrially relevant media has to be investigated, there is a need for methods which can describe the dynamic behaviour and metabolic shifts of the metabolism. For this purpose, different flux estimation strategies can be applied calculating metabolic flux distributions over time. Detailed and reliable ^{13}C MFA, allowing deeper insights into cellular metabolism is still a challenge. A recent study evaluated a set of ^{13}C tracers for their use and informative value in MFA. However, there is still the question, how to solve the problem of isotopic instationarity in typical cultivations. An interesting methodology was recently described using transient ^{13}C labeling experiments and applied to hepatic cells. There are mainly two areas where MFA was successfully applied to mammalian cells, namely cell culture technology as well as toxicology and medicine.

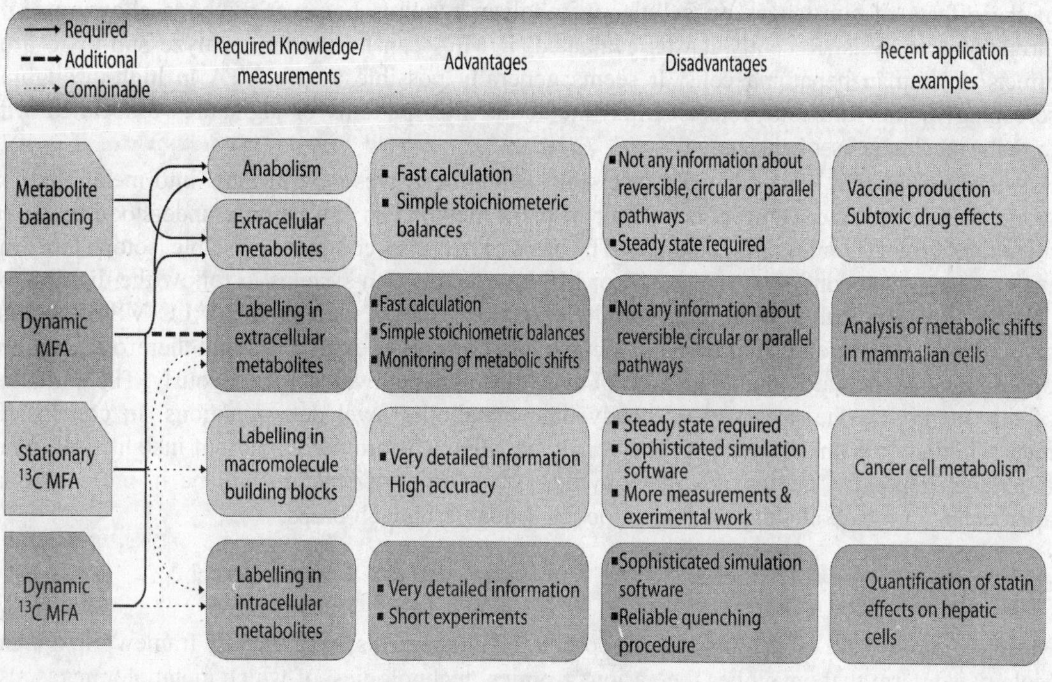

Figure 9.7 Methods of whole cell metabolic flux distribution measurement in mammalian cell systems with required knowledge and measurements and their advantages and disadvantages (taken from Niklas *et al.*, 2010).

In the past decade, metabolic flux analysis (MFA) was employed mainly for the analysis and optimization of cell culture processes, investigating the effects of cultivation conditions, substrates or other factors on cellular metabolism. A recent MFA study evaluated the effects of a glutamine-free medium enhancing vaccine production on the cellular metabolism of MDCK cells observing a more efficient use of nutrients. However, there is still the challenge, to develop easy and widely applicable methods that describe the dynamic and adaptive behaviour in batch or fed-batch cultivations applied in industrial production processes. For this purpose, a time resolved flux estimation strategy can be used which was recently applied to a new human cell line, namely Age1.hn.

An interesting application of MFA in the medical sector has been demonstrated by the study on long-term three-dimensional cultures of rat embryonic brain cells indicating that the applied aggregate cultures could be an interesting system to analyse brain cell metabolism and to find metabolic flux signatures for *in vitro* brain disease models. Several studies in the area of toxicology analyzed hepatic metabolism and the effects of certain compounds on metabolic fluxes in hepatic cells. Transient ^{13}C-flux analysis was applied recently to quantify statin effects on cholesterol synthesis and central metabolism in hepatocytes. This methodology seems very powerful for the analysis of the effects of certain compounds on cellular metabolism but requires sophisticated analytical methods and is very laborious both for analysis as well as modeling and computation. Assessment of the effects of substances on cellular metabolism requires however methods allowing high-throughput analysis. Recently it was evaluated, if MFA can be used to analyze sub-toxic drug effects on human hepatoma cells. It seems generally possible to use MFA in high-throughput screening in the future to detect certain metabolic flux patterns or signatures associated with toxicity mechanisms of drugs.

The measurement of steady-state levels of metabolites gives new insights into metabolic networks at a given time. But real behaviour of plant metabolism can be only understood by determination of the dynamics of metabolism. The basis of MFA is a combination stable isotope labelling under steady-state conditions and NMR or MS-based detection systems to follow the distribution of label. The application of a multi-parallel detection method such as GC-or LC-MS allows the determination of isotope label in many metabolites in a single experiment and therefore gives the opportunity to calculate metabolic fluxes of many different pathways simultaneously. The limitation of this method is the necessity of steady-state metabolite level determinations. In conclusion, metabolomics in combination with stable isotope MFA will provide important insights into plant functional genomics studies. Another obvious use of this information will be in more rational approaches in metabolic engineering of novel, valuable biotech-crops.

System Biology

Metabolomics is said to be a critically important technique in a system biology framework. System biology is a term that envelopes the various '-omics' technologies, of which metabolomics is also one of them. Studies in systems biology aspire to integrate the structures and functions of various levels of encoded information of the organism. If one considers that many proteins, encoded by genes, are in fact enzymes that catalyze chemical reactions, then by extension, metabolomics can be seen as another level of information encoded by the organism but more subject to manipulation by its environment. In a sense, metabolomics represents the meeting of phylogenetics and phonetics.

In conclusion, metabolomics represents the interface between genetic predisposition and environmental influence. The aim of the emerging area of system biology is to investigate the dynamics of all genetic, regulatory, and metabolic processes in a cell and to understand the complexity of cellular networks. It is because of this unique position in the systems biology hierarchy that metabolomics could prove invaluable in our quest to understand the function of genes, to be able to control and/or design novel organisms that may benefit our health or lifestyles, and to understand more fully the molecular physiology of ourselves and that of other organisms.

CHALLENGES AND FUTURE PROSPECTS IN METABOLOMICS

The challenges in metabolomics are multifaceted and analytical technology as well as test system linked. Each biological system offers challenges in terms of complexity of intracellular, cellular and tissue sytems comprising the targeted sample. Ultimately, feasibility of single cell metabolomics and homogeneous set of organellar metabolomics is the answer to understand the metabolism in a metabolomic sense. Till then, somehow and somewhere it reflects some extent of averaging of the metabolite contents at cellular, tissue or organ level. At analytical level, challenges are not only the sum of the challenges/limitations of the technologies but also integrating them all across to derive a normalized version of metabolome. For GC-MS, these include automation of operations like ample preparation, derivatization chemistry and data processing for better throughput and reproducibility, combining multiple analytical technology platforms for the same sample, combined analysis of proteome and transcriptome, profiling of signaling molecules and other compounds occurring in traces along with those present in bulk, increasing accuracy in quantification, combining profiling with flux analysis, identification of unidentified metabolic components from metabolite profiling experiments.

The chromatographic performance (quantified by resolution, selectivity, column efficiency, separation efficiency and peak capacity) of LC is lower than that of GC and CE and it requires significant improvement. By a theoretical calculation, analytical scale LC using a 4.6 × 250 mm column can afford resolvability of maximum 300 compounds in a best-case scenario. In practice, it could hardly be achieved and realistic peak capacities are between 100 and 200 under best conditions for the best case. Thus, currently HPLC technologies are limiting the comprehensive scope of metabolomics. To separate very complex metabolomics mixtures, enhanced resolutions facilitating peak capacities of order of tens of thousands of compounds are necessary. That magnitude of capacities can only be offered, at present, by multidimensional chromatographic methods. Capillary HPLC is being increasingly used for far better peak capacities, however, routine use of such micro-HPLC would require development of better hardware. Capillary LC coupled with electrospray ionization quadropole time-of-flight mass spectrometry offers several advantages but is not being routinely used probably due to prohibitive costs.

NMR has proved exceptionally useful tool for animals but it has not been implemented well for plant metabolomics. The potential of 2D-and hyphenated NMR to increase the number of metabolites that can be resolved and quantified is yet to be realized. Although it would lower the throughput, it would fit into the multi-pass approach. However, NMR aided metabolomics has some inherent limitations like lower sensitivity of measurement that can be improved with spectrometers of higher magnetic field. Solid state NMR methods for insoluble bioorganic constituents like starch, cell wall components, biomembranes and use of labelling together with the state of the art NMR technologies would open many newer avenues for metabolomics. Also, NMR when used in hyphenation/parallel to GC-, CE-and LC-MS would broaden the metabolome coverage.

It would be highly valuable to have an indepth metabolite profiles of all the tissues and treatments that have been analyzed with respect to EST sequencing. It could help *in silico* pairing enzymes with potential substrates and products to comprehend functional association of expression-genomics with metabolic networks. Non-availability of standard compounds is one of the major problems in discerning the metabolite identity. KNApSAcK database (http://kanaya.naist.jp/KNApSAck/KNApSAcK.php) generated from the information collected on more than 18,000 metabolite species pairs covering close to 7500 metabolites and 6300 species allows users to search various aspects of metabolite-species relationships. The database contains chemical diversity of metabolites that originated and propagated through as a concomitant to evolution of species. The growing number of metabolite-species entries in this database would be pivotal to understand metabolite based relationships among the species.

In summation, these are exciting times for metabolomics. It seems as if new advances are being reported almost every week. However, metabolomics is still at an infancy stage of development. This chapter has hopefully given a short introduction about the potentials that metabolomics has to offer for plant and animal research. Metabolomics will become a major player in the investigation of plant metabolism and the phenotypic analysis of many different plant species following environmental and genetic perturbations and what is normal and what is abnormal in human metabolome. This will offer a number of approaches in which metabolomics will be of great use, such as functional genomics, metabolic and genetic engineering or the development of novel biotechnology crops and products. It will also play an outstanding role in phenotyping, determination of novel pathways, cofactor regulation in bio-catalytic redox reactions, fine chemical production, drug production and alternative fuels. In addition, when plant metabolomics will be linked to the field of nutrigenomics, in which role of metabolites in the development of modern-world diseases for example coronary heart diseases or diabetics, it will give the opportunity for selecting crops and food for novel bioactive plant compounds (phytochemicals). It provide invaluable tools for the investigation of the distribution of metabolite concentrations in crops and food and the relationship of those to diseases.

FURTHER READINGS

1. Aristidou A.A., San K.Y. and Bennett G.N. (1994) Modification of central metabolic pathway in *Escherichia coli* to reduce acetate accumulation by heterologous expression of the *Bacillus subtilis* acetolactate synthase gene. *Biotechnol Bioeng.* **(44):** 944-951.
2. Balcarcel R.R. and Clark L.M. (2003) Metabolic screening of mammalian cell cultures using well-plates. *Biotechnol. Prog.* **(19):** 98-108.
3. Bino R.J., Hall R.D., Fiehn O., Kopka J., Saito K., Draper J., Nilkolau B.J., Mendes P., Roessner-Tunali U., Beale M.H., Trethewey R.N., Lange B.M., Wurtele E.S. and Sumner L.W. (2004) Potential of metabolomics as a functional genomics tool. *Trends in Plant. Sci.* **(9):** 418-425.
4. Bonarius H.P., Ozemre A., Timmerarends B., Skrabal P., Tramper J., Schmid G. and Heinzle E. (2001) Metabolic-flux analysis of continuously cultured hybridoma cells using (13)CO(2) mass spectrometry in combination with (13)C-lactate nuclear magnetic resonance spectroscopy and metabolite balancing. *Biotechnol. Bioeng.* **(74):** 528-538.

5. Cameron D.C. and Tong I.T. (1993) Cellular and metabolic engineering. *Appl. Biochem. Biotechnol.* **(38):** 105-140.
6. Davey Matthew P., Burrell Mike M., Woodward F. Ian and Quick W. Paul (2008) Population-specific metabolic phenotypes of *Arabidopsis lyrata* ssp. *Petraea. New Phytologist.* **(177)**: 380-388, **doi**: 10.1111/j.1469-8137.2007.02282.x
7. Deshpande R., Yang T.H. and Heinzle E. (2009) Towards a metabolic and isotopic steady state in CHO batch cultures for reliable isotope-based metabolic profiling. *Biotechnol. J.* **(4):** 247-263.
8. Dixon R.A., Gang D.R., Charllton A.J., Fiehn O., Kuiper H.A., Reynolsds T.L., Tjeerdema R.S., Jeffery E.H., German J.B., Ridley W.P. and Seiber J.N. (2006) Applications of metabolomics in agriculture. *J. of Agric. and. Food. Chem.* **(54):** 8984-8994.
9. Dorsten F.A.V., Daykin C.A., Mulder T.P. and Duynhoven J.P.V. (2006) Metabonomics approach to determine metabolic differences between green tea and black tea consumption. *J. Agric. Food Chem.* **(54):** 6929-6938.
10. Dunn W.B. and Ellis D.I. (2005) Metabolomics: current analytical platforms and methodologies. *Trends in Anal. Chem.* **(24):** 285-294.
11. Edwards J.S. and Palsson B.O. (2000) The Escherichia coli MG1655 in silico metabolic genotype: its definition, characteristics and capabilities. *Proc. Natl. Acad. Sci.* **(97):** 5528-5533.
12. Ensley B.D., Ratzkin B.J., Osslund T.D., Simon M.J., Wackett L.P. and Gibson D.T. (1983) Expression of naphthalene oxidation genes in *Escherichia coli* results in the biosynthesis of indigo. *Science.* **(222):** 167-169.
13. Farmer W.R. and Liao J.C. (1997) Reduction of aerobic acetate production by *Escherichia* coli. *Appl. Environ. Microbiol.* **(63):** 3205-3210.
14. Fiehn O. (2001) Combining genomics, metabolome analysis and biochemical modelling to understand metabolic networks. *Comp Funct Genomics.* **(2):** 155-168.
15. Fiehn O., Kopka J., Dörmann P., Altmann T., Trethewey R.N. and Willmitzer L. (2000) Metabolite profiling for plant functional genomics. *Nat. Biotechnol.* **(18):** 1157-1161.
16. Flores N., Xiao J., Berry A., Bolivar F. and Valle F. (1996) Pathway engineering for the production of aromatic compounds in *Escherichia coli. Nat. Biotechnol.* **(14):** 620-623.
17. Forster J., Famili I., Fu P., Palsson B.O. and Nielsen J. (2003) Genome-scale reconstruction of the saccharomyces cerevisiae metabolic network. *Genome Res.* **(13):** 244-253.
18. German J.B., Roberts M.A. and Watkins S.M. (2003) Genomics and metabolomics as markers for the interaction of diet and health: lessons from lipids. *J. Nutr.* **(133):** 2078S-2083S.
19. Hall R.D. (2006) Plant metabolomics: from holistic hope, to hype, to hot topic. *New phytologist* **(169):** 453-468.
20. Hall R.D., Brouwer I.D. and Fitzgerald M.A. (2008) Plant metabolomics and its potential application for human nutrition. *Physiol. Plant.* **(132):** 162-175.
21. Heinrich R., Rapaport S.M. and Rapaport T.A. (1977) Metabolic regulation and mathematical models, *Prog. Biophy. Mol. Biol.* **(32):** 1-82.
22. Hofmann U., Maier K., Niebel A., Vacun G., Reuss M. and Mauch K. (2008) Identification of metabolic fluxes in hepatic cells from transient 13C-labeling experiments: Part I. Experimental observations. *Biotechnol. Bioeng.* **(100):** 344-354.
23. Jansen Jeroen J., Allwood J. William, Marsden-Edwards Emma, van der Putten Wim H., Goodacre Royston, and van Dam Nicole M. (2009). Metabolomic analysis of the interaction between plants and herbivores. *Metabolomics.* **(5):** 150-161, DOI 10.1007/s11306-008-0124-4
24. Jenkins H., Johnson H., Kular B., Wang T. and Hardy N. (2005) Toward Supportive Data Collection Tools for Plant Metabolomics. *Plant Physiol.* **(138):** 67-77.
25. Kacser H. and Bruns J.A. (1973) The control of flux. *Symp. Soc. Exp. Biol.* **(27):** 65-104.

26. Kallio P.T. and Bailey J.E. (1996) Intracellular expression of vitreoscilla haemoglobin (VHb) enhances total protein secretion and improves the production of a-amylase and neutral protease in Bacillus subtilis. *Biotechnol. Prog.* **(12):** 31-39.
27. Khosla and Bailey J.E. (1988) Heterologous expression of a bacterial haemoglobin improves the growth properties of recombinant *Escherichia coli. Nature.* **(331):** 633-635.
28. Kitano H. (2002) System biology: a brief overview. *Science.* **(295):** 1662-1664.
29. Kluender Christina, Sans-Piche Fre´de´ric, Riedl Janet, Altenburger Rolf, Ha¨rtig Claus, Laue Grit and Schmitt-Jansen Mechthild (2009) A metabolomics approach to assessing phytotoxic effects on the green alga *Scenedesmus vacuolatus. Metabolomics.* **(5):** 59-71, DOI 10.1007/s11306-008-0139-x
30. Lee I.D. and Palsson B.O. (1991) A comprehensive model of human erythrocyte metabolism: Extensions to include pH effects. *Biomed. Biochim. Acta.* **(49):** 771-789.
31. Lee J., Jung K., Choi S.H. and Kim H. (1995) Combination of the tod and the tol pathways in redesigning a metabolic route of Pseudomonas putida for the mineralization of a benzene, toluene, and p-xylene mixture. *Appl. Environ. Microbiol.* **(61):** 2211-2217.
32. Llaneras F. and Pico J. (2007) A procedure for the estimation over time of metabolic fluxes in scenarios where measurements are uncertain and/or insufficient. *BMC Bioinform.* **(8):** 421.
33. Maier K., Hofmann U., Bauer A., Niebel A., Vacun G., Reuss M. and Mauch K. (2009) Quantification of statin effects on hepatic cholesterol synthesis by transient (13)C-flux analysis. *Metab Eng.* **(11):** 292-309.
34. Maier K., Hofmann U., Reuss M. and Mauch K. (2008) Identification of metabolic fluxes in hepatic cells from transient 13C-labeling experiments: Part II. Flux estimation. *Biotechnol. Bioeng.* **(100):** 355-370.
35. Mark R. and Viant (2009) Applications of metabolomics to the environmental sciences. *Metabolomics.* **(5):** 1-2.
36. Metallo C.M., Walther J.L. and Stephanopoulos G. (2009) Evaluation of (13) C. isotopic tracers for metabolic flux analysis in mammalian cells. *J. Biotechnology.* 144 **(3):** 167-174, doi:10.1016/j.jbiotec.2009.07.010
37. Niklas J., Noor F. and Heinzle E. (2009) Effects of drugs in subtoxic concentrations on the metabolic fluxes in human hepatoma cell line Hep G2. *Toxicol. Appl. Pharmacol.* **(240):** 327-336.
38. Niklas J., Schneider K. and Heinzle E. (2010) Metabolic flux analysis in eukaryotes. *Curr. opin. in Biotechnol.* 21 **(1):** 63-69.
39. Oliver S.G., Winson M.K., Kell D.B. and Baganz F. (1998) Systematic functional analysis of the yeast genome. *Trends Biotechnol.* **(16):** 373-378.
40. Palsson B.O. (1987) Making mathematical description of metabolic reaction networks manageable. In: Sideman S, Beyar R, eds. *Activation, Metabolism and Perfusion of the Heart-Simulation and Experimental Models.* Dordrecht/Boston/Lancaster: Martinus Nijhoff pp. 584-618.
41. Palsson B.O., Joshi A. and Ozturk S.S. (1987) Reducing complexity in metabolic networks: Making metabolic meshes manageable. *Fed. Proc.* **(46):** 2485-2489.
42. Quek L.E., Dietmair S., Kromer J.O. and Nielsen L.K. (2009) Metabolic flux analysis in mammalian cell culture. *Metab Eng.* (doi:10.1016/j.ymben.2009.09.002).
43. Rochfort S. (2005) Metabolomics reviewed: a new "omics" platform technology for systems biology and implications for natural products research. *J. Nat. Prod.* **(68):** 1813-1820.
44. Roessner-Tunali U., Lui J., Leisse A., Balbo L., Perez-Melis A., Willmitzer L. and Fernie A.R. (2004) Flux analysis of organic and amino acid metabolism in potato tubers by gas chromatography-mass spectrometry following incubation in 13C labelled isotopes. *Plant. J.* **(39):** 668-679.
45. Rojo F., Pieper D.H., Engesser K.H., Knackmuss H.M. and Timmis K.N. (1987) Assemblage of orthocleavage route for simultaneous degradation of chloro and methylaromatics. *Science.* **(235):** 1395-1398.

46. Santos S.S., Leite S.B., Sonnewald U., Carrondo M.J. and Alves P.M. (2007) Stirred vessel cultures of rat brain cells aggregates: characterization of major metabolic pathways and cell population dynamics. J. *Neurosci. Res.* **(85):** 3386-3397.

47. Savinell J.M. and Palsson B.O. (1992) Network analysis of intermediary metabolism using linear optimization. J. Development of mathematical formalism. *J. Theor. Biol.* **(154):** 421-454.

48. Schripsema J. (2009) Application of NMR in plant metabolomics: Techniques, problems and prospects. Phytochemical analysis published online DOI 10.1002/pca.1185.

49. Schwender J., Ohlrogge J.B. and Shachar-Hill Y. (2003) A flux model of glycolysis and the oxidative pentosephosphate pathway in developing Brassica napus embryos. *J. Biol. Chem.* **(278):** 29442-29453.

50. Schwender J., Ohlrogge J.B. and Shachar-Hill Y. (2004) Understanding flux in plant metabolic networks. *Curr. Opin. Plant. Biol.* **(7):** 309-317.

51. Seger and Sturm S. (2006) Analytical aspects of plant metabolite profiling platforms: current standings and future aims. *J. of Proteome. Res.* **(6):** 480-497.

52. Sidorenko Y., Wahl A., Dauner M., Genzel Y. and Reichl U. (2008) Comparison of metabolic flux distributions for MDCK cell growth in glutamine- and pyruvate-containing media. *Biotechnol. Prog.* **(24):** 311-320.

53. Solanky K.S., Bailey N.J., Beckwith-Hall B.M. and Davis A. (2003) Application of biofluid 1H nuclear magnetic resonance-based metabonomic techniques for the analysis of the biochemical effects of dietary isoflavones on human plasma profile. *Anal Biochem.* **(323):** 197-204.

54. Sweetlove L.J., Last R.L. and Fernie A.R. (2003) Predictive metabolic engineering: a goal for systems biology. *Plant Physiol.* **(132):** 420-425.

55. Trujillo E., Davis C. and Milner J. (2006) Nutrigenomics, proteomics, metabolomics, and the practice of dietetics. *J. Am. Diet. Assoc.* **(106):** 403-413.

56. Villas-Boas G.S., Roessner U., Hansen M. A. E., Smedsgaard J. and Nielsen J. (2007) Metabolome Analysis: An introduction, Wiley-Interscience.

57. Wahl, Y. Sidorenko, M. Dauner, Y. Genzel and U. Reichl (2008) Metabolic flux model for an anchorage-dependent MDCK cell line: characteristic growth phases and minimum substrate consumption flux distribution. *Biotechnol Bioeng.* **(101):** 135-152.

58. Wang Y., Tang H., Nicholson J.K. and Hylands P.J. (2005) A metabonomic strategy for the detection of the metabolic effects of chamomile (*Matricaria recutita* L.) ingestion. *J. Agric. Food. Chem.* **(53):** 191-196.

59. Zahner H. (1979) What are secondary metabolites? *Folia Microbiol.* **(24):** 435-443.

CHAPTER 10

Bioinformatics and *In Silico* Technology

The rapid pace of enhancement in genomic technologies has led to the accumulation of large amount of data. Bioinformatics, as an interdisciplinary subject has provided various tools and techniques for understanding and analyzing the huge datasets. It has not only assisted in making meaning out of the data but has also provided efficient ways of storing and mining of data for specific analysis. Large sequencing initiatives have developed curated databases for providing the sequence and analysis of respective organisms. Agriculture had largely benefited due to such advancements in knowledge, as various plant biologists have been using various genomic data to improve vital traits in plants, thus improving crop production. Large scale comparative genomic analysis has led to the identification of genes and gene families which has enriched our understanding of complicated cellular pathways and mechanisms under various stress conditions. Sequence analysis tools have facilitated the identification of homologs between the close and distant species thus, assisting in annotation of various unknown genes. Also, conserved motifs and signature sequences have been identified using multiple sequence alignment techniques. Phylogenetic analysis has led to the better understanding of various evolutionary events that took place and also hypothesizing the approximate date of the various events. Modeling and structural analysis of various proteins has deduced the importance of the three-dimensional conservation of structural motifs and thus their respective mechanisms of action. Lately, the realization of importance of RNAs has given new dimension to the understanding of gene regulation. Various approaches and algorithms have been developed to identify RNA elements in various plants. Development of various microarray analysis techniques and various algorithms for its analysis has assisted in identifying the simultaneous response of large number of genes under specific stress conditions. Systems biology approaches such as network analysis and pathway simulation have given comprehensive view of various cellular processes related to various responses under stress condition. Programming and scripting languages has led to effortless handling and analysis of large amount of data. Thus, bioinformatics as an interdisciplinary approach has influenced almost every aspect of analysis leading to better understanding of complex questions in agricultural science.

Keywords: Domains, microarray, motifs, networks, phylogeny, sequence analysis, structure, systems biology.

INTRODUCTION

After the discovery of central dogma, biological science has taken a giant leap to decipher the alphabets of life. Biological information of an organism is encoded in the form of long sequence, comprising four letters, also known as its genome. The genome is further divided into discrete units such as genes which codes for proteins and various intergenic regions such as introns and regions that regulate the expression of various genes. The era of genomics (study of genomes) has made computational biology and bioinformatics as one of the main streams of modern biological analysis. The major landmark achieved in this era, is the genome sequencing of large number of organisms ranging from various bacterial species to the complex eukaryotic systems. The culminating example of cogent storage and analysis of biological data was the analysis performed by Gregor Mendel (1822-1884), through which he established the underlying principles of heredity which remain essentially same for all the complex life forms. Mendel analyzed the inheritance pattern in *Pisum sativum* where he could work with only two generations a year, while later researchers chose to work on those species which have a shorter generation time, thus amassing large volume of data. Rapidly growing technologies such as automated DNA sequencing and multiple gene expression tools have played a major role towards the explosive accumulation of biological data in public databases. These accumulated datasets have also presented a unique opportunity to the researchers to answer various unsolved biological questions.

In order to solve conundrum of biological sciences, bioinformatics has emerged as a new discipline which integrates many core subject areas such as mathematics, statistics, physics, chemistry, computer science, cell and molecular biology etc. Earlier, theories of computer sciences have been used essentially for storing and accessing the data, but nowadays, various algorithms and methodologies have been devised for not only efficient storage of data but also for the analysis of such data. Mathematical sciences have come with various novel solutions to solve complex biological problems. Various complex statistical measures have been set for simulating and hypothesizing various biological events. Analysis of nucleotides and proteins sequences, their functional domains and structure of proteins have been greatly assisted by various branches of bioinformatics. Specialized areas such as robotics, graphic designing, 3D visualization have benefited in understanding the protein structures and their conserved motifs. Physical science principles have assisted in realizing real world simulation of biomolecules *in silico*, thus providing great details about their functionality. Various machine learning approaches have been used for searching hidden patterns, signal sequences and understanding the evolutionary pattern of various nucleotide and protein sequences. Clustering of genes on the basis of their expression in multiple-gene-expression technique has led to the learning of minute variations in the gene expression under various conditions. Mysteries of gene regulatory networks and metabolic pathways have been explored using simulations due to development of high throughput computing and algorithms. Thus, with efforts going in the accumulation of genome level data, new tools and techniques in bioinformatics will be required to assist in understanding of the living systems.

The present chapter is an attempt to describe the various tools used in bioinformatics, the various databases which have been generated and their usage. Elaborated tables have also been provided to suggest the various databases which are available online. For brevity sake, related examples have been provided from plant sciences only, same approaches have been used to analyze the genomes of other genera.

BIOINFORMATICS IN AGRICULTURE

Bioinformatics, as a discipline, has influenced all areas of life sciences, with agricultural sciences being no different. Agricultural research communities have been benefited from the spin-off technologies provided by human genome project. The specialized branch known as "genomics" defined as the study of genomes has ameliorated the way of understanding the functional aspects of genes and their interaction with the environment. The most significant breakthrough in the field of genomics in agriculture came from the complete genome sequencing of *Arabidopsis thaliana* in 2000. *Arabidopsis,* a model plant for plant biologists, is a small flowering plant and a member of family, Brassicaceae. Another major landmark in the field of plant genomics came with the completion of rice genome sequencing by international consortium on the rice genome sequencing. Rice is one of the major crops of the tropical region and is considered the next model crop for the plant studies. Comparing genomes of susceptible plant varieties with those of tolerant varieties can assist in cataloguing of useful traits. Plant biologists around the world have started exploring the paragon of useful traits from their respective genomes and post-genomic disciplines such as proteomics and metabolomics have relinquished their functions. Thus, effective knowledge of useful plant traits in various wild varieties can expedite the development of novel varieties that can sustain in today's cacophonous environment. Large numbers of variations have been observed in the genome sizes even in closely related species which might be due to their capability to adapt to various environments. According to an estimate, the smallest genome belong to *Arabidopsis thaliana*, with 125Mbp, whereas the largest reported to date, belongs to *Fritillaria assyriaca*, with 124,852 Mbp. Thus, multiple genome allegory can also highlight the variations in the genome's inter-genomic maps which can trace the evolutionary process leading to the divergence of the genomes. Large scale genome-wide analysis in various plant species have already been undertaken for the identification of gene and gene families in rice, which are playing major role in various processes in the crop plant (Table 10.1).

Table 10.1 Analysis of various gene families in rice.

Gene family	*Function*	*Reference*
Dof	Participate in the regulation of gene expression in processes such as seed storage protein synthesis in developing endosperm	Lijavetzky *et al.*, 2003; Mena *et al.*, 1998; Carbajosa *et al.*, 1997
P450	Encodes large set of Cyt P450 monooxygenases (P450s)	Nelson *et al.*, 2004
Expansin	Cell-wall loosening activity, involved in cell expansion and other developmental events during which cell wall modification occurs	Sampedro *et al.*, 2006
TCS	Signaling system in plants	Pareek *et al.*, 2006
Argonaute	Form the core components that facilitate gene silencing and have been implicated in the initiation and maintenance of the trigger RNA molecules, central to process of RNAi	Kapoor *et al.*, 2008
CBS	Response to various stresses and development	Kushwaha *et al.*, 2009

One of the major conclusions drawn with the help of genome comparisons that have been sequenced is the demonstration of existence of synteny between the cereal genomes. The conservation of gene order and gene content along the genome in various plants is termed synteny. Experiments have shown syntenic relationship between potato and tomato and between various *Brassica* crops and *Arabidopsis*. Also, it is well established that rice has similar genetic makeup with that of barley, millet, sorghum and maize. The knowledge of synteny among the crop plants allows breeders to access all the alleles, thus improving the qualitative traits in the crop plants.

Markers have already been used on an extensive scale in agricultural sciences for the purpose of breeding, study of conservation of the genetic resources and for the verification of various genotypes. Molecular markers are the unique DNA sequences, found in the specific regions of the genome and are linked with the specific gene or traits. Thus, it has been considered that as functional information of genome sequences of model plants is progressively accumulated, listing of markers related to useful traits and diseases will also be intensified.

The betterment in the high-throughput genotyping and gene expression platforms has replenished the concept of expression quantitative trait loci (eQTL) as tool for elucidating the gene regulation in various crop plants. The availability of large scale quantitative expression values along with the high density genotype, eQTL mapping can be realized among various crop plants, thus finding the genomic locations which are likely to regulate the transcript expression. The classical QTL mapping largely focuses on one or few genes, but eQTL mapping provides a platform for simultaneous investigation of several gene expressions and their related phenotype, thus enhancing the probability of finding new genes and gene-families.

TECHNIQUES IN BIOINFORMATICS

Sequence Analysis

Databases

The identification of specific signature, pattern or various homologs pertaining to the sequence under study is termed the analysis of the sequence. As discussed in the introduction, raw nucleotide/protein sequences are stored in various databases for their effective storage, retrieval and analysis. Earlier, databases were used to store raw sequences obtained from various sequencing projects but with the development of algorithms for biological problems, various knowledge based curated databases known as meta-database, have come into the picture. These databases are specific for unique set of information required for some specific analysis such as signaling, promoters, gene structure etc. Some of the sequence databases are mentioned below (Table 10.2).

Table 10.2 List of databases.

Database	*Information*	*Url*
Primary sequence database		
Entrez	Global Query Cross-Database Search System	http://www.ncbi.nlm.nih.gov/sites/gquery

Contd.

GenBank	Nucleotide/protein	http://www.ncbi.nlm.nih.gov/Genbank/
DDBJ	Nucleotide/protein	http://www.ddbj.nig.ac.jp/
EMBL	Nucleotide/protein	http://www.ebi.ac.uk/embl/
Protein databases		
SWISS-PROT	A curated protein sequence database	http://www.expasy.ch/sprot/sprot-top.html
PIR	Protein information resource	http://pir.georgetown.edu/pirwww/
MIPS	Munich information centre for protein sequences	http://mips.gsf.de/
UniProt	Curated protein information	http://www.ebi.ac.uk/uniprot/

Apart from various primary databases which hold sequences of various organisms, scientific initiatives dedicated to sequencing efforts of specific organisms also host databases specific for the organisms (Table 10.3). These databases hold not only raw data but also curated data such as protein sequences, gene structures, etc.

Table 10.3 Databases for specific plant organisms.

Organism	*Url*
Arabidopsis	http://www.arabidopsis.org/
Rice	http://rice.plantbiology.msu.edu
Maize	http://www.maizesequence.org
Populus	http://www.populus.db.umu.se/
Potato	http://solgenomics.net
Beans	http://beangenes.cws.ndsu.nodak.edu/
Castor	http://castorbean.jcvi.org/
Mustard	http://www.brassica-rapa.org/BRGP

Tools for Sequence Analysis

The relatedness or the homology of an unknown sequence can be analyzed by comparing or aligning the sequence with the known sequences present in various databases. The alignment of the sequences not only suggests its homology or similarity with other sequences but also gives essential information about its function, structure and its evolution. Over the years, many methods have been suggested for alignment of nucleotide or protein sequences such as:

- Dot plots
- Global alignment
- Local alignment

Dotplots

This method is basically based on the graphical representation of the alignment between the given two sequences. It was first described by Gibbs and McIntyre (1970). One of the sequences in the alignment is considered the *x*-axis and other sequence is taken as *y*-axis. A dot is used for representing the identity among each character in the alignment. This method is particularly useful in identification of repeats, conserved domains, and frame shifts in the given nucleotide and protein sequences. Analysis performed using dotplot have shed light on the various events related to the genome evolution (Figure 10.1). Over a period of time, many programs have been developed which perform dotplot analysis (Table 10.4).

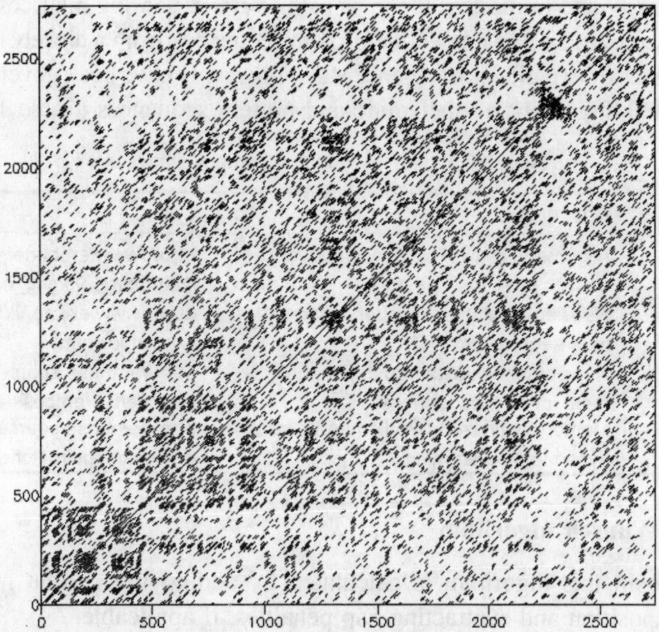

Figure 10.1 Dotplot of rice chromosome 11 nucleotide sequence, plotted using Dotmatcher program of EMBOSS package.

Table 10.4 List of programs which perform the Dot plot analysis.

Program	*Description*	*URL*
Dotmatcher (EMBOSS)	A threshold dotplot of two sequences	http://inn-temp.weizmann.ac.il/cgi-bin/emboss/dotmatcher
Dotpath (EMBOSS)	A non-overlapping wordmatch dotplot of two sequences	http://bioinfo.nhri.org.tw/cgi-bin/emboss/dotpath
Dottup (EMBOSS)	A wordmatch dotplot of two sequences	http://emboss.bioinformatics.nl/cgi-bin/emboss/dottup
Polydot (EMBOSS)	Dotplots of a set of sequences	http://inn-temp.weizmann.ac.il/cgi-bin/emboss/polydot
DotPlot (GCG)	Makes a dot-plot	http://www.life.umd.edu/labs/delwiche/bsci348s/prac/GCGdotplot.html
JDotter	A Java Dot Plot Viewer	http://pgrc.ipk-gatersleben.de/jdotter/
Dotter	A dot-matrix program with interactive greyscale rendering	http://sonnhammer.sbc.su.se/Dotter.html

Global alignment

When two or more nucleotide/protein sequences are aligned over the full length, it is termed global alignment. It was proposed by Needleman and Wunsch (1970). This alignment tends to maximize the regions of similarity and minimizes the gaps using various scoring matrices and gap penalties. It is basically used to compare two nucleotide/protein sequences from a closely related gene family, two homologous genes or two alleles of a gene. Many programs have been developed over the years which perform global alignment of nucleotide and protein sequences (Table 10.5).

Table 10.5 List of global alignment software.

Program	*Description*	*URL*
GAP (GCG)	Alignment of two complete sequences	http://www.embl.de/~seqanal/courses/Hamburg5.99/gcg_course.html
Needle (EMBOSS)	Needleman-Wunsch global alignment of two sequences	http://www.ebi.ac.uk/Tools/emboss/align/index.html
Stretcher (EMBOSS)	Needleman-Wunsch rapid global alignment of two sequences	http://emboss.sourceforge.net/apps/release/6.1/emboss/apps/stretcher.html
Matcher	Memory-optimized Needleman-Wunsch dynamic programming	http://emboss.sourceforge.net/apps/cvs/emboss/apps/matcher.html

Needleman and Wunsch algorithm

The optimal score in this algorithm is calculated by adding the current match score to the previously scored position and subtracting gap penalties, if applicable.

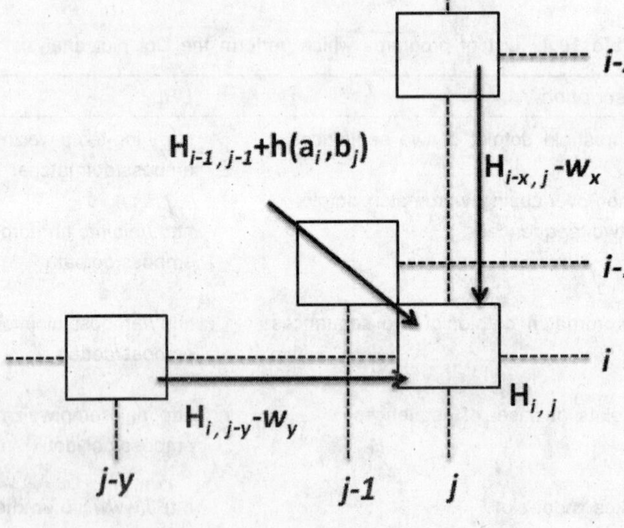

Mathematically, the algorithm can be represented in the following way:

For two sequences **a** = $a_1, a_2 \ldots a_n$ and **b** = $b_1, b_2 \ldots b_n$ where $H_{ij} = H(a_1 a_2 \ldots a_i, b_1 b_2 \ldots b_j)$, then

$$H_{ij} = \max \{ H_{i-1, j-1} + h_{ij}, \quad \max_{x\geq 1} (H_{i-x\, j} - W_x), \quad \max_{y\geq 1} (H_{i, j-y} - W_y), \}$$

where, H_{ij} is the score at position i in sequence **a** and position j in sequence **b**, $h(a_i, b_j)$ is the score for aligning the characters at position i and j, w_x is the penalty for a gap of length x in sequence **a**, and w_y is the penalty for a gap of length y in sequence **b**.

Local alignment

Over the years, dynamic programming algorithm has been vastly used for aligning the two sequences in order to find the homology between the two sequences. Local alignment method is based on the modified dynamic programming algorithm. It was proposed by Smith and Waterman (1981) and is able to find the local common subsequence that is conserved between the two aligned sequences. The scores of the alignment are never allowed to become negative as a zero added when the matrix value reaches the minimum positive value. It is extensively used in the large database searches. Many computational tools have been developed over the years which perform local alignment of nucleotide/protein sequences (Table 10.6).

Table 10.6 List of local alignment tools.

Program	*Description*	*URL*
BLAST	The basic local alignment search tool	http://blast.ncbi.nlm.nih.gov/Blast.cgi
JAligner	Local pairwise sequence alignment software	http://jaligner.sourceforge.net/
YASS	DNA local alignment tool	http://bioinfo.lifl.fr/yass/iedera_proteins/
FASTA	Local search with fast k-tuple heuristic	http://www.ebi.ac.uk/Tools/fasta33/index.html
SSEARCH	Local (Smith-Waterman) alignment with statistics	http://www.ebi.ac.uk/Tools/ssearch/
water	Smith-Waterman dynamic programming	http://www.ebi.ac.uk/Tools/emboss/align/index.html

Multiple sequence alignment (MSA)

Multiple sequence alignment is performed to identify the conserved residues, or motifs within many nucleotide/protein sequences. It not only gives information about the conserved structural or functional domain present with the nucleotide/protein sequences but also emphasize on the evolutionary aspect by reproducing the homologous relationship among the individual residues in a set of nucleotide/protein sequences. MSA is computationally intensive depending on the number of sequences involved in the alignment. Several methods have been proposed in order to obtain the optimal MSA such as: (a) exact method (b) progressive method (e.g., ClustalW) (c) Iterative method (e.g., MUSCLE) (d) consistency based method (e.g., MAFFT) and (e) structure based method (e.g., T-Coffee).

Exact method of obtaining MSA is basically an extension of sequence pair alignment by dynamic programming. This method is computationally intensive considering the comparison of several sequences as memory required for analysis increases exponentially with the number of sequences involved. Progressive method also uses the dynamic programming algorithm to obtain an optimal

MSA, but it is comparatively faster as it starts with the building alignment of most similar pair of sequences and then progressively adding the less similar sequences to initial alignment. The major problem with the progressive method is if there is any error made in the initial alignment, then it may tend to accumulate errors during the progressive addition of the less related sequences. The basic idea behind the iterative approach is to find the suboptimal solution using a progressive alignment approach and then remodel the alignment using dynamic programming approach to find the final optimal solution. In consistency based approach, pairwise alignment scores are used to build the tree which is then used to obtain an optimal MSA. The concept behind the structure based MSA approach is to improve MSA by including the information about the three-dimensional structure of one or more members of the protein sequences involved in the MSA.

MSAs are further used to identify highly conserved portions of the aligned sequences and to generate a scoring matrix which is known as its profile. These profiles include the score for all types of nucleic acid/amino acid substitutions and gaps in each column of the conserved region. The most commonly used method to generate the profile is Hidden Markov Model (HMM), largely known as profile HMM. The profile HMM is the probabilistic model of MSA for a family of nucleotide/protein (Figure 10.2). The profile HMM can be generated for a set of aligned/unaligned sequences and is then used for searching other members of the family. Many MSA databases have been developed (Table 10.7) using tools developed for MSA (Table 10.8). One illustrative example of multiple sequence alignment has been shown in Figure 10.3.

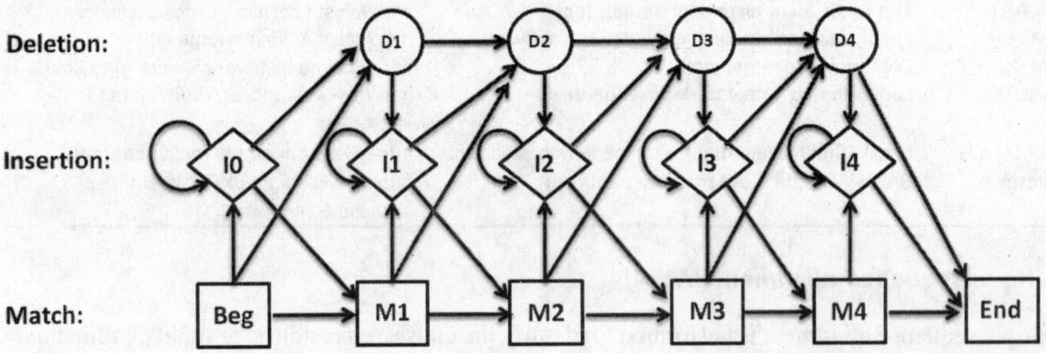

Figure 10.2 The structure of a Hidden Markov Model. The HMM consists of a series of states associated with probabilities (adapted from Krogh et al. (1994)). The "main states" (M1 to M2) are shown in boxes, the "insert states" (I0 to I4) are in diamond-shaped objects and represent insertions, the "deletion states" (D1 to D4) represent gaps in the alignment.

Table 10.7 List of databases obtained using MSA and profile based approach,

Database	*Description*	*URL*
PFAM	Database of protein families	http://pfam.sanger.ac.uk/
SMART	Database of protein families implicated in cellular signaling, extracellular domains, and chromatin function	http://smart.embl-heidelberg.de/
CDD (NCBI)	Database of conserved domains	http://www.ncbi.nlm.nih.gov/Structure/cdd/cdd.shtml

Table 10.8 List of tools for multiple sequence alignment.

Program	*Method*	*URL*
ClustalW	Uses progressive alignment approach	http://www.ebi.ac.uk/Tools/clustalw2/index.html
MUSCLE	Uses iterative approach	http://www.ebi.ac.uk/Tools/muscle/index.html
MAFFT	Uses iterative approach	http://mafft.cbrc.jp/alignment/software/
T-Coffee	Uses both consistency based and structure based approach	http://www.ch.embnet.org/software/TCoffee.html
ProbCons	Uses consistency based approach	http://probcons.stanford.edu/
PRALINE	Uses structure based approach	http://www.ibi.vu.nl/programs/pralinewww/
HMMER	Profile based approach	http://hmmer.janelia.org/
PSI-BLAST	Profile based approach	http://www.ebi.ac.uk/Tools/psiblast/

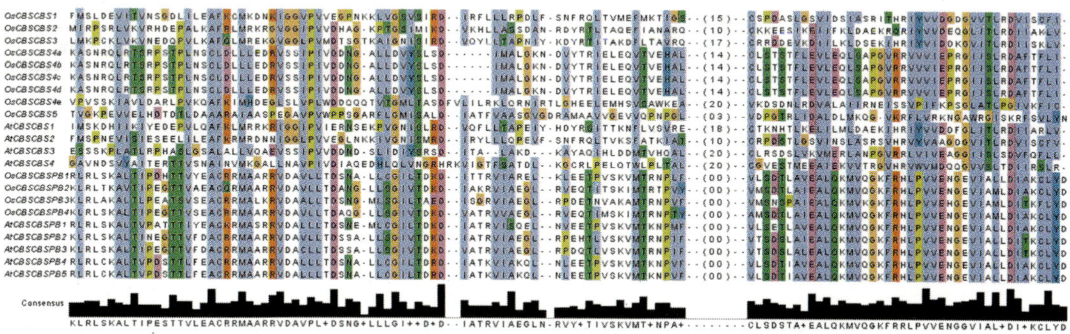

Figure 10.3 An example of multiple sequence alignment performed with MUSCLE and Jalview software showing conserved amino acid residues. The graph underneath depicts the levels of conservation for the respective residue position and the consensus sequence.

Phylogenetic Analysis

Apart from identifying the conserved region of sequences using various approaches of sequences alignment, it is also essential to predict the evolutionary and functional relationship between the sequences. A phylogenetic or evolutionary tree is composed of branches (edges), nodes and leaves with each leaf representing a protein or gene. A node in a tree represents a speciation or divergence event. A branch describes the evolutionary relationship between the nodes and leafs. Trees are of two types: rooted and unrooted. Rooted trees provide full evolutionary meaning in the historic sense since the root of the tree signifies the common ancestor gene. Rooted tree provides information on the relationship between the nodes (Figure 10.4).

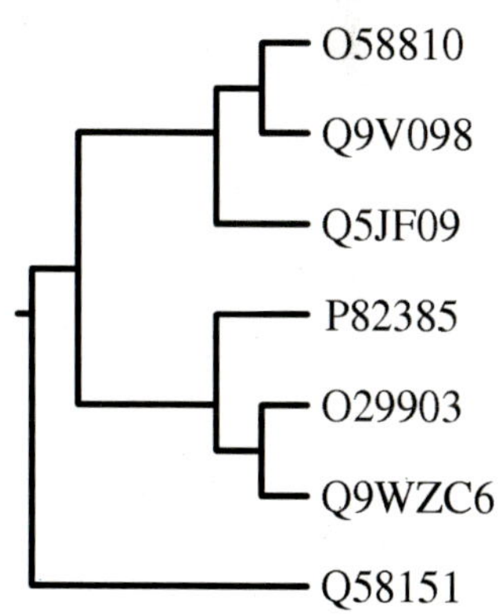

Figure 10.4 The rooted parsimonious tree. The tree was plotted using drawgram program of phylip software.

Over the years, number of tools have been developed for constructing phylogenetic trees (Table 10.9). There are four principle methods of making trees: Distance-based methods, maximum parsimony, maximum likelihood, and Bayesian inference. Distance-based method starts with the analysis of pairwise alignment and uses distance scores to infer the relatedness between all the sequences present. Maximum parsimony is a character-based method in which columns of residues are analyzed in an MSA to identify the tree with the shortest overall branch lengths that can account for the observed character differences. Maximum likelihood and Bayesian inference are model-based statistical approaches in which the best tree is inferred that can account for the observed data.

Table 10.9 List of programs used for phylogenetic analysis.

Program	*Description*	*URL*
ClustalW	Distance matrix/nearest neighbor	http://www.ebi.ac.uk/Tools/clustalw2/index.html
PHYLIP	Maximum parsimony, distance matrix, maximum likelihood	http://evolution.genetics.washington.edu/phylip.html
PAUP	Maximum parsimony, distance matrix, maximum likelihood	http://paup.csit.fsu.edu/
TreeGen	Tree construction given pre-computed distance data	http://www.cbrg.ethz.ch/services/TreeGen
MrBayes	Posterior probability estimation (Bayesian inference)	http://mrbayes.csit.fsu.edu/
TreeFinder	Maximum likelihood, distances, and others	http://www.treefinder.de/

Distance based method

In the distance based method, a tree is constructed using the matrix of pairwise distance between the molecular sequences. The common distance based methods are unweighted pair group methods with arithmetic mean (UPGMA) and neighbor joining (NJ). The UPGMA algorithm is a simple method for tree construction that assumes the rate of change along the branches of a tree is constant and the distances are approximately ultrametric. This method starts by calculating branch lengths between the most closely related sequences, then averaging the distance between the pair or sequence cluster and next sequence or the sequence cluster, and it continues until all the sequences are included in the tree. The most commonly used distance based method is NJ. It searches the minimum pairwise distance according to the distance matrix between the sets of neighbors. It first generates a full tree with all the sequences in a star-like structure with no hierarchy which is followed by pairwise comparisons (to identify two most closely related sequences) which are treated as a single unit. The method identifies the next pair of unit that gives the smallest sum of branch length and it continues to identify the nearest neighbors until all branches are identified.

Maximum parsimony method

Finding the best tree among a set of all the possible trees that requires the least number of nucleic acid/amino acid substitution to explain the observed difference between sequences is the main idea behind this method. According to maximum parsimony theory, having fewer changes to account for the way a group of sequences evolved is preferable to more complicated explanations of molecular evolution. Parsimony analysis assumes that characters are independent of each other. Parsimony algorithms assume that all taxa evolve at the same rate and that all characters contribute the same amount of information.

Maximum likelihood estimation

Maximum likelihood methods are probabilistic, these methods search for the optimal choice by assigning probabilities to every possible substitution in the sequences, and thus maximizing the total probability of the tree. It is the most computationally intensive but most flexible method available till date.

Bayesian inference

In order to model the uncertainty in the complex model, a statistical approach known as Bayesian inference is used. It essentially seeks the probability of a tree conditional on a given MSA. The estimation of the phylogeny in this method is based on the prior information and it uses Markov Chain Monte Carlo (MCMC) to estimate posterior probability distribution.

Structural Analysis of Proteins

Protein plays a major role in all the biological processes which include cell signaling, transport, storage etc. In plants, various membrane proteins such as photoreceptors are essential for various functions in plants. It is well known that linear chain of amino acids folds up to take a three-dimensional structure and their functionality depends on their structure. Experimentally, structure of a protein is analyzed with X-ray crystallography and NMR spectroscopy, but certain proteins are difficult to crystallize. Therefore, computational prediction using homology modeling is being used on a large scale to hypothesize three-dimensional structures of such proteins.

Amino acids are joined by peptide bonds and the core of the protein molecule comprises regular secondary structure, α-helices β-sheets, loops and coils, folded into three-dimensional configurations. A protein molecule can take many conformations due to the rotation of the chain about the backbone C_α atom. The overall structure of protein molecules is assessed using Ramachandran plot. Ramachandran plot is the display of torsional F/Y angle pairs of the polypeptide chain in a given structure. It is used to calculate the allowed backbone conformation of the peptide chain. Over the years, proteins have been classified according to the structure and their sequence similarities. Structurally, proteins are compared on the basis of their secondary structure present and also according to their three-dimensional folds. Various databases hold the information about the conserved secondary structure motifs present till date (Table 10.10) such as SCOP and CATH. SCOP database provides structure classification of proteins on the basis of structures characteristics such as all alpha, all beta, coiled coil etc. CATH (Classifcation, Architecture, Topology and Homology) database provides structure classification on the basis of structure super families.

Table 10.10 List of protein structure databases.

Databases	*Description*	*URL*
PDB	Atomic coordinates of structure as PDB files	http://www.pdb.org/pdb/home/home.do
MMDB (NCBI)	Experimentally resolved structures of proteins, RNA, and DNA	http://www.ncbi.nlm.nih.gov/Structure/MMDB/mmdb.shtml
SCOP	Structural classification of proteins	http://scop.mrc-lmb.cam.ac.uk/scop/
CATH	CATH Protein Structure Classification	http://www.cathdb.info/
3Dee	Database of Protein Domain Definitions	http://www.compbio.dundee.ac.uk/3Dee/
PDBe	EBI Protein Structure Database in Europe	http://www.ebi.ac.uk/pdbe/

Protein Data Bank (PDB) was founded in 1971 and is the repository of all the experimentally determined protein structures (using X-ray crystallography or NMR spectroscopy). Till date, the database has ~ 50,000 protein structures deposited by various research groups worldwide. This database contains three-dimensional atomic coordinate data for various protein structures, citation, primary and secondary structure information as well as experiment (X-ray or NMR) related data. Another web-based database PDBsum, provides the pictorial summary of various key information deposited at PDB (www.biochem.ucl.uk/bsm/pdbsum). This information includes images of the structure; annotated plot of secondary structure of protein, Ramachandran plot derived using PROCHECK for the respective structure and schematic diagram of ligand-protein or protein-DNA interaction. The ligand-protein interaction diagram is generated using LIGPLOT program depicting various hydrogen bonds and non-bonded interactions.

The proteins which share more than 50% identity at the sequence level are said to belong to the same family. A family is considered to preserve its domain structure. Domain is a segment of peptide chain that can fold into a three-dimensional structure irrespective of the presence of other segments in the chain. Many software and web-servers are available to assess and predict the three-dimensional folds in the protein sequence (Table 10.11). Essentially, three basic approaches have been used for predicting the three-dimensional structures of proteins namely: comparative modeling, modeling by threading approach and *ab initio* approach of target structure modeling.

Table 10.11 List of tools for protein structure analysis.

Software	*Description*	*URL*
Secondary	**structure prediction**	
APSSP	Advanced Protein Secondary Structure Prediction Server	http://www.imtech.res.in/raghava/apssp/
Jpred	A consensus method for protein secondary structure prediction at University of Dundee	http://www.compbio.dundee.ac.uk/www-jpred/
JUFO	Protein secondary structure prediction from sequence	http://www.meilerlab.org/web/view.php?section=0&page=6
NetSurfP	Protein Surface Accessibility and Secondary Structure Predictions	http://www.cbs.dtu.dk/services/NetSurfP/
PSIpred	Various protein structure prediction methods at Brunel University	http://bioinf.cs.ucl.ac.uk/psipred/

Contd.

Tertiary structure prediction		
SWISS-MODELAn	Automated knowledge-based protein modeling server	http://swissmodel.expasy.org/
ESyPred3D	Automated homology modeling program using neural networks	http://www.fundp.ac.be/urbm/bioinfo/esypred/
Geno3d	Automatic modeling of protein three-dimensional structure	http://geno3d-pbil.ibcp.fr/cgi-bin/geno3d_automat.pl?page=/GENO3D/geno3d_home.html
Phyre	Automated 3D model building using profile-profile matching and secondary structure	http://www.sbg.bio.ic.ac.uk/~phyre/index.cgi
Fugue	Sequence-structure homology recognition	http://tardis.nibio.go.jp/fugue/
Threader	Protein fold recognition	http://bioinf.cs.ucl.ac.uk/threader/
HMMSTR/ Rosetta	Prediction of protein structure from sequence	http://www.bioinfo.rpi.edu/~bystrc/hmmstr/server.php

In comparative structure modeling (Figure 10.5), it is considered that a template structure with substantial similarity to the target protein is known. Various research groups worldwide have solved many protein structures using X-ray crystallography and NMR spectroscopy, and deposited them into a public database widely known as PDB (www.rcsb.org). In comparative structure modeling, the raw sequence of the protein is first searched into the database for similar proteins with the known structures using BLAST and PSI-BLAST. These known template structures are then aligned to get the profile of the known structures which is used to align the target sequence. This alignment

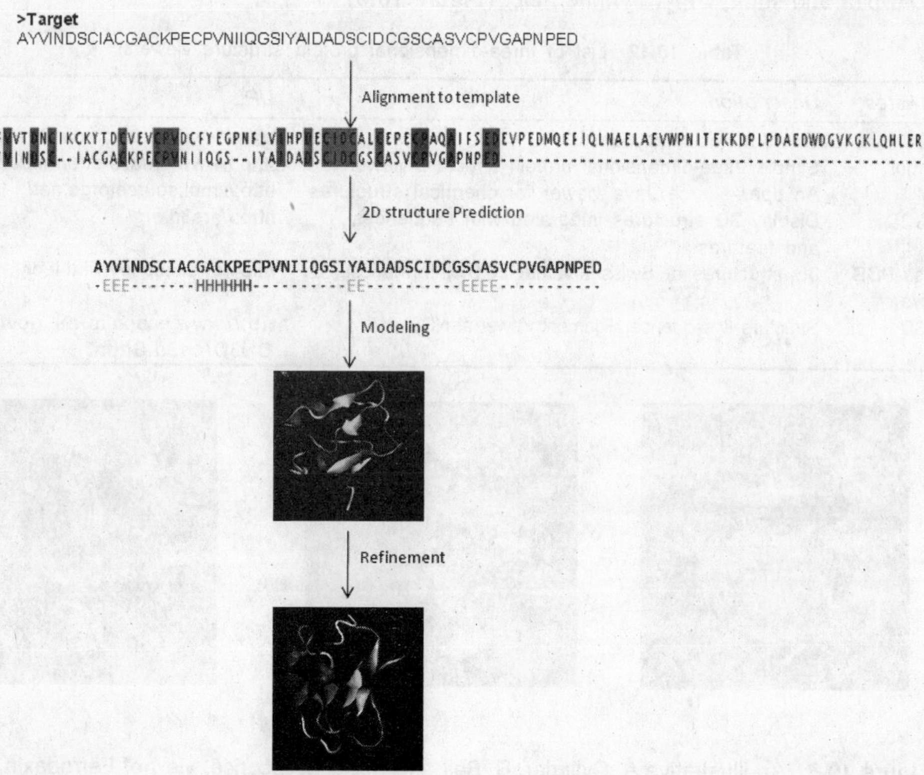

Figure 10.5 A pictorial representation of all the steps of comparative modeling.

is then used for modeling of the target protein sequence using software such as MODELLER, SWISS-MODEL at expasy.

For those proteins where it is difficult to find the known template structures, threading approach is used. In this approach, it is considered that proteins need not to be homologous to the other known proteins whose structure is known but they share common folds due to the convergent evolution. In threading approach, the protein sequence is fragmented and threaded into the library of known folds. Various web-servers are present in the public domain for threading analysis. Three-dimensional protein structure views have been developed over the years for various analyses of protein structures (Table 10.11).

In an another approach, known as *ab initio* approach, also known as template free modeling, it is considered that the target protein does not share significant homology with any of the known protein structure, but lacks in having common folds. The most common strategy which is used for such protein modeling is known as Rosetta method. In this method, the target protein sequence is divided in fragments of nine amino acids and then searched into the PDB database for the known structures. Thus, the complete protein structure is generated using comparison of all the fragments to the structure database.

The three-dimensional structure coordinates of proteins stored in PDB database cannot be assessed and visualized using coordinate points, as connectivity between the atom coordinates is necessary to visualize the protein structure in virtual three-dimensional environments. There are numbers of proteins structure viewers that have been developed over the years (Table 10.12) which allows visual inspection as well as analysis of the proteins macromolecules providing variety of visualizations such as cartoon, ribbon, ball and stick, CPK, cylinder, etc. (Figure 10.6).

Table 10.12 List of three-dimensional protein structure viewers.

Softwares	*Description*	*URL*
VMD	Visual molecular dynamics	http://www.ks.uiuc.edu/Research/vmd/
Rasmol	Simple three-dimensional protein structure viewer	http://www.umass.edu/microbio/rasmol/
Jmol	An open-source Java viewer for chemical structures	http://jmol.sourceforge.net/
SRS 3D	Display 3D structures integrated with sequences and features.	http://srs3d.org/
Swiss-PDB viewer	3D structures at Swiss Institute of Bioinformatics	http://strokespdbv.vital-it.ch/
Cn3D	Structure & sequence alignment viewer at NCBI	http://www.ncbi.nlm.nih.gov/structure/CN3D/cn3d.Shtml

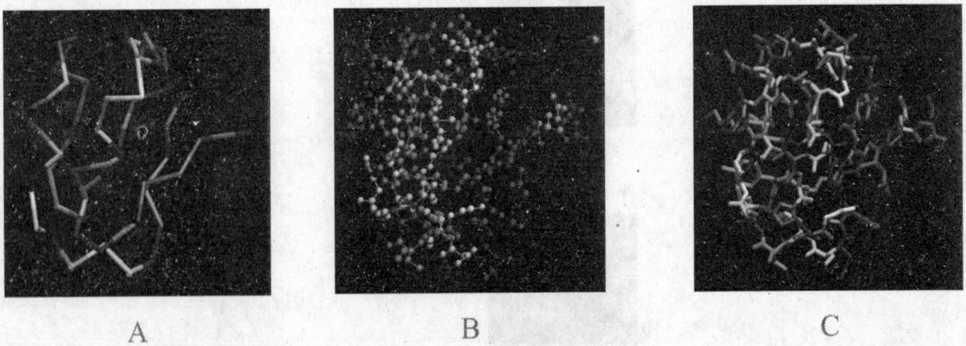

Figure 10.6 An illustrative A. Cylinder, B. Ball and Stick, C. Licorice, view of Ferrodoxin protein molecule using VMD (Source: http://www.bioperl.org/wiki/HOWTO:Beginners).

RNA Analysis

Genome projects have opened a large foreground to understand the complex biological systems with the identification of many novel genes playing role in various processes. It has also revealed the existence of a major class of genes that encodes RNA molecules. These RNA molecules not only play an essential role in transcription and translation but also have been known to play a major role in gene regulation, RNA splicing, RNA editing and catalysis. The major class of small RNAs found in plants are small interfering RNA, microRNA and trans-acting small RNA. The structures of regulatory RNAs determine the functional role played by them. Many computational approaches have been developed to predict the three-dimensional structure of RNA molecules. These structures are considered effective models for their analysis using X-ray crystallography and NMR.

In plants, RNA induced silencing complex comprise siRNAs and miRNAs. miRNAs are the 22-nucleotide long molecules known to play a major role in gene regulation. Various databases dedicated to various classes of RNA have been made available on public domain. Over the years, many software and web-servers have been developed for the analysis of various classes of RNA (Table 10.13 and 10.14).

Table 10.13 List of RNA databases.

Database	*Description*	*URL*
Rfam	A RNA family database	http://rfam.sanger.ac.uk/
ASRP	The Arabidopsis Small RNA Project Database	http://asrp.cgrb.oregonstate.edu/
fRNAdb	A portal site for functional RNAs and non-coding RNAs	http://www.ncrna.org/frnadb/
ncRNAdb	Noncoding RNAs database	http://biobases.ibch.poznan.pl/ncRNA/
GenomeRNAi	RNAi phenotypes	http://rnai2.dkfz.de/GenomeRNAi/

Table 10.14 List of RNA analysis software.

Software	*Description*	*URL*
miRanda200809	An algorithm for finding genomic targets for microRNAs	http://en.bio-soft.net/rna/miRanda.html
RNAsoft	Software for RNA secondary structure prediction and design	http://www.rnasoft.ca/
ESSA	An integrated and interactive tool for analysing RNA secondary structure	http://www.inra.fr/internet/Departements/MIA/T/essa/Doc/essa_home.html
RNAfold	RNA structure prediction algorithm.	http://rna.tbi.univie.ac.at/cgi-bin/RNAfold.cgi
Mfold	MFE RNA structure prediction algorithm	http://mfold.bioinfo.rpi.edu/

Microarray Analysis

The next major advancement in the field of biological sciences after the genome sequencing projects is the development of microarray technology that has enabled assessment of thousands of genes at a time. Many databases have been developed which possess the expression data obtained using various microarray experiments (Table 10.15). In DNA microarray slide, thousands of DNA molecules are chemically bonded to a solid surface. Purified RNA obtained from various tissues is then fluorescently- or radioactively labeled and hybridized to the slide. The intensity of the fluorophore in probe-target hybridization is quantified which tells the relative abundance of the nucleic acid sequence in the target. A matrix is created having all intensity values at its respective spot, with genes represented in the row and samples in the column. The intensity measurements in the matrix are assumed to be directly proportional to the abundance of mRNA that has been transcribed from each gene.

Table 10.15 List of various microarray databases.

Database	*Description*	*URL*
GEO	Gene expression omnibus at NCBI	http://www.ncbi.nlm.nih.gov/geo/
ArrayExpress	Microarray based gene expression data at EBI	http://www.ebi.ac.uk/microarray-as/ae/
SMD	Stanford microarray database	http://smd.stanford.edu/
MIAME	Minimum information about a microarray experiment	http://www.mged.org/Workgroups/MIAME/miame.html
AREX	The Arabidopsis expression database	http://www.arexdb.org/
RMOS	Rice microarray opening site	http://microarray.rice.dna.affrc.go.jp/

The data matrix undergoes a series of preprocessing steps that includes background subtraction in which "noise" is subtracted from the feature intensity and log is taken for all the raw intensity values. This transformation is done to ensure the even spread of features across the intensity range and variability which is to be constant at all the intensity levels. Also, it is considered that the distribution of intensity should be approximately bell-shaped and the experimental errors should be statistically normal. The main purpose behind the data preprocessing is to remove the systematic bias in the data while preserving the variation in gene expression that occurs because of biologically relevant changes in the expression. Then the datasets are subjected to normalization procedure in order to make one sample data comparable to other sample.

Over the years, many normalization methods have been proposed and implemented for the analysis of various microarray data. The simplest way of normalization is known as scale normalization in which the data is simply adjusted to the scale of data range. Another method popularly known as Loess method, usually used in two-color arrays. It performs the many local regressions in overlapping windows and later joins the regressions to form a smooth curve. Quantile normalization method is generally used for affymetrix data and is similar to scale normalization but is more drastic as all of the various quantiles are adjusted in the data. Another approach known as VSN estimates, which is an additive and multiplicative offset and transforms the data to have equal variance for all intensities. It can be used with cDNA or affymetrix data.

After the preprocessing step, the data is subjected to analysis in order to identify various differentially expressed genes. To decide the extent of up-regulated and down-regulated genes, the expression ratios in control and in experimental conditions are calculated and compared followed by choosing the arbitrary cutoff for the final inference. The derived hypothesis is then tested using the above statistical inference to decide the consistency of the differentially expressed genes in one or more experimental conditions. Using *t*-test statistic, *p*-value is calculated which is used for accepting or rejecting the null hypothesis that the control and experimental conditions have equal gene expression values which means there is no differential expression. *t*-test is known to be parametric and assumes that the data distribution is normal but if the data is guided by extreme outliers then non-parametric tests such as Mann-Whitney and Wilcoxon tests which are less influenced by extreme outliers, are considered. Other approaches such as Bayesian statistics is also applied to test the confidence of the inference made from the data. Bootstrap analysis is performed on the data in which the observed scores are compared to the results of repeated measurements to find the false discovery rate estimates. Over the years, many more statistical parameters have been used to analyze the microarray data. To test the data for more than two conditions, the analysis of variance (ANOVA) is used to identify differentially expressed genes which accounts for variance that occurs both within the groups and between the groups.

Clustering analysis is used to identify the pattern of gene expression in the microarray experiment. It is essentially a representation of distance measurement between the genes. There are several methods of clustering of which hierarchical clustering is most commonly used in microarray data analysis. In clustering analysis, the genes or sample profiles are arranged into a tree with similar members appears closer and dissimilar members appear farther. Another machine learning approaches such as K-means clustering and self-organizing maps (SOMs) are also used for microarray data analysis.

The data produced by microarray analysis has very high dimensionality. Therefore, many methods are used for reducing the dimension of the microarray data such as principal component analysis (PCA), individual gene selection, pairwise gene selection and genetic algorithms. In PCA, data of high dimension is projected on the lower dimensional space. In individual gene selection method, genes that rank best between the classes are chosen and used as a classifier while in pairwise gene selection method, pair of genes is chosen that is used as a classifier.

Systems Biology and Network Analysis

With the wealth of information obtained about the various genes due to completion of various genome sequencing projects, attempts are being made to make 'gene networks'. These networks are basically based on graph theory and incorporate information about the various gene interactions. This method is being utilized to build individual gene interactions into pathways thus having a larger overview of cellular processes. These networks can be modeled and simulated in order to understand the basic mechanism of various responses.

Various types of biological network have been extensively worked out and analyzed using various statistical measures such as metabolic network, protein-protein interaction network, signal transduction networks and gene regulatory network. Metabolic networks are the representation of metabolic substrate and products with directed edges joining them. Protein interaction network (PIN) is the network of mechanistic physical interaction between proteins. In another most studied networks, gene regulatory network (GRN), the principle of gene regulation which is, a gene is regulated by the presence of other proteins both as activator and inhibitor is considered. These networks are available in detail in the form of publicly available databases (Table 10.16).

Table 10.16 List of database possessing information in the form of networks.

Database	*Description*	*URL*
KEGG	Kyoto Encyclopedia of Genes and Genomes	http://www.genome.jp/kegg/
EcoCyc	Database for the bacterium *E. coli* K-12 MG1655	http://ecocyc.org/
BNDB	The Biochemical Network Database	http://www.bndb.org/
GO	Gene Ontology relational database	http://www.geneontology.org/
DP	Database of Interacting proteins	http://www.geneontology.org/

Networks are based on the graph theory developed by Euler in the 18th century and are depicted as a set of vertices joined by edges. On the basis of the data available, a biological network can be a directed network or undirected network. In a directed network, interaction between two nodes is defined by a direction while in an undirected network, no specific direction of interaction is defined between the two nodes. Networks are basically defined by certain measures such as degree distribution, clustering coefficient, shortest path or path length, sub-graphs or motifs. A degree k (or connectivity) is the most fundamental characteristic of a node and it gives information about the links one node has with the other nodes. Thus, the probability that a node has k links is defined by its degree distribution P(k). Degree distribution tells the exact nature of the network that is, whether the network is a random network where there is absence of highly connected nodes or if many smaller nodes are held by hubs which is defined by power-law degree distribution. These hubs correspond to the highly central nodes in the network that is, those genes do a large amount of overall regulation. Mostly biological networks are driven by power-law distribution and are largely scale-free networks with great degree of robustness. The clustering coefficient of the network measures the density of triangles in a network.

For biological networks, three network models have been usually considered: random networks, scale-free networks and hierarchical networks. Random network is based on the theory proposed by Paul Erdos and Alfred Renyi and is known as ER model. It starts with N nodes and connects every pair of nodes with probability p, creating a graph with approximately $p(N(N - 1)/2)$ edges distributed randomly. Scale-free nodes are networks with power-law degree distribution: $P(k) \sim k^{-g}$, where k is degree and g is the degree exponent. In networks including metabolic networks, protein interaction network, the scale-free topology and high clustering coexist. Thus, in order to bring modularity, both approaches are combined in a hierarchical manner forming hierarchical network.

Role of Programming Languages and Databases

In bioinformatics, one needs to do diverse tasks ranging from small pattern searching to analyzing huge datasets. Therefore, in order to solve some of the biological problems, programming languages provides an efficient means. Besides having sound knowledge of molecular biology, working knowledge of one of the programming languages provides a great support for complex genome analysis. Various programs written in different languages have not only increased the efficiency, reduced the time complexity but also have given new ways to present the data. Biological databases keep data in diverse formats, thus, a standard software program written is not robust enough to provide linking pipeline between the file formats. Hence, scripting languages act as an interface between various programs written in different programming languages performing sequential parts of the analysis. Scripting languages not only extract information from large datasets with efficiency but also reduce the time for the stipulated task.

There are many programming and scripting languages available till date such as C, C++, Java, Python and many more, but the most preferred scripting language by a bioinformatics analyst is Perl (Practical Extraction and Report Language) due to its highly developed capacities in string handling, text processing, networking, and rapid prototyping. Perl is fairly easy to learn and is extremely successful in sequence analysis pipelines, converting file formats, and extracting information from the output of analysis programs and other text files. Worldwide, various research groups used to maintain their repository of small Perl programs for their reusability in form of Perl modules. In an open source initiative, Bioperl toolkit came into existence in 1995 which has brought together various Perl modules containing generalized routines specific to life-science information in one complete package (http://www.bioperl.org/wiki/Main_Page) (Open Source Initiative 2001). The basic motivation of having this toolkit is focused on the innovative solutions rather than the duplication of the routine work. The open source licence gives everyone a chance to reuse, extend and contribute their own Perl routine to the toolkit. Hence, the task such as parsing and interpreting sequence from EMBL and GenBank format sequence files have become easy and time efficient. Due to the involvement of large number of people in development of the bioperl, it has ventured into new areas including phylogenetics, maps, protein structure, and bibliographic references (Stajich et al. 2002). The complete description of the Perl scripting language and its modules is beyond the scope of this book however literature tutorial in this regard, is available online as shown below: (example 10.1)

```
use Bio::DB::Query::GenBank;
$query = "Arabidopsis[ORGN] AND topoisomerase[TITL] and 0:3000[SLEN]";
$query_obj=Bio::DB::Query::GenBank->new(-db=>'nucleotide',-query => $query );
```

Example 10.1: A script to fetch nucleotide sequence of *Arabidopsis* topoisomerases from Genbank. (Source: http://www.bioperl.org/wiki/HOWTO:Beginners)

As discussed in earlier part of the chapter, research groups around the world have been involved in generating and analyzing biological data obtained from various experiments. The quantity of this data is huge and needs effective storage and efficient means to access this data for further analysis. Web-based databases have been an effective way of storing and sharing this biological data among various scientific communities. Major online databases such as PDB, GenBank (NCBI), Swiss-Prot have been considered major resources nowadays for accessing biological data. Therefore, basic knowledge of database management system (DBMS), its creation and usage is considered an asset for a bioinformatics analyst. This is particularly useful for creation of in-house biological resource for the available data as well as sharing with the data with other research groups worldwide.

Basically, there are two types of database management systems available, namely, flat file indexing system and relational databases. Flat file database is essentially a simple ordered collection of files having a common standard format and are indexed for easy accessibility. The most common example of such database type among the biological database is PDB which has been discussed earlier in the chapter. PDB keeps all the information in standard PDB format and the data can be easily searched using keywords. On the other hand, relational database keeps the information in form of separate tables. Each of the table is given a unique identity and thus all the tables are linked using these identities. Such database allows easy access to all of the data present in the database easily and efficiently. The most common example of the relational database is Entrez at NCBI (http://www.ncbi.nlm.nih.gov/Entrez/). Nowadays, object oriented databases have been used a lot for keeping the biological data because of its capability of handling data as objects rather than as simple tables. Such databases allow storing of the related text data, images and even simple underlying analytical softwares (for online analysis of data) within the same database.

There are many DBMS systems available such as Oracle, PostgreSQL, MySQL etc but the most commonly used database system is MySQL. This is because MySQL is an open source relational database management system and is relatively easy to be set up and used (http://www.mysql.com). The complete description of the MySQL such as how to set up, run and use is beyond the scope of this chapter however lots of literature and tutorial is available online in this regard.

Finally, resources in the area of information technology such as programming languages, algorithms and databases have been the essential part of bioinformatics. This has made the accessibility and analysis of biological data not only an efficient one but has also reduced the time complexity.

Bioinformatics Powered Discoveries in Plant Genomics

The emergence of large scale efforts to understand various plant systems has led to a treasure of information about genes having agronomic importance. Large number of breeding and transgenic approaches has been used to modify the physiological traits of various crop plants and have provided important insights into their role in various environmental conditions. Comparative sequence analysis of genes and gene families has provided valuable insight into the complex origin, evolution and conservation of an important metabolic pathway. In the past, sequence analysis approaches have been utilized to characterize the gene families that play the major role in complex stress tolerance mechanism in rice. These include the monosaccharide transporter gene family, Dof gene family, ERF gene family, Hsp100 gene family, SBP box gene family and CBS domain containing protein family.

Structure analysis of novel serine β-lactamase in plants have shown the conserved structural elements required for the serine protease active center formation and is involved in apoptotic processes through its serine protease and serine/threonine protein kinase activity. Various microarray experiments in plants have shed light of the various aspects of the plant functionality which was difficult to be analyzed earlier. In one of the attempts, novel genes that are regulated by the circadian clock in *Arabidopsis* have been identified. Further, candidate genes have been identified in barley using microarray analysis which play a major role in yield and are of greater agronomic importance in water deficit conditions. In wheat, expression of genes involved in aluminium-tolerance have been analyzed using microarray. Various coordinated plant defense responses have been studied in *Arabidopsis* using microarray.

Sequence analysis has revealed that the origin of miRNA predates the monocot and dicot divergence, as many genes encoding miRNA was found conserved in *Arabidopsis* and rice. Experimental analysis of various miRNA targets has confirmed their role in various major process in *Arabidopsis* such as root development, auxin signaling and oxidative stress regulation. With the availability of transcriptome, proteome, and metabolome data sets, scientific community has started modeling various networks in order to see the complex picture of plant responses. The first dynamic models of plant GRN were proposed for the specification of floral organ and root epidermis cell types in *Arabidopsis*. With the pace of ongoing research, we can hope for answering many questions which have troubled the scientific community for long.

FUTURE PERSPECTIVE AND CONCLUSION

One of the broad goals of the plant biology is to understand the nature of various responses in plants towards environmental conditions. Though large amount of data is available exclusively for plants, but still very little understanding of the system is developed because of the complex nature of gene expression and their regulation. In future, we can expect more data pertaining to genes and gene families and their evolution. One of the major problems the plant research is facing, is the lack of annotation of large number of genes identified. Therefore, effective approaches to annotate these genes is required. Further, development of algorithms to find noncoding RNAs, duplicated blocks of sequences within genome and other genomic features is required. Globally, research communities are generating massive amount of data but an approach to assess the quality and effective storage of such data is also required. Sequence analysis tools should assess the alignments of the target sequence with those in knowledge bases from statistical and biological point of view. Accurate method based on specific criteria is also required for MSA in order to make alignment significant from structure and evolutionary point of view. The three-dimensional structure of protein can be predicted with high confidence when a closely related template is available, but it is still difficult to predict the structure of entirely novel protein structures. Therefore, there is a need for development of tools which can predict three-dimensional structures of complex proteins with higher accuracy and confidence. Efficient methods for simulating and analyzing various metabolic pathways and gene regulatory networks will also help in developing better understanding of the complex plant responses.

FURTHER READINGS

1. A.G.I. (*Arabidopsis* Genome Initiative) (2000) Analysis of genome sequence of the flowering plant *Arabidopsis thaliana. Nature.* **(408):** 796-815.
2. Batra G., Chauhan V.S., Singh A., Sarkar N.K., Grover A. (2007) Complexity of rice Hsp100 gene family: lessons from rice genome sequence data. *J. Biosci.* **(32):** 611-619.
3. Berman H.M., Westbrook J., Feng Z., Gilliard G., Bhat T.N., Weissig H., Shindyalov I.N., Bourne P.E. (2000) The protein data bank. *Nucleic Acids Res.* **(28):** 235-242.
4. Berman H.M., Henrick K., Nakamura H. (2003) Announcing the worldwide Protein Data Bank. *Nature Struct. Biol.* **(10):** 980.
5. Bernstein F.C., Koetzle T.F., Willian G.J.B., Meyer E.F., Brice M.D., Rodger J.R., Kennard O., Shimanouchi T., Tasumi M. (1977) Protein Data Bank: a computer-based archival file for macromolecule structrures. *J. Mol. Biol.* **(112):** 535-542.
6. Bonierbale M., Plaisted R.L., Tanksley S.D. (1988) RFLP maps based on a common set of clones reveal modes of chromosomal evolution in potato and tomato. *Genetics.* **(120):** 1095-1103.
7. Bonnet E., Van de Peer Y., Rouzé P. (2006) The small RNA world of plants. *New Phytol.* **(171):** 451-68.

8. Carbajosa J.V., Moose S.P., Parsons R.L., Schmidt R.J. (1997) A maize zinc-finger protein binds the prolamin box in zein gene promoters and interacts with the basic leucine zipper transcriptional activator Opaque2. *Proc. Natl. Acad. Sci. USA.* **(94):** 7685-7690.
9. Chervitz S.A., Fuellen G., Dagdigian C., Brenner S.E., Birney E., Korf I. (1998) Bioperl: Standard perl modules for bioinformatics. Bio Informatics Technology and Systems (BITS) http://www.bitsjournal.com/bioperl.html.
10. Czelusniak J., Goodman M., Moncrief N.D., Kehoe S.M. (1990) Maximum parsimony approach to construction of evolutionary trees from aligned homologous sequences. *Methods Enzymol.* **(183):** 601-615.
11. Cullis C.A. (2004) *Plant Genomics and Proteomics,* John Wiley & Sons, Inc, pp. 1-22.
12. Felsenstein J. (1981) Evolutionary trees from DNA sequences: a maximum likelihood approach. *J. Mol. Evol.* **(17):** 368-376.
13. Felsenstein J. (1984) Distance methods for inferring phylogenies: A justification. *Evolution.* **(38):** 16-24.
14. Floyd S.K., Bowman J.L. (2004) Gene regulation: ancient micro RNA target sequences in plants. *Nature.* **(428):** 485-486.
15. Gale M.D., Devos K.M. (1998) Plant comparative genetics after 10 years. *Science.* **(282):** 656-659.
16. Guo P-G, Bai G-H, Carver B. (2003) Profiling expression of aluminium-tolerance genes in wheat through microarrays. *Plant and Animal Genome Conference* XI, 11–15 January 2003, San Diego, C.A., p. 265.
17. Huelsenbeck J.P., Ronquist F., Nielsen R., Bollback J.P. (2001) Bayesian inference of phylogeny and its impact on evolutionary biology. *Science.* **(294):** 2310-2314.
18. Johnson D.A., Thomas M.A. (2007) The monosaccharide transporter gene family in ***Arabidopsis*** and rice: a history of duplications, adaptive evolution, and functional divergence. *Mol. Biol. Evol.* **(24):** 2412-2423.
19. Kapoor M., Arora R., Lama T., Nijhawan A., Khurana J.P., Tyagi A.K., Kapoor S. (2008) Genome-wide identification, organization and phylogenetic analysis of Dicer-like, Argonaute and RNA-dependent RNA Polymerase gene families and their expression analysis during reproductive development and stress in rice. *BMC Genomics.* **(9):** 451.
20. Kushwaha H.R., Singh A.K., Sopory S.K., Singla Pareek S.L., Pareek A. (2009) Genome wide expression analysis of CBS domain containing proteins in *Arabidopsis thaliana* (L.) Heynh and *Oryza sativa* L. reveals their developmental and stress regulation. *BMC Genomics.* **(9):** 451.
21. Laskowski R.A. (2001) PDBsum: summaries and analysis of PDB structure. *Nucleic Acids Res.* **(29):** 221-222.
22. Lee D-S, Song H., Kim Y., *et al.* (2003) Identification and characterization of genes responding to temperature stresses in Chinese cabbage using cDNA microarray. *Plant and Animal Genome Conference* XI, 11-15 January 2003, San Diego, C.A., p. 268.
23. Lijavetzky D., Carbonero P., Vicente-Carbajosa J. (2003) Genome-wide comparative phylogenetic analysis of the rice and Arabidopsis Dof gene families. *BMC Evol. Biol.* **(3):** 17-21.
24. Liobikas J., Baniulis D., Stanys V., Toleikis A., Eriksson O. (2006) Identification and analysis of a novel serine â-lactamase-like plant protein by a bioinformatic approach. *Biologia.* **(3):** 126-129.
25. Mena M., Carbajosa J.V., Schmidt R.J., Carbonero P. (1998) An endosperm-specific DOF protein from barley, highly conserved in wheat, binds to and activates transcription from the prolamin-box of a native B-hordein promoter in barley endosperm. *Plant J.* **(16):** 53-62.
26. Mendoza L., Alvarez-Buylla E.R. (2000) Genetic regulation of root hair development in Arabidopsis thaliana: a network model. *J. Theor. Biol.* **(204):** 311-326.
27. Mendoza L., Alvarez-Buylla E.R. (1998) Dynamics of the genetic regulatory network for Arabidopsis thaliana flower morphogenesis. *J. Theor. Biol.* **(193):** 307-319.
28. Millar A.A., Gubler F. (2005) The Arabidopsis GAMYB-like Genes, MYB33 and MYB65. Are microRNA-regulated genes that redundantly facilitate anther development. *Plant Cell.* **(17):** 705-721.
29. Nakano T., Suzuki K., Fujimura T., Shinshi H. (2006) Genome wide analysis of the ERF gene family in Arabidopsis and rice. *Plant Physiology.* **(140):** 411-432.

30. Nelson D.R., Schuler M.A., Paquette S.M., Werck Reichhart D., Bak S. (2004) Comparative Genomics of Rice and Arabidopsis. Analysis of 727 Cytochrome P450 Genes and Pseudogenes from a Monocot and a Dicot. *Plant Physiol.* **(135):** 756-772.
31. Open Source Initiative (2001) The open-source definition. http://opensource.org/docs/definition.html.
32. Pareek A., Singh A., Kumar M., Kushwaha H.R., Lynn A.M., Singla-Pareek S.L. (2006) Whole genome analysis of *Oryza sativa* L. reveals similar architecture of two-component-signaling machinery with Arabidopsis. *Plant Physiology.* **(142):** 380-397.
33. Rohl C.A., Strauss C.E., Misura K.M., Baker D. (2004) Protein structure prediction using Rosetta. *Methods Enzymol.* **(383):** 66-93.
34. Sampedro J., Carey R.E., Cosgrove D.J. (2006) Genome histories clarify evolution of the expansion superfamily: new insights from the poplar genome and pine ESTs. *J. Plant. Res.* **(119):** 11-21.
35. Schaffer R., Landgraf J., Accerbi M., Simon V., Larson M., Wisman E. (2001) Microarray analysis of diurnal and circadian-regulated genes in Arabidopsis. *Plant Cell.* **(13):** 113-23.
36. Schenk P.M., Kazan K., Wilson I., Anderson J.P., Richmond T., Somerville S.C., Manners J.M. (2000) Coordinated plant defense responses in Arabidopsis revealed by microarray analysis. *Proc. Natl. Acad. Sci. USA.* **(97):** 11655-60.
37. Seki M., Narusaka M., Abe H., *et al.* (2001) Monitoring the expression pattern of 1300 Arabidopsis genes under drought and cold stresses by using full-length cDNA microarray. *Plant Cell.* **(13):** 61-72.
38. Simons K.T., Strauss C., Baker D. (2001) Prospects for ab initio protein structural genomics. *J. Mol. Biol.* **(306):** 1191-1199.
39. Stajich J.E., Block D., Boulez K., Brenner S.E., Chervitz S.A., Dagdigian C., Fuellen G., Gilbert J.G., Korf I., Lapp H., Lehväslaiho H., Matsalla C., Mungall C.J., Osborne B.I., Pocock M.R., Schattner P., Senger M., Stein L.D., Stupka E., Wilkinson M.D., Birney E. (2002) The Bioperl toolkit: Perl modules for the life sciences. *Genome Res.* **(12):** 1611-8.
40. Sunkar R., Kapoor A., Zhu J.K. (2006) Posttranscriptional induction of two Cu/Zn superoxide dismutase genes in Arabidopsis is mediated by downregulation of miR398 and important for oxidative stress tolerance. *Plant Cell.* **(18):** 2051-2065.
41. Wang J.W., Wang L.J., Mao Y.B., Cai W.J., Xue H.W., Chen X.Y. (2005) Control of root cap formation by MicroRNA-targeted auxin response factors in Arabidopsis. *Plant Cell.* **(17):** 2204-2216.
42. Wei F., Coe E., Nelson W., Bharti A.K., Engler F., Butler E., Kim H., Goicoechea J.L., Chen M., Lee S., Fuks G., Sanchez-Villeda H., Schroeder S., Fang Z., McMullen M., Davis G., Bowers J.E., Paterson A.H., Schaeffer M., Gardiner J., Cone K., Messing J., Soderlund C., Wing R.A. (2007) Physical and genetic structure of the maize genome reflects its complex evolutionary history. *PLoS Genet.* **(3):** e123.
43. Yang Z., Wang X., Gu S., Hu Z., Xu H., Xu C. (2008) Comparative study of SBP-box gene family in *Arabidopsis* and rice. *Gene.* **(407):** 1-11.

CHAPTER

11

Systems Biology Technology

In 1995, the first full genome sequence became available to the scientific community that has led to usher the genome era. Since then, a number of high-throughput technologies have enabled us to define the molecular parts and catalogs of cellular components. Although, these catalogs are still incomplete, it is now possible to reconstruct, based on this and other information, genome-scale networks of biochemical reactions that take place inside the cells. This process of network reconstruction, followed by the synthesis of *in silico* models describing their functionalities, is the essence of systems biology. Systems biology aims at system-level understanding of biology processes by employing mathematical analysis and computational tools to integrate the information content obtained in experimental biology and to understand biological organism as a 'system'.

Keywords: Systems biology, molecular systems biology, computational systems, biochemical network systems, gene network systems.

INTRODUCTION

There exists a wide gap between the genotype and phenotype in the manifestation of a trait of a biological system. To fill up this gap, research is conducted at different levels—whole organism, cellular, biochemical as well as molecular, i.e., gene and protein levels. Most of these approaches used to study biology have been reductionist in nature. Study of unity and diversity of life forms is done primarily by three approaches:

ONE TO ONE : Hypothesis driven gene by gene approach.

BOTTOM-UP : Thorough understanding of the proteins/genes involved in limited reaction step

TOP-DOWN : Systems biology approach for studying large number of genes coding for hypothetical proteins (unknown function)

Typically, researchers focus only on one component of a biological system at a time—a gene or a protein, for example, gathered data from the individual components is used to understand the functions, whether that system is a tissue, an organ or whole organism. Such a bottom-up approach with collection of data about the individual genes or proteins is often divorced from the context of whole organism. Our understanding of how a genotype influences the phenotype especially during manifestation of agronomically important traits in crops is still not well studied. Recent developments in molecular biology and the huge data developed from sequencing of model organisms such as *Human, Arabidopsis thaliana, rice* and others enable us to draw relationships between genotype and phenotype on large scale and at the level of an organism. However, traditional approach employed by research in molecular biology is a local one, examining and collecting data of a single gene or protein or a reaction at a time. This has enriched significantly our understanding about structure and functions of individual genes and proteins. Of late, genomics approach is actively pursued to analyze the system in totality and as a result, entirely a new class of data is emerging to describe the system. Coupled with revolutionary developments that took place in genome sequencing and high throughput experimental techniques, a new window has opened up for researchers to describe the system. Broad availability of diverse functional genomics data from protein-protein interaction, gene expression, metabolomics, protein localization and regulation studies has enabled prediction of several new genes and finding their biological functions. Organisms enter into complex interactions with environment while consuming matter, energy and information flows during growth and reproduction. All these diverse reactions are regulated genetically with coordination of different signaling, genetic, protein and metabolic networks.

The systems biology can be defined as: *"Systems biology is the application of computational approaches to the understanding of the normal and dysfunctional behavior of cellular systems"* or *"Systems biology can be defined as a biology-based inter-disciplinary study of a field that focuses on complex interactions in biological systems"* or *"a research approach that seeks to describe the overall behavior of a biological system through detailed, quantitative experimentation combined with conceptual or computational modeling of the systems components and their interactions"* or *"the study of biological function that derives from interactions"* or *"Systems biology is the study of biological functions and mechanisms, underpinning inter- and intra-cellular dynamical network, by means of signal- and system-oriented approaches"*.

Systems biology attempts to understand the cellular behavior in terms of spatio-temporal interactions occurring among various cellular components like genes, proteins, enzymes, and organelles. The available molecular and genomic data are however based on static representation of the system. These studies can be extended and a dynamic behavior of the system achieved by modeling and simulation of metabolic reactions underlying various cellular processes occurring in parallel in a system can be understood. Bioinformatics techniques are already available to model and simulate the metabolic behavior of a system *in silico* representing genes, proteins and metabolic pathways in combination with dynamic and simulated environments (Wildermuth, 2000). These powerful computational approaches present a clear picture about a given metabolism in a cell and enable better understanding, for example, the mechanism of a disease. Besides, these bioinformatics approaches facilitate fast and accurate generation of network models through computational prediction and experimental validation. Application of new high-throughput experimental approaches such as metabolic pathway control analysis (or simply metabolomics) attempts to link interacting biochemical pathways to complex networks of genes. Application of computationally robust algorithms can potentially help to answer some of the general questions of crop functional genomics. With the availability of sequence information from model organisms like rice and *Arabidopsis thaliana* and partial annotation of their genomes, it is becoming easier to understand biological regulation of different crop traits at the level of metabolism and even attempt to simulate the systems in context of an object in time and space (analogous to genotype x environment) interaction. Thus, measurement and modeling approaches have already begun to present a big-picture view of biology and may improve drug discovery and development.

SYSTEMS BIOLOGY TECHNOLOGY

Purposes: A systems biology approach means:

(i) Investigating the components of cellular networks and their interactions.

(ii) Applying experimental high-throughput and whole-genome techniques.

(ii) Integrating computational and theoretical methods with experimental efforts.

Associated Disciplines

According to the interpretation of systems biology as the ability to obtain, integrate and analyze complex data from multiple experimental sources using interdisciplinary tools, some typical technology platforms are (Figure 11.1):

(i) Genomics

(ii) Epigenomics/Epigenetics

(iii) Transcriptomics

(iv) Proteomics

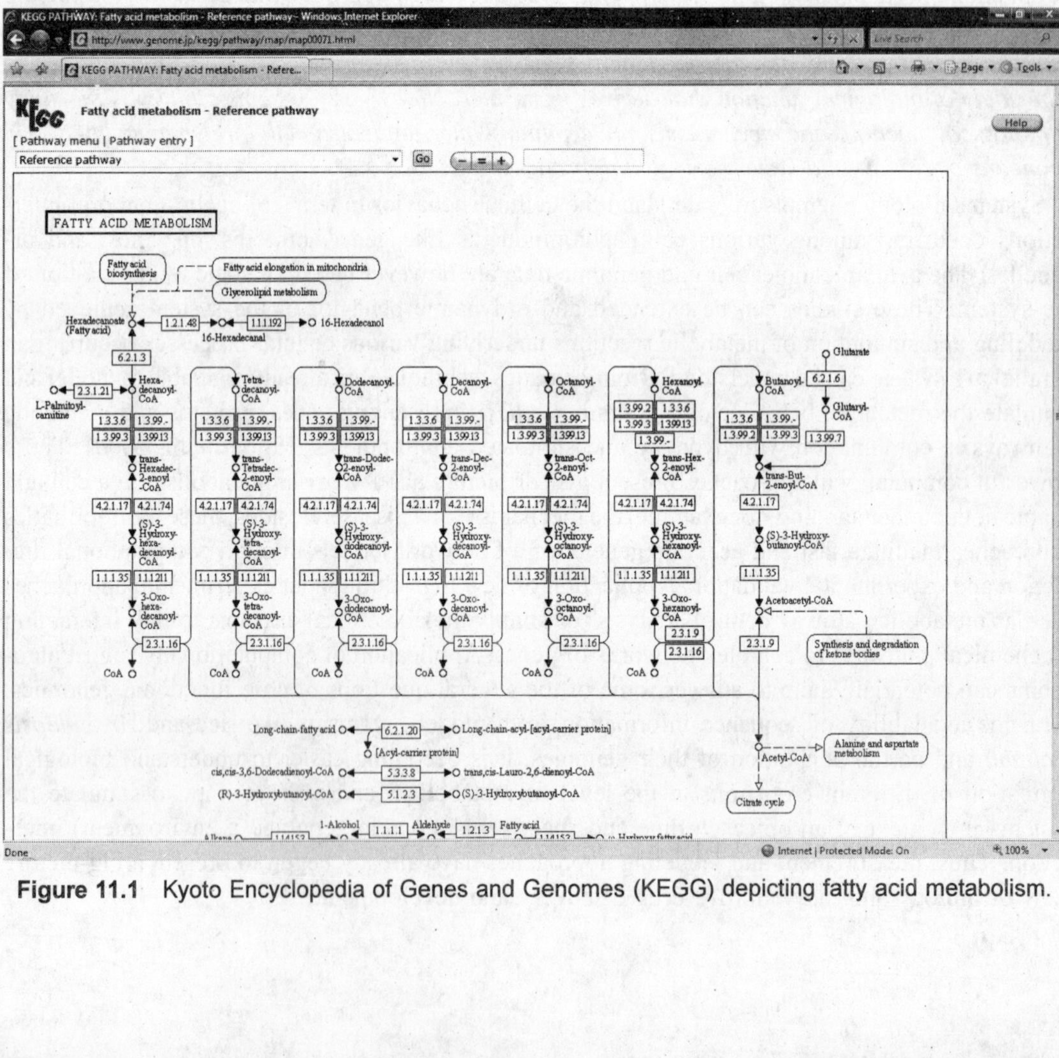

Figure 11.1 Kyoto Encyclopedia of Genes and Genomes (KEGG) depicting fatty acid metabolism.

(v) Metabolomics
(vi) Glycomics
(vii) Lipidomics
(viii) Interactomics
(ix) Mathematical, computational and statistical sciences

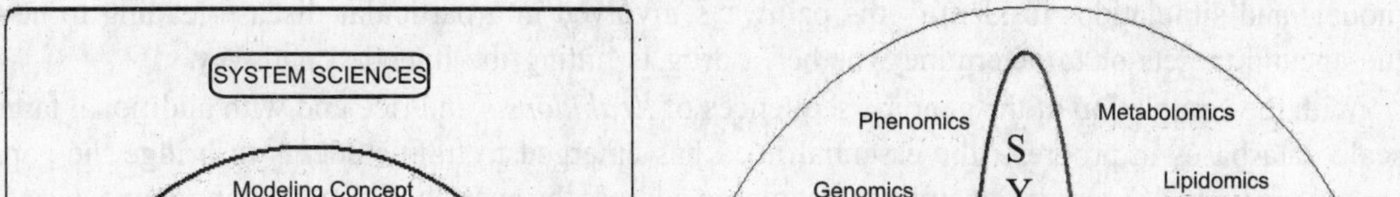

Figure 11.2 The components of systems biology.

Cells respond to environmental changes by reprogramming expression of specific genes throughout the genome. The transcription rate of a particular gene is determined by the interaction of diverse regulatory proteins, transcription activation factor proteins and repressors with specific DNA sequences. How a collection of regulatory proteins (protein-protein interactions) accomplish the task of regulating a set of genes can be described as a regulatory network. Some investigations are beginning to map the regulatory networks that govern gene expression throughout the living cells. For example, a mathematical model of the network of MAP kinase cascade (chiefly forming a network of interacting protein kinases) that transduces regulatory signals from leaf surface to nucleus, where transcription of related resistance genes (R genes) are initiated (Figure 11.2) during pathogenesis of *Alternaria* blight infection in *Brassica juncea*.

Drug discovery approach commonly employed in pharmaceutical industry is similarly reductionist, starting with how potential drug compounds (leads) interact with a drug target tissue in the human body and then moving into *in vitro* models, an approach that is still removed from the ultimate context. Only in clinical trials do potential drugs finally encounter their true context–the patient. Often, it is only at that late point that previously unrecognized effectiveness and toxicity problems become apparent. That's where systems biology comes in. Systems biology tries to bring a big-picture view–context–back to biology and especially drug discovery. Researchers combine data about genes, proteins, and metabolites to generate a comprehensive picture of the connections between the different parts. In the context of drug discovery, the data can be used in computer models and simulations to identify the pathways involved in a particular disease-leading to new therapeutic targets or to determine whether a drug is hitting the intended pathway.

With the completion of the genome sequences of *Arabidopsis* and rice and with additional large scale data bases in progress, the essential need has emerged to train students to bridge the gaps among the widely divergent disciplines in order to address the ever-changing challenges and answer major complex questions in the plant sciences. The enormous quantities of data being generated through genomics, proteomics, protein-protein/DNA interactions and new emerging high through-put technologies represent a new scale and render urgent the need for new systems biology approaches to elucidate the non-linear programs that control plant growth and development.

Genomics and Proteomics

Of late, more has been learnt about various mechanisms underlying the life of plants and this information has enriched our knowledge to better understand the existing gap between the genotype and phenotype. Enormous progress has been achieved from advances in research from genetics, genomics, proteomics and metabolomics. New techniques that build on genomics, such as DNA microarrays (DNA chips) have allowed investigators to identify which genes are turned on or off in a genome in response to an experimental treatment and measure their expression patterns simultaneously. Techniques like microarrays has enabled biologists to measure expression of several genes simultaneously thus paving a way for a paradigm shift in research from one gene/ protein at a time to systems biology. Global study of gene expression has enabled biologists to identify patterns of co-expressed genes/proteins thus enriching our knowledge of mechanisms underlying such complex diseases like diabetes and cancers (for details on this technique, see Chapter 12). The 21st century is otherwise called the "Post-genomic era". By this, it is implied that with the availability of sequence information of major organismal genomes, the next big challenge continues to remain to predict the coded genes and attempt to understand the functions of all gene products.

It is interesting to monitor which genes are being turned on or off during development or in response to a perturbation. Techniques that profile changes in gene expression permit the analysis and identification of patterns of expression levels of thousands of genes simultaneously. In contrast to DNA and RNA, there are currently no techniques available to amplify proteins of low abundance (the equivalent of PCR for DNA) or to identify them with very high-dynamic resolution. Moreover, all of the cells that compose a plant have the same genome, but each cell type has a different collection of proteins. In addition to these cell-to-cell variations in proteomic expression, we must also consider proteomic variation over time. As plant cell matures or responds to an environmental perturbation, its proteome and expressed mRNAs constantly change. Quantitatively measured gene expression data of different organisms is available in databases [such as Serial Expression of Gene

Expression, (SAGE): http://www.ncbi.nlm.nih.gov/SAGE/, Database of The Institute of Genomic Research (TIGR): http://www.tigr.org/tdb/tgi.shtml, UNIGENE: http://www.ncbi.nlm.nih.gov/unigene, dbEST http://www.ncbi.nlm.nih.gov/dbEST/etc.] are excellent transcript databases for accessing genomic resources, expression, map location and other information.

Some popular microarray data analysis and gene expression softwares are:

Expression Profiler (http://www.ebi.ac.uk/microarray-srv/EP/)

GeeSpring (http://www.sigenetics.com/cgi/SiG.cgi/Products/GeneSpring/index.smf)

ArrayMiner (http://www.optimaldesign.com/ArrayMiner/ArrayMiner.htm).

Unlike genome, proteome varies with time and space. There are nearly 30,000 genes in human genome and they can potentially encode 30,000 proteins. However due to alternative splicing and post-translational changes, this number may go up to millions in real terms. Proteomics is acquiring an important role in human health and disease diagnostics, especially in development of protein bio markers and drugs.

It is now widely recognized that proteins generally interact and work together to express a trait rather to act individually. Bioinformatics software tools are available to predict the functional features quantitatively for each protein in a genome. Functionally related proteins interact and form large interaction networks in a cell. Yeast two-hybrid (Y2H) and affinity chromatography, mass spectrometry and 2,D gels are employed for identification protein-protein interactions. Protein-protein interactions can also be predicted computationally using databases like STRING (http://string.embl.de//), DIPTM (http://dip.doe-mbi.ncla.edu/) mitogen activated kinase proteins (MAPKs) are well known mediators in signal transduction connecting perception of the external stimuli to the cellular responses. Molecules that interact among them to form signaling pathways that play a major role in pathogenesis underlying diseases ranging from Alzheimer's disease in humans to fungal diseases in crops.

The activity of many proteins is regulated by interactions with other proteins that form complexes and bring structural modifications. Comprehensive proteomics, therefore, requires not only a list of the protein functions but also a detailed understanding of protein-protein interactions within a cell and protein modifications that regulate function, such as phosphorylation, glycosylation, etc. Methods for the global measurements of various protein modifications, including mass spectrometry and the use of modification-specific antibodies, are only now being developed compared to 2,D Gel separation technique. Protein arrays unlike DNA arrays could not become popular for measuring global expression patterns of proteins. In contrast to genomics in which standardized tools and standards for data storage and sharing are available, the current methodology for handling large proteomics data sets is less uniform and less organized.

Most proteins are also enzymes that catalyze specific chemical reactions. Thus, changes in gene expression are typically accompanied by changes in the levels of many cellular chemicals. The simultaneous measurement of these collective chemical changes is the emerging field of metabolomics. Like proteomic changes, metabolic changes are highly dynamic and require precise high-throughput measurements with enough spatial and temporal resolution to be useful for modeling purposes. As with proteomics, major advances in analytical chemistry are required to allow us to identify and accurately measure thousands of metabolites in a plant. Parallel advances in proteomics and metabolomics are expected to add additional layers of resolution to our ability to integrate all aspects of a biological process. Bioinformatics attempts to store and organize integrated proteomic and metabolomic data in an easy-to-access format are still in their infancy. Thus, there is a real need for software developers and data archivists to establish the tools for creating proteomics and metabolomics databases for use by plant biologists.

Metabolic Pathways

The interdependence of various biochemical processes of metabolism and gene expression can be interpreted and analyzed in terms of complex chemical networks. Metabolic pathways enable easy representation of information of gene regulation and resulting biochemical reactions occurring in cell are stored systematically in databases. A metabolic pathway represents the metabolism of an organism—the biochemical system that synthesizes essential biomolecules such as amino acids, sugars, lipids, vitamins, required energy for the functioning of cells and also secondary and other molecules secreted by cells. Sequencing of genomes of a number of microorganisms, plants and animals including humans has facilitated availability of a few biochemical databases available on world wide web in public domain such as Kyoto Encyclopedia of Genes and Genomes (KEGG: http://www.genome.jp/kegg/; Figure 11.3). It is the most important biochemical pathway database for a comprehensive information relating to reactions, metabolic pathways, enzymes and their coding genes conserved across organisms. For example, KEGG database readily illustrates 9,644 metabolic pathways, 218 reactions and 85 ortholog tables. Other important biochemical databases include-Encyclopedia of *Escherichia coli* K-12 Genes and Metabolism (EcoCyc: http://www.ecocyc.org/), MetaCyc- (http://metacyc.org/). MetaCyc is a database of non-redundant, experimentally elucidated metabolic pathways. MetaCyc contains more than 1,400 pathways from more than 1,800 different organisms. Similarly, RegulonDB is a comprehensive source of transcriptional regulation, operon organization and growth conditions in *Escherichia coli* K-12. BioCyc is another major biochemical database describing about over 450 metabolic pathways and their associated enzymes, from over 150 organisms (http://biocyc.org/). Apart from these, metabolic databases dedicated to all available metabolism of sequenced organisms are also becoming very popular. They include AraCyc (http://www.arabidopsis.org/biocyc/index.jsp) for *Arabidopsis thaliana*, RiceCyc (http://pathway.gramene.org/gramene/ricecyc.shtml). Similarly, HumanCyc-Encyclopedia of *Homo sapiens* genes and metabolism that has contributed enormously in eliciting functions of hundreds of genes underlying mechanisms for important diseases such as cancers. GenPath (http://www.ailab.si/blaz/papers/2001-Medinfo-GenePath.pdf) is a computer-based system that supports the inference of genetic networks from a set of genetic experiments. GenePath implements a framework for reasoning about genetic experiments and hypothesizing genetic networks. Metabolomics approaches enable the parallel assessment of the levels of a broad range of metabolites and have been demonstrated to have great value in phenotyping and diagnostic analyses in agriculture as well as in human health. Analysis of total metabolite profile (so called metabolic flux) is providing means to compare metabolism among various species, in assessment of levels of existing, especially in identification of key enzymes involved in the underlying mechanism of various diseases. This approach is emerging as a promising means of development of biomarkers for early identification of diseases such as cancers. Bioinformatics tools such as Gepasi (www.gepasi.org) and Copasi (www.copasi.org) are wonderful platforms that would enable modeling and simulation of different metabolic reactions occurring in a cell. Metabolomics is fast emerging as an important addition to the tools currently employed in diagnostics, genomics-assisted selection for crop improvement and human health research.

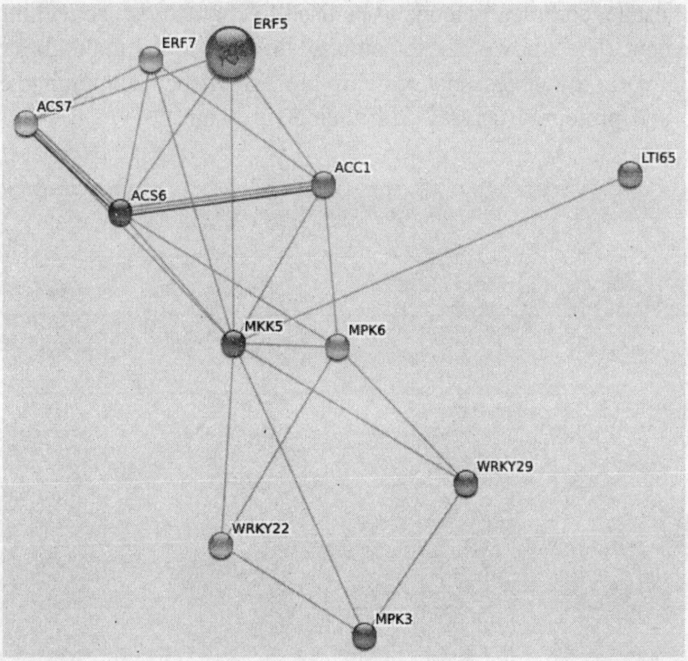

Figure 11.3 MAP kinase 5 interactions with other partner proteins in *Arabidopsis thaliana*. STRING database output.

Gene Networks

Establishing connections among the measured data points and deriving functional linkages from thus formed network of genes and proteins is a stupendous work. The complexity contained in the hub of interacting gene and protein networks can be solved by employing different mathematical algorithms to derive the existing functional links among them. For example Genstruct, a network model that uses human gene expression data collected from a microarray experiment.

Understanding biological networks on a whole-genome scale is a key challenge in modern systems biology. Broad availability of diverse functional genomic data from protein-protein interaction, gene expression, localization, and regulation studies enable fast and accurate generation of network models through computational prediction and experimental validation. Most cellular mechanisms, involve groups of genes or gene products that behave in a coordinated way to perform a specific biological process governed by groups of functionally related genes referred as process-specific networks. Although genomes of several organisms have been sequenced and a wide variety of functional genomic data is available, we are far from exploiting the full potential of these data for discovering such process-function-specific networks. This may be due to lack of accessibility to data and methods and non-availability of suitable bioinformatics tools to analyze them, barriers to incorporating expert knowledge in the network discovery process, and noise and heterogeneity in high-throughput gene data. Integration of data generated from different high-throughput experimental sources with in varied formats is another major challenge faced in data analysis. In general usage, complexity tends to be used to characterize something with many parts in intricate arrangement. The study of these complex linkages is the main goal of network theory based on which networks of genes and proteins are established combining experimental data derived from gene and protein structures with their expression.

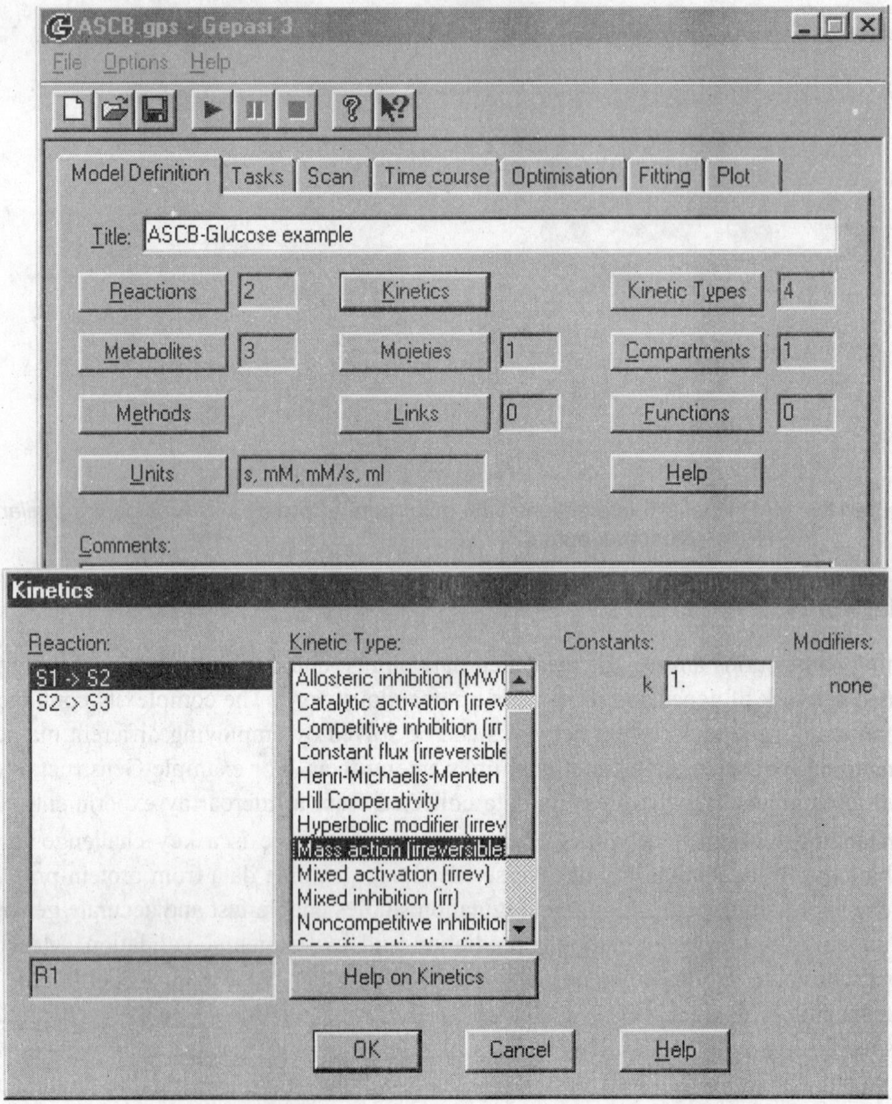

Figure 11.4 Front page view of metabolic pathway modeling software Tool Gepasi.

Gene networks are a group of genes functioning in a coordinated manner to control vital processes in an organism. Each gene network includes several essential components such as groups of genes which form the core of a gene network, proteins encoded by these genes, signal transduction pathways, negative and positive feedback which provide auto-regulation of a system and also low molecular weight compounds. Organization of gene networks is chiefly based on the following principles: 1) there are variety of molecular mechanisms which are responsible for providing feedback regulation of the system, 2) each gene network includes key genes which coordinate the function of other genes in the gene network (Figure 11.4). A single transcription factor can potentially activate many genes via a cassette mechanism and 4) gene networks are auto-regulated via regulatory circuits with positive and negative feed back.

Unlike animals, plants do not have a nervous system but signal communication is achieved by interactions among proteins, genes and other biological molecules facilitated by growth regulators synthesized endogenously. Signaling networks in plants facilitate intake of nutrients, their transport, metabolism, pathogen invasion sensing and defense response. Mitogen activated protein kinases are activated on plant leaf surface upon invasion of external agents such as pathogens and building a cascade of signaling network. The message is transmitted to the transcription zone of corresponding plant disease resistance genes (for example R genes located in the nucleus). Figure 11.5 illustrates the complex network of MAP kinase of protein interaction signaling cascade underlying *Alternaria blight* disease in *Brassica juncea*. The complex organization of gene and protein signaling networks can be represented by employing various bioinformatics algorithms. They permit to describe elementary structure and complex events occurring in pro- and eukaryotic gene networks at different hierarchical levels of organization, i.e. molecular or cellular. GeneNet is a database on structure and functional organization of gene networks (Figure 11.5).

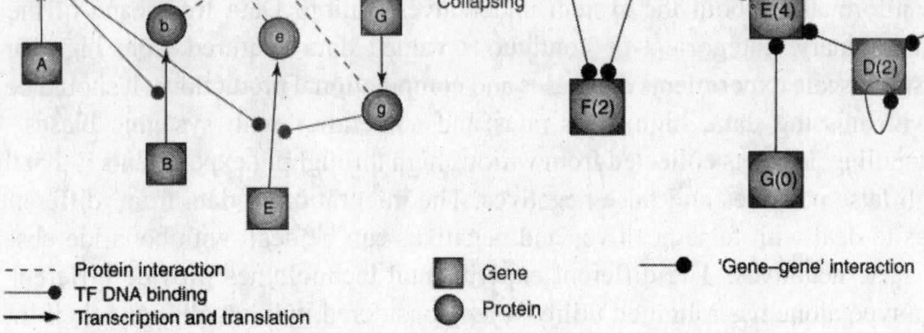

Figure 11.5 A complex network where nodes depict proteins and genes and the ridges represent their interactions (Tegner and Bjorkgren 2008).

Integration of Heterogeneous Experimental Data into Systems Biology

Various computer science based mathematical search algorithms are being actively employed to explore the complex hub of biological networks i.e. in constructing biological networks or protein complexes from integrated data greedy search algorithm applied to a confidence-weighted protein-protein interaction network. The former was specifically targeted towards protein complexes, while the focus on the more general problem of discovering not just physically interacting sets of proteins, but functional or process-specific networks. However recent applications of probabilistic data integration to the related but simpler problem of predicting function of a protein from diverse genomic data have demonstrated that integrated analysis of heterogeneous sources provides a substantial increase in prediction accuracy. Much of the work in function prediction focuses on fusing information from multiple heterogeneous sources for pairs of proteins to make more reliable statements about pair-wise functional relationships. Neural nets have been successfully employed in combination with 2,D gel mass spectrometric analysis in classification of MAP kinases and mapping of protein-protein interaction networks for recognizing and construction of a signaling cascade underlying *Alternaria blight* disease in Brassica juncea. Similarly classification Bayesian networks and variations of this approach have been applied successfully to construct 'functional linkage maps' whose connecting edges represent probabilistic support for a functional relationship between the adjacent proteins. Protein functions are then inferred through 'guilt by association' approach by using Markov Random Field models to propagate known functional annotations through confidence-weighted edges.

There are two major approaches to analyze a system based on measurement of the system and based on computer modeling. Systems biology aims to understand cellular behavior in terms of spatio-temporal interactions occurring among biomolecules such as genes, proteins, metabolites and organelles. As such, a system's behavior is predicted on the integration of measured experimental data collected from various molecular biological, genomic and high-throughput technologies. Integration of the data collected from various experimental sources helps to achieve the important imperatives of systems biology, namely by reduction of dimensionality of acquired global data to yield information about a system's behaviour. Handling data collected from heterogeneous experimental sources poses some serious challenges in analysis and its integration so as to derive a meaningful information about the system under investigation. Data from each of the sources belong to either binary, categorical or continuous valued data acquired from high throughput experiments, small-scale experiments databases and computational predictions. It should be suitable for dealing with missing data, high error rates and sometimes with systemic biases. Another challenge in handling data sets collected from various high throughput experiments is that they have inherently high false positives and false negatives. The integration of data from different experimental sources to deal with false positives and negatives can be dealt with bonafide observations and reducing false negatives. The different experimental technologies provide different insights (and each data type alone has a limited utility when considered individually) and their integration only presents valuable information about a particular cellular process. For example, gene perturbation experiments (e.g. knockouts or RNA interference) reveal relationships between two genes that may imply direct physical interactions or indirect logical interactions.

To address the problems of analysis and integration of data, gathered raw experimental data sets are subjected to normalization and data transformation without allowing the loss of information content (entropy) contained in the data. For integration of heterogeneous data for systems biology, various data integration techniques starting from statistical techniques to computer science protocols are employed. Major statistical techniques widely used are Fisher's X2, Stoffers Z.

Mathematical modeling provides insights into working of different networks regulating a biological system. The temporal dynamics of signaling connecting different molecules are modeled *in silico* to provide a non-intuitive experimental hypothesis regarding the behavior of the regulatory system. *In silico* modeling of signaling networks provides means to organize the known information in a structured manner and analyze it. Combined with experimental data, modeling provides an insight into the intricacies of network behavior and poses us new questions to be answered experimentally. For example, it is now possible more than ever, to visualize a protein of interest and its interactions in the live cells and to study its spatial distribution.

Depending on whether the individual messenger is a genome coded one or not, it has to be eventually activated for stimulating the expression of metabolic enzyme genes for synthesis. Each of these events are subjected to different kind of signal pathways, metabolic pathways and gene regulatory networks. *In silico* analysis provides insights at many levels of working of the signaling networks. Modeling enables to establish quantitative relationships between the variables interacting in the system. As the input and output values of variables in a system can be measured experimentally, the built model enables to estimate quantities of intermediately variables, their interrelationships and even the missing ones. These obtained results can be used to establish a hypothesis which may later be tested experimentally. Also compared to experiments, a model provides the intricacies of a network behavior and may raise new questions which otherwise be verified experimentally in some cases.

Systems Biology Modeling Language (SMBL) is a common, model-based description language for systems biology simulation software. SBML is developed based on defined as a XML markup language. SMBL is often employed in systems biology computational research for access to different databases, analysis and integration of heterogeneous data and its integration in a systems context.

Databases and Resources

As starting point to establish an integrated resource for relevant quantitatively measured experimental data, the following databases/tools have been used.

Proteome Databases and Networking Tools

There is a family of databases aiming at the annotation of complete proteomes of (a) human, mouse and rat (Human Proteome Survey Database; HPSD), (b) G-Protein Coupled Receptor Proteome Database (GPCR PD); (c) *Saccharomyces cerevisisae* (Yeast Proteome Database, YPD) (d) *Schizosaccharomyces pombe* (PombePD), (e) pathological fungi (MycoPathPD), and (f) *Caenorhabditis elegans.*

BIND: A Biomolecular Interaction Network Database (http://bond.unleashedinformatics.com)

BioCyc: BioCyc is a collection of 506 Pathway/Genome Databases. Each database in the BioCyc collection describes the genome and metabolic pathways of a single organism. The two main databases are EcoCyc and MetaCyc databases. EcoCyc is a scientific database for the bacterium *Escherichia coli* K-12 MG1655. MetaCyc describes experimentally elucidated enzymes and metabolic pathways from more than 1800 organisms. MetaCyc does not seek to model the complete metabolic network of any one organism, but to provide a comprehensive collection of experimental pathways. BioCyc contains tools for visualizing and analyzing biochemical data. And also it provides comparative analysis of organisms. These include PathoLogic, Pathway/Genome Editor and Pathway/Genome Navigator. BioCyc can be accessed at www.biocyc.org.

CellDesigner: CellDesigner is a modeling tool of biochemical networks with graphical user interface. The CellDesigner features include-modeling biochemical gene networks, visual representation of biochemical semantics, database connections, direct integration with SMBL ODE Solver and Copasi, etc.

Copasi: COPASI is a software application for simulation and analysis of biochemical networks and their dynamics. COPASI carries out several analyses of the network and its dynamics and has extensive support for parameter estimation and optimization. COPASI provides means to visualize data in customizable plots, histograms and animations of network diagrams. It can be accessed at www.copasi.org.

Cytomer: It is a relational database on organs, tissues, cell types, physiological systems and developmental stages, presently focusing on the human system (www.biobase.de).

Cytoscope: Cytoscope is a project dedicated to building open-source network visualization and analysis software. Cytoscope's roots are in systems biology, where it is used for integrating biomolecular interaction networks with high-throughput expression data and other molecular state information. Although applicable to any system of molecular components and interactions, Cytoscope is most powerful when used in conjunction with large databases of protein-protein, protein-DNA, and genetic interactions that are increasingly available for humans and model organisms. Cytoscope allows the visual integration of the network with expression profiles, phenotypes and other molecular state information, and links the network to databases of functional annotations.

DRTF: A database of rice transcription factors (http://drtf.cbi.pku.edu.cn).

EndoNet is a database on intercellular signaling paths as they are exerted by e.g., hormones to constitute the endocrine network of the human body (http://endonet.bioinf.med.uni-goettingen.de/).

Gepasi: A software tool for metabolic pathway analysis and modeling; http://dbkgroup.org/softw/gepasi.html.

GO: A database containing ontology, gene product, sequence, and manual annotation data; http://www.geneontology.org/GO.downloads.database.shtml.

Gramene: A resource for comparative grass genomics; http://www.gramene.org/about/.

IntAct: IntAct provides a freely available, open source database system and analysis tools for protein interaction data. All interactions are derived from literature curation or direct user submissions and are freely available (http://www.ebi.ac.uk/intact/site/index.jsf).

KEGG: Kyoto Encyclopedia of Genes and Genomes: http://www.genome.jp/kegg/

OMIM: A comprehensive, authoritative, and timely compendium of human genes and genetic phenotypes. The full-text, referenced overviews in OMIM contain information on all known Mendelian disorders and over 12,000 genes. OMIM focuses on the relationship between phenotype and genotype. It is updated daily, and the entries contain copious links to other genetics resources (http://www.ncbi.nlm.nih.gov/omim).

PlanTFDB: A database of integrative plant transcription factor database (http://plntfdb.bio.uni-potsdam.de).

PathoDB is a database on pathologically relevant mutated forms of mammalian transcription factors and their binding sites (http://www.biobase-international.com/index.php?id=pathodb).

PathoSign comprises pathologically relevant mutations of signaling components of mammalian cells (http://pathosign.bioinf.med.uni-goettingen.de/search.jsp?Status=start).

Rice CYC: Oryza *sativa* metabolic pathway database

STRING: A database of known and predicted protein-protein interactions. The interactions include direct (physical) and indirect (functional) associations (http://string.embl.de//).

SYCAMORE: SYCAMORE is a system that provides you with a facilitated access to a number of tools and methods in order to build models of biochemical systems, view, analyze and refine them, as well as perform quick simulations. SYCAMORE is not intended to substitute for expert simulation and modeling software packages, but might interact with those. It is rather intended to support and guide systems biologists when doing computational research. One important function of SYCAMORE is to allow you to build a draft model of your system of interest in such a way that kinetic expressions and parameters are as close to reality as possible. It can be accessed at http://sycamore.eml.org/sycamore/.

TRANSPATH: A database on regulatory network information, mostly in human, mouse and rat cells, originally focusing on signal transduction pathways that aim at gene regulatory molecules (transcription factors), but increasingly expanding to metabolic enzymes and structural proteins as targets (http://www.biobase.de/pages/products/databases.html).

TRANSFAC: A database on transcriptional regulation in eukaryotes, with documentation of transcription factor properties, their genomic and artificial binding sequences, and DNA binding profiles, (http://transfac.gbf.de/srs5/).

Useful Web Resources for Systems Biology Research

The following web resources give more details about systems biology and its current status.

www.systemsbiology.org
www.systems-biology.org

www.sysbio.org/
www.biochemweb.org
www.centerforsystemsbiology.org
www.csbi.mit.edu
www.systembiology.net
www.imsb.ethz.ch/
www.mcisb.org/
www.issb.org/
www.sbi.jp
www.igsb.anl.gov/
www.systemsbiology.fr
www.baliga.systemsbiology.net/
www.ebi.ac.uk/sbo/
www.sbtoolbox.org
www.systemsmicrobiology.org
www.bloodsystemsbiology.org
www.sbcny.org
www.systems-biology.com
www.systemsbiologyireland.org
www.msbf.mpg.de

CONCLUSION

Genome sequences are now available that enable us to determine the biological components that make up a cell or an organism. The new discipline of systems biology examines how these components interact and form networks and how the networks generate whole cell functions corresponding to observable phenotypes.

FURTHER READINGS

1. Bader J.S. (2003) Greedily building protein networks with confidence. *Bioinformatics.* **(19):** 1869-1874.
2. Choi J.K., Kim S.C., Jungmin S. and Sangsoo K. (2004) Cracterization of general transcriptional activity and variability of eukaryotic genes from global expression profiles of human, mouse, rat, fly, plants. www.genetics.org/cgi/content/full/175/1/199.
3. Choi, C., Krull, M., Kel, A., Kel-Margoulis, O., Pistor, S., Potapov, A., Voss, N. and Wingender, E. (2004) TRANSPATH$^{\rangle}$- A high quality database focused on signal transduction. *Comp. Functional Genomics.* **(5):** 163-168.

4. Deng M., Tu Z., Sun F. and Chen T. (2004) Mapping gene ontology to proteins based on protein-protein interaction data. *Bioinformatics.* **(20):** 895-902.
5. Gao G., Zhong Y., Guo A., Zhu Q., Tang W., Zheng W., Gu X., Wei L. and Luo J. (2007) DRTF: a database of rice transcription factors. *Bioinformatics.* **(22):** (10) 1286-1287.
6. Hedges and Olkin I. (1985) Statistical Methods for Meta-analysis Academic Press, Orlando.
7. Jaimovich E., Reyes R., Liberona J.L., Powell J.A. (2000) IP3 receptors, IP3transients, and nucleus-associated Ca2+ signals in cultured skeletal muscle. *American Journal of Physiology - Cell Physiology.* **(278):** C998-C1010.
8. Jansen R., Yu H., Greenbaum D., Kluger Y., Nevan J. Chung S, Emili A, Snyder M,. Greenblatt J.F. and Gerstein M. (2003) A Bayesian networks approach for predicting protein-protein interactions from Genomic Data. *Science.* **(302):** (5644) 449-453.
9. Karaoz U., Murali T.M., Letovsky S., Zheng Y., Ding C., Cantor C.R., Kasif S. (2004) Whole-genome annotation by using evidence integration in functional-linkage networks. *Proceedings National Academy Science USA.* **(101):** 2888-2893.
10. Kenakin, T. (2004) *A Pharmacology Primer: Theory, Application, and Methods,* 1st edn, Elsevier Academic Press, Amsterdam.
11. Kolchanov N.A., Podkolodnaya O.A., Ananko E.A., Ignatieva E. V., Stepanenko I.L.,. Kel-Margoulis O.V., Kel A.E., Merkulova T., Goryachkovskaya T.N., Busygina T.V., Kolpakov F.A., Podkolodny N.L., Naumochkin A.N., Korostishevskaya I.M., Romashchenko A.G. and Overton G.C. (2000) Transcription Regulatory regions database (TRRD): its status in (2000) *Nucleic Acids Research.* 28 **(1):** 298-301.
12. Krull, M., Voss, N., Choi, C., Pistor, S., Potapov, A. and Wingender, E. (2003) TRANSPATH®: an integrated database on signal transduction and a tool for array analysis. *Nucleic Acids Research.* **(31):** 97-100.
13. Lee I, Shailesh V. Date, Alex T. Adai and Edward M. Marcotte. (2004) A probabilistic functional network of yeast genes. *Science.* 306 **(5701):** 1555-1558.
14. Letovsky S, and Kasif S. (2003) Predicting protein function from protein/protein interaction data: a probabilistic approach. *Bioinformatics.* **(19):** (Suppl 1): i197–i204.
15. Marla S.S., Singh V. K., Kumar N., Singhal S., Khan G.T. and Pandey D. (2009) Application of neural networks for classification of *Arabidopsis thaliana* MAP Kinase proteins involved in Alternaria blight disease, AAIDU, Allahabad.
16. Matys V., Fricke E., Geffers R., Gößling E., Haubrock M., Hehl R., Hornischer K., Karas D., Kel A. E., Kel-Margoulis O. V., Kloos D.-U., Land S., Lewicki-Potapov B., Michael H., Münch R., Reuter I., Rotert S., Saxel H., Scheer M., Thiele S. and Wingender E.. TRANSFAC⟩: Transcriptional regulation, from patterns to profiles. *Nucleic Acids Research.* 31, **(1):** 374-378.
17. Meinhardt, T. Prüß, M. Wingender E. (1999) PathoDB - A database that combines pathological data with molecular information Conference: *German Conference on Bioinformatics - GCB.* 212-213,
18. Michael H., Chen X., Fricke E., Haubrock M., Ricanek R. and Wingender E. (2004) Deriving an ontology for human gene expression sources from the CYTOMER® database on human organs and cell types. *In Silico Biology.* **(5):** 0007.
19. Myers, D. Robson, A. Wible, M. A. Hibbs, C. Chiriac, C. L. Theesfeld, K. Dolinski and G.T. Olga (2005) Discovery of biological networks from diverse functional genomic data. *Genome Biol.* **(6):** R114doi:10.1186/gb-2005-6-13-r114.
20. Potapov, A., Liebich I, Dönitz J., Schwarzer K., Sasse N., Schoeps T., Crass T. and Wingender E. (2006) EndoNet: An information resource about endocrine networks. *Nucleic Acids Research.* 34 **(1):** D540-D545.
21. Riaño-Pachón D.M., Ruzicic S., Dreyer I., Mueller-Roeber B. (2007) PlnTFDB: An integrative plant transcription factor database. *BMC Bioinformatics.* **(8):** 42.
22. Schacherer, F., Choi, C., Götze, U., Krull, M., Pistor, S. and Wingender, E. (2001) The TRANSPATH signal transduction database: a knowledge base on signal transduction networks. *Bioinformatics.* **(17):** 1053-1057.

23. Von Mering C., Huynen M., Jaeggi D., Schmidt S., Bork P., Snel B. (2003) STRING: a database of predicted functional associations between proteins *Nucleic Acids Research.* **(1):** 31(1): 258-61.
24. Von Mering C., Krause R., Snel B., Cornell M., Oliver S.G., Fields S., Bork P. (2002) Comparative assessment of large-scale data sets of protein-protein interactions. *Nature*. **(23):** 417(6887): 399-403.
25. Wildrmuth M.C. (2000) Metabolic Control Analysis : Biological applications and Insughs. *Genome Biol.* **(1):** 1031-35.
26. Wingender E., Crass T., Hogan J.D., Kel A. E., Kel-Margoulis O.V. and Potapov A.P. (2006) Integrative content-driven concepts for bioinformatics, "beyond the cell". J. Biosci. **(32):** 169-180.

CHAPTER 12

Microarray Technology

Microarray analysis has emerged in the last few years as a flexible method for analyzing large numbers of nucleic acid fragments in parallel. Its origins can be traced to several different disciplines and techniques. Microarrays can be seen as a continued development of molecular biology hybridization methods, as an extension of the use of fluorescence microscopy in cell biology, as well as a diagnostic assay using capture to solid surface as a way to reduce the amount of analytes needed. The convergence of ideas and principles utilized in these fields, together with technological advancements in preparing miniaturized collections of nucleic acids on solid supports, have all contributed to the emergence of microarray and microchip technologies. This technology promises to monitor the whole genome on a single chip so that researchers can have a better picture of the interactions among thousands of genes simultaneously.

Keywords: Microarrays, differential gene expression, reverse northern, hybridization, oligonucleotide arrays, cDNA arrays.

INTRODUCTION

Gene expression is a highly complex and tightly regulated process allowing a cell to respond dynamically both to environmental stimuli and to its own changing needs. Each cell of an organism usually contains the same set of genes, however there are significant differences in their activation and control. Only a fraction of these genes are expressed in the form of proteins at a particular time and confer unique properties to each cell type. The expression of a single gene can be detected by Northern hybridization where the total RNA of different samples are blotted on a nylon membrane and the expression of a gene of interest is detected by using probes of that particular gene of interest. Single gene expression can also be detected by dot blot technique where the total RNA of different samples (up to 96 samples) are immobilized on nylon membrane and expression of a particular gene in all the samples detected by probe of that particular gene of interest. In the post-genome sequencing era, a large number of gene sequences are known for different organisms, hence there is a need to understand the change that occurring at transcriptome level, i.e., change in the overall transcripts in a cell with respect to time or under different stress conditions. However, the study of transcriptome needs a suitable experimental design and high-throughput instruments. Many techniques are available for the study of transcriptome such as Reverse Northern Blotting (RNB), Serial Analysis of Gene Expression (SAGE), *subtractive hybridization* (SH) or microarray. In this chapter, we have focused on the principles and procedures of microarray.

DNA microarray is defined as an orderly arrangement of DNA fragments representing the genes of an organism and requires specialized robotics and imaging equipment. It is also known as DNA chip, biochip and gene array where thousands of different known genes are spotted on a suitable support and the spot sizes are typically less than 200 microns in diameter. This technique was originally designed to measure gene expression levels, but now it has revolutionized functional genomic analysis. The chronological order of microarray development is summarized in Table 12.1.

Table 12.1 Chronological order of microarray development.

Year	*Brief description of the activity*
1953	Watson and Crick described DNA double helix and their denaturation
1961	Marmur and Doty described DNA renaturation or molecular hybridization
1965	Gillespie and Spiegelman measured the interaction between an RNA molecule and the DNA from which it was transcribed
1966	Khorana and coworkers demonstrated synthesis of complex nucleic acids.
1969	Jones and Robertson discovered *in situ* hybridization
1971	Kleppe provided the primers needed for the polymerase chain reaction (PCR) Engvall and Perlman developed ELISA
1975	Grunstein and Hogness described colony hybridization
1977	Benton and Davis described plaque hybridization
1979	Kafatos introduced dot blot
	Wallace introduced synthetic oligonucleotides as hybridization probes
1987	Wan, Fortuna and Furmanski described tissue microarray technique
1990	Ink-jet spotting methods for *in situ* synthesis of 60-mer oligo spots on glass slides
1991	Photolithographic printing (Affymetrix) developed by Fodor and colleagues
1992	Ward and coworkers introduced multicolor fluorescent labeling techniques in FISH
1992	Kallioniemi and coworkers termed comparative genomic hybridisation (CGH)
1994	First cDNA collections were developed at Stanford University (this was first step toward microarrays)
	Hoheisel and coworkers used multiple libraries for genome analysis
	Hoheisel and coworkers replaced manual procedures by robotics
1995	Quantitative cDNA microarray
1996	Commercialization of oligonucleotide arrays (GeneChip^{Tm} by Affymetrix)
1997	Genome-wide expression analysis in *S. cerevisiae* (yeast)
1998	Kononen and coworkers developed tissue microarray technology
1999	Bulyk and coworkers described DNA–protein interactions in a microarray format
	Mendoza and coworkers developed high-throughput microarray-based ELISA.
2000	Cancer signatures detected
	Ciphergen Biosystems Inc. established protein chip array technology
	de Wildt and coworkers first used antibody arrays to study antibody-antigen interactions
	Afanassiev and coworkers describe protein microarrays on glass slides coated with an agarose film
2001	Zhu and coworkers first used protein microarray to study protein-protein interactions in yeast
2003	Clinical application of microarray
	Rubina and coworkers describe protein microarrays on glass slides coated with polyacrylamide
	Ge developed a universal protein array system (UPA) for quantitative detection of interactions of protein with protein, DNA, RNA and ligand.

Contd.

	Rauch and coworkers redefined CGH as molecular karyotyping
	Angenendt and coworkers developed Multiple Spotting Technology (MIST)
2004	Whole human genome analysis by single microarray
	Kersten and coworkers describe protein microarrays on glass slides coated with nitrocellulose

There are different types of microarrays comprising different types of molecules such as oligonucleotides, cDNAs, clones, PCR products, polypeptides, antibodies and others or tissue sections immobilized at discrete ordered micrometer-to-millimeter-sized locations on the surface of a porous or nonporous insoluble solid support. A microarray works by exploiting the ability of a given mRNA molecule to hybridize specifically to the DNA template from which it originated. For global analysis of gene expression, i.e., for transcriptome analysis, high density microarrays have been developed. Newly annotated genes and novel genes can be analyzed by DNA microarray analysis. A specific location is assigned to each DNA fragment representing a gene on the array. The supports are usually glass microscope slides, silicon chips or nylon membranes. Over 30,000 spots can be placed on one slide through the use of robotic spotters. The spots themselves can be DNA, cDNA, or oligonucleotides. The DNA can be printed or synthesized directly onto the support. Fluorescently labeled DNA or RNA in the sample act as "target", which will hybridize to the complementary spots (probes) on the array. After this, these fluorescent tags are excited by laser of wavelengths 635 nm (for Cy5), 532 nm (for Cy3). Hybridized DNA are identified as glowing spots on the array by exposing the microarray to a scanner, while the spots that do not hybridize will not be visible under the scanner. The microscope and camera work together to create a digital image of the array. The computer program then creates a table that contains the ratios of the intensity of red-to-green fluorescence for every spot on the array (Figure 12.1). In the following text, we describe the basic steps of the making of microarray and the process of hybridization.

CONCEPTS AND PRINCIPLES

Despite the variety of technical solutions that have been developed for performing microarray analysis, all are miniaturized hybridization assays for studying thousands of nucleic acid fragments simultaneously. All microarray systems share the following key components:

- the array, which contains immobilized nucleic acid sequences, or 'targets'.
- one or more labelled samples or 'probes' that are hybridized with the microarray.
- a detection system that quantitates the hybridization signal.

BASIC STEPS IN MICROARRAY TECHNOLOGY

Printing of Microarray

Probe samples are spotted (or printed) on a microscopic glass slide (coated with polylysine) with the help of a microarrayer (or spotter). The polylysine coating is done to enhance binding of DNA/RNA to the plate through electrostatic interactions. Polylysine, which is not fixed to DNA, is blocked in order to avoid target binding. Besides glass slides, specially coated plastic films can also be used as solid support. The spotting process is performed inside a dust- and vibration-free chamber. Evaporation of the samples is further avoided by maintaining high humidity in the

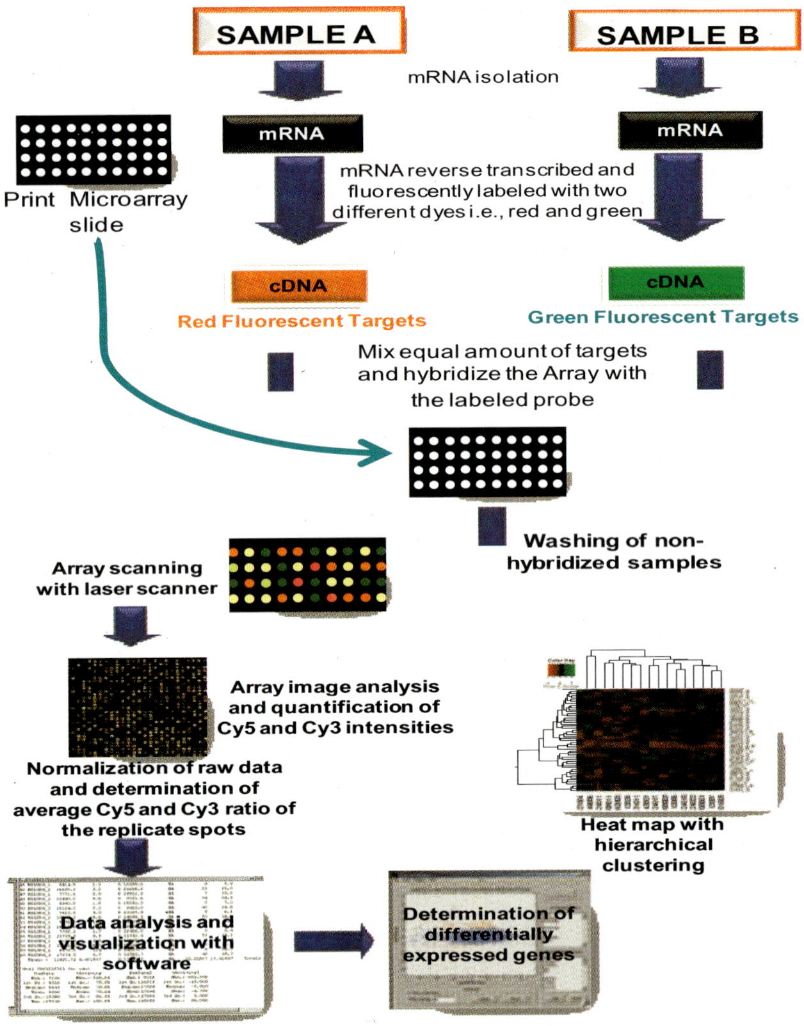

Figure 12.1 Basic steps of microarray Technology: Probes are amplified by PCR and printed on solid support. Total RNA samples extracted from treated and control cells/tissues (Sample A and B) are reverse transcribed and labelled with either Cy3 (green) or Cy5 (red) fluorescent dyes. The samples are combined and hybridised to the microarray. After that washing was done to remove non-hybridized target, laser scanning is carried out and the emissions measured in each colour channel. Specialised software is used to measure intensity ratios to each spot, which are then exported for statistical analysis to identify differentially expressed genes.

chamber. After printing, slides are left at room temperature for 24 h for efficient coupling of printed cDNA. Finally, dried slides are put in a beaker for washing with ethanol followed by air-drying, and stored at room temperature till further use. Prior to hybridization, DNA is denatured to obtain a single strand DNA.

Slide preparation

Microarray slide preparation requires a suitable support so that the probes can be immobilized efficiently. Fabrication is the process of spotting the probes on a suitable support. The support on which the probes have to be spotted should be impermeable to solvent to avoid swelling and shrinking during the experiment. Nitrocellulose membrane provides an excellent support for this purpose as the pores of the membrane provide a larger total surface for binding.

However, reducing the size of spots beyond certain limits or controlling their size and shape on a porous membrane is not possible. Thus, glass or plastic supports are preferred over membrane support because first, these supports have dimensional stability and rigidity, whereas membranes swell in solvent and tend to shrink and distort when dried. Secondly, nucleic acids form a monolayer saturating the surface on glass or plastic and hence the amount of attached DNA is consistent from one region of the array to another. Thirdly, as they are in a monolayer on the surface, the nucleic acids are favorably placed to take part in hybridization reactions. Fourthly, interactions with the solution phase are much faster, because molecules do not have to diffuse into and out of the pores. It has been estimated that the amount of material deposited on the surface of the substrate forming monolayer is equivalent to 10 pmol/mm^2. Therefore, currently, over 50,000 cDNA probes can be spotted onto a 25 × 75 mm slide by robotic printing. Thus, the choice of support is extremely critical determining the success of an experiment.

In this regard, either the presynthesized probes can be spotted or can also be synthesized *in situ* on solid support by high throughput technology, which is described in the following text:

- **Presynthesized Probes:** In this case, the presynthesized probes are covalently crosslinked to the glass slides containing poly-L-lysine using ultraviolet irradiation. The method of application of probes onto the glass slide is a precisely computer-controlled process where a head carrying a pin or pen device is used to pick up small drops of solution containing presynthesized probes from the multiwell plates followed by spotting them on to the surface of glass slide.
- ***In Situ* Synthesis of Probes:** Here, the different probes are directly synthesized on the slide by the process of coupling of nucleotides, which, in turn, is a multistep process. Probes can be synthesized either by using ink-jet fabrication, or flow channels or by light directed fabrication.

  (a) **Fabrication by Ink-Jet Printers:** This technique is based on the principle of ink-jet printers, where the firing solutions of nucleotide reagents are spotted onto the glass surface according to the information of probe sequences feeded in the computer. Computer software is used for moving the pens and substrate as well as for printing four colors for delivering precursors for four different bases. Thus, any set of oligonucleotides can be made and known sequences can thus be placed at any position in the array.

  (b) **Flow Channels and Cells:** In this process, the precursors for the four bases, A, C, G, T are introduced through channels to make 4 broad stripes of the mononucleotides on a square plate. A second set of four nucleotides are laid down in four narrower stripes within each of the monomers to create 16 stripes of dinucleotides. This process is repeated until the oligonucleotides have reached half of probes final length. At this point, the plate is turned 90° and the whole process is repeated. This method is particularly used for making arrays either to those comprising all oligonucleotides of a given length or those comprising all the complements of a target of known sequence. The dimensions of such arrays are determined by the width of the stripes.

(c) **Fabrication by Photolithography:** In this technique of fabrication, the oligonucleotides are synthesized at specific positions on a glass surface by irradiation. Irradiation of glass surface is done by using light of wavelength 365nm. For the addition of bases, photolithographic masks are used for specifically synthesizing probes on a very small area of glass surface. Light is passed through the mask where nucleotide has to be added. When the light is passed through a specific areas on mask, the protecting group on the 5' hydroxyl group of the previously added nucleotide gets activated. The surface is then flooded with the coupling agent for the next base and the process continues till the desired length of the probe is synthesized. This method has the advantage that any sequence can be synthesized at any position in a random fashion within a small area.

Target preparation

Target is a sample for which the transcriptome analysis has to be performed. For the microarray experiment, target sample has to be labeled with fluorescent dyes. mRNA of target sample is reverse transcribed using reverse transcriptase and dNTP mixture containing amino-allyl dCTP into cDNA. Amino-allyl nucleotide is very reactive for coupling with fluorescent dye, cyanine (Cy). Labeling is performed with two dyes Cy3 (green dye) and Cy5 (red dye). One sample is labeled with Cy3, whereas the other sample is labeled with Cy5 for the identification of differentially expressed genes.

Hybridization

Both green and red labelled cDNA (targets) are mixed together and put on the matrix of spotted single strand DNA (probes). The chip is then incubated overnight for hybridization at 60°C under highly humid conditions. At this temperature, DNA strands encounter the complementary strands of the probes on the slide and create double stranded DNA i.e., fluorescent DNA hybridize on the spotted ones. Double stranded DNA thus formed has one unlabelled and other labeled strand. To obtain high quality data, effective hybridization of target is essential. Commercially available cover slips with raised Teflon edging for full contact with arrayed probes (Lifter Slips; Erie Scientific, Portsmouth, NH, USA), hybridization chambers for submerging microarray in water of set temperature (Corning, NY, USA), hybridization solution (Clontech, Palo Alto, CA, USA) etc. are used for effective hybridization. The hybridization rate is increased if the hybridization solution is in motion over the surface of the array i.e., placing the array in a rotating cylinder.

Slide scanning

After hybridization and washing, microarrays are scanned at two different wavelengths corresponding to the absorbance of red and green dye. The signals are analyzed by passing a beam of laser through the microarray slide that excites each spot on the plate and the fluorescent emissions are gathered through a photo-multiplicator tube (PMT) coupled with a confocal microscope. The spot will appear either red or green if the hybridization is stronger with one of the samples. In contrast, the spot on the microarray will appear to be yellow if the intensities of binding of two dyes to target samples are equal. Microscopic detection and quantification of fluorescence images provide the basic array data, but variance is increased by background fluorescence, dust, and spot-to-spot and array-to-array differences in signal intensity. Due to this, complex normalization and correction routines must be applied to the resulting data.

Data analysis

Now there are two images from the same slide corresponding to the two dyes from which we have to calculate the number of DNA molecules in each experimental condition. For any spot on the slide, we measure the signal intensities in the green dye emission wavelength and the red dye emission wavelength. If the mRNA amount used for hybridization is proportional to the amount of fluorescent DNA fixed onto the plate, one can directly calculate the red/green fluorescence ratio. Ratio greater than 1 (red on the image) shows that the gene expression is greater in the sample 2, while ratio smaller than 1 (green on the image) indicates that gene expression is greater in sample 1. These differences in expression can be visualized and interpret using commercially available software (for example, array plot). The signals intensities of the spots are correlated with the concentrations of target mRNA samples. Data mining is conducted by using statistical programs and algorithms to determine whether the gene of interest is up-regulated, down-regulated, or unchanged. Data is then organized using a database and gene annotation can be performed with gene ontology (GO) analysis, clustering analysis and pathways analysis and networking of genes can also be predicted.

To adjust the data for systemic non-biological effects arising from technical variation(s) and measurement, error normalization is essential. The aim is to remove the effect of noise from the data while still maintaining the ability to detect significantly differentially expressed genes. Still, there is no universally accepted method of normalization, but the intensity dependent normalization i.e., local weighted regression is accepted most.

Expression profile clustering

Clustering of expression profiles obtained through arrays can be done at the end of microarray analysis. Genes sharing same expression profile gradually form clusters during phylogenetic analysis. Other complex techniques such as principal component analysis or neuronal networks are also now being used for this purpose. Microarray data is visually presented in a two-dimensional table or "heat-map," each cell of which uses a simple color code to represent the relative transcript expression of a single gene under each of a defined set of experimental conditions. The vertical axis identifies each gene in the collection, whereas the horizontal axis displays each condition or time-point in a time series analysis. Final data is presented in the form of hierarchical clustering, where each column represents the microarray data from one experiment and each row a specific gene. Rigorous experimental design and statistical analysis, together with adequate replication, is critical to draw broad conclusions about the biology of a system based on microarray data. Mostly microarray experiments are designed with only one categorical factor, so paired t-test is used for statistical analysis, but for multiple categorical factors (time and genotype) we require analysis of variance (ANOVA) based methods. B-statistic is an estimate of the odds that the gene is differentially expressed. Commercially available software packages for normalization, statistical analysis and visualization are Cyber-T, SAM, BRB-Array Tools (http://linus.nci.nih.gov/BRB-ArrayTools), QVALUE, Focus, statistical language R, etc.

Microarray data management

As a single chip may contain 30,000 spots of target DNA, there is necessity of uniform system that manages and provides a disbursement point for microarray data. As the proficiency in generating data is overcoming the capacity for storing and analyzing, this data requires standardization of storage and sharing. For public use and dissemination of gene expression data, NCBI has launched the Gene Expression Omnibus (GEO). It has an expression data repository and online resources for the storage and retrieval of gene expression data from any organism or artificial source. GEO will aid in the study of functional genomics by storing vast amounts of data on gene expression profiles derived from multiple experiments using varied criteria and conditions. GEO facilitates cross-validation of data obtained using different techniques and technologies and helps to set standards for further gene expression studies.

Microarray Markup Language (MAML) is developed by Microarray Gene Expression Database (MGED) and is the first attempt to provide a standard platform for submitting and analyzing the enormous amounts of microarray expression data generated around the world. The goal is to facilitate the adoption of standards for DNA-array experiment annotation and data representation, as well as the introduction of standard experimental controls and data normalization methods and also to facilitate the establishment of gene expression data repositories, the comparability of gene expression data from different sources, and data analysis software. MAML is independent experimental platform and provides a framework for describing experiments done on all types of DNA arrays. MAML provides a format that allows analysis of data obtained not only from any existing microarray platforms but also many of the possible future variants, including protein arrays. Additional data set from different experiments available in the Barley Base repository for cereal Gene Chip data (http://barleybase.org/), ArrayExpress (http://www.ebi.ac.uk/arrayexpress/) and Microarray Gene Expression Data Society (http://www.mged.org/) provides an invaluable resource for the scientific community. Different website links related to gene sequences, different techniques, various companies, laboratories and bioinformatics tools are given in Table 12.2.

Table 12.2 List of some representative websites related to microarray.

Types	*Websites*
Gene Sequences	
Cancer Genome Anatomy Project (CGAP)	ncbi.nlm.nih.gov/CGAP
CGAP EST database	ncbi.nlm.nih.gov/dbEST/index.html
Ensemble resources	Ensembl.org
ESTs identified by the Institute of Genomic Research (TIGR)	tigr.org
IMAGE consortium	bio.llnl.gov/bbrp/image/image.html
Incyte	incyte.com
Purchasing UniGene clones	image.llnl.gov/image/htmlidistributors.shtml
Research Genetics	http://www.resgen.com/index.php3
UniGene resources	ncbi.nlm.nih.gov/UniGene

Contd.

Microarray laboratories	
Albert Einstein College of Medicine	sequence:aecom.yu.edu/bioinf/funcgenomic.html
Ed Southern	bioch.ox.ac.uk/rgroups/rgroupslist.asp
Institute of Cancer Research	wyvis.icr.ac.uk
National Human Genome Research Institute (NHGRI)	nhgri.nih.gov/DIR/LCG/15K/HTML
Pat Brown laboratory	cmgm.stanford.edu/pbrown/index.html
Vivian Cheung Laboratory	w95vcl.neuro.chop.edu/vcheung
Company links	
Affymetrix	affymetrix.com
BD Biosciences	bdbiosciences.com
BioRobotics	biorobotics.co.uk
Chroma	chroma.mbt.washington.edu
Ciphergen Biosystems Inc	ciphergen.com
Genometrix	genometrix.com
General Scanning	genescan.com
Gene Logic	genelogic,.com
Hyseq	hyseq.com
Incyte	incyte.com
Luminex® Corporation	luminexcorp.com
Molecular Dynamics	mdyn.com
Molecular Staging, Inc.	molecularstaging.com
Protometrix, Inc.	protometrix.com
Pierce Biotechnology Inc.	searchlightonline.com
RayBiotech Inc.	raybiotech.com
Schleicher & Schuell Bioscience	schleicher-schuell.de/bioscience
SIGMA-ALDRICH Co.	sigmaaldrich.com
Zeptosens AG	zeptosens.com
Zyomyx Inc.	zyomyx.com
Bioinformatics	
ArrayExpress	ebi.ac.uk/arrayexpress
ArrayTrack (NCTR's Center for Toxicoinformatics Array Track)	fda.gov/nctr/science/centers/toxicoinformatics/ArrayTrack
CEBS (Chemical Effects in Biological Systems)	cebs.niehs.nih.gov
CIBEX (Center for Information Biology)	cibex.nig.ac.jp
GEO (Gene Expression Omnibus)	ncbi.nlm.nih.gov/geo
NHGRI Tissue Microarray Project	nhgri.nih.gov/DIR/CGB/TMA
Stanford Link Page	Genomewww4.Stanford.EDU/MicroArray/SMD/restech.html
Tox-MIAMExpress (Toxicogenomics MIAMExpress)	ebi.ac.uk/tox-miamexpress
UCLA Tissue Array Core Facility	genetic.ucla.edu/tissuearray
Whitehead Institute	http://www.wi.mit.edu/nap/features/nap_feature_sabatiniappt.html
Techniques	
BioArray Software Environment – BASE	*base.thep.lu.se*
Bio-IT World	bio-itworld.com
ESF Programme on Integrated Approaches for Functional Genomics	functionalgenomics.org.uk/sections/resources/protein_arrays.htm
Genomics Proteomics	genomicsproteomics.com
Glycominds	http://www.glycominds.com

Contd.

GlycoSuite DB	glycosuite.com
Lab-on-a-chip	lab-on-a-chip.com
NIGMS Consortium for Functional Glycomics	web.mit.edu/glycomics/consortium
Oxford Glycobiology Institute list of publications	bioch.ox.ac.uk/glycob/publications.html
Pharmocogenomics Online	pharmacogenomicsonline.com
The Brown Lab, Stanford University	cmgm.stanford.edu/pbrown
University of New Hampshire Centre for Structural Biology	glycomics.unh.edu

Types of Microarray

Main types of microarrays available commercially are oligonucleotide arrays (GeneChip^{TM} by Affymetrix) and cDNA arrays (BD Biosciences). Other types of microarray are antibody array, protein chip array and tissue array. The following text provides a brief description of these arrays.

Oligonucleotide arrays

In oligonucleotide array (or DNA chip), small oligonucleotide (20~80-mer oligos) or peptide nucleic acid (PNA) probes are synthesized either *in situ* (on-chip) or by conventional synthesis followed by on-chip immobilization (http://www.affymetrix.com). Total 11 to 16 copies of a DNA are spotted for each gene on the array. These DNA fragments have little cross-reactivity with other genes for minimal non-specific hybridization. Still to combat any non-specific hybridization, a second probe identical to the first except for a mismatched base at its centre is placed next to the first. This is termed Perfect Match/Mismatch (PM/MM) probe strategy. To obtain perfect hybridization, any background hybridization with the MM probe is subtracted from the PM probe signal.

Combination of photolithography and combinatorial chemistry is used for the synthesis of diverse sequences of probes. Oligonucleotide array allows the simultaneous generation of thousands of probes relatively quickly on the chip surface of 5-inch square of quartz wafer, which is an ideal substance for adherence of chemicals. This wafer is then washed with a blocking compound, which is then removed by exposure to light. A mask designed with 18-20 micron square windows is laid on top of array and allows ultraviolet light to pass through areas where a specific nucleotide is needed. Exposure of light removes the blocking compound from the probe. The wafer is then washed with a solution of the desired nucleotide that is linked to the same blocking compound and nucleotide attaches to the probes that were exposed to light, while the nucleotide attached with blocking compound ensures that all the probes are protected again. A capping step is added so that probes that did not attach their appropriate nucleotide are not incorrectly synthesized. The process is repeated until all the probes are complete.

In CGH (comparative genomic hybridization), genomic DNA from the patient is labeled with one fluorescent dye while a normal reference sample is labeled with a different dye, and these samples are co-hybridized to the array containing the genomic DNA targets. Chromosomal imbalances across the genome can thus be quantified and positionally defined by analyzing the ratio of the fluorescence of the two dyes along the targets. The availability of clone sets covering the human genome opens the possibility for the widespread use of array CGH for both research and diagnostic purpose. Microarray-based genomic copy-number analysis is now a commonly ordered clinical genetic test for patients and is defined under various names, i.e., “chromosomal microarray” (CMA) and “molecular karyotyping”. CMA, is used for readily available and easy to handle oligonucleotide arrays originally designed for parallel genomewide analysis of over 10000 SNPs.

cDNA Arrays

The principle of this array is same as oligo arrays, but the probes in this case are larger pieces of DNA that are complementary to the genes. PCR using specific primers can be used to amplify specific genes from cDNA to generate the cDNA probes (500~5,000 bases long). A separate PCR reaction must be performed for each gene. cDNA probes can be mechanically spotted onto a glass slide. By using this technology one can display 409,000 spots in an area of 1.28 cm^2. Hence, all 20,000-25,000 genes of Arabidopsis can be displayed on a single slide. Microarray technique is highly sensitive as it can detect mRNAs at level of 1/100,000 or 1/500,000.

There are few distinctions between oligonucleotide and cDNA arrays. First, cDNA arrays eliminate the need for the probe design required for oligonucleotide arrays, while also allowing the entire genome of an organism to be represented on the array easily, making cDNA arrays more useful for the analysis of gene expression on a global level. Oligonucleotide arrays have advantage for their greater hybridization specificity due to PM/MM probe design, resulting in more specific fluorescence detection.

Protein microarray

It is based on the principle of ligand-binding assay that relies on the formation of product with an immobilized capture molecule (target) present in the solution. Protein microarrays are now becoming very popular due to their use in the study of antibody-protein, enzyme-protein, DNA-protein and protein-protein interactions (Figure 12.2). For analysis of protein interactions with other molecules, protein microarrays have various types of molecules immobilized on the slide surface

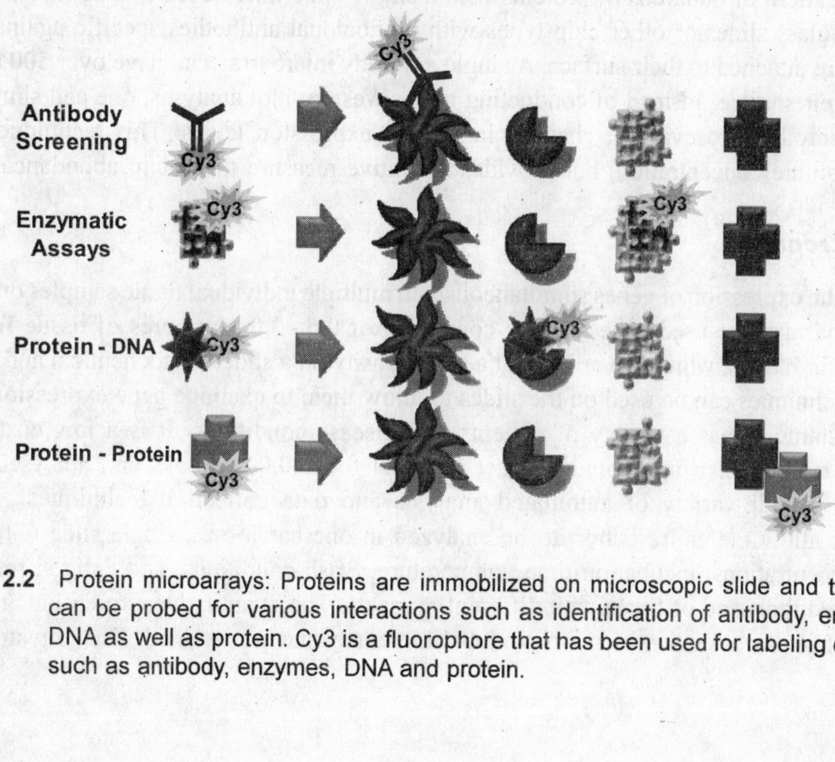

Figure 12.2 Protein microarrays: Proteins are immobilized on microscopic slide and the slide can be probed for various interactions such as identification of antibody, enzymes, DNA as well as protein. Cy3 is a fluorophore that has been used for labeling of target such as antibody, enzymes, DNA and protein.

using a contact spotter or a non-contact microarrayer to act as capture molecules. Aldehyde- and epoxy-derivatized glass surfaces can be used for random attachment of proteins through amines, and coating the glass surface with nitrocellulose, gel pads, or poly-L-lysine achieves a random orientation of the proteins as the proteins are passively adsorbed onto the surface (Figure 12.2). Protein microarrays are of three types, which are described briefly below.

Analytical microarrays

Analytical microarrays are used to measure binding affinities, specificities, and protein expression levels of the proteins in the mixture. In this technique, a library of antibodies, aptamers, or affibodies is arrayed on a glass microscope slide and then probed with a protein solution. Antibody microarrays are the most common analytical microarray. Functional protein arrays are used to study the biochemical activities of an entire proteome in a single experiment i.e., protein-protein, protein-DNA, protein-RNA, protein-phospholipid, and protein-small molecule interactions. In reverse phase protein microarray (RPA), cells are isolated from various tissues of interest and are lysed and then arrayed onto a nitrocellulose slide using a contact pin microarrayer. Slides are then probed with antibodies against the target protein of interest, and the antibodies are detected with chemiluminescent, fluorescent, or colorimetric assays.

Antibody arrays

Antibody microarray is a powerful chip-based technology composed of hundreds of distinct monoclonal antibodies printed at high density on a glass microscope slide enabling to monitor the expression pattern of hundreds of proteins with a single experiment even in a pg/ml range. In this microarray, glass slides or other chip types with monoclonal antibodies specific against proteins of interest are attached to their surface. A single antibody microarray can have over 500 antibodies arrays on their surface. Instead of conducting many Western blot analyses, one can simply use an antibody microarray to evaluate changes in protein expression levels. This technique does not measure absolute concentration, but provides a relative measure of protein abundance.

Tissue microarray

To analyze the expression of genes simultaneously in multiple individual tissue samples on one slide, tissue microarrays are used. The array is composed of 0.6 - 3.0 mm cores of tissue from donor tissue paraffin blocks, which are arrayed at a high density on a slide. Histochemical and molecular detection techniques can be used on the slides to allow them to examine gene expression profiling in disease status across a variety of patients and disease conditions. It is a low cost and high throughput technique, which could produce material for 500,000 assays and analysed per slide block with a wide-variety of automated analysis and data collection techniques. The tissue microarrays allow the entire cohort to be analyzed in one batch on a single slide with identical reagent concentrations, incubation time, temperature, wash conditions, and antigen retrieval and can be reused thousand of times with different reagents. The quantitative expression analysis can be done by H-score system, which is a product of intensity and area stained. The software involved are TMA-Deconvoluter and Stain finder, Tissue Array Data Analysis, Tissue Array Database (TAD), TMAJ, etc.

In this technique, 4-5 micrometer tissue sections are produced using a microtome. Specific areas of interest are selected from paraffin-embedded tissue blocks and are re-embedded into an arrayed blank recipient blocks. Tissue microarray is of different types i.e., cryo-tissue microarray, multi-tissue microarray, progression tissue microarray and prognosis tissue microarray.

Glycomics

Glycans are termed the compounds in which sugar residues are covalently attached with the proteins and biomolecules. An example of carbohydrate microarray is neoglycolipids, spotted onto nitrocellulose and PVD. The neoglycolipids can be probed with proteins of known carbohydrate binding specificity to confirm identification of predicted protein–oligosaccharide interactions. This array technology describes the link of oligosaccharides to the lipid derived from diverse sources, for example, glycoproteins, proteoglycans, glycolipids, whole cells, organs and synthetic oligosaccharides.

APPLICATIONS OF MICROARRAY TECHNOLOGY

DNA microarrays are better than other profiling methods (SAGE, SH, PCR) in the sense that they are easier to use with high-throughput results, and can generate large amount of data in lesser time. They do not require large scale sequencing and allow quantitation of genes for many samples. Thus microarray technique seems to have a significant future in diagnostics. The application of DNA microarray in various fields of research is discussed below in detail.

Changes in Gene Expression Level

With all the techniques to measure gene expression including Northern blotting, differential display, serial analysis of gene expression and dot-blot analysis, the main problem is that they are unsuitable for the parallel testing of multiple gene expression. Southern's method of microarray contains multiple DNA sequences (probes) spotted or synthesized on a relatively small surface allowing simultaneous monitoring of the expression of thousands of genes, thus providing a functional aspect to sequence information in a given sample. This technique seems to be ideal for detection of complex phenotypes and genes whose altered expression underlies complex traits that are located within genetic regions identified by quantitative traits loci (QTL) techniques. However, SNP has allowed polymorphisms to be assayed more quickly and also their relevance to disease to be easily determined. In contrast to the analysis of a single nucleotide polymorphism, gene expression levels are best analyzed with relatively long probes as in microarray. With long probes, it is possible to achieve good yields under stringent hybridization conditions. Also the genomic DNA derived from a normal sample is required for use in the hybridization mixture and whole genome can be used for expression analysis. To detect mutations or polymorphisms in a gene sequence, i.e., change or variation that can occur within a person's DNA sequence, "mutation microarray" analysis is used. Microarrays, in combination with defined mutants, can be used to infer signaling pathways associated with an environmental response i.e., capability to identify common promoter regulatory elements shared by coregulated genes in cell cycle.

DNA microarrays are also used to examine the gene expression changes under various diseases i.e., cancer. Tumor profiling using DNA microarray allows the analysis of the development and the progression of such complex diseases and differential expression in the levels of gene(s) within the same organism under two different conditions or among two different organisms. Microarrays are used to identify inheritable markers used in genotyping tool. Thus information about differences in gene expression between tissue types can help to uncover how our bodies develop sensitivity and which genes are harmful to target for disease therapy. By the microarray technique, gene expression studies can also be done for a subset of genes involved in various metabolic pathways. Microarray expression analysis or expression chip array is used in determining the level, or volume at which a certain gene is expressed and examine changes in gene expression over a given time period i.e., within the cell cycle.

Analysis of Sequence Variation

Sequence variation is best analyzed with the shortest oligonucleotides (<15-mer) that will give specific hybridization to the target site. Multiple genes can be analyzed simultaneously to get a snapshot of the whole transcriptome of a system at a given time point. Treating mRNA transcript abundances as quantitative traits and mapping gene expression QTL for these traits has been pursued in gene-specific ways. Unlike classical quantitative traits, the genetic linkages associated with transcript abundance permits a more precise look at cellular and biochemical processes. Microarray provides powerful tools for the genome-wide correlation of gene transcript levels with physiological responses and alterations in physiological states. It has been applied almost exclusively to a few model species for which the abundant gene sequence data permit the fabrication of whole-genome microarrays. Microarray technique is also used for mapping human genome using DNA polymorphisms, which are further analyzed to give enough analytical power to carry out genetic studies to find the genes associated with common diseases and inherited disease susceptibilities. It can be successfully applied to nonmodel species to generate new insights of comparative and evolutionary significance into animal function.

Drug Discovery (Pharmacogenomics)

The goal of pharmacogenomics is to find correlations between therapeutic responses to drugs and the genetic profiles of patients. Personalized drugs, molecular diagnostics, integration of diagnosis and therapeutics are the long-term promises of microarray technology. One can examine targets for drug discovery and potential diagnostic and prognostic biomarkers for many complex diseases. The use of microarray analysis in drug design and screening allows gene interactions to be studied with compounds that affect the expression of important genes during drug application. After identifying a specific molecular target and the development of a series of small molecule inhibitors, it is necessary to confirm that such inhibitors do indeed act by the desired mechanism of action on their intended target. In addition, identification of potential on-target and off-target effects, and pharmacodynamic markers of these effects is highly beneficial for the subsequent preclinical and clinical studies required for the development of specific drugs.

Toxicological Research (Toxicogenomics)

The goal of toxicogenomics is to find correlations between toxic responses to toxicants and changes in the genetic profiles of the objects exposed to such toxicants. New drug development protocols include genomic and proteomic microarray data obtained during preclinical stages of investigation, but extrapolating this information to humans is not straightforward. However, microarray data can provide greater insight into and better prediction of the performance characteristics of the product as it moves into clinical phases of development. Recent examples of microarray in neurotoxicological research combine toxic drug administration with a genetic knock-out model. Microarray technology has been used to assess toxin induced gene expression abnormalities in cancer biology, hepatotoxicity and drug abuse studies. DNA microarray is also an ideal tool for the identification of bacterial species in a mixed population giving information on both the abundance and identity of the bacteria in a particular environment.

Diagnosis of Disease

Insights into disease have been one of the most beneficial results of microarray technology. Expression chips are used in disease diagnosis, e.g., in the identification of new genes involved in environmentally triggered diseases, i.e., diseases affecting immune, nervous, and pulmonary/respiratory systems. For targeted therapies, identification of genes that are either lost during a disease or typically involved in a cellular function that directly or indirectly prevents the disease from occurring can be done with a microarray. It is also used to diagnose diseases at very early stages, so that therapy could be commenced before the disease can cause any harm. Comparative Genomic Hybridization (CGH) is used to detect any change in the number of copies of a particular gene involved in a disease state. In this array, each spot of target (large pieces of genomic DNA) in the array has a known chromosomal location, and hybridization mixture contains fluorescently labeled genomic DNA taken from both control and diseased tissues.

Molecular karyotyping, can easily and reliably detect unbalanced chromosomal aberrations of various sizes from as little as 250 ng of DNA on a single microarray, based on fluorescence intensity information from clusters of SNPs.

Microarray technology has been widely used in studies identifying new genes or molecular pathways involved in tumor classification, cancer progression and chemotherapy resistance and sensitivity. It allows the rapid identification of genes that are turned on and off in tumor development. Recently a strategy is proposed called SAM (Significance Analysis of Microarrays), which allows the determination of significantly differentially expressed genes between groups of samples analyzed by expression arrays i.e., in early and late stages of cancer.

Microarray technology can be a powerful tool to identify unexpected molecular mediators using animal models that might help in the development of novel targets for improved treatment in Idiopathic Pulmonary Fibrosis (IPF) and asthma. This can provide a large scale of differentially expressed genes, which led researchers to shed further light into transcriptional programs involved in cytokine signaling and apoptosis regulating emphysema, chronic obstructive pulmonary disease (COPD) and pulmonary fibrosis. Furthermore, this technology is already being applied in respiratory clinical pharmacology of complex diseases such as asthma and COPD revealing modern approaches in therapeutic interventions. Finally, it provided scientists with useful information to clarify physiological mechanisms underlying the actions of numerous drugs, elucidate the pathophysiological processes of complex diseases such as IPF, asthma, COPD, lung fibrosis in acute lung injury and pulmonary edema.

With the help of microarray, one can detect viruses and other pathogens from blood samples and thus it can be used as a pathogen detection method. Tissue microarray technology is used for blood cell analysis of patients suffering from red cell disorder and microdissected discs can be used for PCR-based analysis.

Comparative and Evolutionary Biology

Microarray technology is perfectly suited for sub-classifying otherwise indistinguishable diseases using straightforward hierarchical clustering techniques and therefore well suited to situations where just a few genes underpin the condition. This can display pronounced changes in expression related to an imposed change in physiological status or in response to upstream events in a transduction pathway. Microarrays have also been used to identify genes that contribute to enhanced fitness and assess the changes in gene expression. With the help of microarray, transcript screening can be done to find molecular basis of natural variation and genotype to phenotype interaction on an evolutionary scale. Whole genome microarray points toward the environmental responses of organisms that can be addressed on a global scale with differential expression of a common set of genes. Transcript expression data across and between the species shows that closely related species of the same genus may share the expression of many transcripts, whereas distantly related species will have more divergent profiles. Common gene ontology has been developed to provide order in a fragmented functional nomenclature by creating a single listing of attributes to describe objectively gene products in any organism.

Proteomics

Microarray technology can be used efficiently to identify, quantify, and study protein functions from a global perspective. Protein microarrays are suitable for studying protein–protein interactions, enzyme–substrate interactions, protein–DNA interactions, protein-lipid interactions, protein–oligosaccharide interactions, protein–drug interactions, protein-receptor interactions and antigen-antibody interactions simultaneously. Protein microarray is also used in the investigation of kinase activities, serum profiling, neurodegenerative disorders, correlation of cell phenotype with surface markers, identification of chromatin-related proteins as well as mapping of WW domains. This technique is capable of detecting up to 10,000 proteins in parallel. Peptide microarray technology is used for proteome analyses to study molecular recognition events and the identification of biologically active peptides. DNA–protein interaction assays have proven useful in the characterization and identification of DNA binding proteins. Glycomics is used to study protein–carbohydrate interactions in biological processes including normal tissue growth and repair, cell–cell adhesion and inflammation, cell growth, fertilization, viral replications, parasitic infection, tumor-cell motility and progression. Reverse phase protein microarray allows the determination of the presence of altered proteins that may be due to the result of disease. Proteome chips have been used to screen human sera for the presence of autoantibodies or viral specific antibodies.

Analysis of Quantitative Traits

Microarray can also be used to know the response of plants or animals towards traits that are multigene. A good example is response of plants towards environmental stresses such as high temperature or salinity. Several recent studies have indicated the usefulness of microarray technology to understand the response of plants towards salinity. These data have also resulted in prediction of nodal components of stress response pathways in plants.

Assigning Roles to Novel Genes

The most powerful application of microarray technology in biology is to aid in assigning functions to unknown genes. This is especially useful in the post-genome sequencing era. Based on hierarchical clustering, the roles of unknown genes forming a cluster with genes of known function can be predicted.

FURTHER READINGS

1. Anderson K., Potter A., Baban D. and Davies K.E. (2003) Protein expression changes in spinal muscular atrophy revealed with a novel antibody array technology. *Brain.* **(126)**: 2052-2064
2. Angenendt P., Glokler J., Murphy D., Lehrach H. and Cahill D.J. (2002) Toward optimized antibody microarrays: a comparison of current microarray support materials. *Anal. Biochem.* **(309)**: 253-260.
3. Ashburner M., Ball C.A., Blake J.A., Botstein D., Butler H., Cherry J.M., Davis A.P., Dolinski K., Dwight S.S., Eppig J.T., Harris M.A., Hill D.P., Issel-Tarver L., Kasarskis A., Lewis S., Matese J.C., Richardson J. E., Ringwald M., Rubin G.M. and Sherlock G. (2000) Gene ontology: tool for the unification of biology. *Nat. Genet.* **(25)**: 25-29.
4. Baker T.K., Carfagna M.A., Gao H., Dow E.R., Li Q., Searfoss G.H. (2001) Temporal gene expression analysis of monolayer cultured rat hepatocytes. *Chem. Res. Toxicol.* **(14)**: 1 218-1231.
5. Baldi P. and Long A. (2001) A Bayesian framework for the analysis of microarray expression data: regularized t-test and statistical inferences of gene changes. *Bioinformatics.* **(17)**: 509-519.
6. Banerjee S.K., Young H.W., Volmer J.B. and Blackburn M.R. (2002) Gene expression profiling in inflammatory airway disease associated with elevated adenosine. *Am. J. Physiol. Lung. Cell. Mol. Physiol.* **(282)**: 169-182.
7. Barrett T., Xie T., Piao Y., Dillon-Carter O., Kargul G.J., Lim M.K., Chrest F.J., Wersto R., Rowley D.L., Juhaszova M., Zhou L., Vawter M.P., Becker K.G., Cheadle C., Wood W.H., 3rd McCann U.D., Freed W.J., Ko M.S., Ricaurte G.A. and Donovan D.M. (2001) A murine dopamine neuron-specific cDNA library and microarray: increased COX1 expression during methamphetamine neurotoxicity. *Neurobiol Dis.* **(8)**: 822-833.
8. Bartosiewicz M., Penn S. and Buckpitt A. (2001) Applications of gene arrays in environmental toxicology: fingerprints of gene regulation associated with cadmium chloride, benzo(a)pyrene, and trichloroethylene. *Environ. Health. Persp.* **(109)**: 71-742.
9. Bertone P. and Snyder M. (2005) Advances in functional protein microarray technology. *Febs. J.* **(272)**: 5400-5411.
10. Bertucci F., Beranrd K., Loriod B., Chang Y.C., Granjeaud S., Birnbaum D., Ntuyen C., Peck K., Jordan B. (1999) Sensitivity issues in DNA array-based expression measurements and performance of nylon microarrays for small samples. *Hum. Mol. Genet.* **(8)**: 1715-1722.
11. Blanchard A.P., Kaiser R.J. and Hood L.E. (1996) High density oligonucleotide arrays. *Biosensors and Bioelectronics.* **(11)**: 687-690.

12. Boise L.H., González-García M., Postema C.E., Ding L., Lindsten T., Turka L.A., Mao X., Nuñez G. and Thompson C.B. (1993) bclx, a bcl-2-related gene that functions as a dominant regulator of apoptotic cell death. *Cell.* **(74):** 597-608.
13. Brazma A., Hingamp P., Quackenbush J., Sherlock G., Spellman P., Stoeckert C., Aach J., Ansorge W., Ball C.A., Causton H.C., Gaasterland T., Glenisson P., Holstege F.C., Kim I.F., Markowitz V., Matese J.C., Parkinson H., Robinson A., Sarkans U., Schulze-Kremer S., Stewart J., Taylor R., Vilo J. and Vingron M. (2001) Minimum information about a microarray experiment (MIAME)- toward standards for microarray data. *Nat. Genet.* **(29):** 365-371.
14. Brutsche M.H., Brutsche I.C., Wood P., Brass A., Morrison N., Rattay M., Mogulkoc N., Simler N., Craven M., Custovic A., Egan J.J. and Woodcock A. (2001) Apoptosis signals in atopy and asthma measured with cDNA arrays. *Clin. Exp. Immunol.* **(123):** 181-187.
15. Brutsche M.H., Joos L., Carlen-Brutsche I.E., Bissinger R., Tamm M., Custovic A. and Woodcock A. (2002) Array-based diagnostic gene-expression score for atopy and asthma. *J. Allergy. Clin. Immunol.* **(109):** 271-273.
16. Cargill M., Altshuler D., Ireland J., Sklar P., Ardlie K., Patil N., Shaw N., Lane C.R., Lim E.P., Kalyanaraman N., Nemesh J., Ziaugra L., Friedland L., Rolfe A., Warrington J., Lipshutz R., Daley G.Q. and Lander E.S. (1999) Characterization of single-nucleotide polymorphisms in coding regions of human genes. *Nat. Genet.* **(22):** 231-238.
17. Causton H.C., Ren B., Koh S.S., Harbison C.T., Kanin E., Jennings E.G., Lee T., True H.L., Lander E.S. and Young R.A. (2001) Remodeling of yeast genome expression in response to environmental changes. *Mol. Biol. Cell.* **(12):** 323-337.
18. Chambers R.C., Leoni P., Kaminski N., Laurent G.J. and Heller R.A. (2003) Global expression profiling of fibroblast responses to transforming growth factor-beta1 reveals the induction of inhibitor of differentiation-1 and provides evidence of smooth muscle cell phenotypic switching. *Am. J. Pathol.* **(162):** 533-546.
19. Charles P.T., Goldman E.R., Rangasammy J.G., Schauer C.L., Chen M.S. and Taitt C.R. (2004) Fabrication and characterization of 3D hydrogel microarrays to measure antigenicity and antibody functionality for biosensor applications. *Biosens. Bioelectron.* **(20):** 753-764.
20. Cheung V.G., Morley M., Aguilar F., Massimi A., Kucherlapati R. and Childs G. (1999) Making and Reading Microarrays. *Nat. Genet.* 21(1 Suppl): 15-9.
21. Chinnaiyan A.M., Huber-Lang M., Kumar-Sinha C., Barrette T.R., Shankar-Sinha S., Sarma V,J., Padgaonkar V.A. and Ward P.A. (2001) Molecular signatures of sepsis: multiorgan gene expression profiles of systemic inflammation. *Am. J. Pathol.* **(159):** 1199-1209.
22. Cho R.J., Campbell M.J., Winzeler E.A., Steinmetz L., Conway A., Wodicka L., Wolfsberg T.G., Gabrielian A.E., Landsman D., Lockhart D.J. and Davis R.W. (1998) A genome-wide transcriptional analysis of the mitotic cell cycle. *Mol. Cell.* **(2):** 65-73.
23. Chuaqui R.F., Bonner R.F., Best C.J., Gillespie J.W., Flaig M.J., Hewitt S.M., Phillips J.L., Krizman D.B., Tangrea M.A., Ahram M. (2002) Post-analysis follow-up and validation of microarray experiments. *Nat. Genet.* **(32):** 509-14
24. Clark T.A., Sugnet C.W. and Jr. Ares M. (2002) Genomewide analysis of mRNA processing in yeast using splicing specific microarrays. *Science.* **(296):** 907-910
25. Clarke P. A., te Poele R., Wooster R. and Workman P. (2001) Gene expression microarray analysis in cancer biology, pharmacology and drug development: progress and potential. *Biochemical Pharmacology.* **(62):** 1311-1336
26. Clarke P.A., te Poele R., Wooster R. and Workman P. (2001) Gene expression microarray analysis in cancer biology, pharmacology, and drug development: progress and potential. *Biochem. Pharmacol.* **(62):** 1311-1336.
27. Coe B. and Antler C. (2004) Spot your genes- An overview of the microarray. The Science Creative Quaterly. http—www_scq_ubc_ca-wp-content-GeneChip_gif.mht.

28. Cole S.W., Galic Z. and Zack J.A. (2003) Controlling false negative errors in microarray differential expression analysis: a PRIM approach. *Bioinformatics.* **(19):** 1808-1816.
29. Coleman M.A., Miller K.A., Beernink P.T., Yoshikawa D.M. and Albala J.S. (2003) Identification of chromatin-related protein interactions using protein microarrays. *Proteomics.* 3 **(11):** 2101-2107.
30. Crowther D.J. (2002) Applications of microarrays in the pharmaceutical industry. *Curr. Opin. Pharmacol.* 2 **(5):** 551-4.
31. Crystal R.G., Bitterman P.B., Mossman B., Schwarz M.I., Sheppard D., Almasy L., Chapman H.A., Friedman S.L., Jr. King T.E., Leinwand L.A., Liotta L., Martin G.R., Schwartz D.A., Schultz G.S., Wagner C.R. and Musson R.A. (2002) Future research directions in idiopathic pulmonary fibrosis: summary of a National Heart, Lung, and Blood Institute working group. *Am. J. Respir. Crit. Care. Med.* 15 **(166):** 236-246.
32. Delehanty J.B. (2004) Printing functional protein microarrays using piezoelectric capillaries. Methods *Mol. Biol.* **(264):** 135-143.
33. Delehanty J.B. and Ligler F.S. (2003) Method for printing functional protein microarrays. *Biotechniques.* **(34):** 380-385.
34. Doerge R.W. (2002) Mapping and analysis of quantitative trait loci in experimental populations. *Nat. Rev. Genet.* **(3):** 43-52.
35. Dudoit S., Yang Y.H. and Bolstad B. (2002a) Using R for the analysis of DNA microarray data. *R. News.* **(2):** 24-32.
36. Dudoit S., Yang Y.H., Callow M.J. and Speed T.P. (2002b) Statistical methods for identifying differentially expressed genes in replicated cDNA microarray experiments. *Statistica Sinica.* **(12):** 111-139.
37. Eckardt N.A. (2004) Cutting Edge Transcriptome Analysis: It's All about Design. *The Plant Cell.* **(16):** 2249-2251.
38. Eisen M.B. and Brown P.O. (1999) DNA arrays for analysis of gene expression. *Methods Enzymol.* **(303):** 179-205.
39. Eisen M.B., Spellman P.T., Brown P.O. and Botstein D. (1998) Cluster analysis and display of genome-wide expression patterns. *Proc. Natl. Acad. Sci. USA.* **(95):** 14863-14868.
40. Evans A.L., Sharkey A.S., Saidi S.A., Print C.G., Catalano R.D., Smith S.K. and Charnock-Jones D.S. (2003) Generation and use of a tailored gene array to investigate vascular biology. *Angiogenesis.* **(6):** 93–104.
41. Ferea T.L., Botstein D., Brown P.O. and Rosenzweig R.F. (1999) Systematic changes in gene expression patterns following adaptive evolution in yeast. *Proc. Natl. Acad. Sci. USA* **(96):** 9721-9726.
42. Fodor S. (1997) Massively parallel genomics. *Science.* **(277):** 393
43. Fuke S., Betsuyaku T., Nasuhara Y., Morikawa T., Katoh H. and Nishimura M. (2004) Chemokines in bronchiolar epithelium in the development of chronic obstructive pulmonary disease. *Am. J. Respir. Cell. Mol. Biol.* **(31):** 405-12.
44. Fukui S., Feizi T., Galustian C., Lawson A.M. and Chai W. (2002) Oligosaccharide microarrays for high-throughput detection and specificity assignments of carbohydrate-protein interactions. *Nat. Biotechnol.* **(20):** 1011-1017.
45. Garrett M.D. and Workman P. (1999) Discovering novel chemotherapeutic drugs for the third millenium. *Eur. J. Cancer.* **(35):** 2010-2030.
46. Gasch A.P., Spellman P.T., Kao C.M., Carmel-Harel O., Eisen M.B., Storz G., Botstein D. and Brown P.O. (2000) Genomic expression programs in the response of yeast cells to environmental changes. *Mol. Biol. Cell.* **(11):** 4241-4257.
47. Gerhold D., Lu M., Xu J., Austin C., Caskey C.T. and Rushmore T. (2001) Monitoring expression of genes involved in drug metabolism and toxicology using DNA microarrays. *Physiol Genomics.* **(5):** 161-170.
48. Gracey A.Y. and Cossins A.R. (2003) Application of microarray technology in environmental and comparative physiology. *Annu. Rev. Physiol.* **(65):** 231–259.

49. Guo Z., Guilfoyle R.A., Thiel A.J., Wang R. and Smith L.M. (1994) Direct fluorescence analysis of genetic polymorphisms by hybridization with oligonucleotide arrays on glass supports. *Nucleic Acids Res.* **(22):** 5456-5465.

50. Hackett N.R., Heguy A., Harvey B.G., O'Connor T.P., Luettich K., Flieder D.B., Kaplan R. and Crystal R.G. (2003) Variability of antioxidant-related gene expression in the airway epithelium of cigarette smokers. *Am. J. Respir. Cell. Mol. Biol.* **(29):** 331-343.

51. Hakonarson H., Halapi E., Whelan R., Gulcher J., Stefansson K. and Grunstein M.M. (2001) Association between IL-1beta/TNF-alphainduced glucocorticoid-sensitive changes in multiple gene expression and altered responsiveness in airway smooth muscle. *Am. J. Respir. Cell. Mol. Biol.* **(25):** 761-71.

52. Hall D.A., Ptacek J. and Snyder M. (2007) Protein Microarray Technology. *Mech. FAgeing Dev.* 128 **(1):** 161-167.

53. Hall D.A., Zhu H., Zhu X., Royce T., Gerstein M. and Snyder M. (2004) Regulation of gene expression by a metabolic enzyme. *Science.* **(306):** 482-484.

54. Harmer S.L. and Kay S.A. (2000) Microarrays: Determining the balance of cellular transcription. The *Plant Cell.* **(12):** 613-615.

55. Heller M.J. (2002) DNA microarray technology: devices, systems, and applications. *Annu. Rev. Biomed. Eng.* **(4):** 129-53.

56. Howbrook D.N., van der Valk A.M., O'Shaughnessy M.C., Sarker D.K., Baker S.C. and Lloyd A.W. (2003) Developments in microarray technologies. *DDT.* **(8):** 642-651.

57. Hu G.K., Madore S.J., Moldover B., Jatkoe T., Balaban D., Thomas J. and Wang Y. (2001) Predicting splice variant from DNA chip expression data. *Genome. Res.* **(11):** 1237-45.

58. Hu H., Columbus J., Zhang Y., Wu D., Lian I., Yang S., Goodwin J., Luczak C., Carter M., Chen L., James M., Davis R., Sudol M., Rodwell J. and Herrero J.J. (2004) A map of WW domain family interactions. *Proteomics.* **(4):** 643–655.

59. Huang J., Zhu H., Haggarty S.J., Spring D.R., Hwang H., Jin F., Snyder M. and Schreiber S.L. (2004) Finding new components of the target of rapamycin (TOR) signaling network through chemical genetics and proteome chips. *Proc. Natl. Acad. Sci. U S A.* **(101):** 16594-16599.

60. Hueber W., Kidd B.A., Tomooka B.H., Lee B.J., Bruce B., Fries J.F., Sonderstrup G., Monach P., Drijfhout J.W., van Venrooij W.J., Utz P.J., Genovese M.C. and Robinson W.H. (2005) Antigen microarray profiling of autoantibodies in rheumatoid arthritis. *Arthritis Rheum.* **(52):** 2645-2655.

61. Hughes T.R., Mao M., Jones A.R., Burchard J., Marton M.J., Shannon K.W., Lefkowitz S.M., Ziman M., Schelter J.M., Meyer M.R., Kobayashi S., Davis C., Dai H., He Y.D., Stephaniants S.B., Cavet G., Walker W.L., West A., Coffey E., Shoemaker D.D., Stoughton R., Blanchard A.P., Friend S.H. and Linsley P.S. (2001) Expression profiling using microarrays fabricated by an ink-jet oligonucleotide synthesizer. *Nat Biotechnol.* **(19):** 342-47.

62. Ihaka R. and Gentleman R. (1996) R: a language for data analysis and graphics. *Journal of Computational & Graphical Statistics.* **(5):** 299-314.

63. Jones R.B., Gordus A., Krall J.A. and MacBeath G. (2006) A quantitative protein interaction network for the ErbB receptors using protein microarrays. *Nature.* **(439):** 168-174.

64. Kaminski N., Allard J.D., Pittet J.F., Zuo F., Griffiths M.J., Morris D., Huang X., Sheppard D. and Heller R.A. (2000) Global analysis of gene expression in pulmonary fibrosis reveals distinct programs regulating lung inflammation and fibrosis. *Proc. Nat.l Acad. Sci. USA* **(97):** 1778-1783.

65. Kato M., Seki N., Sugano S., Hashimoto K., Masuho Y., Muramatsu M., Kaibuchi K. and Nakafuku M. (2001) Identification of sonic hedgehog-responsive genes using cDNA microarray. *Biochem. Biophys. Res. Commun.* **(289):** 472-78.

66. Katsuma S., Nishi S., Tanigawara K., Ikawa H., Shiojima S., Takagaki K., Kaminishi Y., Suzuki Y., Hirasawa A., Ohgi T., Yano J., Murakami Y. and Tsujimoto G. (2001) Molecular monitoring of bleomycin-induced pulmonary fibrosis by cDNA microarray-based gene expression profiling. *Biochem Biophys Res Commun.* **(288):** 747-751.

67. Kattah M.G., Alemi G.R., Thibault D.L., Balboni I. and Utz P.J. (2006) A new two-color Fab labeling method for autoantigen protein microarrays. *Nat. Methods.* **(3):** 745-51.

68. Kawasaki S., Borchert C., Deyholos M., Wang H., Brazille S., Kawai K., Galbraith D., Bohnert H. J. (2001) Gene expression profiles during the initial phase of salt stress in rice. *Plant. Cell.* **(13):** 889-905.

69. Kerr M.K. and Churchill G.A. (2001) Experimental design for gene expression microarrays. *Biostatistics.* **(2):** 183-201.

70. Ko I.K., Kato K. and Iwata H. (2005) Antibody microarray for correlating cell phenotype with surface marker. *Biomaterials.* **(26):** 687-696.

71. Koike E., Hirano S., Furuyama A. and Kobayashi T. (2004) cDNA microarray analysis of rat alveolar epithelial cells following exposure to organic extract of diesel exhaust particles. *Toxicol. Appl. Pharmacol.* **(201):** 178-85.

72. Kramer A., Feilner T., Possling A., Radchuk V., Weschke W., Burkle L. and Kersten B. (2004) Identification of barley CK2alpha targets by using the protein microarray technology. *Phytochemistry.* **(65):** 1777-84.

73. Krasnova I.N., McCoy M.T., Ladenheim B. and Cadet J.L. (2002) cDNA array analysis of gene expression profiles in the striata of wild-type and Cu/Zn superoxide dismutase transgenic mice treated with neurotoxic doses of amphetamine. *FASEB J.* **(16):** 1379-88.

74. Kricka L.J. and Fortina P. (2001) Microarray Technology and Applications: An All-Language Literature Survey Including Books and Patents. *Clinical Chemistry.* **(47):** 1479-1482.

75. Kupfner J.G., Arcaroli J.J., Yum H.K., Nadler S.G., Yang K.Y. and Abraham E. (2001) Role of NF-kappaB in endotoxemia-induced alterations of lung neutrophil apoptosis. *J. Immunol.* **(167):** 7044-7051.

76. Kusnezow W., Jacob A., Walijew A., Diehl F. and Hoheisel J.D. (2003) Antibody microarrays: an evaluation of production parameters. *Proteomics.* **(3):** 254-64.

77. Laprise C., Sladek R., Ponton A., Bernier M.C., Hudson T.J. and Laviolette M. (2004) Functional classes of bronchial mucosa genes that are differentially expressed in asthma. *BMC Genomics.* **(5):** 21.

78. Lee J.H., Kaminski N., Dolganov G., Grunig G., Koth L., Solomon C., Erle D.J. and Sheppard D. (2001) Interleukin-13 induces dramatically different transcriptional programs in three human airway cell types. *Am. J. Respir. Cell. Mol. Biol.* **(25):** 474-485.

79. Liu T., Dhanasekaran S.M., Jin H., Hu B., Tomlins S.A., Chinnaiyan A.M. and Phan S.H. (2004) FIZZ1 stimulation of myofibroblast differentiation. *Am. J. Pathol.* **(164):** 1315-1326.

80. Lockhart D.J. and Winzeler E.A. (2000) Genomics, gene expression and DNA arrays. *Nature.* **(405):** 827-836.

81. Lonnstedt I. and Speed T.P. (2002) Replicated microarray data. *Statistica Sinica.* **(12):** 31-46.

82. Ma S., Bohnert H.J. (2007) Integration of Arabidopsis thaliana stress-related transcript profiles, promoter structures, and cell-specific expression. *Genome Biol.* **(8):** R49.

83. MacBeath G. (2002) Protein microarrays and proteomics. *Nat. Genet.* 32(Suppl): 526-532

84. MacBeath G. and Schreiber S.L. (2000) Printing proteins as microarrays for high-throughput function determination. *Science.* **(289):** 1760-1763.

85. Macgregor P.F. and Squire J.A. (2002) Application of microarrays to the analysis of gene expression in cancer. *Clinical Chemistry.* **(48):** 1170-1177.

86. McDowell S.A., Gammon K., Bachurski C.J., Wiest J.S., Leikauf J.E., Prows D.R. and Leikauf G.D. (2000) Differential gene expression in the initiation and progression of nickel-induced acute lung injury. *Am. J. Respir. Cell. Mol. Biol.* **(23):** 466-474.

87. Meyers B.C., Galbraith D.W., Nelson T. and Agrawal V. (2004) Methods for transcriptional profiling in plants. Be fruitful and replicate. *Plant Physiol.* **(135):** 637-652.

88. Michaud G.A., Salcius M., Zhou F., Bangham R., Bonin J., Guo H., Snyder M., Predki P.F. and Schweitzer B.I. (2003) Analyzing antibody specificity with whole proteome microarrays. *Nat. Biotechnol.* **(21):** 1509-1512.

89. Miller D.T., Adam M.P., Aradhya S., Biesecker L.G., Brothman A.R., Carter N.P., Church D.M., Crolla J.A., Eichler E.E., Epstein C.J., Faucett W.A., Feuk L., Friedman J.M., Hamosh A., Jackson L., Kaminsky E.B., Kok K., Krantz I.D., Kuhn R.M., Lee C., Ostell J.M., Rosenberg C., Scherer S.W., Spinner N.B., Stavropoulos D.J., Tepperberg J.H., Thorland E.C., Vermeesch J.R., Waggoner D.J., Watson M.S., Martin C.L. and Ledbetter D.H. (2010) Consensus statement: chromosomal microarray is a firsttier clinical diagnostic test for individuals with developmental disabilities or congential anomalies. Am *J. Hum. Gen.* **(86):** 749-764.

90. Morris D.G., Huang X., Kaminski N., Wang Y., Shapiro S.D., Dolganov G., Glick A. and Sheppard D. (2003) Loss of integrin alpha (v) beta6-mediated TGF-beta activation causes Mmp12-dependent emphysema. *Nature.* **(422):** 169-173.

91. Nakajima T., Matsumoto K., Suto H., Tanaka K., Ebisawa M., Tomita H., Yuki K., Katsunuma T., Akasawa A., Hashida R., Sugita Y., Ogawa H., Ra C. and Saito H. (2001) Gene expression screening of human mast cells and eosinophils using high-density oligonucleotide probe arrays: abundant expression of major basic protein in mast cells. *Blood.* **(98):** 1127-1134.

92. Nuwaysir E.F., Bittner M., Trent J., Barrett J.C. and Afshari C.A. (1999). Microarrays and toxicology: The advent of toxicogenomics. *Mol. Carcinog.* **(24):** 153-159.

93. Olman M.A., White K.E., Ware L.B., Cross M.T., Zhu S. and Matthay M.A. (2004) Microarray analysis indicates that pulmonary edema fluid from patients with acute lung injury mediates inflammation, mitogen gene expression, and fibroblast proliferation through bioactive interleukin-1. *J. Immunol.* **(172):** 2668-2677.

94. Park T., Yi S.G., Kang S.H., Lee S.Y., Lee Y.S. and Simon R. (2003) Evaluation of normalization methods for microarray data. *BMC Bioinformatics.* **(4):** 33.

95. Perkowski S., Sun J., Singhal S., Santiago J., Leikauf G.D. and Albelda S.M. (2003) Gene expression profiling of the early pulmonary response to hyperoxia in mice. *Am. J. Respir. Cell. Mol. Biol.* **(28):** 682-696.

96. Petricoin E.F., Hackett J.L., Lesko L.J., Puri R.K., Gutman S.I., Chumakov K., Woodcock J., Jr. Feigal D.W., Zoon K.C. and Sistare F.D. (2002) Medical applications of microarray technologies: a regulatory science perspective. *Nature Genetics Supplement.* **(32):** 474-479.

97. Pirrung M.C., Fallon L. and McGall G. (1998) Proofing of photolithographic DNA syntheisis with 3¢, 5¢-dimethoxybenzoinyloxycarbonyl-protected deoxynucleoside phosphoramidites. *J. Org. Chem.* **(63):** 241-246.

98. Ptacek J., Devgan G., Michaud G., Zhu H., Zhu X., Fasolo J., Guo H., Jona G., Breitkreutz A., Sopko R., McCartney R.R., Schmidt M.C., Rachidi N., Lee S.J., Mah A.S., Meng L., Stark M.J., Stern D.F., De Virgilio C., Tyers M., Andrews B., Gerstein M., Schweitzer B., Predki P.F. and Snyder M. (2005) Global analysis of protein phosphorylation in yeast. *Nature.* **(438):** 679–684.

99. Raitio M., Lindroos K., Laukkanen M., Pastinen T., Sistonen P., Sajantila A. and Syvänen A.C. (2001) Y-chromosomal SNPs in Finn-Ugric-speaking populations analysed by minisequencing on microarrays. *Genome. Res.* **(11):** 471-482

100. Rauch A., Rüschendorf F., Huang J., Trautmann U., Becker C., Thiel C., Jones K.W., Reis A., Nürnberg P. (2004) Molecular karyotyping using an SNP array for genomewide genotyping. *J. Med. Genet.* **(41):** 916-922.

101. Rimm D.L., Camp R.I., Charette L.A., Olsen D.A. and Provost E. (2001) Amplification of tissue by construction of tissue microarrays. *Exp. and Mol. Path.* **(70):** 255-264.

102. Sabbadini M., Barisani D., Conforti E., Marozzi A., Ginelli E., Miserocchi G. and Meneveri R. (2003) Gene expression analysis in interstitial lung edema induced by saline infusion. *Biochim. Biophys. Acta.* **(1638):** 149-156.

103. Sayama K., Diehn M., Matsuda K., Lunderius C., Tsai M., Tam S.Y., Botstein D., Brown P.O. and Galli S.J. (2002) Transcriptional response of human mast cells stimulated via the Fc (epsilon) RI and identification of mast cells as a source of IL-11. *BMC Immunol.* 3 **(1):** 5.

104. Schena M. (2003) *Microarray Analysis. Hoboken*, NJ: Wiley-Liss. p. 630.

105. Schena M., Shalon D., Davis R.W. and Brown P.O. (1995) Quantitative monitoring of gene expression patterns with a complementary DNA microarray. *Science.* **(270):** 467-470

106. Smyth G.K. and Speed T. (2003) Normalization of cDNA microarray data. *Methods.* **(31):** 265-273.

107. Solomon E. and Bodmer W. F. (1979) Evolution of sickle variant gene (letter). *Lancet.* **(1):** 923.

108. Southern E.M. (1975) Detection of specific sequences among DNA fragments separated by gel electrophoresis. *J. Mol. Biol.* **(98):** 503-517.

109. Southern E.M. (2001) DNA Microarrays. History and overview. *Methods Mol. Biol.* **(170):** 1-15.

110. Southern E.M., Case-Green S.C., Elder J.K., Johnson M., Mir K.U., Wang L. and Williams J.C. (1994) Arrays of complementary oligonucleotides for analyzing the hybridisation behaviour of nucleic acids. *Nucleic. Acids. Res.* **(22):** 1368-1373.

111. Speer R., Wulfkuhle J.D., Liotta L.A., and Petricoin E.F. (2005) Reverse-phase protein microarrays for tissue-based analysis. *Curr. Opin. Mol. Ther.* **(7):** 240-245.

112. Spellman P.T., Sherlock G., Zhang M.Q., Iyer V.R., Anders K., Eisen M.B., Brown P.O., Botstein D. and Futcher B. (1998) Comprehensive identification of cell cycle-regulated genes of the yeast *Saccharomyces cerevisiae* by microarray hybridization. *Mol. Biol. Cell.* **(9):** 3273-3297.

113. Stillman B.A. and Tonkinson J.L. (2000) FAST slides: a novel surface for microarrays. *Biotechniques.* **(29):** 630-635.

114. Stoll D., Bachmann J., Templin M.F. and Joos T.O. (2004) Microarray technology: an increasing variety of screening tools for proteomic research. DDT: Targets **(3):** 24-31.

115. Storey J.D. and, Tibshirani R. (2003) Statistical significance for genomewide studies. *PNAS.* **(100):** 9440-9445.

116. Straub T.M. and Chandler D.P. (2003) Towards a unified system for detecting waterborne pathogens. J. *Microbiol. Methods.* **(53):** 185-197.

117. Streelman J.T. and Kocher T.D. (2000) From phenotype to genotype. *Evol. Dev.* **(2):** 166-173.

118. Temple R., Allen E., Fordham J., Phipps S., Schneider H.C., Lindauer K., Hayes I., Lockey J., Pollock K. and Jupp R. (2001) Microarray analysis of eosinophils reveals a number of candidate survival and apoptosis genes. *Am. J. Respir. Cell. Mol. Biol.* **(25):** 425-33.

119. Templin M.F., Stoll D., Schrenk M., Traub P.C., Vohringer C.F. and Joos T.O. (2002) Protein microarray technology. *Trends Biotechnol.* **(20):** 160-166.

120. Tusher V.G., Tibshirani R. and Chu G. (2001) Significance analysis of microarrays applied to the ionizing radiation response. *Proc. Natl. Acad. Sci. U S A.* **(98):** 5116-5121.

121. Tzouvelekis A., Patlakas G. and Bouros D. (2004) Application of microarray technology in pulmonary diseases. *Respiratory Research.* **(5):** 26-44.

122. Tzouvelekis A., Patlakas G. and Bouros D. (2004) Application of microarray technology in pulmonary diseases. *Resp. Res.* **(5):** 26.

123. Vermeesch J.R. and Rauch A. (2006) Reply to Hochstenbach *et al. Eur. J. Hum. Gen.* **(14):** 1063-1064.

124. Vermeesch J.R., Fiegler H., de Leeuw N., Szuhai K., Schoumans J., Ciccone R., Speleman F., Rauch A., Clayton-Smith J., Ravenswaaij C.V., Sanlaville D., Patsalis P.C., Firth H., Devriendt K. and Zuffardi O. (2007) Guidelines for molecular karyotyping in constitutional genetic diagnosis. *Eur. J. Hum. Gen.* **(15):** 1105-1114.

125. Vermeesch J.R., Melotte C., Froyen G., Vooren S.V., Dutta B., Maas N., Vermeulen S., Menten B., Speleman F., Moor B.D., Hummelen P.V., Marynen P., Fryns J.P. and Devriendt Koen (2005) Molecular karyotyping: array CGH quality criteria for constitutional genetic diagnosis. *J. Hist. Cyto.* 53 **(3):** 413-422.

126. Vrana K.E., Freemany W.M. and Aschner M. (2003) Use of microarray technologies in toxicology research. *Neuro Toxicology.* **(24):** 321-332.

127. Vuillemenot B.R., Rodriguez J.F. and Hoyle G.W. (2004) Lymphoid tissue and emphysema in the lungs of transgenic mice inducibly expressing tumor necrosis factor-alpha. *Am. J. Respir. Cell. Mol. Biol.* **(30):** 438-48.
128. Wagner A. (2000) Decoupled evolution of coding region and mRNA expression patterns after gene duplication: implications for the neutralist-selectionist debate. *Proc. Natl. Acad. Sci. USA.* **(97):** 6579-6584.
129. Workman P. (2000) Towards genomic cancer pharmacology: innovative drugs for the new millenium. *Curr. Opin. Oncol. Endocr. Metab. Invest Drugs.* **(2):** 21-25.
130. Workman P. and Clarke P.A. (2001) Innovative cancer drug targets: genomics, transcriptomics and clinomics. *Expert Opin. Pharmacother.* **(2):** 911-915.
131. Xie T., Tong L., Barrett T., Yuan J., Hatzidimitriou G., McCann U.D., Becker K.G., Donovan D.M. and Ricaurte G.A. (2002) Changes in gene expression linked to methamphetamineinduced dopaminergic neurotoxicity. *J. Neurosci.* **(22):** 274-283.
132. Yadav S.K., Pareek S.L.S. and Pareek A. (2006) Transcriptome analysis. *Techniques in Soil Microbiology.* Eds. Varma, A. and Oelmuller. Springer Verlag.
133. Yamanaka Y., Tamari M., Nakahata T. and Nakamura Y. (2001) Gene expression profiles of human small airway epithelial cells treated with low doses of 14- and 16-membered macrolides. *Biochem Biophys. Res. Commun.* **(287):** 198-203.
134. Yang Y.H., Dudoit S., Luu P., Lin D.M., Peng V., Ngai J. and Speed T.P. (2002) Normalization for cDNA microarray data: a robust composite method addressing single and multiple slide systematic variation. *Nucleic Acids Research.* 30 e15.
135. Zhu H., Bilgin M. and Snyder M. (2003) Proteomics. *Annu. Rev. Biochem.* **(72):** 783-812.
136. Zhu H., Bilgin M., Bangham R., Hall D., Casamayor A., Bertone P., Lan N., Jansen R., Bidlingmaier S., Houfek T., Mitchell T., Miller P., Dean R.A., Gerstein M. and Snyder M. (2001) Global analysis of protein activities using proteome chips. *Science.* **(293):** 2101-2105.
137. Zhu H., Hu S., Jona G., Zhu X., Kreiswirth N., Willey B.M., Mazzulli T., Liu G., Song Q., Chen P., Cameron M., Tyler A., Wang J., Wen J., Chen W., Compton S. and Snyder M. (2006) Severe acute respiratory syndrome diagnostics using a coronavirus protein microarray. *Proc. Natl. Acad. Sci. U S A.* **(103):** 4011-4016.
138. Zhu H., Klemic J.F., Chang S., Bertone P., Casamayor A., Klemic K.G., Smith D., Gerstein M., Reed M.A. and Snyder M. (2000) Analysis of yeast protein kinases using protein chips. *Nat. Genet.* 26:283-289.
139. Zuo F., Kaminski N., Eugui E., Allard J., Yakhini Z., Ben-Dor A., Lollini L., Morris D., Kim Y., DeLustro B., Sheppard D., Pardo A., Selman M. and Heller R.A. (2002a) Gene expression analysis reveals matrilysin as a key regulator of pulmonary fibrosis in mice and humans. *Proc. Natl. Acad. Sci. USA.* **(99):** 6292-6297.
140. Zuo J., Young S., Zhu F., Gheyas F., Skeans S., Wan Y., Wang L., Ding W., Billah M., McClanahan T., Coffman R.L., Egan R. and Umland S. (2002.b) Microarray profile of differentially expressed genes in a monkey model of allergic asthma. *Genome Biol.* 3 **(5):** 0020.

CHAPTER

13

Antisense Technology

Antisense RNA and DNA techniques have been developed as a relatively recent approach to the specific modulation of gene expression *in vitro* and *in vivo*. The purpose of this chapter is to lay the foundation of basic concepts and practical uses of antisense technology in medical, veterinary, agricultural sciences and industrial applications.

Keywords: Antisense technology, antisense-oligo-nucleotides, gene silencing, gene expression, phosphorothioates.

INTRODUCTION

Antisense technologies are a suite of techniques that, together, form a very powerful tool for studying gene function (functional genomics) and for discovering new and more specific treatments of diseases in humans, animals and plants (antisense therapeutics). A conventional definition of antisense refers to the laboratory manipulation and/or modification of DNA or RNA so that its components (nucleotides) form a complementary copy of normal, or "sense," messenger RNA (mRNA). The binding or hybridization of antisense nucleic acid sequences to a specific mRNA target will, through a number of different mechanisms, interrupt normal cellular processing of the genetic message of a gene. This interruption, sometimes referred to as "knock-down" or "knock-out" depending upon whether or not the message is either partially or completely eliminated, allows researchers to determine the function of that gene. Three types of anti-mRNA strategies can be distinguished. Firstly, the use of single-stranded antisense-oligonucleotides; secondly, the triggering of RNA cleavage through catalytically active oligonucleotides referred to as ribozymes; and thirdly, RNA interference induced by small interfering RNA molecules (Figure 13.1). The overall goal in introducing an antisense agent into cells either *in vitro* or *in vivo* is to suppress or completely block the production of the gene product. This means that at some point in the transition from DNA sequence to amino acid sequence, the normal transcription and translation apparatus must be affected. Despite the seemingly simple idea to reduce translation by oligonucleotides complementary to an mRNA, several problems have to be overcome for successful application. Accessible sites of the target RNA for oligonucleotide binding have to be identified, antisense agents have to be protected against nucleolytic attack and their cellular uptake and correct intracellular localization have to be achieved. In addition, RNA-cleaving ribozymes, deoxyribozymes and the use of 21-mer double-stranded RNA molecules for RNA interference applications in mammalian cells offer highly efficient strategies to suppress the expression of a specific gene. In this chapter, a survey of the agents employed in antisense technologies will be presented along with a discussion of the various mechanisms they employ to achieve the goal of reducing or eliminating normal processing of a gene of interest.

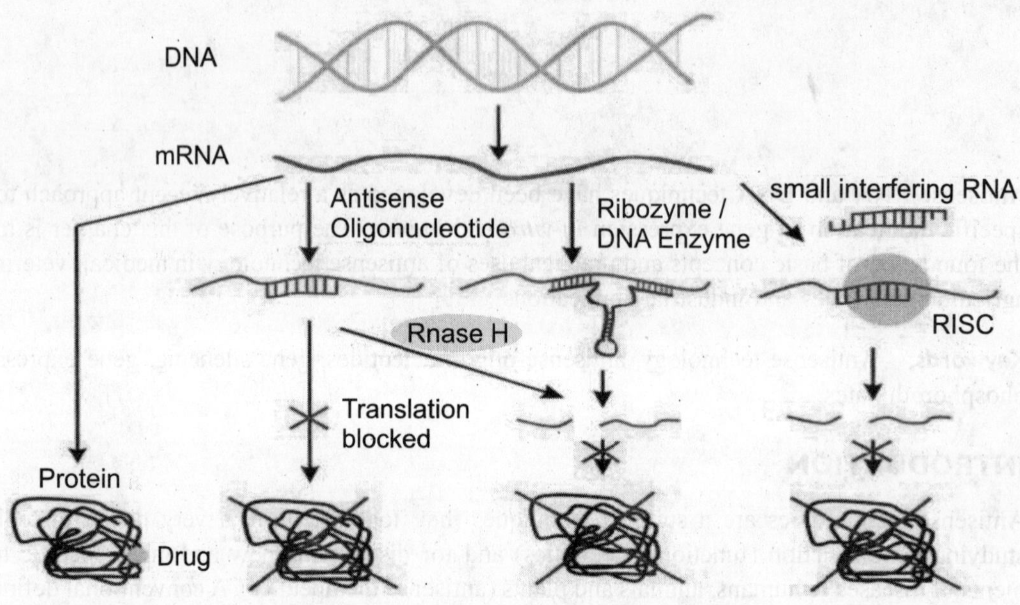

Figure 13.1 Comparison of different antisense strategies. While most of the conventional drugs bind to proteins, antisense molecules pair with their complementary target RNA. Antisense-oligonucleotides block translation of the mRNA or induce its degradation by RNase H, while ribozymes and DNA enzymes possess catalytic activity and cleave their target RNA. RNA interference approaches are performed with siRNA molecules that are bound by the RISC and induce degradation of the target mRNA (Source: Kurreck, 2003).

Among several possible strategies for inactivating a single, chosen gene, the most approved one is antisense technology. This modification does not involve actual subtraction but inactivation of gene or suppressing gene activity. When the DNA strand is normally transcribed, the RNA produced is called sense RNA, complementary to DNA, but if the orientation of gene to be transcribed is reversed with respect to promoter, the RNA transcribed from it would be reversed too, and the RNA produced so has sequence same to that of antisense strand of the normal gene, thus known as antisense RNA (asRNA). The basis of antisense technology is the use of antisense RNA. The gene to be cloned is ligated into the vector in reverse orientation. Thus on transcription, the RNA synthesized is reverse complement of the mRNA transcribed from normal version of gene, and being complementary to each other, they will pair to form a hybrid. Thus this makes mRNA unavailable for translation and the resulting double-stranded RNA molecule is degraded by specific ribonucleases.

Antisense refers to short DNA or RNA sequences, termed oligonucleotides, which are designed to be complementary to a specific gene sequence. The goal is to alter specific gene expression resulting from the binding of the antisense oligonucleotide to unique gene sequences. The antisense effect of a synthetic oligonucleotide sequence was first demonstrated in the late 1970s by Zamecnik and Stephenson (1978). Using nucleotide sequences from the 5′ and 3′ ends of the 35S RNA of Rous sarcoma virus (RSV), Zamecnik and Stephenson identified a repeated sequence of 21 nucleotides (nt) that appeared to be crucial to viral integration. They correctly concluded that the oligonucleotide was inhibiting viral integration by hybridizing to the crucial sequences and blocking them. Simultaneous other groups, notably Tennant *et al.* (1973) and Miller *et al.* (1977) also reported similar effects for synthetic oligonucleotides in other systems. Moreover, Matsukura and colleagues demonstrated that phosphorothioated oligonucleotides were effective hybridons against HIV replication in cultured cells.

The impact of biotechnology on antisense technology is expected to increase dramatically as the links between genetics, protein production and disease are better understood. Currently, antisense technology is used to design therapeutic compounds, which target specific mRNA sequences to obstruct the production of certain disease-causing proteins. Traditional drug therapies focus on a drug's interaction with the disease-causing proteins. However, antisense drug therapies inhibit the production of the disease-causing proteins altogether. Applications of antisense technology in therapeutics are expected to increase substantially as the link between diseases and genes are being discovered. Antisense drug therapies are currently unavailable in Canada. However, there are numerous antisense therapies in development, some of which are in clinical trials, and one of which has been approved for use in the United States.

CONCEPTS

Clearly, the antisense concept derives from an understanding of nucleic acid structure and function and depends on Watson-Crick hybridization. Thus, arguably, the demonstration that nucleic acid hybridization is feasible and the advances in *in situ* hybridization and diagnostic probe technology laid the most basic elements of foundation supporting the antisense concept.

However, the first clear enunciation of the concept of exploiting antisense oligonucleotides as therapeutic agents was in the work of Zameenik and Stephenson in 1978. They had synthesized an oligodeoxyribonuleotide, 13 nucleotides long, which was complementary to a sequence in the respiratory syncytial virus genome. They suggested that this oligonucleotide could be stabilized by 3′ and 5′ terminal modifications and showed evidence of antiviral activity. More importantly, they discussed possible sites for binding in RNA and mechanisms of action of oligonucleotide.

Though less precisely focused on the therapeutic potential of antisense oligonucleotides, the work of Miller and their collaborators during the same period helped establish the foundation for antisense research and reestablish an interest in phosphate backbone modifications as approaches to improve the properties of oligonucleotides. Their focus on methyl phosphotriester-modified oligonucleotides as a potential medicinal chemical solution to pharmacokinetic limitations of oligonucleotides presages a good bit of the medicinal chemistry to be performed on oligonucleotides.

Despite the observations of Miller and Zameenik, interest in antisense research was quite limited until the late 1980s when advances in several areas provided technical solutions to a number of impediments. As antisense drug design requires an understanding of the sequence of the RNA target, the explosive growth in the availability of viral and human genomic sequences provided the information from which "receptor sequences" could be selected. The development of method for synthesis of research quantities of oligonucleotide drugs then supported antisense experiments on both phosphodiester and modified oligonucleotides. The inception of the third key component (medicinal chemistry) forming the foundation of oligonucleotide therapeutics, in fact, is the synthesis in 1969 of phosphorothioate poly rI; poly rC as a mean of stabilizing the polynucleotide. Subsequently, Miller and Ts'o initiated studies on the neutral phosphate analogs, methylphosphonates, and groups at the National Institute of Health and the Food and Drug Administration and the Worcester Foundation investigated phosphorothionate oligonucleotides. With these advances forming the foundation for oligonucleotide therapeutics and the initial studies suggesting *in vitro* activities against a number of viral and mammalian targets, interest in oligonucleotide therapeutic intensified.

PRINCIPLES

In principle, antisense technology is supposed to prevent protein production from a targeted gene. The exact mechanism by which this occurs remains uncertain. Proposed mechanisms include triplex formation, blocking RNA splicing, preventing transport of the mRNA antisense complex into the cytoplasm, increasing RNA degradation, or blocking the initiation of translation (Figure 13.2). Initially, cellular nucleases dramatically reduced the effectiveness of antisense oligonucleotides by rapidly degrading these molecules after administration. These obstacles can be overcome in applications utilizing synthetic oligonucleotides by altering the nature of the phosphodiester bond by replacing oxygen with sulfur. Such modified oligonucleotides are termed phosphorothionates. Delivery of antisense oligonucleotides into target cells or the cell nucleus has been problematic. The variety of viral and non-viral delivery systems previously discussed is currently being explored to overcome this obstacle. Animals treated with antisense oligonucleotides have had significant side effects, some of which have been lethal. Currently, the most problematic aspect associated with antisense technology revolves around the specificity of their action. In some cases, non-specific

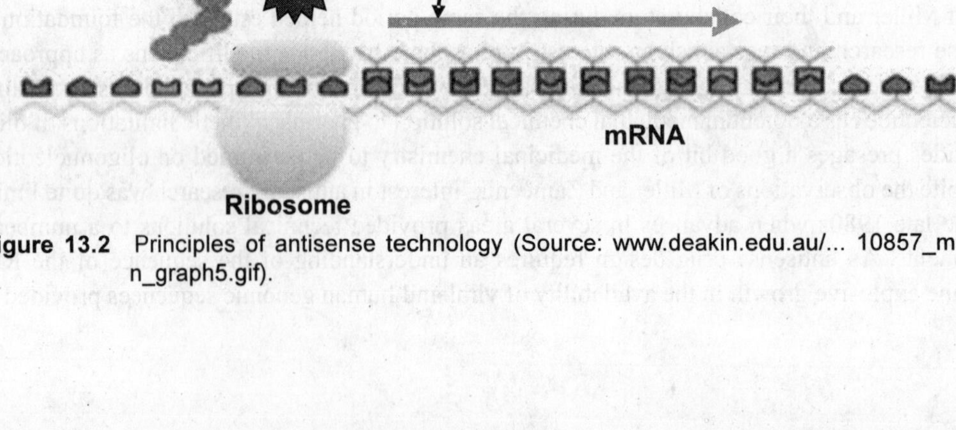

Figure 13.2 Principles of antisense technology (Source: www.deakin.edu.au/... 10857_mru_n_graph5.gif).

antisense sequences, in other words, sequences which do not bind to the targeted gene or RNA, have prevented gene expression to the same degree as their sequence-specific antisense counterparts. This has led to considerable complication in data interpretation and requires detailed and careful data analysis before contemplation of clinical trials. Since antisense technology focuses on preventing gene expression, it has been most widely applied in cancer gene therapy.

ANTISENSE TECHNOLOGY

Antisense technology was first effectively used in plants to alter the levels of various degradative enzymes or plant pigments. The technology was rapidly applied to mammalian cells and in 1992 *Science* named antisense its runner-up in the molecule of the year award.

What is Antisense Technology?

In antisense technology, synthetically-produced complementary molecules seek out and bind to messenger RNA, blocking the final step of protein production. mRNA is the nucleic acid molecule that carries genetic information from the DNA to the other cellular machinery involved in protein production. By binding to mRNA, the antisense drugs interrupt and inhibit the production of specific disease-related proteins. "Sense" refers to the original sequence of the DNA or RNA molecule. "Antisense" refers to the complementary sequence of the DNA or RNA molecule.

How Does Antisense Technology Work?

While traditional drug therapies are based on designing compounds that block or inhibit disease-causing proteins, antisense therapies focus on preventing the production of disease-causing proteins. Antisense drugs are based on small DNA-like or RNA-like constructs that bind to the protein-coding strand of genetic message (mRNA), blocking the translation of the disease-causing protein. By binding to mRNA, antisense drugs prevent the genetic code from being read by the ribosome, which is responsible for translating and manufacturing proteins. Additionally, the bound antisense/mRNA complex is enzymatically degraded so the protein cannot be synthesized (Figure 13.3).

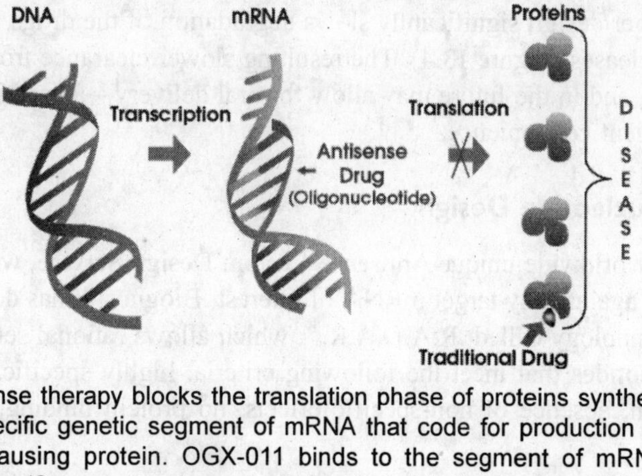

Figure 13.3 Antisense therapy blocks the translation phase of proteins synthesis by binding to the specific genetic segment of mRNA that code for production of a specific disease-causing protein. OGX-011 binds to the segment of mRNA that code for clusterin (Source: employees.csbsju.edu/.../bind/antisense.GIF).

Evolution of Antisense Technology

The first researchers who worked on antisense technology saw the possibilities of new methods of drug design. However, that promise has not yet been fully realized. First-generation drugs have demanded daily, intravenous dosing, and their lower specificity for their target mRNA keeps them from being as potent as is desirable. New developments in the chemistry of antisense give further hope for developing potent, long-lasting antisense therapies that are administered more conveniently. The first antisense constructs studied were based on the natural backbone structure of DNA. These constructs had an extremely high affinity for their target sequences. However, structures based on naturally occurring DNA are subject to swift degradation by nucleases and proved to be unsuitable for therapeutic uses. In an effort to make antisense technology more amenable to therapeutic use, scientists attempted to alter the backbone of the antisense molecules. The first successful backbone chemistry modified the phosphodiester structure in the DNA backbone to a phosphorothioate structure, which increased the construct's stability and made the technology more amenable to therapeutic use. However, these constructs still had plasma half lives of only hours, and the modified DNA backbone decreased the affinity of the antisense molecule to its target mRNA sequence. To increase the stability of the antisense compound, a second-generation chemistry was developed, adding the 2'MOE (2'-methoxyethyl) modification to the oligonucelotide backbone. A further improvement incorporates both first-generation and second-generation chemistries into "gapmers": antisense sequences that have their ends modified with 2'MOE chemistry while retaining at their centers first-generation chemistry. The 2'MOE modified ends protect the construct from degradation, giving significantly improved half life and binding affinity, while the first generation center permits enzymatic degradation of the mRNA/antisense complex. Gapmer second-generation chemistry drugs have increased half-lives of 5- to 10-fold over first-generation chemistry and increased affinity to target mRNA. The improved affinity of second-generation drugs is primarily attributable to their design and composition. Second-generation drugs are composed of both RNA-like and DNA-like nucleotides, while first-generation drugs are entirely DNA-like. Since RNA hybridizes more tightly to RNA than DNA, the second-generation drugs have a greater affinity for their RNA targets and, therefore, greater potency. With increased potency, second-generation drugs are more active at lower doses. Additionally, second-generation chemistry with gapmer design significantly slows degradation of the drugs by protecting the drug from destructive nucleases (Figure 13.4). The resulting slower clearance from the body allows for less frequent dosing, and in the future may allow for oral delivery—a useful feature for long-term use given added patient convenience.

Antisense Oligonucleotide Design

Biognostik offers a worldwide unique Antisense Custom Design Service, which selects optimized antisense sequences against any target mRNA of interest. Biognostik has developed a proprietary sequence design technology called .R.A.D.A.R.®, which allows rational selection of high quality antisense oligonucleotides that meet the following criteria: highly specific, functional *via* a true antisense mechanism, absence of non-specific effects, no protein binding, good cellular uptake

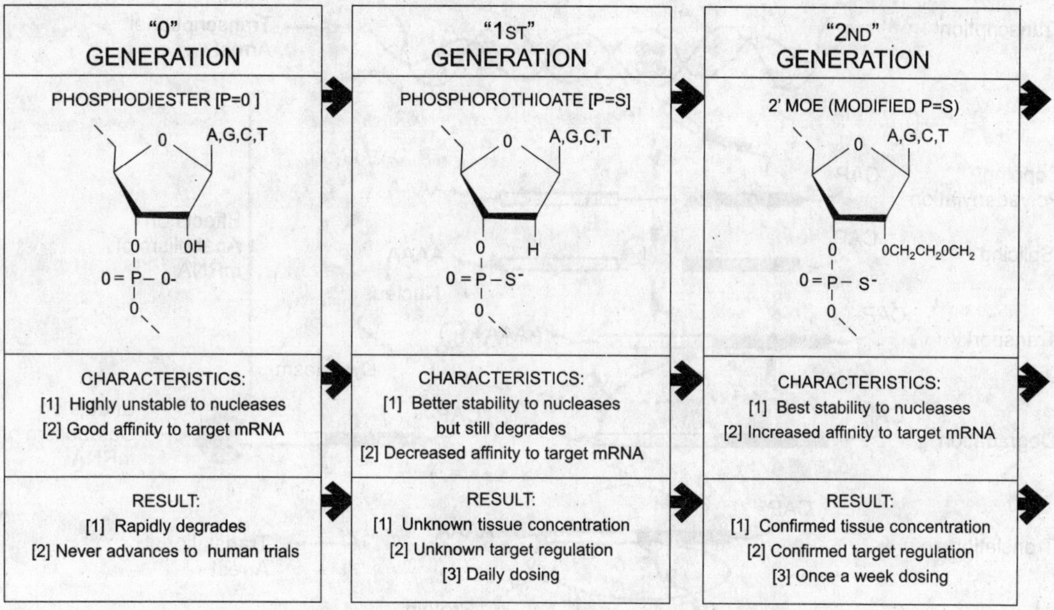

Figure 13.4 Evolution of synthetic antisense oligonucleotides (Source: Crooke, 2004).

pattern and stabilization by phosphorothioate backbone modifications. R.A.D.A.R.® design combines computer aided sequence analysis, molecular modeling and comparison to a core data base in which analysis data of over 3000 antisense sequences are archived.

APPLICATIONS OF ANTISENSE TECHNOLOGY

Antisense technology has potential applications in medical, veterinary, agricultural sciences and industries. Some of the important applications of antisense technology are discussed below.

Medical Applications

Diseases are often connected to the insufficient or excess production of certain proteins. If the production of these proteins is disrupted, many diseases can be treated or cured. Antisense technology is a method that can disrupt protein production. It may be used to design new therapeutics for diseases in whose pathology the production of a specific protein plays a crucial role.

Antisense technology may play a major role in cancer chemotherapy. It is clearly a tool of exceptional value in the fictionalization of genes and their validation as potential targets for cancer therapy. Additionally, there is now substantial voidance that antisense drugs are safe, and a growing body of data showing activity to animal models of human diseases including cancer and suggesting efficacy in patients with cancer. Antisense technology is arguably the most advanced genomically based drug discovery technology. It has been shown to be capable of generating very specific inhibitors, and a significant number of antisense drugs are in development as anticancer agents.

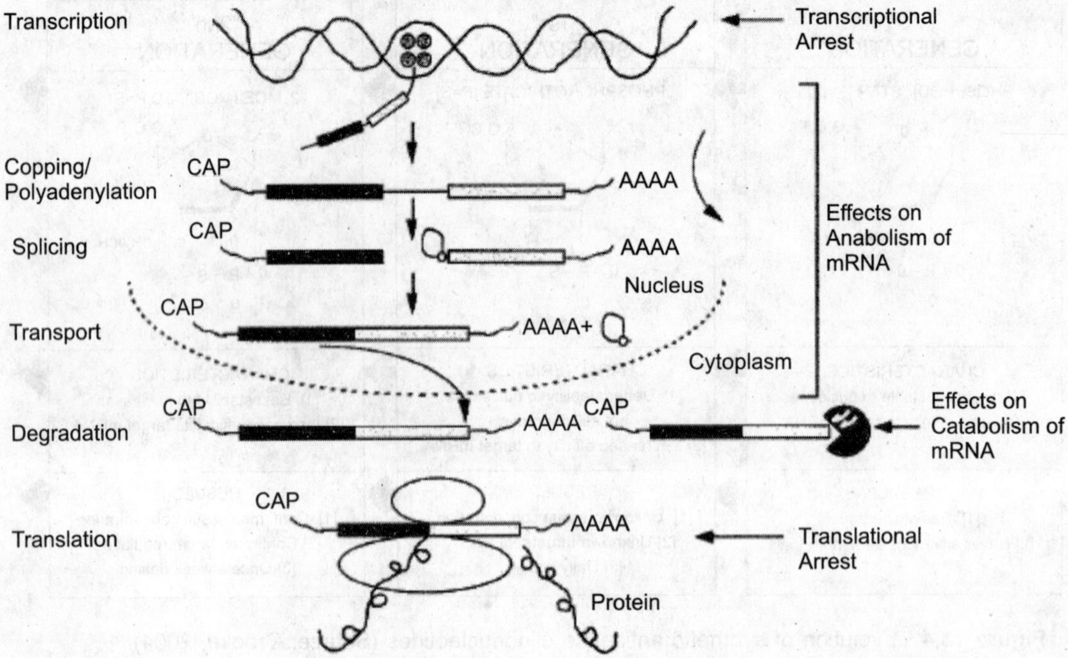

Figure 13.5 Pre-mRNA is transcribed from a gene. It is then processed through a carefully choreographed set of steps to the mature mRNA which is exported to the cytoplasm. These steps include 5' and 3' modifications, (5' cap: 3' poly A) splicing and specific transport activities. Numerous mechanisms of action for antisense drugs have been identified and they affect many steps post transcription and/or enhance cellular degradation of the RNA (Source: Kurreck, 2003).

A number of potential mechanisms by which antisense drugs may work have been identified (Figure 13.5) and they have been partitioned into two broad groups: occupancy only and occupancy activated destabilization. Of the occupancy only mechanism, translation arrest and inhibition of splicing have been most extensively characterized. Occupancy-induced destabilization, as the target RNA, is epitomized by RNaseH degradation of the target RNA, and this mechanism is the most often used and least characterized antisense mechanism.

There are now a number of reports of antisense inhibition of human tumour zenograft and other animal models of human cancers. For many of these studies, appropriate controls, including a variety of mismatched oligonucleotides were used and there is evidence that the effect of the antisense agents were indeed due to an antisense mechanism. Human tumor zenografts have shown that it is feasible to reduce target RNA and protein levels and to induce antiproliferative effects in some of these models. Similar data has been reported by other groups.

Tamoxifen (TAM) is widely used in the treatment and prevention of breast cancer. There is a clear evidence that cytochrome P450 (CYP) 3A enzymes play an important role in TAM metabolism, resulting in metabolites that lead to the formation of TAM–DNA adducts. It has been reported that the effect of CYP3A2 antisense (AVI-4472) exposure on CYP3A2 transcription, enzyme activity, translation, and TAM–DNA adducts, in livers of rats resulted in down-regulation of several CYP genes, suggesting the utility of antisense technology in the redirection of TAM metabolism.

This approach of "metabolic redirection" builds on literature reports implicating the metabolic products of the CYP3A subfamily of enzymes in the genotoxicity of TAM. The utility of antisense phosphorodiamidate morpholino oligomers (PMO) in inhibiting the major CYP3A isoforms in rats and humans has been demonstrated previously.

In the past decade, substantial strides have been made in creating and validating antisense technology. There are several antisense drugs in clinical development that have shown some promise, but only added clinical trials will determine their true value. New generation of antisense drugs are in development and these may offer even more benefits to patients with cancer. If these can be coupled to better target focused decision making deriving from antisense target validation, perhaps even more benefit can accrue. Finally, the therapeutic index of antisense drugs supports their use in combination with traditional cytotoxics drugs or, potentially more exciting, the combination of antisense inhibitors with several different genes.

Antisense oligodeoxynucleotides (ODNs) inhibit target gene expression and are applicable to human diseases including malignancies. Although improvements in ODNs and cellular delivery systems are needed, antisense ODNs hold great promise as a new class of therapeutic agents. Blocking the expression of specific genes with antisense oligonucleotide (ODNs) may promote new therapies for many human diseases. The antisense ODN is usually designed as short (about 20 bp) single-stranded DNA directed to the mRNA of the target gene. Binding to a complementary mRNA sequence followed by prevention of its translation is a basic principle in this strategy. However, a number of mechanisms of antisense ODN actions can produce target gene nonspecific-effects. For example, the sequence can bind to DNA in the nucleus and block the transcription or interact with small molecules and proteins, including the Sp1 transcription factor leading to its activation. Such nonspecific-effects limit the conclusion that can be drawn from the results of the experiments using antisense ODNs. However, gene-specific effects were shown in *in vitro* experiments and animal models. Moreover, clinical trials have shown no remarkable toxicity and suggested therapeutic effects of antisense ODNs in Crohn's disease and malignant lymphoma. Thus, use of antisense ODNs may be still fascinating to explore as a way to treat viral infection, prevent organ allograft rejection, and eradicate malignancies.

Veterinary Applications

Antisense technology has potential applications in veterinary medicine and pharmaceuticals. Transgenic technologies are used for improving milk production and the meat in farm animals as well as for creating models of human diseases. Transgenic animals are used for the production of proteins for medical use. Biotechnology is applied to facilitate xenotransplantation from animals to humans. Genetic engineering is done in farm animals and nuclear transfer technology has become an important and preferred method for cloning animals.

Antisense technology has potential applications in the management of several animal diseases such as foot-and-mouth disease, classical swine fever, avian flu and bovine spongiform encephalopathy. The most important biotechnology-based products consist of vaccines, particularly genetically engineered or DNA vaccines. Gene therapy for diseases of pet animals is a fast developing area because many of the technologies used in clinical trials humans were developed in animals and many of the diseases of cats and dogs are similar to those in humans. RNA interference technology is now being applied for research in veterinary medicine. Molecular diagnosis is assuming an important place in veterinary practice. Polymerase chain reaction and its modifications are considered to be important. Fluorescent *in situ* hybridization and enzyme-linked immunosorbent assays are also widely used. Newer biochip-based technologies and biosensors are also finding their way in veterinary diagnostics. Biotechnology products are approved by the Center for Veterinary Medicine of the FDA. Regulatory issues relevant to animal biotechnology are described. Approximately 108 companies have been identified to be involved in animal biotechnology and are profiled in the report. These are a mix of animal healthcare and biotechnology companies. Share of biotechnology-based products and services in 2007 is analyzed and the market is projected to 2017.

Agricultural Applications

Genetic manipulations of fruit ripening

Controlling the rate of ripening in climacteric fruits is of prime importance in increasing their shelf life. The ripening process in climacteric fruits could not be controlled efficiently by various means such as modern storage facility, cool temperature storage, chemical sprays etc. once the ripening has been initiated. Therefore, molecular genetic approach such as antisense technology could be an ideal approach to control the ripening in climacteric fruits even after the ripening has set in. Ripening is a highly complex final phase of fruit development that involves the expression and regulation of hundreds of genes that can be used for manipulating fruit ripening. Some of the important genes are discussed below.

Genes related to ethylene biosynthesis: Small multi-gene families code for the ACS and ACO enzyme involved in the ethylene biosynthesis. It was observed that tomato fruits of transgenic plant carrying ACS in antisense orientation completely blocked the ripening by decreasing ethylene production to 99%, and these fruits did not ripen without exogenous ethylene. Similarly, anti-ACS apple showed reduced autocatalytic ethylene production and increased shelf life. Tomato fruits from transgenic tomato plants carrying tomato ACO in antisense orientation and melon fruits from transgenic melon plants carrying ACO from melon under the regulation of CaMV35S promoter showed a reduction in ethylene production and delayed ripening.

Genes related to cell wall softening: Several enzymes like polygalacturonase (PG), PME, expansin, cellulose, xyloglucanase etc. are implicated in wall softening during ripening. Transgenic homozygous tomato plants carrying PG gene in antisense orientation showed a reduced PG activity 1% of the normal value. It has been shown that in fruits with antisense PG, the degradation of cellular wall pectins was inhibited (Figure 13.6) but other aspects of maturation, such as ethylene production and lycopene accumulation were not affected. Ripened fruits from transgenic strawberry plants carrying pectate lyase from strawberry in antisense orientation under the expression of CaMV35S were significantly firmer than control fruits and this gene could be an excellent candidate for biotechnological improvement of fruit softening in strawberry. Suppression of Exp1 in tomato lead to firmer fruits as compared to wild type and also substantially inhibited polyuronide depolymerization late in ripening, but did not prevent the breakdown of structurally important hemicelluloses, a major contributor to softening. Antisense suppression of deoxyhypusine synthase in tomato delays fruit softening and alters growth and development. Transgenic strawberry plants carrying antisense pectate lyase cDNA from strawberry under the control of the 35S promoter showed significantly firmer ripened fruits than controls. Highest reduction of softening in these fruits occurred during the transition from the white to the red stage. The postharvest softening of apple fruit was also diminished.

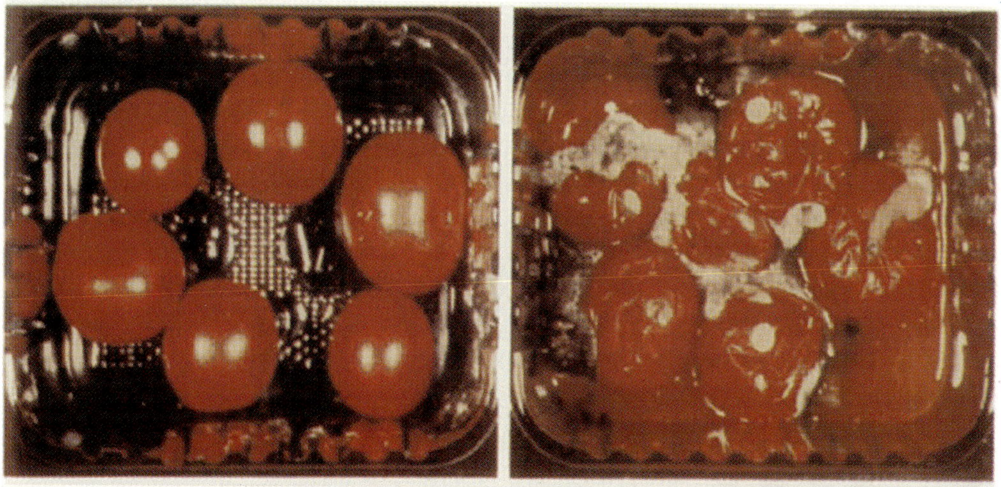

Figure 13.6 Antisense polygalacturonase transgenic tomato (left panel) and wild type (right panel) (Smith *et al.,* 1988).

Genes related to lycopene production: Lycopene possesses beneficial antioxidant properties due to which the researchers aimed to increase its content. Transgenic approaches were employed to increase tomato fruit lycopene content. Suppression of lycopene cyclase (*Lcy*) gene resulted in increased lycopene content in the transgenic tomato fruits. Suppression of *TDET1* (Tomato *DE-ETIOLATED1*) mRNA accumulation by RNA interference (RNAi) specifically in fruits using *TDET1*-derived inverted-repeat constructs driven by three different fruit-specific promoters, P119, 2A11 and TFM7 was shown to enhance the carotenoid and flavonoid content in mature fruit.

Modification of flower colour in decorative plants

Antisense technology can be used for producing decorative plants exhibiting one or more desired phenotypic traits by manipulating genes involved in flavonoid biosynthetic pathway (Figure 13.7a). The class of genes within the flavonoid biosynthetic pathway includes the nucleic acid sequences involved directly in reactions or control of reactions, which synthesize or modify a flavonoid compound whose functions in plants include coloration in flowers, fruits, leaves, and other organs. Examples of flavonoid biosynthetic genes include those for chalcone synthases, chalcone isomerases (CHI), flavanone 3-hydroxylases, dihydroflavonol reductases, flavanone 2-hydroxylases, dihydroflavanol 2-hydroxylases, flavonoid 3'-hydroxylases, flavonoid 5'-hydroxylases, flavonoid glycosyltransferases (including glucosyl transferases such as UDPG: flavonoid 3-O-glucosyl transferase and UDPG: flavonol 7-O-glucosyl transferase, and rhamnosyl transferases), flavonoid methyltransferases (such as SAM:anthocyanidin 3-(p-coumaroyl)-rutinoside-5-glucoside 3',5'-O-methyltransferase) and flavonoid acyltransferases. The biosynthetic pathways of these various pigments have been extensively studied in many different plant species. The chalcones and aurones are products requiring only the initial biosynthetic enzymes, being direct products of the earliest precursors. The flavones and flavonols are intermediate, and the anthocyanins are products requiring substantial modifications from the initial precursors. All of these products are dependent upon the activity of the initial enzyme, chalcone synthase (CHS), which catalyses the production of chalcone from three molecules of malonyl-coenzyme A and one molecule of coumaroyl-coenzyme A.

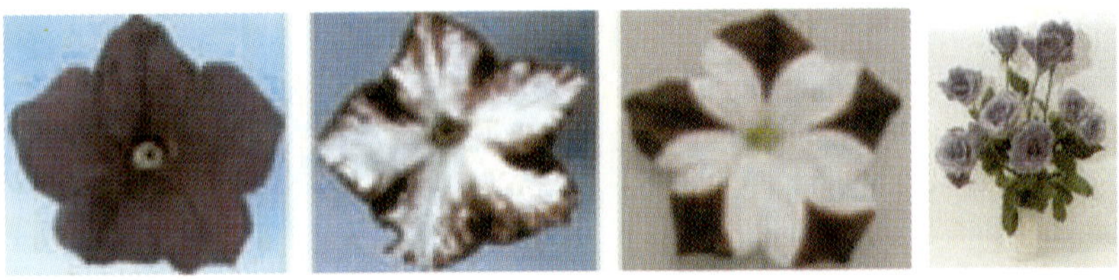

(A) (B)

Figure 13.7 (A) Petunia plants in which genes for pigmentation are silenced. The left plant is wild-type; the right plants contain transgenes that induce suppression of both transgene and endogenous gene expression, giving rise to the unpigmented white areas of the flower. (B) Modified Rosa x hybrida using a gene encoding chalcone synthase to alter the anthocyanin biosynthetic pathway (Source: Souq *et al.*, 1996).

In an effort to search for new flower colour, modified Rosa x hybrida using a gene encoding chalcone synthase to alter the anthocyanin biosynthetic pathway (Figure 13.7b). Enhanced resistance to powdery mildew was observed in GM Rosa x hybrid cv. Carefree Beauty modified with an antimicrobial protein gene. Genetically modified Rosa x hybrida rootstock cv. Moneyway containing rol genes from *A. rhizogenes* showed a threefold improvement in adventitious rooting of cuttings. Recent work on cloning and expression of 1-aminocyclopropane-1-caroxylate synthase from *Rosa* may lead to regulation of ethylene response in plants and potentially a longer vase life for roses, in which ethylene is a hormonal regulator of senescence of most plant organs.

Antisense SAHH gene for resistance against a broad spectrum of viruses in plants

Antisense SAHH gene was used, which conferred resistance against one specific virus. However, if we could inhibit the expression of a gene responsible for a non-essential host cell enzyme required for virus replication, we can get resistance against a broad spectrum of viruses. In one such effort, the enzyme S-adenosyl homocysteine hydrolase (SAUH) was chosen for manipulation. SAHH is responsible for several methylation reactions including 5'-cap mRNA methylation, where S-adenosyl-methionine is used as a methyl donor. If SAHH is inhibited, there will be under-methylation at the 5' end of viral mRNA leading to inhibition of viral replication. SAHH inhibitions have actually been used as antiviral agents and were found to suppress plant viruses in leaf disk assays. In a study reported in 1995, transgenic tobacco plants were produced which expressed antisense RNA against mRNA of a tobacco SAHH gene. This led to the reduction in SAHH level and consequent inhibition of viral replication/infection in the transgenic plants.

Mutant gene for a protein necessary for cell to cell movement of virus in the host plant

In certain viruses (e.g., white colour mosaic virus or WCIMV), there are genes that encode non-virion proteins necessary for cell to cell movement of the virus (but not necessary for viral replication). A mutation in one of these genes may hamper cell to cell movement of the virus. One such approach was used (reported in 1994), where a mutant version of a gene encoding WCIMV-13kDa protein was used for producing transgenic plants. The transgenic plants were found to be resistant to several viruses. The mutant transgene was found to be dominant over the normal gene of virus infecting the transgenic host.

Industrial Applications

Antisense is an important technology for drug discovery and development (Figure 13.8). It is broadly used by the pharmaceutical industry as a tool for functional genomics and as highly specific drugs for a wide range of diseases. Cumulative clinical and preclinical data suggest that antisense technology has the potential to create a new sector of the pharmaceutical industry. After 20 years of technology refinement, antisense is a mature drug discovery and therapeutic platform. Several

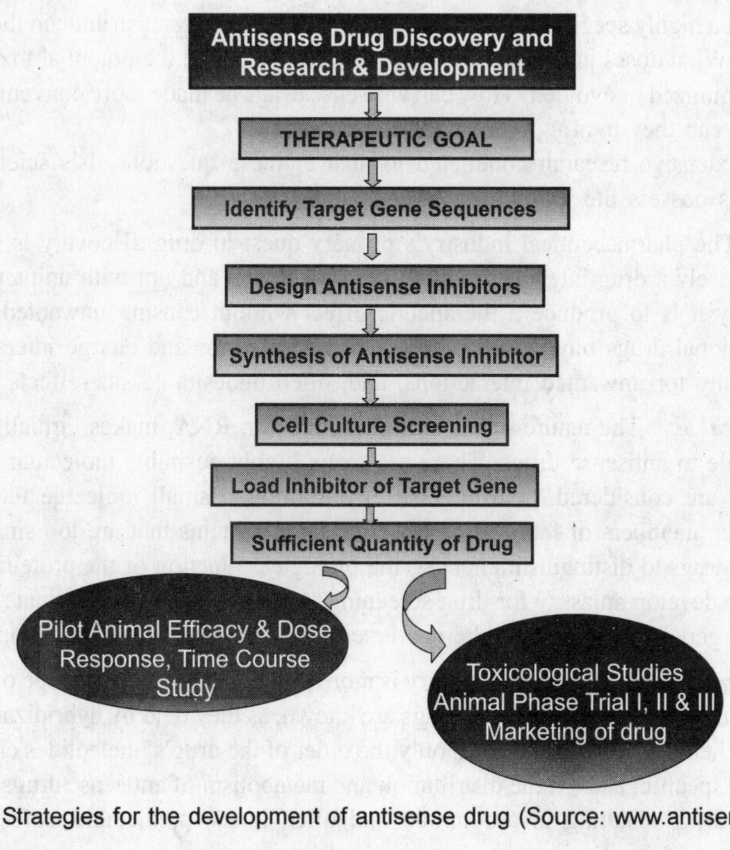

Figure 13.8 Strategies for the development of antisense drug (Source: www.antisense. com).

antisense drugs are now in late stage clinical development with one antisense drug developed by Isis, Vitravene®, marketed in the US and Europe. Antisense inhibitors can target specific aspects of ocular disease processes and have ideal properties as therapies for the eye. Antisense drugs have already been shown to be effective in treating ocular diseases with the commercialization of Vitravene®, approved for the treatment of CMV Retinitis.

With access to Isis Pharmaceuticals' proprietary drug discovery process as illustrated in the Figure 13.8, Antisense Therapeutics Limited can move quickly from drug discovery into developing therapies. Once we have identified a therapeutic application and corresponding gene target, an antisense lead inhibitor compound can be rationally designed within hours suitable for use in research and clinical trials. This compares with traditional drug discovery approaches that can take years to produce such a lead compound. Antisense drug development also benefits from uniform methods of manufacture, formulation and delivery of antisense compounds. At the same time, the explosion of genetic information provided by the completion of the Human Genome Project (HGP) provides a rich resource of information on target genes for the design of antisense drugs. Vitravene is a registered trademark of Novartis AG.

Isis scientists have worked systematically and rigorously to address the questions associated with the development of this new drug discovery platform. Do antisense drugs interact with their RNA targets in a highly specific manner? Where do antisense drugs distribute in the body? Do they get into cells? What doses produce therapeutic effects? What are the potential toxicities, and how can they be minimized or avoided? How can antisense drugs be made more convenient for patients? What diseases can they treat?

Based on extensive research conducted to answer these questions, Isis scientists know that antisense drugs possess the following characteristics:

Specificity: The pharmaceutical industry's primary quest in drug discovery is drug specificity. The more precisely a drug interacts with its intended target, and not with unintended molecules, the more likely it is to produce a therapeutic effect without causing unwanted side-effects. In contrast, traditional drugs bind based on the shape of proteins and charge interactions, creating more opportunity for unwanted interactions, and, often undesirable side-effects.

Broadly applicable: The nature of the antisense receptor, RNA, makes virtually any molecular target accessible to antisense drugs. There are many highly desirable molecular targets for drug discovery that are considered "undruggable" by traditional small molecule technology. These targets are often members of families of closely related proteins that are too similar in structure for traditional drugs to distinguish amongst, the biological function of the protein is unknown, or it is difficult to develop an assay for drug screening. Antisense drugs discriminate between targets based on their genetic sequence, so the universe of potential targets is significantly greater.

Rational design: Antisense drug discovery is more rational than any other type of drug discovery because: (1) the rules for creating these drugs are known, as they bind by hybridization to the target RNA; (2) the chemistry is constant, with only the order of the drug's nucleotides changing to make the drug target specific; and (3) the distribution and metabolism of antisense drugs are very similar from drug to drug, resulting in a common and often times, predictable, safety profile across antisense drugs.

Efficiency: The benefit of a more rational approach to drug discovery is efficiency. The efficiency of antisense results in shortened timelines to identify lead drug candidates in the discovery phase of development. The consistency of the behavior of antisense drugs allows Isis scientists to apply what they learn from the testing of one drug to future drugs, thus reducing the potential for failure in the early stages of development and creating significant competitive advantage for the platform.

Redirection of drug metabolism using antisense technology

The cytochrome P450 (CYP) family is the most catalytically versatile component of the phase I oxidation metabolic pathway and participates in the metabolism of a large majority of drugs used in clinical practice. The inhibition of specific enzymes of this family can significantly alter the disposition and toxicity of substrate drugs by reducing and/or redirecting their metabolism. It is reported that the approaches available for CYP inhibition, with particular emphasis on the potential use of antisense phosphorodiamidate morpholino oligonucleotide strategies to inhibit human CYP3A4. Inter-individual variations of 10- to 50-fold have been reported in the activity of CYP3A4 enzyme, which contributes to the metabolism of more than half of all clinically relevant drugs. The application of antisense technology for inhibition of specific CYP enzymes can provide significant therapeutic benefits, including: (i) reduction of first-pass drug metabolism; (ii) reduction in drug dosage; (iii) selective reduction of toxic metabolites; and (iv) increased oral/topical drug bioavailability. The use of antisense morpholino oligonucleotide strategies to target CYP enzymes may result in safer and more uniform therapeutic applications.

Most pharmaceutical drugs available today interact with one or more proteins. They act to enhance or inhibit the action of a protein or mimic its role thereby bringing about the specified therapeutic effect. To date the pharmaceutical drugs on the market target a total of only about 500 different proteins. Although not all proteins will be suitable targets for therapeutic intervention, there is clearly enormous scope for drug discovery and new therapies in this post-genomic era, considering that the human genome codes for at least 30,000 different proteins. As technologies progress in the medical sciences, newer, more specific and rapid means of drug discovery are emerging—antisense is one of these emerging technologies. The rapid development of antisense technology offers almost unlimited scope for the development of new and highly specific therapeutics. Antisense therapeutics therefore is well positioned to play a significant role in the progression of antisense technology for drug development in human diseases.

CONCLUSION

Antisense technologies have been hailed as one of the best options for gene manipulation to be used in studying gene function and for discovering new and more specific treatments for a wide range of diseases in humans, animals, and plants. However, this success has been mainly restricted to laboratory and research organizations. There has been only one antisense drug in the market, even after almost three decades of research on antisense technologies. Its clinical applications thus far were barred by numerous problems and untrammeled challenges. Despite all the challenges, antisense therapy has held its ground for more than two decades and now it is ready to emerge as a potential tool for gene therapy. With more than a dozen molecules in the clinical development phases, the stage is set for antisense therapy to emerge as a potential option for treatment of a wide range of diseases. The antisense strategy of inhibiting gene expression has tremendous potential in the fields of functional genomics, drug discovery and therapy.

FURTHER READINGS

1. Agrawal S., Goodchild J., Civeira M.P., Thornton A.H., Sarin P.S. and Zamecnik P.C. (1988) Oligodeoxynucleoside phosphoramidates and phosphorothioates as inhibitors of human immunodeficiency virus. *Proc. Natl. Acad. Sci. USA.* 85 **(19):** 7079-7083.
2. Alvarado-Urbina G., Sarhe G.M., Liu W.C., Giller M.F, Duck P.D., Bender R. and Ogilvie K.K. (1981) Automated synthesis of gene fragments. *Science.* 214 **(4518):** 270-274.
3. Arora V. and Iversen P.L. (2001) Redirection of drug metabolism using antisense technology. *Current Opinion in Molecular Therapeutics.* **(3):** 249-257.
4. Ayub R., Guis M., Ben Amor M., Gillot L., Roustan J.P., Latche A, Bouzayen M. and Pech J.C. (1996) Expression of A.C.C. oxidase antisense gene inhibits ripening of cantaloupe melon fruits. *Nat. Biotechnol.* **(14):** 862-866.
5. Baker B and Monia B.P. (1999) Novel mechanisms for antisense-mediated regulation of gene expression. *Biochimica et Biophysica Acta.* **(1489):** 3-18.
6. Barrett J.C, Miller P.S. and Ts'o POP (1974) Inhibitory effect of complex formation with ologodeoxyribonucleotide ethyl phosphotriesters on transfer ribonucleic acid aminoacyiation. *Biochemistry* **(13):** 4897-4906.
7. Bost F., McKay R., Dean N.M., Pota pova O. and Mercola D. (2000) Antisense methods for discrimination of phenotypic properties of closely related gene products: Jun kinase family. *Methods Enzymol.* **(314):** 342-362.
8. Brummell D.A. and Harpster M.H. (2001) Cell wall metabolism in fruit softening and quality and its manipulation in transgenic plants. *Plant Mol. Biol.* **(47):** 311-340.
9. Brummell D.A., Harpster M.H., Civello P.M., Palys J.M., Ben¬nett A.B. and Dunsmuir P. (1999) Modification of expansin protein abundance in tomato fruit alters softening and cell wall polymer metabolism during ripening. *Plant Cell.* **(11):** 2203-2216.
10. Caruthers M.H. (1985) Gene synthesis machines: D.N.A. chemistry and its uses. *Science.* 230 **(4723):** 281-285.
11. Clerq EDe, Eckstein F. and Merigan T.C. (1969) Interferon induction increased through chemical modification of a synthetic polyribonucleotide. *Science.* **(165):** 1137-1139.
12. Crooke S.T. (1998) *Basic Principles of Antisense Therapeutics, Antisense Research and Application,* Springer-Verlag, Berlin, Heidelber, New York, pp. 1-50.
13. Crooke S.T. (2000) Potential roles of antisense technology in cancer chemotherapy. *Oncogens.* **(19):** 6651-6659.
14. Crooke S.T. (2004), Progress in antisense technology. *Annual Review of Medicine.* **(55):** 61-95.
15. Dandekari A.M., Teo G., Defilippi B.G, Uratsu S.L., Passey A.J., Kader A.A., Stow J.R., Colgan R.J. and James D.J. (2004) Effect of down-regulation of ethylene biosynthesis on fruit flavor complex in apple fruit. Transgenic Res. **(13):** 373-384.
16. Devor E.J. (2005) I.D. Tutorial: Antisense Technologies. Integrated D.N.A. Technologies.
17. Dias N. and Stein C.A. (2002) Antisense Oligonucleotides: Basic Concepts and Mechanisms. *Molecular Cancer. Therapeutics.* **(1):** 347-355.
18. Fire A, S.Q. Xu, M.K. Montgomery, S.A. Kostas, S.E. Driver, and C.C. Mello (1998) Potent and specific genetic interference by double stranded R.N.A. in Caenorhabditis elegans. *Nature.* **(391):** 806-811.

19. Gao W., Stein C.A., Cohen J.S., Dutschman G.E. and Cheng Y.C. (1989) Effect of phosphorothioate homo-oligodeoxynucleotides on herpes simplex virus type 2-induced DNA polymerase. *J. Biol. Chem.* **(264):** 11521-11526.
20. Gillespie D. and Spiegelman S. (1965) A quantitative assay for DNA-RNA hybrids with DNA immobilized on a membrane. *J. Mol. Boil.* 12 **(3):** 829-842.
21. Goetz M.P., Knox S.K., Suman V.J., Rae J.M, Safgren S.L., Ames M.M., Visscher D.W., Reynolds C., Couch F.J., Lingle W.L., Weinshilboum R.M., Fritcher E.G, Nibbe A.M., Desta Z., Nguyen A., Flockhart D.A., Perez E. and Ingle J.N. (2007) The impact of cytochrome P450 2D6 metabolism in women receiving adjuvant tamoxifen. *Breast. Cancer. Res. Treat.* 101 **(1):** 113-21.
22. Goodchild J., Agrawal S., Civeira M.P., Sarin P.S., Sun D. and Zamecnik P.C. (1988) Inhibition of human immunodeficiency virus replication by antisense Oligo-deoxynucleotides. *Proc. Natl. Acad. Sci. USA* **(85):** 5507-5511.
23. Gupta S. M., Srivastava S., Sane A.P. and Nath P. (2006) Differential expression of genes during banana fruit development, ripening and 1-MCP treatment: presence of distinct fruit specific, ethylene induced and repressed expression. *Postharvest Biol. Technol.* **(42):** 16-22.
24. Gupta S. M., Srivastava S. Gupta S., and Ahmed Z. (2008) Genetic manipulation of fruit ripening: using antisense mRNA strategies. *J. of Applied Biosciences.* 34 **(2):** 115-123.
25. Gupta S., Kumar N., and Gupta S.M. (2009) Utility of chlorophyllose activity in mango (Mangijera indica) peil for assessing state of ripening. *Natl. Acad. Sci. Lett.* 32 **(182):** 15-17.
26. Hamilton A.J., Lycett G.W. and Grierson D. (1990) Antisense gene that inhibits synthesis of the hormone ehtylene in transgenic plants. *Nature.* **(346):** 284-287.
27. Haseloff J. and W.L. Gerlach (1988) Simple RNA enzymes with new and highly specific endoribonuclease activities. *Nature.* **(334):** 585-591.
28. Heidenreich Olaf, Kang Shin-Heh, Xu Xiao and Nerenberg Michael (1995) Application of antisense technology to therapeutics. *Molecular Medicine Today.* 1 **(3):** 128-133.
29. Herdewijn P. (2000) Heterocyclic modifications of oligonucleotides and antisense technology. *Antisense Nucleic Acids and Drug Development.* **(10):** 117-121.
30. Ito M.K. (2007) ISIS 301012 gene therapy for hypercholesterolemia: sense, antisense, or nonsense? *Ann Pharmacother.* 1 **(10):** 1669-78.
31. Jiménez-Bermúdez S., Redondo-Nevado J., Muñoz-Blanco J., Caballero J.L., López-Aranda J.M. and Valpuesta V. (2002) Manipulation of strawberry fruit softening by antisense expression of a pectate lyase gene, *Plant Physiology.* **(128):** 751-759.
32. Kemmer C., Neubauer P. (2006) Antisense RNA based down-regulation of RNaseE in *E. coli. Microb Cell Fact.* **(12):** 5-38.
33. Knoester M., Linthorst H.J., Bol J.F. and van Loon L.C. (1997) Modulation of stress-inducible ethylene biosynthesis by sense and antisense gene expression in tobacco. *Plant Science.* **(126):** 173-183.
34. Kurreck J. (2003) Antisense technologies: Improvement through novel chemical modifications. *European Journal of Biochemistry.* **(270):** 1628-1644.
35. Marcus-Sekura C.J., Woerner A.M., Zon G. and Quinnan (1987) Comparative inhibition of chloramphenicol acetylttransferase gene expression by antisense oligonucleotide analogues having alkyl phosphotriester, methlyphosphonate and phosphorothioate linkage. *Nucleic Acids Res.* **(15):** 5749-5763.
36. Matsukura M., Shinozuka K., Zon G., Mitsuya H., Reitz M., Cohen J.S. and Broder S. (1987) Phosphorothioate analogs of oligodeoxynucleotides: inhibitors of replication and cytopathic effects of human immunodeficiency virus. *Proceedings of the National Academy of Sciences USA.* **(84):** 7706-7719.
37. Maxon J. and Weaver C. (2007) Antisense therapy: An overview. *Current Topics In Oncology.*
38. Miller P.S., L.T. Braiterman, and POP Ts'o (1977) Effects of a trinucleotide ethyl phosphotriester, Gmp(Et)Gmp(Et)U, on mammalian cells in culture. *Biochemistry.* **(16):** 1988-1996.

39. Neckers L. and whitesell L. (1993) Antisense technology: biological utility and pratical consideration. Am. *J. Physiol.* (265): 1-12.
40. Nielsen P.E. (2005) Systemic delivery: The last hurdle? *Gene Therapy.* **(12):** 956-957.
41. Oeller P.W., Lu M.W., Taylor L.P., Pike D.A. and Theologis A. (1991) Reversible inhibition of tomato fruit senescence by antisense RNA. *Science.* **(254):** 437-439.
42. Redondo-Nevado J., Moyano E., Medina-Escobar N., Caballero J.L. and Muñoz-Blanco J. (2001) A fruit-specific and developmentally regulated endopolygalacturonase gene from strawberry (Fragaria × anaassa cv. Chandler), *J. Exp. Bot.* **(52):** 1941-1945.
43. Richard R. (2000) The application of antisense technology to medicine. *The Ochsner Journal.* **(2):** 233-236.
44. Scherer L.J. and Rossi J.J. (2003) Approaches for the sequence specific knockdown of mRNA. *Nat. Biotech.* **(21):** 1457-1463.
45. Sheehy R.E., Kramer M. and Hiatt W.R. (1988) Reduction of polygalacturonase activity in tomato fruit by antisense RNA. Proc. *Natl. Acad. Sci. USA.* **(85):** 8805-8809.
46. Smith C.C., Aurelian I., Reddy M.P., Miller P.S. and Ts'o POP (1986) Antiviral effect of an oligo (nucleoside methylphosphonate) complementary to the splice junction of herpes simplex virus type I immediate early pre-mRNA 4 and 5. Proc. *Natl. Acad. Sci. USA.* **(83):** 2787-2791.
47. Smith C.J.S., Watson C.F., Ray J., Bird C.R., Morris R. Schuch W. and Grierson D. (1988) Antisense RNA inhibition of polygalacturonase gene expression in transgenic tomatoes. *Nature.* **(334):** 724-726.
48. Smith C.J.S., Watson C.P., MOlTis P.C., Bird C.R., Seymour G.B., Gray J.E., Arnold C., Tucker G.A., Schuch W., Harding S. and Grierson D. (1990) Inheritance and effect on ripening of antisense polygalacturonase genes in transgenic tomatoes. *Plant Mol. Biol.* **(14):** 369-379.
49. Souq F., Coutos-Thevenot P., Yean H., Delbard G., Maziere Y., Barbe J.P. and Boulay M. (1996) Genetic transformation of roses, 2 examples: one on morphogenesis, the other on anthocyanin biosynthetic pathway. *ISHS Acta Horticulturae* 424: II International Rose Symposium (eds. A. Morisot and P. Ricci) pp. 381-388.
50. Srivastava S. and Gupta S.M. (2008) Role of differentially expressed ripening related genes and promoters in banana fruit: identified by mRNA DDRY – *PCR. Res. Environ Life Sci.* 1 **(3):** 81-90.
51. Tennant R.W., J.G. Farrelly, J.N. Ihle, B.C. Pal, F.T. Kenney, and A. Brown (1973) Effects of polyadenylic acids on functions of murine RNA tumor viruses. *Journal of Virology.* **(12):** 1216-25.
52. Thompson J.D. and Gillespie D. (1990) Current concepts in quantitative molecular hybridization. *Clin Biochem.* 23 **(4):** 261-266.
53. Tracie L. Pierce, Anthony R. White, Geoffrey W. Tregear and Patrick M. Sexton (2005) Peptide-Oligonucleotide hybrids in antisense therapy. *Mini-Reviews in Medicinal Chemistry.* **(5):** 41-55.
54. Ts'o P.O., Miller P.S. and Greene J.J. (1983) Nucleic acids alalogs with targeted delivery at the therapeutic agents for development of target oriented anticancer drugs. Raven Press, New York. p. 189.
55. Van der Salm T.P.M., van der Toorn, C.J.G., Bouwer R., ten Cate C.H.H. and Dons H.J.M. (1997) Production of ROL gene transformed plants of Rosa hybrida L. and characterization of their rooting ability. *Molecular Breeding.* **(3):** 39-47.
56. Walder R.Y, and J.A. Walder (1988) Role of RNase H. in hybrid-arrested translation by antisense oligonucleotides. *Proceedings of the National Academy of Sciences USA.* **(85):** 5011-5015.
57. Wan Q, Zhang X.G and Song M. (2007) Fruit-specific RNAi-mediated Restraining Expression of Lcy Gene to Enhance Lycopene Content in Tomatoes. *Chinese Journal of Biotechnology.* 23 **(3):** 29-434.
58. Wang D., Fan J. and Ranu R.S. (2004) Coning and expression of 1-aminocycloproane-1 carboxylate synthase cDNA from rosa (Rosa x hybrida). *Plant. Cell. Rep.* **(24):** 422-429.
59. Wang T.W., Zhang C.G, Wu W., Nowack L.M., Madey E. and Thompson J.E. (2005) Antisense suppression of deoxyhypusine synthase in tomato delays fruit softening and alters growth and development. *Plant Physiol.* **(138):** 1372-1382.

60. Watson J. and Crick F. (1953) Molecular structure of nucleic acids; a structure for deoxyribose nucleic acid. *Nature.* **(171):** 737.

61. Xiangqian L., Gasic K., Camm ie B., Broekaert W. and Korban S.S. (2003) Transgenic rose lines harbouring an antimicrobial protein gene, Ace-AMP1, demonstrate enhanced reistance to powdery mildew (Sphaerotheca pannosa). *Planta.* **(218):** 226-232.

62. Yang S.F. and Hoffman N.E. (1984) Ethylene biosysnthesis and its regulation in higher plants. *Ann. Rev. Plant. Physiol.* **(35):** 155-189.

63. Yoshihiko Tomita (2000) Application of antisense technology to urologic cancers. *Molecular Urology.* 4 **(2):** 55-59.

64. Zamecnik P.C. and M.L. Stephenson (1978) Inhibition of Rous sarcoma virus replication and cell transformation by a specific oligodeoxynucleotide. *Proceedings of the National Academy of Sciences USA.* **(75):** 280-284.

65. Zhang W., Zhang H. and Xing L. (2006) Antisense oligonucleotide of hypoxia-inducible factor-1alpha suppresses growth and tumorigenicity of lung cancer cells A549. *J. Huazhong Univ. Sci. Technolog Med. Sci.* 26 **(4):** 448-450.

66. Zuo S., Luo J., Liu M., Xu L., Dong J., Guo W. and Zou S. (2008) Suppressing effects of down-regulating DNMT1 and DNMT3b expression on the growth of human cholangiocarcinoma cell line. *J. Huazhong Univ. Sci. Technolog. Med. Sci.* 28 **(3):** 276-80.

CHAPTER

14

RNAi Technology

RNA interference (RNAi) is a regulatory mechanism encompassing the various aspects of small double-stranded RNA (dsRNA)-guided gene silencing. It has been developed into a powerful tool to specifically modulate gene expression in a variety of animal and plant cells. These are *LITTLE RNAs but having BIG IMPACT* in the biological system.The RNAi technology has been used not only to understand gene functions but also to develop strategies for therapeutic applications and crop improvements. In this article, we briefly review the mechanism of small RNA mediated silencing. This is followed by a discussion on the development of RNAi as a technology and its applications in the diverse fields of medicine, veterinary science and agriculture.

Keywords: RNA interference, gene silencing, post-transcriptional gene silencing, cosuppression, virus induced gene silencing.

INTRODUCTION

RNA interference (RNAi) is a highly evolutionary conserved process of post-transcriptional gene silencing (PTGS) mediated by small double-stranded RNA (dsRNA). These small RNA (sRNA) molecules act by initiating degradation or translation suppression of mRNA transcripts in a sequence-specific manner. PTGS was first observed as a phenomenon of "co-suppression of gene expression" in an attempt to develop the Petunia plants with Chalcone synthase (CHS) transgene (Figure 14.1). It was later widely studied as an antiviral mechanism in plants (Viral Induced Gene Silencing or VIGS), nematodes, insects and mammals. Using genetically altered strains of the roundworm (Caenorhabditis elegans) scientists in fall of 2000 discovered the machinery of protein factors involved in driving the process. Thus far studies by different research groups have led to an understanding of the basic mechanism and machinery of RNAi. Extensive literature is also available detailing the use of RNAi in addressing problems related to gene functions in various systems, especially plants. Some alternate names of RNA interference are PTGS (Post-Transcriptional Gene Silencing), VIGS (Virus Induced Gene Silencing) and co-suppression in plants, Quelling in fungi, and RNAi in animals. RNAi has since emerged as an excellent technology for identifying and altering gene functions systematically. This knowledge has been exploited to develop the tools for applications in medicine, veterinary science and agriculture.

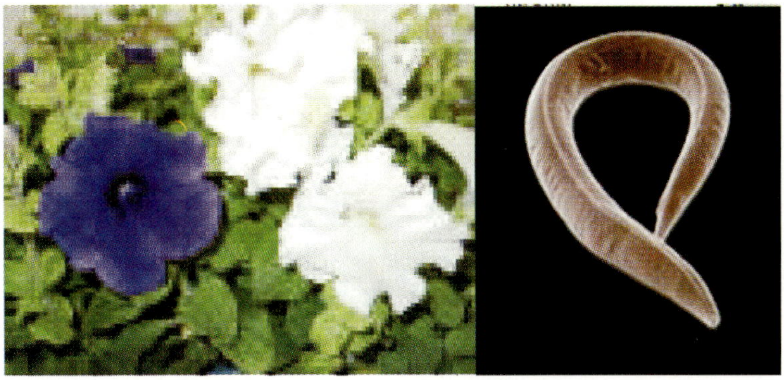

Figure 14.1 Brief history of RNAi using Petunia and Caenorhabditis as model system.

CONCEPTS

The discovery of RNAi was preceded first by observations of transcriptional inhibition by antisense RNA expressed in transgenic plants, and more directly by reports of unexpected outcomes in experiments performed by plant scientists in the United States and the Netherlands in the early 1990s. In an attempt to alter flower colors in petunias, researchers introduced additional copies of *CHS* gene (encoding chalcone synthase), a key enzyme for flower pigmentation into petunia plants of normally pink or violet flower color. The overexpressed gene was expected to result in darker flowers, but instead produced less pigmented, fully or partially white flowers, indicating that the activity of chalcone synthase had been substantially decreased; in fact, both the endogenous genes and the transgenes were downregulated in the white flowers. Soon after, a related event termed *quelling* was noted in the fungus *Neurospora crassa*. Further investigation of the phenomenon in plants indicated that the down-regulation was due to post-transcriptional inhibition of gene expression via an increased rate of mRNA degradation. This phenomenon was called *co-suppression* of gene expression, but the molecular mechanism remained unknown. Not long after, plant virologists working on improving plant resistance to viral diseases observed a similar unexpected phenomenon. While it was known that plants expressing virus-specific proteins showed enhanced tolerance or resistance to viral infection, it was not expected that plants carrying only short, non-coding regions of viral RNA sequences would show similar levels of protection. Researchers believed that viral RNA produced by transgenes could also inhibit viral replication. The reverse experiment, in which short sequences of plant genes were introduced into viruses, showed that the targeted gene was suppressed in an infected plant. This phenomenon was labeled VIGS and the set of such phenomena were collectively called PTGS.

After these initial observations in plants, many laboratories around the world searched for the occurrence of this phenomenon in other organisms. In 1998, Andrew Fire and Craig C. Mello investigating the regulation of muscle protein production in *C. elegans*, observed that neither mRNA nor antisense RNA injections had an effect on protein production, but double-stranded RNA successfully silenced the targeted gene. This was the first report of a potent gene silencing effect after injecting double stranded RNA for which they coined the term RNA interference or RNAi. Fire and Mello were awarded the Nobel Prize in Physiology or Medicine in 2006 for their work.

PRINCIPLES

The discovery of this RNA-based gene-silencing in organisms as diverse as plants, worms and humans suggested that cells must possess evolutionary conserved machinery that mediates the process. In other words, there must be a collection of cellular proteins that recognize and process dsRNAs, then incorporate these small effector molecules into an enzymatic complex that can bind and cleave complementary (target) mRNAs. This machinery has now been well described through the work of many groups, as highlighted in several recent reviews. Cells possess two dedicated ribonuclease (RNase) III enzymes, DROSHA and DICER, which process precursor dsRNAs into smaller intermediates at approximately 20 nucleotides (nt) in length and containing 2-nt 3′ overhangs which are recognized by specific proteins to assemble effector complex (RISC) of gene silencing (Figure 14.2). The cellular sRNAs include a range of specific molecules including siRNAs (small interfering RNAs), miRNAs (microRNAs), piRNAs and 21-mer U-RNAs.

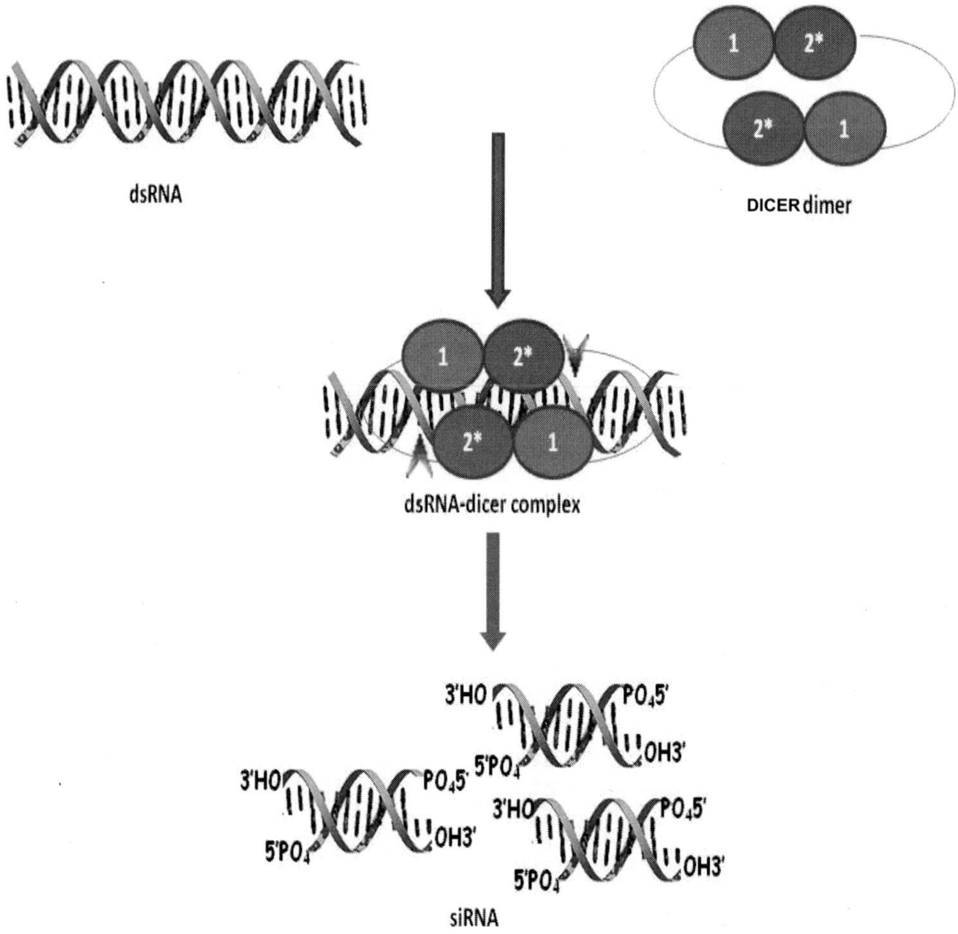

Figure 14.2 Mechanism of DICER action.

RNAi is a two phase process (Figure 14.3) consisting of:

- Initiation of silencing—Involved in generation of mautre siRNA or miRNA
- Effects of silencing—Involved in silencing of target gene

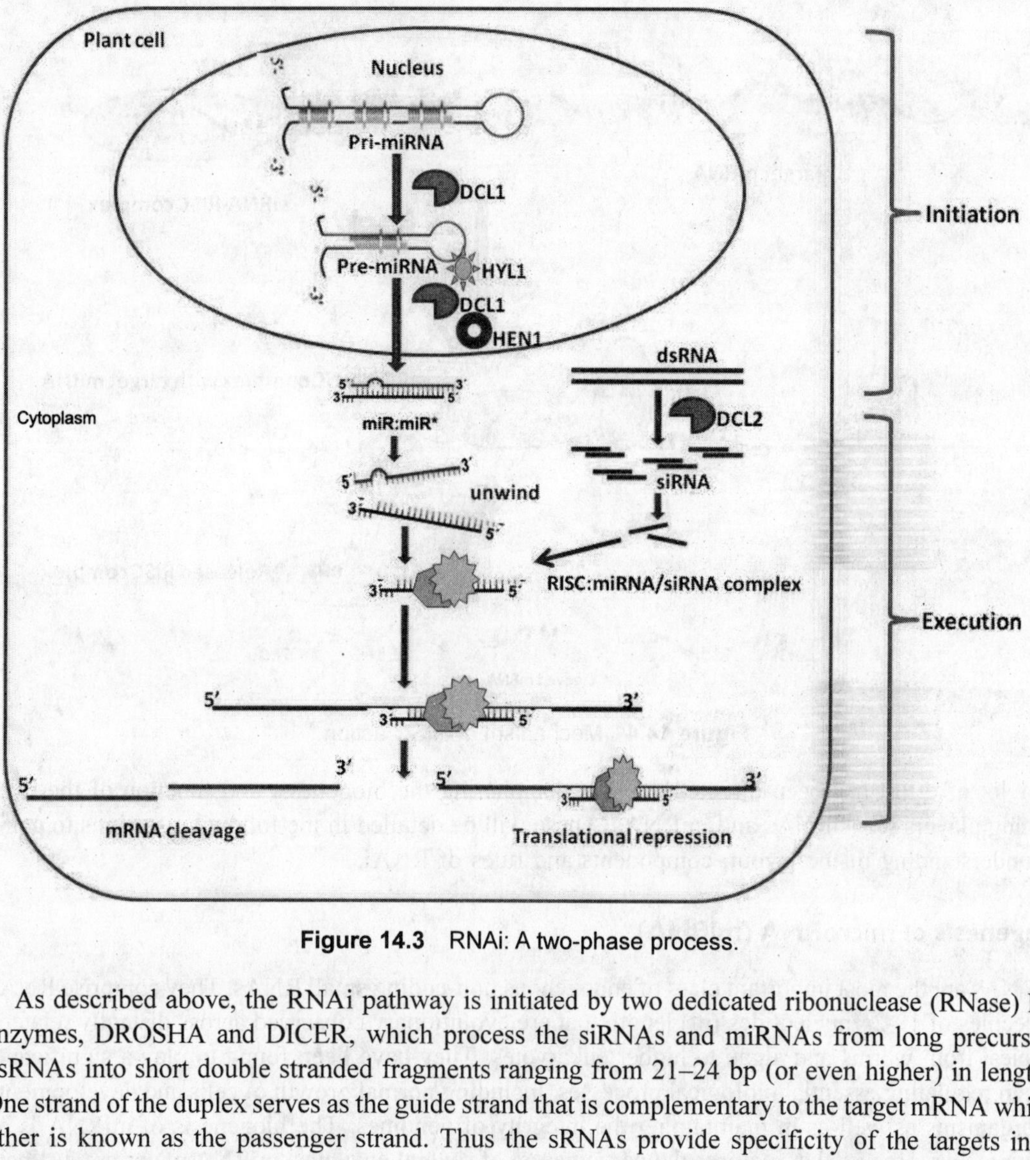

Figure 14.3 RNAi: A two-phase process.

As described above, the RNAi pathway is initiated by two dedicated ribonuclease (RNase) III enzymes, DROSHA and DICER, which process the siRNAs and miRNAs from long precursor dsRNAs into short double stranded fragments ranging from 21–24 bp (or even higher) in length. One strand of the duplex serves as the guide strand that is complementary to the target mRNA while other is known as the passenger strand. Thus the sRNAs provide specificity of the targets in a sequence-dependent manner while the enzymatic machinery called RISC (RNA Induced Silencing Complex) is responsible for the degradation or translation repression of the target mRNA (Figure 14.4). This machinery has now been well described through the work of many groups, as highlighted in several recent reviews. Though the effector complexes of each type of sRNAs are different from each other, the principal slicer component is the ARGONAUTE (AGO) protein.

Multiples isomeric forms of AGO are also present depending on the organisms concerned, ranging from one in *Schizosaccharomyces pombe* to 27 in *C. elegans*. It is not well known how a sRNA is sorted into a specific AGO-RISC. However, a recent study has suggested that sorting may be governed by the first nucleotide residue of the sRNA.

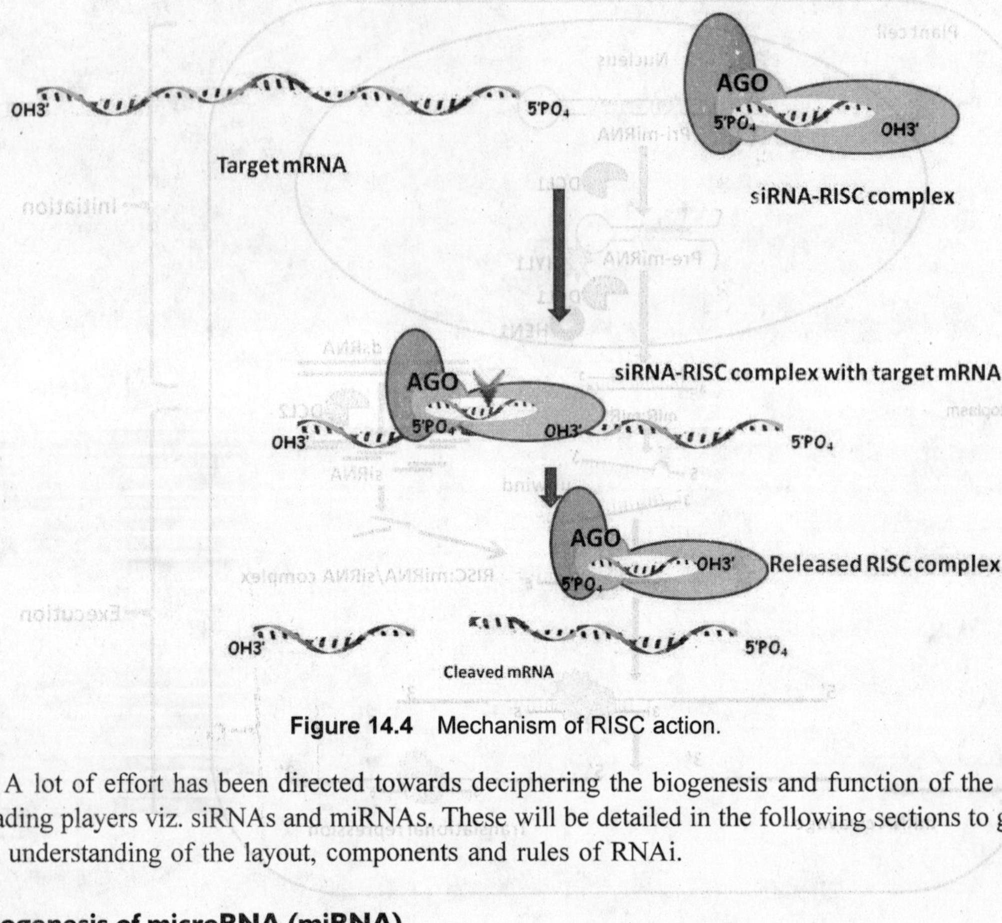

Figure 14.4 Mechanism of RISC action.

A lot of effort has been directed towards deciphering the biogenesis and function of the two leading players viz. siRNAs and miRNAs. These will be detailed in the following sections to gain an understanding of the layout, components and rules of RNAi.

Biogenesis of microRNA (miRNA)

miRNAs are the most important class of endogenous non-coding small RNAs. They comprise RNA molecules of 19-24 nucleotides (nt) length that are evolutionary conserved across distantly related species, from worms and algae to higher eukaryotes. They have been found to play a significant role in regulating essential biological processes, including normal growth of cells and development of organisms as well as in maintaining the integrity of genomes. The biogenesis of miRNA is a multiple-step process that requires the participation of several enzymes. miRNA genes are distinct from the protein coding genes and can exist at any location of a genome, including introns, exons or regions between two protein coding genes. They are transcribed as independent units to primary miRNAs (pri-miRNAs) by RNA polymerase II. They acquire specific hairpin-shaped stem-loop secondary structures that are processed by dsRNA-specific ribonuclease III enzyme, DROSHA to release 60-70 nt precursor miRNAs (pre-miR overhang of 2 nt, are then transported to the cytoplasm by EXPORTIN-5 (Exp5) (a member of the Ran transport receptor family). Once in the cytoplasm, pre-miRNAs are further processed from the end of the hairpin structure stem by DICER in to 20-22 nt long miRNA:miRNA* duplex. The mature miRNA is incorporated into RISC which induces gene silencing by inhibiting the translation machinery in animals and by degradation of the target transcript in plants.

There are several other differences in the biogenesis pathway of plants miRNAs. The processing of pri-miRNAs to pre-miRNAs in plants is mediated by the Dicer-like protein 1 (DCL1) instead of DROSHA. This step also involves cooperation of other proteins like HYPONASTIC LEAVES1 (HYL1), HUA ENHANCER1 (HEN1) and SERRATE (SE). The further cleavage of pre-miRNA to a miRNA:miRNA* duplex is mediated by DCL1 in nucleus and the duplex is transported to cytoplasm by HASTY (HST), the plant ortholog of *exp5* where it gets incorporated into RISC complex.

Biogenesis of siRNA

siRNAs are 21-24 nt long sequences that are generally produced from cleavage of exogenous long dsRNA precursors by the RNase III endonuclease, Dicer or DCL. The exogenous dsRNA may arise as a consequence of viral infection, transposon insertions, and transcription of repeat elements or laboratory manipulations. Each Dicer requires a cognate dsRNA-binding protein (DSRB) to process the precursors into sRNAs *in vivo* and the defects in DSRB activity lead to either incomplete or null processing of the dsRNA. There also exists an endogenous pool of siRNAs that are also processed by the Dicers or DCL but through a process requiring miRNA and RNA dependent RNA polymerase (RdRP), RDR6.

Among the siRNAs various subtypes have been defined including viral siRNAs (vi-si), repeat associated siRNAs (ra-si), transacting siRNAs (ta-si) and natural antisense siRNAs (nat-si). The **vi-si** are the classical siRNAs that are produced by the processing of long dsRNA precursors mainly by DCL4, which are formed in the cell during infection of viruses, especially the RNA viruses. Substrates for Dicer include dsRNA replication intermediates and local base-paired RNA structures of cytoplasmic RNA viruses or overlapping transcripts of gemini-viruses. The sRNA molecules produced are incorporated into the RISC and targeted to the homologous stretches on viral transcripts for destruction by cleavage. The vi-si are utilized by the host as an antiviral defense and have thus been the most well studied class of the siRNAs.

Ra-si, as the name suggests, arise from repeat regions. Transcripts of two canonical repeats like the retrotransposable element AtSN1 and the 5S ribosomal DNA are converted into long dsRNAs by the putative RdRP, RDR2, which are then processed by DCL3 into 24 nt ra-si. The mature siRNAs are then O-methylated by HEN1. These siRNAs are involved in transcriptional gene silencing by methylating DNA and histones on certain retroelements and repeat rich regions. The ra-si pathway also forms a positive feedback loop because methylation of the target loci is essential for the siRNA accumulation.

The **ta-si** arises from endogenous dsRNA precursors that are produced from miRNA cleaved transcripts by the action of RDR6. The precursors are processed by DCL4 into small 24 nt molecules, which then regulate gene expression in a way similar to that of miRNA.

The **nat-si** is a newly defined class of siRNA that includes molecules derived from two convergent and partially overlapping transcripts, at least one of which is induced under specific environments. This class is well exemplified by the constitutively expressed SRO5 transcript that partially overlaps with the salinity inducible P5CDH transcript in antisense orientation. Under salt stress conditions, both transcripts are present and they overlap to create a 760-bp double-stranded region, which is processed by DCL2 to produce a unique 24-nt nat-si.

RNAi TECHNOLOGY

Tuschl's group pioneered the development of RNAi as a technology by demonstrating that exogenously administered siRNAs can down-regulate the target transcripts in a specific manner in mammalian cells. Because of the selectivity and potency of sRNAs for silencing gene expression in eukaryotic cells, RNAi based drugs are emerging as the specialized therapy to treat metabolic disorders and viral diseases as well as to engineer plants with specific traits. Currently at least seven industrial giants are engaged in clinical trials for siRNA or miRNA based antiviral drugs. The lead has, however, been established in the agricultural sector, by the commercial production of PRSV resistant papaya since late 1990s. The immense potential of RNAi based products has revolutionized the pharmaceutical and biotechnology industry and this is reflected by the huge investments directed towards the RNAi market. For the RNAi technology to take deep roots, two fundamental problems namely the design and specific delivery of the sRNAs, need to be solved.

Design of sRNAs

The RNAi technology revolves around the dual aspects of designing specific sRNAs and ensuring their accurate delivery at the intended site(s) of the recipient cells and at the desired time. RNAi can be triggered by two different pathways. The first is a direct approach which involves the delivery of synthetic effector siRNAs to target cells as pre-formed 21 base duplexes. This usually results in potent gene silencing although the effect is transient. The second is an indirect approach in which the sRNAs are produced by intracellular processing of longer RNA hairpin transcripts from exogenously introduced DNA constructs. The longer hairpin or dsRNA precursors are transcribed in the nucleus and then transported to the cytoplasm where they are processed into sRNAs by specific Dicers or DCLs. The DNA-based strategies have the advantage of being stable when introduced in the eukaryotic cell.

Either of the two techniques involves designing the RNA molecules to achieve maximum knockdown of the target transcripts with minimum off-target effects. The optimal sequence of a sRNA molecule is determined empirically by comparing the gene-silencing ability and thermodynamic stability of several candidate duplexes. Elegant studies by several groups have led to the development of specific guidelines or rules to predict the sequence of the sRNA duplex for targeting a specific subset of transcript. Several online tools are also available to assist in designing the synthetic siRNA (http://www.rnaiweb.com/RNAi/RNAi_Web_Resources/RNAi_ToolsSoftware/Online_siRNA_Design_Tools/index.html) or miRNA sequences (http://wmd2.weigelworld.org/cgi-bin/mirnatools.pl) for targeting select mRNA(s).

Delivery of sRNAs

The primary obstacle lies in the delivery of the small molecules to the desired cellular locations at the appropriate time. An appropriate delivery system is also crucial for enhancing the gene-silencing activity and reducing the off-target effects. Various modes of cellular and subcelluar targeting are also reported in literature. The siRNA duplexes and antisense miRNAs (antimiRs) are the main sRNA species that have been used both *in vitro* and *in vivo* to inactivate the endogenous RNAi pathways. The competence of synthetic sRNAs to initiate RNAi is challenged by a number of factors like susceptibility to intracellular exonucleolytic degradation, structural properties of target mRNA, targeting non-specific mRNAs or "off-target effects" and non-specific activation of signaling cascades like innate immune response. Details on each of these aspects are readily available in literature.

Mode of delivery of synthetic sRNAs

It varies from direct uptake to facilitated transport to intracellular production. The direct entry of sRNAs into cells faces the problem of reduced uptake, and hence several different kinds of molecules including proteins, peptides and lipids have been used for transporting them into the cell. A lot of research efforts have been directed towards improving the existing techniques as well as exploring new vehicles of siRNA delivery. The simplest technique probably involves direct transfection of synthetic dsRNAs. An alternate approach involves *in vitro* transcription of DNA oligonucleotides or larger transcripts that can be processed by the sRNA biogenesis machinery of the host. *In vivo* applications however require systemic administration of siRNAs. This has been achieved using intravenous injections, liposomes, lipophilic group conjugates and so on. Recently a nano-particle approach has been developed to carry siRNAs in the cells.

The antimiRNA are synthesized as synthetic locked nucleic acid (LNA)-tagged RNA oligos or on cholesterol support as antagomiRs that contain 2'-OMe phosphoramidites. The endogenous miRNA precursors can also be engineered to produce desired synthetic miRNA or artificial miRNA (amiRNA) targeting completely different transcripts in plant or animal cells. Different types of viral vectors (retroviral or adenoviral) carrying miRNA expressing sequences under constitutive or inducible promoters are also being used for expressing specific miRNAs in desired cell or tissue types.

Sites of delivery of synthetic sRNAs

It can vary from localized to systemic application. In several elegant studies the siRNAs have been directed to specialized tissues to successfully knock down the target genes. This is best exemplified by the sub-retinal delivery of synthetic siRNAs in treating Age related Macular Degeneration (AMD), the intra-nasal delivery of siRNAs to cure respiratory syncytial virus (RSV) infection and the intra-tumoral delivery of siRNAs as an effective anticancer strategy. The strategies for systemic delivery involve production of plasmid or viral vectors to generate and deliver siRNAs. These approaches are more popular as they allow continuous intracellular production of siRNAs enabling sustained gene silencing.

APPLICATIONS OF RNAi TECHNOLOGY

The RNAi induced silencing of gene expression is an excellent tool to modulate biological functions rapidly and consistently. It has thus found numerous applications not only in the understanding of gene functions in model systems but also in clinical and agricultural fields. The *in vivo* delivery of sRNAs and their potential as therapeutic drugs is being extensively explored in human, murine and bovine systems. A few of these studies have already entered clinical trials marking the onset of a drug revolution. The plant world is not left untouched as an equal number of interesting studies in model species like Arabidopsis and tobacco are currently underway to improve plant yields for food, fiber and fuel. A transgenic papaya plant resistant to virus infection, utilizing the siRNA approach, has already been commercialized. In the following section we have attempted to provide an overview of the RNAi applications in different field of science.

Medical Applications

Therapies based on RNAi are currently being developed for fighting viral infections as well as for treating a number of diseases like cancer, neurodegenerative diseases, cardiovascular disorders and metabolic defects. A majority of these studies have been performed *in vivo* with cell cultures or murine models. These findings have also indicated that extreme caution and specific approaches have to be adopted for treating each endogenous cellular malfunction to prevent off target effects, activation of Toll-like receptors (TLRs), type 1 interferon responses and competition with the endogenous RNAi pathway components. It is equally important to determine that the RNAi drugs reach their specific targets in the correct tissues and stay active long enough to fight the disease.

Among the first RNAi drugs to reach patients are formulations aimed at an eye disease called Age-related Macular Degeneration (AMD). The disease is triggered by a protein called VEGF (Vascular Endothelial Growth Factor) that promotes blood vessel growth. These blood vessels often leak leading to clouding and entirely destroying vision. The siRNA based drugs developed to block nascent blood vessel production are currently under clinical trials. Acuity pharmaceuticals have utilized naked or unpackaged short strands of RNA that target VEGF transcripts, while Sirna Therapeutics have developed siRNAs targeting VEGF receptor 1 (Sirna-027). In the absence of the receptor, the protein is not recognized. The advantage is that these drugs can be delivered locally within the eye so that there are no unanticipated, harmful effects elsewhere in the body.

RNAi is also being exploited to selectively eliminate cancer cells without damaging normal cells by targeting gene(s) specifically involved in the growth or survival of the cancer cell. The therapy may involve selective delivery of siRNAs into the cancer cells by transfection. Several studies have been performed in cell cultures or murine models to evaluate the siRNA-mediated knockdown phenotype of oncogenes. The classical studies include downregulation of Bcr/Abl kinase oncogene in Chronic Myeloid Leukaemia cells. Similarly systemic administration of CDP–transferrin-tagged siRNA targeting the EWS–FLI1 fusion oncogene product was demonstrated to inhibit tumour growth in a murine model. Specific combination therapies are also being worked out for knocking down chemo-resistance factors like p53, bcl-2 kinase, p-glycoprotein and so on, to re-sensitize tumour cells to cell death inducing drugs.

Recently it was reported that specific miRNAs, termed oncomiRs, can also function as tumor suppressors or oncogenes. At least 13 miRNAs have been found to be associated with the prognosis and disease progression in chronic lymphocytic leukaemia. This differential expression of specific miRNAs in various tumours can be used as a powerful tool to aid in the diagnosis and treatment of cancer. This is well exemplified by miRNAs such as *let-7*, which negatively regulate the Ras oncogenes, and miR-15 and miR-16, which negatively regulate *BCL2*. RNAi also provides a powerful technique to discover and learn more about genes that trigger or inhibit cancer. Greg Hannon and his group at Cold Spring Harbor Laboratory are attempting to decipher the function of 15,000 genes in a variety of human cancer cell lines. Such efforts might pinpoint the genes never before linked to cancer and generate novel ideas for treatments.

The RNAi technology has helped in the diagnosis and treatment of a number of virus infections. It has been demonstrated that siRNAs have the ability to inhibit the replication or cellular uptake of viruses. This was clearly demonstrated in human cell lines using siRNAs directed against the poliovirus genome, which resulted in resistance of the cells to poliovirus infection. Similarly Song and colleagues showed that siRNAs targeting the gene encoding the death receptor, Fas, could protect mice from liver failure and fibrosis in two models of autoimmune hepatitis. In late 2002, Phillip Sharp and colleagues at MIT demonstrated that the various steps in the HIV life cycle can be interrupted with RNAi molecules in cell cultures. Since then down-regulation of HIV replication and the cellular cofactors required for infection by sRNA duplexes is also being widely studied in established cell lines, as well as in primary peripheral blood lymphocytes. Recently, John Rossi's group at City of Hope Medical Center and Colorado State University has engineered an RNAi therapy aiming at multiple HIV genes by combining RNAi with two other RNA technologies (called ribozymes and RNA decoys) to block HIV's replication and invasion of the immune system. A purely siRNA based strategy for treatment of HIV is developed by Benitec Ltd. by harvesting leucocytes from the peripheral blood, treating them with an anti-HIV shRNA-producing DNA construct and subsequently re-infusing the transfected cells. This gene-therapy-based approach attacking multiple targets of the HIV virus simultaneously is in Phase I trials.

RNAi drugs are being developed to target a host of different respiratory viruses, including SARS, influenza, respiratory syncytial virus and parainfluenza virus. Successful silencing in the lung has been achieved by intra-nasal or intra-tracheal administration of siRNAs. Alnylam, a siRNA company, has set up clinical trials for targeting RSV. Another aspect is promotion of virus replication by specific cellular miRNAs, together with the finding that several pathogenic human viruses encode miRNAs that are important in the virus life cycle. This suggests that technologies that allow the specific inhibition of miRNA function, such as the recently described antagomiR molecules, could have a future role in the treatment of viral induced diseases.

Specific siRNAs are also being used to treat a variety of neurodegenerative disorders like amyotrophic lateral sclerosis (ALS), Spinocerebellar ataxia, and Huntington's disease by selectively suppressing the toxic gain-of-function gene mutations. The strategy employs viral vectors to transport sRNA-making molecules to target cells so that they can get embedded in the cell's machinery to continuously silence the erratic gene.

Recently, RNAi has acquired interest as a potential therapeutic strategy to silence endogenous genes involved in the cause or pathway of metabolic diseases like diabetes. Taniguchi *et al.* (2005)

delivered shRNAs through adenoviral vectors to knock down the expression of insulin receptor substrates, IRS-1 and IRS-2, specifically in the livers of mice to understand the roles of these proteins in hepatic insulin action. Similarly RNAi approach was used to induce silencing of the hepatic PEPCK transcripts. PEPCK is an essential enzyme in gluconeogenesis pathway and is responsible for increased hepatic glucose output. Treatment of diabetic mice with PEPCK siRNA reduced the hepatic PEPCK protein resulting in lowering the blood glucose.

Controlling cholesterol biosynthesis is another area that can benefit from the RNAi approach. Lowering serum cholesterol and LDL levels is important for prevention and management of coronary artery disease and stroke. The strategy involves down-regulating apoB to lower the levels of circulating Low-Density Lipoproteins (LDLs). ApoB is expressed in large quantities in hepatocytes and is essential for the formation and metabolism of LDLs. The identification of miR-122 as a regulator of cholesterol biosynthesis has opened the possibility of utilizing the antagomiR approach as a potential therapeutic agent in cardiovascular diseases.

Thus RNAi has unambiguously become a valuable tool for basic research in medical biology. A few RNAi based drugs are already in the various phases of clinical trials and many more are in pipeline. This has clearly marked the onset of a revolution in the development of novel therapeutic strategies for disorders that have been as yet difficult to treat.

Veterinary Applications

RNAi technology is gaining popularity as a new approach for functional genomics of domestic animals, understanding host-pathogen interaction and treating viral and prion diseases. It is being utilized to reduce the disease susceptibility and enhance the qualitative traits of farm animals.

RNAi has provided the biotechnological tool to probe functional genomics of veterinary animals and potentially generate farm animals that are less susceptible to infectious disease as well better in traits. The classical functional genomics rely mainly upon the standard technique of disrupting a gene by homologous recombination. However, this is difficult and expensive, especially in livestock species where embryonic stem cells have not been isolated. On the contrary, RNAi offers the relatively simple gene specific knockdown tool that is applicable to all cell culture systems. RNAi knockdown experiment in a bovine trophoblast cell line has been used for gene expression profiling of trophoblasts, understanding follicular growth and development as well as early embryogenesis, to study nuclear trafficking pathways in porcine embryos and the functional analysis of genes in porcine granulose cells.

The major thrust is to use RNAi as a potential defense against viral infections in animals. Recently, CSIRO at Australia has launched a program that aims to provide indirect protection for humans against pandemic strains of influenza by using RNAi in poultry. The idea is to establish a real—and impervious—firewall between wild birds and the poultry to prevent the spread of virus. The strategy involves targeting highly conserved genetic regions common to all subtypes and strains of influenza by using siRNAs. The mode of delivery includes introducing siRNAs directly to the birds via drinking water or an aerosol spray for priming their innate RNAi defences to recognize and destroy the virus.

The siRNAs are also being used to target the viral diseases of livestock. The foremost application is in developing a cure for the Foot and Mouth Disease (FMD) that causes huge economic losses not only in India but also worldwide. It has been shown that introduction of shRNA directed against viral structural protein (1D) or polymerase (3D) of FMDV via replication deficient adenoviral vectors has been found to effectively protect swine IBRS-2 cells. It also significantly reduces susceptibility in suckling mouse, guinea pigs and swine to FMDV infection. Two out of three swine treated with FMDV shRNA showed no major clinical disease even after challenged with severe viral dosage. RNAi technology is being developed as a prospective therapy for many other veterinary diseases as well including Bovine viral diarrhea virus (BVDV) using siRNAs targeting the 5′ non-translated (NTR) region and regions encoding the C, NS4B and NS5A proteins, *Peste des petitsruminants* (PPR) and *rinderpest* (RP) using siRNAs targeting the nucleocapsid genes and Feline immunodeficiency virus (FIV) using siRNA targeting FIV gag region. Infection of domestic cats with feline immunodeficiency virus (FIV) has emerged as an important model system for studying human immunodeficiency virus type 1 (HIV-1) infection due to numerous similarities in pathogenesis induced by the two lenti viruses.

Prion diseases of livestock also pose serious threat to human health as they can get transmitted through red meat consumption. *In vitro* and *in vivo* RNAi studies have indicated considerable reduction in bovine prion protein on delivering siRNAs against bovine prion gene (bPRNP). The resultant transgenic livestock is expected to be resistant to prion disease thereby controlling its transmission to humans.

RNAi has been found to be useful tool in designing anti-tick therapy, particularly for veterinary animals. It has proved to be a valuable tool for understanding tick function, comprehending tick-pathogen interface and screening for tick protective antigens to help formulate improved tick-control.

RNAi has also been used to enhance the production trait of farm animals. Several target genes have been identified that are required to be knocked down to enhance the qualitative characters. For example, silencing of myostatin (inhibits lean-muscle growth) or *Socs1* gene might lead to the better development of mammary gland and thus enhanced milk production. Similarly disrupting endogenous spermatogenesis in bulls may improve the success rate of germ cell transplantation.

RNAi also has specific applications in improving bovine reproduction and diminishing calf mortality and morbidity. It can help in understanding the mechanism of genome activation in developing bovine embryos and determining the genes involved in embryo-maternal cross talk. The information gained could be applied to reduce abnormal fetal-maternal interactions and fetal loss in nuclear transfer embryos.

Agricultural Applications

RNAi is an excellent technology for understanding gene functions with an aim to improve the quality of crops. In fact RNA silencing machinery has been found to be activated as a natural defense mechanism of plants against several abiotic and biotic factors. It can thus be used for identifying and adjusting metabolic pathways to enable plants to survive under extremes of environmental fluctuations or pathogen attack.

Metabolic engineering

Improving plant nutritional value: RNAi can prove to be particularly useful in targeting agronomic traits controlled by multigene families in agronomically important plants. It is also useful in knocking of multiple copies of a specific gene, which are normal due to the polyploid nature of majority of the crop plants. Sequences having homology to target gene were used to silence the gene (Table 14.1).

The rice mutant line LGC-1 (Low Glutelin Content-1) is among the first commercially useful cultivar produced by RNAi. It is useful for patients with kidney disease whose protein intake is restricted. The low levels of storage-protein are due to siRNAs directed against the tightly linked glutelin multigene family. Low glutelin content is a relief to kidney patients unable to digest glutenin.

Development of coffee varieties having low caffeine content. Caffeine is a stimulant of central nervous system, the heart muscle and the respiratory system and has a diuretic effect. Theobromine synthase, enzyme involved in biosynthetic pathway of caffeine has been targeted.

By using the RNAi technology, fatty acid composition of soybean has been changed. The content of 18 unsaturated carbon fatty acid has been increased from 18% upto 63%. The strategy was to knock down the gene Fad2, coding for an enzyme catalyzing the reaction C19:1 to C18:2.

Functional RNAi has been implemented to improve the nutritional quality from crops by altering the carbohydrate profile to changing the oil composition. Regina *et al*. (2006) attempted to modify the starch composition of wheat by using hpRNA constructs against an isoform of a starch-branching enzyme that altered the amylose-amylopectin ratio in wheat seeds. This was desirous to reduce the incidence of cardiovascular disease and colon cancer in humans. Inverted repeat against lysine-ketoglutarate reductase/saccharophine dehydrogenase (LKR/SDH) accompanied with over-expression of CordapA, a de-regulated lysine biosynthetic enzyme was used to produce transgenic corn with improved lysine content. Similarly siRNAs directed against the conserved 318-nt sequence of omega-3 fatty acid desaturase (FAD3) gene family have been used to reduce the levels of Ω-linolenic acid (18:3) of soybean that causes instability of the seed oil.

RNAi has also been used to enhance the nutritional quality and improve shelf life of crops. A lot of work in this area has been done on tomatoes. Hairpin targeting photo-morphogenesis regulatory gene (DET1) or lycopene transforming gene (Lycopene cyclase) under fruit specific promoter were used for increasing both carotenoid and flavonoid content of tomatoes. Tomatoes with improved lycopene contents are highly beneficial in preventing cancer and heart diseases. Flavr Savr™ tomatoes with reduced polygalactouronase levels were produced to enhance the shelf life of the fruits. The RNAi technique has also found application in removal of undesirable metabolites from poppy, coffee beans and cotton seed. It has also been used to reduce the lignin levels in forage grasses to facilitate digestion in animals to improve livestock performance.

Table 14.1 Application of RNAi in metabolic engineering.

Trait	*Target gene*	*Host plant*	*Potential benefits*
Enzymatic browning	Polyphenyl oxidase gene	Potato	Extended storage life
Increased stearic	ghSAD-1 and	Cotton	Useful for cooking

Contd.

acid and oleic acid content of seed oil	ghFAD2-1 genes		applications without the need for hydrogenation
Reduced caffeine production	CaMxMt 1 gene	Coffee bean plant	Decaffeinated coffee
Reduced or absent petals	BP1 gene	Oilseed rape	Improved photosynthesis
Increased carotenoid and flavonoid content	DET1 gene	Tomato	Consumer health benefits
Maize quality	Starch branching enzyme	Maize	Up to 50% increase in amylose content
Allergy	Lol p1 and Lol p2	Ryegrass (Lolium spp.)	hypo-allergic ryegrass
Reduced ethylene sensitivity	1-Aminocyclo propane-1-carboxylate oxidase	Tomato	Longer shelf life (slower ripening)
Increased arsenic uptake	ACR2 gene	Arabidopsis	Phytoremediation of soils

Modify plant shape and properties: It is result from heterogeneous expression of miRNA. For example:

- RNAi used to develop a high-lysine maize variant by knockdown Zein (a major seed storage protein (poor in lysine content) gene.
- Blue roses have been created by knocking down the cyanidine gene and introducing the delphinidin gene. The result is spectacular to floral industry. Rose cultivars normally lack a key enzyme for biosynthesis of delphinidin-based anthocyanins that are responsible for violet to blue colour of flower varieties. The strategy involved over-expression of the enzyme flavonoid 3', 5'-hydoxylase and *Iris hollandica* dihydroflavonol 4-reductase (DFR) gene along with the down-regulation of endogenous DFR gene. This was done as the rose enzyme converted the delphinidin compounds into red and yellow pigments resulting in flowers with purple petals. The Iris DFR over-expressing roses exclusively accumulated delphinidin in the petals, and the flowers had blue hues.

Crop protection: Plants resistant to economically important viruses have been engineered and commercially released in the market (Table 14.2). In the late 1990s, a variety of papaya was released in Hawaii that was resistant to Papaya ring spot virus (PRSV). Ever since, different crop plants like barley and turnip have been immunized against a whole range of viruses by using specific constructs that can silence the RNAi suppressors encoded by the plant viruses. Recently Monsanto has prepared two varieties of potato, NewLeaf Plus and NewLeaf Y, which are resistant to Potato leaf roll virus and PVY, respectively (Monsanto, www.research.cip.cgiar.org) for commercial release. Transgenic plants demonstrating resistance to a host of other pathogens like Agrobacterium, bacteria *Erwinia amylovora* or nematodes have been produced using different hpRNA constructs.

- Phytopathogenic DNA viruses can potentially be controlled by RNAi. Complete immunity was reported to Potato virus Y in potato plants. Resistance to the virus was observed in the plants harbouring vectors for the simultaneous expression of both the sense and antisense transcripts of the viral helper-component proteinase (HCPro) gene.
- By using RNAi, barley varieties resistant to BYDV (barley yellow dwarf virus) are developed. Both sense and antisense sequences were cloned under the same promoter separated by an intron. Upon transcription, these sequences form a hpRNA molecule that triggers gene silencing and efficiency of gene silencing varies from 50% to nearly 100%.

Table 14.2 Commercially released genetically engineered plants.

Name of virus	*Family*	*Region targated*	*Results*	*System used*	*Genome*
Potato virus Y	Potyviridae	HC-Pro	Immunity	Potato	RNA
Mungbean yellow mosaic India virus (MY MIV)	Geminiviridae	Bidirectional promoter	Recovery from infection	Vigna mungo (black gram)	DNA
African cassava mosaic virus (ACMV)	Geminiviridae	Replication-associated protein gene	Reduced virus accumulation	Tobacco protoplast	DNA
Tomato yellow leaf curl Sardinia virus	Geminiviridae associated protein gene	Replication-	Poor resistance	Tomato	DNA
Pepper mild mottle virus (PMMoV)	Tobamoviridae	Arbitrary sequence	Block in viral infectivity	Tobacco	RNA
Tobacco etch virus (TEV)	Potyviridae	Arbitrary sequence	No viral-specific symptoms	Tobacco	RNA
Alfalfa mosaic virus (AMV)	Bromoviridae	Arbitrary sequence	Recovery from infection	Tobacco	RNA
Beet necrotic yellow vein virus (BNYVV)	Benyviridae	Coat protein	Tolerance	Tobacco	RNA

Male Sterility: An important issue for hybrid seed production, particularly in species such as oilseed rape, maize and sunflower where the crop is grown from the second generation seed of hybrid plants. In the case of cytoplasmic male sterility, this is achieved by restorer line. Male fertility is restored after hpRNAi-mediated silencing of the Ms45 promoter by expressing the Ms45 gene under a heterologous promoter.

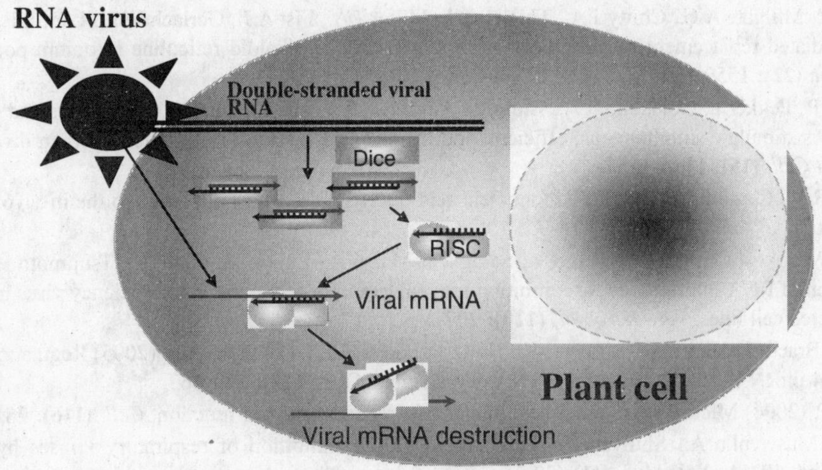

Figure 14.5 Viral RNA degradation induced by RNAi.

Production of biologically important molecules in plants: Another important achievement is the development of plants producing RNAi based vaccines. Influenza virus-specific siRNAs have been over-expressed in plants for introduction into human cells after harvesting to successfully inhibit viral replication (Figure 14.5). Besides, plant-produced antibodies can be used for treating cancer and other inflammatory diseases, however, production in plants causes glycosylation of the Fc region of the antibodies. This might compromise its functional abilities and may also be immunogenic. Green alga, *Lemna*, is being developed as an efficient system to over-express and harvest therapeutic antibodies by silencing two endogenous glycan-transferase enzymes.

CONCLUSION

The RNA-silencing pathways have extensive networks in eukaryotic cells. The study of this mechanism has provided us with tools that can be used not only to understand the basic functioning of biological systems but also for widespread applications from the treatment of diseases to improving the quality of livestock and crop plants. The RNAi industry is currently 30 million in India as per the industry estimates and seeing its potential in the international market, we believe that it will bring a boon in the endogenous sectors as well. The full potential of the siRNAs and miRNAs is yet to be utilized. The near future will witness improvements in the basic understanding and mechanism of RNAi technology. This will undoubtedly have a remarkable impact on the applications in diverse fields of biology.

FURTHER READINGS

1. Akhtar S., Benter I.F. (2007) Non-viral delivery of synthetic siRNAs *in vivo*. *J. Clinical Invest.* **(117):** 3623-3632.
2. Allen E., Xie Z., Gustafson A.M., Carrington J.C. (2005) microRNA-directed phasing during trans-acting siRNA biogenesis in plants. *Cell.* **(121):** 207-221.

3. Allen R.S., Millgate A.G., Chitty J.A., Thisleton J., Miller J.A., Fist A.J., Gerlach W.L., Larkin P.J. (2004) RNAi-mediated replacement of morphine with the nonnarcotic alkaloid reticuline in opium poppy. *Nat. Biotechnol.* **(22):** 1559-1566.
4. Alvarez J.P., Pekker I., Goldshmidt A., Blum E., Amsellem Z., Eshed Y. (2006) Endogenous and synthetic microRNAs stimulate simultaneous, efficient, and localized regulation of multiple targets in diverse species. *Plant Cell.* **(18):** 1134-1151.
5. Anthony R.V., Cantlon J.D. (2007) Ribonucleic acid interference: a new approach to the in vivo study of gene function. *J. Anim. Sci.* **(85):** E18-9.
6. Baba K., Mizukoshi F., Goto-Koshino Y., Setoguchi-Mukai A., Fujino Y., Ohno K., Tsujimoto H. (2007) Application of RNA interference for inhibiting the replication of feline immunodeficiency virus in chronically infected cell lines. *Vet Microbiol.* **(120):** 207-216.
7. Bagga S., Bracht J., Hunter S., Massirer K., Holtz J., Eachus R., Pasquinelli A.E. (2005) Regulation by let-7 and lin-4 miRNAs results in target mRNA degradation. *Cell.* **(122):** 553-563.
8. Bartel D.P. (2004) MicroRNAs: genomics, biogenesis, mechanism, and function. *Cell.* **(116):** 281-297.
9. Bitko V., Musiyenko A., Shulyayeva O., Barik S. (2005) Inhibition of respiratory viruses by nasally administered siRNA. *Nat. Med.* **(11):** 50-55.
10. Borsani O., Zhu J., Verslues P.E., Sunkar R., Zhu J.K. (2005) Endogenous siRNAs derived from a pair of natural cis-antisense transcripts regulate salt tolerance in *Arabidopsis*. *Cell.* **(123):** 1279-1291.
11. Boureau T., ElMaarouf-Bouteau H., Garnier A., Brisset M.N, Perino C., Pucheu I., Barny M.A. (2006) DspA/E, a type III effector essential for *Erwinia amylovora* pathogenicity and growth in planta, induces cell death in host apple and nonhost tobacco plants. *Mol. Plant Microbe Interact.* **(19):** 16-24.
12. Brodersen P., Sakvarelidze-Achard L., Bruun-Rasmussen M., Dunoyer P., Yamamoto Y.Y., Sieburth L., Voinnet O. (2008) Widespread translational inhibition by plant miRNAs and siRNAs. *Science.* **(320):** 1185-1190.
13. Calegari F., Marzesco A.M., Kittler R., Buchholz F., Huttner W.B. (2004) Tissue-specific RNA interference in post-implantation mouse embryos using directional electroporation and whole embryo culture. *Differentiation.* **(72):** 92-102.
14. Calin G.A., Ferracin M., Cimmino A., Di Leva G., Shimizu M., Wojcik S.E., Iorio M.V., Visone R., Sever N.I., Fabbri M., Iuliano R., Palumbo T., Pichiorri F., Roldo C., Garzon R., Sevignani C., Rassenti L., Alder H., Volinia S., Liu C.G., Kipps T.J., Negrini M., Croce C.M. (2005) A MicroRNA signature associated with prognosis and progression in chronic lymphocytic leukemia. *N. Engl. J. Med.* **(353):** 1793-1801.
15. Cao X., Aufsatz W., Zilberman D., Mette M.F., Huang M.S., Matzke M., Jacobsen S.E. (2003) Role of the DRM and CMT3 methyltransferases in RNA-directed DNA methylation. *Curr. Biol.***(13):** 2212-2217.
16. Capodici J., Karikó K., Weissman D. (2002) Inhibition of HIV-1 infection by small interfering RNA-mediated RNA interference. *J. Immunol.* **(169):** 5196-5201.
17. Chan C.S., Elemento O., Tavazoie S. (2005) Revealing posttranscriptional regulatory elements through network-level conservation. *PLoS Comput Biol.* **(1):** e69.
18. Chellappan P., Masona M.V., Vanitharani R., Taylor N.J., Fauquet C.M. (2004) Broad spectrum resistance to ssDNA viruses associated with transgene-induced gene silencing in cassava. *Plant Mol. Biol.* **(56):** 601-611.
19. Chen W., Yan W., Du Q., Fei L., Liu M., Ni Z., Sheng Z., Zheng Z. (2004) RNA interference targeting VP1 inhibits foot-and-mouth disease virus replication in BHK-21 cells and suckling mice. *J. Virol.* **(78):** 6900-6907.
20. Cimmino A., Calin G.A., Fabbri M., Iorio M.V., Ferracin M., Shimizu M., Wojcik S.E., Aqeilan R.I, Zupo S., Dono M., Rassenti L., Alder H., Volinia S., Liu C.G., Kipps T.J., Negrini M., Croce C.M. (2005) miR-15 and miR-16 induce apoptosis by targeting BCL2. *Proc. Natl. Acad. Sci. USA.* **(102):** 13944-13949.
21. Cox K.M., Sterling J.D., Regan J.T., Gasdaska J.R., Frantz K.K., Peele C.G., Black A., Passmore D., Moldovan-Loomis C., Srinivasan M., Cuison S., Cardarelli P.M., Dickey L.F. (2006) Glycan optimization of a human monoclonal antibody in the aquatic plant *Lemna minor*. *Nat. Biotechnol.* **(24):** 1591-1597.

22. Davuluri G.R., van Tuinen A., Fraser P.D., Manfredonia A., Newman R., Burgess D., Brummell D.A., King S.R., Palys J., Uhlig J., Bramley P.M., Pennings H.M., Bowler C. (2005) Fruit-specific RNAi-mediated suppression of DET1 enhances carotenoid and flavonoid content in tomatoes. *Nat. Biotechnol.* **(23):** 890-895.
23. de Almeida R.S., Keita D., Libeau G., Albina E. (2007) Control of ruminant morbillivirus replication by small interfering RNA. *J. Gen. Virol.* **(88):** 2307-2311.
24. de la Fuente J., Kocan K.M., Almazán C., Blouin E.F. (2007) RNA interference for the study and genetic manipulation of ticks. *Trends Parasitol.* **(23):** 427-433.
25. de los Santos T., Wu Q., de Avila Botton S., Grubman M.J. (2005) Short hairpin RNA targeted to the highly conserved 2B nonstructural protein coding region inhibits replication of multiple serotypes of foot-and-mouth disease virus. *Virology.* **(335):** 222-231.
26. Ding H., Schwarz D.S., Keene A., Affar el B., Fenton L., Xia X., Shi Y., Zamore P.D., Xu Z. (2003) Selective silencing by RNAi of a dominant allele that causes amyotrophic lateral sclerosis. *Aging Cell.* **(2):** 209-217.
27. Ding S.W., Voinnet O. (2007) Antiviral immunity directed by small RNAs. *Cell.* **(130):** 413-426.
28. Donnison M., Pfeffer P.L. (2004) Isolation of genes associated with developmentally competent bovine oocytes and quantitation of their levels during development. *Biol. Reprod.* **(71):** 1813-1821.
29. Elmén J., Lindow M., Schütz S., Lawrence M., Petri A., Obad S., Lindholm M., Hedtjärn M., Hansen H.F., Berger U., Gullans S., Kearney P., Sarnow P., Straarup E.M., Kauppinen S. (2008) LNA-mediated microRNA silencing in non-human primates. *Nature.* **(452):** 896-900.
30. Escobar M.A., Civerolo E.L., Summerfelt K.R., Dandekar A.M. (2001) RNAi-mediated oncogene silencing confers resistance to crown gall tumorigenesis. *Proc. Natl. Acad. Sci. USA.* **(98):** 13437-13442.
31. Fairbairn D.J., Cavallaro A.S., Bernard M., Mahalinga-Iyer J., Graham M.W., Botella J.R. (2007) Host-delivered RNAi: an effective strategy to silence genes in plant parasitic nematodes. *Planta.* **(226):** 1525-1533.
32. Flores T., Karpova O., Su X., Zeng P., Bilyeu K., Sleper D.A., Nguyen H.T., Zhang Z.J. (2008) Silencing of GmFAD3 gene by siRNA leads to low alpha-linolenic acids (18:3) of fad3 mutant phenotype in soybean [*Glycine max* (Merr.)]. Transgenic Res. 7. [Epub ahead of print]
33. Frizzi A., Huang S., Gilbertson L.A., Armstrong T.A., Luethy M.H., Malvar T.M. (2008) Modifying lysine biosynthesis and catabolism in corn with a single bifunctional expression/silencing transgene cassette. *Plant Biotechnol. J.* **(6):** 13-21.
34. Fuchs M., Gonsalves D. (2007) Production of virus-resistant transgenic plants two decades after their introduction: lessons from realistic field risk assessment studies. *Annu. Rev. Phytopathol.* **(45):** 173-202.
35. Gitlin L., Karelsky S., Andino R. (2002) Short interfering RNA confers intracellular antiviral immunity in human cells. *Nature.* **(418):** 430-434.
36. Golding M.C., Long C.R, Carmell M.A, Hannon G.J., Westhusin M.E. (2006) Suppression of prion protein in livestock by RNA interference. *Proc. Natl. Acad. Sci. USA.* **(103):** 5285-5290.
37. Gómez-Valadés A.G., Méndez-Lucas A., Vidal-Alabró A., Blasco F.X., Chillon M., Bartrons R., Bermúdez J., Perales J.C. (2008) Pck1 gene silencing in the liver improves glycemia control, insulin sensitivity, and dyslipidemia in db/db mice. *Diabetes.* **(57):** 2199-2210.
38. Haldar J., An D., Alvarez de Cienfuegos L., Chen J., Klibanov A.M. (2006) Polymeric coatings that inactivate both influenza virus and pathogenic bacteria. *Proc. Natl. Acad. Sci. USA.* **(103):** 17667-17671.
39. Hamilton A., Voinnet O., Chappell L., Baulcombe D. (2002) Two classes of short interfering RNA in RNA silencing. *EMBO J.* **(21):** 4671-4679.
40. Hamilton A.J., Baulcombe D.C. (1999) A species of small antisense RNA in posttranscriptional gene silencing in plants. *Science.* **(286):** 950-952.
41. Han J., Lee Y., Yeom K.H., Kim Y.K., Jin H., Kim V.N. (2004) The Drosha-DGCR8 complex in primary microRNA processing. *Genes Dev.* **(18):** 3016-3027.

42. Hannon G.J., Rossi J.J. (2004) Unlocking the potential of the human genome with RNA interference. *Nature.* **(431):** 371-378.

43. Harper S.Q., Staber P.D., He X., Eliason S.L., Martins I.H., Mao Q., Yang L., Kotin R.M., Paulson H.L., Davidson B.L. (2005) RNA interference improves motor and neuropathological abnormalities in a Huntington's disease mouse model. *Proc. Natl. Acad. Sci. USA.* **(102):** 5820–5825.

44. He L., Thomson J.M., Hemann M.T., Hernando-Monge E., Mu D., Goodson S., Powers S., Cordon-Cardo C., Lowe S.W., Hannon G.J., Hammond S.M. (2005) A microRNA polycistron as a potential human oncogene. *Nature.* **(435):** 828-833.

45. Hérard A.S., Besret L., Dubois A., Dauguet J., Delzescaux T., Hantraye P., Bonvento G., Moya K.L. (2006) siRNA targeted against amyloid precursor protein impairs synaptic activity *in vivo*. *Neurobiol. Aging.* **(27):** 1740-1750.

46. Hirano T., Yamauchi N., Sato F., Soh T., Hattori M.A. (2004) Evaluation of RNA interference in developing porcine granulosa cells using fluorescence reporter genes. *J. Reprod. Dev.* **(50):** 599-603.

47. Hofmann J., Szakasits D., Blöchl A., Sobczak M., Daxböck-Horvath S., Golinowski W., Bohlmann H., Grundler F.M. (2008) Starch serves as carbohydrate storage in nematode-induced syncytia. *Plant Physiol.* **(146):** 228-235.

48. Howard K.A., Rahbek U.L., Liu X., Damgaard C.K., Glud S.Z., Andersen MØ., Hovgaard M.B., Schmitz A., Nyengaard J.R., Besenbacher F., Kjems J. (2006) RNA interference *in vitro* and *in vivo* using a novel chitosan/siRNA nanoparticle system. *Mol. Ther.* **(14):** 476-484.

49. Iorio M.V., Ferracin M., Liu C.G., Veronese A., Spizzo R., Sabbioni S., Magri E., Pedriali M., Fabbri M., Campiglio M., Ménard S., Palazzo J.P., Rosenberg A., Musiani P., Volinia S., Nenci I., Calin G.A., Querzoli P., Negrini M., Croce C.M. (2005) MicroRNA gene expression deregulation in human breast cancer. *Cancer Res.* **(65):** 7065-7070.

50. Jacque, J. M., Triques, K. and Stevenson, M. (2002) Modulation of HIV-1 replication by RNA interference. *Nature.* (London) **(418):** 435-438.

51. Jiang M., Milner J. (2003) Bcl-2 constitutively suppresses p53-dependent apoptosis in colorectal cancer cells. *Genes Dev.* **(17):** 832-837.

52. Johnson S.M., Grosshans H., Shingara J., Byrom M., Jarvis R., Cheng A., Labourier E., Reinert K.L., Brown D., Slack F.J. (2005) RAS is regulated by the let-7 microRNA family. *Cell.* **(120):** 635-647.

53. Kahana R., Kuznetzova L., Rogel A., Shemesh M., Hai D., Yadin H., Stram Y. (2004) Inhibition of foot-and-mouth disease virus replication by small interfering RNA. *J. Gen. Virol.* **(85):** 3213-3217.

54. Katsumoto Y., Fukuchi-Mizutani M., Fukui Y., Brugliera F., Holton T.A., Karan M., Nakamura N., Yonekura-Sakakibara K., Togami J., Pigeaire A., Tao G.Q., Nehra N.S., Lu C.Y., Dyson B.K., Tsuda S., Ashikari T., Kusumi T., Mason J.G., Tanaka Y. (2007) Engineering of the rose flavonoid biosynthetic pathway successfully generated blue-hued flowers accumulating delphinidin. *Plant Cell Physiol.* **(48):** 1589-1600.

55. Kim W.J., Christensen L.V., Jo S., Yockman J.W., Jeong J.H., Kim Y.H., Kim S.W. (2006) Cholesteryl oligoarginine delivering vascular endothelial growth factor siRNA effectively inhibits tumor growth in colon adenocarcinoma. *Mol. Ther.* **(14):** 343-350.

56. Kovar H., Ban J., Pospisilova S. (2003) Potentials for RNAi in sarcoma research and therapy: Ewing's sarcoma as a model. *Semin. Cancer Biol.* **(13):** 275-281.

57. Krützfeldt J., Rajewsky N., Braich R., Rajeev K.G., Tuschl T., Manoharan M., Stoffel M. (2005) Silencing of microRNAs in vivo with 'antagomirs'. *Nature.* **(438):** 685-689.

58. Kumar P., Wu H., McBride J.L., Jung K.E., Kim M.H., Davidson B.L., Lee S.K., Shankar P., Manjunath N. (2007) Transvascular delivery of small interfering RNA to the central nervous system. *Nature.* **(448):** 39-43.

59. Kusaba M., Miyahara K., Iida S., Fukuoka H., Takano T., Sassa H., Nishimura M., Nishio T. (2003) *Low glutelin content 1*: a dominant mutation that suppresses the glutelin multigene family via RNA silencing in rice. *The Plant Cell.* **(15):** 1455-1467.

60. Lambeth L.S., Moore R.J., Muralitharan M.S., Doran T.J. (2007) Suppression of bovine viral diarrhea virus replication by small interfering RNA and short hairpin RNA-mediated RNA interference. *Vet Microbiol.* **(119):** 132-143.

61. Lee Y.S., Nakahara K., Pham J.W., Kim K., He Z., Sontheimer E.J., Carthew R.W. (2004) Distinct roles for Drosophila Dicer-1 and Dicer-2 in the siRNA/miRNA silencing pathways. *Cell* **(117):** 69-81.

62. Léonard J.N., Schaffer D.V. (2005) Computational design of antiviral RNA interference strategies that resist human immunodeficiency virus escape. *J. Virol.* **(79):** 1645-1654.

63. Makimura H., Mizuno T.M., Mastaitis J.W., Agami R., Mobbs C.V. (2002) Reducing hypothalamic AGRP by RNA interference increases metabolic rate and decreases body weight without influencing food intake. BMC *Neurosci.* **(3):** 18.

64. Medarova Z., Pham W., Farrar C., Petkova V., Moore A. (2007) *In vivo* imaging of siRNA delivery and silencing in tumors. *Nat. Med.* **(13):** 372-377.

65. Meirelles F.V., Caetano A.R., Watanabe Y.F., Ripamonte P., Carambula S.F., Merighe G.K., Garcia S.M. (2004) Genome activation and developmental block in bovine embryos. *Anim. Reprod. Sci.* 82 **(83):** 13-20.

66. Meister G., Tuschl T. (2004) Mechanisms of gene silencing by double-stranded RNA. *Nature.* **(431):** 343-349.

67. Mi S., Cai T., Hu Y., Chen Y., Hodges E., Ni F., Wu L., Li S., Zhou H., Long C., Chen S., Hannon G.J., Qi Y. (2008) Sorting of small RNAs into *Arabidopsis* argonaute complexes is directed by the 5' terminal nucleotide. *Cell.* **(133):** 116-127.

68. Milhavet O., Gary D.S., Mattson M.P. (2003) RNA interference in biology and medicine. *Pharmacol. Rev.* **(55):** 629-648.

69. Molnár A., Csorba T., Lakatos L., Várallyay E., Lacomme C., Burgyán J. (2005) Plant virus-derived small interfering RNAs originate predominantly from highly structured single-stranded viral RNAs. *J. Virol.* **(79):** 7812-7818.

70. Morrissey D.V., Lockridge J.A., Shaw L. Blanchard K., Jensen K., Breen W., Hartsough K., Machemer L., Radka S., Jadhav V., Vaish N., Zinnen S., Vargeese C., Bowman K., Shaffer C.S., Jeffs L.B., Judge A., MacLachlan I., Polisky B. (2005) Potent and persistent in vivo anti-HBV activity of chemically modified siRNAs. *Nat. Biotechnol.* **(23):** 1002-1007.

71. Nakamura H., Siddiqui S.S., Shen X., Malik A.B., Pulido J.S., Kumar N.M., Yue B.Y. (2004) RNA interference targeting transforming growth factor-beta type II receptor suppresses ocular inflammation and fibrosis. *Mol. Vis.* **(10):** 703-711.

72. Nguyen T., Menocal E.M., Harborth J., Fruehauf J.H. (2008) RNAi therapeutics: an update on delivery. *Current Opinion in Molecular Therapeutics.* **(10):** 158-167.

73. Niu Q.W., Lin S.S., Reyes J.L., Chen K.C., Wu H.W., Yeh S.D., Chua N.H. (2006) Expression of artificial microRNAs in transgenic *Arabidopsis thaliana* confers virus resistance. *Nat. Biotechnol.* **(24):** 1420-1428.

74. Novina C.D., Murray M.F., Dykxhoorn D.M., Beresford P.J., Riess J., Lee S.K., Collman R.G., Lieberman J., Shankar P., Sharp P.A. (2002) siRNA-directed inhibition of HIV-1 infection. *Nature Medicine.* **(8):** 681-686.

75. Novobrantseva T.I., Akinc A., Borodovsky A., de Fougerolles A. (2008) Delivering silence: advancements in developing siRNA therapeutics. *Curr. Opin. Drug. Discov. Dev.* **(11):** 217-224.

76. O'Donnell K.A., Wentzel E.A., Zeller K.I., Dang C.V., Mendell J.T. (2005) c-Myc-regulated microRNAs modulate E2F1 expression. *Nature.* **(435):** 839-843.

77. Ogita S., Zefuji H., Morimoto M., Sano H. (2004) Application of RNAi to confirm theobromine as the major intermediate for caffeine biosynthesis in coffee plants with potential for construction of decaffeinated varieties. *Plant Mol. Biol.* **(54):** 931-941.

78. Okamura K., Ishizuka A., Siomi H., Siomi M.C. (2004) Distinct roles for Argonaute proteins in small RNA-directed RNA cleavage pathways. *Genes Dev.* **(18):** 1655-1666.

79. Paradis F., Vigneault C., Robert C., Sirard M.A. (2005) RNA interference as a tool to study gene function in bovine oocytes. *Molecular Reproduction and Development.* **(70):** 111-121.

80. Parizotto E.A., Dunoyer P., Rahm N., Himber C., Voinnet O. (2004) In vivo investigation of the transcription, processing, endonucleolytic activity, and functional relevance of the spatial distribution of a plant miRNA. *Genes Dev.* **(18):** 2237-2242.
81. Peer D., Park E.J., Morishita Y., Carman C.V., Shimaoka M. (2008) Systemic leukocyte-directed siRNA delivery revealing cyclin D1 as an anti-inflammatory target. *Science.* **(319):** 578-579.
82. Peragine A., Yoshikawa M., Wu G., Albrecht H.L., Poethig R.S. (2004) SGS3 and SGS2/SDE1/RDR6 are required for juvenile development and the production of trans-acting siRNAs in Arabidopsis. *Genes Dev.* **(18):** 2368-2379.
83. Pfister-Genskow M., Myers C., Childs L.A., Lacson J.C., Patterson T., Betthauser J.M., Goueleke P.J., Koppang R.W., Lange G., Fisher P., Watt S.R., Forsberg E.J., Zheng Y., Leno G.H., Schultz R.M., Liu B., Chetia C., Yang X., Hoeschele I., Eilertsen K.J. (2005) Identification of differentially expressed genes in individual bovine preimplantation embryos produced by nuclear transfer: improper reprogramming of genes required for development. *Biol. Reprod.* **(72):** 546-555.
84. Pillé J.Y., Denoyelle C., Varet J., Bertrand J.R., Soria J., Opolon P., Lu H., Pritchard L.L., Vannier J.P., Malvy C., Soria C., Li H. (2005) Anti-RhoA and anti-RhoC siRNAs inhibit the proliferation and invasiveness of MDA-MB-231 breast cancer cells *in vitro* and *in vivo*. *Mol. Ther.* **(11):** 267-274.
85. Powelka A.M., Seth A., Virbasius J.V., Kiskinis E., Nicoloro S.M., Guilherme A., Tang X., Straubhaar J., Cherniack A.D., Parker M.G., Czech M.P. (2006) Suppression of oxidative metabolism and mitochondrial biogenesis by the transcriptional corepressor RIP140 in mouseadipocytes. *J. Clin. Invest.* **(116):** 125-136.
86. Ramon A.L., Bertrand J.R., Malvy C. (2008) Delivery of small interfering RNA. A review and an example of application to a junction oncogene. *Tumori.* **(94):** 254-263.
87. Regina A., Bird A., Topping D., Bowden S., Freeman J., Barsby T., Kosar-Hashemi B., Li Z., Rahman S., Morell M. (2006) High-amylose wheat generated by RNA interference improves indices of large-bowel health in rats. *Proc. Natl. Acad. Sci. USA.* **(103):** 3546-3551.
88. Reynolds A., Leak, D., Boese Q., Scaringe S., Marshall W.S., Khvorova A. (2004) Rational siRNA design for RNA interference. *Nat. Biotechnol.* **(22):** 326-330.
89. Rossi J.J. (2006) RNAi as a treatment for HIV-1 infection. *Biotechniques.* Suppl: 25-29.
90. Scherer L.J., Rossi J.J. (2003) Approaches for the sequence-specific knockdown of mRNA. *Nat. Biotechnol.* **(21):** 1457-1465.
91. Schwab R., Ossowski S., Riester M., Warthmann N., Weigel D. (2006) Highly specific gene silencing by artificial microRNAs in Arabidopsis. *Plant Cell.* **(18):** 1121-1133.
92. Sheehy R.E., Kramer M., Hiatt W.R. (1988) Reduction of polygalacturonase activity in tomato fruit by antisense RNA. *Proc. Natl. Acad. Sci. USA.* **(85):** 8805-8809.
93. Silva J.M., Mizuno H., Brady A., Lucito R., Hannon G.J. (2004) RNA interference microarrays: high-throughput loss-of-function genetics in mammalian cells. *Proc. Natl. Acad. Sci. USA.* **(101):** 6548-6552.
94. Simeoni F., Morris M.C., Heitz F., Divita G. (2005) Peptide-based strategy for siRNA delivery into mammalian cells. *Methods Mol. Biol.* **(309):** 251-260.
95. Song E., Lee S.K., Wang J., Ince N., Ouyang N., Min J., Chen J., Shankar P., Lieberman J. (2003) RNA interference targeting Fas protects mice from fulminant hepatitis. *Nat. Med.* **(9):** 347-351.
96. Soutschek J., Akinc A., Bramlage B., Charisse K., Constien R., Donoghue M., Elbashir S., Geick A., Hadwiger P., Harborth J., John M., Kesavan V., Lavine G., Pandey R.K., Racie T., Rajeev K.G., Röhl I., Toudjarska I., Wang G., Wuschko S., Bumcrot D., Koteliansky V., Limmer S., Manoharan M., Vornlocher H.P. (2004) Therapeutic silencing of an endogenous gene by systemic administration of modified siRNAs. *Nature.* (London) **(432):** 173-178.
97. Sunilkumar G., Campbell L.M., Puckhaber L., Stipanovic R.D., Rathore K.S. (2006) Engineering cottonseed for use in human nutrition by tissue-specific reduction of toxic gossypol. *Proc. Natl. Acad. Sci. USA.* **(103):** 18054-18059.
98. Sutou S., Kunishi M., Kudo T., Wongsrikeao P., Miyagishi M., Otoi T. (2007) Knockdown of the bovine prion gene PRNP by RNA interference (RNAi) technology. *BMC Biotechnol.* **(7):** 44.

99. Taniguchi H., Momiyama Y., Ohmori R., Yonemura A., Yamashita T., Tamai S., Nakamura H., Ohsuzu F. (2005) Associations of plasma C-reactive protein levels with the presence and extent of coronary stenosis in patients with stable coronary artery disease. *Atherosclerosis.* **(178):** 173-177.

100. Ushizawa K., Herath C.B., Kaneyama K., Shiojima S., Hirasawa A., Takahashi T., Imai K., Ochiai K., Tokunaga T., Tsunoda Y., Tsujimoto G., Hashizume K. (2004) cDNA microarray analysis of bovine embryo gene expression profiles during the pre-implantation period. *Reprod Biol. Endocrinol.* **(2):** 77.

101. Vazquez F., Vaucheret H., Rajagopalan R., Lepers C., Gasciolli V., Mallory A.C., Hilbert J.L., Bartel D.P., Crété P. (2004) Endogenous trans-acting siRNAs regulate the accumulation of Arabidopsis mRNAs. *Mol. Cell.* **(16):** 69-79.

102. Voorhoeve P.M., le Sage C., Schrier M., Gillis A.J., Stoop H., Nagel R., Liu Y.P., van Duijse J., Drost J., Griekspoor A., Zlotorynski E., Yabuta N., De Vita G., Nojima H., Looijenga L.H., Agami R. (2006) A genetic screen implicates miRNA-372 and miRNA-373 as oncogenes in testicular germ cell tumors. *Cell.* **(124):** 1169-1181.

103. Wacheck V., Losert D., Gunsberg P., Vornlocher H.P., Hadwiger P., Geick A., Pehamberger H., Muller M., Jansen B. (2003) Small interfering RNA targeting bcl-2 sensitizes malignant melanoma. *Oligonucleotides.* **(13):** 393-400.

104. Wan Q., Zhang X.G, Song M. (2007) Fruit-specific RNAi-mediated restraining expression of Lcy gene to enhance lycopene content in tomatoes. *Chinese Journal of Biotechnology.* **(23):** 429-443.

105. Wilda M., Fuchs U., Wossmann W., Borkhardt A. (2002) Killing of leukemic cells with a BCR/ABL fusion gene by RNA interference (RNAi). *Oncogene.* **(21):** 5716-5724.

106. Wolfrum C., Shi S., Jayaprakash K.N., Jayaraman M., Wang G., Pandey R.K., Rajeev K.G., Nakayama T., Charrise K., Ndungo E.M., Zimmermann T., Koteliansky V., Manoharan M., Stoffel M. (2007) Mechanisms and optimization of *in vivo* delivery of lipophilic siRNAs. *Nature Biotech.* **(25):** 1149-1157.

107. Wu H., Hait W.N., Yang J.M. (2003) Small interfering RNA-induced suppression of MDR1 (P-glycoprotein) restores sensitivity to multidrug-resistant cancer cells. *Cancer Res.* **(63):** 1515-1519.

108. Xia H., Mao Q., Eliason S.L., Harper S.Q., Martins I.H., Orr H.T., Paulson H.L., Yang L., Kotin R.M., Davidson B.L. (2004) RNAi suppresses polyglutamine-induced neurodegeneration in a model of spinocerebellar ataxia. *Nat. Med.* **(10):** 816-820.

109. Xie Z., Johansen L.K., Gustafson A.M., Kasschau K.D., Lellis A.D., Zilberman D., Jacobsen S.E., Carrington J.C. (2004) Genetic and functional diversification of small RNA pathways in plants. *PLoS Biol.* **(2):** E104.

110. Yao J., Ren X., Ireland J.J., Coussens P.M., Smith T.P.L., Smith G.W. (2004) Generation of a bovine oocyte cDNA library and microarray: resources for identification of genes important for follicular development and early embryogenesis. *Physiol. Genomics.* **(19):** 84-92.

111. Ye Z.H., Zhong R., Morrison W.H., Himmelsbach D.S. (2001) Caffeoyl coenzyme A O-methyltransferase and lignin biosynthesis. *Phytochemistry.* **(57):** 1177-1185.

112. Zeng Y., Wagner E.J., Cullen B.R. (2002) Both natural and designed microRNAs can inhibit the expression of cognate mRNAs when expressed in human cells. *Mol. Cell.* **(9):** 1327-1333.

113. Zhou Y., Chan J.H., Chan A.Y., Chak R.K., Wong E.Y., Chye M.L., Peiris J.S., Poon L.L., Lam E. (2004) Transgenic plant-derived siRNAs can suppress propagation of influenza virus in mammalian cells. *FEBS Lett.* **(577):** 345-350.

114. Zinker B.A., Rondinone C.M., Trevillyan J.M., Gum R.J., Clampit J.E., Waring J.F., Xie N., Wilcox D., Jacobson P., Frost L., Kroeger P.E., Reilly R.M., Koterski S., Opgenorth T.J., Ulrich R.G., Crosby S., Butler M., Murray S.F., McKay R.A., Bhanot S., Monia B.P., Jirousek M.R. (2002) PTP1B antisense oligonucleotide lowers PTP1B protein, normalizes blood glucose, and improves insulin sensitivity in diabetic mice. *Proc. Natl. Acad. Sci. USA.* **(99):** 11357-11362.

CHAPTER 15

Hybridoma Technology

Monoclonal antibodies (MAbs) can be produced from hybridoma cells through a technique now popularly known as hybridoma technology. MAbs can potentially be used for many purposes including the diagnosis treatment of disease and the purification of proteins. The hybridoma, being cancer cells, will multiply rapidly indefinitely and will produce large amounts of the desired antibodies. In this chapter, we present the basic concepts and practical applications of hybridoma technology in agricultural, medical, veterinary and industrial applications.

Keywords: Hybridoma technology; hybridomas; monoclonal antibodies, myeloma lymphocytes, HAT.

INTRODUCTION

Hybridoma, a biotechnological tool, is the new path for achieving the goal of complete immunization of human body from infections. Hybridoma technique is a method of creating pure and uniform antibodies (immunoglobulins) against a specific target (antigen). Hybridomas are the hybrid cells of myeloma (cancer) cells with antibody producing cells (lymphocytes) from an immunized donor (animal). The hybrid cell or hybridoma resulting from this fusion has the ability to multiply rapidly and indefinitely *in vitro* and to produce an antibody of predetermined specificity, known as monoclonal antibody (MAb). The technique of producing monoclonal antibodies (MAbs) in specialized cells is now popularly known as hybridoma technology (Figure 15.1). This technology was discovered in 1975 by two scientists, George Kohler of West Germany and Cesal Milstein of Argentina, who jointly with Niels Jerne of Denmark were awarded the 1984 Nobel Prize for physiology and medicine. Kohler (1974) successfully produced a hybridoma by fusing a P3 myeloma cell (resistant to azaguanine) and a lymphocyte (from the spleen of a mouse) immunized against sheep red blood cells. These hybridomas retained the property of immortality of the myeloma cells as well as that of secreting an antibody specific for an unknown antigen, resulting from the fusion of an antibody-secreting cell and a tumour cell. Hybridoma cells are mass-cultured for the production of monoclonal antibodies (MAbs) either *in vivo* in the peritoneal cavity of mice or *in vitro* in large scale culture vessels.

Increased research and accumulation of knowledge in the fields of somatic cell genetics, tissue culture technology and immunology resulted in the development of a technique for *in vitro* production of antibodies. Monoclonal antibody (MAbs) is the first product to move rapidly from the research laboratories through industry to the marketplace. MAbs will find use chiefly as research reagents, diagnostics *in vitro* and *in vivo*, as the therapeutic agents in the purification process and vaccine production. Hybridoma technology is a form of genetic engineering resulting in the production of specific antibodies by specialized tissue culture lines. MAb is an antibody directed against one antigenic determinant or epitope of an antigen. Hybridoma technology has made an impact on many other fields of research such as medical microbiology, parasitology, cell biology, biochemistry and physiology. Furthermore, many diagnostic and therapeutic applications of monoclonal antibodies (MAbs) as well as their use in the biotechnology industry are becoming apparent. The hybridoma technology has already fulfilled the long lasting desire of immunologists for the routine production of monospecific antibody that can be used as immunological reagents.

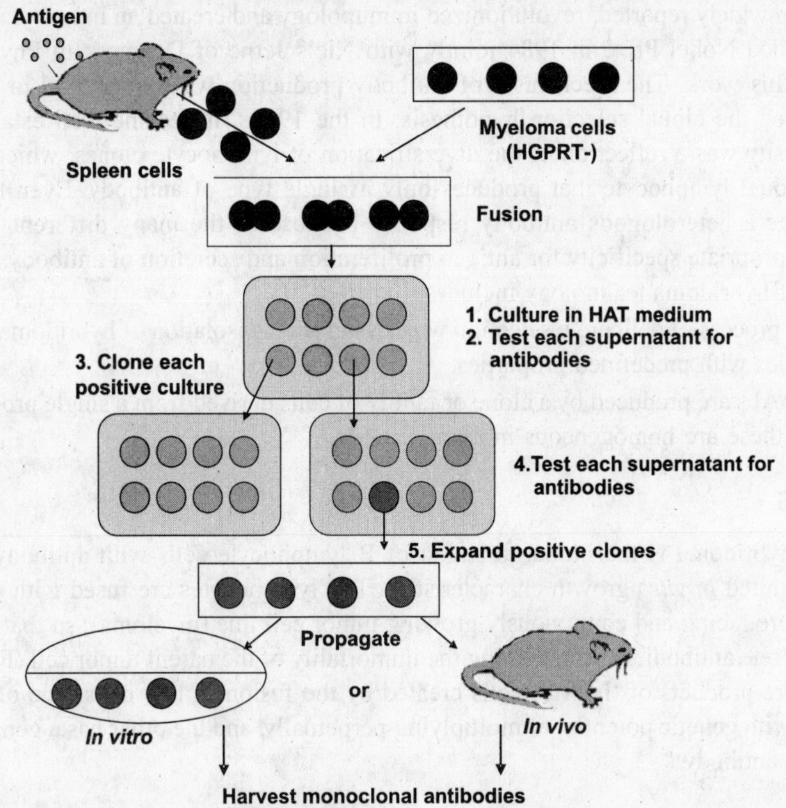

Figure 15.1 Hybridoma technology.

With growing experience, scientists have devised several sophisticated variants of the monoclonal antibody. For instance, they have created some monoclonal antibodies of human rather than mouse origin; human monoclonal antibodies can be used for therapy without risking an immune reaction to mouse proteins. They have also succeeded in "humanizing" mouse antibodies by splicing the mouse genes for the highly specific antigen-recognizing portion of the antibody into the human genes that encode the rest of the antibody molecule. Other monoclonal antibodies have been designed to behave like enzymes. These so-called catalytic antibodies or abzymes speed up, or catalyze selected chemical reactions by binding to a chemical reactant and holding it in a highly unstable "transition state". By, in fact, cutting the proteins to which they bind, such antibodies may be useful for such things as dissolving blood clots or destroying tumor cells.

CONCEPTS

Hybridoma technology, like recombinant DNA technology, is rooted in basic biology and is the result of years of basic research in cell fusion. In 1973, Jeriod Schwaber and Ed Cohen working at the University of Chicago's Liribida Institute were the first to produce antibody-secreting hybridomas by using normal antibody-producing human cells (B cells) and myeloma cells. But it was Kohler and Milstein (1975) working at the medical Research Council Laboratories in Cambridge, UK, who devised and demonstrated a deliberate and rational strategy for the construction of continuous cell lines, which secrete monoclonal antibodies of a desired specificity. That success, which has been widely reported, revolutionized immunology and created an industry. These workers were awarded Nobel Prize in 1984 jointly with Niels Jerne of Denmark in Physiology and Medicine for this work. The mechanism of antibody production was understood in 1975, when Bernet proposed the clonal selection hypothesis. In the 1960s, it became well established that antibody diversity was a reflection of the diversification of lymphocyte clones, which was better than an individual lymphocyte that produces only a single type of antibody. Even homologous antigens induce a heterologous antibody response because of the many different lymphocyte clones with appropriate specificity for antigen proliferation and secretion of antibody.

The concept of hybridoma technology includes:

1. It is the process of deliberate selection which enables the isolation of hybridomas producing antibodies with predefined properties.
2. The MoAbs are produced by a clone or family of cells derived from a single progenitor, that is why these are homogeneous in composition.

PRINCIPLES

The basis of hybridoma is the immortalization of B lymphocyte cells with antibody producing capacity but limited *in vitro* growth characteristics. The lymphocytes are fused with cells from a non-antibody producing and continuously growing tumor cell line (myeloma), so that the hybrids continue to secrete antibodies while gaining the immortality of the parent tumor cell (Figure 15.2). Thus, MAbs are products of 'hybrid' cells created by the fusion of two cells, one of which is a myeloma cell with genetic potential of multiplying perpetually, and the other has a gene that codes for the desired antibody.

HYBRIDOMA TECHNOLOGY

Purpose: The purpose of hybridoma technique is the production of homogeneous antibody against a specific epitope of an antigen *in vitro*. These monoclonal antibodies have wide applications such as:

(a) Research tools for the recognition of specific amino acid sequences of polypeptides.
(b) Diagnostics *in vitro* and *in vivo* for identification and localization of disorders.
(c) Purification of antigens.
(d) Therapeutics for prevention and treatment of diseases.

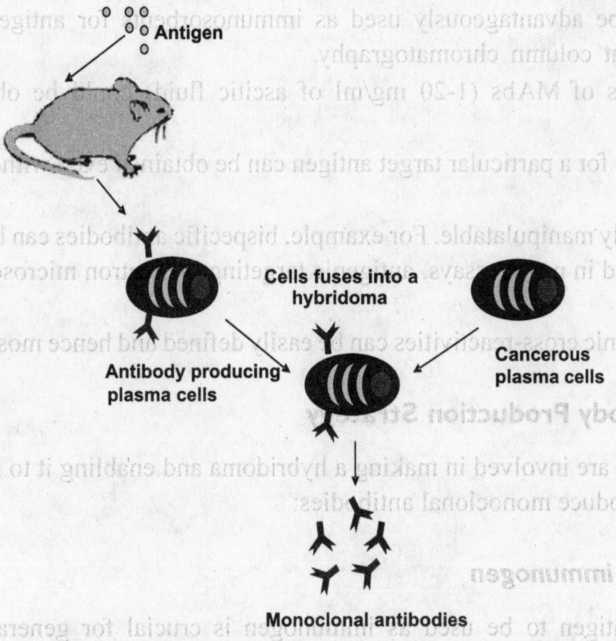

Figure 15.2 Principles of hybridoma technology.

Polyclonal Antiserum Vs. Monoclonal Antibody

Animals respond to an antigenic stimulus by producing a large variety of antibody structures directed against the immunogen. Even a single antigenic determinant is likely to be recognized by a variety of different antibody structures. Thus heterologous mixtures of antibody structures are produced in a polyclonal response, and the populations of antibodies continuously change within the same animal, since each antibody is secreted by all such individual cells into a common blood pool. The composition of polyclonal antibodies will change from day-to-day and from animal to animal. Thus, polyclonal antisera, even when prepared employing well standardized procedures, tend to differ from batch to batch. But MAbs produced by a single clone of cells, which react with a single antigenic determinant, are the most specific biological probes available making possible finer and more sophisticated differences. In 1975, Kohler and Milstein gave the concept of "one lymphocyte-one antibody" in the form of hybridomas. Each lymphocyte produces only one type of antibody, although the isotype may change. The homogeneity, reproducibility and permanent availability of MAbs are the attributes arousing greatest interest in this quickly developing field.

Advantages of monoclonal antibodies

1. Single MAbs are chemically defined, single specificity molecules, and can be used easily for standardization of specific assays.
2. MAbs provide a perpetual source of well defined homogeneous reagents.
3. All the antibodies produced (100%) are active antibodies. Therefore, high specific activity of labelling is possible in radioimmunoassay, enzyme linked immunosorbent assay and fluorescent immunoassay.

4. MAbs could be advantageously used as immunosorbents for antigen purification using immunosorbent column chromatography.
5. Large amounts of MAbs (1-20 mg/ml of ascitic fluid) could be obtained with modest investments.
6. MAbs specific for a particular target antigen can be obtained even without prior purification of antigens.
7. MAbs are easily manipulatable. For example, bispecific antibodies can be prepared from two MAbs and used in novel assays, antigenic targeting in electron microscopy and cytological studies.
8. Distinct antigenic cross-reactivities can be easily defined and hence most useful in diagnosis.

Monoclonal Antibody Production Strategy

Following main steps are involved in making a hybridoma and enabling it to successfully grow in culture medium to produce monoclonal antibodies:

Purity and form of immunogen

The purity of the antigen to be used as immunogen is crucial for generation of monoclonal antibodies. Molecules of low molecular weight (1000 daltons) are poor immunogens and have to be coupled to larger immunogenic molecules. Aggregated and particulate antigens elicit stronger responses. Adjuvants help to achieve stronger responses. The most common carriers are albumins, keyhole limpet haemocyanin, fowl gamma globulin and synthetic polypeptides.

Choice of animals

The choice of the species and strain of the animal used as a source of spleen (donor) for fusion is largely dependent on the myeloma cells available and the origin of the immunogen. Mice are the most common species used for immunization primarily because there are more murine myeloma cell lines available. The BALB/c strain of mice is preferred since the myeloma cell lines available for fusion are derived from this strain.

Immunization procedures

Generally the antigen is injected subcutaneously or into the peritoneal cavity of the animal along with an adjuvant to stimulate the immune system. For most proteins, a dose of 1-50 mg per injection per mouse repeated two or three times is sufficient to evoke a strong antibody response. For soluble antigens, the first injection is given in the presence of the adjuvant and the final booster is given in aqueous solutions. Ten to 14 days afterwards, individual animals are bled and the titre of the antibodies is determined. Animals that show the highest antibody titre are selected and at least 3-4 weeks after the last booster, they are injected i/p with 20-100g of soluble antigen on the first day, and on the following day, they are injected with the same dose intravenously (i/v).

Killing of animal and separation of lymphocytes

Three days after the final dose of antigen has been given intravenously to immunize the animal, the latter is killed. The spleen of the killed animal is removed aseptically and gently disrupted to release the spleen fluid containing lymphocytes and red blood cells. The lymphocytes are separated from the spleen fluid (and red blood cells) by density gradient centifugation, and washed.

Immortalization

The immortalization of antibody producing lymphocytes is the core of hybridoma technology. The purpose of immortalization is to conserve the capability of individual lymphocytes to secrete one single type of MoAb by unlimited *in vitro* growth. This can be done by:

(i) Immortalization by fusion with tumor cells
(ii) Immortalization by infection with a transforming virus
(iii) Immortalization by transfection with tumor or virus derived DNA

Immortalization by Fusion with Tumor Cells

The breakthrough which has become the basis of hybridoma technology was the development of suitable myeloma mutant cell lines that are non-antibody secreting and deficient in the enzyme hypoxanthine quinine phosphoribosy1 transferase (HGPRT) and are able to grow in toxic tissue culture. The enzyme HGPRT is essential for DNA synthesis (by purine salvage pathway) after fusion of these myeloma cells with lymphocytes, metabolic selection in a medium containing HAT (hypoxanthine-aminopterin-thymidine) is accomplished to eliminate the parent myeloma cells and to allow growth of hybridomas which harbour the gene (s) for HGRPT from the parent lymphocytes, i.e., HGPRT myeloma cells die off as aminopterin (a folic acid analogue) blocks the main pathway of DNA synthesis, i.e., *de novo* pathway of DNA synthesis by inhibiting the activity of dihydrofolate reductase. In hybrid cells, spleen cells contribute the functional HGPRT enzyme necessary to overcome the aminoptein block. Lymphocyte parent cells are eliminated due to poor growth *in vitro.*

Fusosen Used

The cell fusion process between amyeloma cella and spleen lymphocytes is usually induced in the presence of polyethylene glycol (PEG-1500). The first fusion experiments were performed with sendai virus as a fusogenic agent. Both regents aggregate the cells which eventually lead to fusion of cells. As compared with UV inactivated sendai virus, PEG increases the number of hybird cells in myeloma fusions because sendai virus has fewer agglutination points on the membrane of B cells. It has recently been shown that hybridization frequencies could be increased by virus by using short electric field pulses of high intensity (electric fusion).

A very recent development, called receptor-directed cell fusion, might be a significant improvement of the fusion process. Lymphocytes carrying antigen-specific antibodies on their surface, are coated with antigen to which avidin is linked. Bioten is bound to the myeloma cell surface. The affinity of avadin for biotin makes the fusion of lymphocytes and mylelomas from a poor efficiency and random process to a controlled and very specific process with high yields. This method is combined with a newly developed hybridization system based on short electric pulses of high intensity.

Condition for Fusion Procedure

Before carrying out the fusion, the following conditions should be met for the mouse system.

- Myeloma cells in the logarithmic growth phase
- Ratio of 2-5 lymphocytes per myeloma cell
- 40% PEG (1000 dal); PEG should be protested for cell toxicity.
- Fusion at 37°C, pH 7.5-8.0, 3 min

Fusion

Membrane fusion consists of 2 distinct stages, cell agglutination, during which the plasma membranes of adjacent cells are brought into close proximity, and the formation of cytoplasmic bridges between cells. These stages are followed by osmotic cell swelling and heterokaryon formation. Polyethylene glycol is used for induction of cells fusion. The mixture of cells is exposed to this fusion promoting agent, but only for few minutes since it is cyotoxic. One minute after exposure of the cells to PEG lipid probes spread from one plasma membrane into the other. Membrane protein mixing does not occur in all systems undergoing fusion. Intercytoplasmic communication begging 1 to 3 min. after dilution of PEG. Water soluble cytoplasmic proteins do not diffuse from one cell to the other until the PEG is removed. Cytoplasmic mixing is optimal at 37°C and is complete at 4h. Cell clumping is maximal within 30 min. and cytoplasmic mixing is almost complete after 40 min.

Immortalization with a Transforming Virus

As an alternative to fusion lymphocytes can be immortalized by a transforming virus. Epstain Barr virus (EBV) is generally used to immortalize human B-lymphocytes. A major problem with EBV transformation is that the cells do not proliferate and / or produce as the hybridomas obtained after fusion. A combination of EBV transformation of human lymphocytes followed by fusion with mouse hybridomas may be a promising technique.

Immortalization with Tumorigenic DNA

Transfection with tumorigenic DNA is a more recent development. Mouse spleen cells have been transfected with DNA from a human leukemia cell line (Reh) in the presence of PEG and DMSO which leads to immortalization of mouse lymphocytes. These last 2 immortalization techniques are attractive alternatives with regard to immortalization of human lymphocytes.

Selection of myeloma cell line

One of the most important points deserving attention during the course of monoclonal antibody production is that just no myeloma lymphocyte be allowed to fuse with normal lymphocyte. The myeloma cell line used must itself not be capable of synthesizing antibody otherwise hybridoma cell line will produce a mixture of antibodies. It is worth noting that in most cases of multiple myeloma there is an overproduction of a particular type of antibody. Such myeloma cell lines that do not produce antibodies are readily available because there are instances where a particular myeloma cell line multiples uncontrollably without antibody production. HPRT-negative myeloma cell line is such an example. Mouse, rat and human myeloma cell lines are available now (Table 15.1).

Table: 15.1 Mouse and rat myeloma lines used for cell fusion.

Name	*Parental tumor**	*Derived from cell lines*	*Phenotype*	
			Ig	*Drug resistance*
Mouse lines				
4 to .2	MPC -11	45.6 TG 1.7	Ig G 2b (K)	6- Thioguanine 1.0 mm Ouabain
P 3-x 63/Ag8	MOPC 21	P 3 k	Ig G1(K)	8- Azaguanine
NSI/1.Ag 4.1	MOPC 21	P 3 –x 63/Ag 8	K (Non-secreted)	8- Azaguanine
FOX- NY	MOPC 21	NS-1	None	8- Azaguanine 2,6 – Diaminopurine
SP 2/0	MOPC 21	P 3-x 63/Ag 8	None	8- Azaguanine
X 63 – Ag 8.653	MOPC 21	P 3 –X 63/Ag	None	8- Azaguanine
Rat Lines				
Y 3- Ag 1.2.3	SR 210	210 – RCY 3 AG 1	(K)	8- Azaguanine
IR 938 F	SR 210	Y3 Ag 1.2.3	None	8- Azaguanine

*MPC – BALB/c mice plasmacytomas ; MOPC – Mineral oil induced tumor cell; SR – Ileocecal immunocytoma tumor cells

The myeloma lymphocytes, before their fusion with normal lymphocytes, are specially selected by growing them in the presence of 8-azaguanine. Most of the cells are killed by the technique, but a few survive. The surviving myeloma lymphocytes are resistant to 8-azaguanine as they have a defect in enzyme Hypoxanthine Phosphorisyl Transferase (HPRT) and are hence called HPRT-negative myeloma lymphocytes.

Fusion of separated lymphocytes with myeloma lymphocytes

After washing, the lymphocytes are mixed with myeloma, and lymphocytes of HPRT-negative cell line. The mixture of the two cell lines is now exposed to polyethylene glycol, a fusion-promoting agent. The latter is cytotoxic and therefore the exposure is limited only to a few minutes. The cells are then washed to make them polyethylene glycol free. The washed cells comprise a mixture of hybridoma cells, unfused lymphocytes and unfused myeloma lymphocytes.

Selection of hybridoma cells

Since the mixture of normal lymphocytes and myeloma lymphocytes contains hybridoma cells, and unfused normal lymphocytes, the hybridoma cells have to be selected from the mixture for further requirements. This is done by using HAT-medium for growth. HAT-medium represents a mixture of hypoxanthine, aminopterin and thymidine. When the said mixture of cells is grown in the HAT-medium, the unfused normal lymphocytes and the unfused myeloma lymphocytes fail to grow. However, the hybridoma cells grow successfully in the HAT-medium because they possess the ability of myeloma lymphocytes to grow *in vitro* and the normal HRPT gene inherited from normal lymphocytes.

Isolation of a monoclonal antibody producing hybridoma cell

If all the hybridoma cells that have been selected using HAT-medium are grown together, a polyclonal antibody mixture would be obtained. Consequently, a single antibody (monoclonal antibody) producing hybridoma cells need to be isolated and grown individually. This is done by diluting a suspension of hybridoma cells to such an extent that individual aliquots contain, on an average, only one cell. Such cells are transferred to separate fresh media for growth. Each mass of hybridoma cells (clone) produced from a single parent hybridoma cell is now examined to determine whether it produces the desired monoclonal antibody. A schematic representation of various steps involved in making a hybridoma is summarized in Figure 15.3.

Cryopreservation of cells

Positive stable hybrids can be stored by freezing them in liquid nitrogen and containing 20-30% FCS and 10% Dimethyl sulphoxide (DMSO) and can be revived wherever required. Ampoules containing hybrids are frozen in a programmable freezer at the rate of 1 DC drop/min. from 40°C to –80°C and then the tubes are transferred into liquid nitrogen, where they can be kept for many years.

Commercial Production of Monoclonal Antibodies (MAbs)

Once the correct hybridoma has been isolated, it can be stored, frozen (cryopreserved) and cultured whenever required. Since the hybridoma is a transferred cell line, it grows readily in culture but the antibody titre is low, say generally 5-10 mg/l. This rate of monoclonal antibody production, which is very low seeing its requirements, has been considerably enhanced using large-scale production methods (Figure 15.4).

Microencapsulation technology

Microencapsulation technology is an interesting method of large-scale production of monoclonal antibodies and has been patented by the Damon Corporation. In this technology, the hybridoma cells, hybridomas, are grown inside hollow microspheres, which are surrounded by a porous membrane. Protected inside the microsphere, the cells multiply and grow to higher densities than is possible with any other culture system. Since the antibody is retained by the membrane, it does

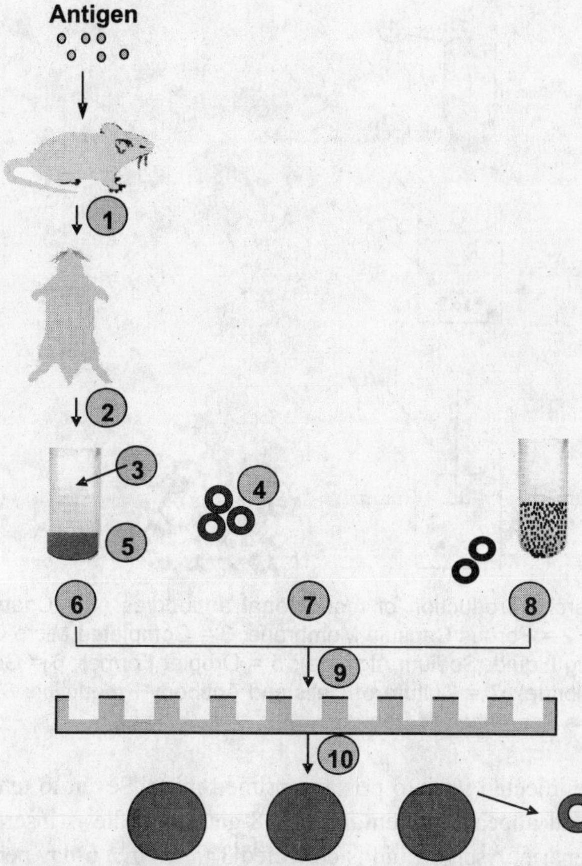

Figure 15.3 Steps involved in making a hybridoma. (1 = Immunization of Mouse with Antigen; 2 = Killing of Mouse and Removal of Spleen; 3 = Splenic Fluid; 4 = Lymphocytes; 5 = Red Blood Cells; 6 = Lymphocytes Purification by Density Gradient Centrifugation; 7 = Fusion; 8 = Myeloma Cells; 9 = Selection Hybrids in Hat Medium; 10 = Cloning and Selection of Hybridoma Cells).

not become contaminated with other immunoglobulins if serum is added in the growth medium. This technology results in the production of 100 mg to one gm of antibody per litre of culture medium and makes large-scale production of monoclonal antibodies (MAbs) commercially feasible.

Ascites-route technology

This technology provides an alternative for MAbs production commercially. In this technique, the hybridoma is grown as cites, as a suspension of tumour cells within the peritoneal cavity of an isogenic species. The ascitic fluid, which is formed following injection of the tumour, generally contains as much as 19.95 gm/L of antibody. This amount is superior to that obtained by the best *in vitro* cultivation technique. Firstly, BALB/C mice that are 6 weeks old are injected i/p with mineral oil, pristane (2, 6, 10, 14-tetramethyl pentadecane) for priming. Two weeks later, hybridoma cells

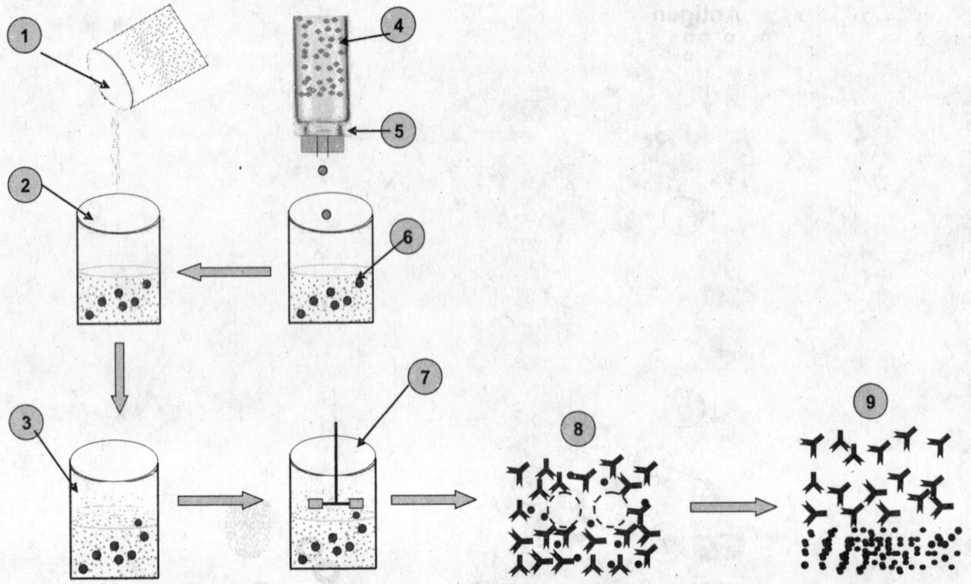

Figure 15.4 Commercial production of monoclonal antibodies (1 = Coating Solution (Poly-Lysine); 2 = Porous Capsule Membrane; 3 = Completed Micro-Capsules; 4 = Cells in Gelling Liquid (Sodium Alginate); 5 = Droplet Former; 6 = Gelled Spheres (Calcium-chloride); 7 = Culture of Cells and Antibody Production; 8 = Release of Antibody; 9 = Separation of Debris).

from selected clones are injected i/p into pristane-primed mice. Seven to ten days after injection, the peritoneal cavities will appear swollen and an 18-gauge needle is inserted into the cavity to collect ascitic fluid in heparin. Ascitic fluid is collected 3 times in a 6-day period. The ascitic fluid is centrifuged (1000 g for 15 min.) to remove cells and fibrin cells. The supernatant is centrifuged again at 52000 g for 10 minutes to remove lipids and small fibrin clots. Antibodies are then precipitated from the supernatants by the addition of an equal volume of saturated ammonium sulphate to the clarified ascitic fluid. The resulting precipitate is dissolved in normal saline (0.85% sodium chloride) and dialysed extensively against normal saline for 12 to 16 hours in cold. The dialysate contains about 80% of antibodies. Some commercial suppliers of monoclonal antibodies use the ascites-route technology, but this technology has considerable disadvantages: (i) it is labour intensive (ii) specific pathogen-free animals required for use and kept quarantined at all times to prevent contamination of the monoclonal antibodies. These disadvantages add generally to the cost of MAbs. In addition, why sacrifice large numbers of laboratory animals when an alternative approach is already available?

Screening Assays for MAbs Activity

The assay system used for the screening of antibody activity in the hybridoma culture supernatants is a key factor that determines success in obtaining the desired MAbs. The main factors to be considered are sensitivity, simplicity, ability to test many samples, speed and reliability. Solid phase radioimmunoassay (RIA) and enzyme linked immunosorbent assay (ELISA) are the frequently used techniques for screening antibody activity in MAbs. ELISA is used commonly for both soluble and cellular antigens. The principle of the ELISA is that in the final step of the assay, the anti-immunoglobulin is enzyme' linked, instead of radio-iodinated. The degree of antibody binding is evaluated by colour development that follows the addition of substrate to the system. The amount of colour developed is proportional to the level of enzyme bound antibody present. ELISA is used for screening the clone supernatants for finding out the isotypes. Although ELISA is somewhat less sensitive than RIA, the handling of samples, colour development and its measurements are faster, especially with automatic scanner that enables the reading, typing and computing of the results of the 96 wells within 1-2 minutes. Another practical advantage of ELISA, especially for the screening procedure is that it allows faster evaluation of results and selection of positive wells based on visual observation.

Problems with Monoclonal Antibody (MAb)

Despite the great promise of MAbs, there are several persistent technical problems to be considered.

1. Obtaining MAbs against certain weak antigens (antigens that do not produce a large immune response) remains difficult.
2. Diagnostic assays employing specific MAbs become ineffective if any alteration in the specific epitope of the target antigen against which the MAbs are made.
3. Low frequency of fusion is a continuing problem in the preparation of hybridomas, as in the stability of the hybridomas and antibodies.
4. Some MAbs are sensitive to small changes in pH, temperature, freezing and thawing and can be inactivated during purification.
5. Another problem being addressed is the development of stable hybridomas for specific species which do not have the preferential loss of the spleen B-lymphocyte chromosomes.
6. MAbs are too specific. Limited MAbs might miss important cross-reactive determinants. This could relate to the animal's immune response to the antigenic stimulus. Polyclonal sera may offer advantage of broad reactivity.
7. It is time-consuming to produce MAbs. The entire process of producing MAbs takes 3-4 months for each fusion experiment. Many of these problems are being alleviated or solved as research with MAbs progresses.

APPLICATIONS OF HYBRIDOMA TECHNOLOGY

There are three main areas in which MAbs are used in human and veterinary medicine. These areas are: (1) immunodiagnostic reagents, either for detection of the causative agents directly in tissues or body fluids or as a reagent used in indirect diagnosis such as serological detection of antibodies to the causative agent, (2) for experimental purposes ranging from molecular dissection of antigenic epitopes to monoclonal anti-idiotype antibody utilized as a vaccine to induce protective immunity and (3) immunoprophylaxis or immunotherapeutics applied to infectious diseases or as a vehicle for delivering toxic substances for example, tumours, or as a tool to identify and locate target tumours. Some of the important applications are discussed.

Medical Applications

Cancer therapy

Immunotoxicology: Generally, most of the tumour (cancer) cells contain additional or new antigens on their surface in comparison to the normal cells from which they are derived. If monoclonal antibodies, which bind to these cancer cells, are isolated, it should be possible to isolate further one or more cancer-specific monoclonal antibody from them. Such antibodies may form the basis of a new form of cancer chemotherapy (Figure 15.5), the immunotoxicology.

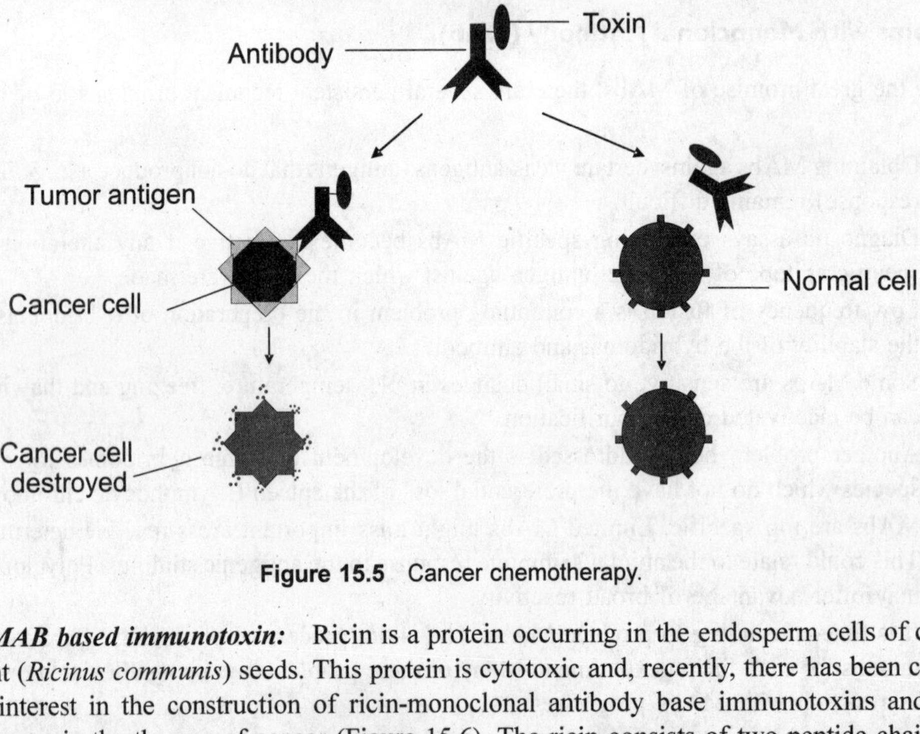

Figure 15.5 Cancer chemotherapy.

Ricin-MAB based immunotoxin: Ricin is a protein occurring in the endosperm cells of castor-oil plant (*Ricinus communis*) seeds. This protein is cytotoxic and, recently, there has been considerable interest in the construction of ricin-monoclonal antibody base immunotoxins and their possible use in the therapy of cancer (Figure 15.6). The ricin consists of two peptide chains, A-chain and B-chain. It is the A-chain of the ricin molecule that enzymatically and irreversibly alters the ribosomes so that they can no longer function and, finally, the sensitive cell to which the ricin has been subjected dies. This toxic A-chain of ricin can be separated from the B-chain and coupled to the monoclonal antibody. This newly created immunotoxin should bind to cancer cells and not normal cells and lead to the death of the former. Since the A-chain of the ricin inhibits protein synthesis and not cell division, it kills even those cells which are potentially harmful but not actively dividing. However, such immunotoxins must be chemically stable in the body; fortunately, studies to date indicate that immunotoxins injected into the body are stable.

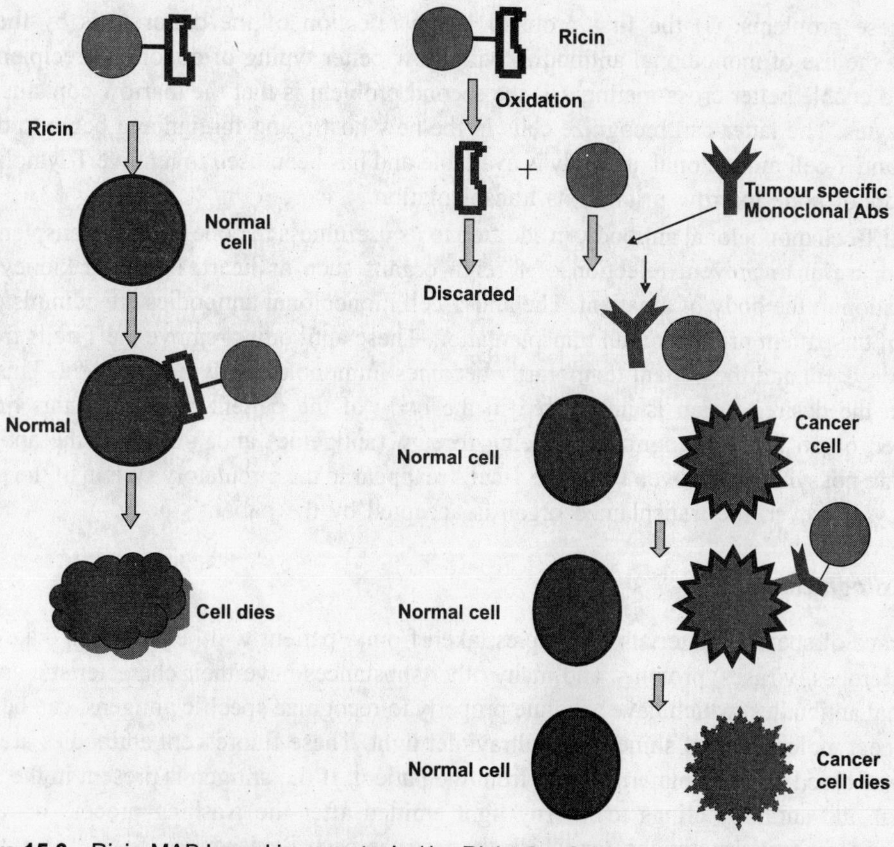

Figure 15.6 Ricin-MAB based immunotoxin (1 = Ricin; 2 = Oxidation; 3 = Discarded; 4 = Tumour-specific MAB; 5 = Immunotoxin).

Radioimmunoassay: Radioimmunoassay is an alternative for cancer therapy. In this, the monoclonal antibody is coupled to a radioisotope such that the cancer cell is killed by irradiation. For this purpose, the radioisotope selected needs to have: (a) high energy so that the target cells are killed; (b) low penetration so that the damage to surrounding tissue be prevented; (c) short half life so that the patient is not a radiation hazard; (d) and the products of radioactive decay stand inert. One isotope, which appears suitable and can be coupled to monoclonal antibodies is "astatine". The half-life of astatine is 13 hours. Unfortunately, astatine has a propensity to be incorporated into bone and this is not desirable. An alternative is "ytrium-90", which has a half-life of 64 hours. Although ytrium-90 is not incorporated into the bone, the β particles, which it, emits, have greater tissue penetration than the α-particles emitted by astatine.

Bone marrow and organ transplantation

There are several diseases where the injection of bone marrow from a healthy individual may be of considerable benefit to a patient. However, there are two main problems associated with bone marrow transplantation and monoclonal antibodies are thought to be significantly helpful in overcoming these problems: (i) the first problem is the rejection of the donor cells by the host. Eventually the use of monoclonal antibodies will allow better typing of donor and recipient lymphocytes to enable better cross-mating; (ii) the second problem is that the marrow contains donor T-lymphocytes. The latter can recognize cells in the new host being foreign and begin to destroy them. An anti T-cell monoclonal antibody is available and has been used to remove T-lymphocytes from the donor bone marrow prior to its transplantation.

The anti T-cell monoclonal antibody, in addition to its usefulness in bone marrow transplantation, has proved useful to prevent rejection of foreign organs such as heart, liver and kidneys after transplantation in the body of a patient. The anti-T-cell monoclonal antibodies are administered in the body of the patient prior to organ transplantation. These antibodies remove the T-cells from the circulatory system and the patient temporarily becomes immunologically incompetent. This is the time when the desired organ is introduced in the body of the patient because at this time the transplanted organ is not recognized as being foreign (antigenic) and, therefore, the antibodies against it are not synthesized even when the T-cells reappear in the circulatory system of the patient. In this way, however, the transplanted organ is accepted by the patient's body.

Disease diagnosis

The presence of specific materials in samples taken from a patient will help doctors diagnose an illness. Microbes, viruses, proteins, and many other substances have their characteristic antigens. Monoclonal antibodies, which have absolute property to recognize specific antigens, can be linked to fluorescent molecules that shine under ultraviolet light. These fluorescent antibodies are added to sample of blood or other material taken from the patient. If the antigen is present in the sample or material, the antibody clings to it. Any light emitted after the washing process betrays the presence of the particular antigen for which the test has been devised.

Infectious diseases: A humanized MAb directed against respiratory syncytial virus (RSC) has been approved in the treatment of premature infants and infants with bronchopulmonary dysplasia. RSV replication was inhibited by palivizumab both *in vitro* and *ex vivo* in tracheal aspirates from infants receiving palivizumab 15 mg/kg.

Parasitic infections: In the field of protozoan and helminthic parasites, MAbs have been used extensively to unravel the relationship between parasite and host. MAbs were used to characterize antigens of *Babesia bovis* and selected MAbs were employed to immunoaffinity-purify *B. bovis* antigen. They further showed that active immunization with one of these purified antigens protected susceptible calves against challenge with virulent *B. bovis* infection. Protozoans studied include those of Plasmodium, Trypanosomes, Leishmania, Theileria and Toxoplasma. Helminths studied include nematodes (*Ascaris* sp., *Onchocerca* sp.), trematodes (*Schistosoma* sp., *Fasciola* sp.) and cestodes (*Taenia* sp. and *Echinococcus* sp.). Monoclonal antibodies were raised against the vaccine strain of *Anaplasma centrale*, which differentiated antigenic differences between cattle vaccinated with *A. centrale* and cattle naturally infected with *A. marginale*.

Bacterial infections: MAbs against bacteria have been used very successfully in classification for diagnostic purposes. The specificity of the MAbs has greatly reduced the cross-reactivity seen using polyclonal sera. Taxonomic studies involving the characterization of evolutionary relationship have been possible. MAbs have been used as structural probes, and the recognition of specific antigens and parts of antigen that can elicit a protective response has been exploited in the preparation of vaccines. Rapid serodiagnostic methods for detection of antigens such as *Neisseria* or *Haemophilus* sp. have been developed. Serotype-specific MAbs have been produced in leptospirosis. Surujballi and Elmgren (2000) produced MAbs suitable for use in a competitive ELISA for detection of specific antibodies to *Leptospira interrogans* serovar pomona. Monoclonal antibody was prepared against *E. coli* 0157 and ELISA specific for this pathogen was developed. This method has proved to be a sensitive and specific technique to detect low number of *E. coli* 0157 in food. Monoclonal antibodies to purified K99 antigen of *Escherichia coli* (*E. coli*) were produced by the hybridoma technique, and a specific clone, NEK99-5.6.12, was selected for propagation in tissue culture. Swiecki *et al.* (2006) developed a variety of isotypes and specificities of MAbs that were able to distinguish *B. anthracis* spores from other Bacillus spores. Recently, LipL32, the major outer membrane protein of pathogenic *Leptospira*, in its recombinant form (rLipL32) was used to immunize BALB/c mice to develop murine MAbs.

Viral infections: In virology, MAbs have been exploited in research and applied areas. This is leading to a better understanding in areas of vaccine formulations, particularly where novel peptide vaccines are being considered. The obvious use of MAbs is in the comparison of viruses from the field MAb panels and is prepared against distinct antigenic sites (epitomes) on viruses and used to examine the possession of these sites in immunoassays. These have an important role in understanding the epidemiology of disease (antigenic variation) and also in monitoring viruses throughout vaccine manufacture (quality control of antigenicity in rabies, polio and influenza vaccines). For example, MAb that distinguish CPV and feline panleukopenia virus have been produced recently. MAbs have been extensively used in studying rinderpest and FMD viruses. Recently, MAbs against several FMDV serotypes have been prepared in European and American laboratories. These have been used as research tools to identify important neutralizing antibodies inducing epitopes and to evaluate the mechanisms by which virus is neutralized *in vitro* and *in vivo*. Two foot-and-mouth disease virus (FMDV) monoclonal antibodies (MAbs) were produced from mice immunized with either FMDV serotype A, subunit (12S) or FMDV serotype 0, whole virus (140S). MAbs produced against 42-kDa major structural proteins of rotavirus could be used for preliminary serotyping of strains from different animal species. MAbs against rabies virus have been employed for molecular characterization of street vaccine and laboratory strains. The use of MAbs against bovine diarrhoea virus in immunofluorescent antibody technique has aided preliminary serological characterization of strains and both indirect and competitive ELISA techniques utilizing MAbs to detect antibodies against the virus in bovine sera. MAbs against bluetongue virus have been used for analysis of serotype and group specific antibodies in cattle and sheep by a MAb blocking (competitive) ELISA and for demonstration of viral antigens in infected tissues. Bovine leukaemia virus infection of cattle is another area where MAb based ELISA system has enabled detection of virus specific serum antibodies. Competitive ELISA using two MAbs was developed and compared with the standard virus neutralization test (VNT) for detecting antibodies against canine distemper virus (CDV) and phocine distemper virus (PDV) in sera from dogs and various species of marine mammals. Monoclonal antibody-based capture ELISA was developed for the diagnosis of rabies suspect specimens. Six clones of monoclonal antibodies (MAbs) to fowl adenovirus (FAV) serotype 1 were produced. All MAbs reacted positively by enzyme-linked immunosorbent assay. A rapid diagnostic strip test for detection of chicken infectious bursal disease (IBD) was developed based on membrane chromatography using high affinity MAbs directed to chicken IBDY. Philippe *et al.* (2007) developed a panel of monoclonal antibodies (MAbs) against the H5Nl avian influenza virus (AIV) and implemented an antigen capture ELISA (AC- ELISA) to detect H5 viral antigen.

In addition, MAbs have been developed against a large number of viruses including rabies virus, foot and mouth disease virus, bovine leukaemia virus and bovine enteric coronavirus. MAbs have been produced against various parasites, including *Trichinella spiralis*, *Babesia bovis* and *Dirofilaria immitis*. MAbs have also been raised against bacterial species, including *Mycobacterium* spp. and *Brucella* spp.

Accurate and rapid diagnosis of infectious agents is of considerable importance in veterinary medicine, particularly when dealing with highly infectious agents such as foot-and-mouth disease virus. MAbs have an important role in the diagnostic laboratory; however, if the antibody is not carefully selected, erroneous diagnosis may result.

Therapeutic monoclonal antibodies

The potential therapeutic application of MAb created a tremendous interest in the medical and pharmaceutical community. A recent survey suggested that over a quarter of all biotech drugs in development are MAbs. Within this group, more than 30 chimeric, humanized, or fully human antibodies account for more than 30 products being routinely used or investigated in the clinic for various indications. The most promising and advanced therapeutic strategies include inhibition of alloimmune and autoimmune reactivity, antitumour therapy, anti-platelet therapy and antiviral therapy. Rabies virus neutralizing human MAbs were evaluated *in vitro* and in a Syrian hamster model as a potential future alternative to rabies immunoglobulin (RIG), which is used for post-exposure prophylaxis. Seven MAbs neutralized a representative rabies virus. In hamsters, one MAb resulted in protection that was comparable to human RIG. Human monoclonal antibodies (HuMAbs) that neutralized rabies virus were developed. The products that obtained marketing approval by the registration authorities in the USA or Europe are discussed in Table 15.2.

Table 15.2 MAbs registered for therapeutic clinical use.

Generic name	*Trade name*	*Company*	*Indication*	*Dose*	*Route*
Muromonab	Orthoclone OKT3	Janssen-Cilag	Renal graft rejection	5 mg per day	Intravenous
Basiliximab	Simulect	Novartis	Renal graft rejection	20 mg direct	Intravenous
Daclizumab	Zenapax	Hoffinan-la Roche	Renal graft rejection	I mg/kg before and 2, 4, 6 and 8 weeks after transplantation	Intravenous
Infliximab	Remicade	Centocer	Rheumatoid arthritis, Crohn's disease	3-10 mg/kg every 4-8 weeks	Intravenous

Contd.

Rituzimab		Genentech-Roche	Lymphoma	375 mg/m2 in four weekly doses	Intravenous
Trastuzuma	Herceptin	Genentech	Metastatic breast cancer	4 mg/kg initially, followed by 2 mg/kg weekly	Intravenous
Abciximab	Reopro	Lilly	Anti-platelet	0.25 mg/kg initially followed by 0.125 mg/kg per min.	Intravenous
Palivizumab	Synagis	Abbot lab	Antiviral	15 mg/kg	Intravenous

Veterinary Applications

The major uses of veterinary pharmaceuticals are as growth promoters, antibacterial agents, and antiparasitic agents. Most animals infected with caprine arthritis-encephalitis virus (CAEV) make antibodies to the p28 major core polypeptide, and these antibodies are used to diagnose CAEV infection. Immunodiffusion and immunoprecipitation assays with sera from animals infected with CAEV, visna virus (VV) and progressive pneumonia virus (PPV) do not differentiate the p28s of these viruses. By Travis *et al.* (1987) have shown that monoclonal antibodies (MAbs) and peptide maps were used to compare p28s from VV, PPV and four CAEV isolates. Advances in antibody engineering have solved many of the problems inherent in traditional sources of antibodies, and about a quarter of all biotechnology-based drugs now in development are antibodies. Recently, Qing *et al.* (2009) have shown antibody-based targeting of (FGF receptor 3) in bladder carcinoma and positive multiple myeloma in mice as potential therapeutic diagnosis agent.

Agricultural Applications

"Molecular farming" is the production of pharmaceutical proteins in transgenic plants and has great potential for the production of therapeutic anti-cancer antibodies and recombinant therapeutic proteins. Plants make fully functional recombinant human or animal antibodies. Cultivating transgenic plants on an agricultural scale will produce almost unlimited supplies of recombinant proteins for uses in medicine. Antibody production on an industrial scale is then possible using plant suspension cell culture in fermenters, or by the propagation of stably transformed plant lines in the field. Recombinant proteins can be produced either in whole plants or in seeds and tubers, which can be used for the long-term storage of both the protein and its production system. This demonstrates the promise of using transgenic plants as bioreactors for the molecular farming of recombinant therapeutics, including vaccines, diagnostics, such as recombinant antibodies, plasma proteins, cytokines and growth factors. The current use of antibody administration for prophylaxis or treatment of infectious diseases in agriculture leads to the development of antibody engineering and "molecular farming" of antibodies in various expression systems. Especially the potential of producing therapeutic antibodies in crops that are routine dietary components of farm animals, such as corn and soybeans, seems to hold promise for future application in the fight against infectious diseases. Plants have many practical and economic advantages over traditional production systems, while edible crops in particular are regarded as among the safest production systems for pharmaceutical proteins.

Yang *et al.* (2005) have prepared monoclonal antibody against hygromycin B phosphotransferase (HPT) that can be used to detect marker protein in genetically modified rice. VH (heavy-chain variable region) and VL (light-chain variable region) genes were amplified by PCR from hybridomas producing MAb-11 and MAb-18, which inhibited Japanese radish acid phosphatase. Galeffi *et al.* (2005) have reported that the cloning and expression of a scFv-alpha HER2 that has been produced in plants using both stable and transient systems in tobacco and Nicotiana benthamiana, which represents a good opportunity for application and use in diagnosis and therapy. Antibodies against large numbers of different antigens, including plant proteins, can be produced by phage selection of singlechain Fv or Fab fragments with recombinant immunoglobulin gene libraries. Using this technology, antibody phage display libraries can be screened against expression products of plant cDNA libraries. Many monoclonal antibodies that are specific for pathogens already exist (Table 15.3), such as tobacco mosaic virus (TMV), and are a resource for pathogen-resistant crop development. These antibodies can be cloned from the hybridoma cell line for use in plant protection. After completing the cloning, the antibody genes have to be modified before they can be expressed in *Escherichia coli*, yeast, insect, mammalian, or plant cells.

Table 15.3 Recombinant antibodies expressed in plants (Source: Rainer *et al.*, 2001).

Year	*rAb format*	*Antigen*	*Cellular location*	*Plant organ*	*Transformed species**	*Maximum yield*	*Reference*
1989	IgG1	Phosphonate ester	ER apoplast	Leaf	*N. tabacum L.*	1.3% TSP	Hiatt *et al.*, 1989
1990	IgM	NP hapten	ER chtoroplast	Leaf	*N. tabacum*	–	Düring *et al.*, 1990
1991	V_H	Substance P (neuropeptide)	Intra-and extra-cellular	Leaf	*N. benthamiana*	1% TSP	Benvenuto *et al.* 1991
1992	scFV	Phytochrome	Cytosol	Leaf	*N. tabacum*	0.1% TSP	Owen *et al.*, 1992
1993	IgG1 Fab	Human creatine kinase	Nucleolus	Leaf	*N. tabacum, A. thaltana*	1.3% TSP	De Neve *et al.*, 1993
1993	scFV	Phytochrome	Apoplast	Leaf	*N. tabacum*	0.5% TSP	Firek *et al.*, 1993
1993	scFV	AMCV	Cytosol	Leaf	*N. benthamiana*	0.1% TSP	Tavladoraki *et al.*, 1993
1994	IgG	Fungal cutinase	Apoplast	Root	*N. tabacum*	0.35% TSP	van Engelen *et al.*, 1994
1994	IgG1	*Streptococus mutans* adhesin	Apoplast	Leaf	*N. tabacum*	7.7 µg/mL plant extract	Ma *et al.*, 1994
1995	IgA/G	*Streptococus mutans* adhesin	Apoplast	Leaf	*N. tabacum*	500 µg/g FM	Ma *et al.*, 1995
1995	IgG	TMV	Apoplast	Leaf	*N. tabacum*	0.3% TSP	Voss *et al.*, 1995
1996	scFV	Cutinase	ER	Leaf	*N. tabacum*	1% TSP	Schouten *et al.*, 1996
1996	IgM	RKN secretion	Apoplast	Leaf	*N.tabacum*	0.01% TSP	Baum *et al.*, 1996
1996	IgM	RKN secretion	Apoplast	Root	*N. tabacum*	0.003% TSP	Baum *et al.*, 1996
1996	scFV	BNYVV	Apoplast	Leaf	*N. benthamiana*	0.1% TSP	Fecker *et al.*, 1996
1996	scFV	Human creatine kinase	Cytoplasm ER	Leaf	*N. tabacum*	0.01% TSP	Bruyns *et al.*, 1996
1996	IgG1 Fab	Human creatine kinase	Apoplast	Leaf	*A. thaliana*	11-13% ICF protein	De Wilde *et al.*, 1996

Contd.

1997	scFV	β-1, 4-Endoglucanse	Cytosol	Root	*S. tuberosum L.*	0.3% TSP	Schouten *et al.*, 1997
1997	scFV	Oxazolone	ER	Leaf	*N. tabacum*	4% TSP	Fiedler *et al.*, 1997
1997	scFV	Oxazolone	ER	Seed	*N. tabacum*	2.6% TSP	Fiedler *et al.*, 1997
1997	scFV	Abscisic acid	ER	Leaf	*N. tabacum*	6.8% TSP	Fiedler *et al.*, 1997
1997	scFV	Abscisic acid	ER	Seed	*N. tabacum*	4% TSP	Phillips *et al.*, 1997
1998	scFV	Oxazolone	ER	Turber	*S. tuberasum*	2% TSP	Artsaenko *et al.*, 1998
1998	Humanized IgG1	HSV-2	Apoplast	Plant	*G. max (L.) Merr.*	–	Zeitlin *et al.*, 1998
1998	mAb	Colon cancer antigen	Apoplast	Leaf	*N. benthamiana*	940 mg/g FM	Verch *et al.*, 1998
1998	scFV	TMV	Apoplast	Leaf	*N. tabacum*	0.006% TSP	Zimmemann *et al.*, 1998
1998	scFV	Atrazine		Leaf	*N. tabacum*	0.014% TSP	Longstaff *et al.*, 1998
1998	scFV	Dihydro-flavonol 4-reductase	Cytosol	Leaf	*P. xhybrida Hort. Vilm-Andr.*	1% TSP	De Jaeger *et al.*, 1998
1999	scFV	38C13 mouse B cell lymphoma	Apoplast	Leaf	*N. benthamiana*	–	Mc Cormick *et al.*, 1999
1999	biscFV	TMV	ER	Leaf	*N.tabacum*	1.65% TSP	Fischer *et al.*, 1999
1999	biscFV	TMV	Apoplast	Leaf	*N. tabacum*	0.064% TSP	Fischer *et al.*, 1999
2000	scFV	TMV	Apoplast membrane	Leaf	*N. tabacum*	8.9 μg/gFM	Schillberg *et al.*, 2000

Note: AMCV, antichoke mottle crinkle virus; BNYVV, beet necrotic yellow vein virus, ER, endoplasmic reticulum; FM, fresh mass; HSV-2 herpes simplex virus-2; ICF, intracellular fluid; RKN, root-knot nematode; TMV, tobacco mosaic virus; TSP, total soluble protein.

**A, Arabidopsis; G, Glycine, N, Nicotiana; P, Penturina; S, Solanum.*

Industrial Applications

Monoclonal antibodies in vaccine production

Antibodies have also been used to immunize against certain diseases in humans and cattle. The most promising outcome is the prospect of developing antimalarial and cancer vaccine in the near future. Monoclonal antibodies that inhibit the *in vitro* multiplication of Plasmodium, and the antigametocyte antibodies that inactivate male gametes have been developed. Monoclonal antibodies that destroy merozoite infected RBCs have also been developed now. Such antibodies may prove useful as vaccines (Table 15.4).

Table 15.4 Antibodies in vaccine production.

Antigen source	*Anti-idiotypic source*	*Species vaccinated*
Streptococcus pneumoniae	Mouse monoclonal	Mouse
E. coli K 13	Mouse monoclonal	Mouse
Trypanosoma cruzi	Rabbit serum	Mouse, rabbit, guinea pig
Hepatitis B surface antigen	Rabbit serum	Chimpanzee

Contd.

Polio virus type II	Mouse monoclonal	Mouse
Rabies virus	Rabbit serum	Mouse
Reovirus	Mouse monoclonal	Mouse
Cytomegalovirus	Mouse monoclonal	Mouse
Human immunodeficiency virus	Rabbit serum	Mouse
Murine sarcoma	Mouse monoclonal	Mouse
Murine bladder tumour	Mouse monoclonal	Mouse
Murine B cell lymphoma	Mouse idiotypic IgM	Mouse
Human melanoma	Rabbit Serum	Mouse
Human T cell lymphoma	Mouse monoclonal	Mouse
Human colon carcinoma	Goat serum	Human
Human colon carcinoma	Human monoclonal	–

Other Biotechnological Applications

Protein purification

Monoclonal antibodies immobilized by coupling to a cyanogen bromide activated chromatography matrix (e.g., sepharose) have proved particularly valuable for the purification of proteins. This is because of their exquisite power of discrimination. Looking for a needle in a haystack and extracting it is not such a problem if one has a magnet, and in monoclonal antibodies we can hope to find a magnet, which will pick up just what we are looking for. This new protein purification technique has at least three advantages over conventional techniques of purification:

(i) Since the monoclonal antibody has unique specificity for the desired protein, the level of contamination by unwanted protein species is usually very low.

(ii) Since the monoclonal antibody-antigen-complex has a single binding affinity, it is possible to elute the required protein (antigen) by washing with buffer.

(iii) Since the capacity of the monoclonal antibody remains unchanged, the concentration of the required protein relative to total protein in a mixture is irrelevant. These are instances where a 97% recovery of interferon was obtained using this technique (immunoaffinity chromatography) when the starting concentration was less than 0.02%. The fact that 5300-fold purification was obtained in a single step highlights the power of the method used, and it is not surprising that the method is being used commercially to purify recombinant derived interferon α_2.

Gene cloning and expression

Recently, it has been studied that the monoclonal antibodies can be utilized in the studies of gene cloning and expression. It is reported that a monoclonal antibody specific for the heavy chain of DR-antigen (coded for by a gene in the major histocompatibility-complex of humans) could be used to precipitate polysomes containing the DR-mRNA from lysates of cells of a human-B-lymphoblastoid line. The monoclonal antibody presumably reacts with the nascent polypeptide chains of DR heavy chain. The researchers found that DR heavy chain is the major product of the cell-free translation of the immunoprecipitated mRNA to construct recombinant plasmids and found that one of a few bacterial transformants expressed DR heavy chain. These results indicate that mRNAs can be enriched greatly by precipitating specific mRNA-containing polysomes with monoclonal antibodies.

Drug targeting

MAbs can be used as vehicles for the delivery of drugs *in vivo*. Conjugates of antibody with drugs are able to bind to an appropriate target cell and the antibody-linked drug is then introduced directly into that cell. This allows higher concentration of the drug to reach the desired site and minimize systemic toxicity. Drugs such as daunamycin, vindesin, methotrexate and adriamycin can be coupled to MAbs. Better survival rates can be observed in experimental mice with lymphomas given daunamycin attached to antilymphoma MAbs compared to those receiving the drug alone. A recombinant chimeric MAb against fibrin coupled to tissue plasminogen activator (tPA) has been used in animal models. Because of its affinity for fibrin, the recombinant protein becomes concentrated in a clot, thereby locally raising the concentration of tPA. This helps in promoting an enhanced lysis of the clot. Such thrombolytic agents would have a crucial role to play in cardiovascular diseases.

Monoclonal antibodies as enzymes (Abzymes)

The use of antibodies as enzymes is described as abzymes. The antibodies may often bind specific ligands (haptens), but may not carry out chemical reactions. By modifying these ligands, antibodies may be generated that will catalyse specific reactions just like enzymes. Production of these abzymes is based on the following two principles: (1) enzymes work by binding the transition state of a reactant better than the ground state, and (2) antibodies that bind to specific small molecules can be produced by coupling this small molecule to a protein carrier and using this protein for immunizing experimental animals.

Abzymes were shown to accelerate the reactions, which they are supposed to catalyse. Some examples of abzymes are given in Table 15.5.

Table 15.5 Antibody with enzymatic activity.

Enzymatic activity of antibody	*Substrate of reaction*	*Acceleration*
Chorismate mutase	Chorismate	1×10^2
Esterase	Hydroxyl ester	1.7×10^2
Esterase	Carboxyl ester	9.6×10^2
		2.1×10^2
Esterase	Carbonate ester	7.7×10^3
Esterase	Coumarin ester	1.5×10^3
Esterase	Carbonate ester	8.1×10^2
Esterase	Carbonate ester	6.3×10^6
		1.2×10^5

Preparation (purification) of medically important products using monoclonal antibodies

Tiny amounts of enzymes and proteins of medical value in a crude preparation have to be extracted in maximum pure form in many cases. Monoclonal antibodies have proved to be useful in high level purification and large-scale preparation of the medically important substances. Immunoaffinity columns containing monoclonal antibodies coupled to cyanogen bromide-activated sepharose, when used for human leucocyte interferon, a product which is 5,000 times richer in interferon, could be obtained from the original crude mixture in a single step.

Monoclonal antibodies for cytogenetic analysis

The technique of ELISA utilizing monoclonal antibodies has also been used for cytogenetic analysis in wheat. Monoclonal antibodies specific to chromosomes 1B, 6A and 6D are already available and those for other chromosomes will become available in future due to proteins coded by chromosomes of all homologous groups. Monoclonal antibodies can be used to enrich the number of aneuploids in a population by rejecting seeds showing high level of reaction with monoclonal antibodies. The major advantage of using monoclonal antibodies is that a very large number of seeds can be examined non-destructively and the chromosome analysis can be greatly reduced, if not eliminated.

Experimental uses of monoclonal antibodies

Cells of immune system: MAbs have been used extensively to characterize various cell populations involved in immune responses of mice and man. The Lyt system of antigens has been developed for functional differentiation of T lymphocytes. Lyb antigens have been used for differentiation of B lymphocytes. Similar studies in domestic animals are in infancy. Krawiec and Muscoplet (1984) developed MAbs specific for canine T lymphocytes and others capable of distinguishing medullary and cortical thymocytes. Davis *et al.* (1984) catalogued about 100 MAbs for their reactivity patterns with bovine, ovine, caprine, porcine, equine and human lymphocytes. Interestingly, interspecies cross reaction was extensive with reagents and limited with others, with mono specificity being relatively rare to some antigens, such as MHC-class I antigen. Lunney (1983) used monoclonal antibody to swine lymphocyte antigen complex to identify and purify *Ia* antigens and to study the immune response to various antigens including a synthetic peptide.

Pregnancy and sex determination: MAbs have been used to detect pregnancy by the presence of progesterone in milk. Using a direct double antibody solid phase enzyme immunoassay it was found that 1-2 pg of progesterone per ml of milk could be detected, which was an excellent assay without extraction or centrifugation of the milk. MAbs to a variety of other hormones have been prepared. Such hormones include somatotropin, human chorionic gonadotropin and bovine and porcine insulin. An interesting and at present controversial application is in the area of embryo sexing. Antibody to H-Y antigen, the male-specific transplantation antigen, has been sought over the years to establish definitely the sex of an embryo.

Molecular structure of antigens: Antigens are defined as substances capable of reacting with antibodies; however, the reactivity with antibody is confined to the antigenic determinants or epitopes present on the antigen molecule. The epitope complements the antigen-binding site of the variable region of the antibody molecule in its configuration. Epitopes of antigens fall into two broad categories-sequential and conformational determinants. Sequential determinants are sequences of amino acids of an unfolded or randomly folded peptide, whereas in conformational epitopes the amino acids are brought into close proximity by the conformation of the antigen; as a consequence, antibody to a true conformational determinant rarely reacts with the unfolded molecule. A considerable number of protein antigens and viruses have been studied in detail with MAbs to determine their epitope structures. The molecular dissection approach has been used with MAbs to select antigenic variants of several viruses of veterinary importance. A single amino acid change-arginine at position 333-Df a glycoprotein in the virulent form of the rabies virus was found to be the only change in non-pathogenic variants. Neutralizing antibodies to antigens such as YP2 antigens in bluetongue virus and foot, and, mouth disease virus YPI antigen and its peptides have been described. MAbs have been found to be useful in dissecting, mapping and identifying the antigenic epitopes of virus proteins that elicit the production of neutralizing antibodies.

Affinity chromatography: Because of their exquisite specificity, MAbs are suitable for use in purification of antigens. This usually entails the immobilization of the MAb on an insoluble matrix, such as agarose beads, by a covalent linking agent, for example cyanogen bromide. The beads with MAb attached can be used either in a batch procedure or in a column chromatography for antigen purification. Antigen purification by affinity has been applied to substances ranging from *Ia* antigens of the swine lymphocyte antigen complex, glycoproteins of herpes viruses, and to antigens of *Trichinella spiralis*.

Inhibition of A1loimmune Reactivity: After successful clinical trials by multicentre transplant study group in 1985, the first license for a MAb was granted by the US Food and Drug Administration for routine use of OKT3 (Muromonab CD3), a murine MAb for the prevention of graft rejection in renal transplant patients. As first-line or in steroid-resistant rejection therapy, OKT3 has proven efficacious and some studies have shown improved graft survival. In the search for more specific immunosuppression with MAb, the interleukin-2 receptor, which is expressed on activated T cells was chosen as a target. Chimeric and humanized MAb boasiliximab (Simulec) and daclizumab (Zenapax) were developed to bind to the interleukin-2 receptor (CD25). These MAbs provide immunosuppression by competitive antagonism of interleukin-2 receptor (CD25) or by elimination of activated T cells.

Inhibition of Autoimmune Reactivity: MAbs have been investigated as a therapeutic approach for the treatment of autoimmune diseases to target elements of the immune response such as T or B lymphocytes, irrespective of their antigen specificity. This approach seeks to suppress excessive immunopathological responses by removing activated cells, blocking their function, or normalizing elevated levels of proinflammatory cytokines. The most encouraging clinical results emerged with TNF-blocking therapies in rheumatoid arthritis and Crohn's disease. TNF is a cytokine produced primarily by activated monocytes and macrophages, with a broad spectrum of biological activities. This enzyme induces vasodilatation, increases vascular permeability, activates platelets, and regulates the production of acute phase proteins, other pro-inflammatory cytokines and mediators of inflammation. TNF is actively produced in various infectious diseases: sepsis, malaria, adult respiratory distress syndrome and AIDS. TNF is also important in autoimmune inflammatory diseases. The cytokine is actively produced at the synovial and mucosal sites of inflammation in rheumatoid arthritis and Crohn's disease. The chimeric (human-mouse) MAb, infliximab (CA2, Remicade), binds to TNF specifically and neutralizes its activity. Administration of infliximab was of substantial clinical benefit in both rheumatoid arthritis and Crohn's disease. The first randomized trial of infliximab on rheumatoid arthritis was reported in 1994.

Anti-platelet Therapy: Acute coronary syndromes and percutaneous coronary interventions share a common pathophysiological mechanism of intimal disruption and platelet aggregation. Glycoprotein IIb/IIIa receptor antagonists, which interrupt the final common pathway of platelet activation and aggregation, have clear benefit as acute therapy. Abciximab (Reo Pro) was the first antagonist to be evaluated in clinical studies. The EPIC trial examined whether an abciximab or placebo would reduce ischaemic complications in high-risk patients undergoing angioplasty (Topol *et al*., 1994). At 30 days there was a 35% reduction of composite death, myocardial infarction and urgent revascularization compared with placebo (8.3 vs 12.8%).

Recent Advancements and Future Prospects of Hybridoma Technology

In recent years, techniques have been developed, which allow production of monoclonal antibodies without hybridomas or even without the help of animals used for providing cells (lymphocytes and myeloma cells). For instance, antibody genes can be isolated from lymphocytes of immunized animals and then cloned and expressed in bacteria. The antibodies produced in bacteria under the control of cloned genes can be screened for binding to specific antigens. Thus, while hybridoma technology can immortalize antibody producing cells, gene technology immortalizes antibody producing genes. Computer graphic techniques are also being used to build specific antigen binding sites in antibodies. Using this approach some designer antibodies of practical value have already been produced. In this latter strategy, genes are not really cloned from lymphocytes, but are instead designed from a repertoire of antibody genes available in a collection.

Somatic cell fusion, as the basis of hybridoma technology is one of the new biology. This together with molecular biology and novel purification technology has become an essential part of the new biotechnologies. These new biologies which go partly hand in hand are reinforcing research efforts to elucidate fundamental biological phenomena. At the same time they are improving the immunochemical detection of foreign proteins. Thus this technique can make impact not only in medical sciences but also in the field of veterinary science, agriculture and animal breeding.

CONCLUSION

Although hybridoma technology has proved useful for the generation of reagent and diagnostic antibodies, the immunogencity of monoclonal antibodies has limited their therapeutic development. This limitation has been largely overcome by the chimerization and humanization of murine monoclonal antibodies. The clinical use of monoclonal antibodies, however, had to wait for advances in genetic engineering. Over the past 15 years, antibody humanization has proved to be a powerful technique to minimize, or even eliminate, the immunogenicity of monoclonal antibodies. Since the basic framework structure of the immunoglobulin variable regions is well conserved among species, humanization technology may be applied beyond rodent antibodies. Non-rodent antibodies, particularly non-mammal antibodies, would recognize antigens (or epitopes) highly conserved between rodents and humans, to which rodents cannot effectively generate antibodies. Thus, the use of non-rodent monoclonal antibodies for humanization could expand the repertoire of antibody-based therapeutics. Currently, over fifty humanized antibodies are being evaluated in a variety of clinical trials. The antigens include cytokines and their receptors, chemokines and their receptors, infectious viruses, microorganisms and their toxins, tumor-specific antigens, growth factor receptors, angiogenic factors, and adhesion molecules. With the advances in genomics and proteomics, the number of target molecules for antibody-based therapeutics is rapidly increasing.

FURTHER READINGS

1. Adams A.N., Barbara D.J. and Clark M.F. (1977) an indirect ELISA using a single antiserum and a general purpose conjugate. *ISHS Acta Horticulturae.* 130: XII International Symposium on Fruit Tree Virus Diseases.
2. Akerstrom B., Brodin T., Reis K. and Bjorck L. (1985) Protein G: A powerful tool for binding and detection of monoclonal and polyclonal antibodies. *J. Immunol.* **(135):** 2589-2592.
3. Alexandra D.B., Stefanie N. and Michael N. (2007) Technology and Production of Murine Monoclonal and Recombinant Antibodies and Antibody Fragments. Series: *Methods in Biotechnology.* **(24):** 93-121.
4. Alexandre S., Charles L., Valentine D., Jean L., Keith V. and Florence C. (2003) Efficacy of rabies immunoglobulins in an experimental post-exposure prophylaxis rodent model. *Vaccine.* 22 **(2):** 244-249.
5. Anilionis A., Wunner W.H. and Curtis P.J. (1982) Amino acid sequence of the rabies virus glycoprotein deduced from its cloned gene. *Comparative Immunology, Microbiology and Infectious Diseases.* 5 **(1-3):** 27-32.
6. Appleton J.A. and Letchwdrth G.J. (1983) Monoclonal antibody analysis of serotype-restricted and unrestricted bluetongue viral antigenic determinants. *Virology.* **(124):** 286-299.
7. Boulain J.C. and Ducancel F. (2004) Expression of recombinant alkaline phosphatase conjugates in *Escherichia coli. Methods in Molecular Biology.* **(267):** 101-112.
8. Boyd J.E. and James K. (1989) Human monoclonal antibodies: Their potential, problems, and prospects. In: *Monoclonal Antibodies: Production and Application.* A. Mizrahi, ed. New York: Alan R. Liss, Inc. pp.1-43
9. Bradbury A., Velappan N., Verzillo V., Ovecka M., Chasteen L., Sblattero D., Marzari O., Lou J.L., Siegel R. and Pavlik P. (2003) Antibody in proteomics. I. *Trends in Biotechnology.* **(21):** 275-281.
10. Brodeur B. and Tsang P. (1986) High yield monoclonal antibody production in ascites. *J. Immunol. Methods.* **(86):** 239-241.
11. Crouch C.F. and Raybould T.J. (1983) Comparison of different antigen preparations as substrates for use in passive hemagglutination and enzyme-linked immunosorbent assays for detection of antibody against bovine enteric coronavirus. *J. Clin. Microbiol.* 18 **(1):** 146-149.
12. Cupit P.M., Whyte J.A., Porter A.J., Browne M.J., Holmes S.D., Harris W.J. and Cunningham C. (1999) Cloning and expression of single chain antibody fragments in *Escherichia coli* and *Pichia pastoris. Letters in Applied Microbiology.* **(29):** 273-277.
13. Davis M.J., Gillaspie A.G., Vidaver A.K. and Harris R.W. (1984) Clavibacter: a new genus containing some phytopathogenic coryneform bacteria, including Clavibacter xyli subsp. xyli sp. nov., subsp. nov. and Clavibacter xyli subsp. Cynodontis sub sp. nov., pathogens that cause ratoon stunting disease of sugarcane and bermudagrass stunting disease. *Int. J. Syst. Bacteriol.* **(34):** 107-117.
14. DiJulio J.E. (2001) Monoclonal antibodies: Overview and use in hematologic malignancies. In P.T. Rieger (ed.), *Biotherapy: A Comprehensive Overview* Sudbury, M.A.: Jones and Bartlett, pp. 283-315.
15. Dyer M.A. and Harbour J.W. (2006) Cellular events in tumorigenesis. In Clinical Ocular Oncology (ed. Singh A.D., Damato B.E., Murphree A.L. and Perry J.D.). Elsevier, London.
16. Elliot M.J., Maini R.N., Feldmann M., Long-Fox A., Charles R., BiJi H. *et al.* (1994) Repeated therapy with monoclonal antibody to tumor necrosis factor alpha (cA2) in patients with rheumatoid arthritis. *Lancet.* 344 **(8930):** 1125-1127.

17. Emanuel P.A., Dang J., Gebhardt J.S., Aldrich J., Garber E.A., Kulaga H., Stopa P., Valdes J.J. and Dion-Schultz A (2000) Recombinant antibodies: a new reagent for biological agent detection. *Biosensors and Bioelectronics.* **(14)**: 751-759.
18. Fernandez I., Zeiser R., Karsunky H., Kambham N., Beilhack A., Soderstrom K., Negrin R.S. and Engleman E. (2007) CD101 Surface expression discriminates potency among murine foxP3$^+$ regulatory T cells. *The Journal of Immunology.* **(179)**: 2808-2814.
19. Franklin S.E. and Mayfield S.P. (2005) Recent developments in the production of human therapeutic proteins in eukaryotic algae. *Expert Opin. Biol. Ther.* **(5)**: 225-235.
20. Franklin W.A., Shpall E.J., Archer P., Johnston C.S., Garza-Williams S., Hami L., Bitter M.A., Bast R.C. and Jones R.B. (1996) Immunocytochemical detection of breast cancer cells in marrow and peripheral blood of patients undergoing high dose chemotherapy with autologous stem cell support. *Breast Cancer Res Treat.* 41 **(1)**: 1-13.
21. Gamble H.R. and Graham C.E. (1984) Monoclonal antibody-purified antigen for the immunodiagnosis of trichinosis. *Am. J. Vet. Res.* **(45)**: 67-74.
22. Gavilondo J.V. and Larrick J.W. (2000) Antibody engineering at the millennium. *Biotechniques.* 29: 128-138.
23. Greenberg H., McAuliffe V., Valdesuso J., Wyatt R., Flores J., Kalica A., Hoshino Y. and Singh N. (1983) Serological analysis of the subgroup protein of rotavirus, using monoclonal antibodies. *Infect Immun.* 39 **(1)**: 91-99.
24. Hiatt A., Cafferkey R. and Bowdish K. (1989) Production of antibodies in transgenic plants. *Nature.* **(342)**: 76-78.
25. Holman P.J., Adams L.G., Hunter D.M., Heck F.C., Nielsen K.H. and Wagner G.G. (1983) Derivation of monoclonal antibodies against Brucella abortus antigens. *Vet Immunol. Immunopathol.* 4 **(5-6)**: 603-614.
26. Hudson P.J. and Souriau C. (2001) Recombinant antibodies for cancer diagnosis and therapy. *Expert Opinion on Biological Therapy.* **(1)**: 845-855.
27. Hudson P.J. and Souriau C. (2003) Engineered antibodies. *Nat. Med.* **(9)**: 129-134.
28. Hwang W.Y. and Foote J. (2005) Immunogenicity of engineered antibodies. *Methods.* **(36)**: 3-10.
29. Kearney J.F., Radbruch A., Liesegang B. and Rajewsky K. (1979) A new mouse myeloma cell line that has lost immunoglobulin expression but permits the construction of antibody-secreting hybrid cell lines. *J. Immunol.* **(123)**: 1548-1550.
30. Kellermann S.A. and Green L.L. (2002) Antibody discovery: the use of transgenic mice to generate human mAbs for therapeutics. *Curr. Opin. Biotechnol.* **(13)**: 593-597.
31. Kipriyanov S.M., Moldenhauer G. and Little M. (1997) High level production of soluble single chain antibodies in small-scale Escherichia coli cultures. *Journal of Immunological Methods.* **(200)**: 69-77.
32. Kohler G. and Milstein C. (1975) Continuous cultures of fused cells secreting antibody of predefined specificity. *Nature.* **(256)**: 495-497.
33. Krawiec D.R. and Muscoplat C.C. (1984) Development and characterization of a monoclonal antibody (Aby 6C6) that distinguishes medullary from cortical thymocytes. *American Journal of_Veterinary Research.* 45 **(3)**: 499-505.
34. Krivi G.G. and Rowold E. (1984) Monoclonal antibodies to bovine somatotropin: Immunoadsorbent reagents for mammalian somatotro-pins. *Hybridoma.* **(3)**: 151-162.
35. Kvalheim G. (1996) Detection of occult tumour cells in bone marrow and blood in breast cancer patients—methods and clinical significance. *Acta Oncol.* **(35)**: 13-8.
36. Lee H.A. and Morgan M.R.A. (1993) Food immunoassays-Applications of polyclonal, monoclonal and recombinant antibodies. *Trends in Food Science & Technology.* **4**: 129-134.
37. Levy R. and Miller R.A. (1983) Biological and clinical implications of lymphocyte hybridomas: tumor therapy with mAbs. *Annu. Rev. Med.* **(34)**: 107-116.

38. Lunney J.K., Osborne B.A., Sharrow S.O., Devaux C., Pierres M. and Sachs D.H.. (1983) Sharing of Ia antigens between species. IV. Interspecies cross-reactivity of monoclonal antibodies directed against polymorphic mouse Ia determinants. *J. Immunol*. 130 **(6): ** 2786-2793.
39. Malley R., De Vincenzo J., Ramilo O. et al. (1998) Reduction of respiratory syncytial virus (RSV) in tracheal aspirates in intubated infants by use of humanized monoclonal antibody to RSV F protein. *J. Infect. Dis*. **(178):** 1555-1561.
40. Maynard J. and Georgiou G. (2000) Antibody engineering. *Annual Review of Biomedical Engineering*. **(2):** 339-376.
41. Meloen R.H., Briaire J., Wortmeyer R.J. and Van Zaane D. (1983) The main antigenic determinant detected by neutralizing monoclonal antibodies on the intact foot-and-mouth disease virus particle is absent from isolated VP1. *Journal of General Virology*. **(149):** 55-63.
42. Molloy J.B., Bock R.E., Templeton J.M., Bruyeres A.G., Bowles P.M., Blight G.W. and Jorgensen W.K. (2001) Identification of antigenic differences that discriminate between cattle vaccinated with Anaplasma centrale and cattle naturally infected with Anaplasma marginale. *International Journal for Parasitology*. 31 **(2):** 179-186.
43. Monzavi-Karbassi B. and Kieber-Emmons T. (2001) Current concepts in cancer vaccine strategies. *Biotechniques*. **(30):** 170-172.
44. Morris J.A. and Ivanyi J. (1985) Immunoassays of field isolates of Mycobacterium bovis and other mycobacteria by use of monoclonal antibodies. *J. Med. Microbiol*. **(19):** 367-373.
45. Peter W.G., Peter J.K., Fiona M. and. Jane O.A. (1986) Monoclonal antibodies to the two most basic papaya proteinases. *Bioscience Reports*. **(6):** 759-766.
46. Philippe B., Mardya S., Vong S., Toyoda T., Aubin J.T., Miller M., Touch S., Sovanne L., Dufourcq J.B., Richner B., Van T.P., Nguyen T.K.T., Limi W., Malik P.J.S. and Vander Werf S. (2007) Influenza A/H5N1 virus infection in humans in Cambodia. *Journal of Clinical Virology*. **(39):** 164-168.
47. Plückthun A., Krebber A., Krebber C. *et al.* (1996) Producing antibodies in Escherichia coli: from PCR to fermentation. In: *Antibody Engineering: A Practical Approach* (McCafferty J., Hoogenboom H., Chiswell D., ed.), Oxford University Press, pp. 203-252.
48. Porath J. (1992) Immobilized metal-ion affinity chromatography. *Protein Expression and Purification*. **(3):** 263-281.
49. Portetelle D., Mammerickx M. and Burny A. (1989) Use of two monoclonal antibodies in an ELISA test for the detection of antibodies to bovine leukaemia virus envelope protein gp51. *J. Virol. Methods*. 23 **(2):** 211-222.
50. Russell P.H. and Alexander D.J. (1983) Antigenic variation of new castle disease virus strains detected by monoclonal antibodies. *Arch. Virol*. 75 **(4):** 243-253.
51. Saliki J.T. and Lehenbauer T.W. (2001) Monoclonal antibody-based competitive enzyme-linked immunosorbent assay for detection of morbillivirus antibody in marine mammal sera. *J. Clin. Microbiol*. **(39):** 1877-1881.
52. Sanz *L*, Cuesta A.M., Compte M. and Alvarez-Vallina L (2005) Antibody engineering: facing new challenges in cancer therapy. *Acta Pharmacol. Sin*. **(26):** 641-648.
53. Schams S,. Menzer C.H., Schallenberger E., Hoffman B., Hahn J. and Hahn R. (1978) Some studiers on pregnant mare serum gonadotrophin (PMSG) and on endocrine responses after application for superovulation in cattle. In: Sreenan J.M. (Hrsg.), *Control of Reproduction in the Cow*. Martin Nijhoff, The Hague, The Netherlands, pp. 122-143.
54. Scott A.L., Diala C., Moraga D.A., Ibrahim S., Redding L. and Tamashiro W.K. (1988) Dirofilaria immitis: biochemical and immunological characterization of the surface antigens from adult parasites. *Exp. Parasitol*. **(67):** 307-323.
55. Sevmis S., Emiroglu R., Karakayali E. et al. (2005) OKT3 treatment for steroid-resistant acute rejection in kidney transplantation. *Transplant Proc*. **(37):** 3016-3018.

56. Shulman M., Wilde C.D. and Köhler G. (1978) A better cell line for making hybridomas secreting specific antibodies. *Nature*. **(276):** 269-270.
57. Sloan S.E., Cathleen H., William W., Michael N., Jesse B., Josh S., Kirk J.R., Robert B.M., Gregory J.B., William D.T. Jr., Charles E.R. and Donna M.A. (2007) Identification and characterization of a human monoclonal antibody that potently neutralizes a broad panel of rabies virus isolates. *Vaccine*. 25 **(15):** 2800-2810.
58. Smith S.J., Lavoie T.B. and Mainhart C.R. (1984) Antigenic regions defined by monoclonal antibodies correspond to structural domains of avian lysozyme. *J. Immunol.* 133 **(1):** 384-393.
59. Surujballi O. and Elmgren C. (2000) Monoclonal antibodies suitable for incorporation into a competitive enzyme-linked immunosorbent assay (ELISA) for detection of specific antibodies to Leptospira interrogans serovar pomona. *Vet. Microbiol.* **(71):** 149-159.
60. Swiecki M.K., Lisanby M.W., Shu F., Turnbough C.L. Jr. and Kearney J.F. (2006) Monoclonal antibodies for *Bacillus anthracis* spore detection and functional analyses of spore germination and outgrowth. *The Journal of Immunology*. **(176):** 6076-6084.
61. Taharaguchi S., Ito H., Ohta H. and Takase K. (2006) Characterization of monoclonal antibodies against fowl adenovirus serotype 1 (FAV1) isolated from gizzard erosion. *Avian Diseases*. 50 **(3):** 331-335.
62. Thiel M.A., Pilkington G.J. and Zola H. (2000) Antibody engineering, in MAbs. *The Basics-From Background to Bench* (Zola H, ed.), BIOS Scientific Publishers Limited, pp. 45-79.
63. Topol E.J. et al. (1994) Randomised trial of coronary intervention with antibody against platelet IIb/IIIa integrin for reduction of clinical restenosis: results at six month. The EPIC investigators. *Lancet*. 343 **(8902):** 881-886.
64. Varshney B.C., Ponnanna N.M., Sarkar P.A., Rehman P. and Shah J.H. (2007) Development of a monoclonal antibody-based co-agglutination test to detect enterotoxigenic *Escherichia* coli isolated from diarrheic neonatal calves. *J. Vet. Sci.* 8 **(1):** 57-64.
65. Wiktor T.J. and Koprowski H. (1980) Antigenic variants of rabies virus. *J. Exp. Med.* 152 **(1):** 99-112.
66. Wong J.Y., Chu D.Z., Williams L.E. *et al.* (2004) Pilot trial evaluating an ^{123}1-labeled 80-kilodalton engineered anticarcinoembryonic antigen antibody fragment (cT84.66 minibody) in patients with colorectal cancer. *Clin. Cancer. Res.* **(10):** 5014-5021.
67. Wright I.G., White M., Tracey-Patte P.D., Donaldson R.A., Goodger B.V., Waltisbuhl D.J. and Mahoney D.F. (1983) Babesia bovis: isolation of a protective antigen by using monoclonal antibodies. *Infect. Immun.* 41. **(1):** 244-250.
68. Xu Z., Tang Q., Song M., Yin W.W. *et al.* (2006) Epidemiological features and analysis on the human rabies in China in 2005. *Dis. Surveill.* **(21):** 360-362.
69. Yang X., Lipchina I., Lifton M., Wang L. and Sodroski J. (2007) Antibody binding in proximity to the receptor/glycoprotein complex leads to a basal level of virus neutralization. *J. Virol.* **(81):** 8809-8813.
70. Yau K.Y., Lee H. and Hall. J.C. (2003) Emerging trends in the synthesis and improvement of hapten-specific recombinant antibodies. *Biotechnology Advances*. **(21):** 599-637.
71. Zhang, Inderpal S., Abhineet S., Xiaochuan F., John N., Angela C. and Saul T. (2005) Infection and immunity, production and characterization of monoclonal antibodies against *Enterocytozoon bieneusi* purified from Rhesus Macaques Quanshun. *Infection and Immunity*. 73 **(8):** 5166-5172.
72. Zhu F., Snezna R. and Thomas L.K. (2005) Rapid detection of *Escherichia coli* O157:H7 by immunomagnetic separation and real-time PCR. *International Journal of Food Microbiology*. 99 **(1):** 47-57.
73. Berghman L.R., Abi-Ghanem D., Waghela S.D. and Ricke S.C. (2005) Antibodies: an alternative for antibiotics? *Poultry Science*. 84 **(4):** 660-666.
74. Birgit K., Lukas B., Eckehard J.K., Patrick G., Zoltan K., Angelika L., Gerald W., Holger E. and Ulrich S. (2002) Large-scale plant proteomics. *Plant Molecular Biology.* **(48):** 133-141.
75. Burnie J. and Matthews R. (2003) The role of antibodies against hsp90 in the treatment of fungal infections. *Drug News Perspect.* 16 **(4):** 205-210.

76. ByTravis C. McGuire, Alberta L.B., William C.D. and William P.C. (1987) Antigenic and structural variation of the p28 core polypeptide of goat and sheep retroviruses. *J. Gen. Virol.* **(68):** 2259-2263.
77. Fischer R. and Emans N. (2000) Molecular farming of pharmaceutical proteins. *Transgenic Res.* 9 **(4-5):** 279-299.
78. Fischer R., Hoffmann K., Schillberg S. and Emans N. (2000) Antibody production by molecular farming in plants. *J. Biol. Regul. Homeost Agents.* 14 **(2):** 83-92.
79. Galeffi P., Lombardi A., Donato M.D., Latini A., Sperandei M., Cantale C. and Giacomini P. (2005) Expression of single-chain antibodies in transgenic plants. *Vaccine.* 23 **(15):** 1823-1827.
80. Gogolewski R.P., Adams D.S., Mc'Guire T.C., Banks K.L. and Cheevers W.P. (1985) Antigenic cross-reactivity between caprine arthritis-encephalitis, visna and progressive pneumonia viruses involves all virionassociated proteins and glycoproteins. *Journal of General Virology.* **(66):** 1233-1240.
81. Griffiths A.D., Williams S.C., Hartley O., Tomlinson I.M., Waterhouse P., Crosby W.L., Kontermann R.E., Jones P.T., Low N.M., Allison T.J. et al. (1994) Isolation of high affinity human antibodies directly from large synthetic repertoires. *EMBO J.* **(13):** 3245-3260.
82. Nissim A., Hoogenboom H.R., Tomlinson I.M., Flynn G., Midgley C., Lane D. and Winter G. (1994) Antibody fragments from a 'single pot' phage display library as immunochemical reagents. *EMBO J.* **(13):** 692-698.
83. Qing J., Du X., Chen Y., Chan P., Li H., Wu P., Marsters S., Stawicki S., Tien J., Totpal K., Ross S., Stinson S., Dornan D., French D., Wang Q.R., Stephan J.P., Wu Y., Wiesmann C. and Ashkenazi A. (2009) Antibody-based targeting of FGFR3 in bladder carcinoma and t(4;14)-positive multiple myeloma in mice. *J. Clin. Invest.* 119 **(5):** 1077-1079.
84. Rainer F., Neil E. and Stefan S. (2001) Achieving plant disease resistance by antibody expression. *Can. J. Plant Pathol.* **(23):** 236-245.
85. Roberson S.M., McGuire T.C., Klevjer-Anderson P., Gorham J.R. and CItEevers W.P. (1982) Caprine arthritisencephalitis virus is distinct from visna and progressive pneumonia viruses as measured by genome sequence homology. *Journal of Virology.* **(44):** 754-757.
86. Schillberg S., Zimmermann S., Zhang M-Y and Fischer R. (2001) Antibody-based resistance to plant pathogens. *Transgenic Research.* **(10):** 1-12.
87. Takata R., Miyamoto Y., Honjoh K., Soeda T., Sakamoto J., Miyamoto T. and Hatano S. (1998) Antibody fragments as inhibitors of Japanese radish acid phosphatase. *Biosci. Biotechnol. Biochem.* 62 **(6):** 1041-1047.
88. Voss A., Niersbach M., Hain R., Hirsch H., Liao Y., Kreuzaler F. and Fischer R. (1995) Reduced virus infectivity in N. tabacum secreting a TMV-specific full size antibody. *Mol. Breed.* **(1):** 39-50.
89. Walter G., Konthur Z. and Lehrach H. (2001) High-throughput screening of surface displayed gene products. *Comb. Chem. High Throughput Screen.* **(4):** 193-205.
90. Yang L.C., Zhang S.X., Pi G.H., Li Y.H., Zhu Z. and Yang X.G. (2005) Preparation of monoclonal antibody against HPT and its application to detecting marker protein in genetically modified rice. *Biomed. Environ. Sci.* 18 **(5):** 321-325.
91. Zimmermann S., Schillberg S., Liao Y.C. and Fischer R. (1998) Intracellular expression of TMV-specific single-chain Fv fragments leads to improved virus resistance in *Nicotiana tabacum. Mol. Breed.* **(4):** 369-379.

CHAPTER 16

Molecular Diagnostic Technology

Molecular diagnostic technology is a major field of science whereby the interacting properties of biomolecules are harnessed for diagnostic purpose. It utilizes properties of molecule-molecule interaction based on their complementarities and affinities. This technology has wide range of applications from detection and identification of pathogens, molecular detection of inherited diseases and gene mutations, resolution and detection of nucleic acids, analysis and characterization of nucleic acids and proteins, prediction of chromosomal structure and chromosomal mutations, quality assurance and quality control in the molecular laboratories, DNA-based tissue typing to molecular oncology and many more. Several of these are discussed in this chapter briefly.

Keywords: Molecular diagnostics, biosensors, radioimmunoassay, ELISA.

INTRODUCTION

Molecular methods have been used increasingly over the past fifteen years to improve the sensitivity and speed of diagnosis of various pathogens of plants, animals and human beings. Advances in modern biotechnology have considerably enhanced the efficiency of available detection systems which utilize various principles of immunology, molecular biology and engineering. The routine use of molecular techniques for disease diagnosis is still limited to the detection of the pathogens and/ or other causative agents of a disease condition. In case of pathogens, which are difficult to culture *in vitro*, the real time molecular methods are more suitable and more sensitive than traditional gold standard diagnostic tests which have been established so far. Prior to the development of recombinant DNA technology, diagnosis of infectious diseases in man and animals were largely dependent on the use of whole pathogens or physically resolved fractions of them.

The success of molecular testing technology contributes to the challenge to define the clinical relevance of each new diagnostic method. Establishing interpretive criteria for molecular tests requires, well-designed clinical studies and in some cases quantitative methods or demonstration of virulence markers. Molecular methods got wider acceptance due to less time involved and simple procedure as compared to conventional methods of diagnosis. The availability of complete genome sequences of large numbers of pathogens will be helpful in understanding of their virulence and host interaction. The modern biotechnological research is mainly concentrated towards the development of improved disease control strategies, based on vaccine and rapid diagnosis. Molecular diagnostic technology has now been used increasingly for the rapid diagnosis and study of the pathogenesis and epidemiology of infectious diseases.

CONCEPTS

The applications of pharamacogenomics/pharmacogenetics in drug development and the practice of medicine are leading the renaissance of molecular diagnostics. The advent of different diagnostics in recent years is mainly due to the availability of gene sequence data and elucidation of different molecular pathways of disease conditions caused either due to genetic aberration or by pathogens. Availability of molecular information of disease conditions has helped pharmaceutical companies to accelerate drug development program. Molecular diagnosis of infectious diseases is a complex process that ideally starts with identification of the causative agent in an appropriate clinical specimen. The slow multiplication or fastidious growth requirements of many important pathogens limit culture-based diagnosis. Methods for rapid detection of infectious bacteria and antimicrobial-resistant pathogens have evolved significantly over the last decade. Many of the new procedures are nucleic acid-based and replace conventional methods. These newly developed diagnostic procedures are superior with respect to turn around time, sensitivity and specificity. Molecular biology has significantly improved diagnosis in the field of clinical virology too. Molecular techniques have revolutionized all domains of virus diagnosis including the rapid identification of emerging or re-emerging viruses. The most striking illustration of the power of molecular techniques concerns blood transmitted viruses like human immune deficiency virus (HIV), hepatitis B virus (HBV) and hepatitis C virus (HCV) for which spectacular progress in the detection and thus in their treatment have been made in recent years. This became possible following the introduction of qualitative and quantitative nucleic acid tests. During the last fifteen years many new human pathogens have been discovered among which eight are viruses with various pathogenicity. Molecular diagnostics have been very rapidly implemented in clinical virology laboratories but the extreme genetic variability of some viruses, especially RNA viruses (which RNA-polymerase have no proof-reading activity), often makes their diagnosis difficult.

PRINCIPLES

Different molecular diagnostic techniques are based on different principles of immunology and molecular properties of biomolecules. Nucleic acid based technology exploits the specific nucleic acid sequences of pathogens. Physical and biochemical properties of specific biomolecules have been exploited for the development of sensitive and specific molecular diagnostics.

Discovery of duplex DNA structure and its complementary rules in 1953 started a new beginning of nucleic-acid based molecular diagnostics of different disease conditions (Table 16.1). The four major techniques that initiated the field and constitute a platform for the development of new technology are enzymatic DNA restriction, nucleic acid hybridization, PCR and fluorescence-based methods. The basic DNA detection methods involve immobilizing sample DNA on a solid phase and probing or hybridizing it with a short strand of labeled target DNA. Because the efficiency of hybridization is dependent on the extent of sequence complemetarity, these techniques are highly specific under appropriate conditions. However, the most important biotechnological advances in DNA detection methodology arose from the development of Polymerase Chain Reaction (PCR). By using PCR, amplified products or amplicons can be detected simply by direct examination in gels. Furthermore, PCR sensitivity can be enhanced by hybridization with a labeled probe. The availability of published whole genome sequencing of pathogens has helped in rapid development of nucleic acid-based diagnostics. Today the major driving forces for developing new diagnostic techniques are reduced hands on-time, faster methods and increased sensitivity. These goals are reached mainly by automating processes and refining detection methods.

Table 16.1 DNA diagnostics timeline (Tsongalis and Silverman, 2006).

Date	*Development*
1953	Discovery of duplex DNA structure and complementarity rules
1957	Phosphonate synthesis of short oligodeoxynucleotides. Triple-stranded nucleic acid complexes are found
1958–1959	Discovery and isolation of DNA polymerases
1960s	Early hybridization techniques and inception of electrochemical DNA detection
1965	Solid-phase oligodeoxynucleotide synthesis. Enzymatic synthesis of short RNAs
1969	*In situ* hybridization
1970	Discovery of restriction enzymes and reverse transcriptase
1975	Southern blotting
1977	Methods for DNA sequencing. First genome (bacteriophage $\Phi \times 174$) is sequenced
1983–1985	First synthesis of modified oligonucleotides
1985	Restriction fragment length polymorphism analysis
1985–1986	Invention and first steps of PCR; thermophilic DNA polymerases
1986	Automated DNA sequencing is pioneered. Development of FISH method
1987–1988	First triplex DNA probes
1988–1991	Origination of first DNA chip conceptions
1990s	Emergence of microelectromechanical systems and DNA nanotechnology
1991	Design of first DNA/RNA mimics: peptide nucleic acid probes/PNA openers. Ligase chain reaction; thermophilic DNA ligases
1992	First methods for whole genome amplification. Strand-displacement amplification
1992–1993	Branched DNA (oligonucleotide dendrimers). Real-time PCR
1993	Discovery of structure-specific endonucleases for invasive-cleavage assays
1994	DNA topological labeling (padlock probes)
1995	First bacteria (*Haemophilus influenzae*) is sequenced
1995–1996	Invention of rolling amplification of circular probes
1996	Molecular beacon probes. First eukaryote (yeast) is sequenced. First applications of DNA chips
1998	Lab-on-a-chip (microfluidics) for DNA analysis
2000	Genomic sequence of fruit fly (*Drosophila melanogaster*)
2000–2001	First versions of human genome sequence

The performance of most nucleic acid-based diagnostic methods is influenced by the purity of the target nucleic acids. Today several platforms for automated DNA extraction exist that ensure a high degree of reproducibility and little hands on time while processing large number of samples (Table 16.2). The advantage of using such methods are that they are fast and remove any undesirable impurities that might create problem following detection. These available automated methods for nucleic acid extraction mostly exploit the high affinity between nucleic acids and silica at defined buffer conditions. On the other hand, protein based molecular techniques utilize the protein-protein interactions. These include immunological assays such as ELISA and Western blot. Further, at present protein microarrays are also available to detect the proteins synthesized by the pathogen.

Table 16.2 Automatic nucleic acid extraction (Barken *et al.*, 2007).

Instrument	*Method*	*No. of samples*	*Time required*
ABI PRISM 6100 nucleic acid PrepStation (Applied Biosystems)	Silica membrane bind/ elute protocols with vacuum processing (RNA and DNA)	Up to 96	30 min
ABI PRISM 6700 automated nucleic acid workstation (Applied Biosystems)	Silica membrane bind/ elute protocols with vacuum processing (RNA and DNA)	Up to 96	90 min
BioRobot EZ1 workstation (QIAGEN)	Silica membrane bind/ elute protocols using magnetic-particle handling (RNA and DNA)	1–6	15–20 min
iPrep Purification instrument (Invitrogen)	Based on a unique, ionizable nucleic acidbinding ligand whose charge can be switched based on the pH of the surrounding medium (DNA)	Up to 12	18 min
KingFisher ML/96 (Thermo Scientific)	Silica membrane bind/ elute protocols using magnetic-particle handling (RNA and DNA)	1–96	20–30 min
MagNA pure compact/LC (Roche Applied Science)	Silica membrane bind/ elute protocols using magnetic-particle handling (RNA and DNA)	1–32	15–40 min
Maxwell 16 Instrument (Promega)	Silica membrane bind/ elute protocols using magnetic-particle handling (RNA and DNA)	Up to 16	30 min
NucliSens miniMAG (BioMérieux)	Silica membrane bind/ elute protocols using magnetic-particle handling (RNA and DNA)	Up to 12	45 min
QIAcube (QIAGEN)	Silica membrane bind/ elute protocols with built in centrifuge (RNA and DNA)	Up to 12	~60 min, user developed protocols
X-Tractor Gene RNA/ DNA Extraction System (Corbett Life Science)	Silica membrane bind/ elute protocols with vacuum processing (RNA and DNA)	8-96	1h

MOLECULAR DIAGNOSTIC TECHNOLOGY

Hybridization Based Diagnostics

Nucleic acid hybridization

Blot transfer hybridization assays are part of molecular diagnostic laboratories. A common way to investigate the sequence of PCR products is hybridization with one or more oligonucleotide probes. Type-specific PCR products can be confirmed with corresponding type-specific probes. In Southern blotting, a PCR product is electrophorosed prior to transfer to a membrane that is subsequently hybridized to a labelled probe (Figure 16.1).

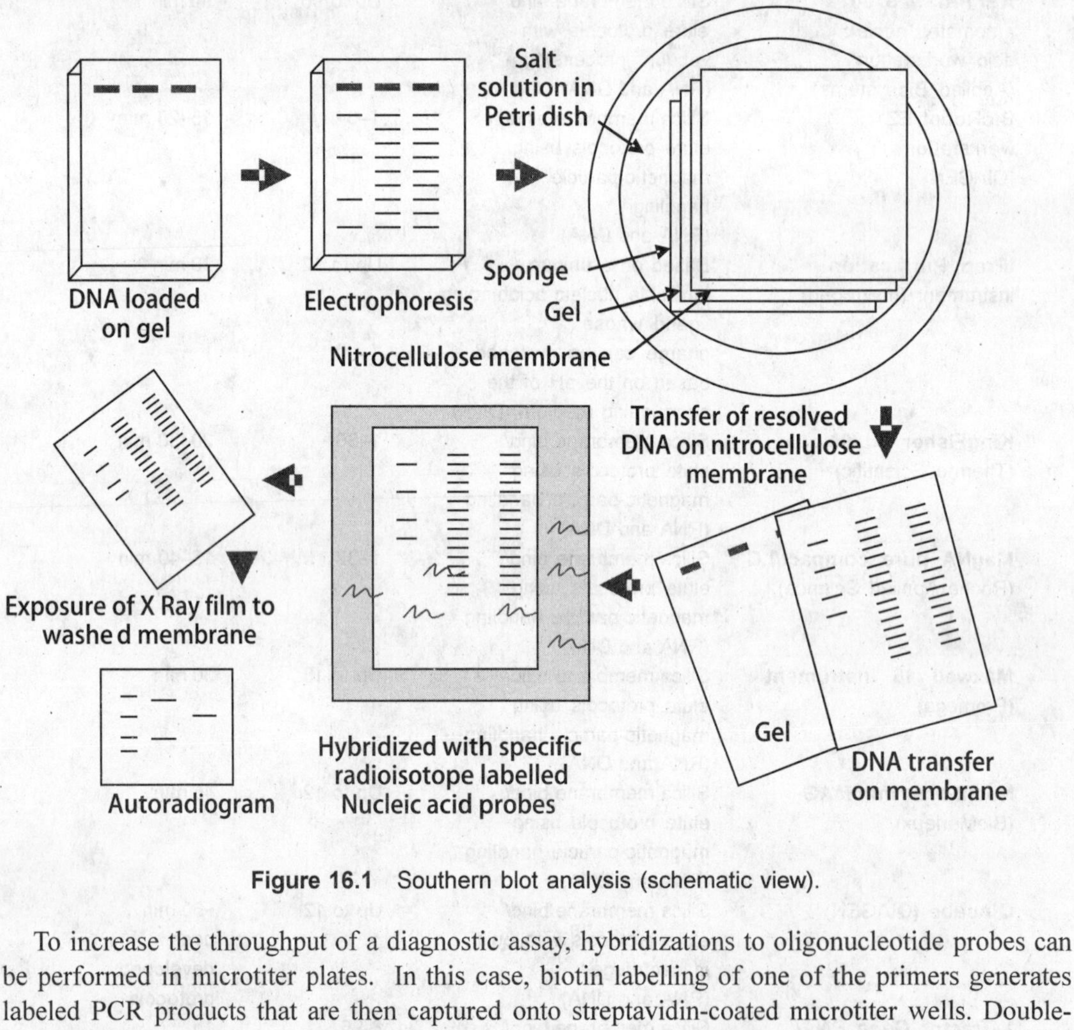

Figure 16.1 Southern blot analysis (schematic view).

To increase the throughput of a diagnostic assay, hybridizations to oligonucleotide probes can be performed in microtiter plates. In this case, biotin labelling of one of the primers generates labeled PCR products that are then captured onto streptavidin-coated microtiter wells. Double-stranded DNA is denatured under alkaline conditions and the unattached strand is removed by washing. A labeled oligonucleotide probe is added, which hybridizes to the captured strand. Hybrids can be detected following binding of conjugate and substrate reaction.

Reverse hybridization also provides an attractive tool for simultaneous hybridization of a PCR product to multiple oligonucleotide probes. This method comprises immobilization of multiple oligonucleotide probes on a solid phase and addition of the PCR product in the liquid phase. Hybridization is followed by a detection stage. The most frequently used reverse hybridization technology comprises a membrane strip containing multiple probes immobilized as parallel lines, called line probe assay (LiPA); line blot assay (LBA) or linear array (LA). A PCR product is generated, usually using biotinylated primers. The double stranded PCR product is denatured under alkaline conditions and added to the strip in a hybridization buffer. After hybridization and stringent washing, the hybrids can be detected by addition of a streptavidin-conjugate and a substrate, generating colour at the probe line, which can be visually interpreted. Reverse hybridization methods are particularly useful for the detection of type specific infections and multiple genotypes.

Several hybridization techniques such as allele specific oligonucleotide (ASO) dot blot, reverse dot blot, amplification refractory mutation (ARMS), and an oligo-ligation assay are available to detect the most common genetic disease in humans. ASO dot-blot is one of the most widely used techniques to diagnose cystic fibrosis. Genomic DNA or cDNA from the patient is amplified by PCR and transferred onto nylon membranes as a "dot-blot". Membranes are hybridized with either a radiolabelled wild type allele specific oligonucleotide (ASO) or mutated ASO under stringent conditions. Following autoradiographic exposure, the combination of oligonucleotide hybridization is observed. Using this combination an ASO dot-blot can clearly distinguish homozygous, heterozygous and wild type subjects. Subsequently, blotting technologies are now being used to detect many human gene sequences. Southern blot transfer assays have become the gold standard for detecting gene arrangements in the immunoglobin heavy and light chain genes and T-cell receptor gene family that have been associated with and often diagnostic for B- and T-cell lymphoma.

Fluorescent *in situ* hybridization (FISH) is another hybridization-based tool that is widely used for identification, visualization, and localization of microorganisms in many fields of microbiology. Initially *in situ* hybridization was performed in bacteria using radioactively labeled rRNA probes. In 1989, Delong *et al.,* reported the first *in situ* hybridization experiment using fluorescently labeled rRNA-directed oligonucleotides probes. It allowed a safer method which simultaneously monitors more than one species in the same sample through the use of multiple probe labeled with different fluorescent dyes with higher sensitivity. FISH is normally based on short nucleotides which are complementary to an rRNA signature sequence and have a fluorescent dye molecule attached to the 3' or, 5'-end. The target DNA in metaphase chromosomes or interphase nuclei is first denatured to separate the complementary strands within the DNA double helix structure. The fluorescently labeled probe of interest is then added to the denatured sample and hybridizes with the target DNA sequence as it reanneals back into a double helix. Signal from the hybridization probe is detected by means of a fluorescent microscope (Figure 16.2).

FISH has obvious advantages as a diagnostic tool as it is simple, sensitive, specific and fast compared to other methods. Improper washing after hybridization can in some cases may result in unspecific binding of probe to non-target organisms or molecules. Sometimes autofluorescence from the target organism may give false results. FISH was primarily a technology performed in the cytogenetics laboratory, but recent development in the chemistries for interphase, FISH can now be suitably used for analysis of paraffin-embedded tissues and other traditional pathology specimen.

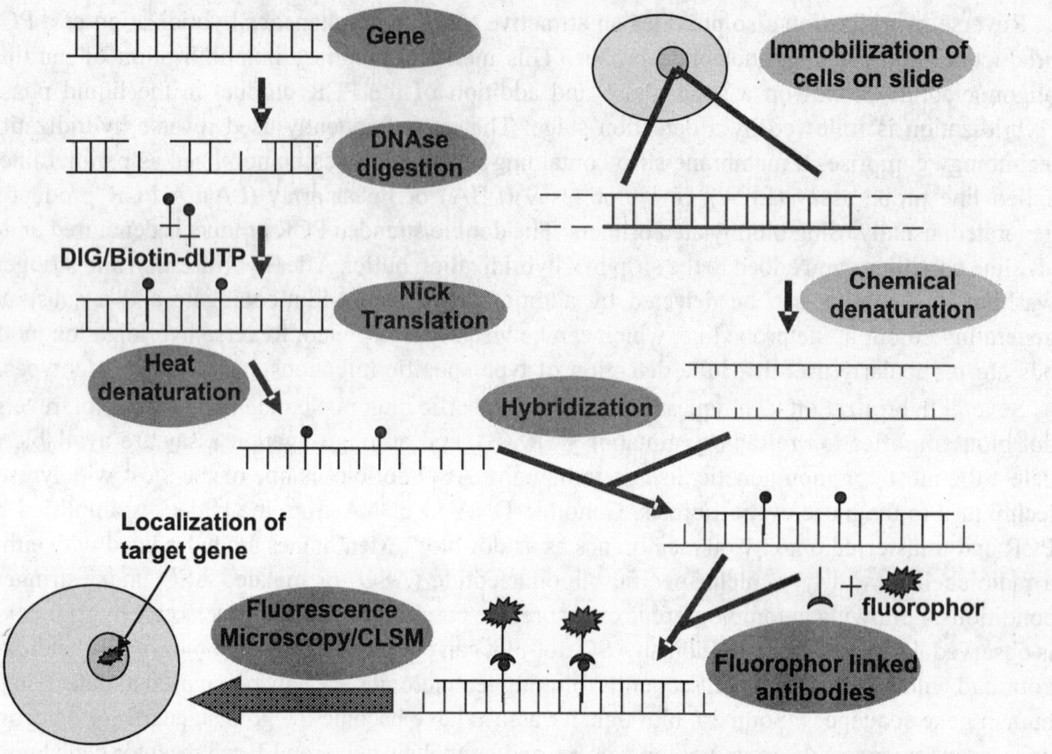

Figure 16.2 Localization of a gene by fluorescent *in situ* hybridization (FISH).

Polymerase chain reaction (PCR)

In the 1970s, nucleic acid hybridization methods were mostly used methods and DNA probes were the powerful tools in molecular diagnostics. Although hybridization methods are highly specific for detecting targets, they are limited by their sensitivity. To get more sensitive and specific methods, Kary Mullis conceived the idea and helped develop polymerase chain reaction (PCR), a technology for rapidly multiplying fragments of DNA in 1983 (Figure 16.3) . In 1985, Saiki and his colleagues first used the new method to detect patient's α-globin gene for diagnosis of sickle cell anaemia. In 1987, Kwok and colleagues identified human immunodeficiency virus (HIV) by using PCR method and this was the first report of the application of PCR in clinical diagnosis of infectious disease. Since then, PCR has become the method of choice for molecular diagnostic analysis because (i) it is easy to perform, (ii) it has an open system that allows the user to easily design assays and control reaction conditions, (iii) it satisfies clinical turn around times, and (iv) it is a universal technology that can be readily applied to multiple applications for genetic, infectious, and neoplastic disease testing. PCR is a powerful tool that allows for the amplification of specific yet small size target sequences that can be analyzed using a variety of methods. Gel electrophoresis as a detection method can be the final step in this four-step analytical process: (i) DNA extraction, (ii) PCR amplification, (iii) restriction endonuclease digestion and (iv) gel electrophoresis.

The introduction of real-time PCR into the field of molecular diagnostics has simplified the quantification of nucleic acids. The first real-time amplification system used ethidium bromide and a mounted CCD camera to monitor PCR amplification in a closed reaction tube. Since then, significant advancements have been made in real-time PCR technology. As a result, this technique now provides an effective tool for disease diagnosis, identification of species, quantifying gene expression, single nucleotide polymorphism (SNP) and so on. Real-time PCR readily allows quantitation of DNA over a broad dynamic range. Different real-time detection chemistries are available commercially. After amplification, the sequence composition of a PCR product can be investigated by restriction enzymes. Digestion of PCR products with restriction endonucleases generates a number of fragments, which can be resolved by gel electrophoresis, yielding a particular banding pattern. This method is straightforward but labor-intensive.

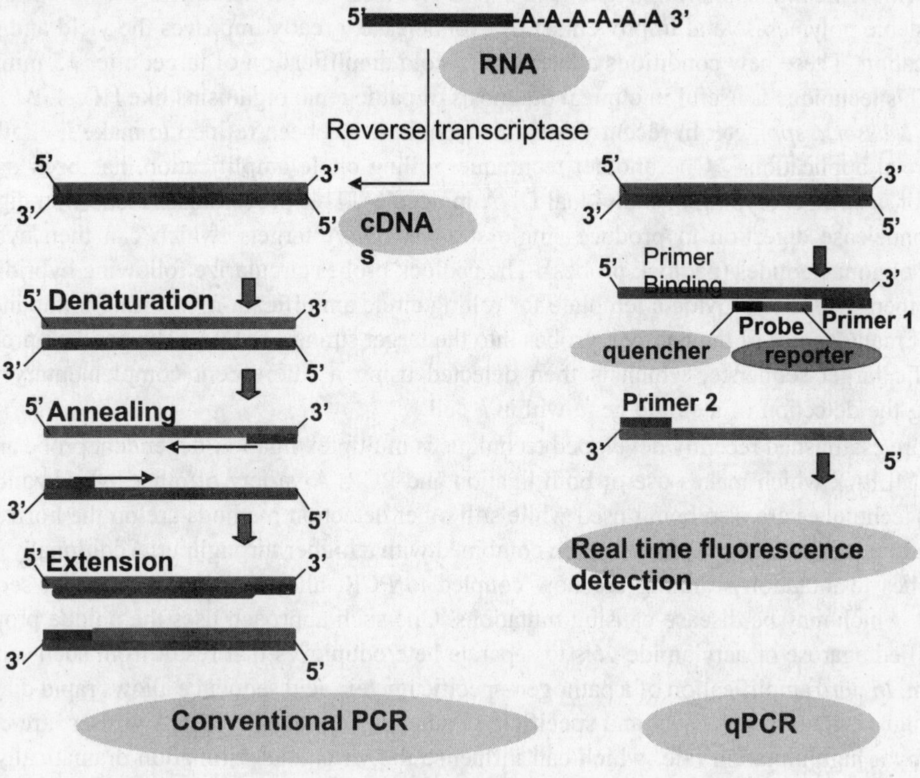

Figure 16.3 Polymerase chain reaction.

Besides PCR, a variety of other nucleic acid amplification techniques have been developed in the mid to late 1980s. These include ligation-mediated amplification and transcription-based amplification like transcription-mediated amplification (TMA), nucleic acid sequenced-based amplification (NASBA), ligase chain reaction (LCR), strand displacement amplification (SDA), linear linked amplification and so on. NASBA is an isothermal amplification technique making use of dual function reverse transcriptase/DNA polymerase, RNA polymerase, RNase H and a T-7 promoter-labelled target specific primer. This technique is widely used for virus detection, most typically using commercial NASBA kits and probe-based chemiluminescent detection of the amplified RNA. This technology is amenable to real-time application. This technique has also been combined with liposome signal amplification technology to develop biosensors for pathogen detection.

LCR is another amplification technique developed shortly after PCR. This technique uses a thermostable DNA ligase and four primers, two adjacent forward primers and their complements. There is typically a gap of 1-3 bases between the adjacent primers, which act as templates for ligation by DNA ligase. DNA ligase is highly specific and intolerant to base mismatches. Thus, this technology holds great promise for SNP detection.

SDA (Strand Displacement Amplification) is another isothermal reaction which makes use of a combination of exonuclease deficient DNA polymerase (Klenow fragment), a restriction endonuclease with a hemiphosphorothioated DNA, and two sets of primers. The incorporation of a thermostable polymerase and improved set of exonuclease, greatly improves the yield and rate of amplification. These new conditions allow a 10^{10} –fold amplification of target after 15 minutes at 60°C. This technique is useful in clinical diagnosis of pathogenic organisms like HIV-1, *M. Tuberculosis, Neisseria spp*., etc. In recent years, this technique has been refined to make it eligible for commercial applications. One another technique, rolling circle amplification, has been used recently for *in situ* genotyping of individual DNA molecules. This process uses restriction digestion and exonuclease digestion to produce single stranded DNA targets, which can then hybridize specific oligonucleotides (padlock probes). The padlock probes circularize following hybridization and are then ligated to provide a template for rolling circle amplification, resulting in the incorporation of many copies of the padlock probes into the target strand of DNA. The padlock probe has a specific target sequence, which is then detected using a fluorescent complementary probe, allowing the detection of a single gene within a cell.

A more established recently developed technique is multiplex ligation-dependent probe amplification (MLPA), which makes use of both ligation and PCR. A variety of other hybridization and blotting techniques are also being used while still other detection methods are on the horizon and promise to provide a more rapid detection combined with a higher throughput. Additionally, newer approaches to mutation scanning are now coupled to PCR, allowing the detection of sequence variants, which may be disease-causing mutations. One such approach uses the unique properties of modified agarose or acrylamide gels to separate heteroduplexes that result from such sequence variation. *In vitro* amplification of a pathogen-specific nucleic acid sequence allows rapid diagnosis with a high degree of sensitivity and specificity. Pathogens, particularly RNA viruses, are characterized by a high mutation rate, which can influence the virus load estimation dramatically. This problem can be overcome by amplification of highly conserved regions of pathogens. Further, Multilocus sequence typing (MLST) is an accurate and highly discriminatory typing system that can be used for any bacterial species. In this method, allele at each locus is defined directly by nucleotide sequencing rather than indirectly from the electrophoretic mobility of their gene products. Sequence data are compared against a central database, accessible via the Internet and each isolate is unambiguously characterized by a series of seven integers. Genotype differentiation has implications in the diagnosis of viral livestock diseases, especially when strains with different pathogenic potential co-circulate in the host population.

PCR technique can be combined with high performance liquid chromatography. A high-capacity low-cost mutation scanning method based on denaturing high-performance liquid chromatography (DHPLC) has been recently introduced. In the first step, a discrete gene sequence is amplified in a 96 well format using PCR machine. In the next step, serial DHPLC analysis of multiple amplicons under conditions optimal for each amplicon is done. HPLC compares two chromosomes as a mixture of denatured and reannealed PCR amplicons. When the PCR amplicon does not contain a mutation, the sense strand and the anti-sense strand of the PCR amplicons are completely complementary to each other. In this case, the molecule is referred to as a homoduplex. When a person is heterozygous for a mutation, the mutant sense and anti-sense strand will not only form a homoduplex, but also heteroduplices with their corresponding wild type sense and anti-sense strands upon renaturation of the denatured PCR product. The physicochemical difference between a homoduplex and heteroduplices can be detected by HPLC using a reverse-phase chromatography column with an affinity for double-stranded DNA. The differential retention of homo- and hetero-duplex DNA on the column after partial denaturation indicates the presence of a mutation. The temperature of the column determines sensitivity, and the optimal temperature is predicted by a mathematical formula based on the amplicon sequence. The output of this formula can be calculated using a computer programme (WAVE Maker, Transgenomic, Omaha, Nebraska, USA). By applying this methodology, single-nucleotide substitutions, deletions, and insertions have been successfully detected within 5-6 minutes using on-line UV or fluorescence monitoring. For diagnosis, usually a single exon of a gene is amplified. When a particular exon has more than one melting domain, the exon is amplified in multiple amplicons. The DHPLC system (WAVE, transgenomic) is equipped with an auto-sampler and is capable of running each PCR amplicon at a pre-determined optimal chromatographic condition. Exons from a particular gene are analyzed in order of increasing melting temperature. DHPLC is a very sensitive analytical method. Therefore, false-positive results can occur if appropriate measures are not taken. By using this molecular technique, small aberrations of the genome sequence of the patients with congenital disorders can be ascertained. This "condition-oriented-PCR primer-embedded-reactor plate" called COPPER plate, system has been developed for more than 20 congenital disorders of human beings.

Sequencing

It is a powerful method for identification of clinical cultures and it is becoming a cheap and attractive method with the introduction of automated procedures as well as the requirement of smaller sample size such as 16S rRNA sequencing in prokaryotes. Rapid sequencing methods of PCR products are also now available for high throughput, thus permitting application in routine clinical analysis. Pyrosequencing is a novel method of nucleic acid sequencing-by-synthesis based on the detection of released pyrophosphate (PPi) during DNA synthesis. The cascades of enzymatic reactions generate visible light. The generated light is proportional to the number of incorporated nucleotides. Pathogen specific genes can be targeted using this method of sequencing.

Biosensor and Immunosensor Based Diagnostics

A biosensor is an analytical device that integrates a biological element on a solid-state surface, enabling a reversible biospecific interaction with the analyte and a signal transducer (Figure 16.4).

The biological element is a layer of molecules qualified for biorecognition such as enzymes, receptors, peptides, single stranded DNA and even living cells are applicable. A biosensor is defined by the International Union of Pure and Applied Chemistry (IUPAC) as a "device that uses specific biochemical reactions mediated by isolated enzymes, immunosystems, tissue, organelles or whole cells to detect chemical compounds usually by electrical, thermal or optical signals". Biosensors intimately couple a biological recognition element (interacting with the target analyte) with a physical transducer that translates the biorecognition event into a useful electrical signal. This category of sensors is based on antigen-antibody binding, nucleic acid hybridization and, receptor-ligand interaction. If antibodies or antibody fragments are applied as biological element the device is called immunosensor. The immunosensors are affinity ligand-based biosensing solid state devices in which the immune-chemical reaction is coupled to a transducer. The fundamental basis of all immunosensors is the specificity of the molecular recognition of antigens by antibodies to form a stable complex. Immunosensors can be categorized based on detection principle applied. The main developments are electro-chemical, optical, and microgravimetric immunosensors. There are four types of immunosensor detection devices: (i) electrochemical (potentiometric, amperometric or, conductometric/capacitative); (ii) optical; (iii) microgravimetric and (iv) thermometric.

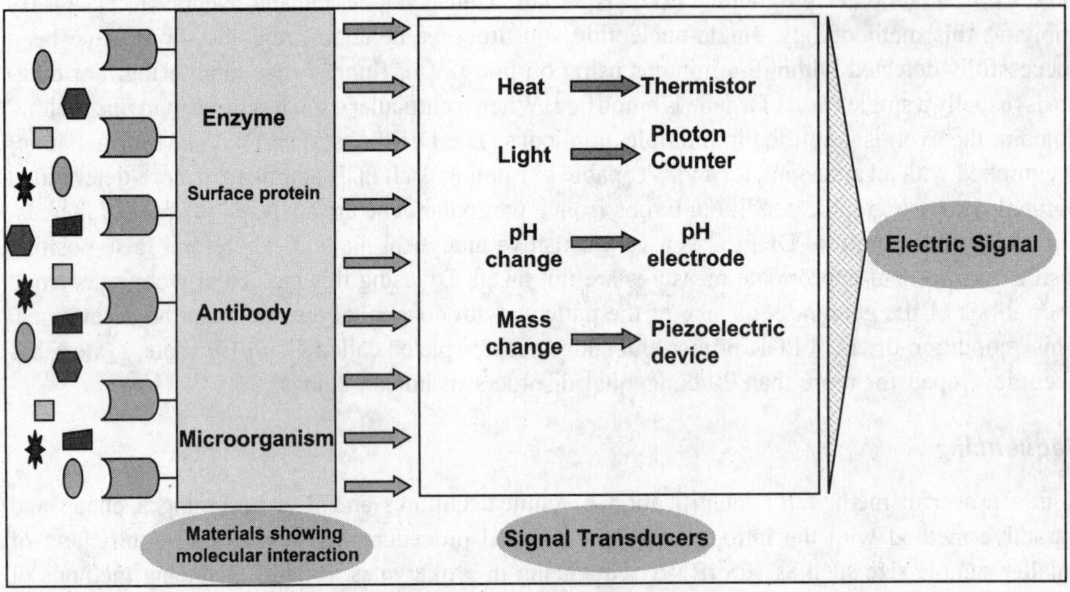

Figure 16.4 Principle of biosensors.

All types can be run on direct and indirect immunosensors. The direct sensors are able to detect the physical changes during the immune complex formation, whereas the latter sensors use signal-generating labels which allow more sensitive and versatile detection modes when incorporated into the complex. There is a great variety of different labels which have been applied in indirect immunosensors. The development of immunoassay technology is a success story especially for the clinical laboratories and still continues to be a vibrant area of research. Many devices are connected with a flow-through cell enabling a flow-injection analysis (FIA) mode of operation. Biosensors combine high analytical specificity with the processing power of modern electronics to achieve high sensitive detection system. There are two different types of biosensors: biocatalytic and bioaffinity-based biosensors. The biocatalytic biosensor uses mainly enzymes as the biological compound, catalyzing a signaling biochemical reaction. The bioaffinity-based biosensor, designed to monitor the binding event itself, uses specific binding proteins, lectins, receptors, nucleic acids, membranes, whole cells, antibodies or antibody related substances for biomolecular recognition. In affinity sensors, the recognition between the analyte in solution and the immobilized biological element is based on an affinity reaction. Biosensors have been developed to detect hybridization of unlabelled DNA using different transduction methodologies.

(A) *Electrochemical detection*: The great advantage of the DNA electrochemical biosensor is that it does not require very expensive components. These are based on the voltametric monitoring of DNA hybridization. Voltametric responses of these indicators are influenced by the result of DNA hybridization. Some electroactive DNA intercalators and minor groove binding substances as redox indicators of the hybridization events are available. A second approach directed to hybridization detection is based on the electroactivity of nucleic acids. Single-stranded and duplex DNA can easily be recognized as the basis of the intrinsic DNA electroactivity (adenosine and guanine) without any redox indicator. Signal of single-stranded DNA obtained at the electrodes differ from those produced by double-stranded DNA, thus making it possible to detect hybridization reactions.

(B) *Piezoelectric detection (mass sensitive devices)*: A useful indicator free detection scheme relies on the use of quartz crystal microbalance (QCM) transducers. The QCM is an extremely sensitive mass-measuring device that allows dynamic monitoring of hybridization events, using an oscillating crystal with the DNA probe immobilized on its surface. The increased mass, associated with the hybridization reaction, results in decrease of the oscillating frequency.

(C) *Optical detection (Surface Plasmon resonance (SPR) based sensing)*: SPR is a widely used optical method for application to biospecific interaction analysis (BIA). By using this method it is possible to monitor real time affinity interaction and to obtain the relative affinity constant (K_A). The SPR phenomenon is influenced by changes in refractive index (RI), occurring when hybridization interaction takes place at the interface (between the immobilized probe and its target in solution). The RI changes influence the resonant angle at which SPR occurs. The recorded signal is expressed as the resonant angle changes vs. time. The hybridization reaction can be followed in real time without the use of any label. Biosensors are extensively used as diagnostic tools, predominantly in point-of-care testing. One such example is the successful commercialization of biosensors for *in vitro* measurement of capillary glucose using various hand-held systems with disposable reagent cartridges. New developments in protein engineering for immunoglobulins (antibody fragments, chimeric antibodies, etc) or in substituting antibodies by alternative binding components (aptamers) or structures (molecular imprinting) will enable changes in the affinity and fine specificity of antibodies as well as expression of fragments as fusion protein coupled to reporter molecules. These developments helped to develop biosensor technology as new molecular diagnostic technique.

Aptamers are single-stranded DNA or RNA oligonucleotides sequences with the capacity to recognize various target molecules with high affinity and specificity. These ligand-binding oligonucleotides mimic properties of antibodies in a variety of diagnostic formats. They are folded into unique overall shapes to form intricate binding furrows for the target structures. Aptamers have advantages over native antibodies to reduce signal-to-noise ratio in diagnostic formats. For example, the standard diagnostic protocol for detecting proteins in blood, urine, saliva, and other body fluids, is the two-antibody sandwich assay. In this assay, a capture monoclonal antibody is used, usually on a solid surface to bind the protein in question. The signal-to-noise ratio of such a single capture step in a mixture of proteins as complex as blood, is never sufficient to provide a useful test. Because of this, a second antibody, either monoclonal or polyclonal, is then used to detect the bound protein. The second antibody is then detected by fluorescence or a colorimetric assay. For such an antibody-based test to be useful in diagnostics, it is essential that these two binding steps be independent so that the background is reduced by the multiplicative specifity of the two steps. It is feasible to use the *in vitro* derived aptamers in such a way that one aptamer can substitute for two antibodies. With arrays of aptamers on a solid surface, blood or any other body fluid can be incubated with this aptamer 'chip'. Proteins will sort themselves out in a manner analogous to affinity chromatography.

Microarray Based Diagnostics

The recent major advances within molecular diagnostics involve high throughput assays. One of the best examples is the introduction of microarrays. Prices of the assays are constantly dropping making them eventually useful tools in the routine clinical laboratory. The development of new simplified detection methodologies and broad application to molecular diagnostics, have rapidly brought microarray technology into the arena of diagnostics. In recent years, new methods of manufacturing microarrays have been developed, which are superceding more traditional spotted array formats. The propagation of novel *in situ* synthesis technologies for oligonucleotides and peptide synthesis on the chip allows distinct microarray designs to be manufactured within days (Figure 16.5). Advancement in the semiconductor materials and electrochemical DNA synthesis are now bringing semiconductor devices to the forefront of microarray technology. DNA microarray popularly known as biochips are composed of a solid support to which the DNA molecules are attached (Figure 16.6).

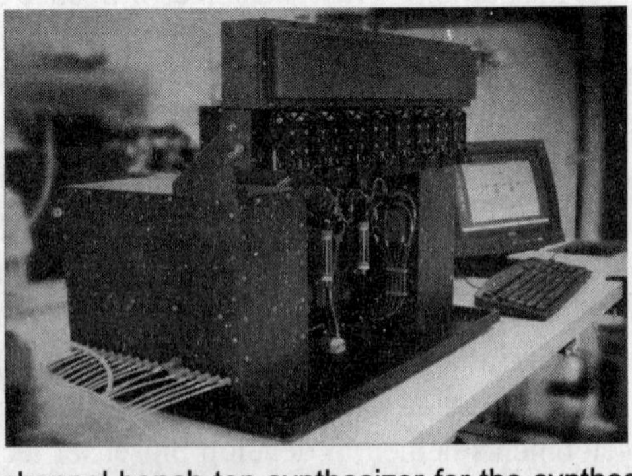

Figure 16.5 An eight-channel bench-top synthesizer for the synthesis of custom oligonucleotide microarrays. (Courtsey: Dill and Mcshea, 2005).

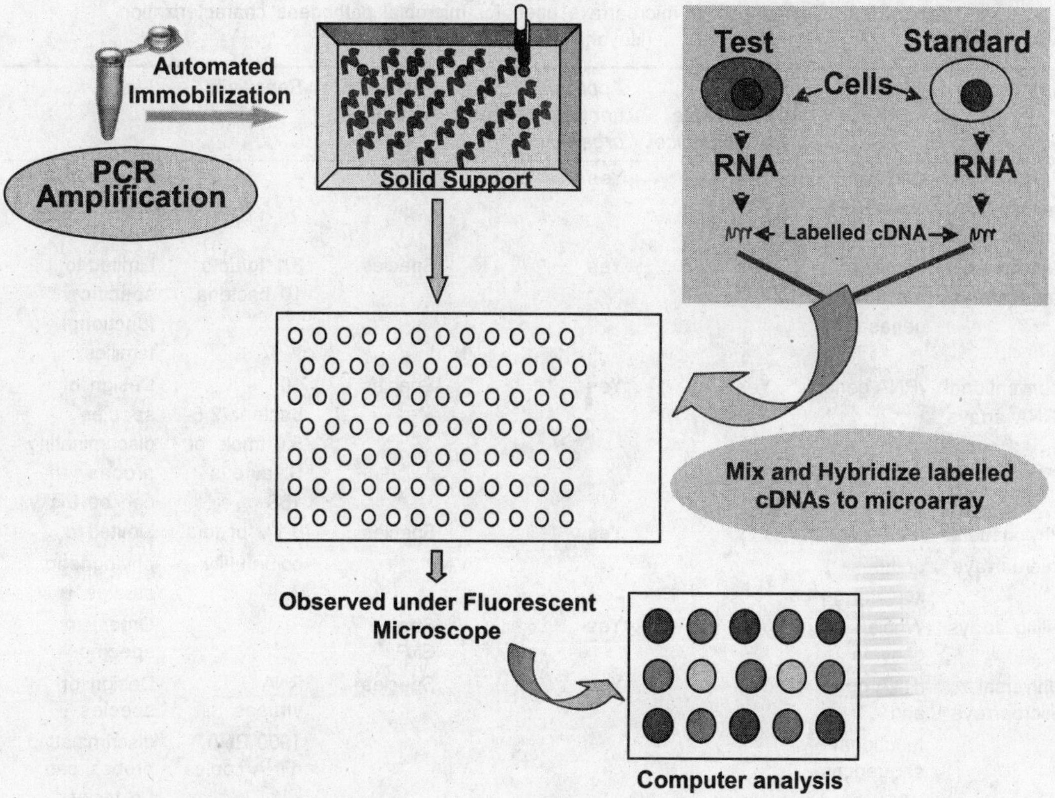

Figure 16.6 DNA microarray.

For spotted oligonucleotide arrays, the chip surface contains activated chemical moieties to couple the oligo to the surface whereas *in situ* synthesis systems use a membrane or a porous reaction layer over the chip surface to support DNA synthesis. Biological materials are bound to these activated materials using varieties of chemistry. Most crucially, these linker and coating chemistries maintain these attachments even after the chemical removal of DNA-protecting groups or hybridization. The means of attachment to the substrate as well as the material/chemistries used do vary. In some cases, it is a direct attachment to some activated groups on the surface of the material used (e.g., epoxy-modified glass slides) or it might simply be a hydrophobic interaction. In other cases, biological glue such as biotin or other hapten ligands, might be used to tether molecules robustly on the surface. There are several types of biochips. The most common are DNA chips, where snippets of DNA ranging from 25 bases (oligonucleotide array) to hundred of bases in length (cDNA arrays) are laid down or synthesized *in situ* on the chip. DNA microarrays for clinical disease diagnosis are now built upon the increasing amount of sequence information available on pathogens (Table 16.3).

Table 16.3 Comparison of microarrays used for microbial pathogens characterization (Huyghe *et al.*, 2009).

Array type	*Target*	*Prior knowledge of sequence*	*Applicable to uncharacterized organisms*	*Highest resolution*	*Sensitivity*	*Limits*
Whole-genome arrays	ORF (and inter-ORF)	Yes	Yes	Strains	–	Organism specific
Functional gene arrays	Family of functional genes	Yes	Yes	Species	3.1 fg/upto 10 bacteria	Limited to specific functional families
Conventional rRNA arrays	rRNA gene	Yes	Yes	Species	10 bacteria/2.5–5.0 fmole of S. aureus 16S	Design of species discriminating probes can be tricky
Phylogenetic microarrays	rRNA gene or house-keeping genes	Yes	Yes	Species	0.1% of total community	Limited to phylognetic studies
Tiling arrays	Whole genome	Yes	Yes	Strains SNP	–	Organism specific
Universal microarrays	rRNA gene and functional sequences	Yes	Yes	Species	RNA viruses: 1900 RNA rRNA copies	Design of species discriminating probes can be tricky
NCHS	Whole genome	No	Yes	Species	To be determined	Inhomogeneous GC content requires use of additives

Basically DNA microarrays are dot-blot hybridization experiments performed in a small and highly parallel format, allowing hybridization to multiple targets in the same assay. They are used to identify or, quantify the amount of a given nucleotide sequence in a sample, by staining the DNA with a fluorophore and subsequently hybridizing the sample to a solid support containing immobilized probes with complementary sequences. The amount of hybridized sample is quantified by signal intensity and the experiments can either be performed individually or comparatively where two samples tagged with two different fluorescent stains are hybridized to the same slide.

Several techniques exist for deposition of probes, but usually they involve immobilization of synthetic oligonucleotide probes or PCR fragments onto glass slides, or they are constructed directly onto the slide by photolithographic methods (in case of the Affymetrix gene chip). DNA chips are divided into two categories 1) spotted arrays and 2) synthesized arrays. *In situ* synthesized arrays are generated by spatially controlled patterning techniques including photolithography, ink-jet synthesis and electrochemical patterning on an electrode array. Detection and labelling methodologies for DNA chips vary widely. Fluorescence labels are available as modified bases or are conjugated chemically after nucleic acid amplification. Another detection method is luminescence. It has advantage of very low intrinsic background. Utilizing enzyme-based luminescence provides some enhancement over fluorescent-based imaging systems. A third detection method is redox enzyme amplification electrochemical detection. Advantages of electrochemical detection include the elimination of the image-analysis step required by all fluorescent or luminescent imaging systems because electrochemical measurement produces a value of current per electrode rather than an image. Neither electrochemical nor luminescent imaging systems suffer from the known problems associated with high resolution fluorescent imaging, namely ozone sensitivity and photobleaching/annealing effects.

In comparison to DNA arrays, gene action can be studied directly, provided that the protein's natural shape and functionality are maintained. This requires novel systems for high-throughput protein expression, which produces sufficient amounts of properly modified and folded molecules. Several peptide and protein chips are available on the marketplace and several systems for performing peptide synthesis *in situ* have been developed (Table 16.4). For larger proteins, *in situ* synthesis is not an option and spotting remains the primary method for making arrays. Additionally, several other types of biochips exist including glycobiology chips as well as organic chemistry-based combinatorial chips. Protein microarrays are constructed from recombinantly expressed, purified and yet functional protein, entailing a range of optimized expression systems. Large number of proteins need to be arrayed at high density, in order to keep them intact and biologically active. Different expression systems are present and are being used having their own merits and difficulties.

Table 16.4 High-throughput protein array techniques and diagnostic applications (Source: Walter *et al.*, 2002).

Techniques	*Advantages*	*Limitations*	*Diagnostic applications*
cDNA clone arrays	Automated colony picking and gridding, direct relation to clone DNA	Cellular protein background, undefined proteins or fragments	Protein expression analysis, protein interaction screening
Protein microarrays	Most sensitive, miniaturized and parallel capture-target assays, analysis of complex samples	Different protein features, no standardized handling native proteins, solid-phase chemistry	Protein expression analysis, molecular identification, quantification, affinity assays
Antibody clone arrays	As cDNA; isolation of antibodies against impure proteins and complex antigens possible	Antigen-coated filters required, sensitivity of detection to be improved by 100–1000-fold	Antibody expression, screening and selection
Antibody microarrays	As protein; robust, standard molecular structure	Limited proteome and marker coverage by antibodies available	As protein; protein marker and expression profiling
Aptamer microarrays	Robust, standard DNA microarray technology, covalent attachment of aptamers to cognate proteins,	Proof-of-concept stage	As antibody

Contd.

	direct protein staining, aptamer specificity optimized by *in vitro* evolution		
PROfusion_ arrays	*In vitro* covalent linkage of a protein to its encoding RNA, self-assembly to surface-bound DNA probes, directed *in vitro* evolution	Proof-of-concept stage	As protein and antibody
Protein nanoarrays	No detectable nonspecific binding of proteins, can be screened by atomic-force microscopy	Proof-of-concept stage	As protein and antibody
Microfluidic arrays (Lab-on-a -Chip)	Optimal surface-to-volume ratio, shorter hybridization times, large binding-signal capacity, readily automated, fast and robust	Proof-of-concept stage	As protein and antibody

A combination of *in vitro* protein expression and direct immobilization on to microtitre plates has been applied commonly called protein *in situ* arrays (PISA) method. High throughput protein array allows the miniaturization and parallel analysis of large numbers of diagnostic markers in complex samples. Using automated colony picking and gridding, cDNA or antibody libraries can be expressed and screened as clone arrays. Proteins can be arrayed either on flat solid phases or in capillary systems (microfluidic arrays). Several formats of microarray are at proof-of-concept stage like antibody-based, aptamer-based, PROfusion ™, nano- and microfluidic arrays (Table 16.5).

Table 16.5 Manufacture of genome-wide arrays showing differences in oligonucleotide length, density and customizability (Source: Dill and Mcshea, 2005).

Manufacturer (method)	*Probe length (length of oligomer)*	*Density (Spot per square cm)*	*Customizable*
ABI (spotting)	60mer	31000	–
Affymetrix (synthesis)	25mer	54000	+
Agilent (synthesis)	60mer	44000	++
Combimatrix (synthesis)	30–50mer	12000 or 90000	+++
GE Codelink (spotting)	30mer	55000	–
Illumina (beads)	50mer	46000	–
Nimblegen (synthesis)	60mer	38000	+++
Home Brew Developed by user	50–70mer	larger fragments Up to 40000	++

Preferred solid phases are modified glass or filter membranes, because of their low fluorescence background. Protein arrays are commonly printed (gridded, spotted) and imaged using the same commercially available automated arrayers and scanners as for DNA arrays. Most imaging systems for protein arrays are fluorescence-based using either direct labeling of ligands or indirect detection via labeled antibodies. Different fluorophores allow multiplexing and differential protein expression profiling. Antibody microarray is becoming a robust format for expression profiling of whole genomes. The microfluidic flow control in lateral flow formats has been evolving dramatically. Sophisticated microcapillary based devices are available for analysis of whole blood sample in clinics (Figure 16.7).

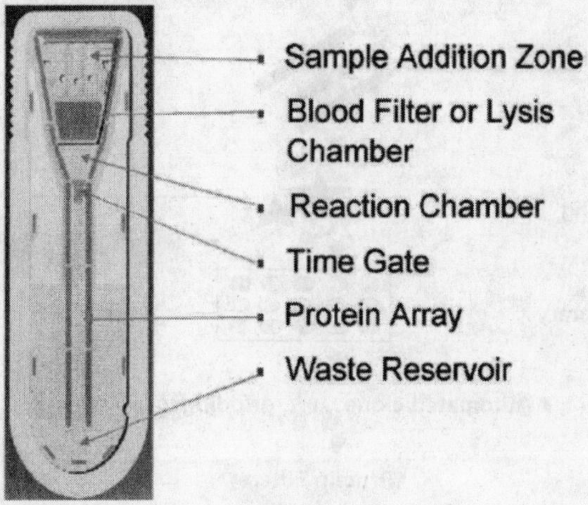

Figure 16.7 Microfluidics protein chip. The blood sample is added at the sample addition zone. The sample enters a filter where red blood cells and plasma are separated by lateral flow. The plasma exits the filter and enters into a high capillarity region termed the sample reaction barrier. The sample reaction barrier helps form the volume of the reaction chamber. In the walls of the sample reaction barrier are grooves that promote the capillary flow of the sample into the reaction chamber, and in doing so, the fluid moves from higher capillarity of the sample reaction barrier to the lower capillarity of the reaction chamber. The sample enters and fills the reaction chamber and the fluid flow is delayed at the area of the time gate. The flow is delayed so that the cardiac marker analytes in the sample can react with the fluorescent antibody conjugates in the reaction chamber to form a reaction mixture. The reaction mixture then flows from the time gate into the protein array. On the protein array are antibodies immobilised in discrete zones and binding of analytes at those zones is detected by a proprietary fluorescent energy transfer detection technology. The movement of fluids in this sophisticated device is enabled by the fundamental properties of fluids at this microscale (Source: Schulte *et al.*, 2002).

Microarray technologies in combination with bioinformatics have the potential to allow the rapid diagnosis of diseases, including mutagenic diseases. This technology is helpful in quantification of whole-genome RNA expression data. This technique is also capable of comprehensive, quantitative RNA expression analysis, with their promise of a global approach to the quantification of gene-expression. Availability of complete genome sequences of different organisms will provide large numbers of drug targets and cause a paradigm shift in medicine. The world of diagnostics and therapeutics is changing towards more complexity. Personalized therapy requires screening and cataloging of patients' gene and protein profile, prior, during and following treatment. Building upon established DNA microarray technology, arrays of purified proteins represent the next level diagnostic tools, allowing direct analysis of gene functions (Figure 16.8).

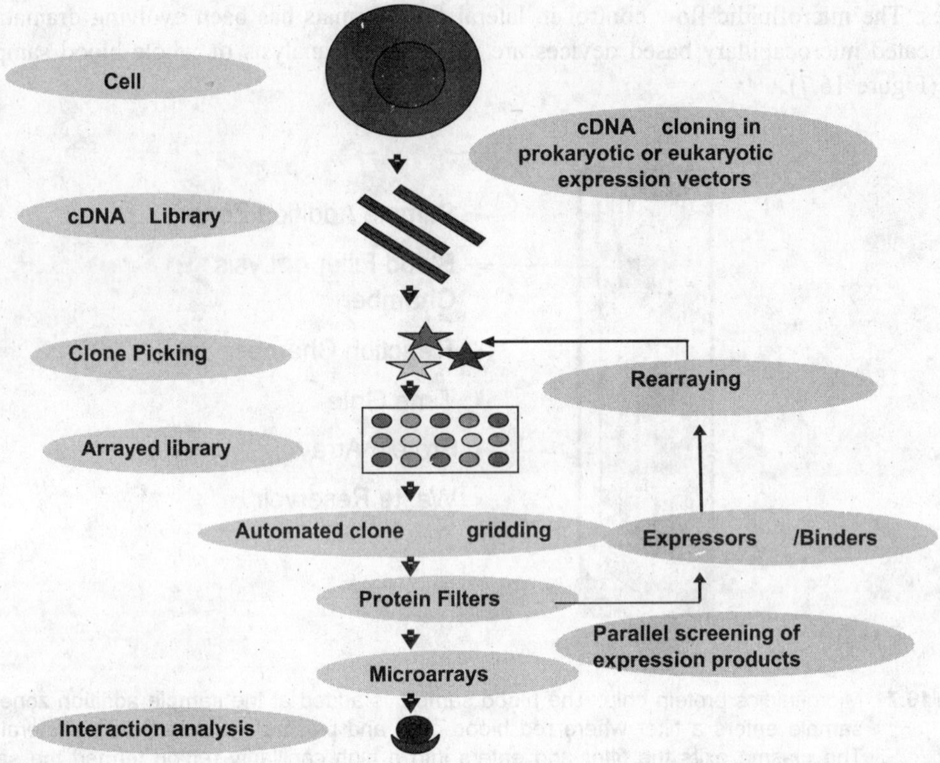

Figure 16.8 High-throughput expression and analysis of unknown proteins using protein microarrays. The arrays are screened for protein expression or ligand binding by incubation with complex molecular mixtures, and protein-expressing or protein-binding clones are subsequently rearrayed into dedicated subset libraries.

Microarray can reveal association between gene-expression signatures and the biology and outcome of disease like identification of clinically significant subtypes of cancers. This technique is already having a major impact on cancer biology, pharmacology and drug development and, with their rapid development, new technologies, method of analysis and applications are emerging continuously. Differential protein profiling has been used as molecular diagnostics for cancer and autoimmune diseases. Proteomic pattern analysis will be applied as a screening tool for cancer in high-risk and general populations. Autoantibodies can be detected for autoimmune disorder by screening of sera of patients or high-risk population by using arrays of large numbers of recombinant proteins of known identity. Microarrays are becoming routine tool for disease diagnosis in high-throughput laboratories because of accumulation of array data deposition in public repositories analysis tools and also due to bulk availability of reagents for microarray analysis.

Nanotechnology Based Diagnostics

Nanotechnology is the creation and utilization of materials, devices, and systems through the control of matter of the nanometer length scale. Nanotechnology has a tremendous potential in molecular diagnostics. Nanomolecular diagnostics is the use of nanobiotechnology in molecular diagnostics and can be termed "nanodiagnostics". Nanotechnology has several potential applications in molecular diagnostics (Table 16.6). Nanobiochips are able to provide label-free detection and are being applied to overcome some of the limitations of biochip technology. Nanoarray chips using the atomic force microscope (AFM) as a readout method optimizes analysis with the advantages like no need for secondary reporter systems, reduction in material used on several thousand molecules can be covered with one test and increased sensitivity with single molecule detection ultimately. Nanoparticle-based protein chip is a sensitive technique being developed for optical detection of nanogold particle-labeled molecules by applying SPR (Surface Plasmon Resonance) and specific molecular binding using rolling circle amplification.

Table 16.6 Nanotechnologies with potential applications in molecular diagnostics (Source: Jain, 2005).

Nanotechnologies	*Applications*
Nanotechnology on a chip	Microfluidic chips for nanoliter volumes: NanoChip Optical readout of nanoparticle labels, NanoArrays, Protein nanoarrays
Nanoparticle technologies	Gold particles, Nanobarcodes, Magnetic nanoparticles: ferrofluids, supramagnetic particles combined with Magnetic resonance imaging (MRI) Quantum dot technology, Nanoparticle probes
Nanopore technology	Measuring length of DNA fragments in a high-throughput manner, DNA fingerprinting, Haplotyping
Cantilever arrays	Multiple combined tests (such as protein and DNA) to be performed on the same disposable chip, Prostate specific antigen binding to antibody
DNA nanomachines for	Nanoparticle-based immunoassays, DNA–protein and nanoparticle conjugates, Nanochip-based single-molecular interaction force assays Resonance light scattering technology
Nanosensors	Living spores as nanodetectors, Nanopore nanosensors, Nanosensor glucose monitor, Optical biosensors: surface plasmon resonance technology, Probes Encapsulated by Biologically Localized Embedding (PEBBLE) nanosensors, Photostimulated luminescence in nanoparticles, Quartz nanobalance DNA sensor, Sensing of Phage-Triggered Ion Cascade

Nanoparticles are typically in the size range of 1-100nm, and can have different shapes and compositions. Nanoparticles are also structurally robust and their physical properties are tailorable by variation of particle size, shape and composition. Several nanoparticles are used in molecular diagnostics. Some of them are gold nanoparticles, quantum dots (QDs) and supermagnetic nanoparticles (Table 16.7).

Table 16.7 Description and advantages of AuNPs, QDs, and superparamagnetic nanoparticles (Azzazy and Mansour, 2009)

Nanoparticle	*Structure*	*Signal detection method(s)*	*Advantages*
AuNPs	Either a dielectric core (normally gold sulfide or silica) enclosed within a thin gold shell (known as nano-shells) or simply a spherical gold nanoparticle.	Several detection methods can be used such as colorimetric, scanometric, electronic and electrochemical, scattered light, surface enhanced Raman scattering.	Optical tenability, Strong optical signal
QDs	Nanocrystals typically composed of a core semiconductor e.g. cadmium selenide (CdSe) which is enclosed in a shell of another semiconductor with a larger spectral bandgap e.g. zinc sulfide (ZnS), A third silica shell can be added to the nanocrystal for water solubility	Fluorescence measurement using a fluorometer, fluorescence microscopy, or wide field epifluorescence microscopy.	Broad excitation range, Narrow emission bands, photostability, optical tunability (control of emission wavelength by size control), multiplexing
Superpara-magnetic nanoparticles	Composed of magnetic metals like iron, or alloys of different metals	Magnetometer	High sensitivity due to detection of subtle modifications in magnetic character.

Gold nanoparticles have been attached onto DNA and Raman-active dyes, which assemble as a sensor surface only in the presence of a complementary target. Gold nanoparticles are particularly good labels for sensors because a variety of analytical techniques can be used to detect them, including optical absorption, fluorescence, Raman scattering, atomic and magnetic force, and electrical conductivity. The detection system also relies on chips dotted with DNA. QDs are nanoscale crystals of semiconductor material that glow, or fluoresce when excited by a light source such as laser. Due to its comparatively broad excitation spectra (from ultraviolet to red) and having narrow emission spectra, a more sensitive assay can be generated using these QDs. Furthermore, these are highly resistant to degradation, and their fluorescence is remarkably stable. The major challenge is that QDs have an oily surface, whereas, the cellular environment is water-based. After modifying the surface chemistries of QDs, it can be specifically attached to biological materials such as cells, proteins, and nucleic acids. QDs can be designed to emit light at any wavelength from the infrared to visible to ultraviolet. This enables the use of large number of colors and thus multiplexed assays can be performed. The organic coatings with short chains of synthetic peptides can be used to disguise QDs so effectively that the cell mistakes them for proteins. This might allow particles to penetrate the cells and light up individual proteins inside.

Magnetic nanoparticles are a powerful and versatile diagnostic tool in biology and medicine. Bound to a suitable antibody, they are used to label specific molecules, structures or, microorganisms. Magnetic immunoassay techniques have been developed in which the magnetic field generated by the magnetically labeled targets is detected with a sensitive magnetometer. Antibodies labeled with magnetic nanoparticle give magnetic signals on exposure to a magnetic field. Antibodies bound to targets can thus be identified as unbound antibodies disperse in all directions and produce no net magnetic signal. CELLTracks^{TM} Technology of immunicon corporation (Huntingdon Valley, PA) is based on magnetic nanoparticles called ferrofluids. Ferrofluid consists of a magnetic core surrounded by a polymeric layer coated with antibodies for capturing cells. Application includes detection of circulating cancer cells in the blood and identification of microorganisms.

Nanomaterials are exquisitely sensitive chemical and biological sensors. Nanosensors with immobilized bioreceptor probes that are selective for target analyte molecules are called nanobiosensors. They can be integrated into other technologies such as lab-on-a-chip to facilitate molecular diagnostics. Their applications include detection of microorganism in different samples, monitoring of metabolites in body fluids and detection of tissue pathology such as cancer. A bioconjugated nanoparticle-based bioassay for *in situ* pathogen quantification can detect a single bacterium within an hour. The nanoparticle provides an extremely high fluorescent signal for bioanalysis and can be easily incorporated in biorecognition molecules such as an antibody. The antibody-conjugated nanoparticles can readily and specifically identify a variety of microorganisms through antibody-antigen interaction and recognition.

A nanotechnology-based technique, SEensing of Phage-Treggered Ion Cascade (SEPTIC), uses a nanowell device with two antenna-like electrodes to detect the electric-field fluctuations which result when a bacteriophage infects a specific bacterium and can thus be used for the identification of the bacterium. Direct, real-time electrical detection of single virus particles can also be achieved with high selectivity by using nanowire field effect transistors. Advances in nanotechnology are providing nanofabricated devices that are small, sensitive and inexpensive enough to facilitate direct observation, manipulation and analysis of single biological molecule from a single cell. Future trends in diagnostic will continue in miniaturization of biochip technology to nano-range.

Antibody Based Diagnostics: Serological Reactions (Serology)

Antigen-antibody interactions *in vitro* (under laboratory conditions) are referred to as serological reactions or serology (so named because they commonly involve patient's serum) (Figure 16.9a). Antigen-antibody interactions were first adapted to laboratory tests to diagnose disease in the late 1800s. At present, they have become a highly sophisticated and often automated discipline of immunology, and are widely used in clinical diagnosis, epidemiology, and basic research. A variety of serological reactions are used in laboratories, the most important and often used ones are: precipitation-test, agglutination-test, fluorescent-antibody technique (immunofluorescence), readioimmunoassay (RIA), and enzyme-linked immunosorbent assay (ELISA).

Precipitation-test (Precipitin-Test)

When soluble antigens and the homologous antibody molecules react, they sometimes form large polymeric macromolecules terminating into visible precipitate (Figure 16.9). The precipitation occurs in two stages: first, the antibodies bind to antigens forming antigen-antibody-complex within a few seconds or minutes, then the constant regions of antibodies of the complexes bind to each other within some hours resulting in the formation of visible precipitate. The formation of precipitate is dependent on the proper relative concentrations of the antigen and antibody molecules in a specific region called the zone of equivalence or zone of precipitating, i.e., the zone of equivalence (or precipitation) defines the region wherein the concentrations of antigen and antibody molecules reach almost equivalence. Precipitation tests are performed either in fluid-fluid precipitation, or gel-gel precipitation. In the former, the solutions of antigen and antibody are layered over each other in a thin tube, whereas the diffusion of antigen and antibody takes place through a semisolid gel (such as agarose). In the latter, mainly applied in the laboratory diagnosis of bacterial infections of humans and important animals, the precipitation tests are also used for many other purposes such as (i) identification of blood or seminal fluid in stains on clothing, weapons, etc.; (ii) postmortem diagnosis of anthrax from a dead or decomposed animal; (iii) detection of food adulteration and (iv) determination of the kind of an animal a mosquito has recently fed on, to help preventing spread of arthropod-borne diseases.

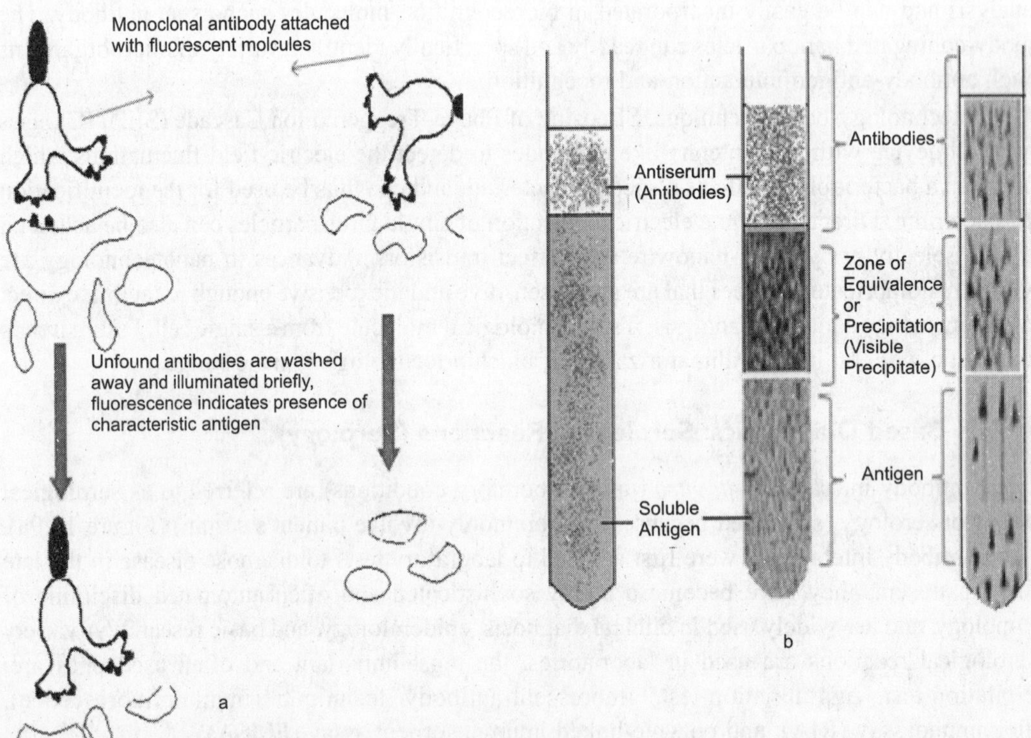

Figure 16.9 (a) Antigen-antibody interactions (b) precipitation-test.

Agglutination-test

In agglutination-test visible clumping or aggregation of cells or particles takes place due to the reaction of surface-bound antigens of such cells or particles with homologous antibodies (Figure 16.10). Pathogens causing many diseases like typhoid fever (*Salmonella typhi*), gonorrhoea (*Neisseria gonorrhoeae*), rickettsial diseases are detected by agglutination-tests; it is probably best known for its use in human red blood cells (RBCs) possess either type A or type B polysaccharide antigens, or both type A and type B polysaccharide antigens or neither of these two antigens on their surface respectively. Blood types are determined by mixing known antisera (anti-A and anti-B antibodies) with a blood possesses type A but not type B antigens on the surface of RBCs; type B blood has the type B but not type A antigens on the surface of RBCs; type AB blood possesses both type A and type B antigens on the surface of RBCs; and type O blood has neither type A nor type B antigens on the surface of RBCs.

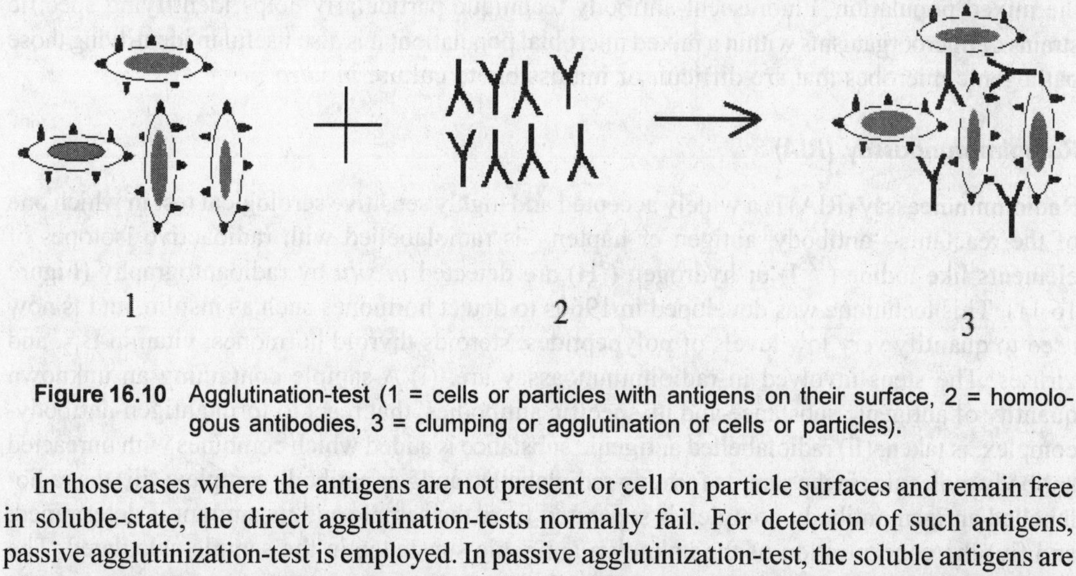

Figure 16.10 Agglutination-test (1 = cells or particles with antigens on their surface, 2 = homologous antibodies, 3 = clumping or agglutination of cells or particles).

In those cases where the antigens are not present or cell on particle surfaces and remain free in soluble-state, the direct agglutination-tests normally fail. For detection of such antigens, passive agglutinization-test is employed. In passive agglutinization-test, the soluble antigens are taken out, are first attached to the surface of one of the carriers like latex beads, polystyrene, particle, red blood cells, and then mixed with patient's serum. Homologous antibodies present in serum attach with antigens present on the surface on the surface of the carrier forming antigen-antibody-complexes that agglutinate. An excellent example of passive agglutination-test using latex beads as carrier is one of the modern pregnancy test; other example is the detection of pathogens like *Haemophilus influenzae* (*Haemophilus meningitis*), *Streptococcus pneumoniae* (pneumonia), *Neisseria meningitides* (meningococcal meningitis), *Treponema pallidum* (Syphilis), Rubella virus (German measles), etc.

Fluorescent-antibody technique (immunofluorescence)

The fluorescent-antibody technique (immunofluorescence) is often used to identify unknown antigens. The technique is based on the behaviour of certain dyes, which fluoresce (glow) when exposed to certain wavelengths of light. Such dyes are: fluorescenin isothiocyanate, which emits an apple-green glow, and rhodamine isothiocyanate, which emits orange-red light. Fluorescent-antibody technique may be direct or indirect. In direct method, known antibody molecules are conjugated (labelled) with a fluorescent dye; the dye-labelled antibodies combine with those microbes that possess complementary antigens on their surface. The mixed microbial population is viewed under fluorescence microscope with an excitation wavelength appropriate for the dye; only dye-labelled antibody attached microbial cells fluoresce and become visible. In indirect method, the initially applied antibody is not labeled (conjugated) with the dye. Instead, a second labeled antibody is applied which binds the fluorescence label to the specific antibody that has already reacted with its complementary antigen present on the surface of the microbial cells in the mixed population. Fluorescent-antibody technique particularly helps identifying specific strains of microorganisms within a mixed microbial population; it is also useful in identifying those pathogenic microbes that are difficult or impossible to culture *in vitro*.

Radioimmunoassay (RIA)

Radioimmunoassay (RIA) is a widely accepted and highly sensitive serological test in which one of the reactants—antibody, antigen or hapten—is radiolabelled with radioactive isotopes of elements like iodine (^{125}I) or hydrogen (^{3}H) are detected *in situ* by radioautography (Figure 16.11). This technique was developed in 1960s to detect hormones such as insulin, and is now used to quantify very low levels of polypeptides, steroids thyroid hormones, vitamin B_{12}, and viruses. The steps involved in radioimmunoassay are: (i) A sample containing an unknown quantity of antigenic substance and its specific antibodies, that react to form antigen-antibody-complex, is taken; (ii) radiolabelled antigenic substance is added which combines with unreacted antibody molecules in the sample forming radiolabelled antigen-antibody complex; (iii) the radio-labelled antigen-antibody-complex is separated from the sample and its amount is determined, and (iv) the concentration of the unknown antigenic substance in the sample calculated. The basis of radioimmunoassay is the competition between a known amount an antigenic substance that is radiolabelled and an unknown amount of the same antigenic substance that is non-radiolabelled for the same antibody. The relative amounts of radiolabelled and non-radiolabelled antigenic substance that bind with the antibody molecules indicated the levels of the antigenic substance in the sample. High levels of antigen-antibody-complex (radiolabelled) indicate a low level of unknown antigenic substance whereas low level of radiolabelled antigen-antibody-complex indicates a high level of unknown antigenic substance in the sample.

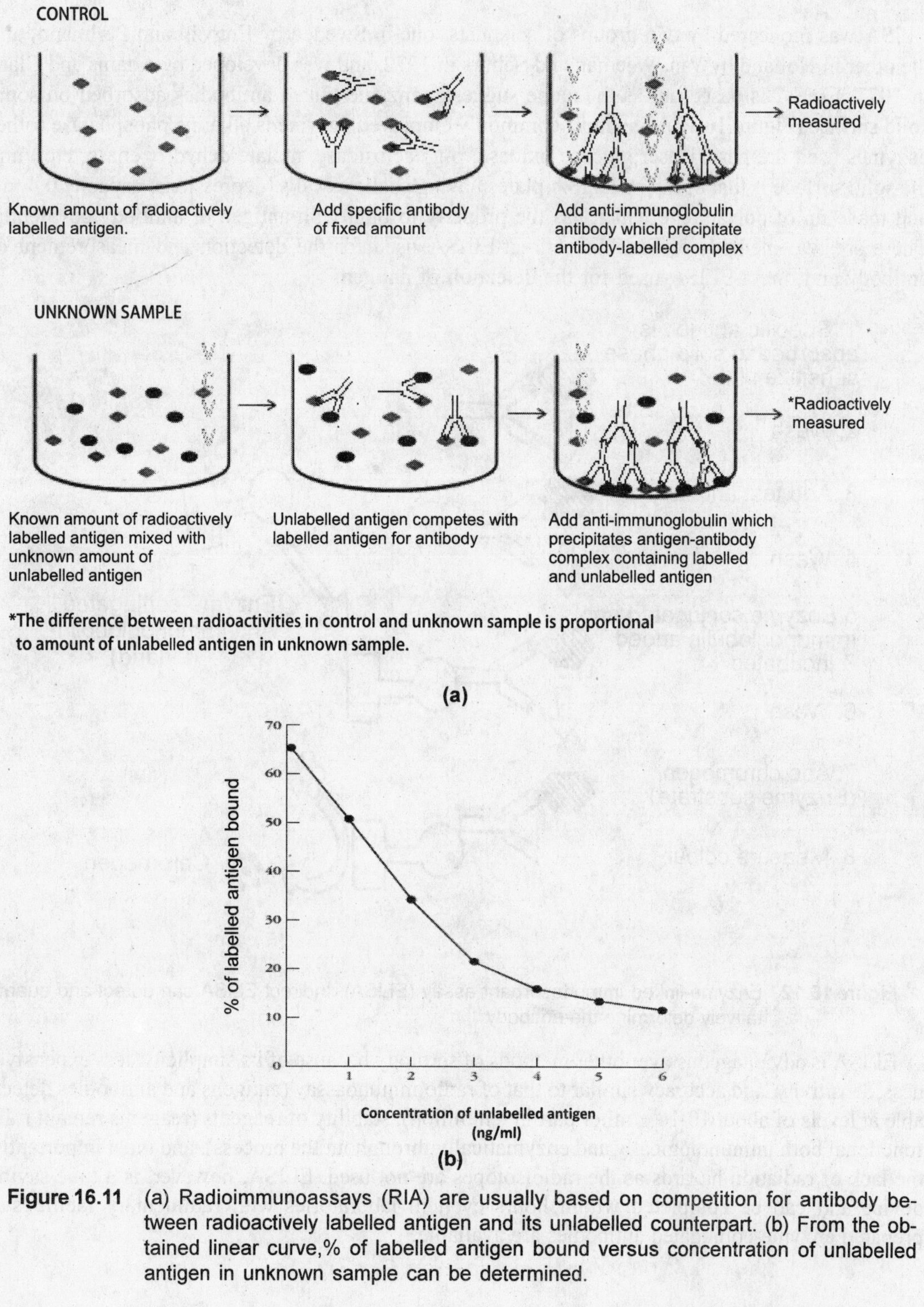

Figure 16.11 (a) Radioimmunoassays (RIA) are usually based on competition for antibody between radioactively labelled antigen and its unlabelled counterpart. (b) From the obtained linear curve,% of labelled antigen bound versus concentration of unlabelled antigen in unknown sample can be determined.

Enzyme-linked immunosorbant assay (ELISA)

ELISA was pioneered by two groups of scientists, one in Sweden by Engvall and Perlmann, and the other in Holland by Van. Weeman and Schurs in 1972, and was developed by Adams and Clark in 1977. ELISA is based on, as the name suggests, enzyme-linked antibodies adsorbed on some solid surface (Figure 16.12). The most commonly employed enzyme is alkaline phosphatase (other enzymes used are peroxidase, glucose oxidase, p-galactosidase, malate dehydrogenase, etc.) and the solid surface is that of micro-ELISA plates having shallow walls (depressions, capacity 0.4 ml) and made up of polystyrene which has the property to bind with antigen or antibody covalently. There are two methods of ELISA: indirect-ELISA used for the detection and measurement of antibody and direct-ELISA used for the detection of antigen.

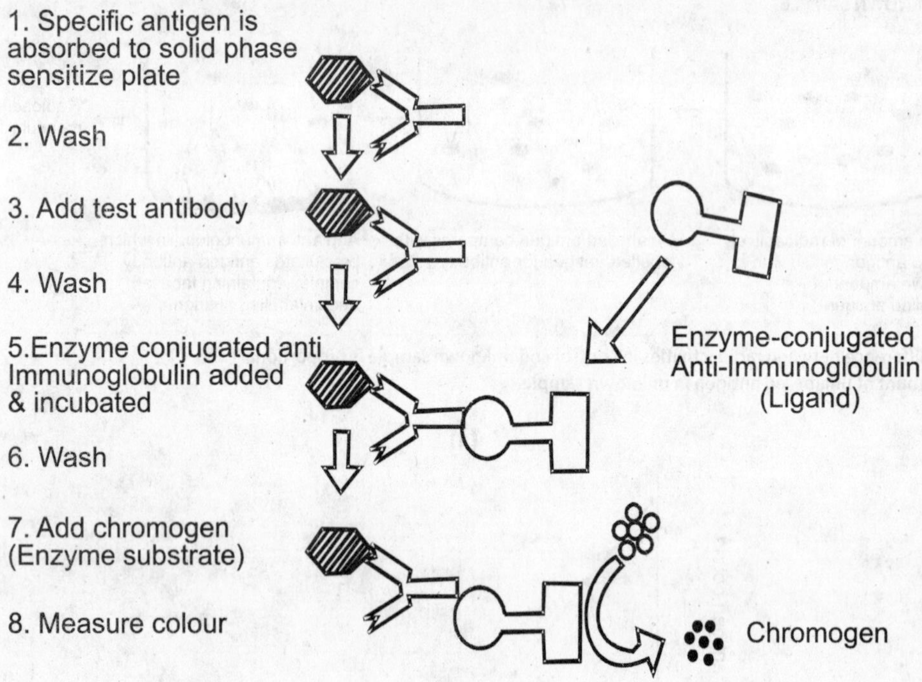

Figure 16.12 Enzyme-linked immunosorbant assay (ELISA). Indirect ELISA can detect and quantitatively determine the antibody.

ELISA is advantageous over other methods of serology because of its simplicity, less expensiveness, sensitivity, and accuracy similar to that of radioimmunoassay (antigens and antibodies detectable at levels of about 10-10 g/ml or part in ten billion), stability of reagents (reagents remain fully functional both immunologically and enzymatically throughout the process), and most importantly, the lack of radiation hazards as the radioisotopes are not used. ELISA, however, is a time saving device and can be completed within hours even in laboratories with rudimentary facilities if prepared enzyme-conjugated antibodies are available.

A majority of ELISA systems now use recombinant antigens for detection of antibodies and as a result, show considerable improvement in sensitivity and specificity. In addition, gene cloning and sequencing has allowed resolution of ELISA systems to provide information on responses to single epitopes or, antibody recognition sites. Antibody based technology: monoclonal antibodies have proved to be invaluable diagnostic reagents that have many applications, from the analysis of cancer cell phenotype and the diagnosis of infections.

Sophisticated techniques are now available to choose high-affinity antibodies and to engineer them to increase their applicability to a range of diagnostic techniques, from ELISA to *in vivo* imaging.

Phage Display: Molecular-evolution studies are important for the generation of new protein diagnostic reagents, and now there are a range of library types such as single-chain Fv fragments (scFvs), Fab synthetic and selection methods appropriate to a particular application. There are different phage display techniques like conventional phage display, selective infective phage (SIP), which are better suited to optimization rather than screening and ribosome display technologies are available.

APPLICATIONS OF MOLECULAR DIAGNOSTIC TECHNOLOGY

Molecular methods are now widely used for epidemiological fingerprinting of microbial/pathogenic isolates affecting public health. Sequence based identification and strain typing, together with the development of tools that can probe for thousands of markers, will allow detailed strain fingerprinting to assist in disease management and control. Molecular methods can be used to identify common viral pathogens not easily detectable by culture or, antigen tests (e.g., Norwalk agent, parvovirus, hepatitis C virus and HIV). Quantitative molecular kits are commercially available for viral load testing to monitor response to therapy of HIV and hepatitis C virus (HCV) infection.

Medical Applications

Molecular diagnostics play an important role in public health worldwide. It facilitates the detection and characterization of diseases, as well as monitors the drug response, and assists in the identification of genetic modifiers and disease susceptibility. Some current uses of nucleic acid tests in the diagnosis of infectious diseases is diagnosis of tuberculosis which can be confirmed in a day rather than 1-2 months as in the past. This is particularly important in tuberculous meningitis, in which the prognosis depends on early treatment. Patient suffering from encephalitis, herpes simplex virus (HSV) can be detected in cerebrospinal fluid (CSF) and no need of brain biopsy. *Chlamydia trochomatis urethritis* can be detected rapidly and specifically by using urine sample and there is no need of urethral or cervical swabs as required in culture method of diagnosis.

Southern blots have been primarily used in linkage analysis for genetic diseases such as cystic fibrosis. Cystic fibrosis is one of the most recessive genetic diseases of human beings caused due to mutations in the cystic fibrosis transmembrane regulator (CFTR) gene. These mutations result in defects in chloride ion transport because CFTR functions as a chloride channel.

A combination of FISH and CSLM (confocal laser scanning microscopy) has been widely used to investigate bacterial biofilms. FISH-based activity measurement could also be applied to biofilms developing in the human body in connection with implants. *In situ* hybridization using peptide nucleic acid (PNA) probes have proven extremely useful for use in a variety of FISH arrays, giving very good signal-to-noise ratio. These molecules also allow hybridization and washing procedures that yield good chromosome images. The DNA mimic, PNA, has been exploited for detection and characterization of nucleic acids based on hybridization properties as well some unique properties offered by its peptide backbone. In most of the cases, PNA hybridizes more strongly to complementary DNA and RNA than do natural deoxynucleotides. PNA-FISH technique has been developed for detection and identification of bacteria in medical diagnostics as well as in environmental analysis. In these cases, PNA probes specific for sequences of the ribosomal RNA of the microorganism are employed and analysis is performed by fluorescence microscopy.

In meningococcal meningitis, *Neisseria miningitidis* can be identified by PCR in culture negative CSF. PCR based detection and typing from clinical specimen can be used for influenza virus. PCR has been used to detect trypanosomes in cattle serum or infected tse-tse flies and *Trypanosoma annulata* in sub-clinical carriers. It has been used to detect *Trypanosoma mutans* in cattle showing parasitemia of less than 0.1%. An additional modification of the PCR that has substantial potential in the diagnostic context is the hybridization of amplification products with tagged specific oligonucleotide probes. In this way, amplicons can be detected using antibodies or other tag-specific reagents. ELISA-based system for DNA detection has been developed for this approach.

Over the past fifteen years, there has been a paradigm shift towards nucleic acid amplification tests in routine diagnosis of infectious diseases. Technical improvements in primer design, nucleic acid extraction, removal of inhibitors, labeling and detection of amplified nucleic acid have increased the sensitivity, specificity and speed of assays. Primers targeting several genes can be combined in a single reaction (multiplex PCR) to detect any of the several alternative pathogens causing common disease syndromes such as community acquired pneumonia, meningoencephlitis, viral diarrhea or intrauterine infections. By using real time assays, it will be possible to identify clinically relevant characteristics of pathogen (for example, methicillin resistance of *Staphylococcus aureus*) or serotype and toxigenicity of *E. coli* either directly in specimens or in early cultures. This technique offers the potential both for simultaneous quantification of several targets and for automation.

Detection of pathogen specific genotype can be carried out using PCR-restriction fragment length polymorphism (PCR-RFLP). PCR-RFLP based diagnosis has been standardized for many pathogens like hepatitis C virus (HCV), *Helicobacter pylori* and Chlamydia *trachomatis* by targeting 5' untranslated region, ure B gene and omp1 gene, respectively.

The DNA microarray formats can be used for many types of applications. In many laboratories, it is used to compare the transcriptome of mutants and wild type species of pathogens or sometimes transcriptome of same pathogenic strain under different environmental cues. There are several applications where the DNA microarray can be used more directly for diagnostic purposes. Gene detection microarrays have recently come to the forefront and are used to detect species specific sequences, virulence island genes and genes encoding antibiotic resistance. DNA arrays have obvious application for identification of infectious agents. This technique further holds potential to provide significant information on other type of diseases like cancer and other life-threatening disorders which are currently classified by immune-histochemical methods.

In cancer diagnosis the progression of mammalian cells towards malignancy involves an accumulation of mutations on both the molecular and chromosomal level. Cancer is generally not caused by a single gene but by multiple genes which are further influenced by environmental factors. Tumor cells harbor specific genetic changes that can be used as molecular markers for cancer diagnosis. These molecular markers can be easily detected using various molecular techniques starting from direct DNA sequencing to biosensor technology. Cancer is a complex syndrome and single molecular marker based detection is not sufficient for early diagnosis. Functional genomics advances help to gather high-throughput genome-wide data, in particular gene expression data from different cancer types. The high throughput molecular methods provide complex profile of genomic alteration, particularly in early stage. These methods might be able to identify molecular subtypes of cancer. A number of biochips are available commercially to diagnose human cancer type mutations. Diagnosis of certain tumor types is easy with the advances in the field of cancer proteomics has made.

Cancer proteomics includes two categories. One is expression proteomic and another is functional proteomics. In expression proteomics, one looks at proteins that are differentially displayed in a given tissue, body fluid or, serum. This approach holds promise for identifying disease markers that could be helpful in early detection and diagnosis of cancer. Cancer arises due to the accumulation of DNA modifications that give cells a selective growth advantage. One common DNA modification is promoter hypermethylation associated with loss of expression of a tumor suppressor gene. Detection of a certain methylation events can be used for early detection of tumors. DNA methylation-based molecular diagnostic assays are particularly attractive because of the stability of the target analyte (DNA) and the potential sensitivity of the assays. The most commonly used methylation assay in research laboratories is methylation-specific PCR. The real-time PCR version has the potential to be used as clinical diagnosis of cancer. The methylation-based markers will play an important role for cancer diagnostics. Traditional genotyping for human diseases including cancer, and detection and identification of infectious agents remain major targets of nucleic acid testing. Other targets include detection of early graft failure, human red blood cells, blood platelets and leukocyte antigen (HLA) typing. Further, preimplatation and foetal testing for both genetic disorders and blood group incompatabilities can be done.

Veterinary Applications

Molecular diagnostic technology has helped to improve diagnosis of important livestock diseases caused by different pathogens. A highly sensitive and specific one-step multiplex RT-PCR assay has been developed and standardized for the simultaneous and differential detection of the most important vesicular viruses like foot-and-mouth disease virus (FMDV), Swine vesicular disease virus (SVDV), and Vesicular Stomatitis Virus (VSV). These animal viruses cause great economic losses in the affected countries. PCR-RFLP technique is useful in identifying economically important traits in domestic animals which is helpful in marker assisted selection (MAS) and breeding program to enhance economic traits. For example, prolificacy related traits in sheep and goats.

Agricultural Applications

Several applications of molecular diagnosis are in vogue in modern agricultural practices. Molecular diagnostic technologies are widely used in detection of several plant pathogens. Several methods are available for rapid, sensitive and specific detection of these plant pathogens. Immunological and DNA-based detection methods are most commonly used. Molecular techniques based on PCR mediated DNA detection are becoming quite popular due to the now commonly available PCR equipment. A number of significant molecular markers have also been detected using genotyping. Markers may be linked (i.e. have a probability of being co-inherited with the trait of interest that is dependent on the genetic proximity of the marker and the gene influencing the trait) or diagnostic (also known as perfect) if the marker is directly associated with the gene that influences the trait. Diagnostic markers have significant advantages that they do not require independent validation for each parental line used in a breeding program and have absolute linkage with the trait being selected. There are several types of markers used by plant breeders. DNA microarrays are applied to unravel gene functions and metabolic pathways in plants by exploiting mutations. A classical approach for elucidating the function of a gene is by mutant analysis. Mutant organisms can be either mutated in the native alleles or may result from the introduction of additional copies of the gene leading to co-suppression or over-expression of the gene in question. Phenotypic analysis of such mutants can then point to the possible function of the gene.

The analysis of pesticide residues is an important concern due to their high toxicity and the serious risk that they represent for the environment and human health. Analysis for pesticides is usually carried out by gas chromatography (GC) or high performance liquid chromatography (HPLC). However, these methods require laborious extraction and clean up steps that increase analysis time and the risk of errors. The development of biosensors is a growing area, in response to the demand for rapid, simple, selective and low cost techniques for pesticides. The main principle of the biosensors developed is based on the correlation between toxicity of a pesticide and a decrease in the activity of a biomarker such as an enzyme. This activity can be registered by employing different transducers, e.g., amperometry, potentiometry, spectrometry, fluorimetry or thermometry for detection of different substrates or products of enzymatic reaction.

Improper package design or temperature abuse during handling may cause fruits and vegetables in modified-atmosphere packages to be exposed to low, injurious O_2 levels associated with the production of fermentation volatiles, quality loss and eventually product breakdown. Excessively low package O_2 also may promote growth of dangerous pathogens (e.g. *Clostridium botulinum*). The detection of ethanol would provide a sensitive technique for low-O_2 injury identification. A commercial ethanol biosensor composed of a chromagen and immobilised enzymes: alcohol oxidase and peroxidase has been tested. Alcohol oxidase catalyses oxidation of ethanol into acetaldehyde and H_2O_2 in the presence of O_2, and peroxidase (an H_2O_2 decomposing enzyme) catalyses oxidation of the chromagen causing a colour change. The onset of low O_2 injury was detected in lightly processed lettuce, cauliflower, broccoli and cabbage modified-atmosphere packages as measured by accumulation of headspace ethanol. Some microorganisms, particularly certain bacteria and fungi, are pathogens that attack crops and cause diseases, sometimes in epidemic proportions. Fungal infection and aflatoxin production can occur at any stage of plant growth, harvesting, drying, processing and storage. Recently an immuno-affinity fluorimetric biosensor was developed for detecting and quantifying aflatoxins, a group of chemically related mycotoxins formed by common fungi (*Aspergillus flavus, A. parasiticus* and *A.nomius*) found in maize, cottonseed, peanuts, and other nuts, grains and spices. Another biosensor has been developed to detect marker volatiles released by potato tubers infested with *Phytophtora infestans*, offering a possible solution to the problem of screening large numbers of seed potatoes for fungal infestation. The biosensor, based on the intact antennae of Colorado potato beetle (*Leptinotarsa decemlineata*), was able to detect one single diseased potato tuber within up to 100 kg potato tubers, offering a promising early warning technique. Insect antennae are very suitable for the construction of highly sensitive biosensors, because of their remarkable sensory abilities.

Industrial Applications

The pharmaceutical industry involved in health care settings felt a paradigm shift in recent years. A wide range of molecular-based detections are available in market today. The scope of molecular testing has expanded rapidly since its introduction in 1980s. From that time, there have been technical innovations together with upgrades, revisions, and modifications, which apply the most exciting elements of molecular biology to the clinical laboratory. Not only has the automated technology revolution had a clear impact on the lives of its users, but it also has stimulated an entire new molecular biology market, which provides new reagents and chemistries for real-time assays.

The markets for high throughput instruments are fast growing along with the growing market for nucleic acid extraction platforms. The market is growing steadily from R&D-based instruments to the diagnostic labeled configurations. Filtration-based procedures have been driving the nucleic acid extraction market; especially platforms that automate such procedures are more common and have been the first to enter the diagnostic market. Advanced molecular diagnostic technology has got several industrial applications too. Rapid diagnosis of a particular disease conditions from a large population of meat and milch animals has helped greatly in the development of meat and milk industry.

Biosensor-based drug residues identification in meat and meat products is possible nowadays. Biosensor technology could also be applied to detect mastitis infection by sensing markers such as enzyme N-acetylglucosaminidase (NAGase) in milk. This enzyme is released into milk as a result of tissue damage when the cow is resisting a clinical intra-mammary infection.

Genomics is revolutionizing our understanding of biological systems and is providing new opportunities for the dairy industry. Genomic approaches are implemented for microbial detection, enumeration, identification and the monitoring of antibiotic-resistant strains. Flow cytometry in combination with an *in situ* hybridization and real-time PCR are two technologies that can be easily implemented for control of microbial quality and safety of milk. Flow cytometry is already in use within the dairy industry and improvements in gene- and mRNA-specific detection of microorganisms using fluorescent probes would enhance this technology beyond simple assessments of bacterial cell counts.

Microarray technology is a relatively new technique that offers diverse and direct applications in milk. Microarrays are presently being developed for comparative genome analyses, strain typing, bacterial community detection and enumeration, gene-expression analysis, and genetic screening. Different molecular diagnostic technologies are now a common practice in many industries for quality control. Microbial contamination of sugar thick juice is common, even under good storage practices, in the sugar industry. Recently, thick juice microflora has been profoundly investigated with molecular tools, encompassing the appiication of 16S rRNA gene clone libraries and Terminal-Restriction Fragment Length Polymorphism (T-RFLP) analysis. In order to be able to detect the different bacteria that may occur in thick juice and may cause thick juice degradation, a DNA array was developed containing detector oligonucleotides for the genera *Bacillus, Kocuria, Staphylococccus,* and *Tetragenococcus,* and the species *Aerococcus viridans, Leuconostoc mesenteroides* and *T. halophilus*. The developed macroarray is considered reliable and sensitive (up to 0.1 pg target DNA) and has potential for monitoring the thick juice microflora during storage.

Currently, DNA array analyses are routinely performed for sugar refineries in order to monitor the microbiological quality of thick juice. Microarray-based drug-candidate is also exploited by pharmaceutical industry. Some toxicogenomics program established at R & D section of the company to predict hepatic toxicity of drug candidates. A reference transcriptional database of 120 paradigm hepatotoxitants was constructed using cDNA microarrays that represent about 3400 rat genes. Three male rats per compound were treated with a single high-dose for 24 hours, and then RNA was prepared from liver. After hybridization of microarrays, distinct gene sets for three different toxicity signatures could be defined–peroxisome proliferators (20 genes), macrophage activators (32 genes) and oxidative stressors (60 genes). The identified sets of marker genes will be used to predict different types of hepatotoxicity to prioritize drug candidates at an early stage of development. Food quality depends directly on the nature of the product, as well as on the handling and storage conditions. Modified atmosphere packaging (MAP) of fresh foods, often in combination with low-temperature storage, has been proven to extend product shelf life by limiting microbial growth. In order to determine the best storage conditions, identification and characterization of the microorganisms which have the ability to grow under these limiting conditions are important. Whole community analysis techniques such as denaturing gradient gel electrophoresis (DGGE), T-RFLP or 16S rRNA gene clone libraries are used increasingly to characterize the predominant microbial flora during MAP storage.

CONCLUSION AND FUTURE PROSPECTS

The molecular diagnostic technologies are bound to play an important role in practice of medicine, public health, pharmaceutical industry, forensics and biological warfare in the 21st century. These include several polymerase chain reaction (PCR)-based technologies, fluorescent *in situ* hybridization (FISH), peptide nucleic acids (PNA), electrochemical detection of DNA, biochips, nanotechnology and proteomic technologies. Initial applications of molecular diagnostics were mostly for infections by pathogens but are now increasing in the areas of genetic disorders, cancer and preimplantation screening. Genetic screening tests, despite some restrictions are a promising area for future expansion of *in vitro* diagnostic market. Molecular diagnostic technology is being combined with therapeutics and forms an important component of integrated health care. These are also involved in the development of personalized medicine based on pharmacogenetics and pharmacogenomics. Currently, there has been a rise in considerable interest for developing rapid diagnostic methods from the point of view of biological warfare agents such as anthrax. The number of companies involved in molecular diagnostics has increased remarkably during the past few years. A major portion of the molecular diagnostic market can be attributed to advances in genomics and proteomics. Biochip and nanobiotechnology are expected to make a significant contribution to the growth of molecular diagnostics in the near future.

FURTHER READINGS

1. Azzazy, H.M.E. and Mansour, M.M.H. (2009) *In vitro* diagnostic prospects of nanoparticles. *Clinica Chimica Acta*. **(403)**: 1-8.
2. Barken, K.B., Haagensen, J.A.J. and Tolker-Nielson, T. (2007) Advances in Nucleic acid-based diagnostics of bacterial infection. *Clinica Chimica Acta.* **(384)**: 1-11.
3. Bustin, S.A. and Dorudi, S. (2002) The value of microarray techniques for quantitative gene profiling in molecular diagnostics. *Trends in Molecular Medicine*. 8 **(6)**: 269-272.
4. Cottrell, S.E. (2004) Molecular diagnostic applications of DNA methylation technology. *Clinical Biochemistry*. **(37)**: 595-604.
5. Delong, E.F., Wickham, G.S. and Pace N.R. (1989) Phylogenetic strains: ribosomal RNA based probes for the identification of single cells. *Science.* **(243)**: 1360-1363.
6. Dill, K. and Mcshea, A. (2005) Recent advances in microarrays. *Drug Discovery Today:Technologies.* 2 **(3)**: 261-266.
7. Eshaque, B. and Dixon, B. (2006) Technology platforms for molecular diagnosis of cystic fibrosis. *Biotechnology Advances*. **(24)**: 86-93.
8. Fernandez, J., Aguero, M., Romero, L., Sanchez, C., Belak, S., Arias, M., and Sanchez-Vizcaino, J.M. (2008) Rapid and differential diagnosis of foot-and-mouth disease, swine vesicular disease, and vesicular stomatitis by a new multiplex RT-PCR assay. *Journal of Virological Methods*. **(147)**: 301-311.
9. Gilbert, G.L. (2002) molecular diagnostics in infectious diseases and public health microbiology: cottage industry to postgenomics. *Trends In Molecular Medicine.* 8 **(6)**: 280-287.
10. Huyghe, A. Francois, P. and Schrenzel, J. (2009) Characterization of microbial pathogens by DNA microarrays. *Infection, Genetics and Evolution.* **(9)**: 987-995.
11. Ikonig,G, Blanco,C, Knowles, N.J., Palma, E.I., Maradei, E. and Piccone, M.E. (2001) Phylogenetic analysis of foot-and-mouth diseases virus isolated in argentina. *Virus Genes*. **(23)**: 175-181.
12. Jain, K.K. (2005) Nanotechnology in clinical laboratory diagnostics. *Clinica Chimica Acta.* **(358)**: 37-54.
13. Jiang T, Minunni, M. and Mascini, M. (2004) Towards fast and inexpensive molecular diagnostic: the case of TP53. *Clinica Chimica Acta*. **(343)**: 45-60.
14. Juste, A. Thomma, B.P.H.J. and Lievens, B. (2008) Recent advances in molecular techniques to study microbial communities in food-associated matrices and processes. *Food Microbiology*. **(25)**:745-761.
15. Kosaki, K., Udaka, T. andOkuyama, T. (2005) DHPLC in clinical molecular diagnostic services. *Molecular Genetics and Metabolism.* **(86)**: 117-123.
16. Kurien, B.T., Scofield, R.H. (2006) Western blotting. *Methods.* **(38)**: 283-293.
17. Luppa, P.B., Skoll, L. and Chan, D.W. (2001) immunosensors-principles and applications to clinical chemistry. *Clinica Chimica. Acta*. **(314)**: 1-26.
18. Marco, M.L. and Wells-Bennik, M.H.J. (2008) Impact of bacterial genomics on determining quality and safety in the dairy production chain. *International Dairy Journal*. **(18)**: 486-495.
19. Mase, M., tsukamoto, K., Imada, T. Imai, K., Tanimura, N., Nakamura, K., Yamamoto, Y., Hitomi, T., Kira, T., Nakai, T., Kiso, M., Horimoto, T., Kawaoka, Y. and Yamaguchi, S. (2005) Characterization of H5N1influenza A virus isolated during the 2003-2004 influenza outbreak in Japan. *Virology. (***332)**: 167-176.

20. Mckeever, D.J. and Rege, J.E.O. (1999) Vaccines and diagnostic tools for animal health: the influence of biotechnology. *Livestock Production Science*. **(59):** 257-264.
21. Molijn, A., Kleter, B., Quint, W. and Doorn, L.J.V. (2005), Molecular diagnosis of human papilloma virus (HPV) infections. *Journal of Clinical Virology*. **(32S):** S43-S51.
22. Monis, P.T. and Giglio, S. (2006) Nucleic acid amplification-based techniques for pathogen detection and identification. *Infection. Genetics and Evolution.* **(6):** 2-12.
23. Neonakis, I.K., Gitti, Z., Krambovitis, E. and Spandidos, D.A. (2008) Molecular diagnostic tools in mycobacteriology. *Journal of Microbiological Methods*. **(75):** 1-11.
24. Nielsen, P.E. (2001) Peptide Nucleic acid: a versatile tool in genetic diagnostics and molecular biology, *Current Opinion in Biotechnology*. **(12):** 16-20.
25. Olvera, A., Busquets N., Cortey M., Deus N.D., Ganges L., Nunez J.I., Peralta B., Toskano J., and Dolz R., (2010) Apply phylogenetic analysis to viral livestock diseases: Moving beyond molecular typing. *The Veterinary Journal.* 184 **(2):** 130-137.
26. Saiz, J.C., Sobrino, F. and Dopazo, J. (1993) Molecular epidemiology of foot-and-mouth disease virus type O. *Journal of General Virology.* **(74):** 2281-2285.
27. Tsongalis, G.J. and Silverman, L. M. (2006) Molecular diagnostics: a historical perspective. *Clinica Chimica Acta*. **(369):** 188-192.
28. Vernet, G. (2004) Molecular diagnostics in virology. *Journal of Clinical Virology*. **(31):** 239-247.
29. Velasco-Garcia, M.N. and Mottram, T. (2003) Biosensor technology addressing agricultural problems. *Biosystem Engineering*. 84 **(1):** 1-12.

CHAPTER

17

Biosensor Technology

Biosensors will have an impact on people's daily lives in the not too distant future since they can fill the very real needs in health care, environmental monitoring and control, agriculture and chemical industries. Biosensors can essentially serve as low-cost and highly efficient devices for this purpose in addition to being used in other day -to-day applications. A biosensor is a sensing device comprising a combination a specific biological element and a transducer. In this chapter, we present the basic concepts and practical applications of biosensors in agricultural, medical, veterinary and industries that will have a marked influence on the development of new biosensing strategies in the next future.

Keywords: Biosensor technology; biodetection technology, affinity signal transducer, bioreceptor.

INTRODUCTION

A biosensor consists of two components, a bioreceptor and a transducer. The bioreceptor is a biomolecule that recognizes the target analyte and the transducer converts the recognition event into a measurable signal. The uniqueness of a biosensor is that the two components are integrated into one single sensor (Figure 17.1).

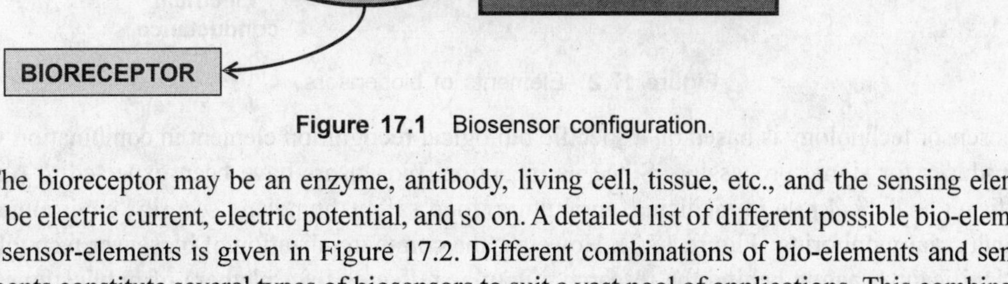

Figure 17.1 Biosensor configuration.

The bioreceptor may be an enzyme, antibody, living cell, tissue, etc., and the sensing element may be electric current, electric potential, and so on. A detailed list of different possible bio-elements and sensor-elements is given in Figure 17.2. Different combinations of bio-elements and sensor-elements constitute several types of biosensors to suit a vast pool of applications. This combination enables one to measure the target analyte without using reagents. For example, the glucose concentration in a blood sample can be measured directly by a biosensor made specifically for glucose measurement by simply dipping the sensor in the sample. This is in contrast to the commonly performed assays in which many sample preparation steps are necessary and each step may require a reagent to treat the sample. The simplicity and the speed of measurements that require no specialized laboratory skills are the main advantages of a biosensor. Depending on the transducing mechanism used, the biosensors can be of many types such as: (i) resonant biosensors, (ii) optical-detection biosensors, (iii) thermal-detection biosensors, (iv) ion-sensitive FET (ISFET) biosensors, and (v) electrochemical biosensors. Details of all these different types will be discussed in this chapter. The electrochemical biosensors, based on the parameter measured, can be further classified as: (i) conductimetric, (ii) amperometric, and (iii) potentiometric.

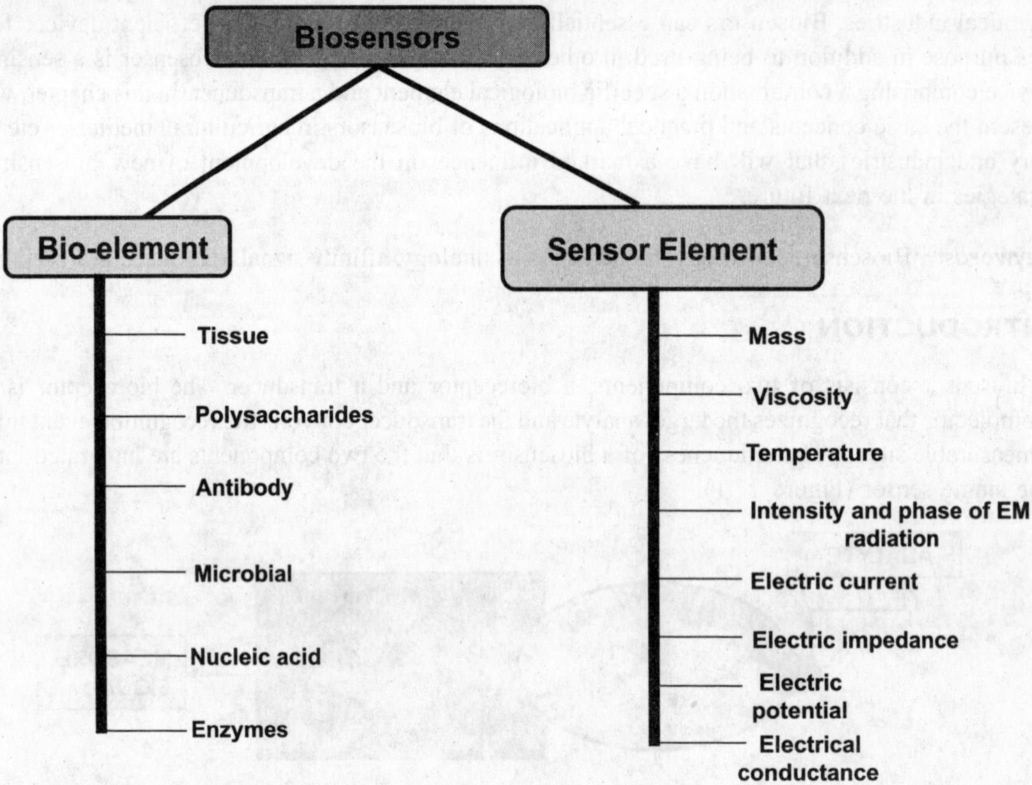

Figure 17.2 Elements of biosensors.

Biosensor technology is based on a specific biological recognition element in combination with a transducer for signal processing. Since its inception, biosensors have been expected to play a significant analytical role in medicine, agriculture, food safety, homeland security, environmental and industrial monitoring (Figure 17.3). However, the commercialization of biosensor technology has significantly lagged behind the research output as reflected by a plethora of publications and patenting activities. The rationale behind the slow and limited technology transfer could be attributed to cost considerations and some key technical barriers. Analytical chemistry has changed considerably, driven by automation, miniaturization, and system integration with high throughput for multiple tasks. Such requirements pose a great challenge to biosensor technology, which is often designed to detect one single or a few target analytes. Successful biosensors must be versatile to support interchangeable biorecognition elements, and in addition miniaturization must be feasible to allow automation for parallel sensing with ease of operation at a competitive cost. A significant upfront investment in research and development is a prerequisite in the commercialization of biosensors. The progress in such endeavors is incremental with limited success, thus, the market entry for a new venture is very difficult unless a niche product can be developed with a considerable market volume.

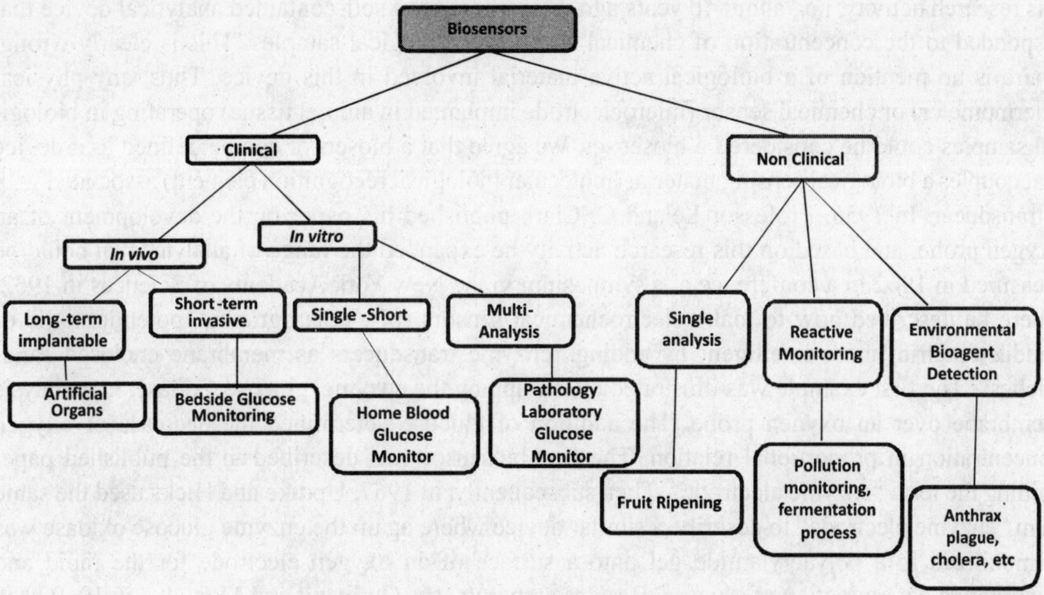

Figure 17.3 Potential applications of biosensors.

Biosensors represent a rapidly expanding field, with an estimated 60% annual growth rate; the major impetus coming from the health care industry (e.g., 6% of the western world is diabetic and would benefit from the availability of a rapid, accurate and simple biosensor for glucose), but with some pressure from other areas, such as food quality appraisal and environmental monitoring. The estimated world analytical market is about £12,000,000,000 year^{-1} of which 30% is in the health care area. There is clearly a vast market but expansion potential as less than 0.1% of this market is currently using biosensors. Research and development in this field is wide and multidisciplinary, spanning biochemistry, bioreactor science, physical chemistry, electrochemistry, electronics and software engineering. Most of this current endeavours concern potentiometric, amperometric biosensors and colorimetric paper enzyme strips. However, all the main transducer types are likely to be thoroughly examined for use in biosensors over the next few years.

CONCEPTS

The history of biosensors started in the year 1962 with the development of enzyme electrodes by the scientist Leland C. Clark. Since then, research communities from various fields such as VLSI, Physics, Chemistry, and Material Science have come together to develop more sophisticated, reliable and mature biosensing devices for applications in the fields of medicine, agriculture, biotechnology, as well as the military and bioterrorism detection and prevention. The vast literature in the last 40 years related to the keyword biosensor reveals without doubt that the scientific field is attractive. Several researchers with different background are involved in this field of research, from chemistry to physics, microbiology and of course electrical engineering. All are deeply involved in several facets of the assembly of the object "Biosensor". Looking at the past also we realize that the concept of biosensor has evolved. For some authors, especially at the beginning of this research activity, i.e., about 40 years ago, biosensor was a self-contained analytical device that responded to the concentration of chemical species in biological samples. This is clearly wrong. There is no mention of a biological active material involved in this device. Thus, any physical (thermometer) or chemical sensor (microelectrode implanted in animal tissue) operating in biological samples could be considered a biosensor. We agree that a biosensor can be defined as a device that couples a biological sensing material (molecular biological recognition element) associated with a transducer. In 1956, Professor Leland C. Clark published his paper on the development of an oxygen probe, and based on this research activity he expanded the range of analytes that could be measured in 1962 in a conference at a symposium in the New York Academy of Sciences in 1962, where he described how to make electrochemical sensors (pH, polarographic, potentiometric or conductometric) more intelligent by adding "enzyme transducers as membrane enclosed sandwiches". The first example was illustrated by entrapping the enzyme, glucose oxidase, in a dialysis membrane over an oxygen probe. The addition of glucose determined the decrease of oxygen concentration in proportional relation. The first biosensor was described in the published paper coining the term "enzyme electrode". Then subsequently, in 1967, Updike and Hicks used the same term "enzyme electrode" to describe a similar device where again the enzyme glucose oxidase was immobilized in a polyacrylamide gel onto a surface of an oxygen electrode for the rapid and quantitative determination of glucose. Besides amperometry, Guilbault and Montalvo in 1969 used glass electrodes coupled with urease to measure urea concentration by potentiometric measurement. There are three so-called 'generations' of biosensors: First generation biosensors, where the normal product of the reaction diffuses to the transducer and causes the electrical response; second generation biosensors; which involve specific 'mediators' between the reaction and the transducer, in order to generate improved response; and third generation biosensors where the reaction itself causes the response and no product or mediator diffusion is directly involved.

PRINCIPLES

A biosensor is based on the use of biological material for its sensing function. The biocomponent specially reacts or interacts with the analyte of interest, resulting in a detectable chemical or physical change. It is an analytical device, which converts a biological response into an electrical signal. The term 'biosensor' is often used to cover sensor devices used in order to determine the concentration of substance and other parameters of biological interest even where they do not utilize a biological system directly. It is an analytical tool or system consisting of an immobilized biological material (enzyme, antibody, whole cell or organelle) in intimate contact with a suitable transducer device. The immobilization of the biological material can, however, be done by adsorption, covalent attachment, cross-linking, physical entrapment or microencapsulation (as described in Chapter 32: Immobilized Biocatalyst Technology). Membranes, in particular, are used as the immobilization support as they allow a thin layer surface of the transducer. A schematic representation of a biosensor is given in Figure 17.1 placed inside a protective as well as selectively permeable membrane. The biological material catalyzes the conversion of analyte or substrate to product. The product is detected through transducer and the signal thus obtained may also be amplified. The signal processing equipment then converts the transducer signal into a suitable display, most commonly the electrical signal. Three main characteristics are important in determining the performance of the biosensors.

(1) **Selectivity:** This characteristic is brought about both by the specificity of the enzymatic reaction towards the substrate and the selectivity of the detector towards the physico-chemical parameter. When the detector directly measures the concentration of the product of the enzymatic reaction, the improvement in selectivity is realized by the addition of a selective membrane between enzymatic reactions and the detector.

(2) **Sensitivity:** Since the response of the biosensor is not linear in all the ranges of substrate concentration, it is necessary to define the range in which the concentration is determined with good precision. The range depends both on the detector type, particular to its detection limit and on the nature of the diffusion and reaction of the enzymatic system.

(3) **Stability:** In addition to the need for general stability of the detector, the stability of the enzyme during measurement or even in storage is crucial. For this, immobilization of the enzyme is not only a way to maintain the enzyme on the detector but also to stabilize its enzymatic activity.

BIOSENSOR TECHNOLOGY

Purpose: It can be used:

1. as an analytical tool in many fields; and
2. for improving the efficiency of technical staff by reducing their workload.

Features of Biosensors

A successful biosensor must possess at least some of the following beneficial features:

1. The biocatalyst must be highly specific for the purpose of the analyses, stable under normal storage conditions and, except in the case of colorimetric enzyme strips and dipsticks, show good stability over a large number of assays (i.e., much greater than 100).
2. The reaction should be as independent of such physical parameters as stirring, pH and temperature as is manageable. This would allow the analysis of samples with minimal pre-

treatment. If the reaction involves co-factors or co-enzymes, these should, preferably, also be co-immobilized with the enzyme.

3. The response should be accurate, precise, reproducible and linear over the useful analytical range, without dilution or concentration. It should also be free from electrical noise.
4. If the biosensor is to be used for invasive monitoring in clinical situations, the probe must be tiny and biocompatible, having no toxic or antigenic effects. If it is to be used in fermenters, it should be sterilisable. This is preferably performed by autoclaving, but no biosensor enzyme can presently withstand such drastic wet-heat treatment. In either case, the biosensor should not be prone to fouling or proteolysis.
5. The complete biosensor should be cheap, small, portable and capable of being used by semi-skilled operators.
6. There should be a market for the biosensor. There is clearly little purpose developing a biosensor if other factors (e.g., government subsidies, the continued employment of skilled analysts, or poor customer perception) encourage the use of traditional methods and discourage the decentralization of laboratory testing.

Mode of Action of Biosensor

The biological component interacts specifically with the analyte, which produces a physical change close to the transducer surface. This physical change may be: (i) heat released or absorbed by the reaction (measured by calorimetric biosensors); (ii) production of an electrical potential due to changed distribution of electrons (potentiometric biosensors); (iii) movement of electrons due to redox reaction (amperometric biosensors); (iv) light produced or absorbed during the reaction (optical biosensors); or (v) change in mass of the biological component as a result of the reaction (acoustic wave biosensor).

The transducer detects and measures this change and converts it into an electrical signal. This signal is necessarily very small, and is amplified by an amplifier before it is fed into the microprocessor. The signal is then processed and interpreted, and is displayed in suitable units. Thus, biosensors convert a chemical information flow into an electrical information flow, which involves various steps such as:

(1) The analyte diffuses from the solution to the surface of the biosensor.
(2) The analyte reacts specifically and efficiently with the biological component of the biosensor.
(3) This reaction changes the physicochemical properties of the transducer surface.
(4) This leads to a change in the optical or electrical properties of the transducer surface.
(5) The change in optical/electrical properties is measured, converted into electrical signal, which is amplified, processed and displayed.

Types of Biosensors

In this section we will discuss some common types of biosensors.

Electrochemical : Electrochemical biosensors are mainly used for the detection of hybridized DNA, DNA-binding drugs, glucose concentration etc. The underlying principle for this class of biosensors is that many chemical reactions produce or consume ions or electrons, which in turn cause some change in the electrical properties of the solution that can be sensed out and used as measuring parameter (Fig. 17.4). Electrochemical biosensors can be classified based on the measuring electrical parameters as: (1) conductimetric, (2) amperometric and (3) potentiometric.

Conductimetric: The measured parameter is the electrical conductance/resistance of the solution. When electrochemical reactions produce ions or electrons, the overall conductivity or resistivity of the solution changes. This change is measured and calibrated to a proper scale. Conductance measurements have relatively low sensitivity. The electric field is generated using a sinusoidal voltage (AC), which helps in minimizing undesirable effects such as Faradaic processes, double layer charging and concentration polarization.

Amperometric: This high sensitivity biosensor can detect electroactive species present in biological test samples. Since the biological test samples may not be intrinsically electro-active, enzymes are needed to catalyze the production of radioactive species. In this case, the measured parameter is current.

Potentiometric: In this type of sensor, the measured parameter is oxidation or reduction potential of an electrochemical reaction. The working principle relies on the fact that when a ramp voltage is applied to an electrode in solution, a current flow occurs because of electrochemical reactions. The voltage at which these reactions occur indicates a particular reaction and particular species. Advantages and disadvantages of various types of electrochemical biosensors are summarized in Table 17.1.

Table 17.1 Comparison of different electrochemical transducers used in biosensors (Source: Cunningham *et al.*, 1998).

Type of energy transducton	*Advantages*	*Disadvantages*
Potentiometric	ISE translation is relatively easy, easily miniaturised	Requires reference electrode, limited linear range, often pH sensitive
Amperometric	Wide variety of biochemical redox mechanisms as basis for signal generation, easily miniaturised, Good dynamic range, controllable by membrane thickness, relatively good sensitivity	Requires a reference electrode Multiple membranes or enzymes may be neccessary for required selectivity and sensitivity
Conductimetric	Easy to fabricate, no reference electrode required, Low frequency/amplitude source	Non-selective unless used in array format

Few classical examples of electrochemical biosensors developed in 1970s have been those of immobilized enzymes (Table 17.2). The electrodes for O_2 and H_2O_2 measurement are common and work on the principle of amperometric determination. For oxygen measurement, a platinum working electrode is polarized- 650 mV with respect to silver-silver chloride reference electrode; for hydrogen peroxide detection, polarity of oxygen electrode is simply reversed. Other species, such as mediators, may also be measured amperometrically by oxidation at a positively polarized electrode.

Table 17.2 Classical examples of electrochemical biosensors (P – Potentiometric, A– amperometric).

Substrate	*Enzyme*	*Species detected*	*Transducer*
Urea	Urease	NH_4	Ammonium ISE (P)
Penicillin	Penicillinase	H	pH electrode (P)
Phenylanine	Phenylalanine	CO_2	CO_2 ISE (P)
Lactate	Lactate oxidase	H_2O_2	Positively polarized Electrode (A)
Glucose	Glucose oxidase	Mediator e.g. Ferrocene Ferricyanide	Positively Polarised electrode (A)
Paracetamol	Acrylacylamidase	p-Aminophenol	Positively Polarized Electrode (A)

Simple enzyme electrode biosensors exhibit a linear response in the range of 10^{-2} to 10^{-4} mol dm^{-3} of substrates, while some electrodes respond to concentrations as low as 5×10^{-7} mol dm^{-3} or as high as 10^{-1} mol dm^{-3}. Some typical examples of enzyme based biosensors are given in Table 17.3.

Table 17.3 Typical enzyme based biosensors.

Substrate	*Enzyme (S)*	*Response time*	*Range*
Glucose	Glucose oxidase	20 S	0.05 – 50 $mmoldm^{-3}$
Cholesterol	Cholesterol oxidase	2-3 min	0 – 0.20 $mmoldm^{-3}$
Penicillin	Penicillinase	25 S	1 – 10 $mmoldm^{-3}$
Amines (meat reshness)	Monoamine oxidase	4 min	50-200 $umoldm^{-3}$
Carbon monoxide	Co: acceptor oxidoreductase	15 S	0 – 65 $umold^{-3}$

Resonant biosensors (acoustic/mechanical sensors): In this type of biosensor, an acoustic wave transducer is coupled with an antibody (bio-element). When the analyte molecule (or antigen) gets attached to the membrane, the mass of the membrane changes. The resulting change in the mass subsequently changes the resonant frequency of the transducer. This frequency change is then measured.

Optical-detection biosensors: The output-transduced signal that is measured is light, for this type of biosensor (Figure 17.5). The biosensor can be made based on optical diffraction or electrochemiluminescence. In optical diffraction based devices, a silicon wafer is coated with a protein via covalent bonds. The wafer is exposed to UV light through a photo-mask and the antibodies become inactive in the exposed regions. When the diced wafer chips are incubated in an analyte, antigen-antibody bindings are formed in the active regions, thus creating a diffraction grating. This grating produces a diffraction signal when illuminated with a light source such as laser. The resulting signal can be measured or further amplified before measuring for improved sensitivity. A most promising biosensor involving luminescence uses firefly Luciferase (Photinus–Luciferin 4-monooxygenase (ATP-hydrolysing), EC 1.13.12.7) to detect the pressure of bacteria in food or clinical samples.

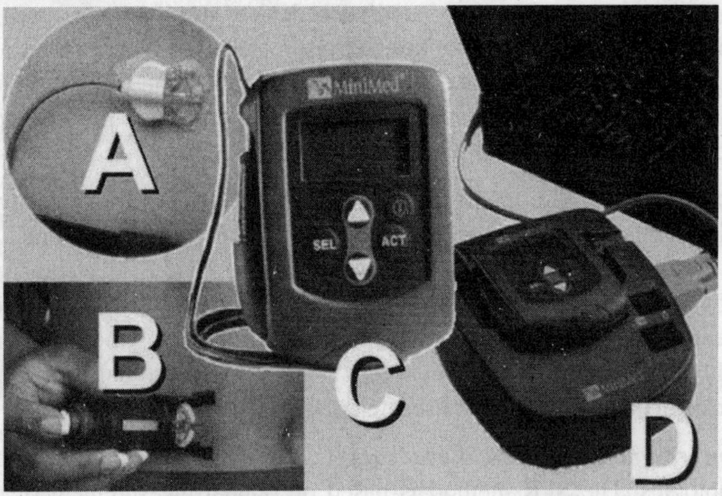

Figure 17.4 Electrochemical biosensors.

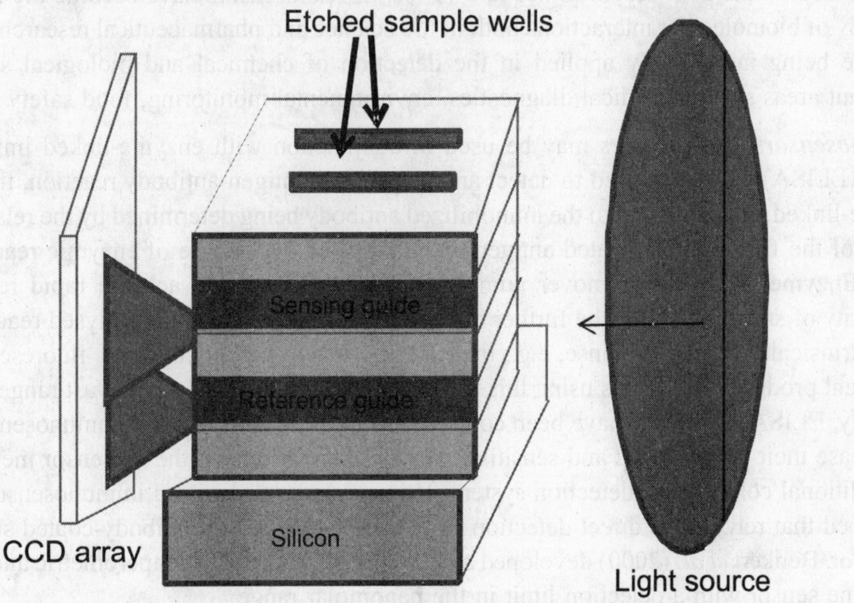

Figure 17.5: Optical-detection biosensors (Source: Cross *et al.*, 2004).

Thermal-detection biosensors (calorimetric sensors): This type of biosensor exploits one of the fundamental properties of biological reactions, namely absorption or production of heat, which in turn changes the temperature of the medium in which the reaction takes place. They are constructed by combining immobilized enzyme molecules with temperature sensors. When the analyte comes in contact with the enzyme, the heat reaction of the enzyme is measured and is calibrated against the analyte concentration. The total heat produced or absorbed is proportional to the molar enthalpy and the total number of molecules in the reaction. The measurement of the temperature is typically accomplished via a thermistor, and such devices are known as enzyme thermistors. Their high sensitivity to thermal changes makes thermistors ideal for such applications. Unlike other transducers, thermal biosensors do not need frequent recalibration and are insensitive to the optical and electrochemical properties of the sample. Common applications of this type of biosensor include the detection of pesticides and pathogenic bacteria.

Ion-sensitive biosensors: These are semiconductor FETs having an ion-sensitive surface. The surface electrical potential changes when the ions and the semiconductor interact. This change in the potential can be subsequently measured. The Ion Sensitive Field Effect Transistor (ISFET) can be constructed by covering the sensor electrode with a polymer layer. This polymer layer is selectively permeable to analyte ions. The ions diffuse through the polymer layer and in turn cause a change in the FET surface potential. This type of biosensor is also called an ENFET (Enzyme Field Effect Transistor) and is primarily used for pH detection.

Surface plasmon resonance (SPR) biosensors: These are based on to label-free optical biosensing technologies. The SPR method is based on optical measurement of refractive index changes associated with the binding of analyte molecules in a sample to biorecognize molecules immobilized on the SPR sensor. Since late 1990s, SPR biosensors have become the main tool for the study of biomolecular interactions both in life science and pharmaceutical research. In addition, they are being increasingly applied in the detection of chemical and biological substances in important areas such as medical diagnostics, environmental monitoring, food safety and security.

Immunosensors: Biosensors may be used in conjunction with enzyme-linked immunosorbent assays (ELISA). ELISA is used to detect and amplify an antigen-antibody reaction, the amount of enzyme-linked antigen bound to the immobilized antibody being determined by the relative concentration of the free and conjugated antigen and quantified by the rate of enzymic reaction (Figure 17.6). Enzymes with high turnover numbers are used in order to achieve rapid response. The sensitivity of such assays may be further enhanced by utilizing enzyme-catalysed reactions, which give intrinsically greater response, e.g., those giving rise to highly coloured, fluorescent or bioluminescent products. Assay kits using this technique are now available for a vast range of analyses. Recently, ELISA techniques have been combined with biosensors to form immunosensors in order to increase their range, speed and sensitivity. In the immunosensor, the biosensor merely replaces the traditional colorimetric detection system. However, more advanced immunosensors are being developed that rely on the direct detection of antigen bound to the antibody-coated surface of the biosensor. Benkert *et al.* (2000) developed a creatinine ELISA and an amperometric antibody-based creatinine sensor with a detection limit in the nanomolar range.

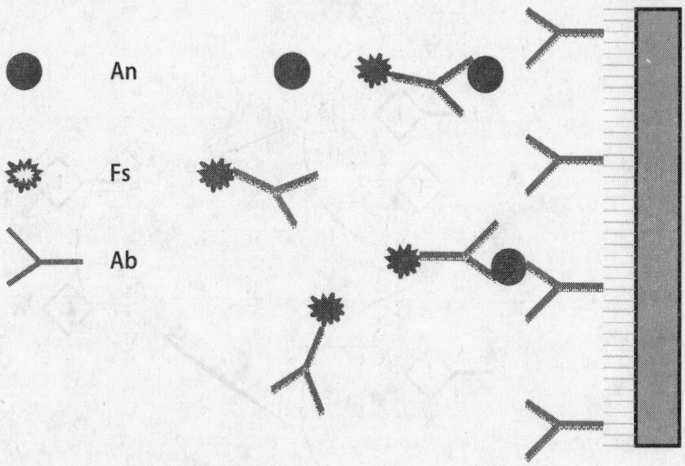

Figure 17.6 Principle of immunosensors (An = Antigen; Ab = Antibody; Fs = Fluorescent substrate).

Bioaffinity sensors: Unlike the enzyme containing biosensors described so far, which measure the concentration of determinants by 'rate' of enzymatic reactions, a new category of biosensors has been evolved, which measures the concentration of determinants on the basis of 'equilibrium binding' and are therefore less sensitive to local concentration changes in the microenvironment and also show high degree of selectivity. Such biosensors have wide versatility because of the use of radiolabelled, enzyme-labeled or fluorescein-labelled substances or the optical systems employing bioluminescence or chemiluminescence. The principle of radiolabelled receptor containing biosensors is elaborated in Figure 17.7. A labeled receptor is weakly bound to the determinant analogue immobilized onto a transducer. When increasing concentrations of the determinant are added, the labelled receptor forms tightly bound complex with determinant and detach from the immobilized determinant analogue. Increasing determinant concentrations can be measured by a reduction in signal of the labeled receptor. An interesting form of this type of biosensor, made for biotin estimation within the detection limit of $10^{-5} - 10^{-8}$ g ml^{-1}, uses the biotin-avidin system in conjugation with an oxygen electrode. Other possibilities are the use of lectins for estimating saccharides hormone receptors, hormone drug receptors, drug and active drug metabolites, antibodies for antigens like drugs and proteins and nucleic acids as gene probes for inherited diseases and finger printing etc.

Whole Cell Biosensors: Biosensors using immobilized whole cell or organelles show characteristically slow response and often react to a broad spectrum of substrates. The latter property is useful in construction of microbial biosensor to perform Ames mutagenesis test. Immobilized *Salmonella typhimurium* revertants are used in conjuction with an oxygen electrode to measure mutagenicity and potential carcinogenicity of various chemicals. Many examples of microbial biosensors to measure biochemical products of cell are given in Table 17.4. A pH electrode with immobilized *Citrobacter ezeundii* is both sensitive (detection limit below 50 mg cm^{-3}) for measurement of cephalosporin and stable for up to 28 days. Similarly, immobilized *Azotobacter vinelandii* containing ammonia electrode exhibits wide sensitivity range ($10^{-5} - 8 \times 10$ mol dm^{-3}) and measures nitrate concentration within 5-10 min.

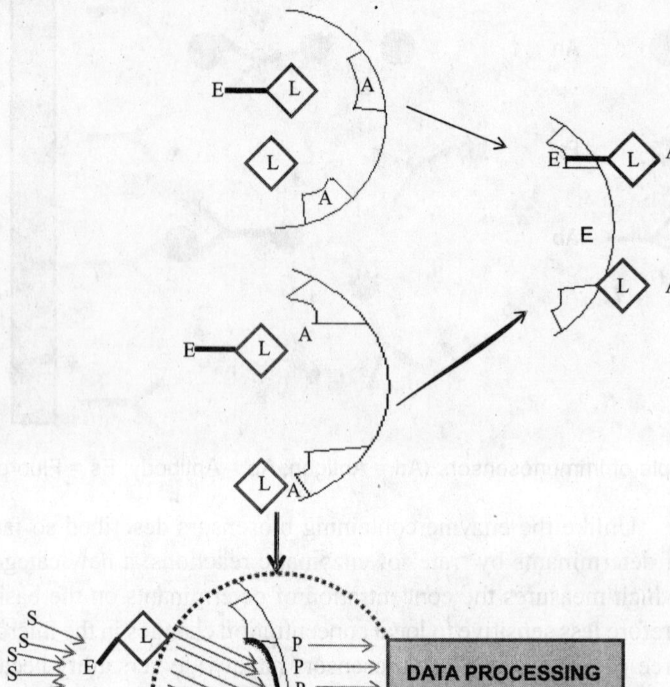

Figure 17.7 Principle of bioaffinity sensors.

Table 17.4 Potential microbial biosensors oxygen electrode as transducers.

Sensor for	*Microbe*	*Response (min)*	*Stability (days)*	*Range*
Assimilable Sugars	*Brevibacterium* Lacto-fermentum	1 -10	10	Linear above 1 ml mol^{-3}
Acetate	*Trichosporon*	6 -10	21	Linear upto 22.5 mg dm^{-3}
Ethanol	*Trichosporon*	10	21	Below 22.5mg dm^{-3}
Glucose	*Pseudomonas*	15 - 20	14	Minimum 2 mg dm^{-3}
Ammonia + NO_2	Mixed culture	4	10	0.1 – 42 mg dm^{-3}
Methane	*Methylomonas Flagellata*	1	20	Upto 6.6 m mol dm^{-3}
Mutagen Screening	*Bacillus subtils*	90-100	-	1.6 mg cm^{-3}

Commercial Potential of Biosensors

Biosensors represent a rapidly expanding economic activity with a vast untapped potential. The estimated world market is approximately $ 25 billion/yr of which 30% is in health care. At present, only 0.1 % of this market is using biosensors. Biosensor market is likely to expand rapidly with the development of low cost, easy to use and durable biosensors. Despite the high number of biosensors under development and also the amount of research literature on this area, few practical systems are currently enjoying market acceptance. However, in other areas such as in food, agriculture, military, veterinary, and the environment, there is a potential market still to be established. A list of commercially available biosensors for the determination of different pollutants is given in Table 17.5.

Table 17.5 Commercially available biosensors (Sara *et al*., 2004).

Instrument	*Biological*	*Transduction element*	*Analyte*	*Company*
BIACORE	Biomolecular interaction	Optical (SPR)	Sulfonamides Pathogens	Biacore AB (Uppsala, Sweden) <http://www.biacore.com>
IBIS	Biomolecular interaction	Optical (SPR)		Windsor Scientific, Ltd. (Berks,UK) interaction<http://www.windsor-ltd.co.uk>
SPR-CELLIA	Whole cells or macromolecules	Optical (SPR)		Nippon Laser and Electronics Lab <http://www.rikei.com>
Spreeta	Biomolecular interaction	Optical (SPR)		Texas Instruments, Inc. (Dallas. USA) <http://www.ti.com>
BIOS-1	Biomolecular interaction	Optical (SPR)		Artificial Sensing Instruments (Zurich, Switzeriand)
–	Immunoreagent	Optical (SPR)		Pathogens Amersham International <http://www.amersham.com>
–	Biomolecular interaction	Optical (SPR)		XanTec Bioanalytics GmbH (Monster, Germany) <http://www.xantec.com>
Kinomics Plasmoon™	Biomolecular interaction	Optical (SPR)		BioTul AG (Munich, Germany) <http://www.biotul.com>
IASys plus™	Antibody or other agent	Optical (SIR) evanescent wave		Affinity Sensors (UK) <http://www.affinity sensors.com>z
REMEDIOS	Whole cells	Optical (bioluminiscence)	Toxicity	Remedios (A berdeen, Scotland) <http://www.remedios.uk.com>
Cellsense	*E.coli* (amperometric)	Electrochemical	Toxicity	Euroclon, Ltd. (Yorkshire, UK) <http://www.euroclone.net/environ_cellsns.htm>
ToxSen™	Biomolecular	Electrochemical interaction		Abtech Scientific, Inc. (Yardley. USA) <http://www.abtechsci.com>
PZ 106 Immunobio-sensor System	Antibodies	Piezoelectric	Pathogens	Universal Sensors (Kinsale, IR) <http://intel.ucc.ie/sensors/universal/>

APPLICATIONS OF BIOSENSOR TECHNOLOGY

Biosensor technology can enable investigators to detect extremely small amounts of chemical or biochemical agents in a biological medium. This technology has many applications, especially in health and medical, agricultural, veterinary and industrial fields. Some of the important applications are discussed below:

Medical and Veterinary Applications

Blood glucose level monitoring for diabetes patients

Biosensors can be used effectively to monitor the glucose levels in diabetic patients (Figure 17.8). These monitoring systems can ease the hassle of controlling diabetes. The glucose monitoring research has been focusing on *in vivo* applications. Scientists are pursuing non-invasive systems for use at home by diabetics based on the direct measurement of the reflection and transmission spectra in the Near Infrared (NIR) Spectrum. Detection can be done non-invasively because skin tissue is quite transparent to the NIR. Presently, glucose needle enzyme electrodes are being successfully tested on lab rats by implanting the sensor and the microflow cannula right below the skin. Researchers are working to modify the sensitivity of the in vivo glucose sensors to be more comparable to the in vitro sensors.

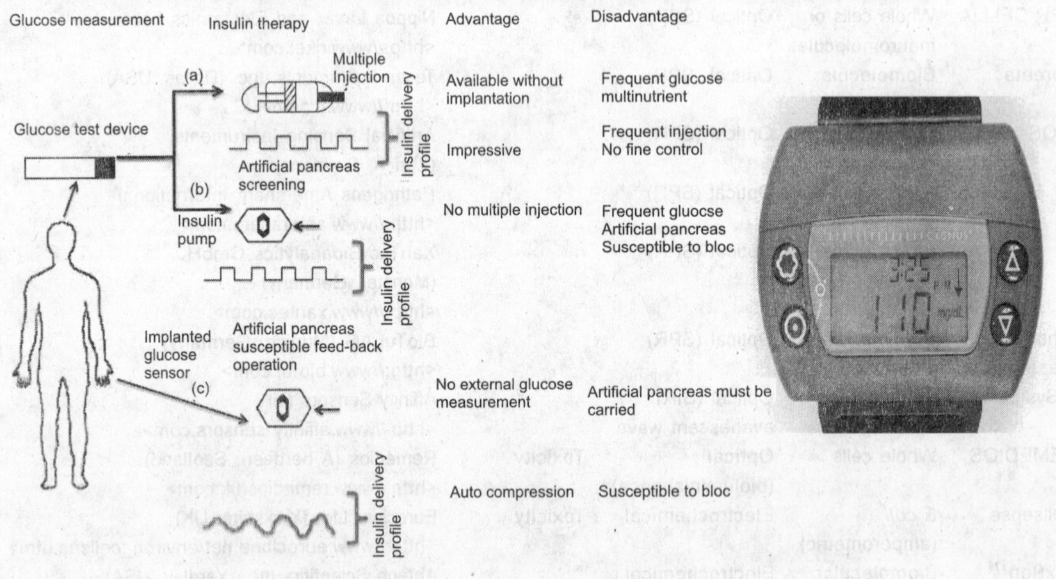

Figure 17.8 Schemes for insulin therapy.

Measurement of metabolites

The initial impetus for advancing sensor technology came from health care area, where it is now generally recognized that measurements of blood gases, ions and metabolites are often essential and allow a better estimation of the metabolic state of a patient. In intensive care units, for example, patients frequently show rapid variations in biochemical levels that require an urgent remedial action. Also, in less severe patient handling, more successful treatment can be achieved by obtaining instant assays. At present, the list of the most commonly required instant analyses is not extensive. In practice, these assays are performed by analytical laboratories, where discrete samples are analyzed frequently using the more traditional analytical techniques.

Novel lactate and pH biosensor for skin and sweat analysis based on single walled carbon nanotubes

Carbon nanotubes (CNTs) are functionalized and employed in an electrochemical cell to serve as a biosensor to specifically detect either lactate or pH in an electrolyte solution of artificial sweat (Figure 17.9). They are functionalized with the carboxyl group (COOH) to detect pH and the enzyme, lactate oxidase (LOX) to detect lactate. All CNT samples are characterized to compare the electrodes before and after functionalization. Fourier transform infrared spectroscopy (FTIR) is used to verify the attachment of both COOH and LOX to the respective carbon nanotubes samples. Scanning electron microscopy (SEM) is then used to examine the structure of the CNT–lactate electrode. Square wave voltammetry proved to be the best template to sense these target analytes. The functionalized CNT–COOH electrode displays a linear response to pH 1–10, with a negative voltage shift corresponding to an increase in pH. Two types of lactate sensors are fabricated, both of which exhibit an increase in current corresponding to an increase in lactate concentration. The functionalized CNT–LOX on a glassy carbon electrode display an amperometric response in the range of 1–4mM lactate. The CNT–LOX on a silicon/indium tin oxide (Si/ITO) substrate display an amperometric response in the range of 0.01–0.05M lactate.

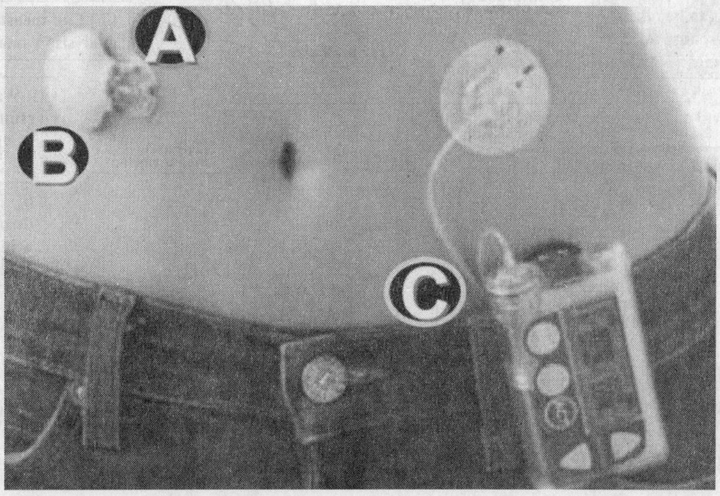

Figure 17.9 Novel lactate and pH biosensor for skin (A & B) and sweat analysis (C).

Biosensors for diagnostics: Among the wide range of applications of biosensors, the most important application is in the field of medical diagnostics, can be conveniently divided into *in vitro* and *in vivo* diagnostics.

In vitro diagnostic

In vitro medical diagnostics has a worldwide market of ~US $9 billion per annum, although strict pre-market approval is required for these diagnostic tests. These *in vitro* diagnostic tests fall in three categories:

(i) Centralized tests in hospitals. These tests conducted in hospitals include tests for glucose, lactate, uric acid, viruses, and a variety of pathogenic microbes. Amperometric biosensor devices for glucose, manufactured in USA, include Satellite G (from MediSense), Glucose Analyser 23A (from Yellow Spring Instruments Co.) and Stat Profile 5 and 6 (from Nova Biomedical). DNA based biosensors are also being developed for the diagnosis of hereditary diseases, viruses and cancer. Significant progress in their development is also expected in future.

(ii) Tests in clinics. Analysers (in the form of portable biosensors) to be used in the nursing homes or private clinics of practising doctors are also being developed for testing glucose, lactate, creatinine and urea. A recent example of these biosensors is the portable I-Stat system, costing US $ 3000, which can make use of unprocessed blood and can be operated by the doctor or a nurse (Figure 17.10).

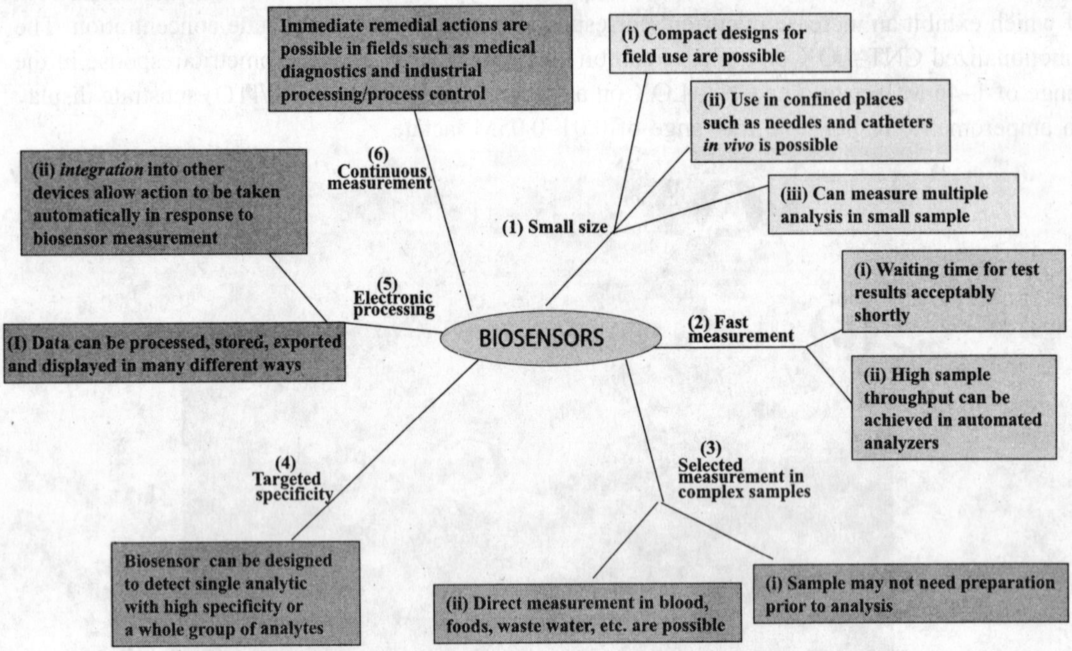

Figure 17.10 Biosensor for medical diagnostics.

This can perform tests for glucose, urea, nitrogen, sodium, potassium and chloride. Similar other biosensors for *in vitro* diagnostics in the clinics are being developed.

(iii) Tests by consumers. Biosensors are now available, which can be used by individuals at their residence without any help from a doctor or a nurse. A popular example is ExacTechTM, blood glucose monitor (from MediSense). Dry reagent tests that measure blood glucose levels colorimetrically (by colour) are also commonly used. In future, consumer tests for pregnancy, ovulation, allergy, cancer and viruses may also become available, although medical approval for some of these consumer tests is difficult, thus delaying the long-term use of such biosensors.

In vivo diagnostics

The most important example of the application of biosensors for *in vivo* diagnostics is the idea of artificial pancreas (permanently implanted in skin of diabetic patients), which continuously monitors *in vivo* level of glucose by a control on the rate of insulin infusion from an implanted minipump, as a potential cure for diabetes. We know that a normal pancreas continuously monitors blood sugar levels and promptly reacts to changes in blood sugar levels by increasing or decreasing the production of insulin. The artificial pancreas system developed in some advanced countries, therefore, consists of a miniaturized biosensor attached with a minipump containing insulin, so that the level of blood sugar is estimated and a desirable quantity of insulin is pumped into the patient's blood. This area of *in vivo* diagnostics is extremely specialized and complex and is affected by difficulties due to allergenicity, bioincompatibility and malfunction. Costs are high and there are legal and ethical barriers to the use of biosensors *in vivo*. These difficulties need to be solved before these devices can be used and *in vivo* diagnostics become popular and widely used.

Agricultural Applications

Pathogen detection in food

As the occurrence of food-borne illness rises, governments are passing stringent regulations for tolerable amounts of contamination in foodstuffs. However, conventional methods of pathogen detection require time-consuming steps to arrive at a useable measurement. This process, usually taking 7 to 10 days, is too long for perishable foods, which usually enters and leaves the marketplace within 2 to 3 days. Biosensor technology can significantly reduce this time as well as detect even smaller amounts of pathogens with fewer false positives. The New Zealand Meat Industry Research Institute is using biosensors to pinpoint the cause of food spoilage. Apparently bacteria in the meat packs release gas and cause the packages to explode in transit. Biosensors have identified eight suspect strains, while conventional innoculation studies have identified only one. The University of Florence has developed a piezoelectric biosensor, which detects the bacteria *Listeria monocytogenes*. This bacterium affects wild and domestic animals and humans causing fever, meningitis and encephalitis. The biosensor was applied to the *Listeria* bacteria diluted in milk and is as sensitive as conventional methods, yet the results can be obtained in less than 15 minutes.

Toxicology tests using biosensors

A variety of pesticides and fungicides that are used for crop protection programmes sometimes reach alarming levels in the atmosphere and become the cause of concern for human health care. These high levels of pesticides and fungicides are often detected through tests conducted on animals. Biosensors are being developed, which will spot dangerous levels of these chemicals in the atmosphere, thus obviating the need of animal testing. Biochips carrying these biosensors are being tested by a British biotechnology company, Zeneca (manufacturer of agrochemicals). These biochips will indicate whether an experimental pesticide has reached a level, which is dangerous for humans, farm animals (including bees and earthworms) and plant life. The biochips as above carry fragments of those genes from an organism, which are switched on due to exposure to high level of toxic chemicals (e.g., some genes that express in liver in humans). They are used to detect specific mRNA derived from these sensitive genes in the cell culture exposed to the chemical. The mRNA synthesized in the cultures exposed to chemical is labelled to facilitate detection. The technique has been successfully used by Zeneca to detect the presence of any fungicide using biosensors with all 6000 genes from yeast. From humans also, 2000 genes known to be activated by toxic drugs or pesticides are being tested to select the best indicators.

Industrial Applications

Drug discovery

Conventionally, drugs are discovered through a time consuming, tedious process. Biosensors have tremendous potential in speeding up this process. Biosensors can detect the interaction between a particular target and a possible drug without using markers or the detection of color changes or fluorescence. Biosensors can quickly measure how well a potential drug binds to a target and by eliminating markers, biosensors eliminate potential causes of interference. Test samples do not need to be purified and can be reused. Biosensors also improve the accuracy of the results and are far less time consuming. For example, Prozac was introduced after 15 years of development, whereas a similar drug took only two trials using biosensing technology. Texas Instruments is marketing a biosensing unit, which can be useful for drug detection. The user simply "paints" some receptors or targets on the top of the device and runs a test. TI has demonstrated applications in "refractive index changes, avidin-biotin binding, antibody-antigen dissociation kinetics, thickness of insulators, refractive index of thin dielectrics, specific detection of small molecules, protein binding, concentrations of analytes, attachment of DNA complements and mixture proportions".

Biosensors for food industry

Various possible applications of biosensors in agriculture include detection of viral, fungal and bacterial diseases; fertilizers and pesticides; even though many of these biosensors will be too expensive to be viable. The most viable use of biosensors in food industry is to include rapid detection of total microbial contaminants and sugar quantification in soft drinks. For instance, in advanced countries, biosensors have been developed to determine the freshness of fish and other food items including beef and other foods. In future, biosensors may be developed for on-line use, where analysis will be carried out on food samples which are removed from the production line if found unsatisfactory. Such an analysis would facilitate real-time control of products during manufacture.

Biosensors for general industry (including fermentation industry)

Biosensors can also be used as analysers for specific chemicals for process control in a variety of industries including pharmaceuticals, chemical and petroleum, mining and construction. Although, the conditions in some of these industries may be too harsh for biological sensors, there is considerable promise in this area. In fermentation industry, biosensors can be used for monitoring the cultured microorganisms producing drugs, hormones, vaccines, single cell proteins, etc. Some biosensors have already been produced for fermentation industry (e.g., Thresh-oldTM from Molecular Devices Corporation). Biosensors can also be developed for alerting workers for the presence of hazardous substances in the industrial atmosphere.

Bioreactor control

Real-time monitoring of carbon sources and dissolved gases in fermentation processes could lead to optimization of the procedure giving increased yields at decreased material cost. While real-time monitoring with feedback control involving automated systems does exist, currently only a few common variables are measured online (e.g., pH, temperature, CO_2, O_2), which are often only indirectly related with the process under control.

Three different methods of controlling a bioreactor are: **(1) Off-line distant:** central laboratory coarse control, with significant time lapse; **(2) Off-line local:** fine control with short time lapse; and **(3) On-line:** real-time monitoring and control.

On-line control: Method 3 is most desirable, which allows the process to follow an ideal pre-programmed fermentation profile to give maximum output. However, many problems exist with on-line measurements including *in situ* sterilization, sensor life-time, sensor fouling, etc. Some of the problems can be overcome if the sensor is situated so that the sample is run to waste, but this causes a volume loss, which can be particularly critical with small volume fermentations.

Off-line control: Although Method 3 may be the ultimate aim, considerable advantage can be gained in moving from Method 1 to Method 2 giving a rapid analysis and thus enabling finer control of the fermentation. The demands of the sensor are perhaps not as stringent in Method 2 as in Method 3.

Benefits of control: The benefits achievable with process-control technology are considerable:

- Improved product quality; reduction in rejection rate following manufacture.
- Increased product yield; process tuned in real time to maintain optimum conditions throughout and not just for limited periods.
- Increased tolerance in quality variation of some raw materials. These variations can be compensated in the process-control management.
- Reduced reliance on human 'seventh sense' to control process.
- Improved plant performance-processing rate and line speed automated, so no unnecessary dead-time allocated to plant.
- Optimized energy efficiency.
- The use of biosensors in industrial process, in general, could facilitate plant automation, cut analysis costs and improve quality control of the product.

Other Biotechnological Applications

Engineering and applications of D1 Subunit of chloroplast in Biosensors for Monitoring Photosystem II-Inhibiting Herbicides

Photosystem II (PSII) is a light driven machine, which supplies our atmosphere with oxygen and, if properly engineered, can be developed into a specific sensor for various pollutants (Figure 17.11).

Its reaction center subunit D1 has long been a target for genetic engineering. It is known to bind a variety of herbicides in a pocket, which is naturally occupied by the plastoquinone molecule QB. Amino acid residues lining this binding niche provides ligands to a diverse set of inhibitors, which can loose or gain affinity upon substitution of certain amino acids. One can exploit this and other properties of the D1 protein by changing the corresponding psbA gene, which is located on the chloroplast genome in algae and higher plants. We have developed fast site-specific and random mutagenesis techniques specifically adjusted for psbA-gene manipulation in the unicellular green alga *Chlamydomonas reinhardtii*. Using these protocols, mutant collections were generated that have the innate potential of becoming an array of sensitive and specific biosensors.

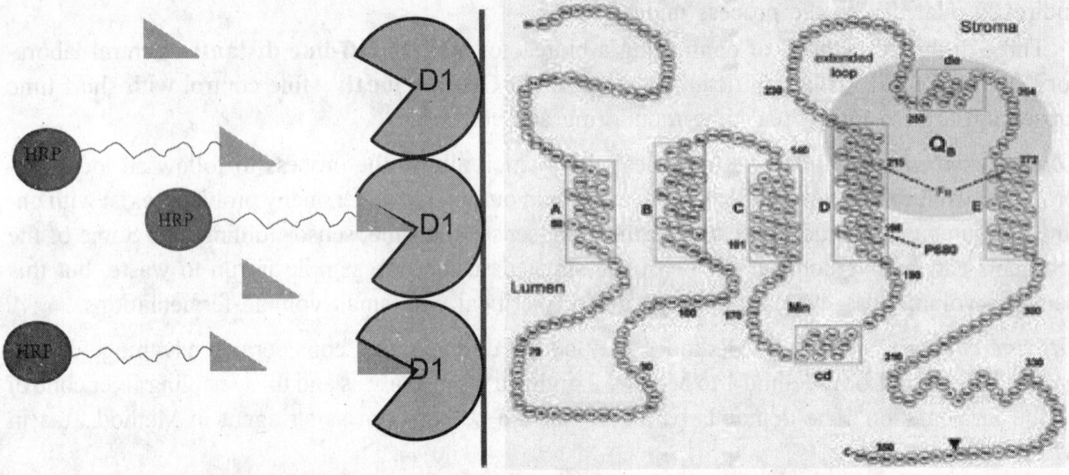

Figure 17.11 Engineering and applications of D1 subunit of chloroplast in biosensors.

Environmental pollution due to toxic chemicals has become one of the world's most serious problems. Among the most widespread pesticides, is photosynthesis inhibiting herbicides, such as atrazine, metribuzin, diuron, bromacil, ioxynil and dinoseb. They all belong to different families but have a common mode of action, i.e., binding specifically to the chloroplast D1 protein with subsequent interruption of the electron and proton flow through Photosystem II. It can be used to evaluate the possibility of application of the natural receptor properties of D1 protein in various biosensor systems for herbicide detection.

Photosystem II biosensors for heavy metals monitoring

The biotesting based on the photosynthetic material is a new and potentially commercially viable method of pollutant detection. The photosynthetic apparatus including photosystem II (PSII) is particularly sensitive to heavy metals. The mechanisms of heavy metals action on photosystem II are well known. The characteristics of different biosensors based on immobilized photosynthetic material are compared and the possibility to use immobilized photosystem II sub-membranes fractions as a tool to monitor environmental sample containing heavy metals (sewage sludge) can be determined.

Biosensors for the detection of hydrogen peroxide

Biosensors can also be used for the detection of analytes such as hydrogen peroxide (H_2O_2). The important areas of H_2O_2 application include industrial (pharmaceutical, food, clinical) and environmental analyses. Its use as an antibacterial agent added to milk and the environmental need to avoid halogenated substances for disinfection purposes makes H_2O_2 an important substance in the food and beverage industry. This has raised extensive demands for establishing protocols for H_2O_2 detection depending on its application. Additionally, it is one of the most important products or substrates of enzyme catalysed oxidation reactions. Besides being a product/substrate of enzymatic reaction, hydrogen peroxide is by itself an important analyte. It plays an important role in natural oxidation processes as it is found in air, solids and water.

Air and water monitoring

Another assay situation that may involve a considerable degree of the unknown is that of environmental monitoring. The primary measurement media here will be water or air, but the variety of target analytes is vast. At sites of potential pollution, such as in factory effluent, it would be desirable to install on-line real-time monitoring and alarm targeted at specific analytes, but in many cases random or discrete monitoring of either target species or general hazardous compounds would be sufficient. The possible analytes include biological oxygen demand (BOD), which provides a good indication of pollution, atmospheric acidity, and river water pH, detergent, herbicides, and fertilizers (organophosphates, nitrates, etc.). Toxicity assays systems are based on the use of luminescent bacteria, *Vibrio fischeri*, to measure toxicity from environmental samples. Bacterial bioluminescence has proved to be a convenient measure of cellular metabolism and consequently, a reliable sensor for measuring the presence of toxic chemicals in aquatic samples. Some bioassay methods are integrated now in biosensors such as the Cellsense, which is an amperometric sensor that incorporates *Escherichia coli* bacterial cells for rapid ecotoxicity analysis. It uses ferricyanine, a soluble electron mediator, to divert electrons from the respiratory system of the immobilized bacteria of a suitable carbon electrode. The resulting current is, thus, a measure of bacterial respiratory activity, and the perturbation by pollutants can be detected as a change in the magnitude of the current.

Military applications

Dip Stick Test: The requirement for rapid analysis can also be anticipated in military applications. The US army, for example, has looked at dipstick tests based on monoclonal antibodies. While these dipsticks are stable and highly specific (to Q-fever, nerve agents, yellow rain fungus, soman, etc.), they are frequently two-step analyses taking up to 20 min to run. Such a time lapse is not always suited to battlefield diagnostics. A particularly promising approach to this unknown hazard detection seems to be via acetylcholine receptor systems. It has been calculated that with this biorecognition system, a matrix of 13-20 proteins is required to give 95% certainty of all toxin detection.

Biosensor technology is also being put to use by the United States military. The US Navy has created underwear woven from conductive polymers that can provide data on the wearer's injuries.

The sensors can recognize when a soldier is bleeding and whether the cut is in a vein or artery, depending on the oxygen content in the blood. The US Army built a pill-sized computer that soldiers can swallow. The computer tracks the health of the soldiers and may detect stress levels (Figure 17.12).

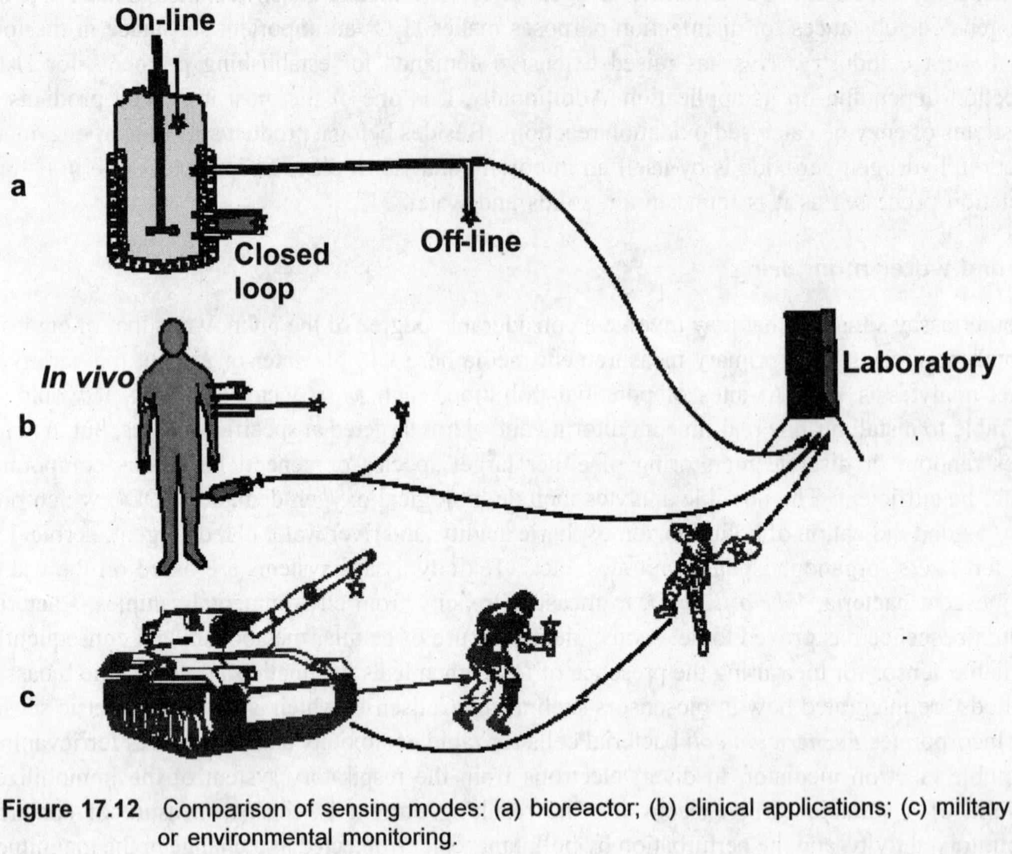

Figure 17.12 Comparison of sensing modes: (a) bioreactor; (b) clinical applications; (c) military or environmental monitoring.

Future Prospects of Biosensor Technology

During the last two decades, advances in microelectromechanical systems (MEMS) have given rise to a whole new class of biosensors, which involve the transduction of mechanical energy and are based on mechanical phenomena. Although there are various technical difficulties for which some solutions exist, still more research efforts are needed in order to find better alternatives. Some of them are as fellow:

(a) **Contamination:** Bioelements and chemicals used in the biosensors need to be prevented from leaking out of the biosensor over time (serious issue for non-disposable ones).

(b) **Immobilization of biomolecules:** To avoid contamination, biomolecules are attached to the transducer as strongly as possible. But the problem with this is that the behavior of enzymes, when absorbed on the surface, is not well understood (reaction of enzymes in free solutions is better understood.

(c) **Sterilization:** If a sterilized probe is used, sensor's biomolecules may be destroyed, whereas if non-sterile probes are used, some compromises are needed.
(d) **Uniformity of biomolecule preparation:** Fabrication of biosensors that can reproduce results need such uniformity.
(e) **Selectivity and detection range:** It should be more selective and the detection range should be large.
(f) **Cost:** Research should be focused on the development of low-cost biosensors. At present, with the threat of bioterrorism omnipresent, the development of faster, reliable, accurate, portable and low-cost biosensors has become more important than ever.
(g) **Multianalyte determination:** Development of sensors capable of determining several analytes simultaneously can represent an interesting tool in environmental monitoring and screening. This configuration allows the reduction in time and sample volume and other reagents required.
(h) **Miniaturization:** In general, there is a growing tendency toward miniaturization of analytical systems since it allows the handling of low-volume samples, a reduction in reagent consumption, waste generation, and increases sample throughput. Taking advantage of miniaturization benefits, sensors and biosensors can become inexpensive and easy-to-handle analytical devices for fast, reliable measurements of chemical species. Miniaturization emerges, thus, as an important aspect of future bioelectronics.
(i) **Network systems:** The future integration of wireless communications systems will generate huge interest, as this will inevitably lead to the emergence of extensive networked multiple autonomous analytical stations in rivers, lakes, wells or even water treatment plants.
(j) **Validation:** Despite the practical advantages of biosensors, they must be able to provide results in real time, simple to use, portable, and cost-effective.
(k) **Bioengineering:** Biosensor sensitivity and selectivity depends essentially on the properties of the biorecognition elements to be used for analyte binding. Genetic engineering provides an elegant way not only for providing unlimited amounts of biorecognition molecules, but also for the alteration of existing properties and supplementation with additional functions. The current generation of biosensors is taking advantage of novel biosensing materials based on gene engineering.

CONCLUSION

Despite the huge potential of biosensors and the ever-increasing number of biosensors developed, commercially available biosensors are being applied to a restricted area of the potential market. In general, biosensors for environmental analysis have several limitations: e.g., sensitivity, response time, and lifetime, which should be improved to make it a competitive analytical tool. The areas of development that are expected to have an impact on biosensor technology are immobilization techniques, nanotechnology, miniaturization, and multisensor array determinations. However, a crucial aspect may be the production of new sensing elements easy to synthesize and with the capability to broaden the spectra of selectivities that can be reached by a biosensor. Improvement in the affinity, specificity and mass production of the molecular recognition components may ultimately dictate the success or failure of biosensor technology. The possibility of tailor binding molecules with predefined properties, such as selectivity, affinity, and stability, is one of the major aims in biotechnology. The development of advanced receptors will allow the analysis of complex samples and *in situ* measurements resolving the responses from the analyte and from nonspecific background effects. Since scientific attention is currently being given to biotechnology, as this review has pointed out, the development of improved molecular recognition elements will be followed by a corresponding enhancement of the biosensor features. From the above viewpoint, it is clear that the future of biosensors will rely on the success of emerging sophisticated micro and nanotechnologies, biochemistry, chemistry, thin-film physics, and electronics. To reach this goal, an important investment in research, expertise, and the necessary facilities is needed. However, as the world becomes more concerned about the impact that environmental contamination may cause on public health and the ecosystem, the demand for rapid detecting biosensors will only increase. Biosensors still need to achieve the confidence of potential users, keeping in mind that the commercialization of new devices will always be the best indicator of the success of a biosensor technology.

FURTHER READINGS

1. Akgol S. and Dinckaya E. (1999) A novel biosensor for specific determination of hydrogen peroxide: catalase enzyme electrode based on dissolved oxygen probe. *Talanta.* **(48):** 363- 367.
2. Akimitsu Kugimiya and Kaori Kohara (2009) Biomimetic sensor for cAMP using an ion-sensitive field-effect transistor. *Materials Science and Engineering.* 29 **(3):** 959-962.
3. Alexander J. Marshall, Duncan S. Young, Jeff Blyth, Satyamoorthy Kabilan and Christopher R. Lowe (2004) Metabolite-sensitive holographic biosensors. *Anal. Chem.* 76 **(5):** 1518-1523.
4. Aston C. (2001) "Biological warfare canaries", Cover story: *IEEE Spectrum.*
5. Bannister J.V. Higgins I.J. and Turner A.P.F. (2001) Development of amperometric biosensors for enzyme immunoassay. Cited in: Blum L. J., and Coulet P.R (ed). *Biosensor Principles and Applications*, Marcel Dekker, Inc. New York.
6. Bardeletti G. Sechaud F. and Coulet P.R. (1991) Amperometric enzyme electrodes for substrate and enzyme activity determinations. Cited in: Blum L. J., and Coulet P. R. (ed). *Biosensor Principles and Applications*, Marcel Dekker, Inc. New York.
7. Bartic C. and Borghs G. (2006) Organic thin-film transistors as transducers for (Bio) analytical applications. *Analytical and Bioanalytical Chemistry.* 384 **(2):** 354-365.
8. Bengt Danielsson (2006) Use of thermal biosensors for specific monitoring and control of bioprocesses. *Annals of the New York Academy of Sciences.* 613 **(10):** 413-414.
9. Benkert Alexander, Frieder Scheller, Werner Schössler, Christian Hentschel, Burkhard Micheel, Olaf Behrsing, Gudrun Scharte, Walter Stöcklein, and Axel Warsinke (2000) Development of a Creatinine ELISA and an Amperometric Antibody-Based Creatinine Sensor with a Detection Limit in the Nanomolar Range. *Anal. Chem.* 72 **(5):** 916-921.
10. Bennetto Dekeyzer D.R. Delaney G.M. Koshy A. Mason J.R. Razak L.A. Stirling J.L. and Thurston C.F. (1987) An amperometric biosensor for laboratory determination of glucose. *Analyst.* **(8):** 22-27.
11. Cardosi M.E. and Turner A.P.F. (1991) Mediated electrochemistry: A practical approach to biosensing. Cited In: Turner, A.P.F. (ed.). *Advances in Biosensors*, Vol. 1. Jai Press Ltd.
12. Carpentier R, Loranger C, Chartrand J and Purcell M. (1991) Photoelectrochemical cell containing chloroplast membranes as a biosensor for phytotoxicity measurements. *Analytica Chimica Acta.* **(249):** 55-60.

13. Cavalcanti A. Shirinzadeh B. Zhang M. and Kretly L.C. (2008) Nanorobot hardware architecture for medical defense. *Sensors.* 8 **(5):** 2932-2958.
14. Corbisier P. Thiry E. and Diels L. (1996) Bacterial biosensors for the toxicity assessment of solid wastes. *Environ. Toxicol. Water Qual.* **(11):** 171-177.
15. Cunningham Alice J. (1998) *Introduction to Bioanalytical Sensors,* 4th edition, Wiley. New York.
16. Davis G (1985) Electrochemical techniques for the development of amperometric biosensors. *Biosensors.* **(1):** 161.
17. Davis J. Huw-Vaughan D. and Cardosi MF. (1995) Elements of biosensor construction. *Enzyme and Microbial Technology.* **(17):** 1030-1035.
18. Diabetes control and complications Trial. *New England Journal of Medicine,* 329 **(14):** 1993. http://diabetes.niddk.nih.gov/dm/pubs/control/.
19. Elena V. Piletska, Sergey A. Piletsky and Regis Rouillon (2006) Application of chloroplast D1 protein in biosensors for monitoring photosystem II-inhibiting herbicides. *Biotechno Logical Applications of Photosynthetic Proteins: Biochips, Biosensors and Biodevices*. Springer, US, pp. 57-68.
20. Fattinger C. Mangold C. Gale M.T. and Schutz H. (1995) Bidiffractive grating coupler: universal transducer for optical interface analytics. *Optical Engineering.* 34 **(9):** 2744- 2753.
21. Fraser D.M. (1994) Glucose biosensors – the sweet smell of success. *Medical Device Technology,* 5 **(9):** 44-47.
22. Guilbault G.G Hock B and Schmid R. (1992) A piezoelectric immunobiosensor for atrazine in drinking water. *Biosenssors Bioelectronics.* **(7):** 411-420.
23. Hendry S.P. Higgins I.J. and Bannister J.V. (1990) Amperometric biosensors. *Journal of Biotechnology.* **(15):** 229-238.
24. Hiep H.M. *et al.* (2007) A localized surface plasmon resonance based immunosensor for the detection of casein in milk. *Sci. Technol. Adv. Mater.* **(8):** 331.
25. Higson S.P.J. Reddy S.M. and Vadgama P.M. (1994) Enzyme and other biosensors: Evolution of a technology. *Engineering Science and Education Journal.* 3 **(1):** 41-48.
26. Holmes D.S. Dubey S.K. and Gangoli S. (1994) Development of biosensors for the detection of mercury and copper Ions. *Environ. Geochem. Health.* **(16):** 229-233.
27. http://www.mdpi.org/sensors/papers/s8052932.pdf.
28. Ivnitski D. Abdel-Hamid I. Atanasov P. and Wilkins E. (1999) Review: Biosensors for detection of pathogenic bacteria. *Biosensors and Bioelectronics.* **(14):** 599-624.
29. Jessica Weber, Arun Kumar, Ashok Kumar and Shekhar Bhansali (2006) Novel lactate and pH biosensor for skin and sweat analysis based on single walled carbon nanotubes. *Sensors and Actuators.* **(117):** 308-313.
30. Kalman A. Caelen I. and Svorc J. (2006) Vitamin and pseudovitamin analysis with biosensors in food products: a review. *J AOAC Int.* 89 **(3):** 819-825.
31. Karube I. (1990) Microbial Sensor. *J. Biotechnol.* **(15):** 255-266.
32. Katchalski T. Soria S. Teitelbaum E. Friesem A.A. and Morowsky G. (2005) Two-photon fluorescence sensors based on resonant grating waveguide structures, *Sensors and Actuators. B.* **(107):** 121-125.
33. Kauffman J.M. and Guilbault G.G. (1991) Potentiometric enzyme electrodes. In: *Biosensor Principles and Applications*. ed. by L. J. Blum and P. R. Coulet, Marcel Dekker Inc., New york, pp. 63-82.
34. Koblitzek M. Masojidek J. Komenda J. Kucera, Pilloton R.T. Mattoo A.K. and Giardi M.T. (1998) A. sensitive photosystem II-based biosensor for the detection of a class of herbicides. *Biotechnology and Bioengineering.* 60 **(6):** 664-669.
35. Kostrzynska M. and Bachand A. (2006) Application of DNA microarray technology for detection, identification, and characterization of food-borne pathogens. *Can. J. Microbiol.* 52 **(1):** 1-8.
36. Lavrik N.V. Sepaniak M.J. and Datskos P.G. (2004) Cantilever transducers as a platform for chemical and biological sensors. *Review of Scientific Instruments.* 75 **(5):** 2229-2253.

37. Lowe C.R. (1985) An introduction to the concepts and technology of biosensors. *Biosensors*. 1 **(1)**: 3-16.
38. Malhotra B.D. Singhal R. Chaubey A. Sharma S.K. and Kumar A. (2005) Recent trends in biosensors. *Current Applied Physics.* **(5)**: 92-97.
39. Mar Masson, Kyusik Yun, Tetsuya Haruyama, Eiry Kobatake and Masuo Aizawa (1995) Quartz crystal microbalance bioaffinity sensor for biotin. *Anal. Chem.* 67 **(13)**: 2212– 2215.
40. Marco M.P. Gee S. and Hammock B.D. (1995) Immunochemical techniques for environmental analysis: I. Immunosensors. *Trends Anal. Chem.* **(14)**: 341-350.
41. Marek Piliarik, Hana Vaisocherová and Jiøí Homola (2009) Surface plasmon resonance biosensing methods in molecular biology. *Methods Mol. Biol*. **(503)**: 65-88.
42. Marquette CA and Blum LJ (2006) State of the art and recent advances in immunoanalytical systems. *Biosensors and Bioelectronics.* **(21)**: 1424-1433.
43. Marrazza G, Chianella I and Mascini M (1999) Disposable DNA electrochemical biosensors for environmental monitoring. *Analytica Chimica Acta.* **(387)**: 297-307.
44. Michael Keusgen (2002) Biosensors: new approaches in drug discovery. *Naturwissenschaften.* **(89)**: 433-444.
45. Newman J.D. and Turner A.P.F. (2008) Historical perspective of biosensor and biochip development. In: *Handbook of Biosensors and Biochips* (Eds. R. Marks, D. Cullen, I. Karube, C. Lowe and H. Weetall) John Wiley & Sons.
46. Northrup M.A. Gonzalez C. *et al.* (1995) A MEMS-based miniature DNA analysis system", in the Proceedings of the 8th International Conference on Solid-State Sensors and Actuators, and Eurosensors IX, Transducers'95, June 25-29, pp. 764-767.
47. Peterson K. (1996) Biomedical applications of MEMS", Electron devices meeting. pp. 239-242.
48. Pohanka M. Jun D. and Kuca K. (2007a) Mycotoxin assay using biosensor technology: review. *Drug Chem. Toxicol.* 30 **(3)**: 253-261.
49. Pohanka M. Skladal P. and Kroca M. (2007b) Biosensors for biological warfare agent detection. Def. *Sci. J.* 57 **(3)**: 185-93.
50. Rasooly A. and Herold K.E. (2006) Biosensors for the analysis of food and waterborne pathogens and their toxins. *J. AOAC Int.* 89 **(3)**: 873-883.
51. Rawson D.M. Willmer A.J. and Turner A.P.F. (1989) Whole-cell biosensors for environment monitoring. *Biosensors.* **(4)**: 299-311.
52. Régis Rouillon, Sergey A. Piletsky. Florent Breton, Elena V. Piletska and Robert Carpentier (2007) Photosystem II biosensors for heavy metals monitoring. *Biotechnological Applications of Photosynthetic Proteins: Biochips, Biosensors and Biodevices*, Springer, US, pp. 166-174.
53. Riedel K. and Kunze G. (1997) Rapid physiological characterization of microorganisms by biosensor technique. *microbiol. Res.* **(152)**: 233-237.
54. Rogers K.R. and Koglin E.N. (1997) Biosensors for environmental monitoring: An EPA perspective. In: *Biosensors for Direct Monitoring of Environmental Pollutants in Field.* ed. by D. P. Nikolelis, U. J. Krull, J. Wang and M. Mascini, Kluwer Publishers, Boston, pp. 335-349.
55. Sanders C.A. Rodriquez M. and Greenbaum E. (2001) Stand-off tissue-based biosensors for the detection of chemical welfare agents using photosynthetic fluorescence induction. *Biosensors and Bioelectronics.* **(16)**: 439-446.
56. Sara Rodriguez-Mozaz, Maria-Pilar Marco. Maria J. Lopez de Alda, and Damià Barcelól (2004) Biosensors for environmental applications: Future development trends. *Pure Appl. Chem.* 76. **(4)**: 723-752.
57. Setford S.J., White S.F. and Bolbot J.A. (2002) Measurement of protein using an electrochemical bi-enzyme sensor. *Biosensors and Bioelectronics*. 17 **(1&2)**: 79-86.

58. Sheppard N.F. and Guiseppi-Elie A. (1998) Enzyme sensors based on conductimetric measurement. In: *Methods in Biotechnology.* Vol. **(6)**: *Enzyme and Microbial Biosensors: Techniques and Protocols*, ed, by A. Mulchandani and K. R. Rogers, Humana Press Inc., Totowa, pp. 157-173.
59. Terry L.A., White S.F. and Tigwell L.J. (2005) The application of biosensors to fresh produce and the wider food industry. *J. Agric. Food Chem.* 53 **(5)**: 1309-1316.
60. Turner A.P.F. (1989) Current trends in biosensor research and development. *Sensors Actuators*. **(17)**: 433-450.
61. Udo Johanningmeier, Ivo Bertalan, Lydia Hilbig, Jana Schulze, Stefan Wilski, Edda Zeidler and Walter Oettmeier (2006) Engineering the D1 Subunit of Photosystem II: Application to Biosensor Technology, *Biotechnological Applications of Photosynthetic Proteins: Biochips, Biosensors and Biodevices*, Springer, US, pp. 46-56.
62. Wang J. and Lin Y. (1993) On-line organic-phase enzyme detector. *Anal. Chim. Acta.* **(271)**: 53-58.
63. Wang J *et al*. (1997) DNA electrochemical biosensors for environmental monitoring: A review. *Analytica Chimica Acta.* **(347)**: 1-8.
64. Watts and Helen J. (1994) Optical biosensor for monitoring microbial cells. *Analytical Chemistry*. 66 **(15)**: 2465-2470.
65. Wise D. and Wingard L. (1991) *Biosensors with Fiberoptics*. Humana Press, Clifton, NJ.

CHAPTER

18 Protein Engineering

Protein engineering is a fascinating mixture of molecular biology, protein structure analysis, computation, and biochemistry, with the goal of developing useful or valuable proteins. *Protein Engineering* will consider the two general, but not mutually exclusive, strategies for protein engineering. The first is known as rational design, in which the scientist uses detailed knowledge of the structure and function of the protein to make desired changes. The second strategy is known as directed evolution. In this case, random mutagenesis is applied to a protein, and selection or screening is used to pick out variants that have the desired qualities. By several rounds of mutation and selection, this method mimics natural evolution. An additional technique known as DNA shuffling mixes and matches pieces of successful variants to produce better results. This process mimics recombination that occurs naturally during sexual reproduction. The rational protein design strategies, including computational methods, the use of non-natural amino acids to expand the biological alphabet, as well as impressive examples for the generation of proteins with novel characteristics. This section focuses on the question of how to design a protein with the desired properties, and examples are chosen to cover a wide range of engineering techniques, such as protein–protein interactions, DNA binding, antibody mimics, and enzymatic activity.

Keywords: Protein folding, α- helix, β-structure, binary patterning, ligand, negative design, TASP.

INTRODUCTION

Why protein engineering? As we know that large number of proteins found in nature, which fold into a variety of different structures and carry out a huge diversity of functions. Protein engineering attempts to design protein structures, including those having particular functions, researchers can improve the knowledge we have about the forces and effects that specify the properties of the folded states of a protein. In addition, control over the design of particular folded state structures will likely lead to new synthetic proteins having the efficiency and specificity of biological proteins. Such applications include therapeutics, sensors, catalysts, and materials. The successful design of proteins is possible even without a complete quantitative understanding of all the forces involved in specifying their structures.

Designing of proteins is non-trivial, however, because of both their complexity and the subtlety of the interactions that specify the folded state. Proteins are macrobiomolecule and having many structural variables specify the folded state, including sequence, backbone topology, and side-chain conformations.

There are two main motivations for doing protein engineering. The first is based upon the assumption that a complete understanding of any natural system depends upon our ability to design a similar artificial system from the first principles. The second motivation is for *de novo* protein design is one of the practical approaches. Therefore, our understanding of natural proteins for their folding pathways, thermodynamic stabilities and catalytic properties is enhanced by our ability to design novel proteins with pre-determined structure and properties. The ability to design proteins *de novo* has the potential to bring a revolution in the field of science and technology ranging from industrial catalyst to biomedical engineering.

Protein design also refers to the effort to design new protein molecules of a desired 3D structure and function. It is a reverse procedure of protein structure prediction and the solution of the problem therefore relies highly on the extent of our understanding of the principle of protein folding. (Figure 18.1).

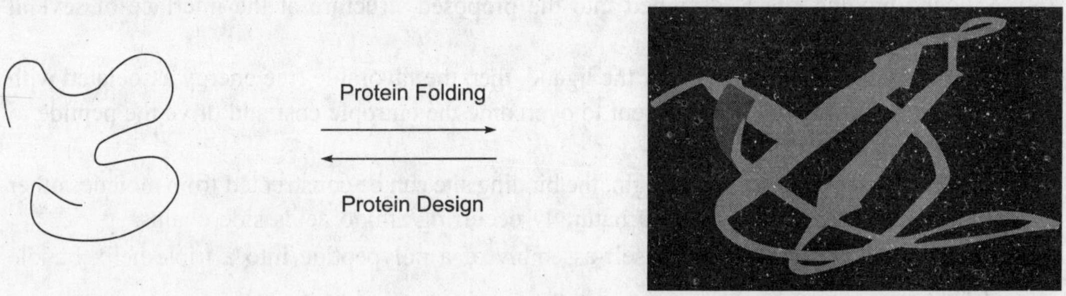

Figure 18.1 Protein design is a reverse procedure of protein folding.

STRATEGIES USED FOR THE DESIGNING OF PROTEIN STRUCTURE

Finding out an amino acid sequence that will adopt a unique and stable three-dimensional structure is the main goal to design a novel protein. The fundamental hurdle to design a novel protein is the conformational entropy of the linear polymer chain which must be overcome. The conformational entropy represents a substantial amount of unfavorable free energy. For a design to succeed the favorable free energy associated with these designed interactions must outweigh the entropic cost of fixing the chain into a unique structure.

Many different strategies have been used to achieve this goal. Most of these strategies have expanded considerable effort to maximize the strength and number of favorable interactions in the designed structure. The entropic cost of folding is reduced by introducing covalent cross-links, which limit the number of conformational states accessible to the chain. Following are the different strategies that have been employed to design novel protein structure:-

Self-Assembly of Modular Units of Secondary Structure

(i) Is the simplest and most direct strategy

(ii) In modular approach a single unit of secondary structure, i.e. α-structure and β-structure is synthesized as an individual segment of polypeptide chain (Figure 18.2).

(iii) β-structures are somewhat less modular than α-structures because individual β-strands are not stable in isolation they must be linked together by inter-strand hydrogen bonds.

(iv) Self-assembly is mediated by non-covalent interactions that are designed into the peptide.

(v) The key advantage of this approach is its simplicity, both at the level of design and at the level of synthesis.

(vi) The key disadvantage of this approach is the stability of structure and repetitive structures.

Ligand-Induced Assembly

(i) Is the second strategy that uses to design novel protein employ a ligand.

(ii) Ligand is the metal ion that induces the assembly of modular protein segments.

(iii) A ligand binding site is designed into the proposed structure at the interface of several interacting segments.

(iv) If the site have a high affinity for the ligand, then the favorable free energy associated with binding the ligand will be sufficient to overcome the entropic cost and drive the peptide to self-assembled.

(v) If the peptide was synthetic in origin, the binding site can be constructed from moieties other than those represented by the 20 naturally occurring amino acids side chains.

(vi) Metal ion-assisted spontaneous self-assembly of a polypeptide into a triple-helix bundle protein.

(vii) Metal-directed protein self-assembly, it utilizes the simultaneous stability, lability and directionality of metal-ligand bonds to drive protein-protein interactions.

(viii) The use of metal coordination to control protein self-assembly is attractive from both structural and functional perspectives: whereas the directionality and symmetry inherent in metal coordination can govern overall supramolecular geometry, the resulting interfacial metal centers may potentially offer new reactivities within biological scaffolds.

(ix) Synthetic metal coordinating functionalities have previously been employed for stabilizing coiled-coil assemblies constructing reactives metal binding sites in protein interiors and tuning the potentials of redox centers, among others.

(x) It was found that in the absence of added metal (i) the helical structures are only marginally stable and (ii) this stability was concentration dependent.

Assembly of Peptides Via Covalent Cross-linking

(i) As we know that the major obstacle in the designing of a novel protein is the conformational entropy of the polypeptide chain. When structures are assembled from several unlinked chains this entropic barrier is all the the more difficult to overcome. Therefore, preorganising the peptides by covalently linking them together is a powerful strategy to direct the formation of a desired structure.

(ii) The disulfide bond is the only bond that is used by the nature to cross-link peptides. If a designed protein is made synthetically, then a variety of other cross-links are also possible. Example: A novel cross-linker called DAB in their initial design of Betabellin, an eight-stranded α-barrel intended to fold with a simple up-and-down topology.

(iii) The covalent bond (also termed a peptide bond) has unique properties that make the protein eminently suited for its role in their structure. The peptide bond has limited rotational freedom because of the partial double-bond character of the amide moiety, while the remaining bonds in the polymer main chain can rotate freely. Therefore, one in every three bonds in the chain is fixed. Because of this constraint, the polypeptide backbone is significantly more structured than typical synthetic polymers, such as polyethylenes and polyesters, which lack such rigidifying elements. Furthermore, the amide bond is equipped with both hydrogen-bond donors and acceptors, allowing the peptide backbone to engage in intricate networks of noncovalent hydrogen-bonding interactions. While these forces are inherently far weaker than the covalent bonds of the polymer chain, the additive effect of a large number of such interactions makes the folded, three-dimensional structures of proteins relatively stable. In fact, some proteins have evolved an unusual stability that allows them to retain their structure under the extreme heat and pressure conditions of deep-sea geothermal vents.

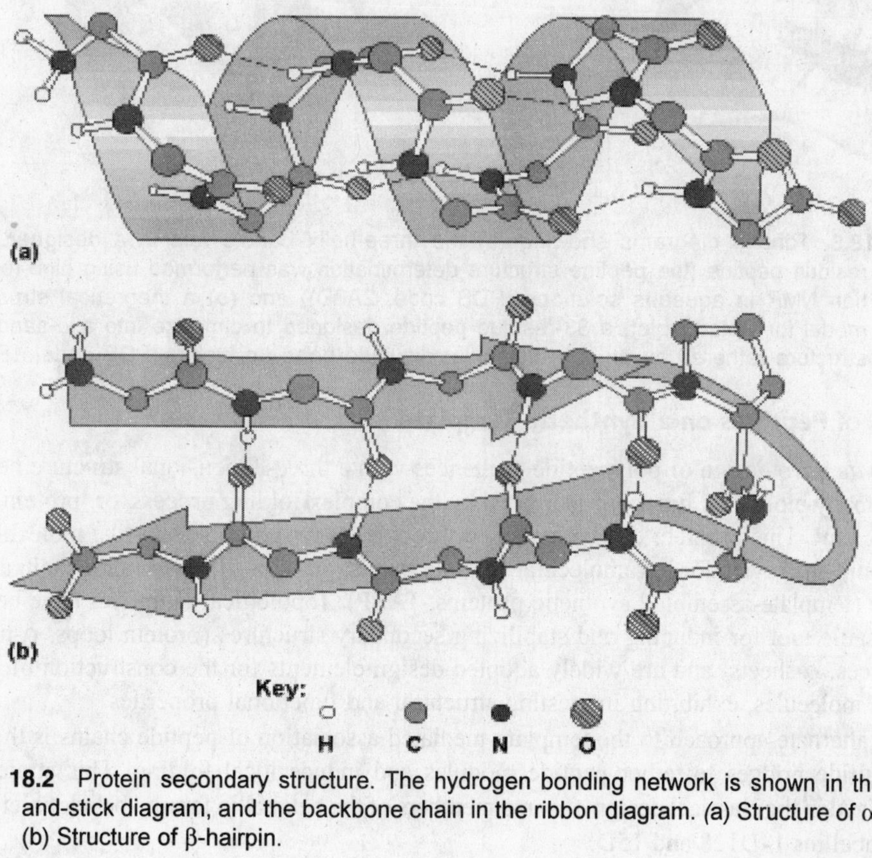

Figure 18.2 Protein secondary structure. The hydrogen bonding network is shown in the ball-and-stick diagram, and the backbone chain in the ribbon diagram. *(a)* Structure of α-helix. (b) Structure of β-hairpin.

(iv) The side chain amino group of lysine or ornithine and the side chain carboxylic acid groups of Glu or Asp can form peptide bonds with each other or with the N-and C- termini of the main chain. Such cross-linking leads to branched structures that are topologicaly quite different from ribosomally produced natural proteins. An advantage of these structure is that the interchain cross-links constrain the position of the chains relative to one another, and thereby reduce the entropic cost of forming a unique structure (Figure 18.3).

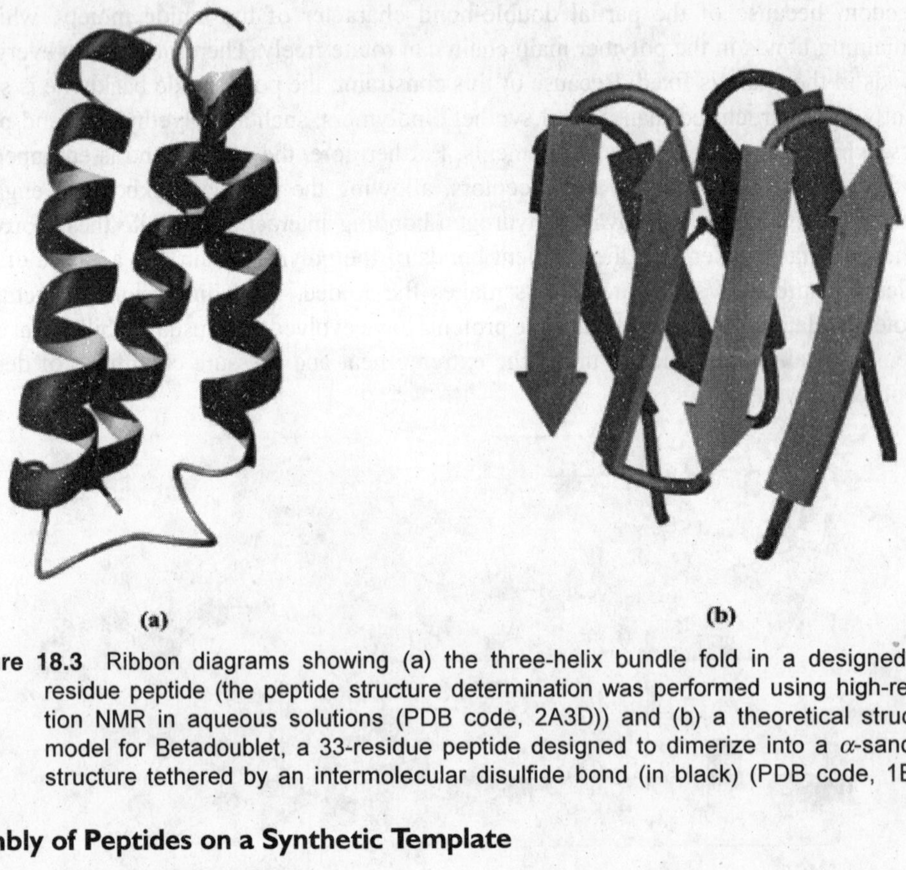

Figure 18.3 Ribbon diagrams showing (a) the three-helix bundle fold in a designed, 73-residue peptide (the peptide structure determination was performed using high-resolution NMR in aqueous solutions (PDB code, 2A3D)) and (b) a theoretical structural model for Betadoublet, a 33-residue peptide designed to dimerize into a α-sandwich structure tethered by an intermolecular disulfide bond (in black) (PDB code, 1BTD).

Assembly of Peptides on a Synthetic Template

(i) The *de novo* design of polypeptide sequences with a three-dimensional structure necessary for many biological functions is limited by the complex folding process, or 'protein folding problem'. This problem can be bypassed through constructing protein-like molecules with a 'built-in' device for intramolecular folding, that is, proteins of non-natural chain architecture (template-assembled synthetic proteins, TASP). Topological templates have become a versatile tool for inducing and stabilizing secondary structures (protein loops, α-turns, α-helices, α-sheets) and are widely adopted design elements for the construction of protein-like molecules, exhibiting interesting structural and functional properties.

(ii) An alternate approach to the template-mediated association of peptide chains is the use of disulfide bridges to tether peptide modules and induce local folding. This strategy was utilized in the classical design of some members of the betabellin family: betadoublet176 and betabellins 14D128 and 15D.

(iii) A less coercive approach to assembled proteins involves metal-mediated association of synthetic modules, whereby strong metal-peptide interactions would drive assembly. Such an approach necessitates the presence of a metal ligand in each interacting subunit and further dictates that such complexes be exchange-inert. Both synthetic peptide assemblies exhibit cooperativity in their denaturation by guanidium hydrochloride, which is a feature associated with compactly folded structures.

Linear Polypeptides that Fold into Globular Structure

(i) Is the ultimate goal in the designing of novel structure of proteins three-dimensional structures without the assistance of templates or covalent cross-links.

(ii) In which a polypeptide folds into its characteristic and functional three-dimensional structure from random coil. Each protein exists as an unfolded polypeptide or random coil when translated from a sequence of mRNA to a linear chain of amino acids. This polypeptide lacks any developed three-dimensional structure (the lef-thand side of the neighboring figure). Amino acids interact with each other to produce a well-defined three-dimensional structure, the folded protein (the right hand side of the figure), known as the native state.

(iii) The first example of a single-chain polypeptide successfully designed to fold into a stable globular structure was the α_4 structure.

(iv) Protein design involves a delicate balance between stabilizing a designed structure and destabilizing competing structure. The process of designing against alternative structure is sometimes called "negative design".

Protein Design by Binary Patterning of Polar and Non-polar Amino Acids

Numerous studies of natural proteins have demonstrated that protein structures are remarkably tolerant to amino acid substitutions. Thus, many different amino acids can encode the information necessary to produce a given three-dimensional structure. We have taken advantage of this tolerance to develop a general strategy for protein design. The strategy—called "the binary code" strategy—is based on the premise that the appropriate patterning of polar and nonpolar residues can direct a polypeptide chain to fold into elements of secondary structure, while simultaneously allowing the burial of nonpolar amino acids in a desired tertiary structure. A designed binary pattern exploits the periodicities inherent in protein secondary structure: α-helices have a repeating periodicity of 3.6 residues per turn, whereas β-strands have an alternating periodicity (Figure. 18.4). Thus, a binary patterned sequence designed to form amphipathic α-helices would place a nonpolar residue at every third or fourth position. In contrast, the binary pattern for an amphipathic β-strand would alternate between polar and nonpolar residues. In the binary code strategy, the precise three-dimensional packing of the side chains is not specified a priori. Therefore, within a library of binary patterned sequences,the identity of the side chain at each polar and nonpolar position can be varied extensively, thus, facilitating enormous combinatorial diversity.

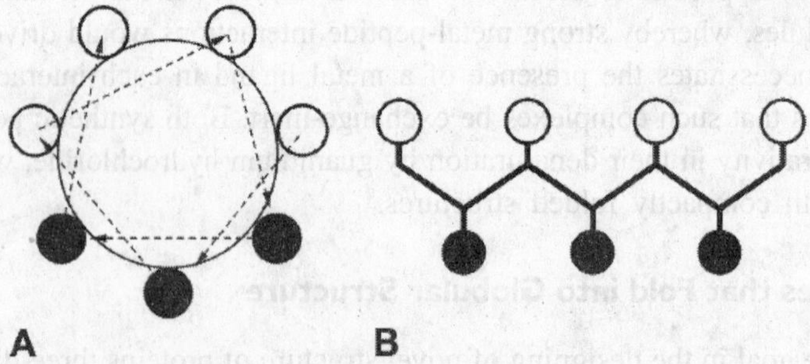

Figure 18.4 The designed binary pattern of polar (○) and nonpolar (•) amino acids for α-helices (A) and β-strands (B) exploits the inherent periodicities of the respective secondary structures. (A) α-helices have a repeating periodicity of 3.6 residues per turn. By placing a nonpolar amino acid at every third or fourth position, an amphipathic helix can be encoded in which one face is polar and the opposite face is nonpolar. Note that this figure shows the positioning of seven amino acids. For longer α-helices, the binary pattern will have to be adjusted to allow the 3.6 residues per turn periodicity to maintain the amphipathic nature the entire length of the helix. (B) β-strands have an alternating periodicity of polar and nonpolar amino acids. This pattern would cause one face of the strand to be polar and the opposite face to be nonpolar.

A combinatorial library of binary patterned proteins is expressed from a combinatorial library of synthetic genes. Each gene encodes a different amino acid sequence, but all sequences within a

First Position	Middle Position: T	C	A	G
T	TTT Phe TTC Phe TTA Leu TTG Leu	TCT Ser TCC Ser TCA Ser TCG Ser	TAT Tyr TAC Tyr TAA Stop TAG Stop	TGT Cys TGC Cys TGA Stop TGG Trp
C	CTT Leu CTC Leu CTA Leu CTG Leu	CCT Pro CCC Pro CCA Pro CCG Pro	CAT His CAC His CAA Gln CAG Gln	CGT Arg CGC Arg CGA Arg CGG Arg
A	ATT Ile ATC Ile ATA Ile ATG Met	ACT Thr ACC Thr ACA Thr ACG Thr	AAT Asn AAC Asn AAA Lys AAG Lys	AGT Ser AGC Ser AGA Arg AGG Arg
G	GTT Val GTC Val GTA Val GTG Val	GCT Ala GCC Ala GCA Ala GCG Ala	GAT Asp GAC Asp GAA Glu GAG Glu	GGT Gly GGC Gly GGA Gly GGG Gly

Figure 18.5 The organization of the genetic code allows sequence degeneracy for polar and nonpolar amino acids to be incorporated into a combinatorial library of synthetic genes by defining the middle position of the codon. For a nonpolar amino acid position, the degenerate codon NTN (N represents a mixture of A, G, T, and C) would encode for Phe, Leu, Ile, Met, or Val incorporation. For positions requiring polar amino acids, the degenerate codon NAN would encode for His, Gln, Asn, Lys, Asp, or Glu incorporation. For the NAN codon, T is excluded from the first base to avoid stop codons.

given library have the same patterning of polar and nonpolar residues. This sequence degeneracy is made possible by the organization of the genetic code (Figure 18.5). The degenerate codon NTN encodes nonpolar amino acids, whereas the degenerate codon NAN encodes polar amino acids (N represents a mixture of A, G, T, and C; see Subheading regarding codon usage). With these degenerate codons, positions requiring a nonpolar amino acid are filled by phenylalanine, leucine, isoleucine, methionine, or valine; whereas positions requiring a polar amino acid are filled by glutamate, aspartate, lysine, asparagine, glutamine, or histidine. (Strategies for the avoidance of stop codons are described in Subheading: The NAN (Polar) Codon).

Design of a Structural Template

Binary patterning can be applied to any amphipathic α-helical or β-stranded segment in a protein. Although our laboratory has focused on *de novo* proteins, the binary code strategy can also be applied to local areas of existing proteins, such as the active site, part of the core, or an interface. For the design of *de novo* proteins, the success of the strategy depends primarily on how well the template is designed. Several factors to consider for template design are presented next.

Binary patterned regions

α-HELICAL DESIGNS

Binary patterning exploits the periodicities inherent in secondary structures.

α-Helices have a repeating periodicity of 3.6 residues per turn (Fig. 18.4A). To design an amphipathic segment of α-helical secondary structure, a binary pattern of P-N-P-P-N-N-P (P represents polar and N, nonpolar) is used. Our initial α-helical design focused on the four-helix bundle motif. In this structure, the hydrophobic face of each of the helices is oriented toward the central core of the bundle, whereas the hydrophilic faces of the helices are exposed to the aqueous environment. The P-N-P-P-N-N-P pattern favors the formation of an amphiphilic α-helical secondary structure that can bury all nonpolar amino acids after formation of the desired tertiary structure. From our designed four-helix bundle libraries, more than 50 proteins have been purified and characterized. All have shown typical α-helical circular dichroism spectra. Moreover, the collection yielded several proteins with native-like properties, such as nuclear magnetic resonance chemical shift dispersion, cooperative chemical and thermal denaturations, and slow hydrogen/deutorium exchange rates.

β-SHEET DESIGN

Amphiphilic β-strands have an alternating periodicity of …P-N-P-N…. Based on this periodicity, a combinatorial library of synthetic genes can be created to encode β-sheet structures. Polar residues will comprise one face of the β-sheet, with nonpolar residues on the opposing face. The sequences in our first library were designed to have six β-strands, with each strand having the binary pattern P-N-P-N-P-N-P. Proteins from this library were expressed from a collection of synthetic genes cloned into *Escherichia coli.* All of the proteins studied in this collection formed a β-sheet secondary structure, having circular dichroism spectra with a characteristic minimum at 217 nm. The β-sheet proteins from this initial library self-assembled into amyloid-like fibrils. The fibrils bury the nonpolar side chains in a hydrophobic core, while exposing polar side chains to solvent. If these same β-sheet sequences are placed in a heterogeneous environment with a polar/nonpolar interface, they form a different structure. For example, at an air/water interface, these proteins self-assemble into flat α-sheet monolayers, with the nonpolar residues pointing up toward air and polar side chains pointing down toward water. Alternatively, at an interface between water and the nonpolar surface of highly ordered pyrolytic graphite, binary patterned α-sheet sequences undergo template-directed assembly on the graphite surface to yield highly ordered structures.

Considerations for the Design of Tertiary Structure

The ultimate success of a designed template is determined by the properties of the proteins it encodes. If the goal is to produce a library of well-folded globular proteins, then the designed template must not only dictate the secondary structure of the protein, but the tertiary structure as well. The template should be long enough to encode well-folded structures, but at the same time be short enough to be accessible to strategies for assembling large libraries of error-free genes. Many proteins from our first generation (74-residue) four-helix bundle library formed fluctuating structures resembling molten globule folding intermediates. To investigate the potential of the binary code strategy to encode collections of native-like tertiary structures, a second-generation library of binary-patterned proteins was prepared. This new library was based on protein 86, a pre-existing sequence from the original 74-residue library. The major change to protein 86 was the addition of six combinatorially diverse residues to each of the four helices, thereby making the second-generation proteins comparable in size to natural four-helix bundle proteins. These 24 additional helix-lengthening residues continued to follow the binary patterning. Characterization of five sequences arbitrarily chosen from this second-generation library showed that all are substantially more stable than the parental protein, 86. In addition, most of them yielded nuclear magnetic resonance spectra that are well dispersed and exhibit well-resolved nuclear Overhauser effect cross peaks, indicative of unique, well-folded tertiary structures. The structures of two of these proteins were determined by NMR and shown to be well-ordered four-helix bundles, as specified by design.

Codon Usage

The degenerate codons NAN and NTN encode polar and nonpolar amino acids, respectively. However, simply using an equimolar mixture of A, C, G, and T at the combinatorial N positions would introduce undesirable traits into the sequence. Most importantly, an unconstrained NAN codon would encode an unacceptably high frequency of stop codons (i.e., 2 out of 16 NAN codons _ 12.5%). Below is a list of considerations we have used in the design of polar and nonpolar codons.

The NAN (polar) codon

1. At the first base of the NAN codon, we use an equimolar mixture of G, C, and A. T is excluded, thereby eliminating the possibility of stop codons and tyrosine. If all bases were included at this first position, then the presence of thymine would give rise to the stop codons TAG or TAA.
2. The mixture of nucleotides at the third base of the NAN codon can be altered to favor some amino acids over others. An equimolar mixture of G, C, A, and T would yield an equal likelihood of histidine, glutamine, asparagine, lysine, aspartate, and glutamate. However, some of the residues of the NAN codon have higher intrinsic propensities than others to form α-helices. By omitting T at the third position, we can favor glutamine, lysine, and glutamate over histidine, asparagine, and aspartate. This matches theses residue's intrinsic propensities to form α-helices.

The NTN (nonpolar) codon

Equimolar mixtures of all four bases at the first and third N positions of the NTN codon would encode six times as many leucines as methionines (i.e., six leucine codons vs one methionine codon). In addition, an equimolar mixture would encode protein sequences in which a quarter of the hydrophobic residues in the interiors would be valine. Because valine has a relatively low α-helical propensity, this may be undesirable for some designs. By altering the molar ratio of the mixture at the first and third N positions, the relative abundance of hydrophobic residues can be altered. For example, in the initial four-helix bundle library, the first base of the NTN codon contained A:T:C:G in a molar ratio of 3:3:3:1 and the third base mixture contained equimolar concentrations of G and C. By biasing the mixture in this way, valine is limited to only 10% of the hydrophobic residues and leucine is represented only three times as frequently as methionine.

Codon usage of the host expression system

The DNA sequences in both the constant and the combinatorial regions of the library should be biased to favor those codons used most frequently in the host expression system. For example, including only C and G (rather than all four bases) in the third position of a degenerate codon biases the library to favor codons preferred by *E. coli*. Codons that are used only rarely in the host expression system, such as CGA, AGA, and AGG (arginine); CTA (leucine); CCC (proline); and ATA (isoleucine) in *E. coli* should be avoided wherever possible, because genes containing rare codons may express poorly.Other (non *E. coli*) expression systems have different codon preferences, and these should be considered in the design.

Assembly of Full-Length Genes

We typically assemble full-length genes from smaller single-stranded oligonucleotides. This is done to minimize the inherent errors (mostly deletions and frameshifts) associated with the synthesis of long degenerate oligonucleotides. Constant regions at the 5'- and 3'-ends serve as sites for the single-stranded oligonucleotides to anneal together and prime enzymatic synthesis (using DNA polymerase) of complementary strands. This strategy allows for a higher yield of error-free genes that correctly encode the desired *de novo* proteins. When synthesizing the semi-random oligonucleotides, some are made as coding (sense) strands and others as noncoding (antisense) strands. Typically, each oligonucleotide is designed to encode an individual segment of binary patterned

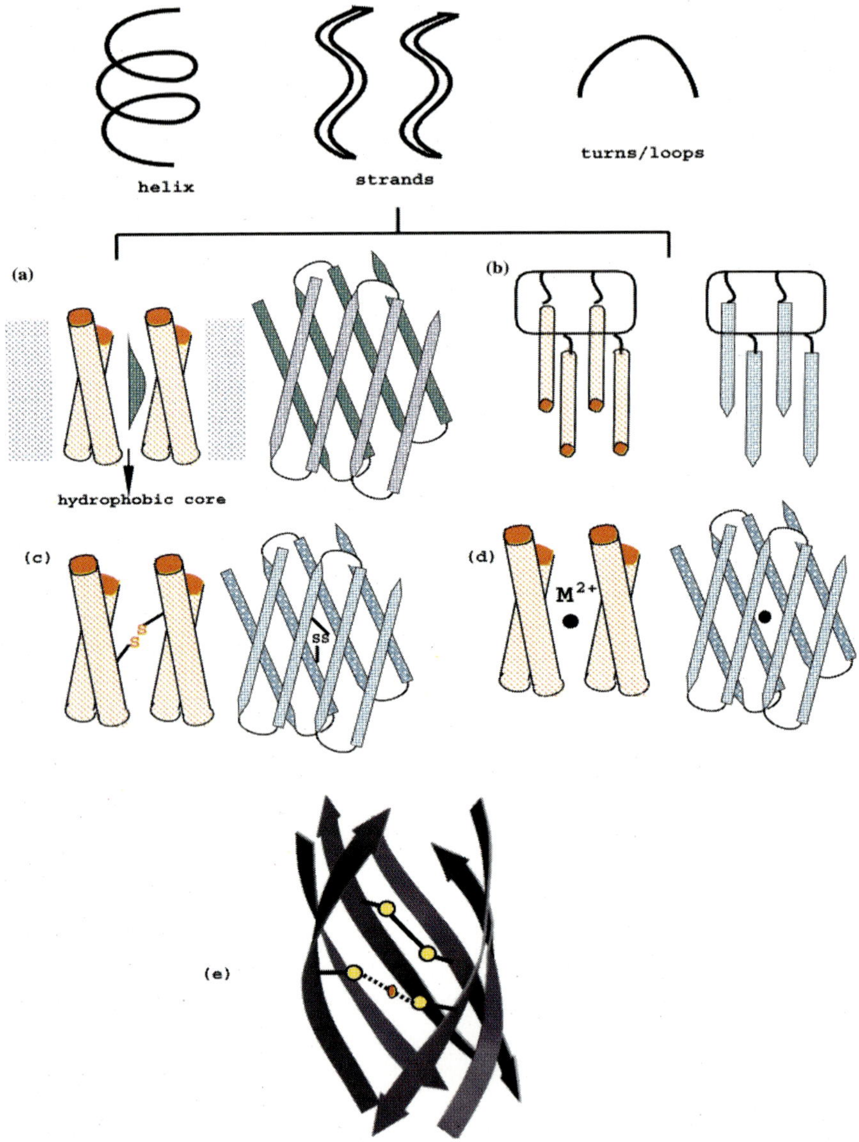

Figure 18.6 Schematic representation of the multiple techniques by which secondary structural elements can be assembled, namely, (a) patterning of residues to form a stable, hydrophobic core (assembly driven by solvent forces), (b) template assisted protein folding (TASP), (c) association of structural units via disulfide links, and (d) metal-mediated assembly. (e) A strategy whereby isolated α-sheets could be assembled to form α-barrels using either disulfide bridging (yellow) or metalion-mediated assembly (red).

secondary structure. Assembly of full-length genes from such segments allows individual α-helices or α-strands to be designed and manipulated as independent modules, thereby enhancing the versatility of the binary code strategy. In the design of our initial four-helix bundle library, four synthetic oligonucleotides were used to construct the full-length gene. Each oligonucleotide was designed to encode a single helix and turn. The turn regions were precisely defined (i.e., not degenerate), thus, allowing them to serve as priming sites for DNA polymerase to synthesize the complementary strands (Figure 18.6).

Various methods for assembling the genes have been used. In some cases, we have made two libraries of half genes, and then ligated them together to produce a library of genes encoding full-length proteins. To ensure correct head-to-tail ligation, nonpalindromic restriction sites can be designed into the constant regions to serve as the ligation sites. Other methods for assembling full-length genes include various polymerase chain reaction strategies (for example, overlap extension), and these have been used in constructing of several of our libraries.

STRATEGIES FOR THE DESIGN OF FUNCTION

Ultimately, the goal of protein design is to produce novel macromolecules that not only fold into predetermined structure, but moreover, possesses interesting and useful functions. Most attempts at the design of function have focused on binding and/or catalysis. To achieve these functions, two very different approaches have been pursued.

(i) "Retrofitting natural proteins to engineer substantial changes in function.

(ii) Designing functional proteins entirely *de novo*.

Most of what follows will focus on the second of these two approaches.

Novel Functions by Retrofitting Natural Proteins

Natural proteins, which have evolved to perform particular biological functions, can now be retrofitted with new activities. The possibility of taking a macromolecule that evolved over billions of years and modifying in to perform a function of our own choosing can be an extremely appealing and profitable enterprise. Nature ahs provided us with many structural scaffolds that are quite robust and able to tolerate a wide variety of sequence modifications. As a result of this tolerance, it is possible to tinker with natural structures and thereby engineer proteins with altered specificities and/or activities. A full summary of successful attempts to modify natural proteins is beyond the scope of this chapter. However, the following examples illustrate the range of possibilities for engineering proteins with altered specificities:

I. Alteration of DNA-binding specificity: *Phage-434 repressor* was changed to recognize the DNA operator site of *phage P-22* in preference to its natural binding site.

II. Alteration of cofactor specificity: Glurathione reductase was changed form an enzyme requiring NADP to one that prefers NAD.

III. Alteration of substrate specificity: Trypsin was changed from a protease that cleaves after lysine and arginine residues to a chymotrypsin like enzyme that cleaves after large hydrophobic residues.

The ability to retrofit natural proteins can extend well beyond modifications that merely alter specificity. Indeed, entirely novel activities can be appended onto the structures of preexisting protein scaffolds. Novel functions engineered into natural proteins include these examples:

1. **Metal binding:** A novel binding site for transition metals was grafted into *E. coli* thioredoxin and a binding site for calcium was introduced into human lysozyme. The calcium site was constructed by replacing Gln_{86} and Ala_{92} with aspartic acid side chains. The resulting metallo lysozyme is both more active and more thermostable than the wild-type enzyme.
2. **Site-specific DNA cleavage:** A 52 residue DNA-binding fragment of the Hin recombinase protein was converted into a sequence specific DNA cleaving protein via the covalent attachment of the iron chelating agent, EDTA.

To date, the most powerful and widely applicable strategy for retrofitting natural protein is the design of catalytic antibodies. Antibodies are ideal proteins upon which to graft novel functions because, in a sense, they have evolved to be retrofitted.Over the past several years. Immunologists and chemists have managed to coax the mammalian immune system into generating antibodies that not only bind specific antigens, but moreover, catalyze a variety of channel reactions. Central to the design of catalytic antibodies has been the use of antigens that resemble the transition state of a reaction. Antibodies raised against transition state analogues can significantly hasten the rate of a chemical reaction by stabilizing the rate determining transition state on a reaction pathway.

De Novo Design of Binding and Catalysis—Early History

The design of novel proteins capable of binding specific ligands was pioneered by the work of Gutte an co-workers. In 1979, they reported the design, synthesis and characterization of a 34 residue peptide that interacts with nucleic acids. The sequence of the peptide was designed to form a $\alpha\alpha\alpha$ structure that would bind the trinucleotide-2-methyl guanine-adenine-adenine, as modeled. In this model, the side chains of Thr_{12} Gln_{14} and Gln_{16} hydrogen bond to the base moieties; Phe_1, Phe_3 and Tyr_5 stack or intercalate with the bases; and Lys_{28} and His_{32} form stabilizing salt bridges with the phosphates of the trinucleotide ligand. A stabilizing salt bridges with the phosphates of the trinucleotide ligand. A disulfide bond connecting $Cys_{10}$with Cys_{13} was included to enhance the stability of the proposed structure.The 34-rsidue peptide was synthesized by the solid-phase method, and both the 34-rsidue monomer and a 68-residue disulfide-linked dimer were isolated.

Incorporation of Binding Sites into *de novo* Proteins

The successful designs of proteins that fold into predetermined structures sets the stage of the eventual design of novel binding sites and catalyze activities. Following the design of α_4, modification of the sequence of this very stable four-helix bundle in order to incorporate metal binding sites, tetrahedral binding site for Zn(II) was chosen. The site is formed by a combination of histidine and cysteine side chains, as is found in several natural proteins such as alcohol dehydrogenase and the zinc finger domains. The particular locations in α_4 most appropriate for the placement of the new His and Cys side chains. A model of the original α_4 protein was uses as the starting structure, and each residue in this structure was replaced to both His and Cys to find combinations of side chains that could form a tetrahedral Zn(II) binding site. The site that was finally chosen is formed by Cys_{21} and His_{25} from the second α-helix and Cys_{47} and His_{51} from the third α-helix. A gene encoding the metal-binding variant of α_4 was constructed and the protein was expressed in *E coli*. Characterization of purified protein demonstrated that:

(i) Zn(II) is bound with a dissociation constant of 2.5 $X10^{-8}$ M;

(ii) the binding site is wholly contained within a single protein monomer;

(iii) the secondary structure of the protein is unchanged upon metal binding;

(iv) Binding of Zn(II) increases protein stability; and

(v) the cysteine sulfahydryls are essential for binding. Furthermore, the absorption spectrum of the Co(II)-substituted protein is consistent with binding to a tetrahedral site formed by two histidine and two cysteine side chains. Zn (II) binding site was also designed by modifying the sequence of α_4. The metal binding variant was synthesized by solid phase methods in both the α_1 context and α_2 context. (As described above, α_4 is a 74 amino acid sequence that folds into a four-helix bundle). In each case, two of the three histidine side chains were incorporated within a single α- helix, while the third His side chain came from the neighboring helix. The binding of Zn (II) to the novel protein occurs with no significant change in secondary structure. However, when metal is bound a number of resonances in the NMR spectrum become sharper and less degenerate. This suggests that Zn(II) binding induces the protein to Assume a more ordered structure that is less like a molten globule and more like the native state of natural proteins.

Construction of novel metallo-proteins has not been limited to α-helical structures, designed a metal binding site into a β-sheet framework, based on the variable heavy domain of immunoglobulin McPC603. Their designed protein, which they call the 'minibody' is 61residue long. The sequence of the designed protein differs from McPC603 in three respects:

(i) Side chains that are buried in the intact McPC603 antibody but would be exposed in the minibody were mutated from nonpolar to polar residues;

(ii) The 7-residue loop connecting β-strands two and three was replaced by two glycines because this loop makes significant contacts with parts of the antibody—present in the minibody;

(iii) A metal binding site was introduced by incorporating these histidines into hypervariable loops H1 and H2. The designed metallo-protein was synthesized by chemical methods (Bianchi *et al.* 1993). Size exclusion chromatography of the purified product showed it to be monomeric and circular dichrosim spectroscopy showed it to be predominantly structure. The minibody binds zinc and the natural metallo-enzyme, is still ~900-fold faster than spontaneous decarboxylation.

Membrane Proteins and Ion Channels

Membrane proteins play an essential role in many biological processes, and the ability to construct novel membrane proteins that possess predetermined structures and "tailor-made" activities is certain to have enormous impact. However, the design of a membrane protein challenges would be designers with obstacles beyond those already encountered in the design of the water-soluble proteins. The interactions that drive the formation of protein structure in membranes differ from those that dominate the folding of water soluble proteins. For example, the hydrophobic effect, which requires proteins in aqueous environments to have nonpolar insides and polar outsides, makes very different demands on proteins immersed in environments that are themselves nonpolar. Furthermore, once an appropriate sequence for a membrane protein is actually designed, constructing the novel protein can be fraught with technical difficulties not encountered in synthesizing and/or expressing water-soluble proteins: Since membrane proteins are not soluble in standard aqueous buffers, they typically form inclusion bodies when expressed *in vivo* or insoluble precipitates when synthesized *in vitro*. Moreover, the transfer of a novel membrane protein from a water-insoluble aggregate into a membrane-like environment will almost certainly require a conformational change that may or may not be kinetically facile.

Despite these challenges, several membrane proteins have been designed and characterized. The synthetic pore proteins, called Synporins, were constructed by using the template-assisted strategy. In one example of this approach, four copies of a 23-residue α-helix were tethered to a carrier template.The sequence of the 23-mer was taken from the δ-subunit of the acetylcholine receptor of *Torpedo callifornica*. The template was a 9-residue peptide originally designed by Mutter and co-workers in 1988 to form a β-strand-turn-β strand with four lysine side chains (two before the turn and two after it), all pointing in the same direction. Thus, when the four 23-mers are attached to this template they are constrained to be parallel to one another. Since the amino acid sequence of the 23-mer can form an amphiphillic α-helix, the Synporin design assume that linkage to the template would direct the formation of a parallel four helix bundle.This model is supported by the results of circular dichroism experiments which show that the structure of the intact 101-residue Synporin is predominantly α-helical. According to the design, the nonpolar side chains of the helices should form an external lipophillic surface, which interacts with the lipid bilayer, while the polar side chains of the helices should form a central pore. Characterization of the synthetic protein shows that it indeed forms ion-channels. These channels:

(i) show single-channel conductance;
(ii) can discriminate between different cations;
(iii) can open and close in the millisecond time range; and
(iv) are sensitive to the local anesthetic channel blockers. Thus, the Synporin molecules reproduce features that are characteristic of the authentic acetylcholine receptor.

In another example of the Synporin strategy, Montal's group constructed an analogue of a calcium channel. This synthetic protein was built on the same template used in the previous study, but the 22-residue α-helical sequence used in this study was taken from the dihydropyridine-sensitive calcium channel. The resulting 97-residue synthetic protein mimics many features of the authentic channel, including the ability to distinguish between enantiomers that act as activators (agonists) or blockers (antagonists).

The occurrence of helical bundle structures in many natural ion channels prompted to design synthetic ion channels comprising simple amphiphillic α-helices. These designed channels differ from those of Montal *et al.*, in two important respects:

(i) The sequences were not based upon the sequences of natural ion channels, but were designed entirely *de novo*; and
(ii) instead of relying upon an artificial template, the synthetic peptides were designed to self-assemble into multimeric structures surrounding a central hydrophilic pore. The "minimalist" approach led to the design of a 23-residue sequence that is extremely simple, but nevertheless captures the essential features of natural ion channels. Repeating sequences composed of only two amino acids (Leu and Ser) were designed to form amphiphillic helices that would assemble into multimeric structures.

Following this work, the synthetic ion channel was preorganized into a four–helix bundle via the template-assisted strategy. A model of the resulting protein, called Tetraphilin. The cross-linked material resembles the original self-assembling material in that both form proton–selective ion channels. However, the cross-linked channels differ from the original channels in three respects: Cross linking:

(i) Increases the life time of the major conductive state by >25-fold;
(ii) Causes channels to form with a linear (rather than higher order) concentration dependence; and
(iii) Causes channel formation to be nearly independent of voltage.

According to this model the parent peptide (without the cross-link) can exist in an equilibrium between the trans-membrane four-helix bundle and an alternative orientation in which the monomeric amphiphilic helices are oriented with their helical axes parallel to the membrane surface. Increasing the concentration of helices or applying a trans-membrane voltage favours the assembly of trans-membrane tetramers and thereby increase pore activity. In the case of tetraphilin,where the four helices are cross-linked to the porphyrin template, the non-productive structure cannot compete with the pore structure. Therefore, the pores have longer lifetimes and are not sensitive to either voltage or peptide concentration. Because the template-assisted strategy constrains the location of the peptides it can direct the molecule towards the desired structure and function.

Membrane proteins are notoriously difficult to work with because of their insolubility in aqueous buffers. Typically, they can only be solubilized in the presence of small-molecule detergents. These protein/detergent complexes are suitable for many purposes, but with few notable exceptions they rarely yield crystal suitable for structure determination by X-ray diffraction. This shortcoming presumably results from a level of disorder imposed by the small detergent molecules surrounding the protein. The peptide called a peptitergent, has the sequence acetyl-EELLKQALQQA QQLLQQAQELAKK-amide. The hydrophilic face of the α-helix contains mostly Gln residue,with Lys and Glu side chains near the N- and C-termini, respectively, to neutralize the helix dipole. The hydrophobic face was designed with alanines projecting from the center, and leucine at the edge, thereby generating a wide that nonpolar surface capable of interacting with and solubilizing, a range of different membrane proteins. The 30A° length of this face is sufficient to cover the membrane –spanning region of the integral membrane proteins. To test the ability of the peptitergent to solubilize membrane protein, experiments were performed using bacterior-hodopsin and bovine rhodopsin, in both cases, small-molecule detergents were diluted away and the peptitergent enabled the protein to remain in solution under conditions where omission of peptitergent led to 100%

precipitation. The crystal structure of the peptitergent (without added membrane protein) was solved and it forms a four-helix bundle. As predicted by the design, the α-helices pack flat surface, suggesting that the observed activity of the peptide reflects the structural features incorporated into its design.

Design of New Protein Materials

Protein like polymeric materials has been designed and constructed both by recombinant methods *in vivo* and *via* synthetic methods *in vitro*. Some of these novel polymers are designed to expand and contract in response to easily manipulated conditions such as temperature, pH or ionic strength. Changes in the length can then be used to achieve mechano-chemical coupling. These polymers have the sequence (Val-Pro-Gly-Xxx-Gly)n ,where Xxx is Val or Glu at ratio of 4:1. (Thus, it contains 4 Glu's per 100 residues). At neutral Ph the glutamates are charged, but when the Ph is lowered to 3, the Glu side chains are converted to neutral groups, thus permitting the hydrophobic collabs or contraction of the polymer. This material is able to pick up and shut down weights that are 1000 times greater than the rate of contacting polymer.

Self-assembly is a theme common to both material science and protein folding. The designed peptide has sequence cyclo [(D-Ala-Glu-D-Ala-Gln)$_2$], which can adopt a flat ring shaped conformation.

At neutral pH the glutamate side chains are negatively charged and the cyclic peptide repel one another. However, at low PH the carboxylate group becomes protonated and repulsion is replaced by inter molecular hydrogen bonding between the flat rings. Thus, acidification of the medium triggers the spontaneous self-assembly of peptide rings into long hollow tubes 100 of nm long and having internal diameter dictated by the size of the cyclic peptide.

EVOLUTIONARY STRATEGIES FOR PROTEIN ENGINEERING

Natural evolution is a process of production of "variants" of a given specimen followed by selection of those best adapted to a specific environmental setting, or to a specific purpose. Natural evolution is the result of genetic mutations or rearrangements resulting in new protein variants within organisms. Antibodies well illustrate the process of evolution: the natural antibody repertoire of an organism represents a large number of variants that are sampled, and those best suited to the purpose of binding a specific ligand are selected from this natural library for further rounds of improvement. Selection of protein variants requires the coupling of genotype and phenotype— given in natural evolution and a requirement hard worked at in the research laboratory where artificial protein evolution is undertaken. Protein engineering tools have undergone a revolution in the past decade as a result of the creation of better-defined large libraries with a variety of strategies for linking genotype and phenotype, which, in turn, have allowed for the development of a host of new approaches to functional screening and selection strategies.

The goal of this chapter is to present some of the main statistical and probabilistic calculations pertinent to protein library creation and to library-based screening and selection strategies in the language of the combinatorial biologist to ensure their ease of application. This chapter also aims to reveal the pertinence of these calculations to the process of library creation and screening.

When designing an experiment in library-based protein engineering, one must counterbalance the scientific value of creating the most diverse protein library with the practical limitations presented by the screening or selection strategies. The statistical and probabilistic questions pertaining to library representation are important, and they vary according to the specific application. We also present tests of experimental biases, to aid in assessing the library quality and the occurrence of biases before or after selection. As we will illustrate, the information revealed by simple analyses of library-based problems can lead to important—and sometimes counter-intuitive—insights, which, in turn, allow rapid improvement of the experimental design and a stronger basis for interpretation of the results.

We first discuss some important parameters related to the design of protein libraries, such as library size, compositional bias, codon degeneracy, and encoded diversity. This is followed by the development of a series of commonly encountered problems, with discussion of the pertinence of addressing each problem and a clear mathematical development. Numerical examples are provided to clarify the application of the formulae. In cases in which the implementation of the mathematical tools is more complex or time consuming, we refer the experimenter to Excel files for input of the appropriate variables. The proposed problems are intended to be general enough to apply to a diversity of library-based systems rather than to any specific subset. It is important to note that many results presented below are suited only when various parameters are sufficiently large or small, and can lead to erroneous conclusions if applied otherwise. Specific conditions are provided. Complementary works on the mathematical treatment of library-based strategies include mathematical modeling of DNA shuffling, specifically treated in the important work of Moore and of Maranas and of Sun, and more recently, Blackburn and colleagues. The latter work also presents a mathematical treatment of library representation for libraries of equiprobable outcomes; we present the same treatment, as a prelude to the treatment of library representation for libraries of nonequiprobable outcomes.

Example: I

Design and Synthesis of Artificial Zinc Finger Proteins

Artificial zinc finger proteins have important applications in biomedical research and in gene therapy, and are novel tools for biochemical and molecular biological investigations. In particular, a (Cys)2(His)2-type zinc finger motif, one of the most common DNA-binding motifs in eukaryotes, presents a versatile and attractive framework for the design of new DNA-binding proteins. The structural analysis of some (Cys)2(His)2-type zinc finger protein–DNA complexes revealed the characteristics of this motif in DNA binding as follows:

1. The zinc finger structure is repeated by the connection with a specific linker.
2. Each zinc finger structure binds to a 3-basepair (bp) subsite of DNA with its α-helix facing toward the major groove.
3. The amino acid residues at four key positions in the α-helix of each zinc finger unit make a 1:1 contact with the DNA bases at specific positions.
4. The overall arrangement of the peptide is antiparallel to the primary interacting strand of DNA.

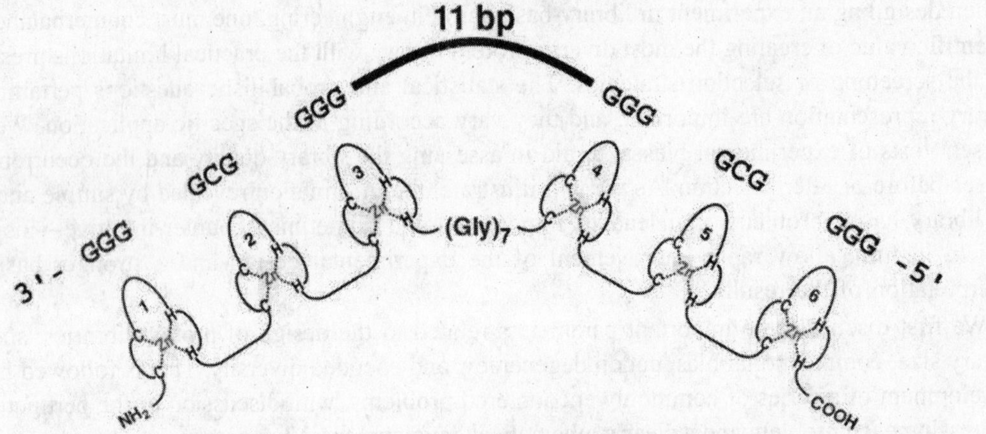

Figure 18.7 Schematic drawing of Sp1ZF6(Gly)7. DNA sequence bent by the six-finger protein is shown above of the figure. The amino acid residues are depicted by their one letter codes.

Because of these features, some artificial zinc finger proteins, for example, long sequence and AT-sequence-binding fingers, have been created successfully. Such a designed DNA-binding protein would be expected to possess a unique binding sequence with high affinity and specificity. In addition, novel zinc finger proteins, such as a DNA-bending finger and a (His) 4-type finger were also designed. These artificial zinc finger proteins offer great promise as useful tools for genetic engineering and genomic-specific transcription switches in the near future.

Strategy of Protein Design

Novel six- and nine-zinc finger proteins, Sp1ZF6 and Sp1ZF9, were created from the three-zinc finger motifs of the transcription factor, Sp1. These proteins were constructed by linking two or three Sp1 zinc finger domains with the Krüppel-type linker (Figures 18.7 & 18.8).

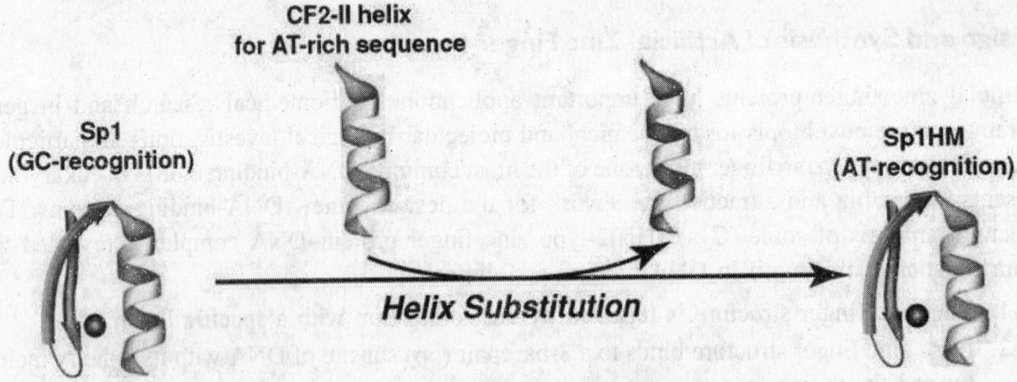

Figure 18.8 Representation of the strategy of helix substitution for alternating between GC and AT recognition.

Example: 2

Monobodies

Monobodies: Antibody Mimics Based on the Scaffold of the Fibronectin Type III Domain. A major goal of protein engineering is to produce novel biomolecules that bind to a specified target. Such molecules would be useful in many biotechnology applications, including diagnosis, therapy, and catalysis. Although there is a vast number of natural proteins that can be exploited for such applications, the approach of engineering novel, useful biomolecules is attractive because it is not limited by the availability of natural biomolecules. The basic architecture of the antibodies, in which variable loops are presented on an essentially constant framework, and the successes of antibody engineering have inspired a number of groups to develop "molecular scaffolds". The main goal of these attempts has been to overcome the disadvantages of antibodies and antibody fragments, including the large size, heterodimeric nature (except for single immunoglobulin domains), low conformational stability, and difficulty in large-scale production while retaining the ability to present multiple peptide segments for target binding. Most of such artificial scaffolds developed to date are based on either fragments of immunoglobulins or small monomeric proteins. We have developed the use of the fibronectin type III domain (FN3) as a molecular scaffold. Fibronectin is a large protein that plays essential roles in the formation of the extracellular matrix and cell-cell interactions. It consists of many repeats of three types (I, II, and III) of small domains. FN3 is a ubiquitous domain, and is estimated to occur in approx 2% of all animal proteins. There are 15 repeating units of FN3 in human fibronectin. We have built our system on FNfn10. FNfn10 is small (94 residues) and monomeric, and it does not contain disulfide bonds. High-level expression of correctly folded FNfn10 in bacteria is straightforward. The three-dimensional structure of FNfn10 is best described as a sandwich similar to that of the antibody variable domain of the heavy chain domain, except that FNfn10 has seven α-strands instead of nine. FNfn10 contains three surface loops on each end, which can potentially be used to present multiple peptide segments. These properties of FNfn10 make it an ideal candidate for a molecular scaffold. We have demonstrated that novel binding proteins (termed monobodies) can be engineered by screening combinatorial libraries of FNfn10 in which residues in surface loops are diversified, and that the resulting monobodies retain the global structure of the scaffold and good conformational stability. Furthermore, because FNfn10 does not require disulfide formation for proper folding and stability, monobodies are compatible with virtually any screening methods, including phage display, peptide–ribonucleic acid fusion, and *in vivo* methods, such as the yeast two-hybrid system. We have also demonstrated that monobodies can be readily used inside living cells. In this chapter, we describe methods for the construction of combinatorial libraries, for library screening using phage display and yeast two-hybrid technologies, and for bacterial production of monobodies.

Example: 3

Engineering Site-Specific Endonucleases

Type II restriction endonucleases are indispensable tools for the site-specific cleavage of DNA. They usually recognize double-stranded DNA sequences, 4 to 8 basepairs (bp) in length. In the presence of Mg2, they cleave the DNA within or adjacent to the recognition site in both strands to produce blunt or sticky ends with a 5'-phosphate and a 3'-OH. Restriction enzymes are among the most specific enzymes known: sequences differing in only 1 bp are cleaved by a factor of 106 more slowly than the canonical recognition sequence. This extreme accuracy results from an intimate interplay between direct (interaction with the bases) and indirect readout (interaction with the sugar-phosphate backbone). Typically, 15 to 20 hydrogen bonds are formed between the restriction enzyme and the bases of the recognition sequence, in addition to numerous van der Waals contacts to the bases and hydrogen bonds to the backbone, some of which are water mediated. This means that recognition is overdetermined and redundant. Any effort to change the specificity of restriction enzymes by rational protein design, therefore, is unlikely to be successful for this reason, because several contacts have to be altered and more than one amino acid residue has to be replaced. In addition, in most restriction enzymes, amino acid residues involved in recognition are located in very close proximity to residues responsible for catalysis. Although this guarantees a tight coupling between recognition and catalysis, it has been a great impediment for protein engineering. Therefore, in retrospect, it is not too surprising that true changes in specificity have not been achieved by rational protein design and that researchers have turned to evolutionary aproaches to achieve changes in specificity of restriction enzymes, both *in vitro* and *in vivo*. However, even with these approaches, thus far, only a reduction of specificity (e.g., BstyI, from RGATCY to preferentially AGATCT) or expansion of specificity (e.g., Eco57I from CTGAAG to CTGRAG) could be achieved. It may well be that restriction enzymes structurally are not sufficiently malleable and that multiple amino acid substitutions would be required for a true change in specificity. This could be a safeguard to prevent unwanted, in most cases deleterious, cleavage of the host genome by restriction enzyme variants that invariably are produced to a small extent in the process of translation. Using the same argument, it can be anticipated that it should be possible to generate variants of restriction enzymes with altered properties that were not counterselected during evolution. Indeed, EcoRI and EcoRV variants with simple amino acid substitutions could be produced that cleave DNA with a modified base or a modified backbone (EcoRV T94V) much better than the wild-type enzyme.

Here, we report how an enzyme related to restriction enzymes, namely the mismatch repair protein, MutH, from *Escherichia coli*, was converted by a single amino acid substitution into a variant with a relaxed specificity. The procedure that was used and is described in detail should be of general applicability. First, the system under study is introduced along with the structural considerations presented that led to the selection of amino acid substitutions required for the desired change in specificity. DNA mismatch repair is one of the most important processes for the correction of replication errors in almost all living organisms; it enhances the fidelity of DNA replication by up to a factor of 1000. In *E. coli*, DNA mismatch repair is initiated by MutS binding to the mismatch, followed by MutL dependent activation of MutH, which nicks the unmethylated (i.e., newly replicated) strand at a hemimethylated d(GATC) site, which may be several hundred basepairs upstream or downstream from the mismatch. The nicked DNA strand is then exonucleotically degraded by one of four exonucleases, assisted by helicase II, up to and beyond the mismatch. The segment removed is subsequently replaced (and repaired) by the action of DNA polymerase III and DNA ligase. MutH is a sequence specific Mg2-dependent DNA endonuclease, with a molecular mass of 28 kDa. It shows sequence similarity with the type II restriction endonuclease Sau3AI , which also recognizes the d(GATC) sequence and cleaves it 5– to the G. However, MutH cleaves only the unmethylated strand, either in a hemimethylated or unmethylated DNA, whereas Sau3AI cleaves both strands regardless of their methylation state. Different from typical restriction endonucleases and from Sau3AI, it is active as a monomer. The determination of the structure of MutH confirmed the relatedness between MutH and type II restriction endonucleases of the PD...D/EXK family. Based on the structural homology between MutH and PvuII, a putative DNA binding and active site of MutH was identified by superposition of monomeric MutH and one subunit of the homodimeric PvuII, comprising, among other residues, Asp 70, Glu 77, and Lys 79.

APPLICATIONS OF PROTEIN ENGINEERING

Medical Applications

Medicinal protein engineering sheds light on this largely unchartered field, covering major strategies for engineering of proteins with predetermined biological properties. It discusses computational approaches to protein design and experimental approaches to protein construction. This volume also explores the tight connection between protein and genetic engineering. It moves researchers beyond experimental protein construction and theoretical protein design to the medicinal applications of engineered proteins. Focusing on the application of protein engineering to medicine, this seminal work outlines the appropriate techniques for studying protein properties and building mathematical engineering models of novel vaccines, diagnostic reagents, and therapeutic treatments. As a truly comprehensive assessment of the medical protein engineering research available and its future implications for disease control and prevention, this is an indispensable reference for biological researchers in this groundbreaking field.

Protein engineering is also being used to create immunotoxins, which are the conjugates of cell binding antibody or antigens, covalently bound to a plant or a bacterial toxin. The procedure of fusion of genes using sequences coding for antibodies and toxic peptides is used to create these immunotoxins. When a patient is treated with the immunotoxins, the antibody or antigen helps in the recognition of the target cells to be killed and the toxin component helps in killing these cells. So immunotoxins are created in such a way that they have two parts- a) a toxin polypeptide or a part of it having toxin activity, called A chain, and b) a cell binding recognition polypeptide or antibody or a part of it having binding site, called B chain, e.g., ricin, a plant toxin has actually been used as a immunotoxin for a study of it's effect on mouse tumour cells.

Rational Design and Protein Engineering of Growth Factors for Regenerative Medicine and Tissue Engineering

Drug designing is another upcoming area in biotechnology. Depending on the mode of action used by the drugs, the drug designing can be modified by blocking the enzyme activity, e.g., Trimethoprim (TMP) is a clinically important antimicrobial drug which inhibits the enzyme dihydrofolate reductase (dHFR) in bacteria and therefore, is used to treat urinary tract infections. However in high concentrations it starts attacking human dHFR thus becoming harmful. Efforts have been made to synthesize TMP, which will have a rigid three-dimensional structure in association with bacterial enzyme dHFR, so that it may not be able to attack human dHFR. Drugs are also being produced by studying the receptor molecules associated with a particular disease and then finding chemicals which can block these receptors. One of the examples is the drug 'Propranolol' which is used to treat heart diseases and hypertension. The two hormones, 'norepinephrine' and 'epinephrine' control the contraction and relaxation of cardiac muscles. These hormones act through the two receptors alpha (α) and beta (β). The drug propranolol blocks the receptor beta (β) and thereby inhibits the activity of hormones which act through a receptor molecule. This relaxes the heart muscle. This drug is being used to treat heart diseases, angina pectoris and high blood pressure. The detailed studies of antimetabolites or inhibitors of DNA synthesis has led to the development of drugs for treating 'cancer', 'gout', 'malaria' and some viral infections like Herpes. Drugs like '6-mercaptopurine' and 'thioguanine' by inhibiting the DNA synthesis and the cell division, are very effective in cancer chemotherapy. Based on the same principle of inhibition of nucleic acid synthesis, the drugs like 'pyramethamine' for malaria, 'trimethoprim' for bacterial infection, and 'acyclovir' for herpes virus infection etc were also developed growth factors provide key instructive cues for tissue formation and repair. However, many natural growth factors are limited in their usefulness for tissue engineering and regenerative applications by their poor retention at desired sites of action, short half-lives *in vivo*, pleiotropic actions and other features. In the present article, we review approaches to rational design of synthetic growth factors based on mechanisms of receptor activation. Such synthetic molecules can function as simplified ligands with potentially tunable specificity and action. Rational and combinatorial protein engineering techniques allow introduction of additional features into these synthetic growth molecules, as well as natural growth factors, which significantly enhance their therapeutic utility.

In Veterinary Sciences

Sulfa antibiotics (sulfonamides) are derivatives of p-aminobenzenesulfonamide that are widely used in veterinary medicine. Foods derived from treated animals may be contaminated with these drugs. However, current immunobased sulfonamide detection methods are unfit for screening of products because they are either too insensitive or specific for a few compounds only. An immunoassay capable of detecting all sulfas in a single reaction would be ideal for screening. For development of a binder capable of binding all sulfas, a protein engineering approach was chosen and the properties of monoclonal antibody 27G3 were improved with mutagenesis followed by selection with phage display. Several different mutant antibodies were isolated. The cross-reaction profile of the best mutant antibody was significantly improved over that of the wild-type antibody: it was capable of binding 9 of the tested 13 sulfonamides within a narrow concentration range and also bound the rest of the sulfas, albeit within a wider concentration range.

Agricultural Applications

Protein engineering in **Bt** *toxins*

The structural similarity of all members of the family of three-domain *Bt* toxins, and the separate roles of the domains in the processes of receptor binding and channel formation, suggested that combining domains from different proteins could generate active toxins with novel specificities.

Transfer of the carbohydrate-binding domain III generated a Cry1Ab-Cry1C hybrid that was highly toxic to armyworm (*S. exigua*), an insect resistant to Cry1A toxins; the presence of the Cry1Ca domain III was sufficient to confer toxicity toward *Spodoptera* (de Maagd et al., 2000). More remarkably, a hybrid Cry protein, containing domains I and III from Cry1Ba and domain II of Cry1Ia, conferred resistance to the lepidopteran pest potato tuber moth (*Phthorimaea operculella*) and to the coleopteran Colorado potato beetle (*Leptinotarsa decemlineata*) when expressed in transgenic potato (Naimov *et al.*, 2003). The "parental" Cry proteins in this hybrid are lepidopteran specific, with no toxicity toward coleopterans such as the potato beetle, demonstrating the creation of a novel specificity.

Mutagenesis of three-domain Cry toxins

Modification of *Bt* toxins by site-directed mutagenesis to increase toxicity toward target pests has been employed as an alternative to the "domain swap" approach. The key role of domain II in three-domain Cry proteins in mediating interactions with insect receptors has been exploited by mutation of amino acid residues in the loop regions of this domain. Mutation of Cry1Ab increased its toxicity toward larvae of gypsy moth (*Lymantria dispar*) by up to 40-fold (Rajamohan *et al.*, 1996), and similar strategies were used to increase the toxicity of Cry3A protein toward target coleopteran pests (Wu *et al.*, 2000). The level to which rational design of toxins is possible is shown by the engineering of toxicity toward mosquito larvae into the lepidopteran-specific toxin Cry1Aa (Liu and 2006). Alternatively, a directed evolution system based on phage display technology for producing toxins with improved binding to a receptor, and thus increased toxicity, has been described (Ishikawa *et al.*, 2007).

Fusion Proteins

Transformation of plants with a gene construct containing a single translationally fused coding sequence encoding two Cry proteins has been used as an alternative to separate constructs (Bohorova *et al.*, 2001), although there is no apparent advantage over simpler methods for introducing two genes. However, addition of sequences from other proteins can be used to introduce extra functionality into Cry toxins. For example, the Gal-binding lectin domain (B-chain) from the ribosome-inactivating protein ricin was fused C terminally to domain III of Cry1Ac (Mehlo *et al.*, 2005), giving a fusion protein that could bind to Gal residues in potential receptors in the insect, in addition to binding to *N*-acetyl galactosamine residues by domain III of the toxin. Expression of the fusion protein in transgenic maize and rice (*Oryza sativa*) plants gave resistance to larvae of stemborers (*Chilo suppressalis*) and leaf armyworm (*Spodoptera littoralis*), whereas plants expressing the unmodified Cry1Ac were susceptible to both insects. Plants expressing the fusion protein were also resistant to a hemipteran pest, the leafhopper *Cicadulina mbila*; the lectin domain may cause this effect because *Bt* toxins are not effective against hemipterans.

Industrial Applications

(a) To create superior enzymes with the capacity to catalyze the production of high value specific chemicals.

(b) In the production of enzymes for large-scale use in the chemical industry.
(c) In the production of biological compounds including synthetic peptides, storage proteins and specific drugs that are superior to the natural ones.

Industrial manufacturing processes often require the use of harsh conditions, specifically toxic chemicals, high temperatures, or extremes in pH. A large portion of biotechnology research is focused on replacing these processes with those mediated by enzymes, that can tolerate these extremes and reduce the use of chemicals, or perform the same reactions under more moderate conditions. Success in these areas of research might mean reduced harm to the environment, lower costs in terms of energy used, less dependence on non-renewable resources and less risk to production employees. Many new techniques for improving the industrial effectiveness of pre-existing enzymes have been made possible since the discovery of PCR. These include DNA sequencing, site-directed mutagenesis and DNA shuffling. Other advances in biotech have led to the development of methods that make it possible to screen large numbers of new recombinant or mutant microorganisms expressing the modified enzymes, and select the best one for a specific application. Large throughput screening has facilitated significant advances in enzyme technology in recent years, since we no longer have to test individual recombinant microorganisms, or their purified enzyme products, one at a time, for improved efficiency of a particular process.

CONCLUSION AND FUTURE PROSPECTS

There are two main motivations for pursuing protein design: (i) design is the ultimate test of our understanding of natural proteins; and (ii) current design efforts represent the first step towards a new generation of novel macromolecules that will have practical applications in industry and biomedicine. Are these motivations justified by the designed proteins described in this chapter? How well has our understanding of natural proteins stood up to the rest of design and how well have current designs laid the ground work for the eventual construction of practical macromolecules? This is not to say that current design demonstrates that we understand all there is to know about proteins. In a sense, the first step—obtaining compact and stable structure—has been easier than expected. However, the difficulty of the second step—the design of uniquely determined interiors—has shown us that there are central features in natural proteins whose importance we did not fully appreciate prior to our attempts to design them.

In terms of the practical goal of designing functionally useful proteins, again the first steps have been remarkably successful while the later steps may be more elusive. It now seems relatively easy to generate macromolecules that possess some low level of activity, as demonstrated by several examples described in the previous sections. However, none of the current generation of novel protein approach the level of either specificity or activity produced routinely by nature. Perhaps our shortcomings here mirror our shortcomings in the design of structure. Perhaps it is easy to produce some activity because it is easy to direct atoms into "more or less" the right place. However, obtaining a level of activity comparable to that produced by nature may require us to pin down the positions of atoms with far greater precision than we are yet capable of doing. Nature's success at making "practical" macromolecules is the product of innumerable trials and errors conducted over 4 billion years.

Protein engineering has proved to be one of the more fruitful technological approaches in industrial biotechnology, being both very powerful and able to generate valuable intellectual property. Protein engineering aims to present examples in which the application of protein engineering has successfully solved problems arising in industrial biotechnology. There is a section on its use to enhance purification of recombinant proteins. The use of protein engineering to modify the activity or the stability of industrial enzymes from lipases to proteases, from carboxypeptidases to glucanases and glucosidases, and from pectin modifying enzymes to enzymes able to degrade recalcitrant compounds is extensively covered. It is shown how areas as diverse as agrofood technology, fine chemistry, detergents, bioremediation and biosensors receive significant contributions from protein and solvent engineering. The application of protein engineering to health care is also covered, from the development of new vaccines to new potential therapeutic proteins. A specific notation is given to protein engineering in the development of target molecules for drug discovery.

FURTHER READINGS

1. Arnold, F. H. and Georgiou, G. (2003) Directed enzyme evolution screening and selection methods. *Methods in Molecular Biology* **(230):** Humana Press, Totowa, NJ.
2. Arnold, F. H. and Georgiou, G. (2003) Directed evolution library creation methods and protocols. *Methods in Molecular Biology.* **(231):** Humana Press, Totowa, NJ.
3. Axe, D. D., Foster, N. W., and Fersht, A. R. (1996) Active barnase variants with completely random hydrophobic cores. *Proc. Natl. Acad. Sci. USA.* **(3):** 5590-5594.
4. Bittker, J. A., Le, B. V., Liu, J. M., and Liu, D. R. (2004) Directed evolution of protein enzymes using nonhomologous random recombination. *Proc. Natl. Acad. Sci. USA.* **(101):** 7011-7016.
5. Bowie, J. U., Reidhaar-Olson, J. F., Lim,W. A., and Sauer, R. T. (1990) Deciphering the message in protein sequences: tolerance to amino acid substitutions. *Science.* **(247):** 1306-1310.
6. Brooks, C. L. 3rd. (2002) Protein and peptide folding explored with molecular simulations. *Acc. Chem. Res.* **(35):** 447-454.
7. Brown, C. L., Aksay, I. A., Saville, D. A., and Hecht, M. H. (2002) Template-directed assembly of a ***de novo*** designed protein. *J. Am. Chem. Soc.* **(124):** 6846-6848.
8. Bryson, J. W., Betz, S. F., Lu, H. S., *et al.* (1995) Protein design: a hierarchic approach. *Science.* **(270):** 935-941.
9. Desjarlais, J. R. and Handel, T. M. (1995) *De-novo* design of the hydrophobic cores of proteins. *Protein Sci.* **(4):** 2006-2018.
10. Dunbrack, R. (2002) Rotamer libraries. *Curr. Opin. Struct. Biol.* **(12):** 431-440.
11. Gassner, N. C., Baase, W. A., and Matthews, B. W. (1996) A test of the "jigsaw puzzle" model for protein folding by multiple methionine substitutions within the core of T4 lysozyme. *Proc. Natl. Acad. Sci. USA.* **(93):** 12,155–12,158.
12. Go, N. (1983) Theoretical studies of protein folding. *Annu. Rev. Biophys. Bioeng.* **(12):** 183-210.
13. Hecht, M. H., Das, A., Go, A., Bradley, L. H., and Wei,Y. (2004) *De novo* proteins from designed combinatorial libraries. *Protein Sci.* **(13):** 1711-1723.
14. Jones, D. T. (1994) De novo protein design using pairwise potentials and a genetic algorithm. *Protein Sci.* **(3):** 567–574.
15. Kamtekar, S., Schiffer, J. M., Xiong, H., Babik, J. M., and Hecht, M. H. (1993) Protein design by binary patterning of polar and nonpolar amino acids. *Science.* **(262):** 1680-1685.

16. Kmiecik, S., and Kolinski, A, (2007) "Characterization of protein-folding pathways by reduced-space modeling". *Proc. Natl. Acad. Sci. U.S.A.* 104 **(30): **12330-5.
17. Kraemer-Pecore, C. M.,Wollacott, A. M., and Desjarlais, J. R. (2001) Computational protein design. *Curr. Opin. Chem. Biol.* **(5)**: 690-695.
18. Lau, K. F. and Dill, K. A. (1990) Theory for protein mutability and biogenesis. *Proc. Natl. Acad. Sci. USA.* **(87)**: 638-642.
19. Lim, W. A. and Sauer, R. T. (1989) Alternative packing arrangements in the hydrophobic core of lambda repressor. *Nature.* **(339):** 31-36.
20. Moffet, D. A. and Hecht, M. H. (2001) *De novo* proteins from combinatorial libraries. *Chem. Rev.* **(101):** 3191-3203.
21. Montal, M., Montal, M. S. and Tomich. J. M. (1990). Synporins–synthetics proteins that emulate the pore structure of biological ionic channels. *Proc. Natl. Acad. Sci. USA.* **(87):** 6929-6933.
22. Moore, G. L. and Maranas, C. D. (2000) Modeling DNA mutation and recombination for directed evolution experiments. *J. Theor. Biol.* **(205):** 483-503.
23. Moore, G. L. and Maranas, C. D. (2002) Predicting out-of-sequence reassembly in DNA shuffling. *J. Theor. Biol.* **(219):** 9-17.
24. Moore, G. L., Maranas, C. D., Lutz, S., and Benkovic, S. J. (2001) Predicting crossover generation in DNA shuffling. *Proc. Natl. Acad. Sci. USA.* **(98):** 3226-3231.
25. Moore, J. C., Jin, H. M., Kuchner, O., and Arnold, F. H. (1997) Strategies for the *in vitro* evolution of protein function—enzyme evolution by random recombination of improved sequences. *J. Mol. Biol.* **(272):** 336-347.
26. Ojeda, P., Garcia, M. (2010) "Electric field-driven disruption of a native beta-sheet protein conformation and generation of a helix-structure". *Biophysical Journal.* 99 **(2):** 595-599
27. P. A., He Y., Chen, Y., Orban, J., Bryan, P. N. (2007) "The design and characterization of two proteins with 88% sequence identity but different structure and function". *Proc. Natl. Acad. Sci. U.S.A.* 104 **(29):** 11963-8
28. Patrick, W. M., Firth, A. E., and Blackburn, J. M. (2003) User-friendly algorithms for estimating completeness and diversity in randomized protein-encoding libraries. *Protein Eng.* **(16):** 451-457.
29. Richardson, J. S. and Richardson, D. C. (1988) Amino acid preferences for specific locations at the ends of alpha helices. *Science.* **(240):** 1648-1652.
30. Riddle, D. S., Santiago, J. V., Bray-Hall, S. T., *et al.* (1997) Functional rapidly folding proteins from simplified amino acid sequences. *Nat. Struct. Biol.* **(4):** 805-809.
31. Robson, B, Vaithilingham A. (2008) Protein folding revisited. Progress in molecular biology and translational science. *Molecular Biology of Protein Folding.* **(84):** 161-202, Elsevier Press/Academic Press.
32. Rosenbaum, D. M., Roy, S., and Hecht, M. H. (1999) Screening combinatorial libraries of *de novo* proteins by hydrogen-deuterium exchange and electrospray mass spectrometry. *J. Am. Chem. Soc.* **(121):** 9509-9513.
33. Roy, S. and Hecht, M. H. (2000) Cooperative thermal denaturation of proteins designed by binary patterning of polar and nonpolar amino acids. *Biochemistry.* **(39):** 4603-4607.
34. Roy, S., Helmer, K. J., and Hecht, M. H. (1997) Detecting native-like properties in combinatorial libraries of ***de novo*** proteins. *Folding Des.* **(2):** 89-92.
35. Roy, S., Ratnaswamy, G., Boice, J. A., Fairman, F., McLendon, G., and Hecht, M. H. (1997) A protein designed by binary patterning of polar and nonpolar amino acids displays native-like properties. *J. Am. Chem. Soc.* **(119):** 5302-5306.
36. Shakhnovich, E. I. and Gutin, A. M. (1993) A new approach to the design of stable proteins. *Protein Eng.* **(6):** 793-800.

37. Sharma, V., Kaila, V. R., and Annila, A. (2009) "Protein folding as an evolutionary process". *Physica A.* 388 **(6):** 851-862
38. Sharma, V., Kaila. V. R. I., and Annila, A. (2009) "Protein folding as an evolutionary process". *Physica A.* 388 **(6):** 851-862.
39. Shea, J. E. and Brooks, C. L. 3rd. (2001) From folding theories to folding proteins: a review and assessment of simulation studies of protein folding and unfolding. *Annu. Rev. Phys. Chem.* **(52):** 499-535.
40. Silverman, J. A., Balakrishnan, R., and Harbury, P. B. (2001) Reverse engineering the (b/a)8 barrel fold. *Proc. Natl. Acad. Sci. USA.* **(98):** 3092-3097.
41. Sun, F. (1999) Modeling DNA shuffling. *J. Comput. Biol.* **(6):** 77-90.
42. Taylor, S. V., Walter, K. U., Kast, P., and Hilvert, D. (2001) Searching sequence space for protein catalysts. *Proc. Natl. Acad. Sci. USA.* **(98):** 10,596-10,601.
43. Wei,Y., Liu, T. I. P., Sazinsky, S. L., Moffet, D. A., and Hecht, M. H. (2003) Well folded ***de novo*** proteins from a designed combinatorial library. *Protein Sci.* **(12):** 92-102.
44. West, M. W.,Wang,W., Patterson, J., Mancias, J. D., Beasley, J. R., and Hecht, M. H. (1999) *De novo* amyloid proteins from designed combinatorial libraries. *Proc. Natl. Acad. Sci. USA.* **(96):** 11,211-11,216.
45. Xiong, H., Buckwalter, B. L., Shieh, H. M., and Hecht, M. H. (1995) Periodicity of polar and nonpolar amino acids is the major determinant of secondary structure in self-assembling oligomeric peptides. *Proc. Natl. Acad. Sci. USA.* **(92):** 6349-6353.
46. Xu, G., Wang, W., Groves, J. T., and Hecht, M. H. (2001) Self-assembled monolayers from a designed combinatorial library of *de novo* â-sheet proteins. *Proc. Natl. Acad. Sci. USA.* **(98):** 3652-3657.

CHAPTER

19

Nano-Biotechnology

Nano-biotechnology is one of the most future-technologies of the 21st century. Nano-biotechnology is becoming established in the interdisciplinary area, supported by a dynamic boom in innovations and will promote close cooperation between the life sciences, physical and chemical science as well as engineering. It is bridging the gap between inanimate and animate nature and aims at understanding the basic principles of biological functional units as well as creating extremely small components at "nano-scale" in a controlled way with technical materials. The convergence of nanotechnology and biomedical sciences opens a wide variety of biological research topics and medical uses at the molecular and cellular level. The real applications can turn around the life cycle of human beings in the years to come.

Keywords: Nano-biotechnology, nanotechnology, nano-scale engineering, molecular engineering, nanoscience.

INTRODUCTION

The nanotechnology has been rightly defined as an area of science, devoted to rational manipulation of atoms and molecules leading to controlled creation of structures in the nanometer (one billionth of a meter) scale size (ranging from 1 to 100 nm), which retain unique properties. The physical and chemical properties of materials can significantly improve or change radically as their size is scaled down to form small clusters of atoms. The unique arrangement, spacing and suitable decoration of molecules may result into improved and unique functional properties.

In other words, Nanotechnology is the design, fabrication and utilization of materials, devices and systems through control of matter on the nanometer length scale and exploitation of novel phenomena and physical, chemical or biological, properties at the nanometer scale. In modern times, the subject of Nanotechnology is now redesignated as "Molecular Nanotechnology" or "Nano-scale Engineering". The properties of materials, when manipulated at quantum or nano scale level, result in production of such novel materials which are lighter, stronger, smarter, cheaper, cleaner and with more precise and defined properties.

Among many other nanomolecules, the colloidal gold, iron oxide crystals, quantum dots, semiconductor nanocrystals, carbon nanotubes and colloidal selenium are only a few examples of nanoparticles, whose size is generally in the range 1 to 20 nm and have potential diagnostic applications in biology and medicine (Figure. 19.1). Besides this, a great amount of structural and functional diversity of protein molecules and their subunits has generated intense interest in designing novel architecture of nanometric dimensions for nanotechnology applications. These nanometric biomolecules have been used significantly in a number of applications including scaffolds for tissue engineering, microelectronics, computation, therapeutics and novel antibacterial agents, peptide nanotubes coupled with silver nanowires for use as degradable casting moulds, peptide scaffolds to support neural growth in damaged optic nerves, development of drug delivery systems and ultra sensitive nano-biosensors and diagnostics for various diseases.

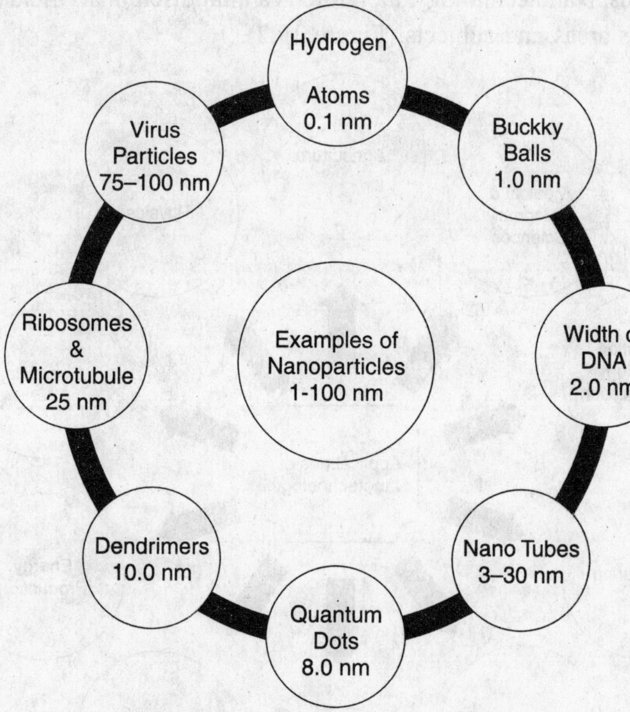

Figure 19.1 Example of nanoparticles.

The small size, surface tailorability, extraordinarily improved solubility and the ability to decorate bio-nanostructures with functional groups has resulted in strong and cooperative interaction of the nanoscale structures with complex biological system. Especially, the protein and peptide based nanostructures have distinct advantages over other inorganic nanoassemblies because these molecules can be easily modified with chemical and biological elements. The molecular self-assembly and fabrication of intact protein molecules, their subunits or even the synthetic peptides have been exploited in a major way to develop improved diagnostics with enhanced sensitivity. Owing to encouraging findings and diverse applications, there has been great interest in engineering peptide and protein-based systems for potential applications in nanosystems and nanodevices development.

Recent advances in the field of modern Structural Biology has resulted in availability of detailed structural information and conformational attributes of proteins and their subunits using techniques like X-ray Crystallography, Nuclear Magnetic Resonance (NMR), Circular Dichroism (CD) Spectroscopy, Confocal Microscopy, Scanning Tunnel Electron Microscopy (STEM), Atomic Force Microscopy (AFM), Scanning Probe Microscope (SPM) and Mass Spectrometry. The coupling of structural information with molecular dynamics studies and nanophysical manipulation techniques has enabled us in elucidating the correlation between protein structure and function. The detailed interrogation of structural properties of protein subunits, supplemented with protein engineering has led to either modification of existing molecules or even creation of entirely new molecules, with all together different and novel properties. These modified nano-biostructures have been increasingly used in developing new generation diagnostics, prophylactics and therapeutics for uplifting living standards. Nanotechnology, therefore is a multidisciplinary field and have made its presence felt in various areas and subjects (Figure 19.2).

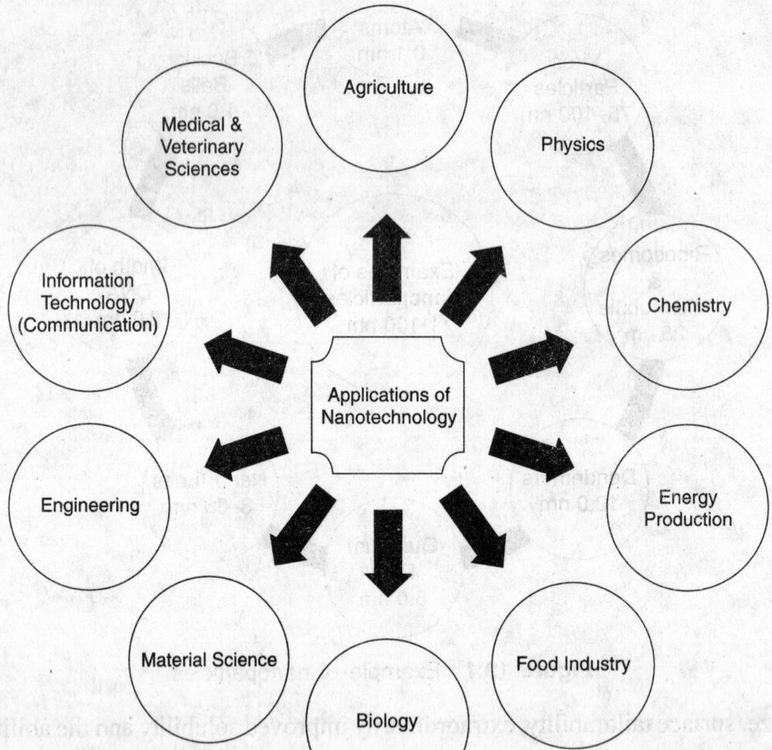

Figure 19.2 Applications of nanotechnology.

CONCEPTS AND PRINCIPLES

As early as in 1831, Michael Faraday first investigated red gold colloids and postulated that the color of gold particles was due to miniaturization of the gold particles. Since then, the gold and silver particles have been used as a colorant material for over 2000 (or 200) years. During the 1950s, the term 'Molecular Engineering' was coined by Arthur Hippel and he hypothesized the possibility of constructing nanomolecular devices. In the year 1959, a renowned Physicist and Nobel Laureate, Richard Feynman envisioned the area of nanotechnology by pointing out that 'there is plenty of room at the bottom'. Later, in the year 1974, the word Nanotechnology was coined by Norio Taniguchi, a material scientist. The scientists during that time were trying to develop miniature chips in electronics. It was the vision of Feynman that he even foresaw the possibility of developing nano machines at the molecular scale.

Then in 2007 came that day when the highest award in science 'The Nobel Prize' was given to Albert Fert and the German Peter Grünberg for developing the giant magnetic resonance technology, which led to miniaturization of the data discs and revolutionized the field of information and communication technology. The following workers have bagged the Nobel prizes for their research in the area of atomic and subatomic particle research:

1. Discovery of Scanning Tunnel Microscope in 1986 : Gerd Binnig and Heinrich Rohrer
2. Development of Traps to isolate atoms and subatomic particles in 1989 : Hans Dehmelt and Wolfgang Paul
3. Developing subatomic particle detectors in 1992 : George Charpak
4. Developing neutron diffraction technique for structure determination in 1994 : Clifford Schull and Bertram Brockhouse
5. Developing methods to cool and trap atoms with the help of Laser Light in 1997 : Steven Chu, Claude Cohen – Tannoudji and William Phillips
6. Developing Giant Magnetic Resonance Technology in 2007 : Albert Fert and Peter Grünberg

In the developing countries also, lot of efforts have been made to welcome the era of nanotechnology and at present, several developing countries have launched national nanotechnology initiatives in order to strengthen their capacity and sustain economic growth. In a recent paper by Buentello *et al.*, (2005), about ten priority areas have been listed which will have a major influence on Nanotechnology. These areas include:

1. Energy storage, production and conversion
2. Agricultural productivity enhancement
3. Water treatment and remediation
4. Disease diagnosis and screening
5. Drug delivery systems
6. Food processing and storage
7. Air pollution and remediation
8. Construction
9. Health monitoring
10. Vector and pest detection and control

The ability to use nanoscience to improve the quality of materials through understanding and refining their nano scale structures is an example of a form of nanotechnology that has been called Incremental Nanotechnology whereas, when the reduction in size of structures leads to step changes in properties, that provide radical new solutions to problems and new commercial opportunities, these types of applications are considered to be Evolutionary Nanotechnology. Besides this, the science of nanotechnology has now touched almost every sphere of mankind. It has made remarkable developments in agriculture, medicine, pharmaceuticals, food sector, and most of the industries are now exploring opportunities to harness the benefits of molecules at the nano scale.

APPLICATIONS OF NANO-BIOTECHNOLOGY

Industrial Applications

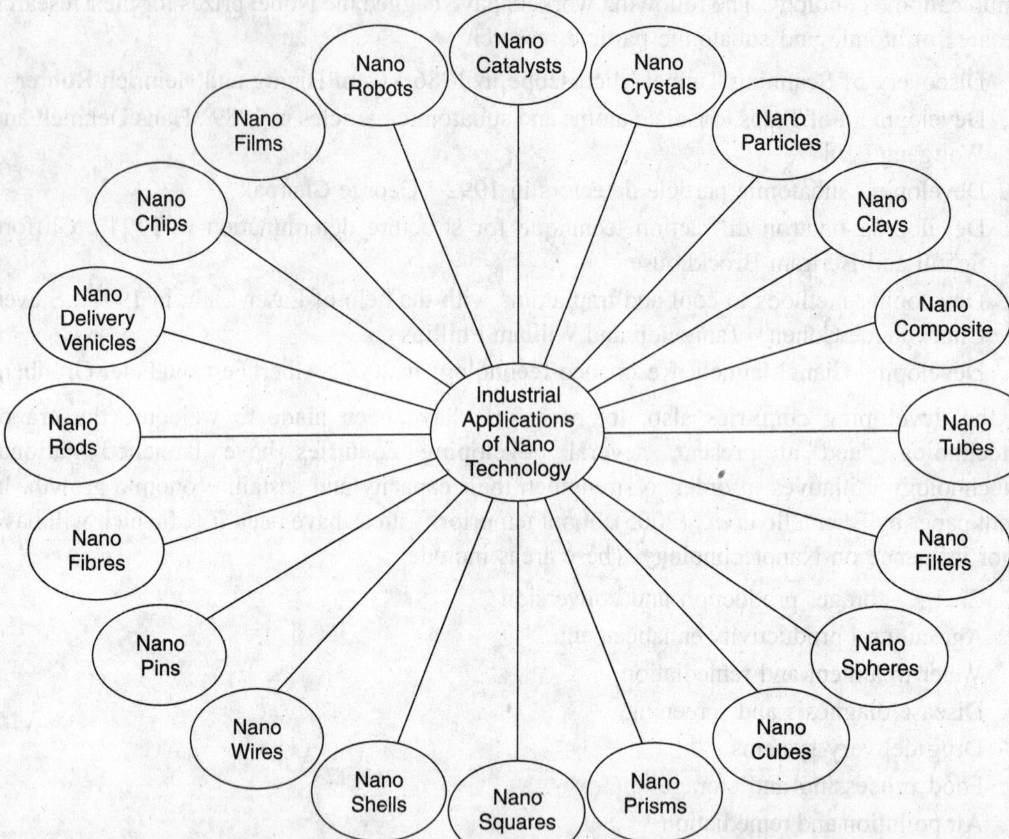

Figure 19.3. Representative examples of industrial nanotechnologies.

Nano fabrics

This is not to say that nanotechnology is a far-off, fuzzy, futuristic technology. It is not. It has already established a beachhead in the economy. The clothing industry is starting to feel the effects of nanotech. As for example scientists are using embedded nanoparticles to create stain-repellent khakis (Figure 19.3).

Nano crystals

Metal nanocrystals might be incorporated into car bumpers, making the parts stronger, or into aluminum, making it more wear resistant. Metal nanocrystals might be used to produce bearings that last longer than their conventional counterparts, new types of sensors and components for computers and electronic hardware (Figure 19.3).

Nanocrystals of various metals have been shown to be 100 percent, 200 percent and even as much as 300 percent harder than the same materials in bulk form. Because wear resistance often is dictated by the hardness of a metal, parts made from nanocrystals might last significantly longer than conventional parts.

Nanocrystals are an ideal light harvester in photovoltaic devices. They absorb sunlight more strongly than dye molecules or bulk semiconductor material, therefore high optical densities can be achieved while maintaining the requirement of thin films. Perfectly crystalline CdSe (expand the term) nanocrystals are also an artificial reaction center, separating the electron hole pair on a femtosecond timescale. Fluorescent nanocrystals have several advantages over organic dye molecules as fluorescent markers in biology. They are incredibly bright and do not photodegrade. Drug-conjugated nanocrystals attach to the protein in an extracellular fashion, enabling movies of protein trafficking. They also form the basis of a high-throughput fluorescence assay for drug discovery.

Nanoparticles

Many vitamins and their precursors, such as carotenoids, are insoluble in water but when they are skillfully produced and formulated as nanoparticles, these substances can easily be mixed with cold water, thereby increasing their bioavailability in the body. Many lemonades and fruit juices contain these specially formulated nanoparticle additives, which often also provide an attractive color to the product. In the cosmetics sector also, nanoparticulate zinc oxide based UV absorbers are being manufactured (Figure 19.3).

Researchers have created nanoparticulate-based synthetic bone by manipulation of calcium and phosphate at the molecular level, which is identical in structure and composition to natural bone made of a calcium and phosphate composite called Hydroxyapatite. This novel synthetic bone will be of immense applications in case of fractures and soft tissue injuries where natural bone is damaged or removed.

Nanostructured materials

Various nanostructured materials like tungsten-carbide-cobalt composite powder is used to make a sintered alloy as hard as diamond, which is in turn is used to make cutting tools, drill bits, armor plate, and jet engine parts. This is one of the impacts of making the things small and to generate such materials with more novel properties and enhance durability of the product (Figure 19.3).

Nanoclays and nanocomposites

Nanoclays has been used in the packaging industry thereby allowing thinner and light weight material to hold the pressure and carbonation inside the beer and soft drink bottles and also increasing shelf life. The nanoclays and nanocomposites have found many applications including flame retardants, barrier film and bottle barriers. They are not only used to improve existing products, but also are extending their reach into those areas which were totally dominated by metal, glass and wood (Figure 19.3).

Nanocomposite coatings

Nanoparticles have been used as coatings on various surfaces to improve their properties. As for example, in the paint industry, this nanocoatings have improved the surface properties of the metals and other surfaces on which these paints are coated. They improve the surface luster and hardness etc. Similarly, the tennis balls coated with nanocomposite mix of butyl rubber, intermingled with nanoclay particles keeps it bouncing twice as long as an old-style ball. The same technology is now being extended to the vehicle tires which would make them lighter and last longer.

Agricultural Applications

Precision farming has been introduced to maximise agricultural outputs by minimizing the inputs at the same time thoroughly monitoring environmental variables and applying targeted action. Precision farming makes use of computers, global satellite positioning systems, and remote sensing devices to measure highly localised environmental conditions thus determining whether crops are growing at maximum efficiency or precisely identifying the nature and location of problems. Parameters governing plant development like seeding, fertilizer applications, chemical and water use can be fine-tuned to lower production costs and potentially increase production thereby benefiting the farmers in terms of increased production.

Precision farming is also aimed to reduce agricultural waste and thus keep environmental pollution to a minimum. In this direction, tiny sensors and monitoring systems based on nanotechnology will have a large impact on future precision farming methodologies. These nanosensors could be distributed throughout the field and will have potential applications in monitoring the soil conditions and crop growth. The precision farming based on smart nanosensors like carbon nanotube sensor or nano-cantilevers will help to trap and measure individual proteins or even small molecules. Nanoparticles or nanosurfaces can be decorated with functional groups or biomolecules like antibodies to trigger an electrical or chemical signal in the presence of a contaminant such as bacteria. In other nanosensor design, the enzymes or dendrimers are used as probes to bind to target chemicals and proteins (Figure 19.4).

Nanotechnology has the potential to enhance agricultural productivity through various ways:

1. By genetic improvement of plants
2. Cellular delivery of various genes and drug molecules
3. Nano-array based gene technologies for targeted gene expression in plants
4. Development of nano-sensors for precision agriculture, early detection of plant pathogens and various contaminants in food
5. Novel smart delivery systems for agro-chemicals, fertilizers and pesticides
6. Better ways and strategies for developing better processing and packaging of food products
7. Information and communication technology in agriculture for monitoring agricultural and food system security

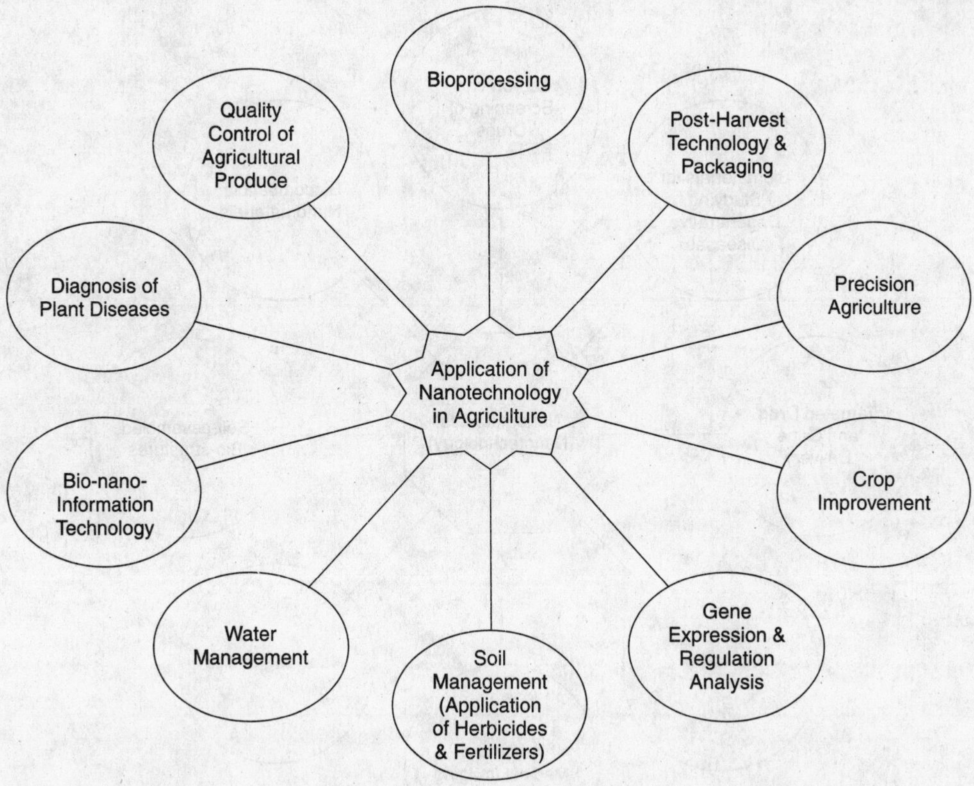

Figure 19.4 Applications of nanotechnology in agriculture.

Medical Applications

The nanomolecules possess certain size dependent properties with respect to optical and magnetic parameters that are usually exploited and manipulated to achieve detectable signals in the development of diagnostics. The basis of developing any nanoparticle-based assay is to generate a measurable signal by binding of a nanoparticle label or probe to the target biomolecule. The nanoparticle label in cases of animal disease diagnostic assays can be either native or recombinant protein, protein subunits, peptides or peptidic dendrimers immobilized on nanoparticles or self-assembled peptidic or protein nanoparticles, which can be used to detect the respective, specific antibody targets. On the contrary, the nanoparticles like colloidal gold, selenium or iron oxide and even the peptidic nanotubes, which are decorated with highly specific purified polyclonal or monoclonal antibodies can be used to detect target protein in the clinical sample. In addition to this, the fluorophore functionalized quantum dots, nanoshells, nanospheres, nanotubes and metal nanoparticles have been successfully utilized as probes for detection of target analyte and pathogens, either in visual assays or those involving fluorescence microscopy or even screening samples in a format, what is called as 'lab-on-chip' screening.

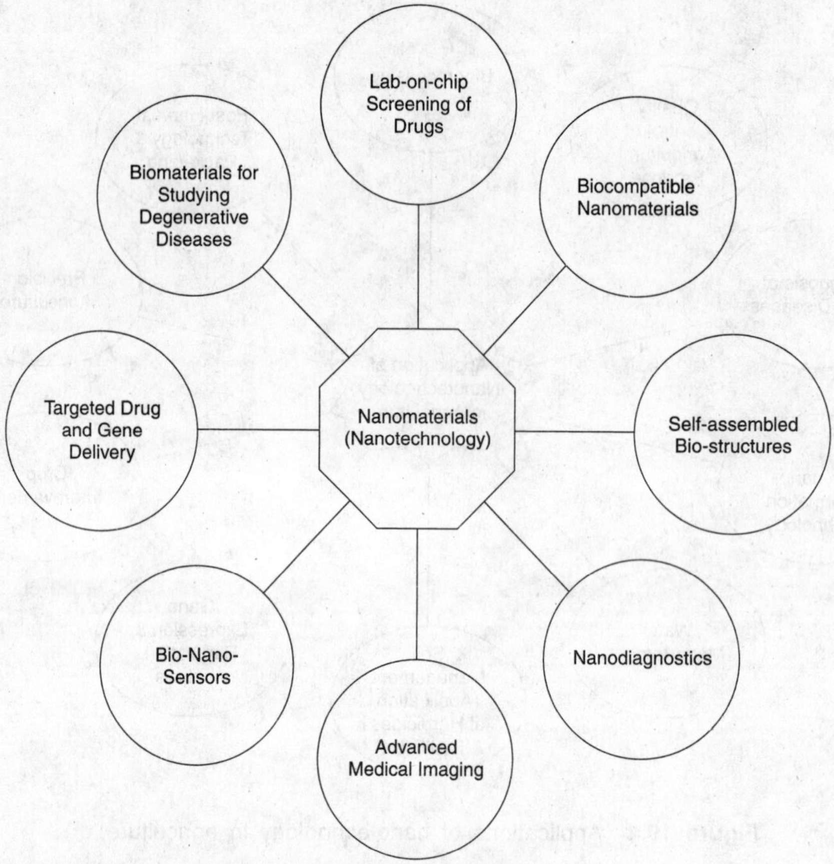

Figure 19.5 Biomedical applications of nanotechnology.

Proteins and Peptidic Nanostructures

The peptide and protein based nanostructures serve as the major molecular scaffold material of the biological world at the nano scale, microscale and even macroscale. To name a few, the self-assembled actin cytoskeleton nanomolecules provide physical rigidity to the cell. Similarly, the self-assembled microtubules serve as nanoscopic protein railways that permit transport of 'cargo' within the cell. Besides this, the proteins like collagen and keratin in skin and nails, respectively, form building blocks for macroscopic structural elements. Additionally, the proteins also constitute building blocks for natural structures possessing unique protection, as for example, silk fibroin, whose ratio of tensile strength to density is about five times higher than that of steel. Similarly, the formation of inorganic biological structures such as bones and teeth and shells of marine animals are an outcome of specific interaction of proteins and peptides with calcium or silicon ions. The protein and peptides also facilitate the biological recognition via receptor-ligand interactions. Thus taken together, the proteins serve both as building scaffold, as well as, functional entities in the biological world and this is the reason why proteins and their peptide fragments has been viewed as potential sources of engineered "Smart Function Materials".

The architecturally engineered peptide and protein nanobiomolecules have found diverse applications in the biomedical research. But in order to successfully integrate these nanostructures into various desired applications, they must be suitably decorated with functional elements such as specific antibodies, receptors, inorganic molecules, fluorophores, dyes and even other functional proteins (Figure 19.5).

Synthesis of Protein and Peptidic Nanosystems

The proteins and peptide fragments can be synthesized either by chemical or biological means. The chemical synthesis, which is the most preferred approach, facilitates incorporating artificial amino acid analogs and generating modified products with groups like nucleic acids (PNAs), sugars (glycopeptides), fluorophores (fluoropeptides) or other small molecules. These artificially synthesized nanomolecules have an edge over cell-based expression systems in the sense that the purified procedures are more straightforward and desired modifications are relatively easy to incorporate. As against this, in the recombinant DNA techniques, the sequence of desired product is encoded as a DNA template that can be modified to generate a library of templates with varied structure, which can then be used to manufacture the desired protein or peptide using inherent protein synthesizing machinery of cells like bacteria or mammalian cells. However, the cell-free protein and peptide synthesis methods are always preferred and beneficial for generating large quantities of desired purified product for suitable applications in therapeutics, as well as, diagnostics.

Decorating Protein and Peptidic Nanosystems with Desired Groups

Various approaches have been in vogue for decorating proteins and peptidic nanostructures. One of the most promising approaches involve the non-covalent hydrogen bonding between bolamphiphile peptidic nanotubes and antibodies through the free amide sites of the nanotube side walls. This engineered decoration of nanomolecules resulted in the formation of antibody-coated nanotubes. In another approach, the affinity of short tripeptide arginine-glycine-glutamate (RGD) to specific cellular ligands is utilized for decoration of nanobiostructures.

In yet another approach, the avidin-biotin (A-B) interactions have been utilized for decorating several nanostructures. The extremely strong interaction (with Kd of 10^{-15}M) between avidin, the egg white and biotin (Vitamin H) is well known. This strongest non-covalent interaction in nature is being largely exploited for various applications such as development of immunoassays, molecular pull down and affinity chromatography procedures. These strong A-B interactions form the basis of functionalizing carbon nanotubes (CNTs) with various biological molecules and for decoration of protein and peptide based nanostructures with antibodies and chemical groups.

Applications of Nano-biotechnology in Diagnostic

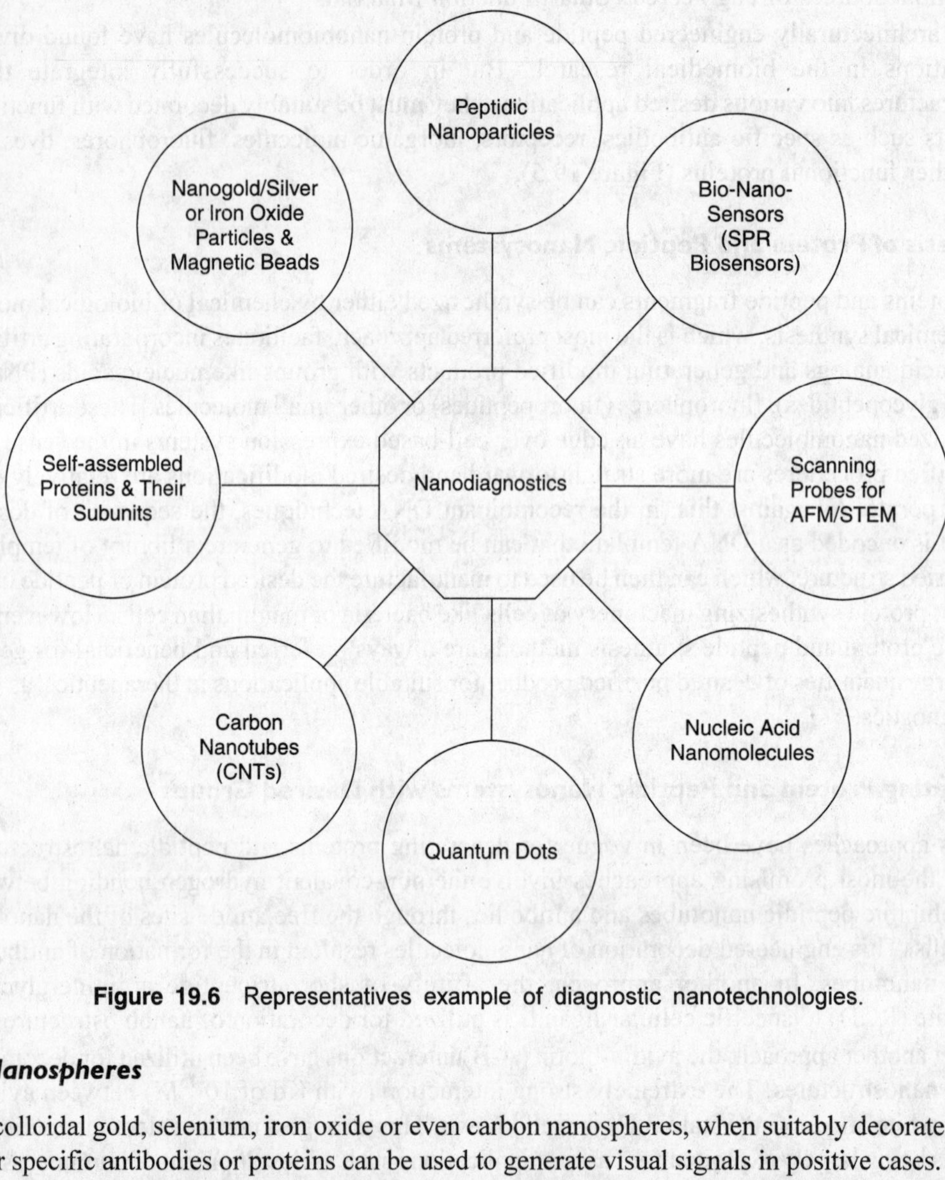

Figure 19.6 Representatives example of diagnostic nanotechnologies.

(i) *Nanospheres*

The colloidal gold, selenium, iron oxide or even carbon nanospheres, when suitably decorated with either specific antibodies or proteins can be used to generate visual signals in positive cases. These functionalized nanospheres are used extensively in development of hand-held assays, owing to unique property of generating a colored signal on aggregation/agglutination with respective specific target analyte. The macroscopic samples of pure gold have only one color, i.e., golden but nanoparticles of gold can show essentially all the colors of the rainbow depending upon the size and shape of nanoparticles formed. The intensity of optical absorption of gold nanoparticles is extraordinarily strong, which means that when suspended in a solution or deposited on a surface, the naked eye can detect very small quantity of these particles. These properties of gold nanoparticles make them suitable as visual indicators and the most appropriate candidate for developing pen-side diagnostic assays (Figure 19.6).

(ii) *Magna nanoparticles*

The magna bead assays are based on the interaction of an analyte with functionalized magnetic beads resulting into generation of magnetic signals, which can easily be detected with the help of magnetometer. This technology is increasingly used in development of assays for the detection of circulating cancer cells and specific microorganisms. Besides this, various kits based on magna bead technology are available for isolation and purification of nucleic acids and proteins and for techniques like Serial Analysis of Gene Expression.

(iii) *Metal nanotubes*

The nanotubes generated using metal ions like selenium and carbon or boron nitrides are used as electrodes, wherein, the open end of single stranded DNA is attached to them. The nucleic acid hybridization with complementary target results into generation of an electrochemical signal. This method has an advantage of detecting target at sensitivity in the atto mole range. It also has the advantage of minimizing the need of amplification of target nucleic acid. The method can be suitably modified to detect any substrate analyte provided the specific enzyme or molecule is attached to the nanotube.

(iv) *Nanowires*

The nanowires are molecular particles of specified shape, which are generated by fabrication of nanoparticles like gold, boron, nickel, selenium, etc. These nanowires allow definite and unique interactions with molecular entities. They can be associated and conjugated with almost any chemical or biological system to allow real-time detection of an analyte. They are most suitably used for *in vivo* diagnosis.

(v) *Nanopores*

The nanopores represent the pores between two membranes having the diameter in nanoscale range. These nanopores are so designed that on passage of electric current they become permeable to only charged molecules like nucleic acids and generate electric signals. These nanopores are used in devising label-less immunoassays. They are reported to have high sensitivity and can detect single base substitutions in DNA molecules.

(vi) *Fluorophore nanoparticles/resonance light scattering (RLS)*

The RLS technique is utilized in generating strong visual signals when incident light is scattered by metallic nanoparticles of uniform size like gold or silver. The high intensity fluorescence signals are sufficient enough to have a million fold increase in sensitivity over presently available detection methods. The RLS technique has been utilized in developing tube based nucleic acid detection assays like LAMP.

(vii) *Nanobarcodes*

The nanobarcodes are principally used for developing multiplexed protein assays and SNP mapping assays. The nanobarcodes are generated by sequential electrochemical deposition of metal ions to provide unique stripping patterns of differential reflectivity when examined by light microscopy. The nanobarcode diagnostics have provided a promising way of producing off-the-shelf, pen-side assays, which can be utilized to interpret results using a portable barcode reader.

(viii) *Nanocapacitors*

The nanocapacitor-based diagnostics measures a change in capacitance when a target DNA or analyte hybridizes with single stranded DNA or enzyme, which is interspersed with nanometallic wires and nanoparticle electrodes to form capacitors. When these probe capacitors are used in assays, they enable label-less detection of target nucleic acids in a sample.

(ix) *PEBBLE nanosensors*

The Probes Encapsulated by Biologically Localized Embedding (PEBBLE) nanosensors are used for real-time inter- and intra-cellular imaging of ions and molecules. The PEBBLE nanosensors are developed by entrapping sensor molecules in a chemically inert matrix via micro-emulsion polymerization process. These nanosensors generate strong electrochemical signals when coming across ionic molecules. At the same time, they are relatively insensitive to protein interferences.

(x) *Ferrofluid nanoparticles*

These ferrofluidic magnetic nanoparticles in liquid samples result in close interaction with the analytes. This is possible because these fluidic magnetic nanoparticles consist of a polymeric layer of a biological substrate with a magnetic core. The molecules with affinity for the target analyte are coated on the outer layer. The separation of ferrofluidic particles bound to analyte is affected by magnetic field. The specially developed ferrofluidic nanoparticles have resulted in making highly sensitive magnetic nanosensors.

(xi) *Surface plasmon resonance (SPR) nanosensors/affinity biosensors*

The biosensors allow detection of affinity-based interactions between biomolecules, as for example, that occurs in antibody-antigen recognition or DNA hybridization. The presence of antigens (target molecules) in an analyte can be verified by binding these molecules to their complementary antibodies (bio-receptors) immobilized onto a biosensor surface. The binding interactions can be very easily measured by sensitive technique like SPR, which is an optical technique that measures the refractive index of very thin layers of materials adsorbed on a metal. It offers the real-time *in situ* analysis of dynamic surface events and is capable of defining rates of adsorption and desorption for surface interactions. The plasmon-plasmon resonance resulting from the interaction of locally adjacent gold nanoparticle label that is bound to a target produces a specific change in optical properties that can be used for diagnosis (Figure 19.7).

The most important challenge in developing a sensitive biosensor is the interaction between inorganic (transducer) and organic materials (e.g., the biological targets), for which extra miniaturization of transducer material using gold, SiO_2 or Ta_2O_5 nanoparticles is desired. Another alternative is formation of self-assembled monolayers (SAMs) by either thiol or silane binding. The multiple antigenic peptides (MAPs) and protein subunits have been reported to possess inherent capacity of forming SAMs, which can be easily exploited to develop sensitive label-less biosensors for detection of specific antibodies.

Using SAMs, the metal surfaces of transducer like platinium and palladium or gold can be very easily modified at nanoscale. The surfaces can be made totally hydrophilic or hydrophobic or functionalized with desired functional groups by a few nanometer thick thiol layer. In addition to this, using mixed SAMs, selective immobilization of biomolecules like antibodies and antigens becomes possible to fabricate the transducer metal surface. These all possibilities reflect that the overall performance of a biosensor can be greatly enhanced by using most appropriate chemistries on the nanoscale.

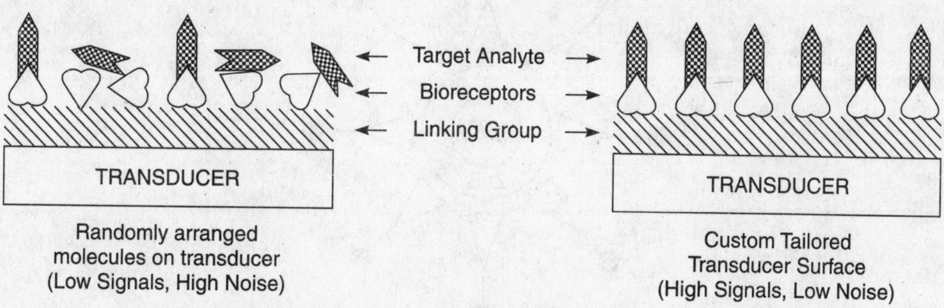

Figure 19.7 Surface Plasmon Resonance (SPR) nanosensors.

(xii) *Nanoshells*

The gold nanoshells provide great sensitivity for the detection of DNA and proteins. The nanoshells can be easily used to label either DNA or protein molecules like protein-A or antibodies, which can then bind to their respective targets. The colloidal gold nanoshells have characteristic red color that changes to bluish purple on colloid aggregation. Silver can be involved in the visualization process and the silver-coated gold nanoparticles (40-100 nm size) have strong light scattering properties, which can be easily detected by standard dark field microscopy with white light illumination. Using this technique, the detection limit of oligonucleotides has been cut down to approximately 10 fmol, which is about 50-fold lower than conventional fluorophore based methods. The gold nanoshells have been utilized to allow direct, rapid and economically feasible analysis of the whole blood samples. The nanoshells possess exceptional biocompatibility, as their behavior is almost identical to that of gold colloids. This property of nanoshells along with tunability (i.e., capability of changing nanoparticle size) of their optical properties allows successful development of highly sensitive immunoassays capable of analyzing multiple antigens simultaneously.

(xiii) *Quantum dots*

The quantum dots (QDs) represent a class of most used and promising nanostructures available for diagnostic applications (Figure 19.8). The QDs are semiconductor nanocrystals, which are characterized by strong light absorbance properties and can be used as fluorescent labels for biomolecules. QDs have a diameter of 2-8 nm and typically composed of a core consisting of a semiconductor material (e.g., CdSe) enclosed in a shell of another semiconductor material (ZnS) with larger spectral band gap. The QDs can be made water soluble and biocompatible by modifying their surface by silanization or coating with thiol containing groups, organic phosphines, dendrons or peptides. The QDs can be easily detected and tracked using different techniques like fluorometry and microscopy such as fluorescence, confocal, total internal reflection, wide-field epifluorescence, atomic force and multiphoton microscopy.

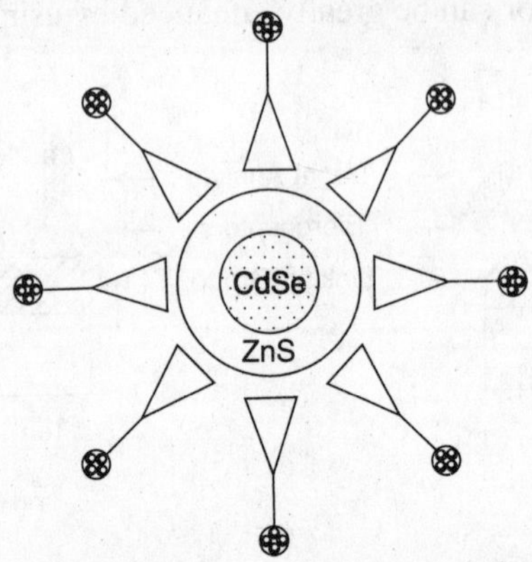

Figure 19.8 Diagrammatic representation of quantum dots (QD).

This group can be either streptavidin, biotin, mercaptoacetic acid, peptide, antibody, recombinant protein, nucleotides, aptamers or peptide nucleic acids (PNAs).

The QDs have found wide applications in diagnostics including detection of prostate specific antigens, acetylcholine, targeting specific P-glycoprotein (Pgp) in transfected Hela cells, for targeting cellular organelles like nucleus and mitochondria in endothelial and carcinoma cells and for targeting the breast cancer markers Her2 on SKBR-3 breast cancer cells. Besides this, the QDs have been a promising tool in *in vivo* imaging applications, wherein, the specific QDs have been detected at target site *in vivo*, using spectral imaging and fluorescence correlation spectroscopy techniques.

Current Status of Nano-biotechnology Research

The current focus of research in the field of nanotechnology is more inclined towards engineering applications. The natural nano-sized molecules such as proteins, nuclides, hydrocarbon, and lipids etc. amalgamated with the fundamental knowledge regarding nano devices, materials, drug design and manufacture of important products presents new dimensions and hopes in this area of research. The science of nanotechnology has its roots in different disciplines of biological sciences like biophysics and biochemistry and also have many relevant technologies in synthesis, assembly, genomics, proteomics, structural biology, toxicology, theoretical biology, biomaterials, bioelectronics, bioinformatics, and biochips.

For nanobiotechnology research at molecular level, there are biochips for disease detection, recognition mechanisms by nanostructure, lipid polymer for drug targeting; at cellular level, there is nano-crystal for fluorescent imaging, immune latex particles and at tissue level, there are multichannel SQUID for magnetic imaging, nano vaccine, and drug delivering. For clinical applications, we have cardiovascular disease diagnostic kits, stent surface material and corneal membrane for regeneration. Each will focus on the novelty for academic excellence and feasibility for industrial mass production. The intended applications include cancer, foot and mouth disease, and gene-modified organism (GMO), all of which have nano-scale limits. Various projects and areas where nanoscience has made its impact include the following:

- Molecular recognition of biomolecules versus nanostructures: design, synthesis, characterization and applications
- Inorganic nano particles as optical catalytic agent
- Nano vaccine delivery system for gene therapy
- Nano magnetic immune latex particles
- A study of purified montmorillonite intercalated 5-ASA composite for inflammatory bowel diseases
- Bifunctional group copolymer as drug delivery system
- Biodegradable nano capsule as a carrier for water soluble drug
- Cardiovascular disease screening and surface modification for STENT
- Infectious keratitis and corneal tissue regeneration by nano stacking
- Rapid nuclide screening kit for colon-rectal cancer
- Data mining for proteomic biochips
- Modified Au nano particles with rolling circle amplification (RCA)
- Protein chip and multifunction optical reader
- Nano scale force mapping for proteomics
- Design, fabrication and applications of biological nano switch
- Fluorescent nano crystal imaging for functional cell studies
- Multichannel quantum dot for SQUID measurement
- Ecological monitoring by nanobiotechnology

CONCLUSION AND FUTURE PROSPECTS

Major applications of Nanotechnology include nanocoating, nucleic acid bioengineering, smart treatment delivery systems, nanobioprocessing, bioanalytical nano-sensors, nanomaterials and bio-selective surfaces and have been identified as some of the potential research areas that would have a significant impact on every field including agriculture. For example, development of low cost sensors for modern diagnostics can detect the presence of foodborne and agriculturally important pathogens, filters for removing undesirable compounds from foods and beverages and also nanoparticles to store flavors in meat and other packaged foods. With advent of hi-throughput experimentation technologies such as DNA & Protein chips (Microarrays) nanotechnology has the potential to miniature and represent a virtual plant or animal cell. Candidate gene studies, fine mapping, pharmacogenomics, linkage mapping, allele specific transcript detection, admixture mapping, clinical diagnostics, forensics, genetic identification are other areas where nanotechnology has made its interference. Increasing advances in the field of nanodiagnostics will allow better clinical diagnostic services, particularly in economically deprived regions and will offer very cost effective assays for diagnosing diseases. However, seeing the present-day progress in the field of research and development of nanotechnology, the advantages that these nanotechnologies offer are too good to dismiss and the concept that the 'World is going NANO' is not too far from becoming a reality.

FURTHER READINGS

1. Akerman M.E., Chan W.C., Laakkonen P., Bhatia S.N. and Luoslahti E. (2002) Nanocrystal targeting *in vivo. Proc. Natl. Acad. Sci. USA.* **(99):** 12617-12621.
2. Chan W.C. and Nie S. (1998) Quantum dot bioconjugates for ultrasensitive, nonisotopic detection. *Science.* **(281):** 2016-2018.
3. Crut A., Geron-Landre B., Bonnet I., Bonneau S., Desbiolles P. and Escude C. (2005) Detection of single DNA molecules by multi color quantum dot end labeling. *Nucleic Acids Res.* **(33):** e98.
4. Fortina P., Kricka L.J., Surrey S. and Grodzinski P. (2005) Nanobiotechnology: The promise and reality of new approaches to molecular recognition. *Trends. Biotechnol.* **(23):** 168-173.
5. Georganopoulou D.G., Chang L., Nam J.M., Thaxton C.S., Mufson E.J. and Klein W.L. (2005) Nanoparticle based detection in cerebral spinal fluid of soluble pathogenic biomarkers for Alzheimers disease. *Proc. Natl. Acad. Sci. USA.* **(102):** 2273-2276.
6. Green R.J., Frazier R.A., Shakesheff K.M., Davies M.C., Roberts C.J., Tendler S.J. (2000) Surface plasmon resonance analysis of dynamic biological interactions with biomaterials. *Biomaterials.* **(21):** 1823-1825.
7. Guler M.O., Soukasena S., Hulvat J.F. and Stupp S.I. (2005) Presentation and recognition of biotin on nanofibers formed by branched peptide amphiphiles. *Nano. Lett.* **(5):** 249-252.
8. Harma H., Soukka T. and Lougren T. (2001) Eropium nanoparticles and time resolved fluorescence for ultrasensitive detection of prostate-specific antigen. *Clin Chem.* **(47):** 561-568.
9. Hartgerink J.D., Bemash E. and Stupp S.I. (2001) Self-assembly and mineralization of peptide-amphiphile Nanofibers. *Science.* **(294):** 1684-1688.
10. Horton M., Khan A. and Maddison S. (2006) Delivering nanotechnology to the healthcare, IT and environmental sectors–a perspective from the 'London Centre for Nanotechnology'. *BT. Technology. Journal.* 24 **(3):** 175-183.
11. Jain K.K. (2003) Nanodiagnostics: Applications of nanotechnology in molecular diagnostics. *Expert. Rev. Mol. Diagn.* **(3):** 153-161.
12. Jain K.K. (2005) Nanotechnology in clinical laboratory diagnostics. *Clin. Chim. Acta.* **(358):** 37-54.
13. Jin T., Fujii F., Sakata H., Tamura M. and Kinjo M. (2005) Amphiphilic P-sulfonatocalix(4)arene-coated CdSe/ZnS quantum dots for the optical detection of the neurotransmitter acetylcholine. *Chem. Commun.* 4300-4302.
14. Kohli P. and Martin C.R. (2005) Smart nanotubes for biotechnology. *Curr Pharma. Biotechnol.* **(6):** 35-47.
15. Larson D.R., Zipfel W.R., Williams R.M., Clark S.W., Bruchez M.P. and Wise F.W. (2003) Water soluble quantum dots for multiphoton fluorescence imaging *in vitro*. *Science.* **(300):** 1434-1436.

16. Lewin M., Carlesso N., Tung C., Tang X.W., Cory D., Scadden D.T. and Weissleder R. (2000) Tat peptide-derivatized magnetic nanoparticles allow *in vivo* packing and recovery of progenitor cells. *Nat. Biotechnol.* **(18):** 410-414.
17. Martin C.R. (1994) Nanomaterials– A membrane based synthetic approach. *Science.* **(266):** 1961-1966.
18. Martin C.R. and Mitchell D.T. (1998) Nanomaterials in analytical Chemistry. *Anal Chem.* **(70):** 322A-327A.
19. Matsumura S., Uemura S. and Mihara H. (2005) Construction of biotinylated peptide nanotubes for arranging proteins. *Mol. Biosyst.* **(1):** 146.
20. Mazzola L. (2003) Commercializing nanotechnology. *Nat. Biotechnol.* **(21):** 1137-1143.
21. McNeil S.E. (2005) Nanotechnology for the biologist. *J. Leucocyte. Biol.* **(78):** 585-594.
22. Michalet X., Pinaud F.F., Bentolila L.A., Tsay J.M., Doose S., Li J.J. (2005) Quantum dots for live cells *in vivo* imaging and diagnostics. *Science.* **(307):** 538-544.
23. Moghimi S.M., Hunter A.C. and Murray J.C. (2005) Nanomedicine: current status and future prospects. *FASEB Journal.* **(19):** 311-330.
24. Nicewarner-Pena S.R., Freeman R.G., Reiss B.D., He L., Penna D.J. and Walton I.D. (2001) Submicrometer metallic barcodes. *Science.* **(294):** 137-141.
25. Nuraje N., Banerjee I.A., Macluspie R.I., Yu L.T. and Matsui H. (2004) Biological bottom-up assembly of antibody nanotubes on patterned antigen arrays. *J. Am. Chem. Soc.* 126 **(26):** 8088-8089.
26. Park S.J., Taton T.A. and Mirkin CA (2002) Assay-based electrical detection with nanoparticle probes. *Science.* **(295):** 1503-1506.
27. Reches M. and Gazit E. (2004) Formation of closed cage nanostructures by self-assembly of aromatic dipeptides. *Nano. Lett.* 4 **(4):** 581-585.
28. Rosi N.L. and Mirkin C.A. (2005) Nanostructures in biodiagnostics. *Chem. Rev.* **(105):** 1547-1562.
29. Salamanca-Buentello F., Persad D.L., Court E.B., Martin D.K., Daar A.S. and Singer P. (2005) Nanotechnology and the developing world. *PLoS Medicine.* 2 **(5):** 0100-0103.
30. Salata O. (2004). Applications of nanoparticles in biology and medicine. *J. Nanobiotechnol.* 2-3.
31. Shim M., Kam N.W.S., Chen R.J., Li Y.M. and Dai H.J. (2002) Functionalization of carbon nanotubes for biocompatibility and biomolecular recognition. *Nano. Lett.* **(2):** 285- 289.
32. Shrivastava S. (2006) Development of synthetic antigens for detection of Peste des petits ruminants (PPR). Ph.D. Thesis submitted to Deemed University, IVRI, Izatnagar.
33. West J.L. and Halas N.J. (2003) Engineered nanomaterials for biophotonics applications: improving sensing, imaging and therapeutics. *Annu. Rev. Biomed. Eng.* **(5):** 285-292.
34. Wu X., Liu H., Liu J., Haley K.N., Treadway J.A. and Larson J.P. (2003) Immunofluorescent labeling ofcancer marker Her2 and other cellular targets with semiconductor quantum dots. *Nat. Biotechnol.* **(21):** 41-46.
35. Yeh H.C., Ho Y.P., Shih L.E.M. and Wang T.H. (2006) Homogenous point mutation detection by quantum dot mediated two-color fluorescence coincidence analysis. *Nucleic Acids Res.* **(34):** e35.
36. Zheng G., Patolsky F., Cui Y., Wang W.U. and Lieber C.M. (2005) Multiplexed electrical detection of cancer markers with nanowire sensor arrays. *Nat Biotechnol.* **(23):** 1294-1301.

SECTION B

Biotechnology for Crop Applications

CHAPTER 20

Molecular Marker Technology in Plants

Molecular markers are used in molecular biology and biotechnology experiments where they identify a particular sequence of DNA. As the DNA sequences are highly specific, they can be identified with the help of the known molecular markers which can find out a particular sequence of DNA from a group of unknown. This chapter deals with the various applications of molecular marker systems and compilation of genetic linkage maps of cultivated plants.

Keywords: Plants molecular markers, genome analysis, RAPD, RFLP, AFLP, SSR, MAS, QTLs.

INTRODUCTION

Molecular markers are heritable differences in nucleotide sequences of DNA from two different individuals, which follow a Mendelian pattern of inheritance. Molecular marker technologies hold great promise in various crop improvement programmes by providing much needed selection precision and acceleration in breeding efforts. Further it also helps in evaluation and management of biodiversity, germplasm banks, providing molecular ID-cards for Intellectual Property Right (IPR) protection of improved varieties and important germplasms. Genome mapping is also one of the important applications of molecular markers. The DNA-based markers have dramatically facilitated the mapping of several plant genomes in the last decade. The linkage between molecular markers and genes controlling valuable agronomic traits (either monogenic or polygenic) accelerates the introgression of these traits via marker assisted selection (MAS), and may be used as a first step towards saturation of the target region of the map for positional cloning.

However, the progress in accepting the molecular markers for efficient use in MAS by the plant breeders has been slow, despite no questions of biosafety and bioethics have been raised against this technology in contrast to the transgenic approach.

GENETIC MARKERS

Variation or polymorphism among the genotypes within a species is the raw material for genome analysis. To be a genetic marker, the marker locus has to show experimentally detectable variation among the individuals in the test population. The variation can be considered at different biological levels, from the simple heritable phenotype for the detection of variation at the single nucleotide. Once the variation is identified and the genotypes of all the individuals in the test population are known, the frequency of recombination events between loci is used to estimate linkage distances between markers for the construction of a linkage map. Target traits or target genes in a segregating population can be identified with the assistance of linked genetic markers to accelerate traditional breeding programmes. This process is known as marker-assisted-selection or MAS.

The most important properties for good quality genetic markers are: (i) highly polymorphic nature, (ii) co-dominant inheritance (which can determine both the homozygous and the heterozygous states of diploid organisms), (iii) frequent occurrence in genome, (iv) selective neutral behaviour (the DNA sequence of any organism is neutral to environmental condition or management facilities), (v) easy availability, (vi) easy and fast assay, (vii) high reproducibility, (viii) no effects of alternate alleles on the plant morphology, and (ix) low or null interaction among markers, allowing the use of many markers at the same time in a segregating population. Three types of markers have been used in genome analysis: morphological markers, protein-based markers and DNA-based markers.

High quality genetic markers, based on the identification of polymorphism in proteins and DNA, have been developed during the last three decades. They are known as molecular markers. These markers have most or all the requisite properties of a good genetic marker. For these reasons, their potential as tools for plant breeding is much greater than that of the morphological markers.

Morphological Markers

Early mapping studies concentrated on discrete traits with simple Mendelian inheritance, such as shape, colour, size or height. Morphological traits often have one to one correspondence with the genes controlling the traits. In such cases, morphological characters (the phenotypes) can be used as reliable indicators for specific genes and are useful as genetic markers on chromosomes. A large number of morphological markers have been studied and mapped for human, mouse, Drosophila, maize, tomato and many other plant and animal species.

Polymorphic, highly heritable morphological traits were some of the earliest genetic markers employed in scientific investigations. Until recently, genetic markers used to develop linkage maps were those affecting morphological characters. These are either macromutations in major genes (wingless flies, hairless mice and dwarf plants) or secondary metabolites (pigments and other secondary metabolites). Macromutations are rare in nature and are deleterious to individuals. In most cases they are expressed only in adult plants. Genes for negative characters such as dwarfism, albinism or other subvital mutants have to be used. Pigments are classes of anthocyanin or flavonoids compounds. They are highly heritable and polymorphic. Genotype and environment interactions generally affect the quality, rather than the type of pigments produced; however, there is an evidence for the selective value of these pigments, which may diminish their utility as genetic markers.

Protein Markers

Proteins are the products of genes. Different alleles of the same gene may produce proteins with different amino acid composition, sizes or modifications. Differences in charge or size can be easily detected using gel electrophoresis and can be used as genetic markers. Protein markers are more specifically allelic variants of several enzymes, so-called isozymes.

In 1959, Markert and Moller introduced the term isozyme to define each one of the possibly many multiple forms of an enzyme existing in the same population of an organism. It is the most commonly used protein marker. Many enzymes can be visualized by using their activity to create a visible product that appears as a band where the enzyme is present. Isozymes often differ in their electrophoretic mobility but have the same enzyme activity. The different forms of isozymes can be detected or visualized typically using electrophoresis in starch gels or polyacrylamide gels. Isozyme linkage maps have been established for several plant species, including important crops such as tomato and rye. Although isozyme numbers are limited and their expressions are often restricted to specific developmental states or tissues, due to the ease of detection by electrophoresis and specific staining, they are used in conjugation with DNA markers.

DNA Markers

A DNA marker is typically a small region of DNA, showing sequence polymorphism in different individuals within a species. A variety of techniques have been developed in the past few years for visualizing the degree of polymorphism. DNA fingerprinting was introduced for the first time by Alec Jeffrey in 1985 to describe the bar-code-like patterns of DNA fragments generated by hybridization of multi-locus probes with genomic DNA fragments, after electrophoretic separation of the latter. DNA fingerprint of an individual is unique and this technique is currently considered to be the ultimate tool for the identification of organisms. Based on the techniques used for detection of polymorphism, DNA markers can be divided into three broad categories: [1] first-generation markers based on hybridization: Restriction fragment length polymorphism, (RFLP), [2] second-generation based on polymerase chain reaction: Sequence-tagged sites (STS); Single strand conformation polymorphism (SSCP); Random amplified polymorphic DNA marker (RAPD); Simple sequence repeat (SSR) or microsatellite; Variable number tandem repeat (VNTR) or minisatellite; Inter simple sequence repeat (ISSR); Random amplified microsatellite polymorphism (RAMP); Amplified fragment length polymorphism (AFLP) and [3] third-generation markers based on DNA sequencing: Single nucleotide polymorphism (SNP); Expressed sequence tag (EST). In hybridization based method, DNA polymorphism is generated by hybridizing the restriction enzyme-digested genomic DNA to a labelled probe (a DNA fragment of known origin or sequence). PCR-based markers involve *in vitro* amplification of particular DNA sequences or loci with the help of specifically or arbitrarily chosen oligonucleotide sequences (primers) and a thermostable DNA polymerase enzyme. The amplified fragments are separated electrophoretically and banding patterns are detected by different methods such as staining and autoradiography. Some of the important marker systems are described below.

Restriction fragment length polymorphism (RFLP)

Restriction endonucleases cut genomic DNA at specific palindromic recognition sequences, generating thousands of fragments (the lengths of which are defined for a particular individual), the number of which depends on the number of recognition sequences in a given genome. If a recognition sequence is present at a distinct genomic location in one individual but not in the other, the enzyme generates differently sized restriction fragments of this locus. This length polymorphism is detected by a DNA probe derived from the same locus and autoradiography (radioactive or chemiluminescence) (Figure 20.1).

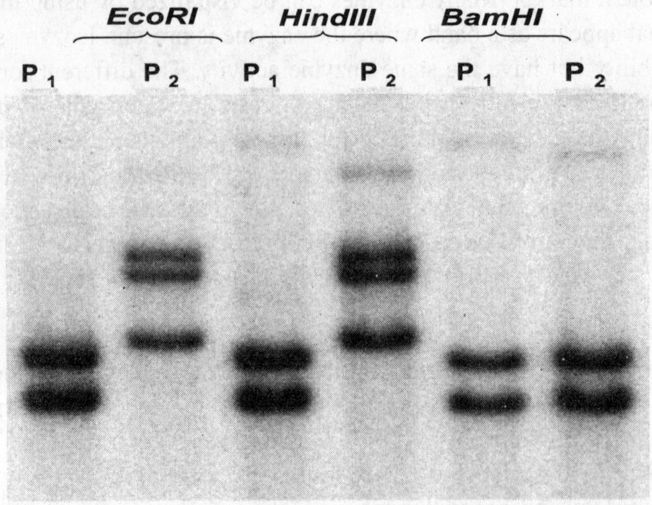

Figure 20.1 RFLPs of parent DNA (P_1 and P_2) digested with *EcoRI, HindIII, BamHI* and probed with a ribosomal DNA.

RFLP markers were used for the first time in the construction of a genetic linkage map in man by Botstein *et al.* (1980). RFLPs, being co-dominant markers, can detect both the homozygous alleles and the heterozygous genotype as DNA fragments from the two homologous chromosomes are detected. They are reliable markers in linkage analysis and breeding, and can easily determine if a linked trait is present in a homozygous or heterozygous state in an individual—an information highly desirable for recessive traits.

Despite their usefulness, the generation of RFLP markers and their application is time consuming and expensive. Firstly, one out of several markers provides a polymorphism. This problem is serious, especially in crosses between closely related cultivated breeding lines. Secondly, for every polymorphic locus tested in a cross, a single experiment has to be performed and this is a formidable task with saturated maps such as those of rice, tomato and maize, with hundreds or more markers. In addition, a large amount of DNA (~5-10 µg) is required for restriction digestion and Southern blotting. The requirement of radioactive isotope makes the analysis relatively expensive and hazardous. Finally, their inability to detect single base changes restricts their use in detecting point mutations occurring within the regions at which they are detecting polymorphism. RFLP markers have been converted into PCR-based markers, which are as follows.

Sequence-tagged Sites (STS)

RFLP markers linked to a desired trait can be converted into PCR-based STS markers based on nucleotide sequence of the probe giving polymorphic band pattern, or amplicons specific to different genotypes (Figure 20.2). Using this technique, tedious hybridization procedures involved in RFLP analysis can be overcome. This approach is useful for studying the relationship between various species. When these markers are linked to some specific traits, for example, the bread wheat grain quality trait, rice blast and bacterial blight diseases, they can be easily integrated into plant breeding programmes for marker-assisted selection of the trait of interest.

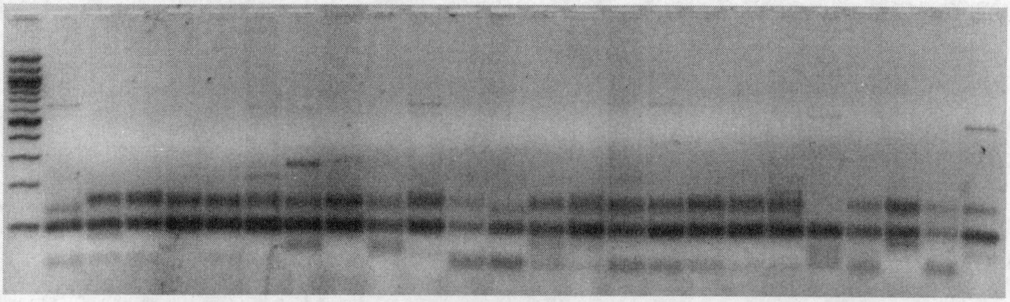

Figure 20.2 STS amplification profiles in a segregating population of wheat.

Single Strand Conformation Polymorphism (SSCP)

This is a powerful and rapid technique for gene analysis, particularly for detection of point mutations and typing of DNA polymorphism. SSCP can identify heterozygosity of DNA fragments of the same molecular weight and can even detect changes in a few nucleotides as the mobility of the single-stranded DNA changes with change in its GC content due to its conformational change.

Random amplified polymorphic DNA (RAPD) markers

Based on the PCR, this method is much faster and cheaper than RFLP analysis and uses only minute amounts of DNA (~20-50 ng). Instead of primers complementary to known sequences, as in normal PCR, randomly generated synthetic oligonucleotides of 9 to 12 bases are used for DNA amplification. This procedure usually amplifies 1 to 10 fragments from a single primer PCR reaction, which are highly polymorphic and can be easily detected on ethidium bromide-stained agarose gels (Figure 20.3). At present, the primers are normally 10bp in length and have a GC content of at least 50% and a low annealing temperature (36°C to 40°C). Unlike typical PCR reactions, a single rather than a pair of primers is used for amplifications. Two correctly oriented primer sites must exist within a limited distance in the genomic DNA for amplification to be successful. Most variations among individuals for RAPDs probably arise from base pair substitutions, or insertion/deletions that modify (or eliminate) the primer site, or insertions in the genomic sequence that changes the intervening length of the DNA between the primer sites, or insertions, which separate the primer sites to a distance that will not permit amplifications. Each of these changes results in the presence or absence of a particular RAPD fragment. For this reason, RAPDs are inherited in a dominant fashion in F_2 populations, exhibiting 3:1 segregation ratios. Analysis of RAPD markers with single, random sequence oligonucleotide primers became popular because of its simplicity and ease. RAPD is now widely used in modestly equipped laboratories. Difficulties with assay reproducibility may be overcome by eliminating variation in DNA concentration, consistent reaction components (including genomic DNA and primers, dNTPs, magnesium, enzyme and buffer) and carefully controlled thermal cycling during amplifications. However, once a marker is found linked to a trait of interest, it is possible to convert the RAPD into a more reproducible PCR assay using techniques such as allele specific PCR or sequence characterized amplified region (SCAR) assays.

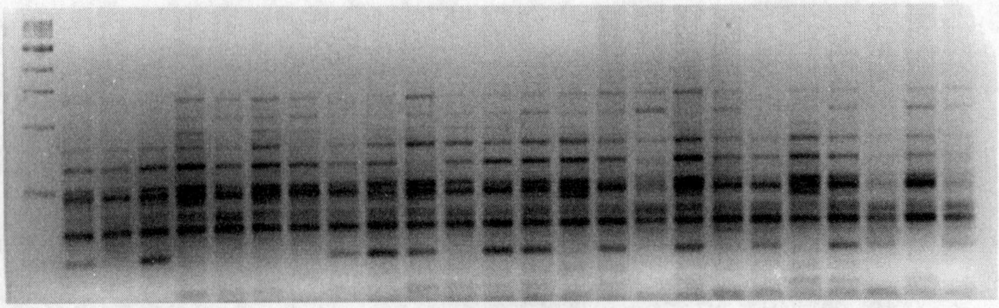

Figure 20.3 RAPD amplification profiles in a segregating population of tomato.

Microsatellites and minisatellites

Litt and Lutty (1989) coined the term microsatellites, while the term minisatellites was introduced by Jeffrey. Both are multi-locus probes creating complex banding patterns and are usually non-species specific, occurring ubiquitously. They essentially belong to the repetitive DNA families. Microsatellites are short tandem repeats (STRs), or simple sequence repeats (SSRs), consisting of 1 to 6 base pair long sequences that are repeated several times, while minisatellites are the tandem repeats with a repeat length of 11 to 60 base pairs. The number of repeats for the microsatellite is usually less than 100. The length variation for SSRs is based on the differences in the number of repeats. Amplifying the tandem arrays and then visualizing them on a agarose or polyacrylamide gel can detect variation in DNA length (Figure 20.4). For minisatellites, the loci that vary in the number of repeat units between genotypes are referred to as variable number of tandem repeats, or hypervariable regions (HVRs) (i.e., numerous loci containing tandem repeats within a genome generating high levels of polymorphism between individuals).

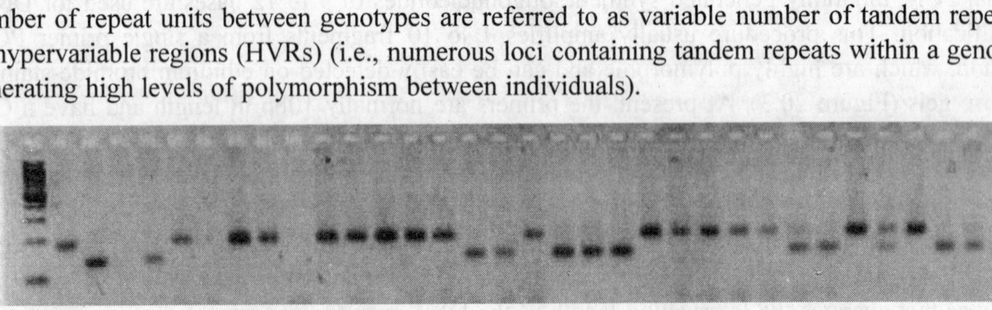

Figure 20.4 Microsatellite amplification profiles in a segregating population of tomato.

There are various methods for identification and development of SSR markers including sequence based methods. For some species, such as human, mouse, soybean, arabidopsis, wheat, barley, maize and rice, a large amount of DNA sequence data has already been accumulated. Microsatellites may be identified by searching through the DNA sequence data bases for sequences containing simple repeats. Primers are commonly designed directly from the sequence data. However, for most plant and animal species, a large effort using hybridization and sequencing is needed to identify microsatellites suitable for use as genetic markers. Hybridization using simple repeats as probes to screen genomic clones can be used to identify the microsatellites. The flanking sequences can be obtained by sequencing the cloned fragments containing microsatellites. Once the microsatellite markers are found, the utility of the markers is high. The SSRs are favoured over minisatellites as the former are evenly distributed in the genome (while the latter are usually confined to the telomeric region), found in abundance and are easier to discover and employ.

The DNA sequences flanking SSRs are known to be conserved in the same manner as those flanking minisatellites as variable number tandem repeats (VNTRs). These unique sequences have been used for designing suitable primers for amplification of the SSR loci. Any such pair of primers, when used to amplify a SSR locus of a number of genotypes, will reveal SSR polymorphism in the form of differences in the length of the amplified product; each length representing an allele at that locus. The length differences are attributed to the variation in the number of repeating units of particular SSR locus. As polymorphism is based on the differences in repeats of simple sequences, polymorphism revealed by SSRs is also termed simple sequence length polymorphism (SSLP) or sequence tagged microsatellite site (STMS). The uniqueness of microsatellites arise from their multi-allelic nature, inherent potential for variation, co-dominant transmission, ease of detection by PCR, relative abundance, extensive genome coverage and requirement of only a small amount of genomic DNA. These properties make microsatellites a valuable source for genetic markers, which provide a common language for collaborative research acting as universal genetic mapping reagents and for the characterization of accessions in plant germplasm collections.

The presence of SSR in plants was first reported by Condit and Hubbel (1991), suggesting their abundance in plant systems. Later, Akkaya *et al.* (1992) reported length polymorphisms of SSR in soybean, which opened a new source of PCR-based molecular markers for other plant genomes. Additionally, it has also been demonstrated that SSRs are highly informative and locus-specific markers in many species. Although SSRs are highly informative, reproducible, co-dominant inheritance and locus specific, they also have several drawbacks including high cost and time required for their development. These are due to the requirement for their isolation *de novo* from most species being examined for the first time. However, despite the initial high cost, once developed, the cost of implementing these markers is greatly reduced. Some modifications of microsatellite markers are as follows.

Inter Simple Sequence Repeat (ISSR) Markers

In this technique, reported by Zietkiewicz *et al.* (1994), primers based on microsatellites are utilized to amplify inter-SSR DNA sequences. Here, various microsatellites anchored at the 3′ ends are used for amplifying genomic DNA, which increases their specificity (Figure 20.5). These are mostly dominant markers, though occasionally a few of them exhibit co-dominance. An unlimited number of primers can be synthesized for various combinations of di-, tri-, tetra- and penta-nucleotides [$4^3 = 64$, $4^4 = 256$] with an anchor made up of a few bases and can be exploited for a broad range of applications in plant species. The frequency of repeats longer than 20 bp have been estimated to occur every 33 kb in plants.

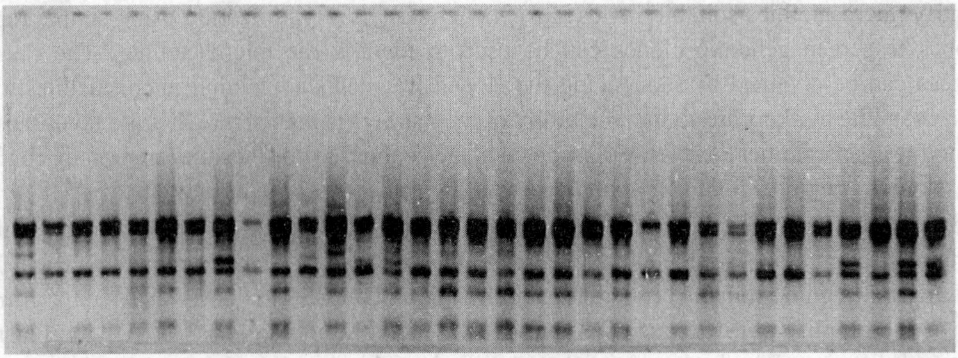

Figure 20.5 ISSR amplification profiles in a segregating population of tomato.

Randomly Amplified Microsatellite Polymorphism (RAMP)

In this PCR-based strategy, genomic DNA is first amplified using arbitrary (RAPD) primers. The amplified products are electrophoretically separated and the dried gel is hybridized with microsatellite oligonucleotide probes. Several advantages of oligonucleotide fingerprinting, RAPD and microsatellite-primed PCR are thus combined—speed of the assay, the high sensitivity, the high level of variability detected and the non-requirement of prior DNA sequence information. This technique has been successfully employed in the genetic fingerprinting of tomato, kiwi fruit and closely related genotypes of *Dioscorea bulbifera*.

Amplified fragment length polymorphism (AFLP)

AFLP is a technique based on the detection of genomic restriction fragments by PCR amplification and can be used for DNA of any origin or complexity. The DNA fingerprints are produced, without any prior knowledge of sequence, using a limited set of generic primers. The number of fragments detected in a single reaction can be 'tuned' by selection of specific primer sets. The technique of AFLP is reliable since stringent reaction conditions are used for primer annealing. AFLP is an ingenious combination of the RFLP and PCR techniques and is useful in detection of polymorphism between closely related genotypes (Figure 20.6). The AFLP procedure involves four major steps:

1. Isolation, restriction of genomic DNA, and ligation of double-stranded oligonucleotide adapters that contain 10-12 arbitrary nucleotides at the 5′ end and the restriction site-specific nucleotides at the 3′ end.
2. Pre-amplification of the restricted fragments using single-stranded primers, complementary to the adapter, in PCR.
3. Selective amplification of pre-amplified fragments using primers with one to three arbitrary selective nucleotides (depending on the genome complexity) added at the 3′ end of the pre-amplification primers.
4. Denaturing PAGE of the PCR products is used to visualize the selectively amplified fragments through autoradiography (by labelling one of the primers with P^{32} or P^{33}) or by silver staining.

AFLP analysis can be applied regardless of the origin and complexity of the genome. Most AFLP fragments correspond to unique positions on the genome and hence can be exploited as landmarks in genetic and physical mapping. AFLPs are useful as tools for DNA fingerprinting and for cloning and mapping of variety-specific genomic DNA sequences. Similar to RAPDs, the bands of interest obtained by AFLP can be converted into STSs. Thus AFLP provides a newly developed, important tool for a variety of applications. Although, the AFLP technique is powerful and reliable in genome mapping and identifying markers closely linked to genes of interest, it has some disadvantages for use in marker-assisted-selection (MAS) and map-based cloning. Their dominant type of inheritance, the intensity of labour involved, and high costs are some of the major limitations to applications of AFLP.

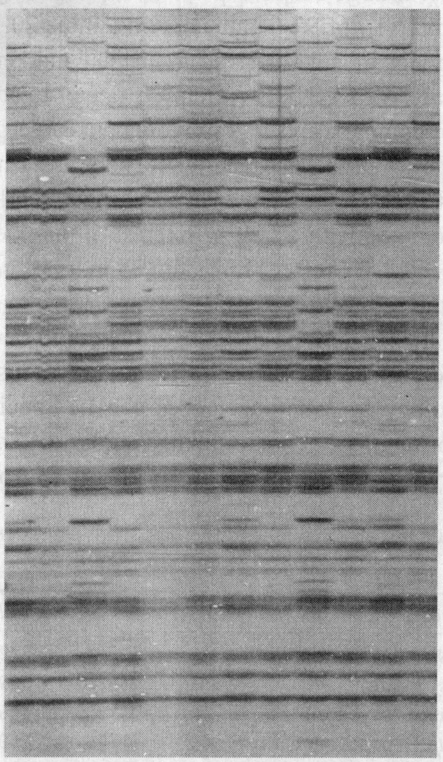

Figure 20.6 AFLP amplification profiles in 12 tomato genotypes.

Single nucleotide polymorphism (SNP)

Single nucleotide polymorphism (SNP) is the ultimate DNA marker consisting of a single base substitution within a given segment of DNA between two individuals. The SNPs are small insertion-deletion (indels) and are the basis of most differences between alleles. They provide an essentially inexhaustible source of polymorphic markers for use in high-resolution genetic mapping of traits, association studies based on candidate genes, and consequently for high throughput molecular marker-assisted-breeding (MAB). The overwhelming attraction towards SNPs is for two main reasons: (a) they offer the potential for the highest density of markers. The relevance of this to MAS is that it should be possible to find an informative marker in the right region in any segregating situation, even if the probability of finding polymorphism at any one SNP locus is low (biallelic nature); and (b) the SNP output is one of the binary type and this presents an easier target for automatic data interpretation. In addition, such data need not be generated by electrophoresis, giving the potential for simpler and cheaper automated analytical platforms.

Expressed Sequence Tags (ESTs)

An EST is a short DNA (~200-500 nucleotides) sequence from a cDNA clone that corresponds to a mRNA. The availability of a large set of expressed sequence tags (ESTs) database (dbEST; http://www.ncbi.nlm.nih.gov/dbEST/dbEST_summary.html; Table 20.1) provides an ample opportunity for systematic development of gene-derived molecular markers for effective use in crop improvement programme. Analysis of ESTs is a simple strategy to study the transcribed parts of genomes, thus rendering even complex and highly redundant large genomes like wheat, barley, maize, chickpea, etc. amenable to large-scale analysis. There are a number of advantages using expressed genes compared with anonymous sequences as genetic markers. First, if an EST marker is found to be genetically associated with a trait of interest, it may be possible that this could be the gene affecting the trait directly. Therefore, EST-derived markers can provide opportunities for gene discovery and enhance the role of genetic markers by assaying variation in transcribed and known-function genes. Second, EST-derived markers are likely to be more highly conserved and therefore may be more transferable between species than anonymous sequence-derived markers. Third, ESTs that share homology to candidate genes can be specifically targeted for genetic mapping and can be useful for aligning genome linkage across distantly related species for comparative analysis. The conserved orthologous set (COS) markers from the sequence databases

Table 20.1 Summary of number of ESTs reported for important plant genomes available in dbEST database (as on August 27, 2010).

Plant species (common name)	*Number*
Arabidopsis thaliana (thale cress)	1,529,555
Zea mays (maize)	2,019,105
Glycine max (soybean)	1,459,936
Oryza sativa (rice)	1,249,124
Triticum aestivum (wheat)	1,071,199
Brassica napus (oilseed rape)	643,884
Hordeum vulgare (barley)	501,620
Gossypium hirsutum (upland cotton)	268,794
Solanum lycopersicum (tomato)	297,069
Sorghum bicolor (sorghum)	209,828
Vigna unguiculata (cowpea)	187,483
Secale cereale (rye)	9,298
Cicer arietinum (chickpea)	34,329
Setaria italica (foxtail millet)	2,451

(unigene derived) of different plant species would be useful for mapping of plant genome, tagging of useful genes and understanding the evolution of genes and genomes. Estimates suggest that 1% to 5% of plant ESTs contains SSRs longer than 18 nucleotides. Thus, the development of EST derived SSR, SNP and COS markers has become commonplace in a wide variety of plant species.

Each of the above molecular marker systems differs not only in principle but also in the type and amount of polymorphism detected. A comparison of the utility of each marker system is summarized in Table 20.2. Out of these, the SSR, EST-derived SSR and SNP markers have all the

Table 20.2 Comparison of main features of different molecular marker systems.

Particulars	*RFLP*	*RAPD*	*ISSR*	*SSR*	*AFLP*	*SNP*
Principle	Restriction Southern blot, hybridization	DNA amplification with random 10-mer primers	Amplification with ISSR primers	PCR amplification of simple sequence repeats using flanking primers	Selective PCR amplification of restriction fragments	Single base differences
Type of polymorphism	Single base changes (Insertion/ Deletion)	Change in binding site(s) of the primer	Base changes (Insertion/ Deletion) in SSR repeat length/no. of motifs	Variations in repeat length/ no. of motifs	Single base changes (Insertion/ Deletion)	Single base changes (Insertion/ Deletion)
Genomic abundance	High	Medium	Very High	Very High	High	Highest
Level of polymorphism	High	Medium	High/Medium	High/very high	High	Highest
Inheritance mode	Co-dominant	Dominant	Dominant/ Co-dominant	Co-dominant	Dominant/ Co-dominant	Co-dominant
Sequence information required	No	No	No	Yes	No	Yes
Reproducibility	Very high	Low	High/Medium	High	Very High	Very High
DNA required per assay	10-200 μg	10-25 ng	50-100 ng	50-100 ng	500 ng-1μg	50-100ng
Development cost	High	Low	Low	High	Medium/High	High
High through-put automat-ion	No	No	No	No	No	Yes
Radioactivity requirement	Yes/No	No	No	No	Yes	No
Main applica-tion	Compara-tive mapping MAS	Fingerprint-ing Diversity analysis	Fingerprinting Diversity analysis	Marker saturation Fingerprinting MAS Tagging	Fingerprint-ing Diversity analysis	Marker saturation Fingerprinting MAS Map based cloning

requisites to be useful in the MAB. However, the cost of development of these markers (SSR and SNP) is quite high due to the need for the availability of sequence information. This is where comparative genomics is useful, as the marker information from one species can be transferred to other closely related species once we understand the synteny and co-linearity of genes between the species.

TILLING—A new technique for detecting polymorphisms

TILLING (Targetting Induced Local Lesions IN Genomes) is a general reverse genetic strategy that works with a mismatch-specific endonuclease to detect induced or natural DNA polymorphisms in genes of interest. With high-throughput TILLING, rapid and low-cost discovery of induced point mutations in populations of chemically mutagenized individuals from diverse organisms becomes possible. Other advantages of TILLING are its independence of genome size, reproductive system or generation time. TILLING yields a traditional allelic series of point mutations, which make it valuable for essential genes, where sub-lethal alleles are required for phenotypic analysis. Current advantages of TILLING have made it an appropriate choice for the detection of both induced and natural variation in several plant species.

The way TILLING works: Basic TILLING method allows for high-throughput identification of single-base-pair (bp) allelic variations. The first step starts with mutagenized seeds obtained from treatment with Ethylmethane sulphonate (EMS). The resulting M_1 plants are self-fertilized and the M_2 generation of individuals is used to prepare DNA samples for mutational screening. The DNA samples are pooled, arrayed on microtiter plates and subjected to gene-specific PCR. Amplification products are incubated with an endonuclease such as CELI, a member of the S1 nuclease family of single strand-specific nucleases. CELI cleaves the 3′ side of mismatched DNA where the heteroduplex between the wild-type and the mutant strands of DNA loops out; homoduplexes are left intact. Cleavage products are electrophoresed using an automated sequencing gel apparatus and gel images are analyzed by examining the gel readout with the aid of a standard commercial image-processing program. Differential double-end labeling of amplification products allows for rapid visual confirmation because mutations are detected on complementary strands and can be easily distinguished from amplification artifacts.

Upon the detection of a mutation in a pool, the individual DNA samples are similarly screened to identify the plant carrying the mutation. This rapid screening procedure determines the location of a mutation to within ±10 bp for PCR products that are 1-kb in size. For mismatch-specific cleavage, several enzymes, including S1 nuclease and T4 endonuclease VII have been used. CELI, a plant-specific extracellular glycoprotein, has been shown to be suitable for genotyping applications because it preferentially cleaves mismatches of all types and has been used to detect heterozygous polymorphisms in DNA pools. Further research showed that comparison of CELI with other single-strand specific nucleases revealed that the endonuclease activity does not differ between these enzymes under optimized conditions. Also, plant extracts performed as well as the highly purified preparations. These results suggest that something in the crude sample either enhances the endonuclease activity of these enzymes at heteroduplex sites or inhibits their activity at the amplicon ends.

In brief, screening is performed on DNAs that have been arrayed in 96-well microtiter plates and pooled eightfold to maximize screening efficiency. Gene specific, fluorescently tagged primers are used to amplify pooled DNA. The amplification products are denatured and allowed to reanneal, generally by heating and cooling. As a result, a mutant strand will often reanneal with a wild-type strand creating heteroduplexes at the site of the mutation or polymorphism. The resultant double-stranded products are digested with CELI, which cleaves one of the two strands at the heteroduplex mismatches. Cleaved products, which are detected on polyacrylamide denaturing gels, identify individuals that have a mutation in the gene of interest. The size of the fragments carrying the 5′ and 3′ fluorescent tags can be used to estimate the position of the mutation within the amplicon.

EcoTILLING: An extension of TILLING is EcoTILLING, which allows natural alleles at a locus to be characterized across many germplasm accessions, enabling both SNP discovery and haplotyping at these loci. This can be done at a fraction of the cost of SNP/haplotyping methods requiring large-scale sequencing. EcoTILLed haplotypes across a range of germplasm can be binned and confirmatory sequencing done on the unique haplotypes. Recent reviews by Henikoff *et al.* (2004) and Stemple (2004) illustrate the broad adoption of these techniques in diverse species, including rice, maize, Lotus, poplar, Brassica, Zebrafish, Drosophila, Caenorhabditis, and rat, demonstrating their broad applicability as a tool for SNP discovery and allele mining. Gilchrist *et al.* (2006) used this method to survey genetic variation of *Populus trichocarpa*.

In addition to allowing efficient detection of mutations, TILLING technology is also ideal for examining natural as well as induced variation. Endonuclease CELI cuts with partial efficiency, making possible to display multiple mismatches in a DNA duplex. Therefore, heteroduplexing DNA of an unknown sequence with that of a known sequence reveals the positions of polymorphic sites. Both nucleotide changes and small insertions/deletions are identified, as well as some repeat number polymorphisms.

Detection of a gene responsible for a mutation is a challenging process. TILLING, a cheap and fast natural polymorphism discovery and genotyping method, has advantages in determining the spectrum of variation and genetic mapping based on linkage association analysis. In TILLING technique, if a mutation is detected in a pool, the individual DNA samples that went into the pool can be individually analyzed to identify the individual that carries the mutation. Once this individual has been identified, its phenotype can be determined. This technique works with good results even if a population contains pre-existing mutations that would compromise SNP discovery by other methodologies.

The TILLING method results in a high-resolution map of mutations in a gene of interest, including silent, missense and truncation mutations. As with other forward and reverse genetics techniques, mutations that would otherwise be silent can be identified. Some genes will not produce overt phenotypes; others could have overlapping functions with other genes that could mask the effects of mutation. Genes like the *puroindolines* and *waxy* have a dominant wild type, requiring homozygosity of any variant to detect a phenotype. In contrast to TILLING, a recent study by Feiz *et al.* (2009) on generated allelic pin mutations by direct phenotyping of an EMS-mutagenized population followed by sequencing. Their results indicated that direct phenotyping was applicable for a single-copy gene conferring a detectable and targeted phenotype. This method may be effective for targeting desired phenotypes, whereas TILLING is more effective for targeting all mutations and genes without detectable phenotypes. The TILLING method allows for the streamlining of the screening–mutation detection part of the investigation, leaving more time for analysis of the candidate mutants by methods appropriate to the gene–trait affected. The production of waxy wheat and hard wheat from TILLING demonstrates that the method is effective and useful for wheat breeding. Other targets, such as starch branching enzymes, starch synthase II and starch synthase III can be TILLed in this TILLING population to produce novel grains with altered starch properties or for functional studies of genes of interest. Background mutations were observed during the production of waxy lines and hard grain lines. Further self-fertilization and hybridization with a wild-type plant can eliminate the undesirable mutations. Information provided in this report is useful for both functional genomics and practical breeding.

CONSTRUCTION OF GENETIC LINKAGE MAPS

The development of molecular marker technology renewed interest in genetic mapping. For a directed use of molecular markers in gene mapping and marker aided selection (MAS), it is essential to construct a high density complete linkage maps. The techniques of genetic mapping and linkage analysis were developed in 1911 by T.H. Morgan and his graduate student Alfred H. Sturtevant and are still used today in much the same way but with far more advanced techniques. The basis of genetic mapping is the phenomenon of "crossing-over" of chromosomes during meiosis, where homologous chromosomes exchange sections of their gene sequence. The tendency of two genes to recombine is used as a measurement of their linkage and distance on a genetic map. For example, two genes that recombine are said to be "linked" and are very close to each other on a genetic map.

A linkage map consists of linkage groups, the number of the group being equal to the number of haploid chromosomes of the species under study. Each linkage group, in turn, consists of genetic markers in a definite order. The distance between any two markers is indicated in centimorgan (cM), which is a function of the extent of recombination between the markers. A number of computer software (Linkage1, G Mendel, Mapmaker, Map manager, and Join map, etc.) are available, which prepare the genetic maps and determine genetic distances based on recombination frequencies. Construction of linkage map involves the following steps:

(1) Identification of the divergent parents
(2) Generation of mapping population
(3) Identification of polymorphic DNA probes and enzyme combinations
(4) Establishing linkage
(5) Identification of linkage groups
(6) Assigning linkage groups to chromosomes

The fast advance in DNA marker technology has facilitated the rapid development of many high-density linkage, physical and consensus maps. In 1986, the construction of the first RFLP-based maps of maize and tomato marked the beginning of a storm of genetic map construction and use. The number of DNA-based marker maps published each year has increased steadily in the past decade. In 1986, only three maps had been published, but since 1993, an average of 30 maps are published each year. DNA-based genetic maps of economically important plant species for more than 60 different genera including monocots, dicots and gymnosperms have been published. A list of these molecular genetic maps, (Table 20.3) the mapping populations, the number and types of markers, the genetic length of these maps and references of some of the economically important

Table 20.3 Summary of published DNA based marker maps of economically important plants.

Common name/ Botanical name	Population used[#]	Marker Type*	No. of mapped loci	Map Length (cM)	Reference
Alfalfa (*Medicago sativa* L.)	F_2 (MqK93 × McW2)	RFLP, RAPD isozyme morphology	89	659	Kiss *et al.* 1993
	F_2 (W2xiso × USDA PI440501)	RFLP (cDNA)	108	467.5	Brummer *et al.* 1993
	BC_1 (Noninbred parents)	RFLP RAPD	153	659	Echt *et al.* 1994
	F_1 (consensus map of 2 BC population)	RFLP, SDRFs	88	443	Brouwer & Osborn 1999
	F_2 (spp. *quasifalcata* × spp. *coreulea*)	RFLP, RAPD, isozyme, morphology, seed protein	868	754	Kalo *et al.* 2000
	2 F_1 (Mercedes 4.11 & Magali 2)	AFLP, SSR	339, 350	3045, 2649	Julier *et al.* 2003
	F_2 (Jemalong × DZA315)	RAPD, AFLP, genes, isozyme	289	1225	Thoquet *et al.* 2002
(*Medicago truncatula* L.)	F_2 (ecotypes A17 × A20)	EST, BAC, RGA	288	513	Choi *et al.* 2004
	F_1 (*M. sativa subsp. falcata* × *M. sativa subsp. sativa*)	SDA, BAC, SSR	286	624	Sledge *et al.* 2005
Banana (*Musa acuminate* Colla)	F_2 (F1 hybrid 'SFB5'; SF265 × Banksii)	RFLP, isozyme, RAPD	90	606	Faure *et al.* 1993
	Composite map of 2 populations	RFLP,RAPD, isozyme, SSR, AFLP	373	1227	http://wwww.cirad.fr
Barley (*Hordeum vulgare* L.)	DH (Proctor × Nudinka)	RFLP	154	1091	Heun *et al.* 1991
	DH (Igri×Franka, *H. vulgare* spp. Vada × H. vulgare *spp.* Spontaneum *line1B-87)*	RFLP	226	1453	Graner *et al.* 1991
	DH (Steptoe × Morex)	RFLP, isozyme, RAPD, morphology, SAP, diseasse	295	1250	Kleihofs *et al.* 1993
	DH (Harrington × TR306)	RFLP	898	1060	Kasha *et al.* 1994
	Consensus map (7 maps)	RFLP, others	587	1087	Langridge *et al.* 1995
	DH (Proctor × Nudinka)	AFLP	118	1096	Becker *et al.* 1995
	Consensus map (4 maps)	RFLP, others	880	-	Qi *et al.* 1996
	RIL (L 94 × Vada)	AFLP	566	1062	Qi *et al.* 1998
	DH (Proctor × Nudinka)	AFLP	511	2673	Castiglioni *et al.* 1998
	F_2 (Ko A × Mokusekko)	RFLP	222	1389	Miyazaki *et al.* 2000
	DH (H vulgare var. Lina × H. spontaneum Canada Park)	SSR	242	1173	Ramsay *et al.* 2000
	F_2 (Lerche × BGRC41936), DH (Igri × Franka)	SSR	57	840	Pilen *et al.* 2000
	F_2 *(H. Chilense)*	RAPD, SSR, RFLP, STS	123	694	Hernandez *et al.* 2001
	DH (OWB Dom × OWB Rec)	RAPD, SSR, RFLP	720	1387	Costa *et al.* 2001
	RI (Azumamugi × Kato Nakate Gold)	AFLP, STS	272	926	Mano *et al.* 2001
	DH (*H vulgare* var. Lina × *H. spontaneum* Canada Park)	IMP	88	-	Chang *et al.* 2001
	3 DH- Consensus (Igri× Franka; Steptoe × Morex; OWB Dom×OWB Rec)	SSR	76	-	Thiel *et al.* 2003
	2 DH- Consensus (Igri× Franka; Steptoe × Morex)	SSR	127	-	Li *et al.* 2003

Contd.

	3 DH- consensus (OWB Dom×OWB Rec. Steptoe × Morex; Lina× HS92)	SNP, RFLP, AFLP, SSR	1237	1211	Rostoks *et al.* 2005
	3 DH- Consensus transcript map (Igri × Franka; Steptoe × Morex; OWB Dom × OWB Rec)	SSR	185	1109	Varshney *et al.* 2006
	Consensus map (Igri × Franka', 'Steptoe × Morex', 'OWB$_{Rec}$ × OWB$_{Dom}$', 'Lina × Canada Park', 'L94 × Vada' and 'SusPtrit × Vada')	SSR	775	1068	Varshiney *et al.* 2007
	3 DH- Consensus transcript map (Igr i× Franka; Steptoe × Morex; OWB Dom×OWB Rec)	EST derived-RFLP, SNP	1032	118.3	Stein *et al.* 2007
	3 DH- Consensus transcript map (Igri × Franka; Steptoe × Morex; OWB Dom×OWB Rec)	SNP	220	1136	Kota *et al.* 2008
Bean (*Phaseolus vulgaris* L.)	BC XR-235-1-1' × ('Calima' × 'XR-235-1-1')	RFLP, isozyme, seed protein, flower colour	244	1200	Vallejos *et al.* 1992
	F_2 (BAT93 × Jalo EEP558)	RFLP, RAPD, isozyme, disease resistance, morphology	152	827	Nodari *et al.* 1993
	BC_1 ('Ms8E02' × 'Corel') × 'Corel')	RFLP, RAPD, SCAR< morphology	157	567.5	Adam-Blodon *et al.*1994
	RIL (PC-50 × XAN-159)	RFLP, morphology	181	426	Jung *et al.* 1997
	Consensus map-RI (BAT93 × Jalo EEP558 (BJ)	RFLP, RAPD, isozyme, morphology	563	1226	Freyre *et al.* 1998
	$F_{2:4}$ (OAC Seaforth × OAC 95-4)	RFPD, RAPD, SSR, AFLP	114	-	Tar'an *et al.* 2002
	2RI population (DOR364 × G19833) (BAT93 × JaloEEP558)	SSR	100(78+22)	1720	Blair *et al.* 2003
Cotton (Gossypium spp.)	F_2 (*G. hirsutum* L. × *G . barbadense* L.)	RFLP	705	4675	Reinisch *et al.* 1994
	F_2 (*G. hirsutum* L. × *G . barbadense* L.)	RFLP, RAPD	355	4766	Kohel *et al.* 2001
	DH (*G. hirsutum* L.× *G .barbadense* L.)	SSR, RAPD	489	3315	Zhang *et al.* 2002
	F_2 & F_3 (*G. hirsutum* L. × *G. hirsutum* L.)	RFLP	284	1503	Ulloa *et al.* 2002
	F_2 (*G. nelsonii.* × *G. australe*)	AFLP	176	773	Brubaker & Brown 2003
	F_2 (*G. nelsonii.* × *G. australe*)	AFLP	213	931	Brubaker & Brown 2003
	BC_1 (*G. hirsutum* L.× *G. barbadense* L.)	AFLP, SSR, RFLP	888	4400	Lacap *et al.* 2003
	F_2 (*G. hirsutum* L. × *G. barbadense* L.)	SRAP	237	3031	Lin *et al.* 2003
	BC_1 (*G. hirsutum* L.× *G. barbadense* L.)	SSR	642	5644	Han *et al.* 2004
	F_2 (*G. hirsutum* L.× *G. barbadense* L.)	RFLP	2584	4448	Rong *et al.* 2004
	F_2 (*G. tomentosum*×*G. raimondii*)	RFLP	763	1493	Rong *et al.* 2004
Coton (Gossypium spp.)	BC_1 (*G. hirsutum* L.× *G. barbadense* L.)	AFLP, SSR, RFLP	1160	5519	Nguyen *et al.* 2004
	F_2 (*G. hirsutum* L. × *G. barbadense* L.)	AFLP, SSR, RFLP	392	3287	Mei *et al.* 2004
	F_2 (*G. hirsutum* × *G tomentosum*)	RFLP	589	4259	Waghmare *et al.* 2005
	F_2 (*G. hirsutum* L.× *G. barbadense* L.)	SRAP, SSR, RAPD	566	5142	Lin *et al.* 2005
	RIL (*G. hirsutum* L. cv. TM1 × *G barbadense* L. Pima 3-79.)	EST-SSR	193	1277	Park *et al.* 2005
	BC_1 (*G. hirsutum* L. × *G barbadense* L.)	SSR	442	4331	Song *et al.* 2005
	DH (*G. hirsutum* L. × *G .barbadense* L.)	SSR	444	3263	Song *et al.* 2005
	BC_1 (*G. hirsutum* L. × *G .barbadense* L.)	SSR	907	5060	Hen *et al.* 2006
	RIL (*G. hirsutum* L. × *G. barbadense* L.)	SSR	433	2126	Frelichowski *et al.* 2006
	F_2 (*G. arboretum* × *G . herbaceum*)	RFLP	275	1147	Desai *et al.* 2006
	F_2 (*G. hirsutum* L.× *G . barbadense* L.)	SRAP, SSR, RAPD, REMAP	1029	5472	He *et al.* 2007
	BC_1 (*G. hirsutum* L. × *G .barbadense* L.)	SSR	1790	3426	Guo *et al.* 2007

Contd.

	F_2 (*G. arboreum* L.) Jianglingzhongmian × Zhejiangxiaoshanlüshu	SSR	267	2508.7	Ma *et al.* 2008
Cucumber (*Cucumis sativus* L.)	F_2 (Gy14 × 432860)	RFLP, RAPD, isozyme, morphology, disease-resistance	58	766	Kennard *et al.* 1994
	F_2 (*C. sativus* × *C. hardwickii* (R) Alef.)	RFLP, RAPD, isozyme, morphology, disease-resistance	70	480	Kennard *et al.* 1994
	F_2 (G421 × H-19)	RAPD, morphology	80	600	Serquen *et al.* 1997
	Consensus-2 maps(within *C. sativus*) & (*C. sativus* × *C. sativus* var. *hardwickii*)	RFLP, RAPD, isozyme, morphology, disease-resistance	255,197	-	Braden *et al.* 2001
	F_2 & RI (G421 × H-19)	SSR, SCAR, AFLP, RAPD, SNP, morphology	131	706	Fazio *et al.* 2003
	F_2 (PW0832 × PW0801)	SRAP, ISSR	62	992.2	Yeboah *et al.* 2007
	F_2 (S94 × S06)	SRAPs, RAPDs, SSRs, SCARs, ISSRs, STS	173	1016	Guan *et al.* 2008
Cucurbita (*Cucurbita pepo*)	F_2 (*C. pepo* × *C. moschata*)	RAPD	28	-	Lee *et al.* 1995
	BC (*C. pepo* L. yellow streighneck A0449 × *C. moschata* Duchesne ex Lam Nigerian Local)	RAPD, morphology	153	1954	Brown & Myers 2002
	$2F_2$ (Pumpkin–Crookneck; *C. pepo* subsp. *pepo* × *C. pepo* subsp. *ovifera;* O5 × CV)	RAPD, AFLP. SSR, morphology	333 & 323	2140, 2234	Zraidi *et al.* 2007
	Consensus map of Zraidi et al. 2007	RAPD, AFLP	62	-	Zraidi *et al.* 2007
	$2F_2$ (Pumpkin–Crookneck; *C. pepo* subsp. *pepo* × *C. pepo* subsp. *ovifera*; O5 × CV)	SSR	177	1008.6	Gong *et al.* 2008 Gong *et al.*
	Updated map of Zraidi et al. 2007 using	RAPD, AFLP, SSR, SCAR, morphology	659	1936	Gong *et al.* 2008
Foxtail Millet (Setaria italica)	F_2 (B100 × A10)	RFLP	160	964	Wang *et al.* 1998
Maize (*Zea mays L.*)	RIL (T232 × CM37)	RFLP	334	1460	Burr *et al.* ***1988***
	F_2 (CO159 × T × 303)	RFLP	215	-	Gardiner *et al.* 1993
	F_2 (CO159 × T × 303)	RFLP	92	-	Chao *et al.* 1994
	Consensus $F_2/F_{5\text{-}6}$ (10 × F_2, 1252 × F_2)	ESTs, RFLP	275	1765	Causes *et al.* 1996
	F_2 (T × 303 × CO159)	ESTs, RFLP, SSR	1736	1727	Davis *et al.* 1999
	RIL (B73 × Mo17)	AFLP	1539	1178	Vuylsteke *et al.* 1999
	F_2 (D32 × D145)	AFLP	1355	1376	Vuylsteke *et al.* 1999
	F_2 (B73 × A7)	AFLP	246	2057	Castiglioni *et al.* 1999
	RIL (B73 × Mo17)	MITE-HBr	213	1092	Casa *et al.* 2000
	F_2 (T1 × T2)	SSR	310	-	Marsan *et al.* 2001
	RIL (B73 × Mo17)	SSR	978	4906	Sharopova *et al.* 2002
	Intermated RI (B73 × Mo17)	RFLP	180	5917	Lee *et al.* 2002
	2RI population (B73 × Mo17) (F2 × F252)	RFLP, cDNA, SSR, SNP	1454 (1056+398)	1825, 1862	Falque *et al.* 2005
	IBM2 2005 neighbors (Several mapping zpopulations)	Genetic + BAC	>34, 581	-	http://maizegbo.org/neighbors.php
Oat (*Avena sativa* L.) 'Cc7050-CAV4490')	F_2/F_3 (*A. atlantica* 'M66/3' × *A. hirtula*	RFLP	192	614	O'Donoughe *et al.* 1992
(2×)	F_2 (*A. Strigosa* Shreb × *A. wiestii* Sleud)	RFLP	208	2416	Rayapaty *et al.* 1994
(2×)	RIL (*A. byzantina* cv Kanota × *A. sativa* cv Ogle)	RFLP	561	1482	O'Donoughe *et al.* 1995

Contd.

(6×)	RIL –consensus (Kanota × Ogle; Clintland64 × IL86-5698)	AFLP, RFLP	300	2351	Jin *et al.* 2000
(6×)	RIL (Kanota × Marion)	AFLP, RFLP	178	736	Groh *et al.* 2001
	RIL –consensus (Ogle × TAM O-301)	RFLP, AFLP, RAPD, STS	441	2049	Portyanko *et al.* 2001
(6×)	F_2 (*A. Strigosa* CI3815 × *A. wiestii* CI1994)	RFLP	181	880	Krener *et al.* 2001
(2×)	RIL (Ogle-CI9401 × MAM17-5)	RFLP, AFLP, SSR	510	1396.7	Zhu & Keeppler 2003
(6×)	RIL –consensus (Kanota × Ogle; Clintland64 × IL86-5698)	RFLP, AFLP, RAPD, SSR, isozyme	1166	1890	Wight *et al.* 2003
(6×)	RIL (MN841801 × Noble-2)	RFLP, AFLP, SSR, SCAR	230	1509	Portyanko *et al.* 2005
Papaya (*Carica papaya* L.)	F_2 (Sunrise × UH356)	RAPD	62	999	Sondur *et al.* 1996
	F_2 (Kapoho × SunUp)	AFLP, virus coat protein, morphology	1501	3294.2	Ma *et al.* 2004
	F_2 (AU9 × SunUp)	SSR, morphology	707	1069.9	Chen *et al.* 2007
Rye (*Secale cereale* L.)	F_2 (DS2 × RXL10)	RFLP	50	-	Devos *et al.* 1993
	IBL (DS2 × RXL10)	RFLP, isozyme, RAPD, morphology, physisology	60	350	Philipp *et al.* 1994
	F_2 (E × R)	RFLP, RAPD	99	-	Loarce *et al.* 1996
	F_2 (synthetic I0.1 lines I-lines×a genebank acc.)	RFLP, RAPD	92	760	Senft & Wricke 1996
	F_2 (P87 × P105)	RFLP	88	660	Korzun *et al.* 1998
	Consensus-(13 mapping populations)	RFLP, isozyme, gene loci	413	-	Borner & Korzun 1998
	F_2 (P87 × P 105)	RFLP, SSR, others	183	1063	Korzun *et al.* 2001
	F_2 (UC-90 × E-line) (King II×Imperial)	RFLP, SSR, others	184	727	Ma *et al.* 2001
	F_2 (DS2 × RXL10)	RFLP, RAPD, others	282	1140	Masojc' *et al.* 2001
	F_2 (synthetic I0.1 lines)	AFLP	71	215 (total 1100)	Saal & Wricke 2002
Rye (*Secale cereale* L.)	F_2 (DS2 × RXL10)	RFLP, AFLP, RAPD, Protein loci, morphology	480	1386	Bednarek *et al.* 2003
	Consensus -F_2 (P87 × P105; N6 × N2; N7× N2; N7 × N6)	SSR	99	1111, 1087, 1109, 1111	Kheleskina *et al.* 2004
	F_2 (541 × Ot1-3)	RAPD, SSR, STS, SCAR, ISSR	148	1401.4	Milczarski *et al.* 2007
Soybean (*Gylcine max* L.)	F_2 (*G. max* × *G. soja*)	RFLP	135	1200	Keim *et al.* 1990
	F_2 (*G. max*; × A81-356022 × *G. soja* Sieb. & Zucc; PI 468916)	RFLP	252	2147	Diers *et al.* 1992
	F_2 (*G. max* × *G. soja*)	RFLP, RAPD, isozyme, classical	383	-	Shoemaker & Olson 1993
	RIL (BSR-101× PI437.654)	RFLP, RAPD, AFLP	840	3441	Keim *et al.* 1997
	Consensus map of 3 pop.; 2F_2 (*G. max* × *G. soja*) & (Clark × Harosoy); RI (Minsoy × Noir)	RFLP, AFLP, SSR, RAPD, isozyme, classical, others	1423	-	Cregan *et al.* 1999
	RIL (consensus) (Minsoy × Noir 1, Minsoy × Archer, Archer × Noir 1, Clark × Harosoy, & A81-356022 × PI468916)	RFLP, AFLP, SSR, RAPD, isozyme, classical, others	1849	2523.6	Song *et al.* 2004

Contd.

	F_2 (consensus) (Misuzudaizu × Moshidou	RELP, AFLP, SSR, STS, RAPD, morphology	1277	3080	Xia *et al.* 2007
	RIL (Minsoy × Noir 1, Minsoy × Archer, Evans × PI 209332)	Sequence based genic marker	1141	2388.6	Chio *et al.* 2007
Vigna (*Vigna* spp.)	F_2 (*IT2246-4* × *TVNI963*)	RFLP, cDNA, RAPD,	>90	684	Fatokun *et al.* 1993
	F_2 (*V .angularis* × *V. nakashimae*)	RFLP, RAPD, morphology	132	1250	Kaga *et al.* 1996
	F_2 (*V .angularis* × *V. umbellata*)	RFLP, RAPD, morphology	189	1702	Kaga *et al.* 2000
	F_2 (*V.radiata* × *V. radiata var.sublobata*; Madagascar)	RFLP, cDNA, pest locus	172	1570	Menacio-Hautea *et al.* 1993
	F_2 (*V.radiata* × *V. radiata var.sublobata*; Australia)	RFLP, RAPD, morpholoy	110	758.3	Lambrides *et al.* 2000
	RIL (*V.radiata* × *V. radiata var.sublobata*; *Australia*)	RAPD, morphology	115	691.7	Lambrides *et al.* 2000
	RIL (*V.radiata* cv.Berken × *V. radiata* spp.*sublobata*, ACC41)	RFLP	255	737.9	Humphery *et al.* 2002
	RIL (*V.ungivulata*, *IT84S* × *V. ungiculata*, 524B)	RFLP, RAPD, AFLP, morphology, biochemical	181	972	Menendez *et al.* 1997
	RIL (*V.ungiculata*, *IT84S* × *V. ungiculata*, 524B)	RFLP, RAPD, AFLP, morphology, biochemical	440	2670	Ouedraogo *et al.* 2002
	BC_1F_1 (BC48 × TC221)	RF:P, AFLP, morphology	148	783	Chaitieng *et al.* 2006
White clover (*Trifolium repens* L.)	F2 (intercross of 4th & 5th generation inbred genotypes carrying a S_f mutation)	SSR, AFLP	135	825	Jones *et al.* 2003
	F_1 (Double pseudo-testcross; 364/7 × 6525/5)	EST-SSR	493	1144	Barrett *et al.* 2004
	F_1 (Double pseudo-testcross; GA43 × SRVR)	SSR	415	1877	Zhang *et al.* 2007

 # Abbreviations: $F_{x=}$ selfed generation, RIL = recombinant inbred line; DH = double haploid; B = baccross genration; IBL = inbre backcross line

*** Abbreviations: BAC = bacterial artificial chromosome; RFLP = restriction fragment length polyorphism; SCAR = sequence characterized amplified region; ISSR = inter simple sequence repeat; AFLP = amplified fragment length polmorphism, RAPD = random amplified polymorphic DNA; SSR = simple sequence repeat; STS = sequence tagged site; SNP = single nucleotie polymorphism; EST-SSR = expressed sequence tag derived simple sequence repeat; RGA = resistance gene analogue; SDRF = single-dose restriction fragment; MITE-HBr = miniature inverted repeat transposable element-Heartbreaker; IMP = Inter-MITE polymorphism; SRAP = sequence-related amplified poly morphism; REMAP = retrtransposon-microsatellite amplified polymorphism.**

plants are presented in Table 20.3. A detailed map holds the opportunity for the identification of DNA markers for quick evaluation of large population. The molecular marker will help in the plant breeding programme to identify and tag novel/gene(s)/QTLs and adopt MAS for improvement of simply inherited qualitative traits as well as complex quantitative traits.

CONCLUSION

Recent advances and development in genome research have resulted in the generation of large data set of DNA and protein sequences from different organisms. Therefore, to use this large data set of sequence information, there is an urgent need to develop a synergism among plant biologists of various hues—genomists, molecular biologists, bioinformatics, geneticists, physiologists and agronomists to solve crop specific problems. A comprehensive resource for genomic and gene-derived markers has been developed for a number of plant species. The widespread application of these molecular markers in a variety of studies will have far reaching implications relevant to crop improvement. Molecular maps of different species have also been developed and some of the important genes have been mapped. This information along with the advancement of new tools/ technologies will increase our knowledge in planning the breeding strategies and will create an avenue for crop improvement.

FURTHER READINGS

1. Adam-Blondon A., Se vignac M. and Dron M. (1994) A genetic map of common bean to localize specific resistance genes against anthracnose. *Genome.* **(37):** 915-924.
2. Akkaya M. S., Bhagwat A. A. and Cregan P. B. (1992) Length polymorphisms of simple sequence repeat DNA in soybean. *Genetics.* **(132)**: 1131-1139.
3. Armour J. A. L. Neumann R., Gobert S. and JeflYeys A. J. (1994) Isolation of human simple repeat loci by hybridization selectionl. *Human. Mol. Gen.* **(3)**: 599-605.
4. Barrett B., Griffiths A., Schreiber M., Ellison N., Mercer C., Bouton J., Ong B., Forster J., Sawbridge T., Spangenberg G., Bryan G., Woodfield D. (2004) A microsatellite map of white clover. *Theor. Appl. Genet.* **(109):** 596-608.
5. Becher R. (2007) EST-derivėd microsatellites as a rich source of molecular markers for oats. *Plant Breed.* **(126):** 274-278.
6. Becker J., Vos P., Kuiper M., Salamani F. and Heun M. (1995) Combined mapping of AFLP and RFLP markers in barley. *Mol. Gen. Genet.* **(249):** 65-73.
7. Bednarek P. T., Masoc' P., Lewandowska R. and Myoeków B. (2003) Saturating rye genetic map with amplified fragment length polymorphism (AFLP) and random amplified polymorphic DNA (RAPD) markers. *J. Appl. Genet.* **(44):** 21-33.
8. Bernatzky R and Tanksley S. D. (1986) Towards a saturated linkage map in tomato based on isozymes and random cDNA sequences. *Genetics.* **(112):** 887-898.
9. Bhattramakki D and Rafalski A. (2001) Discovery and application of single nucleotide polymorphism markers in plants. In: Henry R. J. (ed.) *Plant Genotyping: The DNA Fingerprinting of Plants.* CABI Publishing. Oxon. U.K. pp. 179-192.
10. Blair M. W., Pedraza F., Buendia H. F., Gaitán-Solís E., Beebe S. E., Gepts P. and Tohme J. (2003) Development of a genome-wide anchored microsatellite map for common bean (*Phaseolus vulgaris* L.). *Theor. Appl. Genet.* **(107):** 1362-1374.
11. Börner A. and Korzun V. (1998) A consensus linkage map of rye (*Secale cereale* L.) including 374 RFLPs, 24 isozymes and 15 gene loci. *Theor. Appl. Genet.* **(97):** 1279-1288.

12. Botstein D., White R. L., Skolnick M. and Davis R. W. (1980) Construction of a genetic linkage map in man using restriction fragment length polymorphisms. *Am. J. Hum. Genet.* **(32):** 314-331.
13. Bradeen J. M., Staub J. E., Wye C., Antonise R. and Peleman J. (2001) Towards an expanded and integrate linkage map of cucumber (*Cucumis sativus* L.). *Genome* **(44):** 111-119.
14. Bretting P. K. and Widrlechner M.P. (1995) Genetic markers and plant genetic resources management. *Plant Breeding Reviews* **(13):** 11-86.
15. Casa A. M., Brouwer C., Nagel A.,Wang L., Zhang Q., Kresovich S. and Wessler S. R. (2000) The MITE family Heartbreaker (Hbr): molecular markers in maize. *Proc. Natl. Acad. Sci. USA.* **(97):** 10083-10089.
16. Castiglioni P., Ajmone-Marsan P., van Wijk R., Motto M. (1999) AFLP markers in a molecular linkage map of maize: codominant scoring and linkage group distribution. *Theor. Appl. Genet.* **(99):** 425-431.
17. Castiglioni P., Pozzi C., Heun M., Terzi V., Muller K. J, Rohde W. and Salamini F. (1998) An AFLP-based procedure for the efficient mapping of mutations and DNA probes in barley. *Genetics.* **(149):** 2039-2056.
18. Causse M., Santoni S., Damerval C., Maurice A., Charcosset A., *et al.* (1996) A composite map of expressed sequences in maize. *Genome.* **(39):** 418-432.
19. Chaitieng B., Kaga A., Tomooka N., Isemura T., Kuroda Y. and Vaughan D. A. (2006) Development of a black gram [*Vigna mungo* (L.) Hepper] linkage map and its comparison with an azuki bean [*Vigna angularis* (Willd.) Ohwi and Ohashi] linkage map. *Theor. Appl. Genet.* **(113):** 1261-1269.
20. Chang R. Y., O'Donoughue L.S. and Bureau T. E. (2001) Inter-MITE polymorphism (IMP): a high throughput transposon-based genome mapping and fingerprinting approach. *Theor. Appl. Genet.* **(102):** 773-781.
21. Chao S., Baysdorfer C., Herediadiaz O., Musket T., Xu G. and Coe E. H. (1994) RFLP mapping of partially sequence leaf cDNA clonesin maize. *Theor. Appl. Genet.* **(88):** 717-721.
22. Chen C., Yu Q., Hou S., Li Y., Eustice M. *et al.* (2007) Construction of a sequence-tagged high-density genetic map of papaya for comparative structural and evolutionary genomics in brassicales. *Genetics.* **(177):** 2481-2491.
23. Chen X., Salamini F. and Gebhardt C. (2001) A potato molecular function map for charbohydrate metabolism and transport. *Theor. Appl. Genet.* **(102):** 284-295.
24. Choi H. K., Kim D., Uhm T., Limpens E., Lim H., Mun J. H., Kalo P., Penmetsa R. V., Seres A., Kulikova O. *et al.* (2004) A sequence-based genetic map of Medicago truncatula and comparison of marker colinearity with *M. sativa. Genetics.* **(166):** 1463-1502.
25. Choi Ik-Y., Hyten D. L., Matukumalli L. K., Song Q. (2007) A soybean transcript map: Gene distribution, haplotype and single-nucleotide polymorphism analysis. *Genetics.* **(176):** 685-696.
26. Condit R. and Hubbell S. P. (1991) Abundance and DNA sequence of two-base repeat regions in tropical tree genomes. *Genome.* **(34):** 66-71.
27. Cordeiro G. M., Casu R., McIntyre C. L., Manners J. M. Henry R. J. (2001) Microsatellite markers from sugarcane (*Saccharum* spp.) ESTs cross transferable to erianthus and sorghum. *Plant Sci.* **(160):** 1115-1123.
28. Costa J. M., Corey A., Hayes P. M., Jobet C., Kleinhofs A., Kopisch-Obusch A., Kramer S. F., Kudrna D., Li M., Riera-Lizarazu O. and Sato K. *et al.* (2001) Molecular mapping of the Oregon Wolfe Barleys: a phenotypically polymorphic doubled-haploid population. *Theor. Appl. Genet.* **(103):** 415-424.
29. Cregan P. B., Jarvik T., Bush A. L., Shoemaker R. C., *et al.* (1999) An integrated genetic linkage map of the soybean genome. *Crop Sci.* **(39):** 1464-1490.
30. Davis G. L., McMullen M. D., Baysdorfer C., Musket T., Grant D., Staebell M., Xu G., Polacco M., Koster L., Houchins K., Chao S. and Coe E. H., Jr. (1999) A maize map standard with sequenced core markers, grass genome reference points, and 932 ESTs in a 1736-locus map. *Genetics.* **(152):** 1137-1172.
31. Decroocq V., Fave M. G., Hagen L. Bordenave L. (2003) Development and transferability of apricot and grape EST microsatellite markers across taxa. *Theor. Appl. Genet.* **(106):** 912-922.
32. Desai A., Chee P. W., Rong J., May O. L. and Paterson A. H. (2006) Chromosome structural changes in diploid and tetraploid a genomes of *Gossypium. Genome.* **(49):** 336-345.

33. Devos K. M., Atkinson M. D., Chinoy C. N., Francis H. A., Harcourt R. L., Koebner R. M. D., Liu C. J., Masojc P., Xie D. X. and Gale M. D. (1993) Chromosomal rearrangements in the rye genome relative to that of wheat. *Theor. Appl. Genet.* **(85):** 673-680.
34. Diers B. W., Mansur L., Imsande J. and Shoemaker R. C. (1992) Mapping of *Phytophthora* resistance loci in soybean with restriction for genetic analysis that is appropriate to the needs of fragment length polymorphism markers. *Crop Sci.* **(32):** 377-383.
35. Echt C. S., Kidwell K. K., Knapp S. J., Osborn T. C. and McCoy T. J. (1994) Linkage mapping in diploid alfalfa (*Medicago sativa*). *Genome.* **(37):** 61-71.
36. Edwards K. J., Barker J. H. A., Daly A., Jones C., Karp A. (1996) Microsatellite libraries enriched for several microsatellite sequences in plants. *Biotechniques.* **(20):** 758-760.
37. Epplen J., Ammer H., Epplen C., Kammerbauer C., Mitreiter R., Roewer L., *et al.* (1991) Oligonucleotide fingerprinting using simple repeat motifs: a convenient, ubiquitously applicable method to detect hypervariability for multiple purposes, *In* Burke T., Dolf G., Jeffreys A. J. and Wolff R. (ed.), *DNA Fingerprinting: Approaches and Applications*. Birkha¨user Verlag, Basel. p. 50-69.
38. Eujayl I., Sledge M. K., Wang L., May G. D., Chekhovskiy K., Zwonitzer J. C. and Mian M. A. (2004) *Medicago truncatula* EST–SSRs reveal cross-species genetic markers for *Medicago* spp. *Theor. Appl. Genet.* **(108):** 414-422.
39. Falque M., Décousset L., Dervins D., Jacob A. M, Joets J., Martinant J. P., Raffoux X., Ribière N., Ridel C., Samson D., Charcosset A. and Murigneux A. (2005) Linkage mapping of 1454 new maize candidate gene Loci. *Genetics.* **(170):** 1957-1966.
40. Fatokun C. A., Danesh D., Menancio-Hautea D. I. and Young N. D. (1993) A linkage map for cowpea [*Vigna unguiculata* (L) Walp] based on DNA markers (2n = 22). *In Genetic maps 1992. A Compilation of Linkage and Restriction Maps of Genetically Studied Organisms. Edited* by J.S. O'Brien. Cold Spring Harbor Laboratory Press, Cold Spring Harbour, N.Y. pp. 6256-6258.
41. Faure S., Noyer J. L., Horry J. P., Bakry F., Lanaud C. and Gonza lez de Leon D. (1993) A molecular marker-based linkage map of diploid bananas (*Musa acuminata*). *Theor. Appl. Genet.* **(87):** 517-526.
42. Fazio G., Staub J. E. and Stevens M. R. (2003) Genetic mapping and QTL analysis of horticultural traits in cucumber (*Cucumis sativus* L.) using recombinant inbred lines. *Theor. Appl. Genet.* **(107):** 864-874.
43. Frelichowski Jr J. E., Palmer M. B., Main D. *et al.* (2006) Cotton genome mapping with new microsatellites from Acala 'Maxxa' BAC-ends. *Mol. Gen. Genomics.* **(275):** 479-491.
44. Freyre R., Skroch P. W., Geffory V., Adam-Blondon A. F., Shirmohamadali A., Johnson W. C., Llaca V., Nodari R. O., Periera P. A., Tsai S. M., Tohme J., Dron M., Nienhuis J., Vallejos C. E. and Gepts P. (1998) Towards an integrated linkage map of common bean for Development of a core linkage map and alignment of RFLP maps. *Theor. Appl. Genet.* **(97):** 847-856.
45. Gardiner J. M., Coe E. H., Melia-Hancock S., Hoisington D. A. and Chao S. (1993) Development of a core RFLP map in maize using an immortalized F_2 population. *Genetics.* **(134):** 917-930.
46. Gong L., Stift G., Kofler R., Pachner M. and T. Lelley Microsatellites for the genus *Cucurbita* and an SSR-based genetic linkage map of *Cucurbita pepo* L. (2008) *Theor. Appl. Genet.* **(117):** 37-48.
47. Graner A., Jahoor A., Schondelmaier J., Siedler H., Pillen K., Fischbeck G., Wenzel G. and Herrmann R. G. (1991) Construction of an RFLP map of barley. *Theor. Appl. Genet.* **(83):** 250-256.
48. Groh S., Zacharias A., Kianian S. F., Penner G. A., Chong J., Rines H. W. and Phillips R. L. (2001) Comparative AFLP mapping in two hexaploid oat populations. *Theor. Appl. Genet.* **(102):** 876-884.
49. Guan, Y., Chen Q., Pan J., Li Z., He H., Wu A., Song R. and Cai R. (2008) Construction of a BAC library from cucumber (*Cucumis sativus* L.) and identification of linkage group specific clones. *Progress in Natural Science.* **(18):** 143-47.
50. Gupta P. K. and Varshney R. K. (2000) The development and use of microsatellite markers for genetic analysis and plant breeding with emphasis on bread wheat. *Euphytica* **(113):** 163-185.
51. Gupta P. K, Roy J. K. and Prasad M. (2001) Single nucleotide polymorphisms: a new paradigm for molecular marker technology and DNA polymorphism detection with emphasis on their use in plants. *Curr. Sci.* **(80):** 524-535.

52. Gupta P. K, Varshney R. K. and Prasad M. (2002) Molecular markers: principles and methodologies. In: Jain S. M., Brar D. S. and Ahloowalia B. S. (eds.) *Molecular Techniques in Crop Improvement,* Kluwer Academic Publishers, Dordrecht, The Netherlands, pp. 9-54
53. Gupta P. K. and Rustgi S. (2004) Molecular markers from the transcribed/expressed region of the genome in higher plants. *Funct. & Integr. Genomics.* **(4):** 139-162.
54. Gupta P. K. and Varshney R. K. (eds.) (2004) *Cereal Genomics*. Kluwer Academic Publishers, Dordrecht, The Netherlands, pp. 639
55. Han Z.-G., Guo W.-Z., Song X.-L. and Zhang T.-Z. (2004) Genetic mapping of EST-derived microsatellites from the diploid *Gossypium arboreum* in allotetraploid cotton. *Mol. Gen. Genomics.* **(272):** 308-327.
56. He D. H., Lin Z. X., Zhang X. L. *et al.* (2007) QTL mapping for economic traits based on a dense genetic map of cotton with PCR-based markers using the interspecific cross of *Gossypium hirsutum* x *Gossypium barbadense*." *Euphytica.* **(153):** 181-197.
57. Helentjaris T, Slocum M, Wright S, Schaeffer A. and Nienhuis J. (1986) Construction of genetic linkage maps in maize and tomato using restriction fragment length polymorphisms. *Theor. Appl. Genet.* **(72):** 761-769.
58. Hernandez P., Dorado G., Prieto P., Gimenez M. J., Ramirez M. C., Laurie D. A., Snape J. W. and Martin A. (2001) A core genetic map of Hordeum chilense and comparisons with maps of barley (*Hordeum vulgare*) and wheat (*Triticum aestivum*). *Theor. Appl. Genet.* **(102):** 1259-1264.
59. Heun M., Kennedy A. E., Anderson J. A., Lapitan N. L. V., Sorrells M. E. and Tankslet S. D. (1991) Construction of a restriction fragment length polymorphism map of barley (*Hordeum vulgare*). *Genome.* **(34):** 437-447.
60. Hittalmani S., Foolad M. R., Mew T. V., Rodriquez R. L. and Huang N. (1995) Development of PCR based marker to identify rice blast resistance gene, *Pi 2(t)* in a segregating population. *Theor. Appl. Genet.* **(91):** 9-14.
61. Hongtrakul V., Huestis G. M. and Knapp S. J. (1997) Amplified fragment length polymorphism as a tool for DNA fingerprinting sunflower germplasm: genetic diversity among oilseed inbred lines. *Theor. Appl. Genet.* **(95):** 400-407.
62. Humphry M. E., Konduri V., Lambrides C. J., Magner T., McIntyre C. L., Aitken E. A. B. and Liu C. J. (2002) Development of a mungbean (*Vigna radiata*) RFLP linkage map and its comparison with lablab (*Lablab purpureus*) reveals a high level of colinearity between the two genomes. *Theor. Appl. Genet.* **(105):** 160-166.
63. Jain S. M, Brar D. S. and Ahloowalia B. S. (eds.), (2002) *Molecular Techniques in Crop Improvement.* Kluwer Academic Publishers, Dordrecht, pp. 616.
64. Jeffrey A. J., Wilson V. and Thein S. L. (1985) Hypervariable 'minisatellite' regions in human DNA. *Nature.* **(314):** 67-73.
65. Jin H., Domier L. L., Shen X. and Kolb F. L. (2000) Combined AFLP and RFLP mapping in two hexaploid oat recombinant inbred populations. *Genome.* **(43):** 94-101.
66. Jones K. C., Levine K. F., Banks J. D. (2002) Characterization of 11 polymorphic tetra-nucleotide microsatellites for forensic applications in California cec (*Cervus elaphus canadensis*). *Mol. Ecol. Notes.* **(2):** 425-427.
67. Jones E., Hughes L., Drayton M., Abberton M., Michaelson-Yeats T., Bowen C. and Forster J. (2003) An SSR and AFLP molecular marker-based genetic map of white clover (*Trifolium repens* L.). *Plant Sci.* **(165):** 531-539.
68. Kaga A., Ishii T., Tsukimoto K. and Tokoro E. (2000) Comparative molecular mapping in Ceratotropis species using and interspecific cross between azuki bean (*Vigna angularis*) and rice bean (*V. umbellata*). *Theor. Appl. Genet.* **(100):** 207-213.
69. Kaga A., Tomooka N., Egawa Y., Hosaka K. and Kamijima O. (1996) Species relationships in the subgenus *Ceratotropis* (genus Vigna) as revealed by RAPD analysis. *Euphytica.* **(88):** 17-24.

70. Kaló P., Endre L., Zimányi G., Csanádi G. and Kiss G. B. (2000) Construction of an improved linkage map of diploid alfalfa (*Medicago sativa*). *Theor. Appl. Genet.* **(100):** 641-657.
71. Keim P., Schupp J. M., Travis S. E., Clayton K. and Zhu T. *et al.* (1997) A high-density soybean genetic map based on AFLP markers. *Crop Sci.* **(37):** 537-543.
72. Kennard W. C., Poetter K., Dijkhuizen A., Meglic V., Staub J. E., Havey M. J. (1994). Linkages among RFLP, RAPD, isozyme, diseases resistance, and morphological markers in narrow and wide crosses of cucumber. *Theor. Appl. Genet.* **(89):** 42-48.
73. Khlestkina E. K., Than M. H., Pestsova E. G., Roder M. S., Malyshev S. V., Korzun V. and Börner A (2004) Mapping of 99 new microsatellite-derived loci in rye (*Secale cereale* L.) including 39 expressed sequence tags. *Theor. Appl. Genet.* **(109):** 725-732.
74. Kiss G. B., Csanádi G., Kálmán K., Kaló P. and Ökrész L. (1993) Construction of a basic genetic map for alfalfa using RFLP, RAPD, isozyme and morphological markers. *Mol. Gen. Genet.* **(238):** 129-137.
75. Kleinhofs A., Kilian A., Saghai-Maroof M. A., Biyashev R. M., Hayes P. M., Chen F. Q., Lapitan N., Fenwick A., Blake T., Kanazin V. et al. 1993 A molecular, isozyme and morphological map of barley (*Hordeum vulgare*) genome. *Theor. Appl. Genet.* **(86):** 705-712.
76. Koebner R. M. and Summers R. W. (2003) 21st century wheat breeding: plot selection or plate detection? *Trends Biotechnol.* **(21):** 59-63.
77. Kohel R. J., Yu J., Park Y.-H. and Lazo G. R. (2001) Molecular mapping and characterization of traits controlling fiber quality in cotton. *Euphytica.* **(121):** 163-172.
78. Lacape J.-M., Nguyen T.-B., S. Thibivilliers, *et al.* (2003) A combined RFLP-SSR-AFLP map of tetraploid cotton based on a *Gossypium hirsutum* x *Gossypium barbadense* backcross population. *Genome.* **(46):** 612-626.
79. Lagercrantz U., Ellegren H. and Andersson L. (1993) The abundance of various polymorphic microsatellite motifs differs between plants and vertebrates. *Nucleic Acids Res.* **(21):** 1111-1115.
80. Lambrides C. J., Lawn R. J., Godwin I. D., Manners J. and Imrie B. C. (2000) two genetic linkage maps of mungbean using RFLP and RAPD markers. *Aust. J. Agric. Res.* **(51):** 415-425.
81. Langridge P., Karakousis A., Collins N., Kretchmer J. and Manning S. (1995) A consensus linkage map of barely. *Mol. Breed.* **(1):** 389-395.
82. Lee M., Sharopova N., Beavis, W. D., Grant D., Katt M., Blair D. and Hallauer A. (2002) Expanding the genetic map of maize with the intermated B73 × Mol7 (IBM) population. *Plant Mol. Biol.* **(48):** 453-461.
83. Lee Y. H., Jeon H. J., Hong K. H. and Kim B. D. (1995) Use of random amplified polymorphic DNA for linkage group analysis in an interspecific cross hybrid F_2 generation of *Cucurbita. J. Kor. Soc. Hortic. Sci.* **(36):** 323-330.
84. Li J. Z., Sjakste T. G., Roeder M. S. and Ganal M. W. (2003) Development and genetic mapping of 127 new microsatellite markers in barely. *Theor. Appl. Genet.* **(107):** 1021-1027.
85. Lin Z., He D., Zhang X. *et al.* (2005) Linkage map construction and mapping QTL for cotton fibre quality using SRAP, SSR and RAPD. *Plant Breed.* **(124):** 180-87.
86. Lin Z., Zhang X., Nie Y., He D. and Wu M. (2003) Construction of a genetic linkage map for cotton based on SRAP. *Chinese Science Bulletin.* **(48):** 2063-2067.
87. Litt M. and Lutty J. A. (1989) A hypervariable microsatellite revealed by *in vitro* amplification of a dinucleotide repeat within the cardiac muscle actin gene. *Am. J. Hum. Genet.* **(4):** 397-401.
88. Loarce Y., Hueros G. and Ferrer E. (1996) A molecular linkage map of rye. *Theor, Appl. Genet.* **(93):** 1112-1118.
89. Lörz H. and Wenzel G. (Eds.) (2005) *Molecular Marker Systems in Plant Breeding and Crop Improvement*. Springer-Verlag, Berlin, Heidelberg, pp. 476.
90. Ma X-X., Zhou B-L., Lü Y-H., Guo W-Z., Zhang T-Z. (2008) Simple sequence repeat genetic linkage maps of A-genome diploid cotton (*Gossvpium arboreumv*). *J. Integr. Plant Biol.* **(50):** 491-502.

91. Ma H., Moore P. H. Liu Z., Kim M. S., Yu Q., Fitch M. M, M., Sekioka T., Paterson A. H. and Ming R, (2004) High-density linkage mapping revealed suppression of recombination at the sex determination locus in papaya. *Genetics.* **(166):** 419-436.

92. Ma X-F Wanous M, K., Houchins K., Rodriguez Milia M. A., Goicoechea P. G, Wang Z. *et al.* (2001) Molecular linkage mapping in rye (*Secale cereale* L.). *Theor. Appl. Genet.* **(102):** 517-523.

93. Mano Y., Kawasaki S., Takaiwa F. and Komatsuda T. (2001) Construction of a genetic map of barley (*Hordeum vulgare* L.) cross 'Azumamugi' ´ 'Kanto Nakate Gold' using a simple and efficient amplified fragment-length polymorphism system. *Genome.* **(44):** 284-292.

94. Market C. L. and Moller F. (1959) Multiple forms of enzymes: tissue ontogenetics and species specific pattern. *Proc. Natl. Acad. Sci. USA.* **(47):** 753-763.

95. Marsan P, A., Gorni C., Chittò A., Redaelli R., van Vijk R., Stam P. and Motto M. (2001) Identification of QTLs for grain yield and grain-related traits of maize (*Zea mays* L.) using an AFLP map, different testers, and cofactor analysis. *Theor. Appl. Genet.* **(102):** 230-243.

96. Masojc' P., Myoekòw B. and Milczarski P. (2001) Extending a RFLP-based genetic map of rye using random amplified polymorphic DNA (RAPD) and isozyme markers. *Theor. Appl. Genet.* **(102):** 1273-1279.

97. Mei M., Syed N. H., Gao W., *et al.* (2004) Genetic mapping and QTL analysis of fiber-related traits in cotton (*Gossypium*). *Theor. Appl. Genet.* **(108):** 280-291.

98. Meksem K. and Kahl G. (2005) *The Handbook of Plant Genome Mapping: Genetic and Physical Mapping.* Wiley-VCH Verlag GmbH, Weinheim.

99. Menacio-Hautea D., Fatokun C. A., Kumar L., Danesh D. and Young N. D. (1993) Comparative genome analysis of mungbean (*Vigna radiata* L. Wilczek) and cowpea (*V unguiculata* L. Walpers) using RFLP mapping data. *Theor. Appl. Genet.* **(86):** 797-810.

100. Menendez C. M., Hall, A. E. and Gepts P. (1997) A genetic linkage map of cowpea (*Vigna unguiculata*) developed from a cross between two inbred, domesticated lines. *Theor. Appl. Genet.* **(95):** 1210-1217.

101. Merdinoglu D, Butterlin G, Bevilacqua L, Chiquet V, Adam-Blondon AF, Decroocq S. (2005) Development and characterization of a large set of microsatellite markers in grapevine (*Vitis vinifera* L.) suitable for multiplex PCR. *Mol Breed.* **(15):** 349-366.

102. Milczarski P., Banek-Tabor A., Lebiecka K., Stojalowski S., Myoekow B. and Masoc' P. (2007) New genetic map of rye composed of PCR-based molecular markers and its alignment with the reference map of the DS2 ´ RXL 10 intercross. *J. Appl. Genet.* **(48):** 11-24.

103. Miyazaki C, Osanai E., Saeki K., Hirota N., Ito K., Ukai Y., Konishi T. and Saito A (2000) Construction of a barley RFLP linkage map using an F2 population derived from a cross between Ko A and Mokusekko 3. *Barley Genet Newslett.* **(30):** 41-43.

104. Mohan M., Nair S., Bhagwat A., Krishna TG., Yano M., Bhati CR. and Sasaki T. (1997) Genome mapping, molecular markers and marker assisted selection in crop plants. *Mol. Breed.* **(3):** 87-103.

105. Morgante M. and Olivieri A M. (1993) PCR-amplified microsatellites as markers in plant genetics. *Plant J* **(3):** 175-182

106. Mun J. H., Kim D. J., Choi H. K., Gish J., Debelle F., *et al.* (2006) Distribution of microsatellites in the genome of *Medicago truncatula*: a resource of genetic markers that integrate genetic and physical maps. *Genetics.* **(172):** 2541-2555.

107. Nguyen T.-B., Giband M., Brottier P., Risterucci A.-M. and Lacape J.-M. (2004) Wide coverage of the tetraploid cotton genome using newly developed microsatellite markers," *Theor. Appl. Genet.* **(109):** 167-175.

108. Nodari R. O., Tsai S. M., Gilbertson R. L. and Gepts P. (1993) Towards an integrated linkage map of common bean. II. Development of an RFLP-based linkage map. *Theor. Appl. Genet.* **(85):** 513-520.

109. O'Donoughue L. S., Kianian S. F., Rayapati P. J., Penner G. A., Sorrells M. E Tanksley S. D., Phillips R. L., Rines H. W., Lee M., Fedak G., Molnar S. J., Hoffman D., Salas C. A., Wu B., Autrique E. and Van Deynze A. (1995) A molecular linkage map of cultivated oat. *Genome.* **(38):** 368380.

110. O'Donoughue L. S., Wang Z., Röder M., Kneen B., Leggett M., Sorrells M. E., and Tanksley S. D. (1992) An RFLP-based linkage map of oats based on a cross between two diploid taxa (*Avena atlantica ′ A. hirtula). Genome.* **(35):** 765-771.

111. Orita M., Iwahana H., Kanazawa H., Hayashi K. and Sekiya T. 1989 Detection of polymorphism of human DNA by gel electrophoresis as single strand conformation polymorphisms. *Proc. Natl. Acad. Sci. USA.* **(86):** 2766-2770.

112. Ouedraogo J. T., Gowda B. S., Jean M., Close T. J., Ehlers J. D., Hall A. E., Gillaspie A. G., Roberts P. A., Ismail A. M., Bruening G., Gepts P., Timko M. P., Belzile F. J. (2002) An improved genetic linkage map for cowpea (*Vigna unguiculata* L.): combining AFLP, RFLP, RAPD, biochemical markers, and biological resistance traits. *Genome.* **(45):** 175-188.

113. Paglia G. P., Olivieri A. M. and Morgante M. (1998) Towards second generation STS (sequence tagged sites) linkage maps in conifers: A genetic map of Norway spruce (*Picea abies* K.). *Mol. Gen. Genet.* **(258):** 466-478.

114. Park Y.-H., Alabady M. S., Ulloa M. *et al.* (2005) Genetic mapping of new cotton fiber loci using EST-derived microsatellites in an interspecific recombinant inbred line cotton population. *Mol. Gen. Genomics.* **(274):** 428-441.

115. Parsons B. J., Newbury J. H., Jackson M. T. and Ford L. B. V. (1997) Contrasting genetic diversity relationships are revealed in rice (*Oryza sativa* L.) using different marker types. *Mol. Breed.* **(3):** 115-125.

116. Phillips R.L. and Vasil I.K. (eds.), (1994) *DNA-Based Markers in Plants*. Kluwer Academic Publishers, Dordrecht. pp. 383.

117. Phillips R.L. and Vasil I.K. (eds.), (2001) *DNA-Based Markers in Plants.* Kluwer Academic Publishers, Dordrecht. pp. 512.

118. Philipp U., Wehling P. and Wricke G. (1994) A linkage map of rye. *Theor Appl. Genet.* **(88):** 243-248.

119. Pillen K., Binder A., Kreuzkam B., Ramsay L., Waugh R., Forster J. and Leon J. (2000) Mapping new EMBL-derived barley microsatellites and their use in differentiating German barley cultivars. *Theor. Appl. Genet.* **(101):** 652-660.

120. Portyanko V. A., Chen G., Rines H. W., Phillips R. L., Leonard K. J., Ochocki G. E. and Stuthman D. D. (2005) Quantitative trait loci for partial resistance to crown rust, *Puccinia coronata,* in cultivated oat, *Avena sativa* L. *Theor Appl. Genet.* **(111):** 313-324.

121. Portyanko V. A., Hoffman D. L., Lee M. and Holland J. B. (2001) A linkage map of hexaploid oat based on grass anchor DNA clones and its relationship to other oat maps. *Genome* **(44)**, 249-265.

122. Powell W. Machray G.C. and Provan J. (1996) Polymorphism revealed by simple sequence repeats. *Trends Plant Sci.* **(1):** 215-222

123. Prasad, M., Varshney, R. K., Kumar, A., Balyan, H. S., Sharma, P. C, Edwards, K. J., Singh, H., Dhaliwal, H. S., Roy, J. K. and Gupta, P. K. (1999) A microsatellite marker associated with a QTL for grain protein content on chromosome arm 2DL of bread wheat. *Theor. Appl. Genet.* **(99):** 341-345

124. Prasad, M., Varshney, R. K., Roy, I. K., Balyan, H. S. and Gupta, P. K. (2000) The use of microsatellites for detecting DNA polymorphism, genotype identification and genetic diversity in wheat. *Theor. Appl. Genet.* **(100):** 584-592.

125. Prasad, M., Kumar, N., Kulwal, P. L., Roeder. M. S., Balyan, H. S., Dhaliwal. H. S. and Gupta, P. K. (2003) QTL analysis for grain protein content using SSR markers and validation studies using NILs in bread wheat. *Theor. Appl. Genet.* **(106):** 659-667.

126. Qi X., Stam P. and Lindhout P. (1996) Comparison and integration of four barley genetic maps. *Genome.* **(39):** 379-394.

127. Qi X., Stam P. and Lindhout P. (1998) Use of locus-specific AFLP markers to construct a high-density molecular map in barley. *Theor. Appl. Genet.* **(96):** 376-384.

128. Rafalski J. A. and Tingey S. V. (1993) Genetic diagnostics in plant breeding-RAPDs: microsatellites and machines. *Trends Genet.* **(9)**: 275-280.

129. Ramsay L., Macaulay M., Ivanissevich D. S., MacLean K., Cardle L., Fuller J., Edwards K. J., Tuvesson S., Morgante M., Massari A. *et al.* (2000) A simple sequence repeat-based linkage map of barley. *Genetics.* **(156):** 1997-2005.

130. Rayapati P. J., Gregory 1. W., Lee M. and Wise R. P. (1994) A linkage map of diploid *Avena* based on RFLP loci and a locus conferring resistance to nine isolates of *Puccinia coronata* var. *avenae. Theor. Appl. Genet.* **(89):** 831-837.

131. Reinisch A. J., Dong J.-M., Brubaker C L., Stelly D. M., Wendel J. F. and Paterson A. H. (1994) A detailed RFLP map of cotton, *Gossypium hirsutum x Gossypium barbadense*: chromosome organization and evolution in a disomic polyploid genome. *Genetics.* **(138):** 829-847.

132. Richardson T., Cato S., Ramser J., Kahl G. and Weising K. (1995) Hybridization of microsatellites to RAPD: a new source of polymorphic markers. *Nucleic Acids Res.* **(23):** 3798-3799.

133. Riera-Lizarazu O., Vales M. I. and Phillips R. L. (2001) A compendium of molecular genetic maps of cultivated plants. *In* R.L. Phillips, and I.K. Vasil (eds.), *DNA-Based Markers in Plants*. pp. 463-497. *Advances in Cellular and Molecular Biology of Plants*. Kluwer Academic Publishers, Dordrecht.

134. Rong J. K., Abbey C; Bowers J. E., *et al.* (2004) A 3347-locus genetic recombination map of sequence-tagged sites reveals types of genome organization, transmission and evolution of cotton (*Gossypium*). *Genetics.* **(166):** 389-417.

135. Rostoks N., Mudie S., Cardle L., Russell J., Ramsay L., Booth A., Svensson J., Wanamaker S., Walia H., Rodriguez E., Hedley P., Liu H., Morris J., Close T., Marshall D. and Waugh R. (2005) Genome-wide SNP discovery and linkage analysis in barley based on genes responsive to abiotic stress. *Mol. Gen. Genomics.* **(274):** 515-527.

136. Roy J. K., Prasad M., Varshney R. K., Balyan H. S., Blake T. K., Dhaliwal H. S., Singh H., Edwards K. J., and Gupta P. K. (1999) Identification of a microsatellite on chromosome 6B and a STS on 7D of bread wheat showing association with pre-harvest sprouting tolerance. *Theor. Appl. Genet.* **(99):** 336-340.

137. Saal B. and Wricke G. (2002) Clustering of amplified fragment length polymorphism markers in a linkage map of rye. *Plant Breed.* **(121):** 117-123.

138. Senft P. and Wricke G. (1996) An extended genetic map of rye (*Secale cereale* L.). *Plant Breed.* **(115):** 508-510.

139. Serquen F.C., Bacher J. and Staub J. E. (1997) Mapping and QTL analysis of a narrow cross in cucumber (*Cucumis sativus* L.) using random amplified polymorphic DNA markers. *Mol. Breed.* **(3):** 257-268.

140. Sharopova N., McMullen M. D., Schultz L., Schroeder S., Sanchez-Villeda, H., Gardiner J., Bergstrom D., Houchins K., Melia-Hancock S., Musket T., Duru N., Polacco M., Edwards K., Ruff T., Register J. C., Brouwer C., Thompson R., Velasco R., Chin E., Lee M., WoodmanClikeman W., Long M. J., Liscum E., Cone K., Davis G. and Coe E.H. Jr. (2002) Development and mapping of SSR markers for maize. *Plant Mol. Biol.* **(48):** 463-481.

141. Shoemaker R.C. and Olson T. C. (1993). Molecular linkage map of soybean (*Glycine max* L. Merr.). *In:* S.J. O' Brien *Genetic. Maps: Locus Maps of Complex Genomes*. Cold Spring Lark. 1996. Genetic mapping of agronomic traits using recombinant. Harbor Laboratory Press, Cold Spring Harbor, New York; pp. 6.131-6.1381

142. Sledge M. K., Ray I. M. and Jiang G. (2005) An expressed sequence tag SSR map of tetraploid alfalfa (*Medicago sativa* L.). *Theor. Appl. Genet.* **(111):** 980-992.

143. Sondur S. N., Manshardt R. M. and Stiles J. I. (1996) A genetic linkage map of papaya based on randomly amplified polymorphic DNA markers. *Theor. Appl. Genet.* **(93):** 547-553.

144. Song Q. J., Fickus E. W. and Cregan P. B. (2002) Characterization of trinucleotide SSR motifs in wheat. *Theor. Appl. Genet.* **(104):** 286-293.

145. Song Q. J., Marek L. F., Shoemaker R. C. *et al.* (2004) A new integrated genetic linkagc map of the soybean. *Theor. Appl. Genet* **(109):** 122-128.

146. Song X., Wang K., Guo W., Zhang J. and Zhang T. (2005) A comparison of genetic maps constructed from haploid and BC1 mapping populations from the same crossing between *Gossypium hirsutum* L. and *Gossypium barbadense* L. *Genome.* **(48):** 378-390.

147. Stein N., Prasad M., Scholz U., Thiel T., Zhang H., Wolf M., Kota R., Varshney R. K., Perovic D., Grosse I. and Graner A. (2007) A 1,000-loci transcript map of the barley genome: new anchoring points for integrative grass genomics. *Theor. Appl. Genet.* **(114):** 823-839.

148. Stuber C. W., Polacco M. and Senior L. M. (1999) Synergy of empirical breeding, marker-assisted selection and genomics to increase crop yield potential. *Crop Sci.* **(39):** 1571-1583.

149. Tanksley S. D. (1993a) Molecular markers in plant breeding. *Plant Mol. Biol. Rep.* **(1):** 3-8.

150. Tanksley S. D. (1993b) Mapping Polygenes. *Annu. Rev Genet.* **(27):** 205-233.

151. Tanksley S. D. and Orton T. J. (1983) *Isozymes in Plant Genetics and Breeding*. Amsterdam: Elsevier Science.

152. Tanksley S. D. and Rick C. (1980) Isozyme gene linkage map of the tomato: application in genetics and breeding. *Theor. Appl. Genet.* **(57):** 161-170.

153. Tar'an B., Michaels T. E. and Pauls K. P. (2002) Genetic mapping of agronomic traits in common bean. *Crop Sci.* **(42):** 544-556.

154. Thiel T., Michalek W., Varshney R. K., Graner A. (2003) Exploiting EST databases for the development of cDNA derived microsatellite markers in barley (*Hordeum vulgare* L.). *Thear. Appl. Genet.* **(106):** 411-422.

155. Thoquet P., Ghérardi M., Joumet E. P., Kereszt A., Ané J. M., Prosperi J. M. and Huguet T. (2002) The molecular genetic linkage map of the model legume *Medicago truncatula*: an essential tool for comparative legume genomics and the isolation of agronomically important genes. *BMC Plant Bioi.* **(2):** (2 January 2002).

156. Ulloa M., Meredith Jr. W.R., Shappley Z.W. and Kahler A. L. (2002) RFLP genetic linkage maps from four F2.3 populations and a joinmap of *Gossypium hirsutum* L.," *Theor. Appl. Genet.* **(104):** 200-208.

157. Vallejos C. E., Sakiyama N.E. and Chase C. D. (1992) A molecular-marker based linkage map of *Phasealus vulgaris* L. *Genetics.* **(131):** 733-740.

158. Varshney R. K, Grosse I., Haehnel U., Siefken R., Prasad M., Stein N., Langridge P., Altschmied L. and Graner A. (2006) Genetic mapping and BAC assignment of EST-derived SSR markers shows non-uniform distribution of genes in the barley genome. *Theor. Appl. Genet.* **(113):** 239-250.

159. Varshney R. K., Graner A. and Sorrells M. E. (2005) Genic microsatellite markers in plants: features and applications. *Trends in Biotech.* **(23):** 48-55.

160. Varshney R. K., Marcel T.C., Ramsay L., Russell J.R., Roder M., Stein N., Waugh R., Langridge P., Niks R. E. and Graner A. (2007) A high density barley microsatellite consensus map with 775 SSR loci. *Thear. Appl. Genet.* **(114):** 1091-1101.

161. Villariel C. P., Resurreccion A. P., Constantino S. V., Robeniol J. M. and Bennet J. (1994) Conversion of RFLP markers to sequence tagged sites for chromosome 1 of rice. *Rice Genet. Newl.* **(11):** 120-123.

162. Vos P., Hogers R., Bleeker M., Reijans M., Van de Lee T., Homes M., Frijters A., Peleman P., Kuiper M. and Zabeau M. (1995) AFLP: a new technique for DNA fingerprinting. *Nucleic Acids Res.* **(23):** 4407-4414.

163. Vuylsteke M., Mank R., Antonise R., Bastiaans E., Senior M. L., Stuber C. W., Melchinger A. E., Lübberstedt T., Xia X. C., Stam P., Zabeau M. and Kuiper M. (1999) Two high-density AFLP_ linkage maps of *Zea mays* L.: analysis of distribution of AFLP markers. *Theor. Appl. Genet.* **(99):** 921-935.

164. Wang Z., Weber J. L., Zhong G. and Tanksley S. D. (1994) Survey of plant short tandem DNA repeats. *Theor. Appl. Genet.* **(88):** 1-6.

165. Wang Z. M., Devos K. M., Liu C. J., Wang R. Q., Gale M. D. (1998) Construction of RFLP-based maps of foxtail millet, *Setaria italica* (L.) P. Beauv. *Theor. Appl. Genet.* **(96):** 31-36.

166. Waghmare V. N., Rong J., Rogers C. J., Pierce G. J., Wendel J. F. and Paterson A. H. (2005) Genetic mapping of a cross between *Gossypium hirsutum* (cotton) and the Hawaiian endemic, *Gossypium tomentosum. Theor. Appl. Genet.* **(111):** 665-676.

167. Weeden N., Zamir N. and Tadmore Y. (1988) Application of isozyme analysis in pulse crops. In: *World Crops: Cool Season Food Legumes*, ed. Summerfield R. Amsterdam: Nijhoff. pp. 979-987.

168. Wehling P., Schmidt Stohn G. and Wricke G. (1985) Chromosomal location of esterase, peroxidase and phosphogluco mutase isozyme structural genes in cultivated rye (*Secale cereale* L.) *Theor. Appl. Genet.* **(70):** 377-382.

169. Weising K., Nybom H., Wolff K. and Meyer W. (1995) *DNA Fingerprinting in Plants and Fungi*. CRC Press, Boca Raton, Florida.

170. Weising K., Nybom H., Wolff K. and Kahl G. 2005 *DNA Fingerprinting in Plants: Principles, Methods, and Applications.* 2nd ed. CRC Press, Boca Raton, Florida, USA, pp. 444.

171. Welsh J. and McClelland M. (1990) Fingerprinting genomes using PCR with arbitrary primers. *Nucleic Acids Res*. **(18):** 7213-7218.

172. Werner J.E., Finkelstein R.R. (1995) Arabidopsis mutants with reduced response to NaCl and osmotic stress. *Physiol. Plant*. **(93):** 659-666.

173. Whitkus R., Doebley J. and Wendel J, F. (1994) Nuclear DNA markers in systematics and evolution. In: Phillips R.L. and Vasil I.K. (eds), *DNA-Based Markers in Plants,* Kluwer Academic Publishers, The Netherlands, pp. 116-141.

174. Wight C.P., Tinker N A., Kianian S. F.,. Sorrells M. E, O'Donoughue L. S., Hoffman D. L., Groh S., Scoles G. J. *et al.* (2003) A molecular marker map in 'Kanota' ´ 'Ogle' hexaploid oat (*Avena* spp.) enhanced by additional markers and a robust framework. *Genome.* **(46):** 28-47.

175. Williams J. G. K., Kubelik A. R., Livak K. J; Rafalski J. A. and Tingey S.V. (1990) DNA polymorphism, amplified by arbitary primers are useful as genetic markers. *Nucl. Acids. Res*. **(18):** 6531-6535.

176. Winter P. and Kahl G. (1995) Molecular marker technologies for plant improvement. *World. J. Microbiol. Biotechnol*. **(11)**: 438-448.

177. Wright S. (1943) Isolation by distance. *Genetics* **(28):** 114-138.

178. Xia Z., Tsubokura Y., Hoshi M. *et al.* (2007) An integrated high-density linkage map of soybean with RFLP, SSR, STS, and AFLP markers using a single F_2 population. *DNA Res*. **(14):** 257-269.

179. Yeboah M. A., Xuehao C., Feng C. R., Liang G. and Gu M. (2007) A genetic linkage map of cucumber (*Cucumis sativus L*) combining SRAP and ISSR markers. *African J. of Biotech*. **(6):** 2784-2791.

180. Yong G. Y., Glenn R. B. and Saghai Maroof M. A. (1996) Isolation of a superfamily of candidate disease-resistance genes in soybean based on a conserved nucleotide-binding site. *Proc. Natl. Acad. Sci. USA.* **(93):** 11751-11756.

181. Zane L., Bargelloni L., Patarnello P. (2002) Strategies for microsatellite isolation: a review. *Mol. Ecology.* **(11):** 1-16.

182. Zhang J., Guo W. and Zhang T. (2002) Molecular linkage map of allotetraploid cotton (*Gossyptum hirsutum L.* x *Gossypium barbadense* L.) with a haploid population. *Theor. Appl. Genet*. **(105):** 1166-1174.

183. Zhang Y., Sledge M. K. and Bouton J. H. (2007) Genome mapping of white clover (*Trifoltum repens* L.) and comparative analysis within the Trifolieae using cross-species SSR markers. *Theor. Appl. Genet*. **(114):** 1367-1378.

184. Zheng K., Huang N., Bennett J. and Khush G. S. (1995) PCR based marker assisted selection in rice breeding. IRRI. Discussion Paper Series, No.12. International Rice Research Institute. P.O. Box 933, Manila, Philippines.

185. Zhu S. and Kaeppler H. F. (2003) Identification of quantitative trait loci for resistance to crown rust in oat line MAM 17-5. *Crop Sci*. **(43):** 358-366.

186. Zietkiewicz E., Rafalski A. and Labuda D. (1994) Genome fingerprinting by simple sequence repeat (SSR) anchored polymerase chain reaction amplification. *Genomics*. **(20):** 176-83.

187. Zraidi A., Stift G., Pachner M., Shojaeiyan A., Gong L., Lelley T. (2007) A consensus map for *Cucurbita pepo. Mol. Breed.* **(20):** 375-388.

CHAPTER

21 Marker Assisted Selection Technology

Molecular markers are DNA based markers which are either coding or noncoding sequences in nature, and that assist in crop breeding programmes. The restriction fragment length polymorphism (RFLP) was the first DNA based marker to be used successfully in crop improvement followed by others like AFLP, SSR, DarT, and SNPs. For significant use in plant breeding programmes, molecular markers essentially need to be present in abundance in the genome and be polymorphic in nature, amongst the various other salient features required. These markers help in effective utilization of germplasm and improve and genetic gains more precisely and efficiently by using marker assisted selection (MAS). MAS application strategies in plant breeding includes development of suitable mapping population, linkage analysis and development of linkage map using suitable markers, QTL identification and QTL-marker association analysis, validation of marker-QTL association and then integration of MAS in plant breeding process. MAS aids plant breeding in numerous ways, namely by marker assisted backcrossing, marker assisted background selection, linkage drag in gene introgression, marker assisted gene pyramiding, marker assisted recurrent parent selection and early generation marker assisted selection. MAS is more efficient over phenotypic selection alone, however, theoretical and analytical investigations reveal maximum selection efficiency for quantitative traits by use of a combination of molecular and phenotypic information. A more detailed picture on molecular markers, its essential properties, use of MAS and its different strategies in breeding and some successful stories are discussed in the chapter.

Keywords: Marker assisted selection; molecular breeding; association mapping; QTL; marker-traits.

INTRODUCTION

Plant breeding principles, in its conventional form, basically concentrate around phenotypic selection of superior plant phenotypes in the form of improved cultivars for commercial cultivation to fulfill the requirements of human beings, animals and industrial products. Variations that either already exist in nature or induced using hybridization or recombination or mutation have been the basis of selection. Classical approaches of plant breeding have been enormously successful in increasing production and productivity of most of the crops; however, the success rate has been variable. Exploitation of hybrid vigour in the form of hybrids in many self- as well as cross-pollinated crops has been an excellent example of the application of classical tools of plant breeding in improving yield and other vital parameters. Utilization of dwarfing genes in breeding strategies led to significant increase in production and productivity of rice and wheat, sparking off "Green

Revolution' and making it possible to feed millions of people across the world. Thus, it was universally demonstrated that conventional plant breeding has been successful in the past in improving the production and productivity of cultivated crop plants. However, application of this methodology which involves crossing of genotypes followed by selection of the superior recombinants from among the several segregating progenies is often laborious and time consuming. Further, genotype x environment interactions and the linkage drag (tight linkage of the undesired loci with the desired loci) have often made the strategies difficult to implement or achieve the desired objectives in an efficient manner.

Intensive research on genomics over the last few decades led to identification of an array of DNA-based markers, popularly called "molecular markers". These molecular markers include: (i) hybridization-based markers such as restriction fragment length polymorphism (RFLP), (ii) PCR-based markers: random amplification of polymorphic DNA (RAPD), amplified fragment length polymorphism (AFLP) and microsatellite or simple sequence repeat (SSR), and (iii) sequence-based markers: single nucleotide polymorphism (SNP). Molecular markers can be expressed DNA regions (coding sequences) or DNA segments that have no known coding function (non-coding sequences). Most of the molecular markers have been developed either from genomic DNA libraries (e.g., RFLPs and SSRs) or from random PCR amplification of genomic DNA (e.g. RAPDs) or both (e.g., AFLPs). These DNA markers can be generated in large numbers and can prove to be very useful for a variety of purposes relevant to crop improvement. Excellent reviews are available providing in detail the characteristics of different molecular markers, means of detection of polymorphism, and utility for various purposes in molecular genetics and plant breeding. For instance, molecular markers have been utilized extensively for the preparation of saturated genetic maps of several crop species. Their association with genes/QTLs (Quantitative Trait Loci) controlling the traits of economic importance has also been utilized in some cases for molecular marker-assisted selection (MAS). Other uses of molecular markers include gene introgression through backcrossing, germplasm characterization, genetic diagnostics, characterization of transformants, study of genome organization and phylogenetic analysis. MAS is an approach where DNA sequences linked to target traits are used as selection unit, and has been developed to avoid the problems connected with conventional plant breeding. Thus, the criterion of selection is changes form phenotype based selection to selection based on DNA sequence, either directly or indirectly. Molecular markers are unaffected by the conditions in which the plants are grown and are detectable in all stages of plant growth. In this way, the selection of target traits can be achieved indirectly using molecular markers that are closely linked to underlying genes or that have been developed from the actual gene sequences.

The development of molecular markers for plant breeding applications was first popularized in the early 1980s when isozyme markers were used to speed up the introgression of monogenic traits from exotic germplasm into a cultivar background. The restriction fragment length polymorphism (RFLP) was the first DNA based marker and was subsequently used in crop improvement including theoretical issues related to marker-assisted backcrossing (MABC) for improvement of qualitative traits. Theoretical basis for the application of MAS have been addressed subsequently, including the optimization of MABC systems and strategies to pyramid favorable alleles through recurrent crossing schemes. These theoretical studies have greatly contributed to our understanding of many fundamental issues of genetics regarding the development of MAS systems such as population type, sample size, genome size, and marker number. Considering the significance of molecular markers in plant breeding, extensive research programmes that aim at developing effective markers system, identifying markers linked genomic regions of interest have been conducted worldwide. Molecular markers that are associated with economically important traits have been identified and/or used for MAB in several plant species, including maize, rice, wheat, barley, tomato, potato, sunflower, pea, bean, rye, millet, cotton, soybean, sorghum, cowpea, tobacco, turnip rape, cauliflower, sunflower, alfalfa, carrot, sugarcane, sugar beet, and grape.

CATEGORIES OF DNA BASED MARKERS

Based on the location, genomic region from where a marker is derived and functional properties of the marker region, DNA-based markers can be broadly divided into two broad categories.

Random DNA Markers (RDMs)

Majority of the markers derived and used in the past were from the genomic DNA, and therefore could belong to either the transcribed or the non-transcribed part of the genome. The molecular markers derived from anonymous regions of the genome are called random DNA markers (RDMs), which may or may not be developed from the polymorphic site in gene or may not be developed from a gene.

Genic Molecular Markers (GMMs)

GMMs are developed from coding sequences like expressed sequence tags (ESTs) or from fully characterized genes and frequently such markers have been assigned known functions. Based on the site of polymorphism and effects on phenotypic variation, GMMs can be further divided into gene targeted markers and functional markers:

(i) Gene-targeted markers (GTMs): GMMs are those markers which have been derived from polymorphisms within genes, however not necessarily involved in phenotypic trait variation. For example, it may be based on the polymorphisms in un-translated regions (UTRs) of EST sequences.

(ii) Functional markers (FMs): FMs are derived from polymorphic sequences or sites within genes and, thus, more likely to be causally involved in phenotypic trait variation (e.g., candidate gene-based molecular markers). The FMs, depending on the involvement in the phenotypic trait variation, are further classified into two subgroups: (a) indirect functional markers (IFMs), for which the role for phenotypic trait variation is indirectly known, and (b) direct functional markers (DFMs), for which the role for the phenotypic trait variation is well proven.

SALIENT FEATURES OF MOLECULAR MARKERS

When individuals have different sequences in the DNA at a particular chromosome region such that the individuals can be distinguished, the molecular marker is said to be polymorphic. The markers follow the same rules of inheritance as genes, which allow them to be placed on genetic maps, and represent their genetic locations, order and relative distances pictorially on a chromosome. The markers thus act as "sign posts" at many locations along the chromosome. Linkage maps can be generated that have molecular markers covering all the chromosomes, at reasonably close proximity to each other. To be of significance to plant breeding programmes, molecular markers should have the following salient features:

- Genomic abundance and even distribution throughout the genome
- High level of polymorphism
- Co-dominant inheritance (discrimination of homozygous and heterozygous states)
- Unambiguous identification of alleles
- Selectively neutral behavior (no pleiotropic effects)
- Easy access to the markers
- Easy and fast assay (e.g., by procedure amenable to automation)
- High reproducibility
- Possibility of exchanging data between laboratories
- Marker development at reasonable cost

Salient characteristics of some widely used molecular marker systems are as follows.

- **Simple Sequence Repeat (SSR) or microsatellite markers** Need a small amount of medium quality DNA, but for characterization studies, should be high quality; PCR based, so cheap and easy to run; require much discovery and optimization for each species before use; do have multiple alleles (co-dominant) and are very repeatable.
- **Amplified Fragment Length Polymorphisms (AFLP)** Combine restriction, adapters, and PCR to generate many polymorphisms per run; needs a small amount of very high quality DNA; expensive, slow, laborious; cannot be mechanized nor scaled up; do not require much discovery and optimization for each species before use; do not have multiple alleles (dominant), but you get many loci per run.
- **Diversity Array Technology (DArT)** Relies on hybridization to previously defined clones; needs a small amount of very high quality DNA; can be mechanized and you get many loci per run; do not have multiple alleles (dominant); require much discovery and optimization for each species before use; require special equipment to visualize; generally better to outsource.
- **Single Nucleotide Polymorphism (SNP)** Are a change in the sequence of one base in the DNA (or, occasionally, a small insertion or deletion into the sequence of the DNA); are the most basic polymorphism type; you are looking at the actual change, not a change in amplification or restriction pattern caused by it; need a small amount of medium quality DNA, but for characterization studies, should be high quality; can be mechanized, and are many different ways to visualize the differences; do not have multiple alleles (dominant); require much discovery and optimization for each species before use; require special equipment to visualize; often better to outsource; if many SNPs are run simultaneously, the cost per SNP is many times cheaper than any other marker type; may be functional markers (within genes of interest).

The availability of sequence data of expressed DNA has enabled the development of markers that are physically associated with coding regions of the genome. Expressed Sequence Tags (ESTs) are the result of sequencing complementary (cDNA) clones and the information generated is generally stored in databases. These sequences can then be used for designing primers to readily generate polymorphic markers. The raw sequence information will also aid in screening for the occurrence of microsatellite sequences (EST-SSR) or single nucleotide polymorphisms (EST-SNP), after which markers can be developed that are targeted to transcribe regions of the genome. Complementary DNA can also be used as template for subsequent direct marker generation, for example through AFLP technology (cDNA-AFLP). cDNA-AFLP is commonly used in the identification of genetic polymorphisms between contrasting phenotypes under controlled conditions in order to facilitate the construction of linkage maps, or to identify candidate genes. In diversity studies, the application of cDNA-AFLP should be limited to the identification and comparison of specific gene-related patterns, as in general cDNA differences may be caused by differences in the developmental stage of plants and the environmental conditions rather than by existing DNA polymorphisms. Several other techniques such as Sequence-Related Amplified Polymorphism (SRAP), Target Region Amplification Polymorphism (TRAP) have also proved to be useful in detecting functional polymorphisms. In case gene sequence data are available, markers can be developed for particular (groups of) genes. This is the case, for example, in a recently developed strategy for analyzing groups of resistance genes — Resistance Gene Homologue Polymorphism (RGHP). With this methodology, groups of resistance genes are targeted by PCR using primers aimed at conserved domains of resistance genes, such as the Leucine Rich Repeat (LRR) or the Nucleotide Binding Site (NBS), both involved in resistance mechanisms.

RELEVANCE OF MOLECULAR MARKERS IN PLANT BREEDING

There are several ways in which molecular markers can help plant breeders to achieve the desired objectives of the breeding programmes. The following is a non-exhaustive list of areas where marker systems can play a very important role in terms of effective utilization of germplasm, speeding-up of breeding process or to improve the genetic gains.

(i) Effective utilization of genetic resources through precise characterization, quantification and identification of genetic variation from all available sources. DNA markers are now seems to be an indispensable tool for characterizing genetic resources and providing breeders with more detailed information to assist in selecting parents.

(ii) Tagging, cloning, and introgressing genes and/or Quantitative Trait Loci (QTL) useful for enhancing the target trait using marker technologies. Markers have significant role in identifying rare recombinants with minimum linkage drag and recovering recurrent parent genotypes in back cross breeding programme.

(iii) Manipulating (differentiating, selecting, pyramiding, and integrating) genetic variation in breeding populations.

(iv) Markers techniques can also help plant breeding programs through assisting plant variety protection as well as in distinctness, uniformity, and stability (DUS) testing processes.

(v) Assessment of purity of cultivar especially markers can help to ensure the purity of hybrid cultivars.

(vi) DNA markers have been and can be used to define heterotic groups that can be used to exploit heterosis (hybrid vigour). It is also possible to predict the heterosis using molecular markers, thus, time and resources involved in generating more number of crosses and further their evaluation could be avoided. It is true that molecular markers based prediction of heterosis is not conclusive so far, yet it is expected that further investigation particularly in functional markers system may help accurate prediction of heterosis in future.

MARKER ASSISTED SELECTION (MAS): HOW DOES IT ENHANCE PLANT BREEDING PROGRESS?

The rapid development of molecular techniques has opened up sources of genes to plant breeding that were not available previously through conventional breeding, creating a lot of excitement about marker-assisted selection (MAS). MAS is an approach where DNA sequences linked to target traits are used as selection unit, and has been developed to avoid the problems connected with conventional plant breeding. The opportunity to select desirable lines based on genotypes rather than phenotype was extremely attractive to breeders; analyzing plants at the seedling stage, screening multiple traits that would normally be epistatic with one another, minimizing linkage drag, and rapidly recovering a recurrent parent's genotype were just a few of the attractions of MAS. MAS is particularly helpful in cases of simple but important characters that are difficult to assay such as resistance to pathogens, insects and nematodes, besides quality parameters, and some quantitative traits.

The process involves two steps: validation of the particular marker in different genetic backgrounds and then exploitation of validated markers in breeding operations. This analysis is simpler in case of qualitative traits as compared to quantitative traits where genotype x environment interaction plays a significant role. It is projected that the SNP assays would reduce the unit cost per assay thereby increasing the number of assays possible and would become a widespread tool of MAS in crop improvement.

Whenever reliable markers are available, MAS can be used to pyramid several resistance genes into a single host genotype and to estimate the presence of quality and agronomically important gene blocks. The use of marker data together with phenotypic evaluations provides instruments suitable for more effective breeding. Integrating molecular marker technologies such as MAS into breeding programmes could become increasingly important in the coming years, to realize genetic gains with greater speed and precision. MAS applications in plant breeding become meaningful and justified in six broad situations:

(i) Early, quick and precise selection of a trait that is difficult to phenotype or has complex/low inheritance.

(ii) Traits whose selection depends on specific environments or developmental stages that influence the expression of the target phenotype.

(iii) Maintenance of the specific donor trait in backcross breeding with minimum linkage drag from the donor parent.

(iv) Where recessive alleles are desirable and require to be restored during backcrossing or for speeding up backcross breeding in general.
(v) Pyramiding of various genes which are difficult to phenotype in presence of the other trait.
(vi) Selection of appropriate parents with diverse alleles.

BASIC REQUIREMENTS FOR MAS APPLICATION IN CROP IMPROVEMENT

MAS is a selection procedure based on the specific DNA sequences whose inheritance can be monitored easily, already mapped and located within the target gene or QTL or tightly linked to the target gene/QTLs. Its successful application to assist breeder while dealing with the improvement of a monogenic, oligogenic or a polygenic trait depend on several factors. These factors are:

(i) Availability of a genetic map with an adequate number of uniformly-spaced polymorphic markers to accurately locate desired QTLs or major gene(s).
(ii) There must be a close linkage between the QTL or a major gene of interest and adjacent markers. The success of MAS by and large depends on the localization of marker with respect to the target gene. The most desirable situation for MAS is when the molecular marker is located within the gene of interest. The localization of microsatellite markers within the *opaque2* gene is an excellent example of this situation. Another situation encountered in breeding populations where markers are in linkage disequilibrium (LD) with the gene of interest throughout the population. LD is the tendency of certain combination of alleles to be inherited together. Selection using these markers can be called LD-MAS. In the third situation, the marker is in linkage equilibrium (LE) with the gene of interest throughout the population. LE is in fact a random association of alleles at different loci and equals the product of allele frequencies within haplotypes, meaning that at random combination of alleles at each locus its haplotypes (combination of alleles) frequency has equal value in a population. This is the most difficult and challenging situation for applying MAS.
(iii) There must be adequate recombination between the markers associated to the trait(s) of interest and the rest of the genome.
(iv) Adequate infrastructural facilities particularly for high-throughput genotyping and manpower support to analyze a large number of plants in a time and cost-effective manner.

MAS STRATEGIES IN PLANT BREEDING

Considerable progress has been made in the development of molecular markers since the discovery of the first marker system in 1980. Now different types of molecular markers are available which can be used in mapping/tagging of genes/ QTL controlling important agronomic traits in all major crops. Molecular markers closely associated with desirable traits are being utilized to increase the efficiency and effectiveness of conventional breeding by indirect selection of the desirable plants in segregating populations. Molecular markers are now widely used to track loci and genome regions in several crop-breeding programmes, as markers tightly linked with a large number of agronomic and disease resistance traits are becoming available as output of the research works undertaken in different laboratories across the continents. MAS application strategies in plant breeding includes development of suitable mapping population, linkage analysis and linkage map using suitable markers, QTL identification and QTL-marker association analysis, validation of marker-QTL association and then integration of MAS in plant breeding process.

Mapping Populations

A population used for gene mapping is commonly called a mapping population. Mapping populations are usually obtained from controlled crosses. Decisions on selection of parents and mating design for development of mapping population and the type of markers used depends upon the objectives of experiments, availability of markers and the molecular map. The parents of mapping populations must have sufficient variation for the traits of interest at both the DNA sequence and the phenotype level. The variation at DNA level is essential to trace the recombination events. The more DNA sequence variation exists, the easier it is to find polymorphic informative markers. When the objective is to search for genes controlling a particular trait, genetic variation of trait between the parents is important. If the parents are greatly different at phenotypic level for a trait, there is a reasonable chance that genetic variation exists between the parents, although uncontrolled environmental effects could create large phenotypic variation without any genetic basis for the effects. However, lack of phenotypic variation between parents does not mean that there is no genetic variation, as different sets of genes could result in the same phenotype.

Selection of parents for developing mapping population is critical to successful map construction. Since a map's economic significance will depend upon marker-trait association, as many qualitatively inherited morphological traits as possible should be included in the genetic stocks chosen as parents for generating mapping population. Consideration must be given to the source of parents (adapted vs exotic) used in developing mapping population. Chromosome pairing and recombination rates can be severely disturbed (suppressed) in wide crosses and generally yield greatly reduced linkage distances. Wide crosses will usually provide segregating populations with a relatively large array of polymorphism when compared to progeny segregating in a narrow cross (adapted x adapted). To have significant value in crop improvement programme, a map made from a wide cross must be collinear (i.e., order of loci similar) with map constructed using adapted parents.

Types of Mapping Populations

Different types of mapping populations that are often used in linkage mapping are: (i) F_2 population; (ii) F_2 derived F_3 (F_2:F_3) populations; (iii) backcross inbred lines (BILs); (iv) doubled haploids (DHs); (v) recombinant inbred lines (RILs); (vi) near-isogenic lines (NILs) and (vii) chomosomal segment substitution lines (CSSLs).

Based on contrasting characteristics or phenotypic polymorphisms, parents are selected and crossed to develop segregating mapping populations (Figure 21.1). Another type of mapping population is an "association mapping panel" which consists of diverse lines from the natural populations or germplasm collections which can be employed for identifying marker-trait associations through association mapping or linkage disequilibrium (LD) mapping.

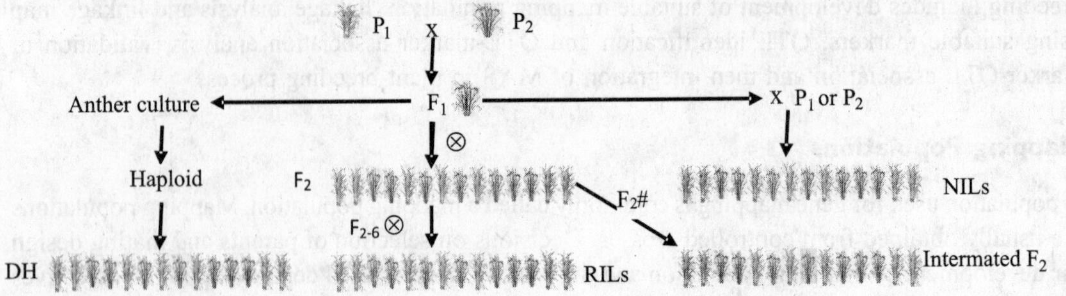

Figure 21.1 Generalized scheme for mapping population development.

The choice of a mapping population could vary based upon the objectives of the experiment, the timeframe as well as resources available for undertaking genotyping, phenotyping and QTL analysis. While selecting parents for generating mapping populations, DNA polymorphisms among parental lines, purity of the self-breeding parental lines in terms of true breeding nature, fertility of the hybrids generated by crossing parental lines and exclusions of individuals with translocation, and in polyploidy species, the monosomic individuals or individuals containing partial chromosomes should be ensured.

Size of the Mapping Population

The size of the mapping population for QTL analysis depends on several factors, including the type of mapping population employed for analysis, genetic nature of the target trait, objectives of the experiment, and the resources available for handling a sizable mapping population in terms of phenotyping and genotyping. Relatively small population is required when the objective is to generate molecular map, however, fine mapping experiments require significantly large size of population. The development of high density marker map can be achieved with as few as 200 plants but fine mapping with objective to clone a gene requires over 1000 plants. While analysis of large number of individuals (~500 or more) would enable detection of even QTLs having small effects on the target trait, from the practical point of view, the basic purpose of QTL mapping would be largely served if one can detect the QTLs with major effects. This would require, in general, a mapping population of a size of 200-300 individuals. The population size also depends on the type of the mapping population used. More individuals are required when F_2 populations are used when compared with back cross (BC) or double haploid (DH) populations. It is because, the F_2 population contains more marker genotypes and to ensure detection of each genotype, a greater number of individuals are required. In general F_2 population size should be doubled compared to BC in order to obtain the same mapping accuracy.

Linkage Mapping

The main goal of genetic mapping is to detect neutrally inherited markers in close proximity to the genetic causatives or genes controlling the complex quantitative traits. Genetic mapping can be done mostly in two ways: (1) using the experimental populations (also referred to as "biparental" mapping populations) that is called QTL-mapping as well as "genetic mapping" or "gene tagging," and (2) using the diverse lines from the natural populations or germplasm collections that is called LD-mapping or "association mapping."

The genetic segregation ratio at maker locus is jointly determined by the nature of marker (dominant/codominant) and types of mapping populations (Table 21.1). Therefore, a thorough understanding of the nature of markers and mapping population is crucial for any mapping projects. Markers such RFLPs, microsatellites and CAPS etc. are co-dominant in nature, while AFLP, RAPD, ISSR are often scored as dominant markers. Mapping populations such as RILs and DHs equalize marker type because of fixation of parental alleles at marker locus in homozygous condition. These population results in 1: 1 segregation ratio at marker locus irrespective of genetic nature of markers, while an F_2 population segregates in 1: 2: 1 ratio for a codominant marker and in 3:1 ratio for dominant marker. Depending upon the segregation pattern, statistical analysis of marker data will vary.

Table 21.1 Genetic segregation ratio at marker locus in different marker–population combinations.

Marker	*Nature*	*Genetic Segregation Ratio*					
		F_2	*RILs*	*DHs*	*NILs*	*Backcross Popn.*	
						B_1	*B_2*
RFLP	Co-dominant	1 : 2 : 1	1 : 1	1 : 1	1 : 1	1:1	1:1
RAPD	Dominant	3 : 1	1 : 1	1 : 1	1 : 1	1:0	1:1
AFLP	Dominant	3 : 1	1 : 1	1 : 1	1 : 1	1:0	1:1
Microsatellites	Co-dominant	1 : 2 : 1	1 : 1	1 : 1	1 : 1	1:1	1:1

By screening the mapping population using polymorphic markers (popularly called 'genotyping'), we can analyze the segregation patterns for each of the markers. The segregation patterns are usually in consonance with the type of mapping population used. The genotypic data is then analyzed using statistical package such as MAPMAKER or JOINMAP for construction of a linkage map in order, indicating the relative genetic distances between them, and assigning them to their linkage group on the basis of recombination values from all pair-wise combinations between the markers.

To perform whole genome QTL scan, it is desirable to have a saturated marker map. In such map, markers are available for each chromosome from one end to the other, and adjacent markers are spaced sufficiently close that recombination events only rarely occur between them. For practical purpose, this is generally considered to be less than 10 recombination per 100 meiosis, or a map distance of less than 10 centiMorgans (cM). As few as 50 markers can be used where genome size is small whereas manifold more markers are required when analysing individuals with large genome size.

QTL Mapping

A QTL is defined as 'a region of the genome that is associated with an effect on a quantitative trait'. Conceptually, a QTL can be a single gene, or it may be a cluster of linked genes that affect the trait. QTL may be located on one region of the genome or it may be dispersed on different regions across the genome depending on the nature of the trait. Most of the important agronomic characters like yield and yield components (grain number, grain weight), plant height, days to flowerings and tolerance to abiotic stresses in general are controlled by many genetic factors. However, the number of genes and their interactive effects controlling the expression of quantitative traits are poorly understood. A number of methods for mapping QTLs, and estimating their effects have been suggested and investigated. Further, quantitative trait modifying factors (QTMFs) have been identified as those loci which affect quantitative traits through epistasis in contrast to QTLs which have relatively large phenotypic effects independent of the genetic background.

QTL mapping studies have been reported in most crop plants for diverse traits including yield, quality, disease and insect resistance, abiotic stress tolerance, and environmental adaptation. Advances in genomics will further accelerate the acquisition of knowledge of genomic regions influencing an array of quantitative traits, and that, in turn, will directly impact the future strategies for crop improvement.

The molecular maps when fully integrated will have several roles: (i) to provide a focal point and hub for data derived from the perspectives of myriad disciplines of each crop, (ii) to constitute a vital two-way avenue connecting plant breeding and plant molecular biology, (iii) to contribute essential information for the positional closing of genes, (iv) to facilitate considerable and directed expansion of a crop's gene pool through comparative mapping of related and correlated taxa, (v) to accelerate identification and incorporation of useful genes into cultivars, and (vi) to contribute important clues towards understanding the biological basis of complex traits and phenomena important to crop improvement.

Random mating populations are more difficult for QTL mapping, because linkage disequilibrium is key to detecting QTLs with markers. It is essential to develop a suitable experimental mapping population, as explained in above section, using parental lines that are highly contrasting phenotypically for the target trait. Another important requirement is that these parental lines should be genetically divergent; this is important to enhance the possibility of identifying a large set of polymorphic markers that are well-disturbed across the genome. To fulfill the second criterion, one may have to carry out molecular polymorphism survey across a set of potentially useful lines so as to identify the most suitable ones for generation of mapping population.

With the availability of different types of markers, it is now easy to identify and map sufficient number of markers per chromosome. However, only a small fraction of these markers might be linked to genomic regions that influence the trait of interest. Where such linkage occurs, the marker locus and QTL will co-segregate. Therefore, the basic principle of determining whether a QTL is linked to a marker is to partition the mapping population into different genotypic classes based on genotypes at the marker locus, and to apply statistics to determine whether the individuals of one genotype differ significantly from the individuals of other genotype with respect to the trait being measured. Situations where genes fail to segregate independently are said to be in LD. QTL analysis, thus, depends on LD. The molecular markers in QTL mapping basically used; i) to identify the regions of chromosome that affect the trait of interest and ii) to analyze the effect of the QTL on the trait, i.e., how much of the variation for the trait is caused by a specific region? And nature of gene action associated with the QTL, and which allele is associated with the favourable effect.

Salient Requirements for QTL Mapping

- A mapping population generated from phenotypically contrasting parents
- Molecular marker based saturated linkage map
- Reliable phenotyping of mapping population for the trait of interest
- Comprehensive statistical packages that can analyze the marker data in combination with phenotypic data for QTL detection.

Factors that Influence QTL Mapping

QTLs are statistically inferred from the data generated in an experiment. However, statistical influence does not always indicate biological significance due to multiple test problems associated with QTL mapping. The following factors affect the power of QTL mapping:

- Number of genes controlling the target trait(s) and their genome positions.
- Distribution of genetic effects and existence of genetic interactions.
- Heritability of the trait.
- Number of genes segregating in a mapping population.
- Type and size of mapping population.
- Density and coverage of markers in the linkage map.
- Statistical methodology employed and significance level used for QTL mapping.

Phenotyping of mapping population

The target quantitative traits have to be phenotyped as precisely as possible with minimum amount of missing data. The power to resolve the QTL location is limited first by sample size, quality of the phenotyped data and then by genetic marker coverage of the genome. Often, the number of individuals in a sample might appear to be large, but missing data or skewed allele frequencies in the population cause the effective sample size to diminish, thus sacrificing statistical power. Sometimes, it may be necessary to sacrifice population size in favour of data quality, and this trade off means that only major QTL can be detected. Phenotyped data is typically pooled over environments and replications to obtain a single quantitative trait value for the line. To be more precise in phenotyping data, it is also preferable to measure the target trait (s) in experiments conducted over locations or years to have a better understanding of the QTL x environment interaction, if any.

Statistical methods for QTL mapping

The basic objective in QTL mapping is to detect QTL, while minimizing the occurrence of false positives (Type I errors, that is, declaring an association between a marker and QTL when in fact one does not exist). Precise marker-QTL/trait association analysis depends on the quality of the phenotyped and genotyped data of the mapping population, size of the mapping population and saturated linkage map evenly covering all the chromosomes of the genome. Data on marker-QTL/ trait association are often performed by the following approaches.

Single Marker Approach

Single marker approach is the simplest method for QTL analysis, sometimes also referred to as the single factor analysis of variance (SF-ANOVA) or single point analysis. SF-ANOVA is done for each marker locus independent of information from loci. F-test provides evidence whether differences, between marker locus genotype classes are significant or not. Although computationally simple, serious limitation of this approach is confounding of the effect of one QTL by many others that influence the trait. Another serious limitation is that a QTL with major effect and loose linkage cannot be distinguished from a QTL with minor effect and tight linkage.

Simple Interval Mapping (SIM)

SIM approach needs a molecular genetic map and utilizes, in a single analysis, information from all the markers of a linkage group, thus permitting detection of QTL in each interval (described as a bin) lying between any two flanking markers that individually may show no association with the trait. Presence of putative QTL is estimated if the log of odds ratio (LOD) exceeds a critical threshold. The formulae for calculating significance levels appropriate for interval mapping have been developed and fit well when the genome size, number of chromosomes, number of marker intervals, and the overall false positive rate desired are given. SIM has been the most widely used approach as it can be easily accessed through statistical packages such as MAPMAKER/QTL. By using tightly linked markers for analysis, it is possible to compensate for recombination between markers and QTL, thereby increasing the probability of statistically detecting the QTL, and providing an unbiased estimate of QTL effect. However, when multiple QTLs are segregating in a cross, SIM fails to take into account genetic variance caused by other QTLs. In such a case, SIM suffers essentially from the same shortcomings as of single marker analysis approach.

Composite Interval Mapping (CIM)

CIM and multiple-QTL model or marker QTL marker analysis (MQM) combine interval mapping for a single QTL in a given interval with multiple regression analysis on marker associated with other QTL. CIM is thus an extension of interval mapping with some selected markers also fitted in the model as cofactors to control the genetic variation of other possibly linked or unlinked QTL. Using the appropriate unlinked markers can partly account for the segregation variance generated by unlinked QTL, while the effects of linked QTL can be reduced by including markers linked to the interval of interest. When two QTL are closely linked in coupling phase, i.e. two decreasing (or increasing) alleles are linked together, the marker between the two QTL will show the highest *t*- or *f*-value for single marker analysis because of the additivity of two linked QTL. As a result, a false QTL will be declared to be located between the two real QTL, which is called a 'ghost QTL'. Ideally when we test an interval for a QTL, we would like to have our test statistic independent of the effects of possible QTL at other regions of the chromosome to avoid 'ghost' QTL. This test can be constructed by using a combination of interval mapping with multiple regression. Largely because of the linear structures of the locations of genes on chromosomes, multiple regression analysis has a very important property in that the partial regression coefficient of a trait on a marker is expected to depend only on those QTL, which are located on the interval bracketed by the two neighboring markers and to be independent of any other QTL if there is no crossing over and epistasis. It considers a marker interval plus a few other well-chosen single marker in each analysis, so that *n*-1 tests for interval-QTL associations are performed on a chromosome with *n* markers. The advantages of CIM are (i) mapping of multiple QTLs can be accomplished by the search in one dimension, (ii) by using linked markers as cofactors, the test is not affected by QTL outside the region, thereby increasing the precision of QTL mapping, and (iii) by eliminating much of the genetic variance by other QTL, the residual variance is reduced, thereby increasing the power of detection of QTL. CIM is more powerful than SIM.

Multiple Interval Mapping (MIM)

MIM is a multiple-QTL oriented method combining QTL mapping analysis with the analysis of genetic architecture of quantitative traits through a search algorithm to search for number, positions, effects, and interaction of significant QTL. In general, there are three different approaches for multiple interval mapping: (i) maximum likelihood using EM include multiple interval mapping and sequential testing to search model space, (ii) multiple imputation uses Bayesian log posterior odds and sequential testing and pair wise plots to search, and (iii) Markov Chain Monte Carlo (MCMC) employs Markov chain sampling to search model space. MIM allows one to infer the location of QTLs to positions between markers, makes proper allowance for missing genotype data, and can allow interactions QTLs. Model selection is the principal problem in multiple QTL methods, the chief concern is the formation of appropriate criteria for comparing models. MIM consisted of four components:

(i) An evaluation procedure to analyse the likelihood of the data given a genetic model (number, position and epistasis of QTL)
(ii) A search strategy to select the best genetic model in the parameter space
(iii) An estimation procedure to estimate all parameters of interest in the genetic architecture of the quantitative traits (number, positions, effects and epistasis of QTL; genetic variances and covariances explained by QTL effects) given the selected genetic model
(iv) A prediction procedure to estimate or predict the genotypic values of individual based on the selected genetic model and estimated genetic parameters for MAS.

Bayesian Mapping

Bayesian methodology has become popular in QTL mapping because of the availability of simulation based MCMC algorithms. MCMC provides an approach for achieving number analytical goals that are otherwise difficult to achieve. In Bayesian analysis everything is treated as an unknown variable with a prior distribution. A variable can be classified into one of two classes: observable and unobservable. Bayesian mapping allows the use of prior knowledge of QTL parameters and the posterior variances and credibility intervals for the estimated QTL parameters is automatically obtained. With MCMC approaches, it is possible to perform linkage analysis with any number of marker loci, multiple trait loci and multiple genomic segments. At the same time, these approaches allows the use of pedigrees of arbitrary size and complexity. In addition to mapping the loci, Bayesian reversible jump MCMC approaches allows one to estimate the number of loci and associated individual locus model parameters as well as *covariate* effects in a joint linkage and oligogenic segregation analysis.

Bulk Segregant Analysis (BSA)

Replacing individual genotyping by selecting only the individuals from the high and low tails of the population distribution (selective genotyping) or DNA analysis in pools of the selected individuals (pooled DNA analysis) was proposed for QTL analysis and for testing of linkage between markers and a major gene. This concept is referred to as tail analysis, bulk segregant analysis or selective DNA pooling and is an effective solution to reduce costs associated with genotyping large mapping populations. As reducing the size of a QTL mapping population will decrease the detection power and increase the QTL confidence interval, as well as the risk of detecting false QTL, selective genotyping can save much more cost than using smaller population sizes while maintaining the same mapping power as the large populations.

Major gene controlled traits can be selectively genotyped through bulk segregant analysis. Briefly, individuals are selected so that two groups of individuals have contrasting phenotype, i.e. resistant versus susceptible plants, or early versus late maturity with a randomizes genetic background for other traits. Molecular markers that detect polymorphism between the groups may be linked to the character and this possibility then be tested in a segregating population. The genotyping in this approach becomes very simple since it relies on just two DNA pools each of plants from one or other of the phenotypic extremes. The pools that have been used in plants usually consist of 10-15 individuals taken from as large a population as possible. This approach has already been successfully used for mapping trait which have contrasting phenotypic identity (such as resistant versus susceptible) in many plants.

Association Mapping or LD Mapping

Linkage mapping methods most frequently used so far are largely based on segregating populations derived from two parental lines, although some of them may be modified to use multiple populations simultaneously. Although such segregating populations are easy to create, they come with a number of disadvantages. First, the amount of segregating genetic variation within the population is limited, because at most two alleles per locus can segregate in a diploid species, where in the absence of allele polymorphisms between the parents no QTL can be identified. Secondly, the genetic background within which mapping studies take place are generally not representative of the backgrounds used in elite germplasm. Thirdly, the relatively low number of generations after maximum LD, where the maximum LD is reached in the F1, implies a reduced number of sampled meiosis within designated population, leading to relatively long stretches of chromosome being in LD. Consequently, the characteristics size of confidence intervals for QTL locations is between 10 and 20 cM. In addition, germplasm resources and breeding populations that have been accumulating in breeding programmes with available phenotypic information cannot be used so that genetic mapping and breeding are usually two separate, independent procedures.

The problems associated with segregating population based linkage mapping can be addressed using an approach called association mapping. Association mapping has been defined in many ways and has also been referred to as 'association genetics', 'association studies' and linkage disequilibrium mapping'. The general characteristics of this field of genetics involve the use of unstructured or loosely structured population that are both phenotypically and genotypically characterized to detect statistical associations between genetic polymorphism and heritable traits variation. As the fundamental aim of genetics is to connect genotype to phenotype, association mapping seeks to identify specific functional variants (i.e. loci, alleles) linked to phenotypic differences in a trait, to facilitate detection of trait causing DNA sequence polymorphisms and/or selection of genotypes that closely resemble the phenotype.

LD mapping or association mapping can be exploited to identify QTL using collections of germplasm, cultivars and all available genetic and breeding materials, by which molecular dissection of complex traits can be more closely linked up with the plant breeding programme. LD mapping shares much in common with the field of what is commonly known as quantitative trait loci (QTL) mapping. Both attempt-via statistical inferences to detect co-segregation of polymorphic genetic markers with genes underpinning trait variation. However, the two differ in terms of some key properties which have implications for the applications of each of these areas of study. LD is also known as gametic phase disequilibrium, gametic disequilibrium and allelic association. Simply stated, LD is the 'non-random association of alleles at different loci'. The terms linkage and LD are often confused. Linkage refers to the correlated inheritance of loci through the physical connection on a chromosome, whereas LD refers to the correlation between alleles in a population. LD mapping takes advantage of events that created association in the relatively distant past. Assuming many generations and therefore meiosis have elapsed since these events, recombination will have removed association between a QTL and any markers not tightly linked to it. LD mapping thus allows for much finer mapping than standard biparental cross approaches. LD analysis has the potential to identify a single polymorphism within a gene that is responsible for the difference in phenotype and is perfectly suited for sampling a wide range of alleles from germplasm collections with high resolution.

For marker trait association, differences in both phenotype and allele frequency can be identified in a group of cultivars that are derived from a common ancestral gene pool. The development of saturated linkage maps and highly informative microsatellite and SNP markers in plants makes it possible to systematically survey marker trait association on a whole genome scale. An important advantage of LD mapping strategies is the straightforward utilization of large amounts for historical phenotypic data that are available for mapping efforts at no or little extra costs.

Analysis of QTL Effects on Genotype

Once QTL are detected, the next step is to estimate the genotypic effect of the QTL and to localize the QTL to precise genomic region. The interval mapping approach is superior to the ANOVA approach in terms of both localization and estimation of the effects of QTL. However, the reliability in terms of estimation of the QTL effects depends on the linkage between marker(s) and QTL, the number and type of progeny evaluated, and the heritability of the trait. From multiple regression analysis, one can also obtain a value which gives the presence of the total genetic variance explained by all of the markers. The R^2 value for the line is considered to be the amount of total genetic variation that is explained by the specific molecular marker. Statistical packages are now also available that offer means to analyze the QTL x environment interactions.

The most commonly used statistical packages for QTL analysis are MAPMAKER/QTL, QTL Cartographer, PLABQTL, QTL Mapper and Qgene. Most of these statistical packages yield essentially similar QTL locations and gene effects on a given set of data, while there could be slight variation in the confidence intervals. Nonparametric statistics or association-based approaches to identify QTLs and to calculate empirical critical (threshold) values for declaring significant QTLs will further refine QTL mapping.

Validation of Marker-trait Association

Establishment of highly significant marker-trait associations is one of the prerequisites for MAS. Demonstrated linkages between target traits/genes and molecular markers are traditionally based on genetic mapping experiments and it is important to confirm that these associations are consistent in mapping as well as in breeding populations. Thus, validations of markers-QTL association in different populations are important for successful application of MAS because, genetic mapping results obtained from specific crosses cannot be used for MAS for the same traits in different crosses. Non-transferability of marker-trait association in breeding populations may be because of (i) multigenic nature of inheritance of quantitative traits. Genes are only segregating at loci where two parents are genetically different and thus can be mapped using the population derived from these two parents. For a randomly selected mapping population, the parents will have a strong chance to share identical alleles at some of the genetic loci. There is high probability that segregating genes in any breeding population could be different from the genes already mapped. (ii) multiple alleles at a locus work in the same way to complicate MAS, because mapping parents could have alleles that are different from those of breeding populations. Interaction among these multiple alleles will modify marker trait associations when different allele combinations are considered. (iii) genotype x environment interaction could make the specific environment based establishment of marker-trait association. Thus, QTL markers identified using a single mapping population may not be automatically used directly in unrelated populations without marker validation and/or fine mapping. Therefore, marker-trait association must be validated, in representative parental lines, breeding populations and phenotypic extremes before it can be used for routine MAS, particularly for QTL with relatively small effects.

APPLICATION OF MARKER-TRAIT ASSOCIATION IN PLANT BREEDING

Advancement in genomics has not only helped in efficient understanding of structural and functional aspects of many plant genomes but also provided practical feasible platform for manipulation of genomes for crop improvement. It has provided new tools such as molecular markers for discovering and tagging novel alleles/genes or chromosomal regions useful for improvement of agronomically important traits and for manipulating those genes in breeding programmes through MAS, i.e., selection of phenotypic traits indirectly using markers that are closely linked to the traits or developed from the gene related sequences. MAS influence plant breeding process in many ways:

Marker Assisted Backcrossing (MAB)

Marker-assisted backcrossing (MAB) is the process of using the results of DNA tests to assist in the selection of individuals to become the parents in the next generation of a genetic improvement program. It is an approach that has been developed to avoid problems connected with conventional plant breeding by changing the selection criteria from selection of phenotypes towards selection of genes/QTL that control traits of interest, either directly or indirectly. There are three levels of selection in which markers may be applied in backcross breeding (Figure 21.2).

1. In the first level, markers may be used to screen for the target trait, which may be useful for traits that have laborious phenotypic screening procedures or controlled by recessive alleles. Incorporation of recessive *opaque2* mutant in the background of normal endosperm maize is the most suitable example of this category.
2. The second level of selection involves selecting backcross progeny with the target gene and tightly-linked flanking markers in order to minimize linkage drag. This is referred to as 'recombinant selection'. This is the most required task in backcross breeding programme while using wild relatives such as *Glysine soja* in soybean or *Lycopersicon pennellii* in tomato or any other wild relatives or otherwise undesirable plant as donor parent for transferring disease/pest resistance, tolerance to environmental extremes any other desirable trait(s).
3. The third level of MAB involves selecting backcross progeny (that have already been selected for the target trait) with 'background' markers. In other words, markers can be used to select against the donor genome, which may accelerate the recovery of the recurrent parent genome. With conventional backcrossing, it takes a minimum of five to six generations to recover the recurrent parent. Data from simulation studies suggests that at least two but possibly three or even four backcross generations can be saved by using markers. Again, conversion of normal endosperm maize into quality protein maize (QPM) can be cited as an example where several markers are used to recover the background of normal maize while retaining recessive *opaque2* gene using foreground selection.

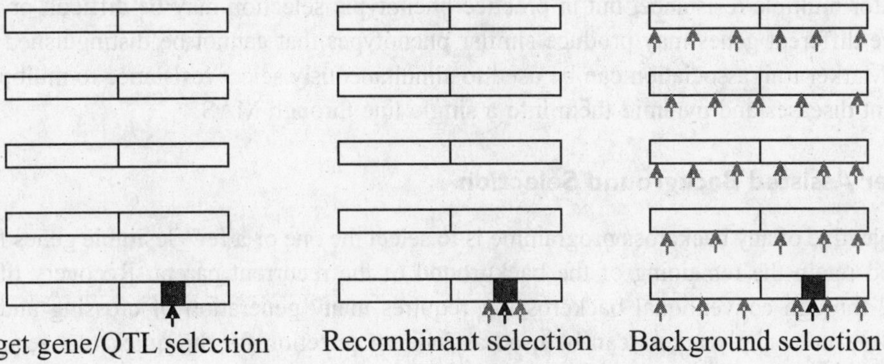

Figure 21.2 Three levels of selection during marker-assisted backcrossing.

Marker Assisted Foreground Selection

There are several approaches using molecular markers to select an associated target gene or allele (foreground selection). Foreground selection can be used for gene introgression from one genetic background to another and pyramiding multiple alleles/genes to a genotype from multiple donors as well. The simplest way to introgress a target allele or gene is to sue one closely linked marker. However, the most complicated approach is to integrate foreground selection with background selection using multiple markers for target locus and many others for covering entire genome.

Single Marker Based Selection

The reliability of MAS based introgression of a trait (foreground selection) largely depends on the co-localization of the markers and the target gene. Marker and trait must be in close proximity, i.e., there must be a tight linkage if only one marker is used in selection which is located on either side of the target gene. If the marker is part of the target trait genomic sequence, the situation becomes more satisfying in terms of MAS efficiency and genetic gain.

Selection using Flanking Markers

To reduce false positives in MAS, flanking markers or multiple markers around the target region should be used simultaneously. The three-marker system where marker in the middle preferably intragenic or co-segregating with the gene is used to indicate the presence of the target gene whereas other two flanking markers ensure the absence of the undesirable chromosome segment from the donor parent. This is in fact, a MAS based selection procedure of desirable individuals where recombination has taken place between the target gene locus and the marker loci.

MAS using Multiple Markers

MAS has inherent potential to support simultaneous selection of multiple traits/genes in breeding programme where multiple markers are used as reference points of selection. In some cases multiple pathogen races (such as multiple races of bacterial leaf blight in rice) are used to identify plants for multiple resistance, but in practice phenotypic selection may be difficult or impossible because different genes may produce similar phenotypes that cannot be distinguished from each other. Marker trait association can be used to simultaneously select resistance to multiple races of different diseases and pyramid them into a single line through MAS.

Marker Assisted Background Selection

The objective of any backcross programme is to select the one or a few desirable genes from donor line and retain the remaining of the background of the recurrent parent. Recovery of the background through conventional backcrossing requires many generation of crossing and selection. However, molecular markers can be used as indirect selection for the quick recovery of genetic background of recurrent parent. Selection targeted for the recovery of the remainder of the genome excluding the target gene(s), i.e., genetic background, is called background selection. The background selection aims at the whole genome screening using linked molecular markers. In segregating population, each chromosome represents a random combination of two parental chromosomes. So we have to know the parental combination of each chromosome in order to do whole genome selection, i.e., the entire genome has to be covered by molecular markers.

Linkage Drag in Gene Introgression

When transferring a single gene from the donor into the genetic background of a recurrent parent by repeated backcrossing, genetic linkage will cause fragments of the donor genome surrounding the target gene to be 'dragged' along, which is called linkage drag, a persistent problem in plant breeding. In traditional BC programme, the linked segments usually remain large for many generations not because recombination had not occurred in these regions, but because there is no effective way to identify recombinant individuals. Usually, it is by chance that such recombinants are occasionally selected in classical breeding programme which contribute to reduction in size of the donor segment. With high density molecular maps it is possible to directly select individuals that have experienced recombination near the gene of interest.

Marker Assisted Gene Pyramiding

Pyramiding is the process of simultaneously combining multiple genes/QTLs together into a single genotype that has been identified in multiple parents. This is possible through conventional breeding but extremely difficult or impossible at early generations. Using conventional phenotypic selection, individual plants must be phenotypically screened for all traits tested either, using artificially created or naturally existed environment supporting biotic or abiotic stresses, or using biochemical and physiological assays as the case may be. Therefore, it may be very difficult to assess plants from certain population types (e.g., F_2) or for traits with destructive bioassays. DNA markers may facilitate selection because DNA marker assays are non-destructive and markers for multiple specific genes/QTLs can be tested using a single DNA sample without phenotyping. The most widespread application for pyramiding has been for combining multiple disease resistance genes in order to develop durable disease resistance (Figure 21.3). The gene pyramiding may be of two

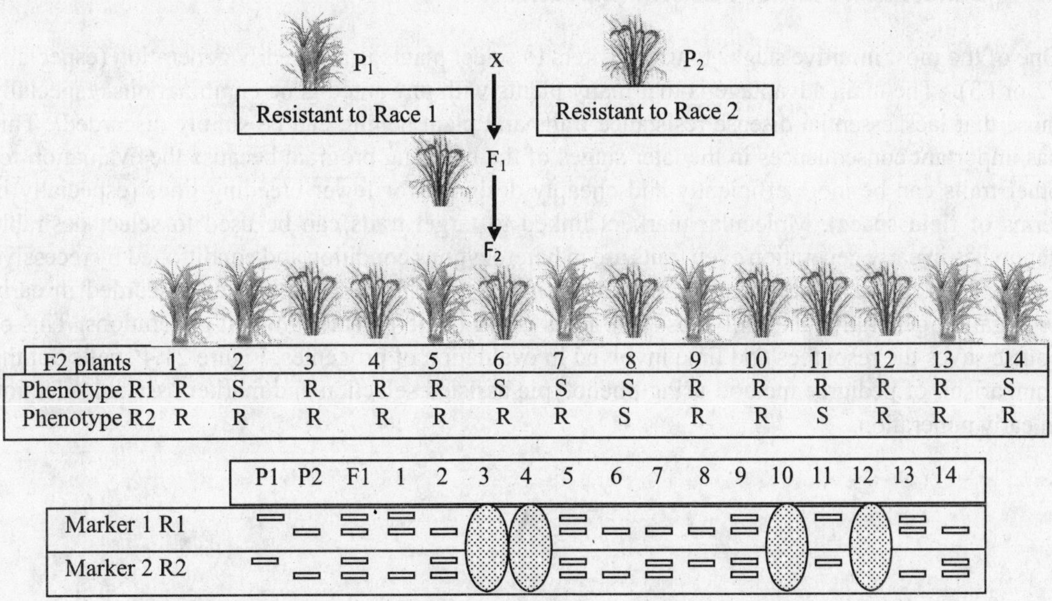

Figure 21.3 Marker assisted pyramiding of two disease resistance genes.

types: i) pyramiding genes affecting a specific traits. For example pyramiding of different genes responsible of bacterial leaf blight resistance in rice, and (ii) pyramiding of favourable genes for different traits in a single genotype. For example, simultaneous introgression of genes for bacterial leaf blight and blast resistance in a rice genotype.

Marker Assisted Recurrent Selection (MARS)

Recurrent selection is one of the selection procedures to combine favourable alleles distributed among different source germplasm. MARS involves crossing in selected individuals at each cycle of crossing and selection. In this way, desirable alleles can be brought into the breeding scheme from many different sources. This technique has been applied to sunflower, soybean, and maize to bring desirable alleles at several target loci into single elite lines. Further analyzed the prospects for genome-wide selection (GWS) for improving quantitative traits in maize was analyzed, and it was concluded that this approach effectively avoids issues pertaining to the number of QTL controlling a trait, the distribution of effects of QTL alleles, and epistatic effects due to genetic background. Genome-wide or genomic selection also relies on MAS and is under evaluation for the feasibility of incorporating desirable alleles at many loci that have small genetic effect when used individually. In this approach, breeding values can be predicted for individual lines in a test population based on phenotyping and whole-genome marker screens. These values can then be applied to progeny in a breeding population based on marker data only, without the need for phenotypic evaluation. Modeling studies indicate that this method can lead to considerable increases in the rates of genetic gain by accelerating the breeding cycles. The MARS/GWS strategy is presently being implemented by CIMMYT in over 40 biparental populations in Africa, Asia, and Latin America.

Early Generation Marker Assisted Selection

One of the most intuitive stages to use markers to select plants is at an early generation (especially F2 or F3). The main advantage is that many plants with unwanted gene combinations, especially those that lack essential disease resistance traits and plant height, can be simply discarded. This has important consequences in the later stages of the breeding program because the evaluation for other traits can be more efficiently and cheaply designed for fewer breeding lines (especially in terms of field space). Molecular markers linked to target traits can be used to select desirable genotypes in early generation even traits are in heterozygous condition and conditioned by recessive genes. Thus, using MAS in early generation, many undesirable lines can be discarded in early segregating generation and only desirable lines could be perpetuated in next generations. This of course saves the resources and time involved in evaluation of progenies. Figure 21.4 spells out the comparison of pedigree method using phenotypic assisted selection and marker assisted selection in early generation.

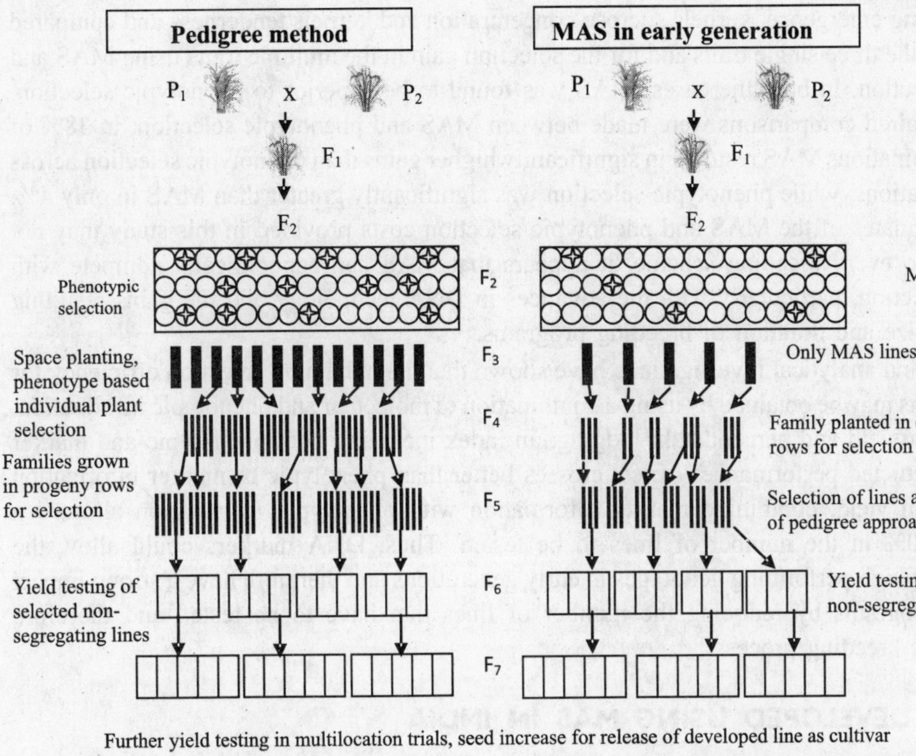

Figure 21.4 Comparison of pedigree and MAS in early generation, selection scheme.

Efficiency of MAS

Application of MAS basically lies in its potential to improve the plant breeding process. It has therefore emerged as an important strategy for increasing selection gains with respect to phenotypic selection alone and quantitative genetic theory suggests that the effectiveness of MAS is inversely proportional to the heritability of a given trait. In this context, theoretical approach to estimate the probability of selecting one or more superior genotypes by MAS and define a parameter to estimate the cost efficiency of MAS relative to phenotypic selection was developed. Depending on the selection pressure, the genotypic superiority target and the trait heritability, it is estimated that a breeder using phenotypic selection must test 1.0 to 16.7 times more progeny than a breeder using MAS to be assured of selecting one or more superior genotypes. Thus, using MAS, the resources needed can be substantially minimized to accomplish a selection goal for a low to moderate heritability trait when the selection goal and the selection intensity are high. When MAS is applied, the selection intensity can be increased to exclude inferior genotypes in case the heritability is high.

The efficiency of MAS and phenotypic selection for the simultaneous improvement of quantitative traits involved in seedling emergence and quality characteristics were compared in three different sweet corn populations. They used five markers per QTL for selection of genomic regions affecting seedling emergence, kernels sucrose concentration and kernels tenderness and compared gain in each of the three single traits and for the selection gain in the multiple traits using MAS and phenotypic selection. In both the cases, MAS was found to be superior to phenotypic selection. A total of 52 paired comparisons were made between MAS and phenotypic selection; in 38% of the paired combinations MAS resulted in significantly higher gains than phenotypic selection across the three populations, while phenotypic selection was significantly greater than MAS in only 4%. Even if the estimates of the MAS and phenotypic selection costs provided in this study may not be applicable to every breeding scheme, it appears that MAS can economically compete with phenotypic selection, particularly with the advances in DNA technology and the gains resulting from reduced size and duration of breeding programs.

Theoretical and analytical investigations have shown that the maximum selection efficiency for quantitative traits may be obtained by using a combination of molecular and phenotypic information. For maize grain yield and percent stalk lodging, an index including both phenotypic and marker information predicted performances of test crosses better than phenotypic or marker information alone. For grain yield, combining marker information with phenotypic information allowed a reduction of 40% in the number of lines to be tested. Thus, DNA markers could allow the identification of high performing genotypes in early generations and therefore have a strong impact on breeding programs by reducing the number of lines that have to be tested and therefore accelerating the breeding process.

CULTIVARS DEVELOPED USING MAS IN INDIA

The success of MAS in the recent past is evident from the fact that a large number of cultivars involving several crops have been produced through MAS and released for commercial cultivation; in wheat alone about a dozen cultivars have been released for commercial cultivation in USA and Canada. In India, the first product of MAS was a downy mildew resistant pearl-millet hybrid HHB-67-2 developed at ICRISAT.

In rice, MAS has been successfully exploited for pyramiding different genes for bacterial leaf blight and blast diseases. 'Pusa 1460', is a new version of 'Pusa Basmati 1' developed by Indian Agricultural Research Institute. This variety developed by pyramiding bacterial leaf blight (BLB) resistance genes (xa13 & Xa21) in the background of 'Pusa Basmati 1' through marker assisted backcross breeding. Similarly another variety namely 'RP BIO 226' developed by Directorate of Rice Research using MAS. 'RP BIO 226' is developed by marker assisted pyramiding of three BLB resistance genes (*Xa21*, *xa13* and *xa5*) in the genetic background of an elite fine grained rice variety, Samba Mahsuri. Two high yielding BLB susceptible indica rice cultivars ADT43 and ASD16, popular among farmers and consumers across South India were introgressed with the three BLB resistance genes *xa5*, *xa13* and *Xa21* using functional markers. Thirty pyramided genotypes with two or three resistance genes exhibited high levels of resistance against two predominant *Xanthomonas oryzae* isolates of South India. Twelve pyramided genotypes (*xa5* + *xa13* + *Xa21*) were found to be significantly high yielding with desirable agronomic characteristics and the selection efficiency of the present markers was hundred percent. Three rice blast resistance genes, namely *Pi1*, *Piz5* and *Pita* have been pyramided in a susceptible rice variety, CO39 using RFLP and PCR-based markers for durable blast resistance.

In maize, MAS has been used successfully in conversion of normal maize lines into quality protein maize (QPM). The QPM converted lines were crossed and the first QPM hybrid namely "Vivek QPM 9" has been developed and released for cultivation. Besides, QPM versions of six elite inbred lines, which are the parents of three single-cross hybrids, PEHM2, Parkash and PEEHM5 have been recently developed by the Maize Genetics Unit, IARI, New Delhi, through the ICAR Network Project on Molecular Breeding. In addition, the Maize Genetics Unit at IARI, also developed maize genotypes with resistance to Turcicum leaf blight and Polysora rust through MAS, under an ICAR Network Project on Gene Pyramiding.

In wheat, the leaf rust resistance genes Lr24 and Lr28 were the first two genes pyramided through MAS in India in 2003-04 in the variety HD 2329, which has been followed up with PBW 343 pyramided with the same two genes at IARI, New Delhi. Now there are large number of combinations in different trials having components of Lr24, Lr28, Lr9, Lr19 and adult plant resistance genes like Lr48. The genes Lr24, Lr28 and Lr9, Lr37 have been pyramided in the genetic background of popular cultivar WH147 in various combinations using validated molecular markers for these genes. Pyramided lines with gene combinations Lr24+Lr28,Lr24+Lr37,Lr28+Lr37 in the genetic background of WH147 and gene combinations Lr24+Lr28+Yr15 in the background of high yielding cultivar HD2687 have been produced using molecular markers.

CONCLUSION

Despite significant success already achieved in many cases, as discussed above, there are still several limitations in effectively using MAS in crop improvement. Some of these limitations include: (i) reliability and accuracy of QTL mapping; (ii) loose association between marker(s) and gene/QTL in many cases; (iii) effect of the genetic background; (iv) QTL x environment interactions; (v) application gap between research laboratories and plant breeding institutes; (vi) knowledge gap between plant breeders and molecular biologists. Most of these limitations will be overcome during the next decade, so that MAS will become an integral component of conventional plant breeding. With the collective efforts of the broad community of scientists committed to plant biology and crop improvement, molecular plant breeding will further expand its contributions and impacts to meet global needs for sustainable increases in agricultural productivity.

FURTHER READINGS

1. Babu R., Nair S.K., Kumar A., Venkatesh S., Sekhar J.C., Singh N.N., Srinivasan G. and Gupta H.S. (2005) Two-generation marker-aided backcrossing for rapid conversion of normal maize lines to quality protein maize (QPM). *Theor. Appl. Genet.* **(111):** 888-897.
2. Babu R., Nair S.K., Prasanna B.M., and Gupta H.S. (2004) Integrating molecular assisted selection in crop breeding-Prospects and challenges. *Current Sci.* **(87):** 607-619.
3. Bernardo R. and Yu J. (2007) Prospects of genomewide selection for quantitative traits in maize. *Crop Sci.* **(47):** 1082-1090.
4. Collard B.C. and Mackill D.J. (2008) Marker assisted selection: an approach for precision plant breeding in the twenty-first century. *Philos. Trans. R. Soc. Lond. Ser. B. Biol. Sci.* **(363):** 557-572.
5. Cooper M., Smith O.S., Graham G, Arthur L., Feng L. and Podlich D.W. (2004) Genomics, genetics, and plant breeding: a private sector perspective. *Crop Sci.* **(44):** 1907-1913.

6. Dudley J.W., Saghai Maroof M.A. and Rufener G.K. (1992) Molecular marker information and selection of parents in corn breeding programs. *Crop Sci.* **(32):** 301-304.
7. Eathington S.R., Crosbie T.M., Edwards M., Reiter R.S. and Bull J.K. (2007) Molecular markers in a commercial breeding program. *Crop Sci.* **(47):** S154-S163.
8. Goodman M.M. (2004) Plant breeding requirements for applied molecular biology. *Crop Sci.* **(44):** 1913-1914
9. Gupta H.S., Agrawal, P.K., Mahajan, V., Bisht G.S., Kumar A., Verma P., Srivastava A., Saha S., Babu R., Pant M.C. and Mani V.P. (2009) Quality protein maize for nutritional security: rapid development of short duration hybrids through molecular marker assisted breeding. *Current Sci.* **(96):** 230-237.
10. Heffner E.L., Sorrells M.E. and Jannink J.L. (2009) Genomic selection for crop improvement. *Crop Sci.* **(49):** 1-12.
11. Melchinger A.E. (1990) Use of molecular markers in breeding for oligogenic disease resistance. *Plant Breed.,* **(104):** 1-19.
12. Moose, S.P. and Mumm, R.H. (2008) Molecular plant breeding as the foundation for 21st century crop improvement. *Plant Physiol.* **(147):** 969-977.
13. Prasanna B.M., Pixley K., Warburton W.L. and Xie C-X. (2010) Molecular marker assisted breeding options for maize improvement in Asia. *Mol. Breed.* **(26):** 339-356.
14. Ribaut J.M. and Betran J. (1999) Single large-scale marker-assisted selection (SLS-MAS). *Mol Breed.* **(5):** 531-541.
15. Stuber C.W., Polacco M., and Senior M.L. (1999) Synergy of empirical breeding, marker-assisted selection, and genomics to increase crop yield potential. *Crop Sci.* **(39):** 1571-1583.
16. Sundaram R.M., Vishnupriya M.R., Biradar S.K., Laha G.S., Reddy G.A., Shobha Rani N, Sarma N.P., and Sonti R.V. (2007) Marker assisted introgression of bacterial blight resistance in Samba Mahsuri, an elite indica rice variety. *Euphytica.* **(160):** 411-422.
17. Xu, Y. (2009) *Molecular Plant Breeding.* CABI, Oxfordshire, UK. p. 734.

CHAPTER 22

Plant Transgenic Technology

Transgenic technology has provided important tools for sustainable development of agriculture and forestry and can be of significant help in meeting the food needs of a growing and increasing urbanized population. The potential benefit of transgenic plants is the applications for which they are being developed, the new traits being introduced. Transgenics have potential to reduce usage of insecticides, improve quality and tolerance to stress, and function as edible vaccine and biosensors.

Keywords: Transgenic technology, transgenesis, plant transformation, genetically modified plants, genetically engineered plants, cisgenesis.

INTRODUCTION

Plant transgenic technology, also called plant genetic transformation, is defined as an *in vitro* gene transfer technique for transferring refined desirable gene(s) across taxonomic boundaries into plant from other plants, animals and microbes, or even to introduce artificial, synthetic or chimeric genes into plants. The technique thus involves recombinant DNA techniques allowing artificial insertion of gene(s) to plants (excluding insertion of genes through pollination), its subsequent stable integration into the plant genome, and expression of foreign gene. The inserted gene sequence is known as transgene and the plant developed after a successful gene transfer is known as transgenic plant (or genetically modified plant or GM plant or genetically engineered plant).

The transgenes are introduced into plant cells, tissues, or organs by a variety of methods, which includes biological vector-mediated transformation, or direct gene transfer mechanisms. The transgene once introduced into the plant genome by any of these methods is expressed in plants. This allows production of new plant variety, which is usually normal in appearance and differs from the parent only with respect to the function of the inserted transgene. This directed genetic engineering of plants requires that gene(s) of interest introduced into plant cells are capable of regenerating into intact plants and that the gene carries with it a selectable marker so that the transformed plant cells can be isolated from a large population of untransformed normal cells. Finally, the transformed plant cell must retain its capacity to regenerate.

The aim of plant transgenic technology is to create diversity of plants serving human needs and hence to benefit producers, processors and consumers. This involves improving production stability, giving nutritional benefits to the consumers, reducing environmental impacts of intensive agriculture, decreasing dependency on hazardous and expensive chemicals to overcome biotic stresses, providing sufficient food in order to meet the demand of growing population, overcoming problems of malnutrition, increasing yield from limited resources, providing access to food for small-scale farmers in developing nations, using non-food crops as renewable sources of oil, starch and other raw materials for industry, detoxifying hazardous compounds, sensing environmental pollution, increasing the amount of land available to cultivate crops, increasing the availability of polymers, pharmaceuticals and vaccines and increasing the understanding of the role and behavior of plant genes. Thus the plant transgenic technology offers opportunities to introduce genes conferring resistance to insects, viruses, bacteria, fungi, herbicides and abiotic stress factors. Besides the strategy also aims to increase nutritional content of plants, manipulate biochemical pathway of flower pigmentation, delay fruit ripening, increase shelf-life, modify plant products, augment sweetness, alter lignin content of trees, increase efficiency of crop production, sense pollution and introduce male sterility. Another major goal for production of transgenic plants is related to 'molecular farming', i.e., the use of transgenic plants as bioreactors (or biofactories) for the production of nutraceuticals, therapeutic agents, antigens, monoclonal antibody (McAb) fragments, vaccines, biopolymers, etc. Transgenic plants are also produced for identification of regulatory sequences for many genes, using gene constructs with overlapping deletions. Thus, plant transgenic technology has been used to produce a variety of crop plants to date, primarily with the above-mentioned 'market-led' traits. This chapter deals with various techniques used for plant transformation and the applications of transgenic plants.

CONCEPTS AND PRINCIPLES

For genetic manipulation of plants, a suitable plant transformation vector, plant explant and a source of transgene (exogenous DNA) are required. General procedure for vector construction and recombinant DNA preparation used for plant transformation remains essentially the same as discussed in the chapter on Recombinant DNA Technology. In brief vector construction involves cloning of gene of interest under the control of a strong and organ specific plant promoter to allow high-level expression of cloned gene in plants. CaMV 35S promoter of cauliflower mosaic virus is the promoter of choice for dicots and promoters of genes encoding maize ubiquitin and rice actin allow high-level expression of cloned gene in monocots. Targeting of the protein to appropriate cellular compartment may be helpful in stabilizing the protein. Though signals for membrane targeting, protein folding, oligomerization and N-glycosylation are highly conserved in animals and plants, while expressing bacterial proteins targeted to ER, a plant-specific ER-targeting sequence is preferred. Likewise for expression of protein in chloroplast, chloroplast plant transformation vectors harboring chloroplast sequences are used. In expression vectors optimized translation start site context is created and the codons are altered to suit the expression of prokaryotic genes in a plant. After vector construction (i.e., formation of recombinant vector DNA), it is transformed into a suitable host (biological system such as Agrobacterium or plant viruses), which then transfers the recombinant DNA into target explant, or exogenous DNA is directly transferred into target explant (protoplasts / cells / calli /auxillary nodes, etc.), the choice of which is dependent on the method used for plant transformation. Once selected, the explant is surface sterilized and transformed with DNA by any of the plant transformation methods described below. The targeted explants are finally transferred to selection medium for selection of transformants exploiting the property of plant selection marker gene present on plant transformation vectors. Assay of reporter gene products can also be done to determine the extent of expression of the cloned gene. A suitably transformed explant is then regenerated into a plant (putative transformant), which is acclimatized to environmental and soil conditions and transferred to field. Following transformation and plant regeneration, F_0 and progeny plants are analyzed to ensure stable integration and proper functioning of the transgene using techniques such as PCR amplification and Southern hybridization.

PLANT TRANSGENIC TECHNOLOGY

Vector Mediated and Direct Methods of Plant Transformation

A variety of techniques are available for easy and successful transformation of almost all the plant species, which provide the basis for the advances in plant biotechnology. These techniques fall into two main categories, namely, vector-mediated gene transfer and direct DNA transfer. Vector-mediated gene transfer involves plant vectors, e.g., *Agrobacterium tumefaciens*, *A. rhizogenes* and plant viruses, for the transfer of genetic information to plants from other organisms, viz. bacteria, fungi and animals as well as between plants. Direct DNA transfer, also called, vectorless gene transfer does not employ any biological vector and are species and genotype independent. These methods serve as simple and effective means for the introduction of foreign DNA into plant genomes and were developed to overcome the initial difficulties in monocot (grasses and cereals) transformation by Agrobacterium. However, now Agrobacterium-mediated gene transfer in monocot species is also possible. These techniques include direct gene transfer by physical means and direct gene transfer by chemical means. Physical gene transfer methods, also called DNA-mediated gene transfer (DGT), are based on direct delivery of naked DNA to the plant cells. This subcategory includes microprojectile bombardment, electroporation, microinjection, silicon carbide whiskers, ultrasonication, U.V. laser microbeam irradiation and liposome-mediated transformation. On the other hand, chemical gene transfer methods employ direct gene transfer with the aid of chemical agents, for example, calcium phosphate and polycations. In the following sections, a detailed description of successful transformation methods is provided.

Agrobacterium tumefaciens plant transformation

Agrobacterium tumefaciens, a Gram negative pathogenic soil bacterium, has played a significant role in the development of plant transgenic technology. It has natural gene transfer capability to plant cell and has long been exploited to introduce DNA into plants. Initially, it was believed that only dicots, gymnosperms and a few monocot species could be transformed by this bacterium, but later this view was totally changed as many 'recalcitrant' species not included in its natural host-range such as monocots and fungi could also be transformed. The simple *in vivo* transformation of tissue in intact plants by cocultivation and the 'agrolistic' methods to transform recalcitrant plants are the two novel technical achievements related to *Agrobacterium*. Combined with powerful vectors such as bacterial artificial chromosome, very large DNA fragment can be transformed into the plant genome by *Agrobacterium*. In present times, *Agrobacterium* is successfully employed for the transformation of almost all the plant families and accounts for ~ 80% transgenic plants produced so far.

Characteristics of pTi favoring its use as plant transformation vector: The property of natural tendency of gene transfer to plants comes from the genes present on tumor-inducing plasmid (pTi) of *Agrobacterium*, which catalyze the natural transfer of T-DNA (i.e., transferred DNA) to plants leading to the formation of crown gall tumor. The transfer of T-DNA to plants demonstrates certain important facts for the practical use of *Agrobacterium* in plant transformation. First, the tumor formation is a consequence of transformation process of plant cells, which results from transfer and integration of T-DNA into plant genome and the subsequent expression of T-DNA genes including auxin, cytokinin and opine synthesizing genes. Thus, the disarming of the T-DNA to remove tumor-inducing genes prevents pathogenecity or oncogenecity associated with *Agrobacterium* and also increases the space for insertion of exogenous DNA. Secondly, any foreign DNA placed between the T-DNA borders can be transferred to plant cells, no matter where it comes from. Thirdly, while growing *A. tumefaciens in vitro*, opine synthesizing and catabolizing genes may also be deleted from pTi. Rather other nitrogen and carbon sources required for their growth can be supplied in the medium. This also increases the insert capacity. Finally, the T-DNA genes are transcribed only in plant cells and do not play any role during the transfer process. Thus the genes essential for the transfer of T-DNA (i.e., *vir* genes) need not be present on the same vector and can be supplied *in trans*. These facts have allowed the construction of pTi-based vectors and bacterial strain systems that can be employed for plant transformation in order to acquire a particular trait.

Manipulations for the construction of pTi-based vectors: By exploiting the above facts, pTi-based vectors have been constructed through certain manipulations of wild-type pTi.

(i) Size reduction pathogenicity prevention and biological containment: For recombinant DNA experiments, a much smaller version is preferred, so large segments of DNA that are non-essential for a cloning vector are removed. Thus genes governing auxin and cytokinin production (the oncogenes) as well as opine synthesizing genes may be deleted from the T-DNA in a process called disarming of T-DNA. Besides these opine catabolizing genes may also be deleted. The *tra* loci may also be deleted to prevent conjugative ability thereby facilitating biological containment.

(ii) Introduction of origin of replication for multiplication in *E. coli* (shuttle vector system): pTi cannot replicate in *E. coli*, hence the convenience of perpetuating and manipulating pTi carrying inserted DNA sequences in these bacteria does not exist. Therefore, in developing pTi-based vectors, an *E. coli* origin of replication must be added. As *E. coli* and *Agrobacterium* both are Gram-negative bacteria, a broad host-range origin of replication may also be employed, which allows replication in both *E. coli* and *Agrobacterium*.

(iii) Insertion of selection marker gene(s): Selection marker gene(s) such as an antibiotic resistance gene(s) conferring antibiotic resistance to plants is inserted into plant transformation vector. As the selection marker gene is prokaryotic in origin, it is put under the control of plant (eukaryotic) transcriptional signals (promoter and termination polyadenylation sequence) to allow its efficient expression in plants.

(iv) Insertion of multiple cloning site or polylinker: A multiple cloning site is added to facilitate insertion of the cloned gene into the region between T-DNA border sequences (Right Border RB and Left Border LB). This will allow the transfer of cloned gene into plants.

Classes of pTi-based vectors: The *vir* gene products may be supplied in *cis* as well as *trans* and depending on this, two vector systems, *viz.* cointegrate or *cis* vector system and binary or *trans* vector system, have been developed. Cointegrate vector system comprises a single large plasmid formed by homologous recombination of two plasmids in an agrobacterial cell. These two plasmids are the *E. coli* plasmid (cloning vector, or cointegrate cloning vector) and the disarmed helper pTi. The cloning vector harbors plant selectable marker gene(s), polylinker site for insertion of exogenous DNA, RB, *E. coli* origin of replication, bacterial selectable marker gene and homologous sequences. The disarmed pTi is deletion derivative of wild-type pTi and comprises *vir* genes, origin of replication (*Agrobacterium*), LB and DNA sequences to serve as sites for homologous recombination. After all the manipulations, the cloning vector is introduced into an agrobacterial cell harboring helper pTi, where the cloning vector recombines with helper pTi and the entire cloning vector is integrated into helper pTi by homologous recombination to form a recombinant pTi, called cointegrate vector. Following recombination, the cloning vector becomes the part of disarmed helper pTi, which provides the *vir* genes necessary for the transfer of T-DNA to the host plant cells. Best-known example is pGV2260. The strategy used for cointegrate construction and a general vector map of a cointegrate vector are given in Figure 22.1.

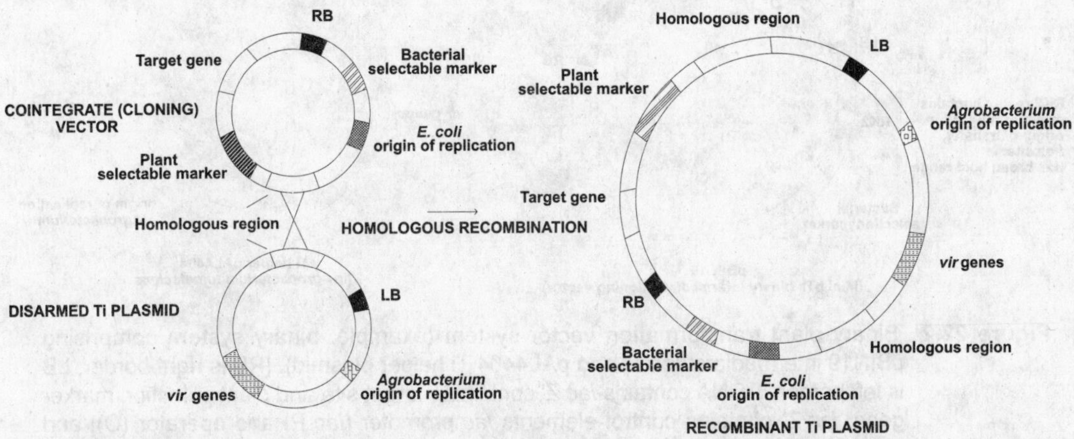

Figure 22.1 Cointegrate vector system for plant transformation. [RB and LB are right border and left border sequences].

The cointegrate vector system, however, suffers from certain drawbacks, e.g., large size and difficulty in handling, manipulation and insertion (relative to binary vectors). Moreover, the requirement of homologous sequences limits the integration of *E. coli* plasmid into limited number of pTi. However, once formed, this plasmid is stable in *Agrobacterium*. To overcome the problems associated with cointegrate vectors, binary vector system has been developed. It is a two-vector system comprising a pair of plasmids, viz, mini-Ti (or intermediate vector; iv) and helper Ti. In mini-Ti, disarmed T-DNA flanked by RB and LB contains plant selection marker gene and a site for insertion of exogenous DNA. It is a shuttle vector capable of replication both in *Agrobacterium* and *E. coli*, and also contains bacterial selection marker gene. Examples of some commonly used mini-Ti vector are pBIN19, pGREEN, pBI101, pBI121 and pCAMBIA, etc. The helper strain acts as recipient of mini-Ti and harbors a modified (defective or disarmed) pTi that contains a complete set of *vir* genes but lacks T-DNA. It is however capable of autonomous replication in *Agrobacterium*. Example of a commonly used helper is pAL4404. As mini-Ti lacks *vir* genes, it is incapable of catalyzing the transfer and integration of T-DNA region into recipient plant cells, rather it requires the help of helper Ti. Thus all the cloning steps are carried out in *E. coli* and then mini-Ti is introduced into *Agrobacterium*, where the helper supplies the *vir* functions *in trans* to catalyze the transfer of T-DNA from mini-Ti to plant cell. This binary vector system is unstable in *Agrobacterium* as compared to cointegrate vector and is susceptible to be lost from the cell. However, as compared to cointegrate vectors, binary vectors exhibit several advantages and hence serve as the most commonly used vectors for plant transformation. This includes small size, ease of handling, manipulation and introduction into host, higher frequency of introduction (10^{-1} as compared to 10^{-5} in cointegrate vector) and a broad range, i.e., capability of being introduced into any *Agrobacterium* host due to non-requirement of sequence homologies. The binary plant transformation system is shown in Figure 22.2.

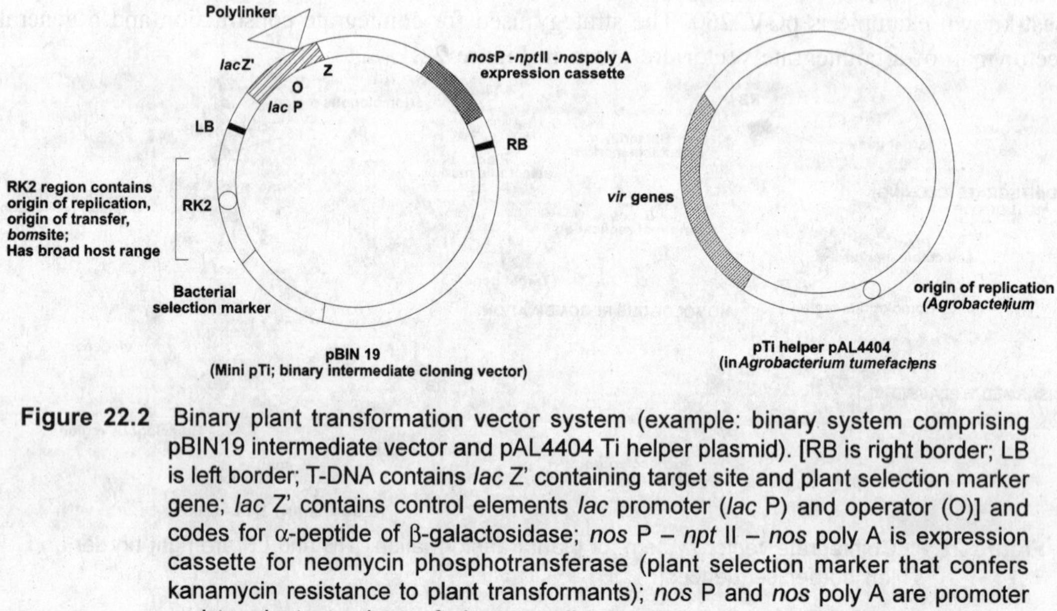

Figure 22.2 Binary plant transformation vector system (example: binary system comprising pBIN19 intermediate vector and pAL4404 Ti helper plasmid). [RB is right border; LB is left border; T-DNA contains *lac* Z' containing target site and plant selection marker gene; *lac* Z' contains control elements *lac* promoter (*lac* P) and operator (O)] and codes for α-peptide of β-galactosidase; *nos* P – *npt* II – *nos* poly A is expression cassette for neomycin phosphotransferase (plant selection marker that confers kanamycin resistance to plant transformants); *nos* P and *nos* poly A are promoter and terminator regions of plant nopaline synthase, respectively; *lac* Z' contains polylinker or multiple cloning site (MCS); *vir* genes encode virulent proteins responsible for catalyzing T-DNA transfer; intermediate vector contains broad host range origin of replication, and is capable of multiplication both in *E. coli* and *A. tumefaciens*, while helper P^{Ti} contains only *A. tumefaciens* origin of replication.

Either of these two vectors, i.e., binary or cointegrate vectors, are employed can be employed for plant transformation. The gene of interest for the required trait is inserted into the polylinker site lying with T-DNA portion of the vector and a recombinant vector is constructed. This recombinant vector is then employed for transformation of plant explant. This can be achieved simply by coculture (or cocultivation) of recombinant vector harboring *Agrobacterium* with various explants, such as protoplasts, leaf discs and the tissues in whole plants. The protocol is standardized for an individual plant species. A general protocol of cocultivation is summarized in Figure 22.3.

Besides agroinfection/agroinoculation (integrating non-*Agrobacterium* factors such as the systematic virus infection) and agrolistics (the biolistic method for gene transfer) can also be employed. Some of the plant viruses (e.g., mastre viruses) are not mechanically transmissible and hence cannot be effectively introduced into the plant cells. By this technique, *Agrobacterium* can also introduce a complete copy of a viral genome the isolated plant cells or whole plants. In this manner, it is possible to generate transiently transformed cell lines, or transgenic plants carrying an integrated recombinant viral genome and the viral symptoms are visible within two weeks of inoculation.

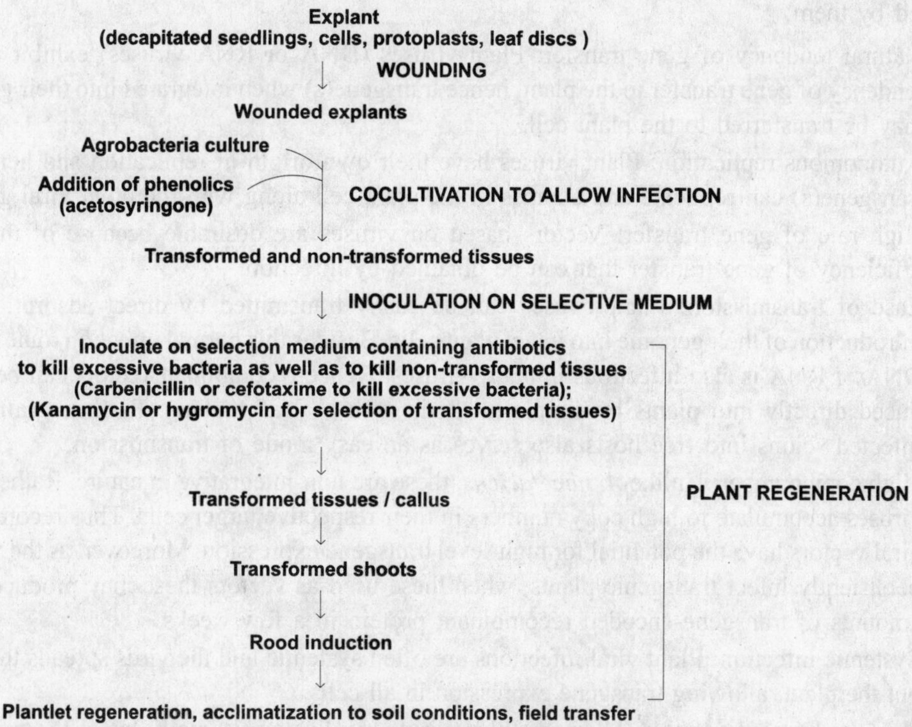

Figure 22.3 Protocol for *A. tumefaciens*-mediated transformation of plant explants.

Transformation by Agrobacterium rhizogenes

Agrobacterium rhizogenes is a soil-borne plant pathogenic bacterium, the infection of which causes proliferation of secondary roots at a wound site of higher plants. This prolific root growth, also called hairy root disease, occurs due to transfer of T-DNA from a large bacterial plasmid (the root inducing or Ri plasmid) to plant cells. The T-DNA of Ri plasmid is analogous to the pTi of *A. tumefaciens*. Due to natural gene transfer ability, similar to *A. tumefaciens*, *A. rhizogenes* also finds place in plant transformation. Several *A. rhizogenes* based vectors are now available. When foreign DNA is introduced into T-DNA region, it can be carried via the Ri plasmid into host plant cells, making it a natural vector for rapid introduction of genes into higher plants. Further it is reported that *Agrobacterium* containing both Ri plasmid and a disarmed pTi can frequently cotransfer both of them. If such a dual system is used, no drug resistance marker on the T-DNA is necessary for selection of transformants. In contrast, the transformants can be easily selected on the basis of hairy root formation in the target tissue, thereby indicating cotransfer of recombinant T-DNA. Intact plants are then regenerated by manipulation of phytohormone in culture medium.

Transformation by Plant Viruses

Plant viruses also exhibit natural tendency of gene transfer to plants and thus have the potential for use as stable plant transformation vectors. This probability is speculated due to several properties possessed by them:

(i) Natural tendency of gene transfer: Plant viruses (DNA or RNA viruses) exhibit natural tendency of gene transfer to the plant, hence transgene(s) when integrated into their genome may be transferred to the plant cell.

(ii) Autonomous replication: Plant viruses have their own origin of replication and hence the transgene(s) can replicate and express in the plant cell along with the other viral genes.

(iii) High rate of gene transfer: Vectors based on viruses are desirable because of the high efficiency of gene transfer that can be obtained by infection.

(iv) Ease of transmission: Plant viruses can be easily transmitted by direct adsorption and introduction of their genome into intact plant cells. Besides this normal infection route, naked DNA or RNA is also infectious in many viruses. Hence recombinant vectors can be introduced directly into plants by simple methods such as leaf rubbing. Further, grafting an infected scions into free hosts also serves as an easy mode of transmission.

(v) High copy number: Unlike *A. tumefaciens*, these are non-integrative in nature. Rather these viruses accumulate to high copy numbers in their respective target cells. Thus recombinant viral vectors have the potential for high-level transgene expression. Moreover, as the viruses persistently infect transgenic plants, when these used as vectors these may produce large amounts of transgene-encoded recombinant protein in a few weeks.

(v) Systemic infection: Plant viral infections are often systemic and the virus spreads throughout the plant, allowing transgene expression in all cells.

(vii) No risk of position effects: All known plant viruses replicate episomally, hence the transgene they carry is not subject to the position effects that often influence the expression of integrated transgenes.

(viii) Biological containment: Plant viruses neither integrate into the plant genome, nor are transmitted through seeds (germ line). This is advantageous in terms of biological containment of the virus.

Characteristics of plant virus-based vectors: By exploiting these properties of plant viruses, plant viruses-based vectors have been created, which possess characteristics such as:

(i) Small size: The genome size should be as small as possible. This involves deletion of non-essential genes. Note that small size allows easy handling during isolation and manipulation, increases the chances of occurrence of unique restriction site for cloning and increases the space for insertion of exogenous DNA.

(ii) Non-pathogenicity: Genes conferring pathogenicity are deleted. This further leads to size diminution and increase in the insert capacity.

(iii) Ease of transmission: The vector should have a broad host range, ease of mechanical transmission and high rate of seed transmission.

(iv) High insert capacity: The vector should have the potential to carry additional genetic information since there are strict packaging limitations. Thus viruses whose capsids are filamentous or rod shaped, or viruses that possess a multipartite genome, or a helper or satellite component, offer the potential for carrying exogenous DNA.

(v) Expression of transgene(s) in plant cell: Virus stability as a vector depends on the fact that genetic material must be able to be manipulated in such a way that these are expressed in the plant.

(vi) Retention of the capability of natural infection: There should not be any loss of infectivity of viruses.

Plant viruses used for plant transformation: Certain plant viruses (DNA and RNA plant viruses) having the above-mentioned biological characteristics have been assessed for their plant transformation capability. These include DNA viruses [e.g., cauliflower mosaic virus (CaMV) and gemini virus (GV) including begamoviruses and mastreviruses] and RNA viruses [e.g., tobacco mosaic virus (TMV) and potato virus X (PVX)]. Besides their use as plant expression vector, certain plant viruses have also been developed to present short peptides on their surfaces. Epitope-display systems based on alfalfa mosaic virus, cowpea mosaic virus, potato virus X and tomato bushy stunt virus have been developed as a potential source of vaccines, especially against animal viruses. In the case of DNA viruses, *Agrobacterium*-mediated transient or stable transformation with T-DNA containing a partially duplicated viral genome can lead to the 'escape' of intact genomes, which then replicate episomally. The latter process known as 'agroinfection' or 'agroinoculation' provides a very sensitive assay for gene transfer. More recently, the *Agrobacterium*-mediated delivery of viral genomes has been enhanced through a process called 'magnifection', in which amplification of the vector occurs in all infected leaves.

Transformation by microprojectile bombardment

Microprojectile bombardment, also called 'biolistics', 'particle gun', 'particle bombardment', 'gene gun', and 'bioblaster' is an equipment used to introduce transgene into plant cell suspensions, callus cultures, meristematic tissues, immature embryos, protocorms, coleoptiles and pollen in a wide range of different plants including monocots and conifers. This method was developed at the time when monocots were considered intractable to *A. tumefaciens*-mediated transformation due to inappropriate wound responses and hormonal differences between dicots and monocots. This method has also opened the possibility of delivering transgenes into organelles such as chloroplasts and mitochondria. Note that this is not possible with *A. tumefaciens*-mediated transformation procedure, as it targets the DNA only into the nucleus of plant cells. Thus microprojectile bombardment serves as one of the most important alternatives to *A. tumefaciens* based DNA delivery systems for plants. Today microprojectile bombardment is the method of choice in most of the laboratories and is routinely used to create transgenic monocot as well as dicot plants.

Principle: When small high-density particles (microprojectiles) are accelerated to high velocity, these particles acquire sufficient kinetic energy and can penetrate cells and membranes. When DNA-coated microprojectiles are used, these particles penetrate the outer cell layers and target the DNA into the cells.

Equipment design: After its first development in 1987, today biolistic devices have become much more sophisticated and advanced. The basics of all of these designs remain the same and involve coating of DNA into small dense microparticles followed by their high velocity acceleration towards a target tissue. Thus the microprojectile bombardment equipment comprises high-pressure source, microprojectiles, macrocarriers, stopping screen, vacuum pump and baffles/vents/meshes, the details of which as follows:

(i) High-pressure source for propulsion of microprojectiles: Three different sources are used for generation of high-pressure, which provides the propelling force for targeting microprojectiles to target tissues. These include chemical explosion (use of gun powder), discharge of compressed air and helium shock. The gun powder-driven system employs nail-gun cartridges. This blast system from the gun powder cartridge is not only dangerous, but also leads to uncontrolled generation of dirty gases and debris within the apparatus thereby necessitating frequent cleaning of the chamber. Moreover, polyethylene macrocarrier as well as stopping plate have to be discarded after each transformation process. However, pressure cannot be regulated, which may lead to target variation and non-reproducibility of results after transformation. As a consequence of these drawbacks, this system has been abandoned. Today, the most common system is helium-driven system. Helium being a light gas expands faster and is superior to gases such as nitrogen or compressed air. This leads to better dispersal of microparticles resulting in more uniform field of transformation. It is more effective, safer and cleaner than gun powder-driven system. Another advantage of using a helium-driven system is that it reduces drag on microparticles. The pressure thus generated is monitored by pressure gauge and is used to accelerate the DNA-coated microparticles with high velocity and kinetic energy sufficient to penetrate the target cell. Note that helium-driven system is functional in pressure ranging from 600-2,400 psi, but ~ 1,000 psi is optimal. Pressure below 600 psi is suboptimal for transformation and above 2,400 psi though there is an increase in velocity but gas shock impacting biological target also increases.

(ii) Microprojectiles/microparticles: Small high-density microparticles are used for carrying coated DNA. Note that low-density microparticles may have the ability to penetrate cell walls but their reduced momentum reduces the efficiency of penetration. Ideally these microparticles have good initial affinity for the DNA, yet are able to freely release it once in the cytoplasm, or nucleus of the target cell. Moreover, these microparticles are small enough to enter the plant cell without too much damage, yet large enough to have the mass to penetrate the cell wall and carry an appropriate amount of DNA on its surface into the interior of the plant cell. As such, gold or tungsten microparticles are used for coating of DNA. These microparticles are spherical in shape ranging in diameter from ~ 0.5 – 2 mm, or about the size of some bacterial cells. As a rule of thumb, microparticles are roughly $1/10^{th}$ the diameter of cell. Gold microparticles offer certain advantages as compared to tungsten microparticles. These are biologically inert and do not produce cytotoxic effects. Moreover, these are more uniform in size than tungsten microparticles and allow size optimization for a cell type. Furthermore, gold microparticles do not attack the DNA bound to them. Because of their properties described above, FDA has approved gold microparticle as human therapeutic agent. One problem while using gold microparticles is that these tend to agglomerate irreversibly in aqueous suspensions over a period of time, i.e., these are unstable. This problem is however overcome by preparing them at the time of use. On the contrary, tungsten microparticles are somewhat cytotoxic and over time these catalytically degrade DNA bound to them. As compared to gold microparticles, tungsten microparticles tend to be heterogeneous in size, as a consequence of which size optimization for a cell type is a problem. Moreover, tungsten microparticles are subject to surface oxidation, which can alter their DNA binding capacity. However, the cost of gold particles may limit their accessibility and the tungsten particles being more affordable are sufficient for most studies. Besides gold and tungsten, other microparticles reported with some success include glass needles, silica and dried cells of *E. coli* and *A. tumefaciens* (biological capsules).

(iii) Macrocarrier/Macroprojectiles/Flying disk: Many particle guns utilize a macrocarrier to support or carry the microparticles. These are accelerated under high-pressure carrying the microparticles towards the target explant. In the path, a stopping plate usually retains the macrocarrier, whereas the microparticles continue along their course to reach the target explant. The macrocarriers are of different types. For gun powder-driven system, cylindrical, high-density polyethylene macroprojectiles are used, while for helium-driven system, circular Kaplon membranes are the best. Membranes require very little time to come up to speed, hence short flight distance is required. The less massive membrane can be stopped with a screen, rather than Lexan disk as in the case of polyethylene macrocarriers. As a result more microparticles can be delivered without any associated high velocity 'debris', which can be generated from the macrocarrier or stopping screen.

(iv) Rupture disc: Some designs of gene gun include plastic rupture disc, which is fitted in a rupture disc holder and placed at appropriate position in equipment chamber. This rupture disc bursts due to passage of high-pressure gas and allows it to hit the macrocarrier loaded with DNA-coated microprojectiles. These have a pressure cut-off valve and are available for 450, 650, 1100 and 1350 psi, etc.

(v) Stopping screen or plate: These are metallic plates with a small opening at the center. This blocks the movement of macrocarrier ahead of it, while DNA-coated microparticles travel through the opening and penetrate the cell wall and membrane of the target explant.

(vi) Vacuum pump: Microprojectiles are rapidly decelerated as these pass through gas (helium exerts reduced drag on microparticles as compared to any other gas). Hence, in most cases, the microparticles are accelerated under partial vacuum in a vacuum chamber to reduce drag due to gas. As gas can transmit potentially damaging shock wave, evacuation of the chamber by vacuum pump reduces the severity of gas shock. Standard vacuum gauge reading inside the chamber is 25 – 29" Hg.

(vii) Shock absorbers: Acoustic shock/gas blast is reduced by positioning of baffles/vent/meshes between microprojectile launch site and target explant.

Procedure for microprojectile bombardment: PDS-1000/He device (BioRad) is the most commonly used device in most of the laboratories. This biolistic transformation system uses an evacuated sample chamber that positions the target cells directly in the path of DNA-coated tungsten or gold particles traveling at a velocity of 1100 mph (Figure 22.4). Another example of gene gun, Helios gene gun (BioRad), is a hand-held device and uses low-pressure helium to accelerate DNA-coated microparticles from the interior of a small plastic cartridge towards the target explant. Various steps involved in PDS-1000/He transformation system are:

(i) Preparation of microparticle suspension: Gold or tungsten microparticles are suspended in sterile water (30 mg / 500 µl) and vortexed briefly. These microparticles are then washed once in 70% ethanol and twice in absolute ethanol. Finally, the microparticles are suspended in sterile water and while vortexing slowly these are aliquoted into very small volume (50 µl each) in clean tubes for storage at 4°C (gold), or – 20°C (tungsten). This preparation is good for 2-3 months.

(ii) Preparation of DNA-coated microparticles (precipitation of DNA on microparticles): At the time of use, one tube of microparticle (prepared in first step) is taken and water is discarded by brief spin (15 s). With slow and continuous vortexing, 5 – 10 µl of DNA (1 – 2 mg / ml), 50 ml of 2.5 M $CaCl_2$ and 20 µl of 0.1 M spermidine free-base are added in the mentioned order. Spermidine protects DNA from degradation and / or prevents conformation changes in DNA. The DNA-coated microparticles are spun at 10,000 rpm for 10 s in cold and supernatant is removed to the maximum possible extent. The microparticles are washed with ethanol and resuspended in 60 volumes of ultra pure ethanol, vortexed very briefly at low speed and the tube is then kept on ice till required. This preparation should be used within a few hours of preparing.

(iii) Application of DNA-coated microparticles on macrocarrier membrane: Macrocarrier membrane, stopping screen and macrocarrier holder are soaked in ethanol for 15 min. Ethanol is removed and the apparatuses are air-dried under the laminar flow hood. Caution is taken to avoid touching of these apparatuses while drying. On the other hand, the DNA-coated microparticles are briefly sonicated/vortexed/suspended with the help of tip and 10 ml of suspension is immediately but slowly released on the center of macrocarrier without touching its surface. The drop is allowed to air dry under laminar flow hood. The particle density used is such that it does not significantly damage the cells.

(iv) Setting of macrocarrier and rupture disc holders in PDS assembly: The stopping screen is placed in the assembly followed by macrocarrier in the macrocarrier holder. Rupture disc is rinsed once in isopropanol (optional) and placed into rupture disc holder.

(v) Steps for using PDS-1000/He: Helium cylinder is unlocked and the first stage meter reading is set to more than 2200 psi. The PDS assembly is then switched on and 'vent' switch is kept at 'on' position. Then second stage pressure regulator is opened and the pressure is kept at least 200 psi more than the grade of rupture disc used. For example, if 1350 psi rupture disc is used, the meter should read at least 1,550 psi. The rupture disc holder containing rupture disc is placed at appropriate position and tightened into the PDS assembly. Then macrocarrier holder with fitted metallic stopping screen and macrocarrier is mounted in the PDS launch chamber in the required slot. The Petri dish that contains the target to be transformed is then placed under the assembly in the desired slot and the door of the chamber is closed. The chamber is then evacuated to 25-29″ Hg and held as such during transformation. When the helium pressure builds up to a required value, the 'fire switch' is turned on and kept in position till a 'phut' sound is heard in the launch area indicating the bursting of plastic rupture disc. During this shot, released gas accelerates the macrocarrier with the DNA-coated microparticles on its side. The distance between rupture disc and macroprojectile launch site is called gap distance. Propelled under high-pressure, the DNA-coated microprojectiles pass the stopping screen and penetrate plant cell walls and membranes, while stopping screen holds back the macrocarrier. The distance between macroprojectile launch site and stop screen is called macroflight distance or macroprojectile

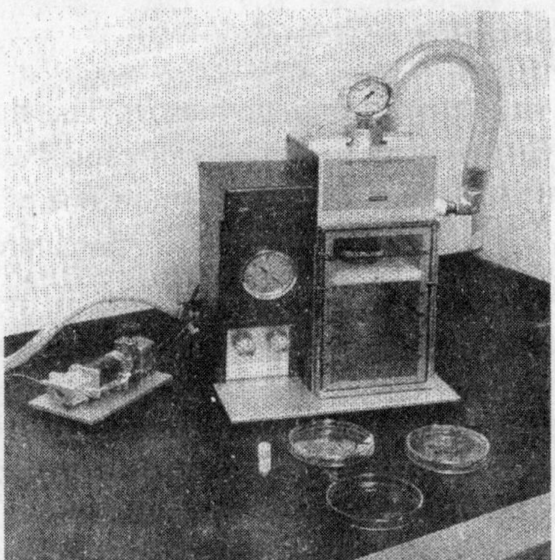

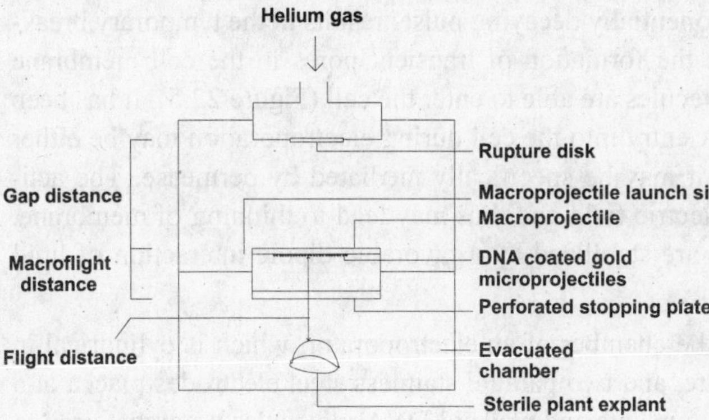

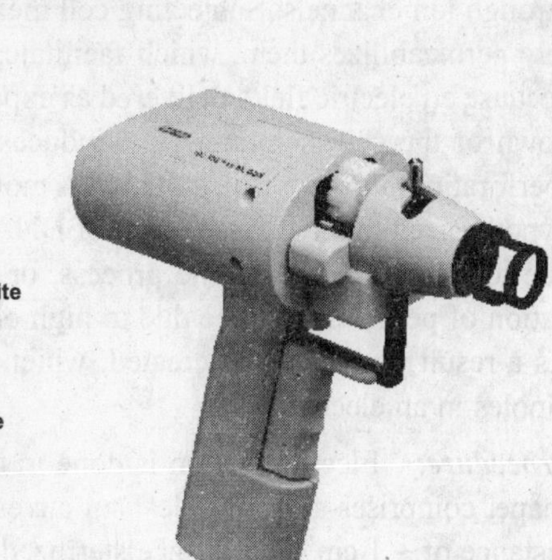

Figure 22.4 Design of gene gun.

flight distance and the distance that the microparticles have to travel to reach the target cells is called target distance. Once inside a cell, the DNA is removed from the microparticles and integrates into plant genome in some cells. After the shot the 'fire switch' is switched off and the vacuum is quickly released. This step is important and should be performed within 2 s of fire. The door is opened after release of entire vacuum. The Petri plate containing target explant on suitable media is removed. It is estimated that ~ 10,000 transformed cells are formed per bombardment if proper considerations are taken into account. The macrocarrier assembly and rupture disc holder are also removed and dismantled. The PDS assembly is wiped with ethanol and switched off. Helium cylinder is closed with the help of key and its closure is ensured by noticing that needles on both the meters of pressure gauges attached to He cylinder have fallen towards zero.

Transformation by electroporation

Electroporation is a direct physical method of gene transfer. This method is suitable for both the monocot and dicot plant cells and protoplasts. Initially protoplasts were used for transformation, which employs a difficult plant regeneration system but now one of the advantages of the system is that intact plant cells and tissues such as callus culture, immature embryos and inflorescence, can also be used. However, the plant material may require specific treatments, such as pre- and post-electroporation incubation in high-osmotic buffers. In many cases, the target cells are wounded, or penetrated with enzymes in order to facilitate gene transfer. However, presently electroporation using organized and easily regenerable tissues such as immature embryos is possible, and immature rice, wheat, and maize embryos can be easily transformed without any form of pretreatment.

Principle: Cell membrane is an electric capacitator and the current cannot pass across it except through ion channels. Subjecting cell membranes to electrical pulses of high field strength reversibly permeabilizes them, which facilitates uptake of even macromolecules such as DNA. This is because an electric field, delivered as exponentially decaying pulse, results in the temporary breakdown of the cell membrane and induces the formation of transient pores in the cell membrane (perforation) through which the DNA molecules are able to enter the cell (Figure 22.5). It has been hypothesized that the mechanism of DNA entry into the cell during electroporation may be either due to unspecific membrane process, or it may be specifically mediated by permease. The activation of permease may be due to high electric field and thus may lead to thinning of membrane. As a result pores may be created, which are stabilized by a favorable dipole interaction of lipid dipoles in an electric field.

Procedure: Electroporation is done in the chamber of an electroporator, which is cylindrical in shape, comprises a disposable 1 ml cuvette, and two parallel stainless steel electrodes placed at a distance of ~ 1 cm. The surface sterilized explants and plasmid DNA molecules are transferred to cuvette containing electroporation buffer, which is kept in the electroporator and electrodes are inserted into it. This is followed by delivery of a single exponential decaying pulse (shock of desired voltage) by discharge of a capacitator across the cell. Usually an electric field with a relatively high initial field strength (1-1.5 kV) with a low capacitance, and hence a short decay time is used. After pulse delivery, cuvettes are kept on ice for 10-15 min. Explants are taken out, rinsed in medium, and plated on MS medium with appropriate selection pressure.

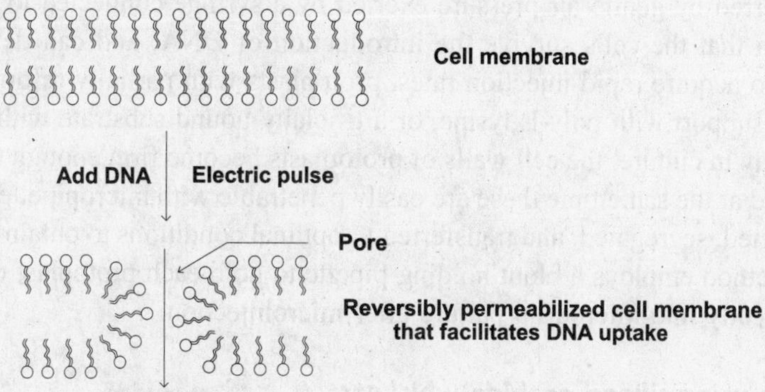

Figure 22.5 Principles of electroporation.

Transformation by microinjection

Microinjection is a direct physical approach for mechanical introduction of DNA into a specific target under microscopical control. The possible targets in plants include defined cells within a multicellular structure such as embryo, ovule or meristem. Both intact cells and protoplasts can be employed for insertion of foreign DNA by this technique. The introduction of DNA is so precise that besides intracellular injection, direct intranuclear injection is also possible.

Principle: Microinjection involves injection of an appropriate volume of biological sample directly into the cytoplasm or nucleus of cell with the aid of gentle air pressure applied to the capillary through a syringe (or micropipette) (Figure 22.6).

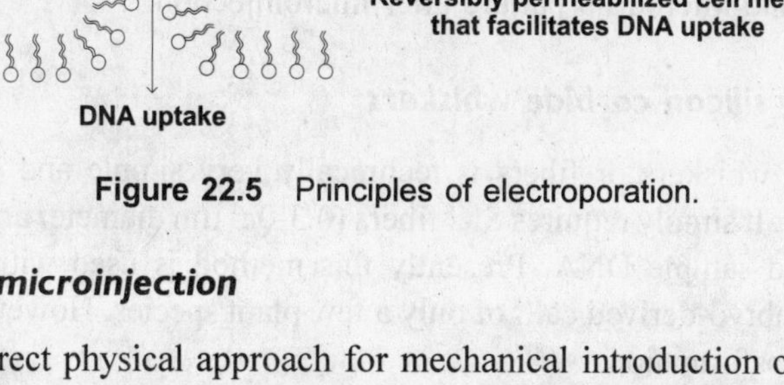

Figure 22.6 Technique of microinjection.

Procedure: Microinjection uses a glass capillary needle (or micropipettes) with a tip diameter ranging from 0.5-10 μm for precise transfer of the DNA into the cytoplasm or the nucleus of a recipient target cell or protoplast tightly held or immobilized on solid support (i.e. glass cover slips or slides imprinted with numbered squares) and performed under phase contrast microscope. The immobilization of the recipient cells is done by using methods such as agarose embedding, agar embedding, poly-L-lysine treatment of glass surfaces, and suction holding with the aid of a micromanipulator that positions the holding pipette to hold the cell in position. The capillary is filled from the tip with the biological sample, and directed into immobilized cells. An appropriate sample volume is transferred by gentle air pressure exerted by a syringe connected to the capillary. The procedure is such that the cells survive the introduction of DNA, and can develop further into clones. In order to acquire rapid injection rates, protoplasts with partially reformed cell walls are attached to solid support with poly-L-lysine, or artificially bound substrate without damaging the cells. After one day in culture, the cell walls of protoplasts become firm enough to provide support and protection and at the same time these are easily penetrable with micropipettes. Each protoplast is then microinjected, segregated, and transferred to optimal conditions to obtain transformed cells. An alternative method employs a blunt holding pipette to hold each protoplast under suction, and segregating it directly into microdrop culture after microinjection.

Transformation using silicon carbide whiskers

Transformation by SiC whiskers or fibers is technically very simple and does not require any sophisticated equipment. It simply requires SiC fibers (0.3-0.6 μm diameter and 10-100 μm length), vortex, target tissue and sample DNA. Presently this method is used with cells in suspension culture, embryos and embryo-derived calli of only a few plant species. However, the method offers a great potential for transformation.

Principle: SiC fibers apparently act as microinjection needles facilitating DNA delivery. SiC forms microscopically small needles that can perforate plant cell walls and plasmalemma by forceful intercellular collisions during vortexing. This allows the DNA adsorbed to them to gain access inside the cell by diffusion.

Procedure: In this method, DNA, SiC whiskers and plant tissue are mixed in a suitable buffer in a microfuge tube. This mixture is vortexed to facilitate cellular penetration by enhancing frequency and forceful intercellular collisions during which, DNA adsorbed on them diffuses into the cell.

Transformation by ultrasonication

The latest method developed for plant transformation uses ultrasound to facilitate the uptake of DNA into plant cells. By this technique, versatile cell types such as plant protoplasts, cells in suspension and intact pieces of plant tissues can be readily transformed. Furthermore, the equipment for ultrasound transformation is simple, cheap and multifunctional. This method holds prospects for substantial applications in plant transformation.

Principle: Ultrasonication involves permeabilization of membrane leading to DNA uptake. Two hypotheses have been proposed to explain its mechanism. First, the violent collapse of activation bubbles, generating high pressure and temperature shock waves possibly causes localized rupture of plasmalemma, and lead to uptake of exogenous DNA. The second hypothesis predicts the existence of critical hydrostatic pressure at which the intrinsic membrane potential is sufficiently high to induce mechanical breakdown of membrane (60-100 MPa) in a hyperbaric chamber. Consequently, it is possible that either the high oscillating pressure generated by the ultrasonic field, and / or the high pressure shock waves originating from collapse cavitation could produce such higher hydrostatic pressures that reversible membrane breakdown to occur allowing the passage of DNA.

Procedure: The plant tissue is suspended in few milliliters of sonication medium in a microfuge tube. Plasmid DNA (and possibly carrier DNA) is added to the tube. After rapid mixing, the samples are ready for sonication. A microtip, generally tapered, is immersed 2-3 mm into sonication medium, and pulses of ultrasound of selected intensity and duration are delivered to the tube by ordinary machines such as homogenizers. In the process, reversible membrane damage takes place, which serves as a route for DNA diffusion.

Laser microbeam irradiation-mediated DNA uptake

In this method finely focused laser beam is used for introducing transgenes into the whole plant cells. This technique is an ideal tool for manipulation of cell components and organelles due to several advantages associated with it. This technique can also be used for genetic manipulation of plant tissue, individual cells, protoplasts and organelles as well as cells with hard walls. Laser beam can be used inside the tissues, cells and organelles, thereby increasing the rate of transformation and the speed of operation. Laser beam intensity can be widely controlled and optical manipulation is very flexible. Wide choice for laser wavelength and pulse width is other advantage. The method permits selective fusion in a part of a subcellular organelle present inside a single living cell. Finally, it has the ability to transfer cytoplasmic material.

Principle and procedure: Plant cell transformation by laser microbeam irradiation is based on the delivery of high-energy light pulses focused through a microscope phase contrast objective onto regions of the target tissue of less than 1 μm in diameter. A continuously adjustable optical attenuator placed in the light path controls the laser energy. The beam can be focused very accurately so that the targeted area can be finely controlled. It is suggested that the focused high energy removes components from the plant cell walls or perforate self-healing holes of defined dimensions in the plant cell wall and membrane, which allow DNA uptake through passive diffusion. By creating an osmotic gradient between the target cells and an external hypotonic buffer, the efficiency of the technique for plant transformation can be increased.

Lipofection

Liposomes are closed, self-sealing, solvent-filled vesicles bound by a single bilayer and possess many properties similar to those of biological membranes. These serve as ideal carrier systems and are now used to deliver exogenous DNA into plant protoplasts. This use of liposomes as a transformation or transfection system is called lipofection.

Principle: Liposomes represent special type of lamellar phase in which water is self-contained and the lipid molecules are disposed of in bimolecular layers attached by their non-polar interfaces. These are easy to manipulate. Their lipid contents can be varied, and many substances may be trapped inside the interlamellar spaces. Owing to their properties, a wide variety of molecules including DNA can be encapsulated within their aqueous interior, and can be delivered to cells in a biologically active form via endocytosis or membrane-membrane fusion (Figure 22.7).

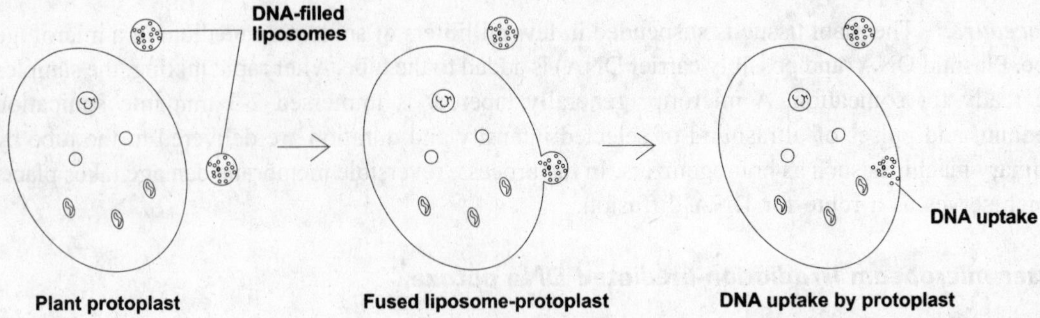

Figure 22.7 Fusion of DNA-filled liposomes with protoplast and DNA uptake.

Procedure: A stable water-in-oil emulsion is produced in a screw-capped glass tube by brief sonication of phospholipid (phosphatidyl serine/phosphatidyl choline/phosphatidyl glycerol) plus an aqueous buffer (Tris/HEPES/phosphate buffer) containing DNA to be packaged in a large volume of organic solvent (diethyl ether/isopropyl ether). The sonicator is purged with inert gas to keep the preparation sterile. The phases are reversed subsequently by evaporation of the organic solvent (reversed phase evaporation; REV) using rotary evaporator till a viscous gel is obtained. The system is vortexed briefly to promote breakdown on gel, and then vacuum is increased to 500-600 mm Hg. At this point encapsulation of DNA is complete, and the preparation is stable for months at inert atmosphere and 4°C. These liposomes with encapsulated or internalized DNA then serve as carrier of DNA, when incubated for ~ 30 min with plant protoplasts, transfer DNA into them by either direct fusion with the naked plasma membrane, or through endocytosis of the liposome. At the end of incubation the cells are washed with buffer, and plated on growth medium.

Liposome strategy is also useful for transferring DNA into vacuoles of walled plant cells. The targeting of DNA to vacuole is done for delivering the encapsulated DNA into the cytoplasm. This strategy is advantageous because the liposome protects the DNA from being damaged by the acidic pH and proteases present in the vacuole. To achieve this, DNA is encapsulated into liposome and pressure injected into the vacuole. Another way is to construct liposomes from material compatible with the lipids of the tonoplast, encapsulate DNA into it, and allow liposome-tonoplast fusion.

Direct gene transfer by chemical means

Some chemical agents can also facilitate direct gene transfer. Examples of such methods are Ca-phosphate coprecipitation, polycation-mediated transformation and application of dimethylsulphoxide (DMSO) along with polycations.

Calcium phosphate coprecipitation (Ca-DNA coprecipitation): In this method, DNA is mixed with $CaCl_2$ solution and isotonic phosphate buffer to form a DNA-calcium phosphate coprecipitate (also called Ca-DNA coprecipitate). On contact with protoplasts, protoplast/Ca-DNA complex is formed. Note that instead of protoplasts, other actively dividing cells can also be used. In order to encourage the endocytic uptake of the coprecipitate, the protoplast/Ca-DNA complex is treated with polyvinyl alcohol and high pH calcium. A physiological shock with DMSO can also increase the efficiency of transformation to a certain extent. Upon several hours of incubation, the Ca-DNA coprecipitate is transferred across the plasma membrane in a calcium requiring process. The protoplasts are washed and then implanted on fresh culture medium. Relative success depends on high DNA concentration and its apparent protection in the coprecipitate. This method was first used for transformation of tobacco leaf protoplast.

Polycation-mediated DNA uptake: Direct DNA uptake by protoplasts can be stimulated by using extremely hydrophilic, high molecular weight, long chain polycations such as polyethylene glycol (PEG) with or without metal ions such as Zn^{2+}, Li^{+}, Cs^{+}, Rb^{+}, K^{+}, Na^{+}, Ca^{2+} or Mg^{2+}. When placed in a solution, PEG removes 'free water', i.e., molecules that interact with charged (usually ionic) molecules soluble in water. Both protoplast membrane and DNA are normally negatively charged, hence have a tendency to repel each other due to charge repulsion, thereby limiting the interaction between the two. PEG at very high concentration seems to minimize this charge repulsion effects, and stimulate DNA uptake by endocytosis without any gross damage to protoplasts. Under PEG concentration ranging from 15-25%, ionic macromolecules such as DNA no longer stay in solution and precipitate out. PEG probably increases the adsorption of DNA to the surface, and enhance DNA uptake as a result of the interaction of PEG at the following levels: (i) protection of the exogenous DNA against nuclease degradation (ii) increase in the permeability of plasma membrane. However, the mechanism of cross-membrane transport in presence of PEG is still to confirm. The technique can be applied virtually to every protoplast system and for transfer of even small quantities of DNA. PEG also enhances efficiency of transformation by electroporation, liposome-mediated gene transfer and Ca-DNA coprecipitation procedures. Other polycations such as poly-L-lysine/poly-L-ornithine/DEAE-dextran (diethyl amino ethyl-dextran)/polybrene (hexamidethrine bromide) also work on the same principle as that of PEG. Polybrene possesses lesser toxicity as compared to PEG and is widely used in plant transformation.

Further improvement in the method involves the use of a polycation (which increases the adsorption of DNA to the surface), followed by a brief treatment with 25-30% DMSO, which increases membrane permeability and hence enhance DNA uptake.

Chloroplast Transformation

Chloroplast transformation is an important technique in plant transformation and is effectively used for obtaining transgenic plants.

Procedure: Microprojectile bombardment is the main strategy for introducing recombinant DNA into plastids. The vectors used are designed specifically for chloroplast transformation. Thus a basic chloroplast expression vector for single transgene contains two expression cassettes, one for selection of transformants (e.g., *aad* A for spectinomycin resistance; betaine-aldehyde dehydrogenase gene) and another for expression of transgene. Transgene is kept under the control of chloroplast specific regulatory sequences, *viz.* promoter and ribosome binding site of *psb* A, which ensures proper transcription and translation of the transgene, respectively. Regions of chloroplast

DNA (CpDNA) flank these two expression cassettes. After introduction into the chloroplast, homologous recombination occurs between the plastid sequences on the vector and those on the genome (Figure 22.8).

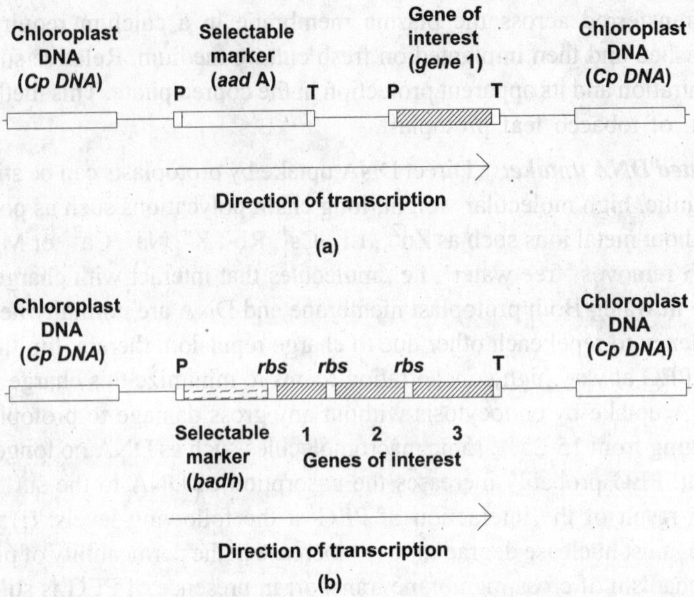

Figure 22.8 Vectors for chloroplast transformation. (a) A construct designed for the expression of one gene of interest (*gene* 1). Vector contains two expression cassettes, one for the gene of interest and the other for selectable marker gene (shown here is *aad* A conferring spectinomycin resistance). Each gene is driven by promoter (P) and terminator (T) sequences. Chloroplast DNA (*Cp DNA*) flanks the two expression cassettes and plays role in homologous recombination for site-specific integration into chloroplast genome. (b) A construct designed for the expression of multiple transgenes (*genes* 1, 2 and 3). The complete polycistronic unit or operon [comprising selectable marker gene (shown here is *badh*, which codes for betaine-aldehyde dehydrogenase), and three genes of interest] is driven by single promoter and terminator sequences. Each transgene is preceded by ribosome binding site (rbs) to ensure efficient translation. Chloroplast DNA (*Cp DNA*) flanking the two expression cassettes catalyze that plays role in homologous recombination for site-specific integration into chloroplast genome.

Advantages: The chloroplast transformation technique offers opportunities for creating crops that are both environment-friendly and more efficient. Various advantages of the technique are:

(i) No risk of cross-pollination: In many crop species, chloroplasts display only maternal inheritance so there is no danger of any gene transfer to related weedy species through pollen.

(ii) High-level gene expression: Through chloroplast transformation, very large transgene copy number may be obtained. Transgene insertion may occur into a single genome contained within an individual chloroplast. However, by using several rounds of selection during the plant regeneration process, it is possible to develop a homoplasmic population of chloroplasts (where all the chloroplasts are transformed). As there may be as many as 100 chloroplasts per cell, each containing up to 100 copies of the genome, there may be as many as 10,000 copies of the transgene per cell.

(iii) Synthesis of biologically active protein: There is a tremendous potential in chloroplast transformation for very high-level gene expression and synthesis of active proteins because chloroplast correctly folds and cross-links protein expressed from exogenous DNA.

(iv) No risk of gene silencing: As the integration of recombinant vector into the chloroplast genome occurs by homologous and site-specific integration, any problems associated with random insertion into the nuclear genome are avoided. This is in contrast to that observed with the methods mentioned above where non-homologous and random integration into nuclear genome takes place. Thus, gene silencing is not a problem during chloroplast transformation.

In Planta Transformation

The above-described plant transformation methods involve the use of cells or explants as transformation targets, and also require an obligatory tissue culture step for the regeneration of whole fertile transgenic plants. These extensive periods of tissue culture have several drawbacks, such as loss of time (typically many months), tendency of induction of somaclonal variations (i.e., the variation in plants derived from tissue culture) and requirement of space and labor. Considerable interest has therefore been taken in developing transformation methods that minimize or obviate the need for tissue culture steps. Thus recently *in planta* transformation systems have been developed in which DNA is introduced either by *Agrobacterium* or by direct transfer methods into intact plants, with no need for plant regeneration under tissue culture conditions. Such *in planta* transformation methods have been demonstrated to work in a limited number of plant species, opening up the possibility of widespread application to crop improvement.

Techniques for in planta transformation

In planta transformation protocols are of two types, viz., germ line transformation and meristem transformation. Germ line transformation is done at an appropriate time in the life cycle of plant so that the DNA becomes incorporated into cells that will contribute to the germ line. Thus DNA is transformed directly into the germ cells themselves, often around the time of fertilization, or into the very early plant embryo. However, the germ line transformation techniques are not reproducible, hence an alternative is to introduce DNA directly into meristems *in planta,* followed by the growth of transgenic shoots. Some commonly used methods for *in planta* transformation are as follows:

(i) ***DNA imbibition:*** The first *in planta* transformation system involved imbibing *Arabidopsis thaliana* (model dicot plant) seeds overnight in an *Agrobacterium* culture followed by germination. This resulted in a large number of transgenic plants containing T-DNA insertions. In case of *A. thaliana*, probably its small size and its ability to produce over 10,000 seeds per plant are advantageous. Generally *in planta* transformation methods have a very low efficiency, and low reproducibility. These limitations have so far prevented *in planta* techniques from being widely adopted for other plant species.

(ii) ***Floral dip:*** This is an extremely simple and popular technique in which at the time of fertilization, plants with young flowers are dipped (with or without a vacuum being applied) into a culture of *Agrobacterium*, which also contains a surfactant. The plant is subsequently allowed to set seed, whereupon a small proportion of the seeds produced are transgenic. This technique was used with *Arabidopsis* flowers, but the efficiency was very low and the transformed plants thus obtained were chimeric. However, the vast number of seeds produced resulted in acceptable overall transformation efficiency.

(iii) ***Vacuum infiltration:*** A more reliable method for *in planta* transformation is vacuum infiltration in which the bacteria are vacuum-infiltrated into flowers or ovules.

(iv) ***Incubation in DNA:*** This approach has potential for the recovery of transgenic cereals and grain legumes. Dry embryos are split off from the endosperm creating a giant wound across scutellum. As the tissues are dry, cell contents do not leak out. These are incubated in DNA solution. A microenvironment is created in the open cell that enables *in vitro* transcription, translation and replication.

(iv) ***Macroinjection:*** This method involves the injection of naked DNA solution (5-10 μl) with the aid of micropipettes into the developing floral tillers of plants such as rye tillers and post-fertilization cotton flowers. Within the floral tillers are archesporial cells that give rise to pollen in the developing sac by two meiotic cell divisions. It is suggested that such large cells are capable of taking up large molecules of DNA. Using this procedure, a plasmid harboring *npt* II gene was introduced into the tillers of rye plants and two kanamycin-resistant plants were obtained. However, these experiments were not reproducible.

(v) ***Incubation of DNA with cut pistil:*** This method is based on the fact that if DNA is applied to the cut pistil, it will reach zygote and hence seed. The plant produced from this seed will be transgenic.

(vi) ***Inoculation of cut apical shoots:*** Meristem transformation is achieved simply by severing apical shoots at their bases, followed by inoculation of the cut tissue with suspension. Using this process, transgenic *Arabidopsis* plants have been recovered from the transformed shoots at a frequency of about 5%. In rice, explanted meristem tissue has been transformed using *Agrobacterium* and particle bombardment, resulting in the proliferation of shoots that were regenerated into transgenic plants.

APPLICATIONS OF PLANTS TRANSGENIC TECHNOLOGY

The widespread application of conventional agricultural technologies such as herbicides, pesticides, fertilizers and tillage, etc. has resulted in severe environmental damage in many parts of the world. This demands the development of strategies to prevent or reduce their application. An effective strategy in this direction is the development of transgenic plants. Thus with the development of a variety of gene transfer techniques, a wide range of plants are transformed with foreign genes for the acquisition of useful quality traits such as insect-resistance, herbicide-tolerance, abiotic stress-tolerance (e.g., salt and drought-tolerance), disease-resistance, high nutritional quality (e.g., changing amino acid and lipid content, augmentation of sweetness), high yield potential, delayed ripening, enhanced ornamental value (e.g., new petal coloration) and edible vaccines, etc. Besides, plants have been developed as bioreactors for the large-scale production of important foreign proteins such as polymers, antibodies, antigens, and therapeutics. In this section, the applications of plant transformation in various fields are presented.

Development of Insect-Resistant Plants

Infestation of crop plants by insects in the field and to harvested products in transit or storage leads to heavy economical losses every year. Moreover, the routinely used insecticide application (often six to eight times during a growing season) to prevent these insects is not a cost-effective, environment-friendly and specific strategy. Due to health concerns and environmental impact registration of many promising chemical pesticides has been limited. Hence, genes for pest-resistance carefully deployed in crops to avoid selecting for future pest resistance provides alternative opportunities to reduce the use of chemical pesticides in many important crops. In addition, lowering the contamination of our food supply by pathogens that cause food safety problems (e.g., mycotoxins) would be beneficial to farmers and consumers alike. In this field of transgenics, extensive research has been done and several transgenic plants have been developed that are capable of producing functional insecticide, and are intrinsically resistant to insect predators. These transgenic plants do not need to be sprayed with costly, and hazardous chemical pesticides, and the cost of maintaining such insect-resistant crops is lower than that for non-resistant crops. These transgenic plants are usually highly specific in action, and act on a limited number of insect species. Moreover, these biological insecticides are also non-hazardous to humans and other higher animals. In many cases, they have also benefited the environment because of reduced pesticide usage or by providing the means to grow crops with less tillage.

Different strategies employed for generation of insect-resistant transgenic plants include introduction of genes encoding the following through recombinant DNA technology: (i) an insecticidal protoxin (Bt toxin or Cry protein encoded by *cry* gene) produced by one of several subspecies of *Bacillus thuringiensis*, and (ii) proteins that protect plants against a variety of insects, which exert their action by interfering with insect development, for example, protease inhibitors, α-amylase inhibitors, lectins, cholesterol oxidase, tryptophan decarboxylase and avidin. A summary of various transgenic strategies used to develop insect-resistant plants is presented in Table 22.1. It is significant to note that a range of insecticidal crystal proteins has been isolated and characterized from *B. thuringiensis* strains, and presently Bt technology is the most effective and the safest mode for the control of plant pests, and hence the best choice for pest control. The practical results obtained with *Bt*-crops have demonstrated that these are safe and beneficial, and few of the *Bt*-transgenic plants have been commercialized. A modified *cry* 3A gene was introduced in potato to provide resistance against Colorado beetle. In 1995, this crop became the first transgenic insect-resistant crop to reach commercial production, as NewLeaf™ potato marketed by Monsanto. The same company also released the first commercial transgenic, insect-resistant cotton and maize under the trade names Bollgard® and YieldGard™, respectively. Three transgenic *Bt* cotton hybrids containing lepidopteran specific Bollgard® *Bt* gene, *cry*1 Ac, offered protection against all the major species of Indian bollworms, *viz*, *Helicoverpa armigera*, *Pectinophora gossypiella*, *Earias vittella*, and *E. insulana*. Maize YieldGard™ expressed *cry* 1Ab and was resistant to the European corn borer.

Table 22.1 Insecticidal genes used to engineer pest resistance in plants.

S. No.	*Genes*	*Encoded protein*	*Origin (plant or bacteria)*	*Target insects*	*Transformed plants*
		Cry proteins (Bt toxin) from *Bacillus thuringiensis*			
1	*cry* genes (e.g. *cry* 1Ac)	Bt toxin	*Bacillus thuringiensis*	Lepidoptera, Diptera, Coleoptera	Cotton, corn, soybean
		α-amylase inhibitors from plants			
2	*a-AI-Pv*	α-amylase inhibitor	Common bean	Coleoptera	Azuki bean, pea, tobacco
3	*WMAI-I*	α-amylase inhibitor	Cereals	Lepidoptera	Tobacco
4	*14K-CI*	Bifunctional serine protease and α-amylase inhibitor	Cereals		Tobacco
		Protease inhibitors from plants			
5	*c-II*	Serine protease	Soybean	Coleoptera, Lepidoptera	Oilseed rape, poplar, potato, tobacco
6	*CMe*	Trypsin	Barley	Lepidoptera	Tobacco
7	*CMTI*	Trypsin	Squash	Lepidoptera	Tobacco
8	*CpTI*	Trypsin	Cowpea	Coleoptera, Lepidoptera	Apple, lettuce, oilseed rape, potato, rice, strawberry, sunflower, sweet potato, tobacco, tomato, wheat
9	*14K-CI*	Bifunctional serine protease and α-amylase	Cereals		Tobacco
10	*MTI-2*	Serine protease	Mustard	Lepidoptera	Arabidopsis, tobacco
11	*OC-1*	Cysteine protease	Rice	Coleoptera, Homoptera	Oilseed rape, poplar, tobacco
12	*PI-IV*	Serine protease	Soybean	Lepidoptera	Potato, tobacco
13	*Pot PI-I*	Proteinase	Potato	Lepidoptera, Orthoptera	Petunia, tobacco
14	*Pot PI-II*	Proteinase	Potato	Lepidoptera, Orthoptera	Birch, lettuce, rice, tobacco
15	*KTi3, SKTI*	Kunitz trypsin	Soybean	Lepidoptera	Potato, tobacco, tomato
16	*PI-I*	Proteinase	Tomato	Lepidoptera	Alfalfa, tobacco, tomato
17	*PI-II*	Proteinase	Tomato	Lepidoptera	Tobacco, tomato
		Plant enzymes			
18	*bch*	Chitinase	Bean	Homoptera, Lepidoptera	Potato
19	*pod*	Anionic	Tobacco	Lepidoptera,	Sweet gum, tobacco,

Contd.

		peroxidase		Coleoptera, Homoptera	tomato
20	*tdc*	Tryptophan decarboxylase	*Catharanthus roseus*	Homoptera	Tobacco
			Plant lectins		
21	*GNA*	Lectin	Snowdrop	Homoptera, Lepidoptera	Grapevine, oilseed rape, potato, rice, sweet potato, sugarcane, sunflower, tobacco,
22	*p-lec*	Lectin	Pea	Homoptera, Lepidoptera	Potato, tobacco
23	*WGA*	Agglutinin	Wheat germ	Lepidoptera, Coleoptera	Maize
24	*Jacalin*	Lectin	Jack fruit	Lepidoptera, Coleoptera	Maize
25	*Rice lectin*	Lectin	Rice	Lepidoptera, Coleoptera	Maize
			Others		
26	*Avidin*	Avidin	Chicken eggs	Coleoptera	Corn
27	*Cholesterol oxidase*	Cholesterol oxidase	Streptomyces	Coleoptera (*Anthonomus grandis grandis*)	Tobacco, Cotton

Development of Disease-Resistant Plants

Several plant pathogenic fungal or bacterial infections result simultaneously, or as a consequence of infestation of plants by insects, which often result in extensive damage, and loss of crop productivity accounting to enormous economic losses. In present times, chemical agents such as fungicide or bactericide are used for the control of fungi or bacteria, respectively. However, the application of chemicals is disadvantageous because these may persist in the environment, and may pose threat to animals or humans. To circumvent these problems associated with the application of chemicals, fungal- or bacterial pathogen-resistant transgenic plants have been developed as a simple, inexpensive, effective, and environment-friendly non-chemical means. In this direction, several approaches have been tested, which involves expression of gene products that are grouped into five categories:

(i) Gene product that is directly toxic to pathogens or that reduces their growth. These include pathogenesis-related proteins (PR proteins), e.g., hydrolytic enzymes (chitinases, glucanases), antifungal proteins (osmotin- and thaumatin-like), antimicrobial peptides (thionins, defensins and lectin), ribosome inactivating proteins (RIP), and phytoalexins.

(ii) Gene products responsible for destruction or neutralization of a component of the pathogen arsenal, e.g., polygalacturonase, oxalic acid and lipase.

(iii) Gene products that can potentially enhance the structural defenses in the plant, e.g., elevated levels of peroxidase and lignin.

(iv) Gene products releasing signals that can regulate plant defenses, e.g., production of specific elicitors, hydrogen peroxide (H_2O_2), salicylic acid (SA), and ethylene (C_2H_4).

(v) Resistance gene (R) product involved in the hypersensitive response (HR) and in interactions with avirulence (Avr) factors. In a very recent study, *BAA* 1 gene encoding the fruit bromelain has been used to successfully transform *Brassica rapa*, which conferred enhanced resistance to the soft rot pathogen *Pectobacterium carotovorum* spp. *carotovorum*. Some common examples of disease-resistant transgenic plants using any of these strategies are listed in Table 22.2.

Table 22.2 Plant species genetically transformed to enhance resistance to fungal diseases.

S. No.	*Gene product*	*Plant species engineered*	*Resistance against*
	Expression of hydrolytic enzymes		
1.	Alfalfa glucanase	Alfalfa	*Phytophthora megasperma*
2.	Baculovirus chitinase	Tobacco	*Alternaria alternata*
3.	Barley chitinase	Wheat	*Blumeria graminis and Puccinia recondita*
4.	*Trichoderma harziamum* endochitinase	Apple	*Venturia inaequalis*
5.	Tobacco chitinase	Peanut	*Cercospora arachidicola*
6.	Tomato chitinase	Canola	*Cylindrosporium concentricum and Sclerotinia sclerotiorum*
	Expression of PR proteins		
7.	*Aspergillus giganteus* antifungal protein	Wheat	*Blumeria graminis and Puccinia recondita*
8.	Pea PR-10 gene	Potato	*Verticillium dahliae*
9.	Pea defense response gene, defensin	Canola	*Leptosphaeria maculans*
10.	Potato osmotin like protein	Potato	*Phytophthora infestans*
11.	Rice *Rir* 1b defense gene	Rice	*Magnaporthe grisea*
12.	Rice thaumatin-like protein (TLP)	Wheat	*Fusarium graminearum*
13.	Tobacco PR-1a	Tobacco	*Peronospora tabacina* and Phytophthora parasitica
	Expression of antimicrobial proteins, peptides, or compounds		
14.	Alfalfa defensin	Potato	*Verticillium dahliae*
15.	Antifungal (killing) protein from virus infecting *Ustilago maydis* (dsRNA)	Wheat	*Ustilago maydis* and *Tilletia tritici*
16.	Arabidopsis thionin	Arabidopsis	*Fusarium oxysporum*
17.	*Bacillus amyloliquefaciens* barnase (RNase)	Potato	*Phytophthora infestans*
18.	Barley ribosome inactivating protein (RIP)	Tobacco	*Rhizoctonia solani*
19.	Barley RIP	Wheat	*Blumeria graminis*
20.	Chloroperoxidase from *Pseudomonas pyrocinia*	Tobacco	*Colletotrichum destructivum*
21.	Human lysozyme	Tobacco	*Erysiphe cichoracearum*
22.	Human lysozyme	Carrot	*Erysiphe heraclei* and *Alternaria dauci*

Contd.

23.	Mistletoe thionin viscotoxin	Arabidopsis	*Plasmodiophora brassicae*
24.	Onion antimicrobial protein	Geranium	*Botrytis cinerea*
25.	Radish defensin	Tomato	*Alternaria solani*
26.	Sarcotoxin peptide from *Sarcophaga peregrina*	Tobacco	*Rhizoctonia solani*, *Pythium aphanidermatum*, and *Phytophthora nicotianae*
27.	Synthetic antimicrobial peptide	Tobacco	*Colletotrichum destructivum*
28.	Synthetic cationic peptide chimera	Potato	*Fusarium solani and Phytophthora cactorum*
29.	Synthetic magainin-type peptide	Tobacco	*Peronospora tabacina*
	Expression of phytoalexins		
30.	Alfalfa isoflavone *O*-methyltransferase	*Alfalfa*	*Phoma medicaginis*
31.	Grape stilbenes (Resveratrol) synthase	Barley	*Botrytis cinerea*
32.	Peanut resveratrol synthase	Alfalfa	*Phoma medicaginis*
	Inhibition of pathogen virulence products		
33.	*Collybia velutipes* oxalate decarboxylase	Tomato	*Sclerotinia sclerotiorum*
34.	Pear polygalacturonase inhibiting protein	Tomato	*Botrytis cinerea*
35.	Wheat oxalate oxidase	Poplar	*Septoria mustiva*
	Alternation of structural compounds		
36.	Wheat germin (no oxalate oxidase activity)	Wheat	*Blumeria graminis*
	Regulation of plant defense responses		
37.	Arabidopsis *NPR* 1 protein	Arabidopsis	*Peronospora parasitica*
38.	Bacterial enzymes generating salicylic acid	Tobacco	*Oidium lycopersicon*
39.	*Phytophthora infestans* elicitor (β-cryptogein)	Tobacco	Phytophthora parasitica
40.	*Talaromyces flavus* glucose oxidase	Cotton	*Rhizoctonia solani* and *Verticillium dahliae*
41.	Tobacco catalase	Potato	*Phytophthora infestans*
	Expression of combined gene products		
42.	Barley chitinase + β-1, 3-glucanase, or chitinase + RIP	Tobacco	*Rhizoctonia solani*
43.	Rice chitinase + alfalfa glucanase	Tobacco	*Cercospora nicotianae*
44.	Tobacco chitinase + β-1, 3-glucanase	Tomato	*Fusarium oxysporum*
45.	Tobacco chitinase + β-1, 3-glucanase, osmotin	Carrot	*Alternaria dauci, Alternaria radicina,* and *Erysiphe heraclei*

Development of Virus-Resistant Plants

Plant viruses often cause considerable crop damage with significant reduction of plant yields. Therefore, in the absence of effective chemical treatments, plant breeders have attempted to transfer naturally occurring virus resistance genes from one plant cultivar to another. However, resistant cultivars often revert to virus sensitivity, and resistance to one virus does not necessarily confer resistance against other similar viruses. Plants also exhibit certain natural viral resistance mechanisms, for example, blockage of viral transmission, prevention of establishment of virus and bypassing of viral symptoms. Genetic engineering has also been used to develop non-conventional types of virus-resistant transgenic plants. Such virus-resistant transgenic plants will benefit farmers, as well as the environment by a reduction in the use of pesticides. The type of interaction between transgenic sequences and virus life cycles is categorized into two groups: those involving the synthesis of viral proteins, and those involving viral RNA. Based on these two types of interactions, various strategies have been developed for raising virus-resistant plants. These include application of viral coat protein (CP-mediated resistance), antisense RNA for viral coat protein, *RNase* III gene, antiviral plant protein, virion specific antibodies, and non-viral gene products such as ribosome inactivating proteins which blocks protein synthesis, 2′, 5′ oligoadenylate synthetases, which interfere with replication and ribozymes, which cleave viral genomes causing them to be degraded by cellular enzymes (Table 22.3). Using the strategy of viral coat protein, transgenic papaya plants resistant to papaya ringspot potyvirus have been commercialized and grown in Hawaii. Zucchini yellow mosaic virus and watermelon mosaic virus resistant 'Freedom II' squash plants have also been produced using this strategy.

Table 22.3 Transgenic plants engineered to have viral coat protein-mediated protection against vira infection.

S. No.	*Source of coat protein*	*Transgenic plant*
1.	Alalfa mosaic virus	Alfalfa, tobacco, tomato
2.	Arabis mosaic virus	Tobacco
3.	Beet necrotic yellow vein virus	Sugar beet
4.	Cucumber mosaic virus	Cucumber, tobacco
5.	Cymbidium ringspot virus	Tobacco
6.	Grapevine chrome mosaic virus	Tobacco
7.	Maize dwarf mosaic virus	Sweet corn
8.	Papaya ringspot virus	Papaya, tobacco
9.	Plum pox virus	Tobacco
10.	Potato aucuba mosaic virus	Tobacco
11.	Potato leaf-roll virus	Potato
12.	Potato virus S	Potato
13.	Potato virus X	Potato, tobacco
14.	Potato virus Y	Potato, tobacco
15.	Rice stripe virus	Rice
16.	Soybean mosaic virus	Tobacco
17.	Tobacco mosaic virus	Tobacco, tomato
18.	Tomato mosaic virus	Tomato
19.	Tomato rattle virus	Tobacco

Contd.

20.	Tomato streak virus	Tobacco
21.	Tomato spotted wilt virus	Tobacco
22.	Watermelon mosaic virus II	Tobacco
23.	Zucchini yellow mosaic virus	Muskmelon, tobacco

Development of Herbicide-Tolerant Plants

Two strategies in common use for controlling weeds are tillage (ploughing) and application of herbicides. However, these are not effective strategies. Extensive tillage may lead to soil erosion thereby causing a serious loss of water content. Many herbicides are unable to discriminate between weeds and crop plants, some have to be applied early before the establishment of weeds and some persist in the environment due to their non-biodegradable nature. Besides these drawbacks, chemical herbicides incur heavy expenditure and despite their application on crop plants ~ 10% of global production is lost per year through weed infestation. Thus to overcome these drawbacks, herbicide-resistant plants have been developed. Several strategies have been envisioned to develop herbicide-tolerant plants, which are based on any one of the following: (i) endowment of plants with the capability to metabolically inactivate the herbicide, (ii) inhibition of herbicide uptake, (iii) overproduction of the target protein, (iv) detoxification of herbicide, and (v) inability of herbicide-sensitive target protein to bind to a herbicide. One of the most common strategies used for the development of herbicide-tolerant transgenic plants is overexpression of herbicide resistant target protein in crop plants. Thus resistant plants have been developed for herbicide glyphosate, which acts as an inhibitor of an enzyme 5-enol pyruvyl shikimate-3-phosphate synthase (EPSPS) involved in the shikimate pathway for aromatic amino acid biosynthesis. Using this strategy, 'Round-Up Ready' soybean plants resistant to Round-Up™ herbicide (glyphosate) were grown in the U.S. by Monsanto Co. These transgenic soybean plants contained gene encoding Roundup®-tolerant enzyme (CP4-EPSPS). Other strategies for the development of herbicide tolerant plants include mutation of the target gene, inactivation of the herbicide using a single gene from a foreign source (e.g., bromoxynil tolerance through nitrilase-encoding gene from soil bacteria *Klebsiella ozaenae*), enhanced plant detoxification and increased superoxide dismutase level. A list of herbicide-tolerant transgenic crops in the field is given in Table 22.4.

Table 22.4 Engineering herbicide-resistant transgenic plants.

S. No.	*Herbicide*	*Class of herbicide*	*Mode of action of herbicide*	*Transgene of resistance in crops*	*Development*	*Companies*	*Crops*
1.	Glyphosate (Roundup)	Glycine	Inhibits enzyme EPSPS involved in aromatic amino acid biosynthesis	*Agrobacterium* CP4-*epsps* resistant gene	Overproduction of EPSPS Effect of inhibition of EPSPS by herbicide is overcome its overproduction	Monsanto	Soybean, Rape, Tomato
				Glyphosate oxidoreductase	Detoxification (or degradation)	Monsanto	Maize, Rape,

Contd.

				gene	of this herbicide by glyphosate oxidoreductase		Soybean
2.	Phosphinothricin (Basta), (Liberty), (Glufosinate)	Phosphinic acid	Inhibits glutamine synthase, an important enzyme involved in ammonia assimilation, and regulation of nitrogen metabolism	*bar* gene from *Streptomyces hygroscopicus* cr *pat* gene from *S. viridochromogenes*	Detoxification (or degradation) of this herbicide by phosphinothricin acetyltransferase	Hoechst / AgrEvo / Aventis, Novartis / Syngenta	Maize, Rice, Wheat, Cotton, Rape, Potato, Tomato, Sugar beet
3.	Chlorsulphuron	Sulphonylurea	Noncompetitively inhibit acetolactate synthase involved in the biosynthesis of branched amino acids	Mutant plant acetolactate synthetase selected from tissue culture	Altered enzyme is herbicide insensitive	DuPont – Pioneer Hi-Bred	Rape, Rice, Flax, Tomato, Sugar beet, Maize
4.	Arsenal	Imidazolinone	Noncompetitively inhibit acetolactate synthase involved in the biosynthesis of branched amino acids	Mutant plant acetolactate synthetase selected from tissue culture	Altered enzyme is herbicide insensitive	American Cyanamid	-
5.	Atrazine (Lasso)	S-triazines	Targets Q_B of photosystem II	Mutant plant chloroplast *psb* A gene or Q_B gene or introduction of gene for glutathione-S-transferase	*psb* gene encodes chloroplast protein D-1; Mutant psb protein is insensitive to the action of herbicide; Glutathione-S-transferase detoxifies atrazine	DuPont, Ciba Geigy / Novartis	Soybean
6.	Bromoxynil (Buctril)	Nitriles	Inhibits photosynthesis	Bacterial nitrilase gene	Detoxification (or degradation) of this herbicide by nitrilase	Calgene	Cotton, Rape, Potato, Tomato, Tobacco
7.	2, 4-D	Phenoxy-carboxylic acids	Action liked indole acetic acid (synthetic	*tfd* A gene from Alcaligenes	Detoxification (or degradation) of this herbicide	Schering / AgrEvo	Maize, Cotton, Tobacco

Contd.

	auxin); Decrease acetate metabolism		by oxygenase	

Development of Abiotic Stress-Tolerant Plants

Plants have evolved various physiological strategies to evade several stresses such as high-levels of light, U.V. irradiation, heat, high salt concentrations, oxidative stress or drought. Taking advantage of these strategies, several transgenic plants resistant to abiotic stresses have been generated, some of which are discussed below. A list of various abiotic stress tolerant transgenic plants is provided in Table 22.5.

Table 22.5 Engineering abiotic stress-tolerant transgenic plants.

S. No.	*Transgene*	*Encoded product*	*Crop plant (host)*	*Stress tolerance*
1.	Mitochondrial Mn-SOD	Mn-SOD	Alfalfa and tobacco chloroplasts	Drought, Ozone
2.	Mn SOD	Mn-SOD	Canola	Aluminium
3.	Chloroplast Cu /	Cu / Zn-SOD	Tobacco chloroplast	High light, chilling
4.	Cytosolic Cu / Zn-SOD	Cu / Zn-SOD	Tobacco cytosol	Acute ozone exposure
5.	Fe-SOD (Arabidopsis)	Fe-SOD	Tobacco	Acute ozone exposure
6.	*Apx* 1	Ascorbate peroxidase	Tobacco	Oxidative stress
7.	GST / GPX	Glutathione *S*-transferase with glutathione peroxidase	Tobacco	Oxidative stress
8.	*Nt* 107	Glutathione *S*-transferase	Tobacco	Cold, salinity
9.	*Par* B	Glutathione *S*-transferase	Arabidopsis	Aluminium toxicity, oxidative stress
10.	*Nt pox*	Glutathione peroxidase	Arabidopsis	Aluminium toxicity, oxidative stress
11.	*Glutathione reductase* (*E. coli*)	Glutathione reductase	Tobacco cytosol	Paraquat
12.	*MsFer* (alfalfa)	Ferritin	Tobacco	Oxidative damage caused by excess iron
13.	*E. coli bet* A	Choline dehydrogenase	Tobacco cytosol	Salt
14.	*bet* A / *bet* B	Choline dehydrogenase with betaine aldehyde dehydrogenase [Glycine betaine osmoprotectant]	Tobacco	Chilling, salt
15.	*bet* A	Choline dehydrogenase [Glycine betaine osmoprotectant]	Rice	Drought, salt
16.	*A. globiformis cod* A	Choline oxidase	Arabidopsis chloroplast	Salt, chilling, freezing, heat, strong light
17.	*cod* A	Choline oxidase	Rice	Salt, chilling

Contd.

18.	*cox*	Choline oxidase	Tobacco, *Brassica napus*	Drought, salt
19.	Mothbean *P5 CS*	Pyrroline carboxylate synthetase [Proline osmoprotectant]	Tobacco	Salt
20.	*P5 CS*^{F127A} (feedback inhibition insensitive)	Pyrroline carboxylate synthetase [Proline osmoprotectant]	Tobacco	Salt
21.	Anti-ProDH	Proline dehydrogenase Proline osmoprotectant]	Arabidopsis	Salt, freezing
22.	*E. coli mt1D*	Mannitol-1-phosphate dehydrogenase [Mannitol osmoprotectant]	Arabidopsis	Salt
23.	*E. coli mt1D*	Mannitol-1-phosphate dehydrogenase [Mannitol osmoprotectant]	Tobacco	Salt
24.	Apple *s6pdh*	Sorbitol-6-phosphate dehydrogenase [Sorbitol osmoprotectant]	Tobacco	Oxidative stress
25.	Apple *s6pdh*	Sorbitol-6-phosphate dehydrogenase [Sorbitol osmoprotectant]	Persimmon	Salt
26.	Yeast *tps1*	Trehalose-6-phosphate synthase [Trehalose osmoprotectant]	Tobacco, Potato	Drought
27.	*E. coli ots* A + *ots* B	Trehalose-6-phosphate synthase with Trehalose-6-phosphate phosphatase [Trehalose osmoprotectant]	Tobacco	Drought
28.	Ice plant *imtl*	Myo-inositol *o*-methyltransferase [D-Ononitol osmoprotectant]	Tobacco	Drought, Salt
29.	*B. subtilis sac* B	[Fructans osmoprotectant]	Tobacco	Drought
30.	*B. subtilis sac* B	[Fructans osmoprotectant]	Sugar beet	Drought
31.	*GS2*	Chloroplastic glutamine synthetase [Glutamine osmoprotectant]	Rice	Salt, chilling
32.	*Osm* 1 - *osm* 4 (protein accumulation)	[Osmotin osmoprotectant]	Tobacco	Drought, salt
33.	Annexin like protein	Annexin like protein	Brassica	Water deficit, salinity
34.	*lea*	Late embryogenesis abundant protein	Arabidopsis	Cold
35.	*CBF* 1	CRT / DRE element binding protein	Arabidopsis	Cold
36.	Glycerol-3-phosphate acyl-transferase	Glycerol-3-phosphate acyl-transferase	Tobacco	Cold

Contd.

37.	*Antifreeze gene from fish*	Antifreeze protein	Tobacco, Potato	Cold
38.	*apx* 1	Ascorbate peroxidase	Arabidopsis	Heat
39.	*AtHSF 1*	Heat-shock transcription factor HSF1::GUSfusion	Arabidopsis	Heat
40.	*Hsp 101*	HSP100 class heat-shock protein	Arabidopsis	Heat
41.	*Hsp 70*	HSP70 class heat-shock protein	Arabidopsis	Heat
42.	*Hsp 17.7*	SmHSP small heat-shock protein family	Carrot	Heat
43.	*TLHS 1*	Class I sm HSP	Tobacco	Heat

Engineering oxidative stress-tolerant plants

Several abiotic stresses such as salt, freezing, drought, exposure to pollutants as ozone, SO_2, are responsible for the generation of reactive oxygen species (ROS) in plant cells. These molecules result in oxidative stress by damaging membranes, membrane bound structures and macromolecules including proteins and nucleic aids, especially in the mitochondria and chloroplast. Thus plants engineered to tolerate ROS (i.e., oxidative stress) can withstand such environmental stresses. This can be easily accomplished by targeting oxygen radical scavengers such as superoxide dismutase (SOD) and oxidized glutathione.

Engineering salt and submergence stress-tolerant plants

The growth of many plants is severely impaired by either drought or high salinity. Moreover, a large fraction (~ one-third) of the world's irrigated land is laden with excessive salt and has become unsuitable for growing crops. Thus the development of crops with an inbuilt salinity-resistance can stabilize annual production and use of marginal lands for cultivation. The resistance to salt stress is best achieved by increase in cellular accumulation of osmoprotectants (or osmolytes), for example, sugars, alcohols, proline, glycine betaine and quaternary ammonium compounds etc. A list of osmoprotectants used to engineer salt-tolerant plants is provided in Table 22.5. Another strategy is compartmentalization of salts into vacuole by overproduction of Na^+/H^+ antiport protein.

Engineering cold and heat stress-tolerant plants

Different plants vary enormously in their ability to withstand cold and freezing temperatures. Most tropical plants have virtually no capacity to survive freezing conditions. On the other hand, many temperate plants can survive a range of freezing temperatures from – 5 to – 30°C, depending upon the species. Plants from colder regions routinely withstand temperatures even lower than this. Considering this difference, efforts were made to engineer cold stress-tolerant plants. In this direction, several cold-induced proteins have been identified in different plant species. These include 'late embryogenesis abundant' (LEA) proteins and 'cold responsive' (COR) proteins. Both these proteins contribute directly to freezing tolerance by mitigating the potentially damaging effects of dehydration associated with freezing. Overexpression or ectopic expression of these cold-induced proteins could therefore be a possible route to the specific engineering of cold or freezing stress-tolerance. There are some examples of the expression of cold-induced proteins in transgenic plants. For example, constitutive expression of small, hydrophilic, chloroplast-targeted COR protein COR15a in *Arabidopsis* improved the freezing tolerance of chloroplasts frozen *in situ* and of protoplasts frozen *in vitro*. Other strategy is based on engineering plants with the overexpression of a common regulatory protein. Note that several cold tolerance-related genes form COR regulon, where all the cold tolerance-related genes contain a similar regulatory element in their promoters (CRT/DRE element), which is bound and activated by CBF1 transcription factor. Thus by overexpressing *CBF* 1 gene, the entire group of COR regulon will be induced. In this direction, transgenic *Arabidopsis* plants carrying a CaMV 35S promoter :: CBF 1 gene construct have been produced. These plants express a number of *COR* genes, and have been shown to be freezing-tolerant. A yet another strategy involves the application of antifreeze gene from cold-water fish or spruce budworm or overwintering plants.

Similar to cold/freezing tolerance, heat-shock proteins (Hsp) are inducible by heat-stress. Note that some Hsp proteins that are molecular chaperones involved in protein folding are constitutively expressed. In a way analogous to cold/freezing tolerance strategies, individual heat-shock proteins have been transformed into plants in order to enhance heat-tolerance. Similar to CBF 1, heat-shock transcription factor (HSF) also binds and activates the promoter element (heat-shock element; HSE) contained in all the heat-shock genes. Thus, fusion of *AtHSF* 1 gene to N- or C- terminus of the *gus* A reporter gene was used for *Arabidopsis* transformation and the transgenic plants expressed heat-shock proteins constitutively, and demonstrated enhanced thermo-tolerance.

Improvement of Plant Nutritional Content

Upgradation of plant nutritional content can be done in a variety of ways, e.g., increase the amino acid content (specifically met and lys) of seed storage proteins, modify lipid (or fatty acid) composition of both edible and non-edible oil producing crops so that the oil becomes better suited for intended end use, synthesize vitamin E, and β-carotene and increase the levels of available iron etc. Such modifications increase the nutritional status of foods, and may help to improve human health by addressing malnutrition, under-nutrition and micronutrient deficiencies. Traditionally plant nutritional improvement was achieved by plant breeding, but these approaches were difficult, slow and intrinsically limited by the existing genetic content and cross-breeding strains. Presently, genetic engineering strategies are being routinely adopted for obtaining nutritionally enriched plants which are given below.

Improvement of amino acid (or protein) content of seed storage proteins

Seed storage proteins are used as sources of both carbon and nitrogen during seed germination and are the major protein source for most of the world's population. However, most often these seed storage proteins are deficient in one or the other essential amino acids. Cereals are usually deficient in lys. Rice, though has higher lys compared to other cereals, has low protein content. Recently genetic engineering techniques are being employed to alter the amino acid composition of seed storage proteins, and hence to improve their nutritional quality. This also decreases the need for amending grains with costly feed supplements. Engineering plant with a gene that encodes a seed protein rich in a particular amino acid can be used as a strategy to enrich its own seed proteins with the amino acids it lacks. For example, lupine, a grain legume used as feed for cattle, pigs and chickens lacks met and cys. Thus lupine has been successfully engineered to express sunflower seed albumin, a rich source of sulfur containing amino acids met and cys. The protein was stable in rumen, and was available for digestion and absorption in the lower gut. These transgenic lupine plants when used as rat feed as sole nitrogen source, rats made significantly greater weight gains. Similarly seed-specific 2S albumin gene from Brazil nut (*Bertholletia excelsa*) has been used to transform several plant species, e.g., *Vicia*, tobacco, alfalfa, *Trifolium*, etc. to increase met or sulfur content. One novel way to increase the lys content of seeds is to increase the production of lys in transgenic plants by deregulating lys biosynthesis pathway. Lys has been overproduced by cloning lys feedback insensitive genes for dihydrodipicolinic acid synthase and aspartokinase from *Corynebacterium* and *E. coli*, respectively. Nutritional enhancement in potato by deploying a non-allergenic seed albumin gene *ama* I derived from the plant *Amaranthus hypochondriacus* has also been reported.

Alteration of fatty acid composition

Rapeseed (canola), soybean, palm and sunflower accounts for ~ 75% of worldwide plant oil production and for most part, these oils consist of fatty acids such as palmitic, stearic, oleic, linoleic and linolenic acids. In addition, some vegetable oils contain fatty acids with conjugated double bonds. This is in contrast to the more usual case in which the typical polyunsaturated fatty acids of plant seed oils contains double bonds that are separated by methylene groups. Different types of fatty acids, viz., saturated fatty acids, or fatty acids with conjugated double bonds or polyunsaturated fatty acids (PUFA), are required for different applications. Besides chain length is also significant in different applications. For example, for use as drying agents in paints and inks, oils used should be such that less oxygen is required for the polymerization reactions occurring during drying, hence oils containing conjugated double bonds (i.e., methylene interrupted double bonds) are most suitable. This is because the presence of conjugated double bonds increases the rate of oxidation (in contrast to PUFA). Production of shortening, margarine, and confectionery goods requires large amounts of stearate. Thus, for application of fatty acids for different purposes, its degree of unsaturation and chain length should be modified. This modification is easily done in plants by genetic engineering. In this direction, a number of canola and other transgenic plants with modified fatty acid content and composition have been created that produced oils with better cooking and nutritional properties, or for better suitability in detergents, soaps, cosmetics, lubricants and paints. A list of enzymes targeted for engineering plants with altered lipid content and compositions is provided in Table 22.6.

Table 22.6 Genetically engineered plants with altered lipid content and composition.

S. No.	Gene	Source	Trait	Crop
1.	Acetyl-CoA carboxylase	Rapeseed, *Triticum aestivum*, Alfalfa	Increased seed oil	Canola
2.	Antisense stearoyl-ACP desaturase	*Brassica rapa*	Increased strearic acid	Canola
3.	Lauryl acyl carrier protein (ACP) thioesterase	*Umbellularia californica*	Increased lauric acid	Canola
4.	Oleate hydroxylase	*Ricinus communis*	Increased ricinolic acid	Canola
5.	Palmitoyl-ACP desaturase	*Coriandrum sativum*	Increased petroselinic acid	Canola

Enhancement of α-tocopherol (vitamin E)

Several studies have demonstrated that dietary supplement with a lipid soluble antioxidant vitamin E (400 International units) results in a decreased risk for cardiovascular diseases and cancer, assists in immune function, and prevents or slows a number of degenerative diseases in humans. The oils extracted from seeds have a relatively high-level of total tocopherols, but in most of the cases the fraction of α-tocopherol is not high enough. In an example of sunflower oil, which contains high-fraction of α-tocopherol, a large dietary intake (~ 400 g/day) is required to obtain sufficient amount of vitamin E. To avoid the problem of huge consumption, an alternative approach is to engineer plants with γ-tocopherol methyltransferase and homogentisic acid prenyltransferase.

Enhancement of β-carotene

β-carotene, a common carotenoid pigment normally found in plant photosynthetic membranes, is the precursor of vitamin A. But a few plants, including rice, are poor sources of several nutrients and vitamins, including vitamin A. Traditional breeding methods have been unsuccessful in producing crops containing a high vitamin A concentration and most national authorities rely on expensive and complicated supplementation programs to address the problem. To overcome this problem, transgenic approach was developed to engineer plants with inbuilt β-carotene pathway. For example, *Agrobacterium*-mediated transformation was used to transform rice with geranyl geranyl diphosphate (GGDP) (the progenitor of vitamin A in rice endosperm) in a research funded by Rockefeller Foundation, Swiss Federal Institute of Technology and European Community Biotech Program. Three genes of vitamin A biosynthesis pathway (viz., phytoene synthase: *psy*, phytoene desaturase: *crt*, and lycopene β-cyclase: *lcy*) were fused to transit peptides for targeting encoded proteins into the plastids. The encoded enzymes catalyze the biosynthesis of β-carotene from GGDP (PSY converts GGDP to phytoene, CRT causes desaturation of phytoene to lycopene and LCY catalyzes cyclization of lycopene to form β-carotene). For plant transformation, *psy* and *lcy* genes were isolated from daffodil (*Narcissus pseudomarcissus*) and cloned separately under glutelin promoter (i.e., promoter of rice seed storage protein). The *crt* gene isolated from bacteria *Erwinia uredovora* was put under the control of CaMV 35S promoter. The *psy* and *crt* genes were introduced on a construct lacking selectable marker. The *lcy* gene was part of a separate construct that contained a selectable marker. All three genes were expressed in endosperm (major part of the rice grain) and the frequency of insertion of all the three genes into the genomic DNA, and their subsequent expression was quite high. Thus the engineered rice produced β-carotene, which after ingestion by mammals could be converted to vitamin A. This strategy facilitated the eventual development of transgenic strains of rice that not only produced high-levels of β-carotene, but could also be easily manipulated so that these no longer contained antibiotic resistance marker genes. This β-carotene producing transgenic rice was transformed with gene encoding an iron storage protein ferritin (from bean), which allowed overexpression of this protein in endosperm of rice. As this transgenic rice was yellow or golden color, it was named 'golden rice'. Preliminary studies indicated that this golden rice synthesized enough β-carotene to provide individuals with more than the minimal daily requirement of vitamin A. Moreover, in contrast to vitamin A, excess dietary β-carotene had no harmful effects. Unfortunately production was too low, and normal serving of rice (300 g) provided a few percentage of daily diet. Further transformation of rice with phytase gene from *Aspergillus fumigatus* fungus, or overexpression of endogenous cysteine-rich metallothionein protein (e.g., cysteine peptidase having opposite effect to phytic acid) has been reported to favor efficient iron absorption. Another example is that of Beta Sweet® carrot produced at Texas A & M University, which contained inbuilt β-carotene biosynthesis pathway to combat cancer (β-carotene is also a potent cancer-fighting antioxidant). The transgenic carrot contained ~ 50% more β-carotene than normal carrot. The color of this carrot was dark maroon-purple due to addition of another antioxidant, anthocyanin (most common flower pigment belonging to the class of flavonoids). Its taste was similar to wild-type carrots, but had a very crispy texture, which was easier to chew.

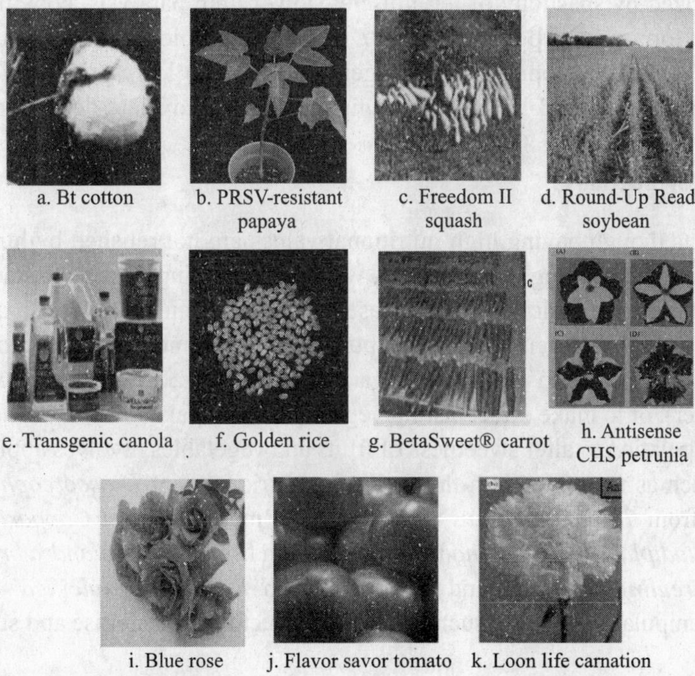

Figure 22.9 Examples of some transgenic plants.

Enhancement of iron content

Iron deficiency is the most common nutritional disorder that causes anemia in pregnant women and young children. According to WHO estimates, iron deficiency affects ~ 30% of world's population, and the problem is most severe where vegetable-based diets are the primary food source. Although a number of crops are rich in iron, its absorption is often prevented by the presence of phytic acid. Hence, iron fortification of cereal grains or food crops is required. As a first step toward developing food crops with a high enough level of iron to prevent iron deficiency anemia, cloning of gene encoding ferritin (an iron storage protein found in animals, plants, and bacteria that carries up to 4,500 iron atoms in its central cavity formed from the interaction of 24 monomeric ferritin subunits) was done. Rice was transformed with ferritin encoding genes from soybean and a gene encoding an enzyme that facilitates iron availability in the human diet. These transgenic rice plants contained 2-4 times the levels of iron normally found in non-transgenic rice. Another example is that of double transgenic golden rice, which was designed to prevent and treat vitamin A and iron deficiencies.

Overcome oxalic acid-induced nutritional stress

Some green leafy vegetables (e.g., *Amaranthus*, spinach, rhuburb) are rich sources of vitamins and minerals but these contain oxalic acid, a nutritional stress factor. This is because oxalate chelates calcium, and precipitation of calcium oxalate in kidney leads to hyperoxaluria and destruction of renal tissues. Similarly, consumption of *Lathyrus sativus* (chicken vetch) causes neurolathyrism, which is characterized by spasticity of leg muscles, lower limb paralysis, convulsions and death. This is the result of formation of β, N-oxalyl, L-α, β-diamino propionic acid (ODAP), a neurotoxin, from oxalic acid. Hence development of transgenic plants with low oxalic acid content may be beneficial. This can be achieved by genetic manipulation using oxalate decarboxylase gene.

Modification of sweetness

Some food products though having high nutritional values are not relished by human beings, and need to be made more appetizing. Furthermore, with the increasing health consciousness, a desire to get products having lesser calories has increased. Thus transgenic plants with a modification of sweetness (taste) have been generated. The purpose of this modification can be varied. For example, the purpose can be to prepare a sugar substitute (e.g., low calorie sweetener or non-digestible sweetener), or to make sweet tasting vegetables more palatable and with longer shelf life. Thus genetic manipulation to alter sweetness of fruits and vegetables involves application of sweet-tasting proteins such as monellin from the fruit of an African plant *Dioscoreophyllum cumminsii* Diels, thaumatin from *Thaumatococcus danielli* Benth, mabinlin from *Capparis masakai* Levl, pentadin from *Pentadiplandra brazzeana* Baillon, brazzein from *Pentadiplandra brazzeana* Baillon, curculin from *Curculingo latifolia* and miraculin from *Richadella dulcifica*. Other strategies include genetic manipulation using 1-sucrose : sucrose fructosyl transferase and sucrose phosphate synthase.

Modification of starch content and composition

The starch found in potatoes and most other crop plants consists of 20-30% straight chain amylose having α-1, 4 linkage, and 70-80% branched chain amylopectin having α-1, 6 linkage. For many industrial applications it is useful to have starch that is highly enriched in either amylose or amylopectin. By changing the activities of ADP – glucose pyrophosphorylase, starch synthase and branching enzyme, amylose/amylopectin ratio and hence the physical and chemical properties of starch can be greatly influenced. The modification of starch content and composition can be achieved by the antisense inhibition of starch branching enzyme to get high amylose content and low amylopectin content, overexpression of plastidic ADP-glucose pyrophosphorylase (AGPase) to accumulate more starch, and antisense inhibition of AGPase to reduce starch content, antisense inhibition of plastidic ATP/ADP-transporter protein (AADP) to reduce starch content and a reduced level of amylose/amylopectin ratio, sense expression of AADP to produce plants with higher starch and a higher amylose/amylopectin ratio.

Genetic Manipulation of Flower Pigmentation

Traditional breeding techniques have long been used to create thousands of new varieties of flowers differing from one another in color, shape and architecture. However, these techniques are slow, tedious and are limited by gene pool of a particular species. Now uniquely colored flowers have been developed by manipulation of genes encoding enzymes involved in anthocyanin and carotenoid biosynthetic pathway. This is achieved by genetic manipulation using genes encoding chalcone synthase, dihydroflavonol-4-reductase, β-carotene ketolase and delphinidin. Thus antisense CHS petunia plants have produced flowers with pale corolla pigmentation (white) instead of normal pink flowers. Similarly petunia plants have been transformed with maize dihydroflavonol-4-reductase to produce unique brick red-orange flowers and β-carotene ketolase from unicellular algae *Haematococus pluvialis* has been expressed in tobacco flowers to produce pink flowers. Australian company Florigene and Japanese company Suntory used CSIRO's gene silencing technology and created a blue rose. The strategy involved three steps: silencing of endogenous dihydroflavonol reductase (DFR) responsible for red color, insertion of delphinidin gene from pansy (responsible for production of blue pigment) and replacement of rose *dfr* gene with iris *dfr* gene.

Delaying of Post-Harvest Softening and Discoloration of Fruits

The major problem faced by the food industry is post-harvest softening and discoloration of fruits and vegetables during marketing and transport. Due to unacceptability by consumers, food industry has to invest a lot in the addition of food additives to prevent their discoloration and ripening. However, the safety of some of these food additives, especially sulfites, is questionable. It was therefore planned to engineer plants in such a way that the fruits and vegetables have increased shelf-life (i.e., long-term storage without discoloration as well as delayed ripening or softening). In this direction, the strategies adopted include antisense inhibition of polyphenol oxidase, pectin methylesterase, polygalacturonase (PG) and pectate lyase. Transgenic tomato plants constitutively expressing antisense pg gene were the first transgenic plants developed by antisense RNA technology to be commercialized in U.S.A. (released into the market in 1994 by Calgene) under the trade name 'Flavr Savr'. Other strategies include antisense inhibition of expansin and cellulose. Furthermore antisense inhibition of ethylene producing enzymes such as S-adenosyl synthetase, 1-amino cyclopropane-1-carboxylic acid (ACC) synthase and 1-amino cyclopropane-1-carboxylic acid oxidase, inhibition of ethylene biosynthesis by expression of malonyl ACC transferase, or glutamyl ACC transferase or bacterial ACC deaminase have also been reported to increase fruit shelf-life or to delay fruit ripening.

Delaying Flower Discoloration, Wilting and Senescence

Similar to food industry, flower industry also suffers from extensive economic losses due to premature wilting of flowers. The strategy used for delaying wilting and senescence is inhibition of ethylene production. In an example, Melbourne based company Florigene Pvt. Ltd. had produced transgenic long-life carnations by antisense inhibition of ACC synthase. The genetically eternal transgenic flowers neither required expensive refrigeration, nor silver thiosulfate or EthylBlock compound. Yet another strategy is overexpression of superoxide dismutase.

Detoxification of Toxic Metals

Toxic metals such as Hg, Pb, Cd and Se pose a great threat to environment and mankind. To overcome the associated problems, systems for detoxification and/or chelation of such toxic compounds are required. Presently, phytoremediation, i.e., the use of green plants to remove, contain, or render harmless environmental pollutants, offers an effective, environmentally nondestructive, and cheap remediation method. However, the use of genetic engineering to modify plants for metal uptake, transport, and sequestration has opened up new avenues for enhancing efficiency of phytoremediation. Thus, genes encoding phytochelatin synthase or glutathione synthetase (i.e., enzymes responsible for the synthesis of a metal chelator, phytochelatin) have been transferred to plants for improved metal uptake and sequestration. Plants have also been engineered to detoxify toxic metals. For example, transgenic plants containing genes for bacterial detoxifying enzymes have been used for bioremediation of contaminated soils. Thus in a study, *Arabidopsis* plants engineered with *mer* A gene encoding mercuric reductase were found to be capable of growing on mercurium contaminated soils. These plants were found to be 50 times more tolerant to mercury than wild-type plants. Further the introduction of *mer* B gene encoding organomercurial lyase into *Arabidopsis* plants led to generation of plants, which were 10 times more tolerant to mercury than *mer* A plants.

Increase Yield of Plant and its Components

It is desirable to increase the yield of plant or its components for maximal exploitation of plant biomass for any application. Theoretically, this may be achieved by a number of ways as exemplified below.

Increasing iron availability

Though iron is present in significant amounts on the surface of the earth, its availability for plant growth is often limited. At physiological pH, under aerobic conditions, iron is sparingly soluble in the soil solution and hence it is not readily available to plants. Therefore, some plants have developed mechanisms to acquire iron from the soil, for example, by secreting iron-binding phytosiderophores, which are linear hydroxy- and amino-substituted iminocarboxylic acids, such as mugineic acid and avenic acid. Mugineic acid family phytosiderophores are natural iron chelators that graminaceous plants secrete from their roots to solubilize iron in the soil. Rice plants, which secrete very low amount of mugineic acid, are highly susceptible to growth inhibition from iron deficiency. Thus by engineering rice plants to increase the secretion of mugineic acid, their capability to take up iron can be enhanced, which further increases the plant yield. This has been achieved by transforming rice plants with a 11 kbp fragment of barley genomic DNA containing two *naat genes*, *naat* A and *naat* B, encoding subunits of nicotianamine aminotransferase (NAAT), an enzyme responsible for catalyzing amino group transfer of nicotianamine (an intermediate in the biosynthesis of mugineic acid phytosiderophores).

Increasing photosynthesis

In order to increase yields, photosynthesis is perhaps the most obvious target for genetic intervention because it determines the rate of carbon fixation, and hence the overall size of the organic carbon pool. Strategies used for increasing photosynthetic activity include the modification of light-harvesting phytochromes, and key photosynthetic enzymes. Attempts have been made to introduce components of the energy-efficient C4 photosynthetic pathway into C3 plants, which lose a proportion of their fixed carbon through photorespiration. In this direction, maize gene encoding phosphoenol pyruvate carboxylase of C4 pathway has been transferred into several C3 plants including potato and rice. This manipulation increased the overall level of carbon fixation. Transgenic rice plants expressing pyruvate orthophosphate dikinase and NADP-malic enzyme have also been produced.

Increasing oxygen content

Oxygen is an essential substrate for plant respiratory metabolism. The amount of available O_2 may limit a number of plant biochemical reactions. Thus, to increase O_2 concentration inside a plant, an O_2 sequestering protein may be provided where needed. To achieve this, the gene encoding a dimeric Hb has been engineered from a Gram-negative bacterium *Vitreoscilla* into tobacco.

Manipulating lignin content and composition of trees

The presence of lignin in forest trees is a major impediment in obtaining cellulose for pulp and paper industry. Presently lignin is usually removed from cellulose by harsh physical and chemical treatments, which are expensive and environment damaging. High lignin also decreases nutritional value of forage crops that are used for cattle feed. Thus the strategy for optimal utilization of plant biomass in pulp and paper industry and as nutritious cattle feed is to alter lignin content and composition. In this direction, lignin down-regulation has been successfully obtained by antisense inhibition of any one (or more) of the lignin biosynthetic genes in plants. Thus transgenic plants with altered lignin content and composition have been obtained by single or multiple gene constructs encoding enzymes such as *O-methyltransferase* (*omt*), ferulate 5-hydroxylase (*f5h*), cinnamoyl

CoA O-methyltransferase (*ccoaomt*), cinnamoyl CoA reductase (*ccr*), or cinnamyl aldehyde dehydrogenase (*cad*), etc.

Obtaining bioenergy

The potential of bioenergy crops depends on optimization of dry matter and energy yield per area of land and obtaining efficient conversion. The economics and efficiency of conversion of plant biomass into bioethanol, a liquid fuel, can be significantly enhanced by genetically engineering bioenergy crops for better yield, amenability to bioprocessing and cell wall digestion. This involves altering biochemical composition of plants, modifying plant stature and architecture, increasing capacity to produce harvestable yield, decreasing lignin content and ameliorating negative biotic and abiotic stresses. In this direction, overexpression of cellulases, endoglucanases, exoglucanases and glucosidases or down-regulation of lignin biosynthetic pathway genes in biomass crops are useful strategies.

Reversible Male Sterility in Plants

Heterozygous individuals often are healthier and stronger than homozygous ones, and the only way to guarantee heterozygosity in plants is to make sure that self-pollination cannot occur. For most crop plants it was very tedious or practically impossible to exclude selfing. To exclude self-pollination, it would be good to introduce male sterility in plants. Progeny from such plants are then expected to be 100% heterozygous (assuming these were pollinated with pollen from an unrelated variety). Strategies used to introduce male sterility include expression of barnase, and several genetically modified crops with barstar and barnase are available. A closely related approach is called 'terminator technology'. This technology is, however, criticized as a way for companies to protect and enforce their patents.

Transgenic Plants as Biosensors

Rapid technological development is inevitably associated with many environmental problems which primarily include pollution of soil, water and air. In many cases, the presence of contamination is difficult to assess. It is even more difficult to evaluate its potential danger to the environment and humans. Despite the existence of several whole organism-based and cell-based models of sensing pollution and evaluation of toxicity and mutagenicity, there is no ideal system to make a quick and cheap assessment. In this respect, transgenic organisms that can be intentionally altered to be more sensitive to particular pollutants are especially promising. One of the important advantages of transgenic biosensors is the ability to customize the assay in accordance with monitoring needs. This not only makes transgenic biosensors more sensitive to a particular pollutant, but also allows for easy scoring. Another big advantage of a customized transgenic assay is the ability to understand changes at the molecular level.

Transgenic plants represent an ideal system for biomonitoring genotoxic pollutants, since these can be grown at the site of pollution or potentially dangerous sites. Plants are ethically more acceptable and aesthetically more appealing than animals as sensors of environmental pollution.

Transgenic plant biomonitors used for the evaluation of genotoxicity are relatively cheap and simple in use. The assays used in the past decade were based on the restoration of the transgenes α-glucuronidase (*uid* A or *gus*) and luciferase activity in model plants transformed with non-active forms of these marker genes. The current visible marker of choice is green fluorescent protein (GFP) from the Pacific jellyfish (*Aequorea victoria*). GFP has the unique property of fluorescing green when excited by blue or U.V. light. A DNA construct containing a specific inducible promoter could be fused to GFP and then transferred into a plant for biomonitoring.

It is possible that in the near future, transgenic plants could provide constant, landscape-level data on environmental hazards. Transgenic plants could also be used as biosensors to monitor radioisotope levels around nuclear power plants or to detect jet fuel contaminants at military bases. These could also disclose the presence of certain unwanted and especially dangerous substances in the environment of which presently there is no good way of monitoring. Transgenic plants may be used to evaluate the genotoxicity of chemical and radiological compounds. Plant biosensors also offer the potential to monitor expansive areas of land using satellite remote sensing to detect the biosensor output.

Molecular Farming or Application of Plants as Bioreactors

Another major goal for raising transgenic plants is their use as bioreactors (or biofactories) for production of speciality chemicals and pharmaceuticals. Some common examples are production of high value compounds such as biopolymers, vaccines, recombinant antibodies, therapeutic agents, nutraceuticals, hormones and industrial enzymes, etc. This area is described as molecular farming (or biofarming). Plant system is relatively more advantageous as compared to recombinant microbial system because of ease of growth and transformation, high-level expression and high yield, rapid scale-up, stability of exogenous DNA, formation of biologically active proteins, ease of storage and distribution and above all safety and economic viability.

Only problem while using transgenic plants for large-scale production of high value products is their purification from an enormous amount of harvested transgenic plant. However, this is easily achieved either by expressing foreign protein at a high-level or by ensuring its expression in a manner that facilitates its purification. These strategies include chloroplast targeting of foreign protein, directing the foreign protein to cell apoplast thereby facilitating its exudation or fusing foreign protein to plant oleosins. In view of various advantages of plant system, considerable attention has been drawn in using transgenic plants as bioreactors for the large-scale production of biopolymers, vaccines, therapeutic proteins, nutraceuticals, hormones and industrial enzymes.

Biopolymer production

Owing to the above advantages of using plants as bioreactors and to overcome the problems associated with the fermentative production of biopolymer poly (3-hydroxy butyric acid) (PHB), which is used in the synthesis of biodegradable plastics (bioplastics), research has been conducted to produce this biopolymer in plants. As plant lack enzymes involved in PHB biosynthesis, engineering plants with these genes from some other source (e.g., bacteria) may be a useful strategy. It is speculated that plant seeds may be a potential source for plastics that could be produced and easily extracted. In *Alcaligenes eutrophus*, PHB is synthesized from acetyl CoA in three enzyme-catalysed steps (encoded by genes in a single operon). These are 3-ketothiolase, acetyl CoA reductase, and poly (3-hydroxy butyric acid) synthase. Thus, to produce transgenic *A. thaliana* plants, genes for each of these three enzymes were isolated, cloned separately into a plasmid and targeted to chloroplast.

Large-scale production of antibodies, antibody fragments and therapeutic agents

As already mentioned, crops have unmatched opportunities of biomass production. Besides the common advantages of exploiting plants as bioreactors, certain other advantages are as follows: (i) As biopharmaceuticals are intended for human use, these should be biologically active (proper post-transcriptionally and post-translationally processed). Hence, eukaryotic proteins can be properly expressed in plants. (ii) The production in transgenic plants significantly reduces the risk of mammalian viral contamination in comparison to the ones produced in animal cells grown in culture. There is no danger from mammalian cells and tissue culture medium that might be contaminated with infectious agents. (iii) Cultivation on large-scale is inexpensive. The cost benefit analysis has revealed that antibodies production costs ~ 5,000 per g from hybridoma cell culture, \$ 1,000 per g from transgenic bacteria and \$ 10 – 100 per g from transgenic plants. Thus, the exploitation of transgenic plants is envisaged for producing large quantities of biomolecules of therapeutic use to combat various diseases in developing countries, in a convenient, effective and inexpensive way. In this direction, various antigens, antibodies, antibody fragments, hormones, enzymes and therapeutic proteins, etc. have already been expressed successfully in plants and have been shown to retain their native functional forms. Note that the antibodies produced in plants are called plantibodies. Plants producing recombinant sIgA against the oral pathogen *Streptococcus mutans* generated and these plantibodies are being commercially developed as the drug CaroR$_x$™, marketed by Planet Biotechnology Inc. Various other examples of transgenic plants used for the production of antigens, antibodies, antibody fragments and therapeutic agents are given in Tables 22.7, 22.8 and 22.9.

Table 22.7 Some antigens produced in transgenic plants.

S. No.	*Antigen*	*Host Plant*
1.	(4-hydroxy-3-nitrophenyl) acetyl	Tobacco
2.	Abscissic acid	Tobacco
3.	Abscissic acid	Pea
4.	Artichoke mottled crinkle virus	Tobacco
5.	B-cell lymphoma	Tobacco
6.	Beet necrotic yellow vein virus coat protein	Tobacco
7.	Cell surface protein from mouse	Tobacco
8.	Dihydrofolate reductase (DHFR)	Petunia
9.	Fungal chitinase	Tobacco
10.	Gibberellin	Tobacco
11.	*Herpes simplex* virus	Soybean
12.	Human cancer cell surface antigen	Pea
13.	Human carcinoembryonic antigen	Tobacco

Contd.

14.	Human creatine kinase	Tobacco
15.	Oxazolone	Tobacco
16.	Phosphonate ester	Tobacco
17.	Phytochrome	Tobacco
18.	Root rot nematode surface glycoprotein	Tobacco
19.	Stolbar phytoplasma membrane protein	Tobacco
20.	*Streptococcus mutans* cell surface antigen SA I / II	Tobacco
21.	TMV	Tobacco

Table 22.8 Some antibodies and antibody fragments produced in transgenic plants.

S. No.	*Antibody*	*Antigen*	*Host Plant*
1.	Fab; IgG (κ)	Human creatine kinase	Arabidopsis
2.	IgG	Glycoprotein B of *Herpes simplex* virus	Soybean
3.	IgG (κ)	Transition stage analog	Tobacco
4.	IgG (κ)	Fungal cutinase	Tobacco
5.	IgG (κ) and IgG/ hybrid	*S. mutans* adhesin	Tobacco
6.	IgM (λ)	NP (4-hydroxy-3-nitrophenyl) acetyl hapten	Tobacco
7.	Single chain Fv	Phytochrome	Tobacco
8.	Single chain Fv	Artichoke mottled crinkle virus coat proteint	Tobacco
9.	Single chain Fv	Abscissic acid	Tobacco
10.	Single chain Fv	Nematode antigen	Tobacco
11.	Single chain Fv	β-glucuronidase, β-1, 4 endoglucanase	Tobacco
12.	Single chain antibody fragment	Atrazine, Paraquat	Tobacco
13.	Single domain (dAb)	Substance P	Tobacco

Table 22.9 Therapeutic recombinant proteins (biopharmaceuticals) produced in transgenic plants.

S. No.	*Protein*	*Application*	*Host Plant(s)*
1.	α-Tricosanthin	HIV therapy	Tobacco
2.	Angiotensin-1-converting enzyme	Hypertension	Tobacco, tomato
3.	Angiotensin-1 converting enzyme	Hypertension	Tobacco, tomato
4.	Collagen Human	Tissue repair	Tobacco
5.	Factor XIII (A-domain)	Bleeding	Tobacco
6.	Glucocerebrosidase	Gaucher disease	Tobacco
7.	Hirudin Leech	Anticoagulant	Canola
8.	Human α-antitrypsin	Cystic fibrosis, Liver disease, Haemorrhage	Rice
9.	Human α-interferon	Hepatitis C and B	Rice, turnip
10.	Human aprotinin	Trypsin inhibitor for transplantation surgery	Corn
11.	Human enkephalins	Anti-hyperanalgesic by opiate activity	Thale Cress, canola
12.	Human epidermal growth factor	Wound repair/Control of cell proliferation	Tobacco

Contd.

13.	Human erythropoietin	Anemia	Tobacco
14.	Human granulocyte-macrophage colony stimulating factor	Neutropenia	Tobacco
15.	Human growth hormone	Dwarfism, Wound healing	Tobacco
16.	Human hemoglobin	Blood substitute	Tobacco
17.	Human hirudin variant C	Anticoagulant	Tobacco, canola, Ethiopain mustard
18.	Human homotrimeric collagen I	Collagen synthesis	Tobacco
19.	Human protein C	Anticoagulant	Tobacco
20.	Human serum albumin	Liver cirrhosis	Potato, tobacco
21.	Interleukin-2, 4, 10, 12, 18	Antiviral, anticancer	Potato, tobacco
22.	Lactoferrin	Antimicrobial	Potato tubers, rice, tobacco
23.	Lysozyme	Antimicrobial	Rice
24.	Pancreatic lipase	Exocrine pancreatic deficiency	Tobacco, maize
25.	Synthetic elastin	Tissue repair	Tobacco

Edible vaccine production

The development of vaccines is essential to effectively combat infectious diseases and to overcome increased occurrence of antibiotic-resistant pathogens. Many vaccines developed through conventional ways are administered through injections, which require trained personnel. Moreover, the application of antigens for inducing oral tolerance requires production of the human antigens in large amounts, which is generally difficult to achieve by conventional means. Furthermore, traditionally produced vaccines are expensive to produce and package. These vaccines are costly and are not available for widespread distribution in the developing countries of the world, where infectious diseases are still the primary cause of death. These vaccines are destroyed (or denatured) rapidly due to lack of physical infrastructure such as roads and refrigeration. Thus, to eliminate and simplify the process of vaccine production on large-scale, vaccine administration, and vaccine dissemination in developing countries, a relatively newer concept of edible vaccines was developed. These edible vaccines represent production of protective antigens in transgenic plants, such that eating raw fruits or vegetables can induce neutralizing antibodies and trigger immune response to pathogen. Thus food crops can play significant new roles in promoting human health by serving as vehicles for both production and delivery of vaccines. In contrast to traditionally produced vaccines, edible vaccines offer several advantages such as large-scale and fail-safe mode of immunization, ease of administration, vast applicability, ease of storage and transport, cost-effectiveness and ethical acceptance.

The strategy of edible vaccines was first used for the production of surface protein antigen A (*spa* A) from *Streptococcus* in tobacco. In 1992, Charles Arntzen and coworkers expressed hepatitis B surface antigen (HBsAG) in tobacco, and an accumulation of 0.01% of soluble protein level has been reported. Since then several other plants are being considered as effective vaccine delivery systems. These include potato, banana, papaya, tomato, lettuce, carrot, peanut, cucumber, rice, wheat, soybean and corn (Table 22.10).

Table 22.10 Antigens expressed in plants for the production of edible vaccines.

S. No.	*Antigen*	*Causal organism/disease*	*Host Plant*
1.	Capsid protein epitope	Mink enteritis virus	Cowpea
2.	c-Myc	Cancer	Tobacco
3.	CT-B toxin	Cholera	Potato
4.	ET-B	Travellers diarrhea	Potato
5.	Foot and mouth disease antigen	Foot and mouth disease	Cowpea
6.	Gp41 peptide	HIV-1	Cowpea
7.	Haemagglutinin	Influenza	Tobacco
8.	Hepatitis B surface antigen	Hepatitis B	Tobacco, potato
9.	Human cytomegalovirus glycoprotein B	Human cytomegalovirus	Tobacco
10.	Malarial antigens	Malaria	Tobacco
11.	Norwalk virus antigen	Gasterointestinal distress	Tobacco, potato
12.	Rabies virus glycoprotein	Rabies	Tomato, tobacco, spinach
13.	Spike protein	Piglet diarrhea	Tobacco

CISGENESIS

As the transgene comes from another unrelated plant or even from an entirely different kingdom, there is possibility of not only bringing in desirable characteristics from other varieties of the plant, but also of adding undesirable characteristics from them. Thus, due to the fear of mingling of genetic material between species that cannot hybridize by natural means, several public concerns and strict regulatory mechanism, plant transformation using its own genetic material or gene(s) from species with which it can intercross or able to breed conventionally (cisgenes) has gained much significance. This process is known as cisgenesis or intragenesis and the plant transformants thus obtained are called cisgenic plants. Plants genetically modified by cisgenesis are very similar to those generated by conventional breeding with respect to plant fitness and no risk of unwanted plant invasives. Moreover, in contrast to conventional breeding, cisgenesis offers several advantages such as potentiality to create new varieties quickly and in cost-effective manner. Furthermore, as only selected beneficial genes are transferred and not other genes located nearby on the chromosome, it is expected that the cisgenic plants would receive wide public acceptance and less regulation.

CONCLUSION

With depleting natural resources and changing global climate, conventional agricultural practices alone are unable to sustain the quality and quantity of the produce. With advent of modern biotechnology, newer tools permitting gene transfer across the species, transgenics, opened an avenue for solving the age old problem. Genetically modified crops can be produced by several ways, be it a physical or chemical delivery method of inserting gene of choice. The aim of gene transfer is breeding crops with improved traits, as well as molecular farming, the production of pharmaceuticals, therapeutic molecules or specialty chemicals for industry. Transgenics have the potential to reduce usage of insecticides, herbicides and weedicides, improve tolerance to stress, and function as edible vaccines. Like any known technology, genetic manipulation of crop genome has its advantages and disadvantages. Potential risks associated with GM crops include gene flow, allergenic, toxic anti-nutritional effects, use of antibiotic resistance marker genes (ARMGs), undesirable evolutionary traits and change in biodiversity. Though genetic engineering is known as simple extension of conventional breeding, the developed crops are analyzed and evaluated for the potential risks by following the protocols mentioned in the Codex Alimentarius Commission Report. The Cartagena Protocol of Biosafety is internationally acknowledged as it harmonizes the issues of international regime in relation to GM crops.

FURTHER READINGS

1. Aida R., Yoshida T., Ichimura K., Goto R. and Shibata M. (1998) Extension of flower longevity in transgenic torenia plants incorporating ACC oxidase transgene. *Plant Sci.* **(138):** 91-101.
2. Antonelli N.M. and Stadler J. (1990) Genomic DNA can be used with cationic methods for highly efficient transformation of maize protoplasts. *Theor. Appl. Gen.* 80 **(3):** 395-401.
3. Apse M.P., Aharon G.S, Snedden W.A. and Blumwald E. (1999) Salt tolerance by overexpression of a vacuolar Na^+/H^+ antiport in *Arabidopsis. Sci.* **(285):** 1256-1258.
4. Arntzen C.J. (1997) Edible vaccines. *Public Health Rep.* **(112):** 190- 197.
5. Ayub R., Guis M., Amor M.B., Gillot L., Roustan J.P., Latche A., Bouzayen M. and Pech J.C. (1996) Expression of ACC oxidase antisense gene inhibits ripening of cantaloupe melon fruits. *Nature Biotechnol.* **(14):** 862-866.
6. Bachem C.W.B., Speckmann G.J., vander Linde P.C.G., Verheggen F.T.M., Hunt M.D., Steffens J.C. and Zabeau M. (1994) Antisense expression of polyphenol oxidase genes inhibits enzymatic browning in potato tubers. *Biotechnol.* **(12):** 1101-1105.
7. Baker S.S., Wilhelm K.S. and Thomashow M.F. (1994) The 5'-region of *Arabidopsis thaliana cor* 15a has *cis*-acting elements that confer cold-, drought- and ABA-regulated gene expression. *Plant Mol. Biol.* 24 **(5):** 701-713.
8. Bent A.F. (2000) *Arabidopsis in planta transformation*, uses, mechanisms, and prospects for transformation of other species. *Plant Physiol.* **(124):** 1540-1547.
9. Bizily S.P., Rugh C.L. and Meagher R.B. (2000) Phytodetoxification of hazardous organomercurials by genetically engineered plants. *Nature Biotechnol.* **(18):** 213-217.
10. Bohmert K., Balbo I., Kopka J., Mittendorf V., Nawrath C., Poirier Y., Tischendorf G. and Trethewey R.N. (2000) Transgenic *Arabidopsis* plants can accumulate polyhydroxybutyrate to up to 4% of their fresh weight. *Planta.* **(211):** 841-845.
11. Bohmert K., Balbo I., Steinbuchel A., Tischendorf G. and Willmitzer L. (2002) Constitutive expression of the β-ketothiolase gene in transgenic plants. A major obstacle for obtaining polyhydroxybutyrate-producing plant. Plant Physiol. **(128):** 1282-1290.
12. Bouzayen M., Hamilton A., Picton S., Barton S. and Grierson D. (1992) Identification of genes for the ethylene-forming enzyme and inhibition of ethylene synthesis in transgenic plants using antisense genes. *Biochem. Society Trans.* **(20):** 76-79.
13. Brien J.O. and Lummis S.C. (2000) An improved method of preparing microcarriers for biolistic transfection. Brain Res. Protocols. **(10):** 12-15.
14. Caboche M. (1990) Liposome-mediated transfer of nucleic acids into plant cell. *Physiol. Plant.* **(79):** 173-176.

15. Caima P.G., McCole L.M., Klein T.M. and Kerr P.S. (1996) Fructan accumulation and sucrose metabolism in transgenic maize endosperm expressing a *Bacillus amyloliquefaciens sac* B gene. *Plant Physiol.* **110:** 355-363.

16. Cebadera E. [* | In-line.WMF *] and Camara M.(2007) Plants as biofactories: edible vaccines production. *J. Biotechnol.* 131 **(2):** S43-S44.

17. Chabaud M., Boisson-Dernier A., Zhang J., Taylor C.G., Yu O. and Barker D.G. (2006) *Agrobacterium rhizogenes*-mediated root transformation. In: *Medicago Truncatula.* handbook version. pp. 1-8.

18. Chakraborty S., Chakraborty N. and Datta A. (2000) Increased nutritive value of transgenic potato by expressing a non-allergenic seed albumin gene from *Amaranthus hypochondriacus. Proc. Natl. Acad. Sci. U.S.A.* 97 **(7):** 3724-29.

19. Chang S.S., Park S.K. and Kim B.C. (1994) Stable genetic transformation of *Arabidopsis thaliana* by *Agrobacterium* inoculation *in planta*. *Plant J.* **(5):** 551-558.

20. Chen T.H.H. and Murata N. (2002) Enhancement of tolerance of abiotic stress by metabolic engineering of betaines and other compatible solutes. *Curr. Opin. Plant Biol.* **(5):** 250-257.

21. Clough S.J. and Bent A.F. (1998) Floral dip: a simplified method for *Agrobacterium-mediated* transformation of *Arabidopsis thaliana. The Plant J.* 16 **(6):** 735-743.

22. Comai L., Facciotti D., Hiatt W.R., Thompson G., Rose R.E. and Stalker D.M. (1985) Expression in plants of a mutant *aro* A gene from *Salmonella typhimurium* confers tolerance to glyphosate. *Nature*. **(317):** 741-744.

23. Courtney-Gutterson N., Napoli C., Lemieux C., Morgan A., Firoozabady E. and Robinson K.E.P. (1994) Modification of flower color in florist's chrysanthemum: production of a white-flowering variety through molecular genetics. *Biotechnol*. **(12):** 268-271.

24. Crossway A., Oakes J.V., Irvine J.M., Ward B., Knauf V.C. and Shewmaker C.K. (1986) Integration of foreign DNA following microinjection of tobacco mesophyll protoplasts. *Mol. Gen. Genet*. **(202):** 179-185.

25. Curtis I.S. and Nam H.G. (2001) Transgenic radish (*Raphanus sativus* L. var longipinnatus Bailey) by floral-dip method – plant development and surfactant are important in optimizing transformation efficiency. *Transgenic Res*. **(10):** 363-371.

26. Curtis R.I. and Cardineau C.A. (1990) Oral immunization by transgenic plants. World patent application, WO 90/02484.

27. Daniell H., Kumar S. and Dufourmantel.N. (2005) Breakthrough in chloroplast genetic engineering of agro-nomically important crops. *Trends Biotechnol*. **(23):** 238-245.

28. De la Penna A., Lörz H. and Schell J. (1987) Transgenic rye plants obtained by injecting DNA into young floral tillers. *Nature*. **(325)**: 274-276.

29. Dekker J. and Duke S.O. (1995) Herbicide-resistant field crops. *Adv. Agron.* **(54):** 69-116.

30. Eapen S. and D'Souza S.F. (2005) Prospects of genetic engineering of plants for phytoremediation of toxic metals. *Biotechnol Adv*. 23 **(2):** 97-114.

31. Falco S.C., Guida T., Locke M., Mauvais J., Saunders C., Ward R.T. and Webber F. (1995) Transgenic canola and soybean seeds with increased lysine. *Biotechnol*. **(13):** 577-582.

32. Faus I. (2000) Recent developments in the characterization and biotechnological production of sweet-tasting proteins. Appl. Microbiol. *Biotechnol*. **(53):** 145-151.

33. Feldman K.A. and Marks M.D. (1987) *Agrobacterium*-mediated transformation of germinating seeds of *Arabidopsis thaliana* – a non-tissue culture approach. *Mol. Gen. Genet*. **(208):** 1-9.

34. Fischer R., Stoger E., Schillberg S., Christou P. and Twyman R.M. (2004) Plant-based production of biopharmaceuticals. *Curr. Opin. Plant Biol*. **(7):** 152-158.

35. Fitchen J.H. and Beachy R.N. (1993) Genetically engineering protection against viruses in transgenic plants. *Annu. Rev. Microbiol*. **(47):** 739-763.

36. Geigenberger P. (2003) Regulation of sucrose to starch conversion in growing potato tubers. *J. Expt. Bot.* 54 **(382):** 457-465.

37. Gilbert J., Jordan M., Somers D.J., Xing T. and Punja Z.K. (2006) Engineering plants for durable disease resistance. In: *Multigenic and Induced Systemic Resistance in Plants*, Springer, U.S.A., pp. 415-455.

38. Gleba Y., Marillonnet S. and Klimyuk V. (2004) Engineering viral expression vectors for plants: the 'full virus' and the 'deconstructed virus' strategies. *Curr. Opin. Plant Biol.* **(7):** 182-188.

39. Goto F., Yoshihara T., Shigemoto N., Toki S. and Takaiwa F. (1999) Iron fortification of rice seed by the soybean ferritin gene. *Nature Biotechnol.* 17 **(3)** 282-86.

40. Grimsley N.H. (1990) Agroinfection. *Physiol. Plant.* **(79):** 147-153.

41. Haigler C.H., Singh B., Zhang D., Wang S.H., Wu C., Cai W.X., Hozain M., Kang W., Kiedaisch B. and Strauss R.E. (2007) Transgenic cotton over-producing spinach sucrose phosphate synthase showed enhanced leaf sucrose synthesis and improved fiber quality under controlled environmental conditions. *Plant Mol. Biol.* 63 **(6):** 815.

42. Hain R., Stabel P., Czernilofsky A.P., Steinbib, H.H., Herrera-Estrella L. and Schell J. (1985) Uptake, integration, expression and genetic transmission of a selectable chimeric gene by plant protoplasts. *Mol. Gen. Genet.* 199 **(2):** 161-168.

43. Hellens R., Mullineaus P. and Klee H. (2000) A guide to *Agrobacterium* binary Ti vectors. *Trends Plant Sci.* **(5):** 446-451.

44. Hess D. (1987) Pollen based techniques in genetic manipulation. *Int. Rev. Cytol.* **(107):** 169-190.

45. Hiatt A. (1990) Antibodies produced in plants. *Nature*. **(344):** 469-470.

46. Hilder V.A. and Boulter D. (1999) Genetic engineering of crop plants for insect resistance - a critical review. *Crop Prot.* **(18):** 177–191.

47. Hoffman F. (1996) Laser microbeams for the manipulation of plant cells and subcellular structures. *Plant Sci.* **(113):** 1-11.

48. Holm P.B., Olsen O., Scnorf M., Brinch-Pedersen H. and Knudsen S. (2000) Transformation of barley by microinjection into isolated zygote protoplasts. *Transgenic Res.* **(9):** 21-32.

49. Holmberg N., Lilius G., Bailey J.E. and Bülow L. (1997) Transgenic tobacco expressing *Vitreoscilla* hemoglobin exhibits enhanced growth and altered metabolite production. *Nature Biotechnol.* **(15):** 244-247.

50. John M. and Keller G. (1996) Metabolic engineering in cotton: biosynthesis of polyhydroxybutyrate in fiber cells. *Proc. Natl. Acad. Sci., USA.* **(93):** 12768-12773.

51. Jouanin L., Bonadé-Bottino M., Girard C., Morrot G. and Giband M. (1998) Transgenic plants for insect resistance. *Plant Sci.* **(131):** 1-11.

52. Jung Y.J., Su. Choi C., Park J.H., Kang H.W., Choi J.E., Nou I.S. and Lee S.Y. (2008) Overexpression of the pineapple fruit bromelain gene (BAA) in transgenic chinese cabbage (*Brassica rapa*) results in enhanced resistance to bacterial soft rot. *Electronic J. Biotechnol.* 11 **(1):** 1-8.

53. Kasuga M., Liu Q., Miura S., Yamaguchi-Shinozaki K. and Shinozaki K. (1999) Improving plant drought, salt, and freezing tolerance by gene transfer of a single stress-inducible transcription factor. *Nature Biotechnol.* **(17):** 287-291.

54. Khammuang S., Dheeranupattana S., Hanmuangjai P. and Wongroung S. (2005) *Agrobacterium*-mediated transformation of modified antifreeze protein gene in strawberry. Songklanakarin *J. Sci. Technol.* 27 **(4):** 693-703.

55. Kikkert J.S. (1993) The Biolistic® PDS-1000 / He device. Plant Cell Tissue Organ Cult. 33 **(3):** 221-226.

56. Klee H.J., Hayford M.B., Kretzmer K.A., Barry G.F. and Kishore G.M. (1991) Control of ethylene synthesis by expression of a bacterial enzyme in transgenic tomato plants. *Plant Cell* **(3):** 1187-1193.

57. Kloti A., Iglesias V.A. and Wunn J. (1993) Gene transfer by electroporation into intact scutellum cells of wheat embryos. *Plant Cell Rep.* **(12):** 231-243.

58. Kovalchuk I. and Kovalchuk O. (2008) Transgenic plants as sensors of environmental pollution genotoxicity. *Sensors*. **(8):** 1539-1558.
59. Ku M.S.B., Agarie S., Nomura M., Fukayama H., Tsuchida H., Ono K., Hirose S., Toki S., Miyao M. and Matsuoka M. (1999) High level expression of maize phosphoenol pyruvate carboxylase in transgenic rice plants. *Nature Biotechnol*. **(17):** 76-80.
60. Kumar G.B.S., Ganapathi T.R. and Bapat V.A. (2004) Edible vaccines: current status and future prospects. *Physiol. Mol. Biol. Plants*. 10 **(1):** 37-47.
61. Lee J.H., Hubel A. and Schoffl F. (1995) Derepression of the activity of genetically engineered heat shock factor causes constitutive synthesis of heat-shock protein and increased thermo-tolerance in transgenic *Arabidopsis. Plant J.* **(8):** 603-612.
62. Lucas W.J., Lansing A., deWet J. R. and Walbot V. (1990) Introduction of foreign DNA into walled plant cells via liposomes injected into the vacuole: a preliminary study. *Physiol. Plant*. **(79):** 184-189.
63. Lucca P., Hurrell R. and Potrykus I. (2001) Genetic engineering approaches to improve the bioavailability and the level of iron in rice grains. *Theor. Appl. Genet*. **(102):** 392-397.
64. Ma J.K., Hikmat B.Y. and Wycoff K. (1998) Characterization of a recombinant plant monoclonal secretory antibody and preventive immunotherapy in humans. *Nature Med*. **(4):** 601-606.
65. Ma J.K.C., Drake P.M.W. and Christou P. (2003) The production of recombinant pharmaceutical proteins in plants. *Nature Rev. /Genet*. **(4):** 794-805.
66. Maliga P. (2004) Plastid transformation in higher plants. *Annu. Rev. Plant Biol*. **(55):** 289-313.
67. Mann V., Harker M., Pecker I. and Hirschberg J. (2000) Metabolic engineering of astaxanthin production in tobacco flowers. *Nature Biotechnol*. **(18):** 888-892.
68. Marillonnet S., Thoeringer C., Kandazia R., Klimuyk V. and Gleba Y. (2005) Systemic *Agrobacterium tumefaciens*-mediated transfection of viral replicons for efficient transient expression in plants. *Nature Biotechnol*. **(23):** 718-723.
69. Mason H.S., Lam D.M.K. and Arntzen C.J. (1992) Expression of hepatitis surface B antigen in transgenic plants. *Proc. Natl. Acad. Sci., U.S.A.* 89 **(24):** 11745-11749.
70. Molvig L., Tabe L.M., Eggum B.O., Moore A.E., Craig S., Spencer D. and Higgins T.J.V. (1997) Enhanced methionine levels and increased nutritive value of seeds of transgenic lupins (*Lupinus angustifolia* L.) expressing a sunflower seed albumin gene. *Proc. Natl. Acad. Sci., U.S.A.* **(94):** 8393-8398.
71. Murphy D.J. (1996) Engineering oil production in rapeseed and other oil crops. *Trends Biotechnol*. **(14):** 206-213.
72. Nagatani N., Honda H., Shimada T. and Kobayashi T. (1997) DNA delivery into rice cells and transformation using silicon carbide whiskers. *Biotechnol. Techniques*. **(11):** 471-473.
73. Negruitiu I., Shillito R., Potrykus I., Biasini G. and Sala F. (1987) Hybrid genes in the analysis of transformation conditions. I. Setting up a simple method for direct gene transfer in plant protoplasts. *Plant Mol. Biol.* **(8):** 363-373.
74. Park S.H., Pinson S.R.M. and Smith R.Z.H. (1996) T-DNA integration into genomic DNA of rice following *Agrobacterium* inoculation of isolated shoot apices. *Plant Mol. Biol*. **(32):** 1135-1148.
75. Peñarrubia L., Kim R., Giovannoni J., Kim S.H. and Fischer R.L. (1992) Production of the sweet protein monellin in transgenic plants. *Biotechnol*. **(10):** 561-564.
76. Perlak F.J., Oppenhuizen M., Gustafson K., Voth R., Sivasupramanian S., Heering D., Corey B., Ihrig R.A. and Roberts J.K. (2001) Development and commercial use of Bollgard cotton in the U.S.A. – early promises versus today's reality. *Plant J.* **(27):** 489-501.
77. Perlak F.J., Stone T.B. and Muskopf Y.M. (1993) genetically improved potatoes: protection from damage by Colorado potato beetles. *Plant Mol. Biol*. **(22):** 313-321.

78. Pogue G.P., Lindbo J.A., Garger S.J. and Fitzmaurice W.P. (2002) Making an ally from an enemy: plant virology and the new agriculture. *Ann. Rev. Phytopathol.* **(40):** 45-74.

79. Porta C. and Lomonossoff G.P. (2002) Viruses as vectors for the expression of foreign genes in plants. Biotechnol. *Genetic Engg.* **(19):** 245-291.

80. Punja Z.K. (2001) Genetic engineering of plants to enhance resistance to fungal pathogens - a review of progress and future prospects *Can. J. Plant Pathol.* **(23):** 216–235.

81. Quinn J.P. (1990) Evolving strategies for the genetic engineering of herbicide resistance in plants. *Biotechnol. Adv.* **(8):** 321-333.

82. Raghuwanshi A., Singh R.K. and Jain R.K. (2004) The golden rice: five years after.' *Physiol. Mol. Biol. Plants.* 10 **(1):** 1-5.

83. Rastogi S. and Dwivedi U.N. (2006) Down-regulation of lignin biosynthesis in transgenic *Leucaena leucocephala* harboring O-methyltransferase gene. *Biotechnol. Prog.* **(22):** 609-616.

84. Rastogi S. and Dwivedi U.N. (2008) Manipulation of lignin in plants with special reference to O-methyltransferase. *Plant Sci.* **(174):** 264-277.

85. Rastogi S. and Pathak N. (2009) *Genetic Engineering*. Oxford Univ. Press, India.

86. Regierer B., Fernie A.R., Springer F., Perez-Melis A., Lissel A., Koehl K., Willmitzer L., Geigenberger P. and Kossmann J. (2002) Starch content and yield increase as a result of altering adenylate pools in transgenic plants. *Nature Biotechnol.* **(12):** 1256-1260.

87. Rigano M.M., Alvarez M.L., Pinkhasov J., Jin Y., Sala F., Arntzen C.J. and Walmslcy A.M. (2004) Production of a fusion protein consisting of the enterotoxicogenic *E. coli* heat-labile toxin B subunit and a tuberculosis antigen in *Arabidopsis thaliana. Plant Cell Rep.* **(22):** 502-508.

88. Rishi A.S., Nelson N.D. and Goyal A. (2001) Molecular farming in plants: a current perspective. *J. Plant Biochem. Biotechnol.* **(10):** 1-12.

89. Roxas V.P., Smith R.K., Allen Jr. E.R. and Allen R.D. (1997) Overexpression of glutathione S-transferase/ glutathione peroxidase enhances the growth of transgenic tobacco seedlings during stress. *Nature Biotechnol.* **(15):** 988-991.

90. Saalbach I., Pickardt T.,. Waddell D.R, Hillmer S., Schieder O. and Müntz K. (1995) The sulphur-rich Brazil nut 2S albumin is specifically formed in transgenic seeds of the grain legume *Vicia narbonensis*. *Euphytica.* 85 **(1-3):** 181-192.

91. Sakamoto A. and Murata N. (2002) The role of glycine betaine in the protection of plants from stress: clues from transgenic plants. *Plant Cell Env.* **(25):** 163-171.

92. Sanford J.C., Klein T.M., Wolf E.D. and Allen N. (1987) Delivery of substances into cells and tissues using a particle bombardment process. *J. Particle Sci. Techniques* **(6):** 559-563.

93. Savidge B., Weiss J.D., Wong Y.H.H., Lassner M.W., Mitsky T.A., Shewmaker C.K., Post Beittenmiller D. and Valentin H.E. (2002) Isolation and characterization of homogentisate phytyltransferase genes from *Synechocystis* sp. PCC 6803 and *Arabidopsis*. *Plant Physiol.* **(129):** 321-332.

94. Schwall G.P., Safford R., Westcott R.J., Tayal A., Shi Y.C., Gidley M.J. and Jobling A.S. (2000) Production of very-high-amylose potato starch by inhibition of SBE A and B. *Nature Biotechnol.* **(18):** 551-554.

95. Sévenier R., Hall R. D., vander Meer I.M., Hakkert H.J.C., vanTunen A.J. and Koops A.J. (1998) High level fructan accumulation in a transgenic sugar beet. *Nature Biotechnol.* **(16):** 843-846.

96. Sheehy R.E., Kramer M. and Hiatt W.R. (1988) Reduction of polygalacturonase activity in tomato fruit by antisense RNA. *Proc. Natl. Acad. Sci., U.S.A.* **(85):** 8805-8809.

97. Shillito R.D., Saul M.W., Pazkowski J., Muller M. and Potrykus I. (1985) High efficiency direct gene transfer to plants. *Biotechnol.* **(3):** 1099-1103.

98. Shintani D. and Della Penna D. (1998) Elevating the vitamin E content of plants through metabolic engineering. *Sci.* **(282):** 2098-2100.

99. Slater A., Scott N.W. and Fowler M.R. (2004) Techniques for plant transformation. In: *Plant biotechnology* (eds. A. Slater, N.W. Scott and M.R. Fowler), Oxford Univ. Press, NY, pp. 55-78.

100. Smith C.J.S., Watson C.F., Ray J., Bird C.R., Morris P.C., Schuch W. and Shah D.M. (1988) Antisense RNA inhibition of polygalacturonase gene expression in transgenic tomatoes. *Nature*. **(334):** 724-726.

101. Stuiver M.H. and Custers J.H.H.V. (2001) Engineering disease resistant plants. *Nature*. **(411):** 865-868.

102. Takahashi M., Makanishi H., Kawasaki S., Nishizawa N.K. and Mori S. (2001) Enhanced tolerance of rice to low iron availability in alkaline soils using barley nicotianamine aminotransferase genes. *Nature Biotechnol*. **(19):** 466-469.

103. Tanaka Y., Tsuda S. and Kusumi T. (1998) Metabolic engineering to modify flower color. *Plant Cell Physiol*. 39 **(11):** 1119-1126.

104. Taylor N.J. and Faquet C.M. (2002) Microparticle bombardment as a tool in plant science and agricultural biotechnology. *DNA Cell Biol*. **(21):** 963-977.

105. Töpfer R., Gronenborn B., Schell J. and Steinbiss H.H. (1989) Uptake and transient expression of chimeric genes in seed-derived embryos. *The Plant Cell*. **(1):** 133-139.

106. Trieu A.T., Burleigh S.H. and Kardailsky L.V. (2000) Transformation of *Medicago truncatula* via infiltration of seedlings or flowering plants with *Agrobacterium*. *Plant J*. **(22):** 531-541.

107. Ussuf K.K., Laxmi N.H. and Mitra R. (2001) Proteinase inhibitors: Plant-derived genes of insecticidal protein for developing insect-resistant transgenic plants. *Curr. Sci*. 80 **(7):** 847-853.

108. VanderKrol A.R., Lenting P.E. and Veenstra J. (1988) An antisense chalcone synthase gene in transgenic plants inhibits flower pigmentation. *Nature*. **(333):** 866-869.

109. Veluthambi K., Gupta A.K. and Sharma A. (2003) The current status of plant transformation. *Curr. Sci*. **(84):** 368-372.

110. Ye X., Al-Babili S., Klöti A., Zhang J., Lucca P., Beyer P. and Potrykus I. (2000) Engineering the provitamin A (b-carotene) biosynthetic pathway into (carotenoid-free) rice endosperm. *Sci*. 287 **(5451):** 303-305.

111. Yusibov V. and Rabindran S. (2004) Plant viral expression vectors: history and new developments. In: *Molecular Farming: Plant-made Pharmaceuticals and Technical Proteins* (eds. R. Fischer and S. Schillberg), John Wiley & Sons Inc., NY, pp. 77-89.

112. Zhang H.X. and Blumwald E. (2001) Transgenic salt-tolerant tomato plants accumulate salt in foliage but not in fruit. *Nature Biotechnol*. **(19):** 765-768.

113. Zhang J., Kueva N.Y., Wang Z., Wu R., Ho T.H. and Nguyen H.T. (2000) Genetic engineering for abiotic stress resistance in crop plants. *In vitro Cell. Dev. Biol. – Plant*. **(36):** 108-114.

114. Zhang L.J., Cheng L.M. and Xu N. (1991) Efficient transformation of tobacco by ultrasonication. *Biotechnol*. **(9):** 996-997.

115. Zhu Y.L., Pilon-Smits E.A.H., Jouanin L. and Terry N. (1999) Overexpression of glutathione synthetase in Indian mustard enhances cadmium accumulation and tolerance. *Plant Physiol*. **(119):** 73-79.

116. Zupan J.R., Muth T.R., Draper O. and Zambryski P.C. (2000) The transfer of DNA from *Agrobacterium tumefaciens* into plants: a feast of fundamental insights. *The Plant J*. 23 **(1):** 11-28.

CHAPTER

23

Bioinoculant Technology

Government initiatives to reduce the use of agro-chemicals including pesticides renewed the interest in microbial inoculants to enhance soil productivity, and biological control of insect pests, plant diseases and soil-borne pathogens. Microbial interactions play very important roles in sustainable agriculture mainly through integrated nutrient management. A conservative estimate for biologically fixed nitrogen in India accounts to 4.20 million tonnes per year, which at the current price of urea works out to Rs. 4410 crore every year. Currently, there are numerous inoculants in the market, not only for N_2 fixation and nutrient release, but also for biocontrols and bioremediations. Various microbial inoculants being commercially produced in India by various government/semi-government or private agencies include: *Rhizobium, Bradyrhizobium, Azospirillum, Azotobacter, Bacillus megaterium, Bacillus polymyxa*, mycorrhizal inoculants and *Pseudomonas* as Plant Growth Promoting Rhizobacteria (PGPR) and biocontrol agent. Application of PGPR is one of the best approaches along with conventional breeding in the management of abiotic stresses in crop production. New environment-friendly, genetically-modified, microbial inoculants are being produced commercially and used for protecting plants from disease and insects and to promote plant growth. These new products are expected to bring down the use of biocides and chemical fertilizers. This chapter deals with an overview of microbial inoculants aimed at nutrient, disease and pest management, and the concept and application of mixed bioinoculants.

***Keywords*:** Abiotic stress, biofertilizer, biopesticides, soil productivity, organic decomposers.

INTRODUCTION

With the advent of green revolution or high input agrotechnologies in India, we achieved self-reliance in food production. At the same time, modern Indian agriculture is getting more and more dependent upon the steady supply of synthetic inorganic fertilizers and pesticides that are products of fossil fuels. There is a growing concern about the excessive dependence on the supply of chemical fertilizers and pesticides, and adverse effects of indiscriminate use of these synthetic inputs on soil productivity and environmental quality. The cumulative effect of environmental degradation due to application of agro-chemicals resulted in a declined food production during the last two decades. The food grain production has stagnated at 1.5 %. To overcome the adverse effects, there is a need to develop new strategies to ensure further growth in agricultural output. Adapting a strategy of integrated nutrient supply by using a combination of chemical fertilizers and pesticides with organic manures, biofertilizers and biopesticides, soil can be protected from further impoverishment. The concept of sustainable agriculture also urges the utilization of an array of techniques as organic farming, application of bioinoculants and mixed or inter-cropping. Bioinoculants have been gaining increased attention and interest among those concerned with developing environment-friendly, safe and integrated crop management (ICM) compatible approaches and tactics for both fertilizer and pest management. Bioinoculants are the live microbial cells of single species or consortium of different microbial isolates that are applied to the soil or treated with plant/seed materials in order to improve the plant health. Acceptance of bioinoculants may also follow the current trend towards organic farming, the introduction of more effective biologically based products with a broader spectrum of biological effect and better activity against the key target organisms. Broadly, bioinoculants include biofertilizers and biopesticides. Biofertilizers are live cells of beneficial microbial isolates that provide necessary nutrients (nitrogen, phosphorous etc.), excrete growth promoting compounds and enhance the yield and production. While biopesticides are live microbial isolates or their metabolic products that eradicate or kill known insect pests of crops. The beneficial free living rhizobacteria, usually referred to as plant growth promoting rhizobacteria (PGPR) are defined by three intrinsic characteristics: (i) they must be able to colonize the root, (ii) they must survive and multiply in microhabitats associated with the root surface, in competition with other microbiota, at least for the time needed to express their plant growth promotion or protection activities, and (iii) they must promote plant growth (Kloepper *et al.*, 1989). Plant beneficial bacteria are discussed in this review under different sections based on their plant growth promoting or disease and insect pest controlling traits.

BIOINOCULANTS FOR BIOFERTILIZATION

Biofertilizers are live formulations of agriculturally beneficial bacteria and fungi, which on application to seed, root or soil can fix atmospheric nitrogen or solubilize phosphorus and oxidize sulphur in the soil by their biological activity and help to improve the soil health. Microbes involved in the formulations also secrete various growth promoting substances like hormones, vitamins and amino acids. Crops have to be provided with chemical fertilizers repeatedly to replenish the loss of nitrogen utilized for crop growth. On the other hand, biofertilizers supply the nitrogen continuously throughout the entire period of crop growth in the field under favorable conditions. The continuous use of chemical fertilizers adversely affects the soil structure, while biofertilizers when applied to soil improve the soil structure, microbial life, soil fertility, stability and reduce pollution. Biofertilizers are not the substitute for chemical fertilizers, but used to improve the inorganic fertilizers use efficiency supplemented by low cost inoculants to the extent possible. Biofertilizers may be broadly classified into nitrogen fixing biofertilizers and phosphate solubilizing and mobilizing biofertilizers.

Nitrogen Fixing Bioinoculants

Nitrogen is the most limiting nutrient for increasing crop production. Only few prokaryotic microbes are capable of fixing atmospheric nitrogen directly through biological process. The concept of microbial inoculation started with legume-*Rhizobium* inoculants first patented by Nobe and

Hiltner in 1896. In developed countries like USA, UK and France, once biofertilization was restricted to nitrogen fixing *Rhizobium*, while in Brazil, China and India, it has been diversified to a large number of bacteria and fungi that promote plant health. Major microorganisms used as nitrogen fixing bioinoculants are listed in Table 23.1.

Table 23.1 Nitrogen fixing bioinoculants and their target crops.

S. No.	*Bioinoculant*	*Target crop*
1.	*Rhizobium* (symbiotic)	Legume: chickpea, red gram, pea, lentil, black gram Oilseed legumes: soybean, groundnut Forage legumes: clover, lucerne Tree legumes: leucaena
2.	*Azospirillum* (associative)	Rice, wheat, vegetables, sugarcane
3.	*Azotobacter* (free living)	Rice, wheat, sugarcane, cotton, sorghum, maize
4.	*Gluconacetobacter*	Sugarcane
5.	Cyanobacteria (oxygenic phototrophs)	Flooded rice
6.	*Azolla* (symbiotic)	Flooded rice

Annual biologically fixed nitrogen is estimated at 175 mt of which 75% is accounted for terrestrial fixation. From the average values of biologically fixed nitrogen in legumes, cereals, oilseeds, fibres, horticultural and fodder crops, a conservative estimate for biologically fixed nitrogen in India amounts to 4.20 million tonnes per year which at the current prices of urea works out to Rs. 4410 crore every year. Considering that biological nitrogen fixation efficiencies are at least twice that of fertilizer urea nitrogen, the corresponding monetary benefits would also be twice as much. Extrapolation of the benefits of biofertilizer consumption of 13,000 tonnes per year (taking into consideration the average yield, nitrogen (N) and phosphorous (P) saving benefits observed in AICRP-BNF centres all over India in the last 20 years) show that inoculation benefits amount to about N and P inputs of 0.32 and 0.13 million tonnes, respectively, equivalent to a monetary benefit of Rs. 600.2 crore per annum.

Rhizobium-Legume Symbiosis

A classical example of nitrogen fixation is the symbiosis between leguminous plants and bacteria of the genus *Rhizobium.* The seat of symbiosis is within the nodules that appear on the plant roots where the two organisms interact in such a way to influence and coordinate the expression of both prokaryotic and eukaryotic genes. Beijerinck was the first to isolate and cultivate the bacterium responsible for nodulation and he named it *Bacillus radicicola* which is now placed in the genus *Rhizobium*. A typical rhizobial cell is small to medium sized (0.5 to 0.9 × 1.2 × 3.0 μm), Gram-negative rod, motile when young. The cells exhibit characteristic presence of copious amount of α-hydroxy butyrate granules forming 40-50% of the cell dry weight that can easily be observed by using stains specific for metachromatic granules. Most of the rhizobial strains produce sticky gum-like substance of varying composition. They grow better in glutamate supplemented media than nitrate or ammonium ion supplemented media. Rhizobial growth is also influenced by the presence of other inorganic cations. Cells of *R. trifoli*, grown under calcium deficient medium become swollen and vacuolated. *R. trifoli, R. leguminosarun* and *R. meliloti* are grouped into fast growing acid producing *Rhizobium* that utilizes most of the carbohydrates as carbon sources. *Bradyrhizobium japonicum* and cow pea rhizobia are grouped into slow growing rhizobia which are more fastidious in their carbon source as well as vitamin requirements. They can utilize mannitol, arabinose, xylose, galactose, fructose, sodium citrate and rarely dextrin as carbon source and vitamins like thiamin, biotin and calcium pantothenate.

Rhizobium is found as a free-living organism in the soil but does not fix atmospheric nitrogen in that state. Only after its association with a leguminous plant and after the formation of root nodules, it fixes atmospheric nitrogen in the nodules. At present, 36 rhizobial species distributed among seven genera of rhizobia are recognized based on the polyphasic approach. The genera *Azorhizobium*, *Bradyrhizobium* and *Mesorhizobium*, which have been included in the family Rhizobiaceae, are now included in the new families Azorhizobiaceae, Bradyrhizobiaceae and Phyllobacteriaceae, respectively in the forthcoming second edition of the Bergey's Manual of Systematic Bacteriology. The revised family Rhizobiaceae has two genera, *Rhizobium* and *Sinorhizobium*, and is genotypically related to Bartonellaceae, Brucellaceae and Phyllobacteriaceae. Families Azorhizobiaceae and Bradyrhizobiaceae are closely related to each other, but are distant from other families in the group based on 16S rDNA sequence alignment. In addition to reorganization at family level, the genus *Rhizobium* has also been extensively revised. Bacterial isolates from nodules of *Aspalathus carnosa* and *Machaerium lunatum* have been identified as *Burkholderia*. Subsequently, *Ralstonia taiwanensis* has been identified in the nodules of Mimosa from China and *Ralstonia eutropha* in Mimosa nodules from India based on polyphasic taxonomic approach. *Rhizobium*-legume symbiosis contributes significantly to the total biological nitrogen fixation. The amount of nitrogen fixed by some of the legumes is listed in Table 23.2.

Table 23.2 Symbiotic nitrogen fixation by plants.

Plant	*kg of nitrogen/ha*
Tropical/sub-tropical legumes	
Cowpea	73-354
Pigeon pea	168-280
Green gram	61-342
Soybean	1-168
Groundnut	77-124
Clover	100-150
Lentil	34-320
Cluster bean	37-196
Temperate legumes	
Broad bean	45-552
Garden bean	52-77
Lupin	145-208
Lucerne	184-463
Chickpea	85-100
Fenugreek	44
Non-legumes	
Casuarinas	52
Alnus	139

Azospirillum

Azospirillum belongs to α-proteobacteria that resides in close association with plant roots and exhibits loose associative or endophytic nitrogen fixation in C_4 plants. It is a Gram-negative bacterium that fixes atmospheric nitrogen under low concentration of dissolved oxygen (< 8 mm) using a high affinity terminal oxidase. *Azospirillum brasilense, A. lipoferum, A. amazonense, A. halopraeferens* and *A. irakense* are the most commonly used species for inoculation. *A. lipoferum* is known to produce siderophores when grown in iron deficient medium. Certain *Azospirillum* species offer protection to cotton plant against *Fusarium oxysporum*. They colonize cortex cells without causing cell collapse and may accelerate water uptake and minerals by roots. *A. brasilense* cells are able to aggregate under certain environmental conditions, leading to the formation of flocs that affect the dispersal and survival of these bacteria in soil. *Azospirillum* has been found to colonize, promote growth and increase the yield of numerous plant species. N_2-fixation may be one of the minor mechanisms involved in plant growth promotion by *Azospirillum*. Despite very little importance of this mechanism to plants, the role of N_2-fixation in rhizo-competence, survival in soil and interactions of *Azospirillum* with other rhizosphere bacteria has been overlooked.

The capacity of a bacterium to fix N_2 may improve its survival as compared to non-fixing strains. The success of an *Azospirillum* inoculant in promoting plant growth will largely depend on its survival in the hostile soil environment and on its movement towards the host plant both in bulk soil and in the rhizosphere. Inoculation of *Azospirillum* results in increasing the numbers of root hairs, their length and density due to the release of phytoharmones like IAA, synthesized through several tryptophan dependent IAA biosynthetic pathways and indole 3-acetamide (IAM) pathway through a Trp independent route. Bhaskara Rao and Charyulu (2005) have reported increase in various plant growth parameters, viz., plant height, dry weight, and N content of shoot, root, and grain yield of faxtail millet due to inoculation of three strains of *A. lipoferum* either alone or in combination with nitrogen fertilizer (40 kg N/ha).

Azotobacter

Azotobacter is a free-living diazotroph isolated from soil and water. *Azotobacter* nitrogenase is oxygen-sensitive, but the extremely high respiration rate of *Azotobacter* soaks up free oxygen within the cells and protects the nitrogenase. *Azotobacter* species are Gram-negative, aerobic soil-dwelling bacteria. There are around six species in the genus, some of which are motile by means of peritrichous flagella, others are not. They are typically polymorphic, i.e. of different sizes and shapes. Their size of the cells ranges from 2-10 μm long and 1-2 μm wide. Inoculation with efficient strains of *Azotobacter* increased the yield of brinjal, tomato, cabbage and onion by 2-40% and in sorghum, maize and cotton in the range of 9-71%. The organism fixes atmospheric nitrogen in the range of 2-15 mg nitrogen/g of carbon source. The ability of *Azotobacter* to synthesize auxins, vitamins and antifungal antibiotics that suppress pathogens, is well recognized.

Cyanobacteria

Cyanobacteria are both unicellular and multicellular filamentous bacteria. They fix atmospheric nitrogen in differentiated specialized structures called heterocyst. All heterocystous cyanobacteria are aerobic photodiazotrophs. However, the non-heterocystous cyanobacteria fix much less nitrogen aerobically than they could fix anaerobically or microaerobically. The aerobic filamentous heterocystous as well as colonial forms represent the common flora of arable lands and are considered to be important in nitrogen economy of rice cultivation. The most common filamentous heterocystous species include *Anabaena, Anabaenopsis, Aulosira, Calothrix, Cylindrospermum, Fischerella, Hapalosiphon, Mastigocladus, Nostoc, Scytonema, Scytonematopsis, Stigonema, Tolypothrix, Westiella* and *Westiellopsis* and the unicellular or colonial are the species of *Aphanothece, Chroococcidiopsis, Cyanothece, Dermocarpa, Gloeothece, Myxosarcina, Synechoococcus, Synechocystis* and *Xenococcus*. The non-heterocystous filamentous forms capable of nitrogen fixation are species of *Oscillatoria, Trichodesmium, Microcoleus, Pseudanabaena, Plectonema* and *Lyngbya*.

In suitable conditions, for example, on the surface of bare moist earth in the tropics, they may add valuable amounts of nitrogen to the soil. In the tropics where paddy rice is grown, the whole nitrogen requirements of the rice crop may be provided by these cyanobacteria. Many studies have been reported on the use of dried cyanobacteria to inoculate soils as a means of aiding fertility, and the effect of adding cyanobacteria to soil on rice yield was first studied in the 1950s in Japan. The average of the results from all these studies has shown an increase in grain yield of 15-20% in field experiments. It has been suggested that the cyanobacteria introduced as a result of bacterization can establish themselves permanently if inoculation is done consecutively for 3-4 cropping seasons. As many as 23 consecutive rice crops have been successfully grown from soils unfertilized with nitrogen at the International Rice Research Institute in Manila, Philippines. In these soils, the nitrogen came from the cyanobacterial fixation.

The basic method of mass production involves a mixture of nitrogen fixing cyanobacteria in shallow trays or polythene lined pits filled with water kept in open air, using clean, sieved farm soil as a carrier material. To each pit, 10 kg soil and 250 g single super phosphate is added and water is filled up to a height of 12-15 cm. Starter culture, a mixture of *Anabaena, Nostoc, Aulosira* and *Tolypothrix*, is inoculated in each multiplication unit. Malathion (5-10 ml per tank) or carbofuran (3% granules, 20 g per tank) is also added to prevent insect breeding. In hot summer months, the cyanobacteria form a thick mat over the surface after 10-12 days of growth in open sun. The contents are allowed to dry and the dried flakes are collected, packed and used to inoculate rice fields. The basic advantage of this technology is that farmers after getting the soil based starter culture can produce the biofertilizer on their own with minimum additional inputs. An inoculum of 10-12 kg is considered sufficient to inoculate one hectare of paddy field 3-4 days after transplantation.

Tamil Nadu state in India has been particularly successful in propagating and using cyanobacteria as a valuable renewable resource in rice cultivation on commercial basis. In this programme, naturally growing cyanobacteria including species of *Anabaena, Aulosira, Nostoc, Cylindrospermum, Gloeotrichia, Lyngbya, Chroococcus, Wollea, Aphanothece, Calothrix, Gloeocapsa, Plectonema* and *Microcystis* are propagated in the rice fields by adding 50 kg of P_2O_5/ha about a month before the planting of rice. Phosphate stimulates growth of cyanobacteria.

Another approach has been developed by Farmers Training Centre at Aduthurai by which even small farmers can prepare their own cyanobacteria inoculum. This approach involves artificial multiplication (either single species or composite mixtures of various species of cyanobacteria) in shallow metal troughs lined with polythene and containing fine so 10 kg, superphosphate 250 g, and rice bran or sawdust 250 g (source of molybdate). These troughs are filled with water up to 2" to 6". Acidity is corrected by adding about 50 g of lime. 25 g of 3% carbofuran granules are applied which prevents the attack of aphids and mosquitoes on multiplying cyanobacteria. These troughs are then inoculated with 250 g of powered soil-based cyanobacterial culture.

Azolla

The genus *Azolla* established by Lamarck (1983) is a small aquatic to semi-aquatic heterosporus leptosporangiate fern. The plant has deeply bilobed leaves. Each leaf has dorsal and ventral lobe. The dorsal lobe is exposed to air and contains chlorophyll. It has an algal symbiont *Anabaena* within the central cavity. *Azolla-Anabaena* symbiotic system has proved to be a potential N-source in water logged rice ecosystem which is most effective when ploughed into the soil. The natural floating 'nitrogen factory' consists of two plants, the water fern *Azolla* and a nitrogen fixing cyanobacterium *Anabaena azollae* Strasburger, living together in symbiotic association. *Azolla-Anabaena* symbiosis is the only plant cyanobacterial symbiosis used as biofertilizer in agriculture.

The seven extant species of *Azolla* are grouped under two sections, viz., EuAzolla and Rhizosperms based on megaspore floats and glochidia. There are different genotypes of *Azolla*, viz., *A. pinnata, A. caroliniana, A. filiculoides, A. mexicana, A. microphylla* and *A. rubra*. Among them, *A. pinnata* is native to India with high sporulating nature but highly sensitive to temperature above 25°C. *A. caroliniana* is a pest and disease tolerant genotype while *A. filiculoides* is producing higher biomass but non-sporulating. Recently, several *Azolla* hybrids have been developed by crossing megasporocarp and microsporocarps. TNAU has developed an *Azolla* hybrid called TNAU-1 (*A. microphylla* X *A. pinnata*), which has high adaptability in rice ecosystem. *Azolla* is readily decomposed to NH_4^+ that is used by rice plant. *Azolla* application is known to increase the rice yield by 0.5 to 2.0 t/ha. Nitrogen content of rice receiving *A. mexicana* was reported to be 10-35 kg/ha higher than control.

BIOINOCULANTS FOR IMPROVED P-SUPPLY

Phosphorous (P) is the second most limiting plant nutrient after nitrogen, as approximately 95-99% of it is present in the form of insoluble phosphates. Phosphorous is absorbed by the plant primarily as the monovalent phosphate ion ($H_2PO_4^{2-}$) and less readily as divalent phosphate ion ($H_2PO_4^{2-}$). The general availability of soluble orthophosphate ion exist as H_2PO^{4-} > $H_2PO_4^{2-}$ > PO_4^{3-}. Phosphate availability to plant depends on soil pH. At low pH of 4 to 5, there occurs relative abundance of H_2PO^{4-} ions while decrease in acidity of soil increase $H_2PO_4^{2-}$ ion followed by PO_4^{3-}. At high pH, phosphorous get fixed on reaction with calcium while at lower pH it reacts with iron or aluminium ions. P-deficiency is alleviated by massive application of pi fertilizers currently estimated to be 40 million metric tonnes per year worldwide. Only 10-15% of the phosphorous introduced by the way of fertilizers is acquired by the plants and remaining is transformed into insoluble form like oxyapatite, hydroxyapatite, carbonate apatite and fluoroapatite in neutral and alkaline soil and hydroxy phosphates of iron and aluminium as dufreenite, strengite and avriate in acidic soils. The release of fixed and poorly soluble form of P is an important aspect for increasing soil fertility. The available P in soil solution is increased by both phosphate solubilization and mobilization.

PHOSPHATE SOLUBILIZING BIOINOCULANTS

Being a part of rich rhizosphere microbial diversity, P-solubilizing bacteria play an important role in the dissolution of insoluble phosphate from soil and allowing sustainable use of phosphate fertilizer. Development of commercial P-solubilizing bioinoculants has resulted in the highly efficient, low cost and environmentally safe technologies used by the agro-industries worldwide. Goenadi *et al.* (2000) reported 9-day old culture supernatant of *Aspergillus niger* BCC F194 isolated from tropical acid soils on Moroccan Rock Phosphate (MRP) to have highest P solubility (2.5 g/ L MRP), thus decreasing the dependency of concentrated sulphuric acid treatment.

Various mechanisms like lowering pH by acid production, ion chelation and exchange reactions in the growth environment have been traditionally associated with P-solubilization by microorganisms. Production of low molecular weight organic acid and their ability to form stable metal complexes were linked with microbial phosphate solubilization. Gram-negative bacterial isolates are considered good phosphate solubilizers, probably because of the involvement of direct oxidation of glucose into gluconic acid. Low molecular weight organic acids, mainly gluconic acid (GA) and ketogluconic acids (KGA), are produced in the periplasm of Gram-negative bacteria by direct oxidation pathway of glucose (DOPG) enzymes, i.e., glucose dehydrogenase (GDH) and gluconate dehydrogenase (GADH). P solubilizing potential of Gram-negative isolates belong to *Serratia marcescens, Pantoea agglomerans*, and *P. dispersa* have been recently studied. *Pantoea ananatis* and *Pantoea agglomerans* strains isolated from iron rich soil samples, showed their potential on mineral phosphate solubilization Selvakumar *et al.* (2008) isolated a cold tolerant *Pantoea dispersa*1A that solubilized 17.9 µg of P_2O_5 ml^{-1} day^{-1} at 15°C in NBRIP broth. Inorganic P-solubilization by *Pantoea agglomerans* was also linked to a mechanism involving both gluconic acid production and proton extrusion as a consequence of NH_4^+ uptake.

VAM: PHOSPHATE MOBILIZING BIOINOCULANTS

Vesicular Arbuscular Mycorrhiza (VAM) is the most abundant kind of mycorrhiza described as a universal plant symbiosis. About 80 % of all terrestrial plant species form VAM symbiosis and approximately 95% of world's present species of vascular plants belongs to families that are characteristically mycorrhizal, including roots of angiosperms, gymnosperms and pteridophytes. However, certain crop plants belonging to cruciferae, brassicaceae, chenopodiaceae and caryophyllaceae do not form symbiosis with VAM fungi. The term vesicular and arbuscular is derived from characteristic structures, i.e., branched hyphae or arbuscles that are formed within the root cortical cells and vesicles or swollen lipid storage organs. VAM fungi are members of class zygomycota that contains one order, Glomales, encompassing six genera and approximately 150 species. Soil analysis from various ecosites of India has demonstrated the occurrence of five types of VAM fungal genera viz *Glomus, Sclerocystis, Gigaspora, Acaulospora* and *Endogene*. The association between plant and VAM fungi is a functional symbiosis in which the mycorrhizal fungus is obligatory or facultatively dependent on host photosynthates and energy. The fungal mycelium that extends from root surfaces into soil matrix captures nutrients from soil solution and mobilizes them to plants. Mycorrhizal roots are more efficient in nutrient uptake than non-colonized roots. The extended hyphae are able to draw nutrients from more distance or inaccessible supplies of nutrients regions than the root can reach. It is estimated that nearly 25-30% of phosphatic fertilizer can be saved through inoculation with efficient VAM fungi and yield is also improved. VAM fungal association results in increased P-nutrition and the plants accrue other benefits like increased protection from environmental stress including cold, salinity, drought, pollution and reduction in incidence of root diseases. VAM fungi symbiosis results in increased heavy metal tolerance at certain specific soil pH value. AM fungi increased the shoot uptake of heavy metals in slightly contaminated soil while in severely contaminated soil could reduce shoot metal concentration and protect the plants against harmful effects of metals.

MIXED MICROBIAL CONSORTIUM FOR BIOFERTILIZATION

Use of mixed biofertilizers containing a consortium of N fixers, P solubilizers and PGPR (plant growth promoting rhizobacteria) has been found to promote the growth of cereals, legumes and oilseeds better than their individual application. For example, inoculation of consortia of *Azospirillum,* PSB and PGPR on rice variety 'white ponni' in the presence of 75% N and P, recorded 13% higher grain yield than with 100% N and P, besides saving 25% N and P. *Rhizobium*, RBG 314 and P solubilizer, AMT 1001, the promising and compatible combination developed in Andhra Pradesh gave 15% increase in yield of black gram variety LBG 20. Chilli is an important crop of great commercial value in Andhra Pradesh. *Azospirillum* strains were developed and inoculated on chillies which yielded 25% yield increase over 100% RDF (recommended dose of fertilizers) and 30% over 75% RDF. Bioinoculants (*Azotobacter* + *Azospirillum*) improved the yield of okra, tomato and brinjal by 13.5-20.0% over farmers practice and 8.5-14.3% over recommended dose of fertilizers. Most significantly the apparent Fertilizer Use Efficiency (FUE) increased in the case of nitrogen by 6-15% for nitrogen, 10-22% for phosphorus, 13-28% for potassium and 2.7-5.0% for sulphur. On an average, they represent an increase in the yield of 16.6% over farmer's practices and 11.3% over RDF due to the use of bioinoculants. Average increase in FUE due to inoculants was 11.3% in the case of N, 14.2% in the case of P, 20% in the case of K and 3.6% in the case of S. In vertisols of Maharashtra, inoculation of *Azotobacter* and PSB on black gram, soybean and pigeon pea increased the seed yields significantly by 150-250 kg/ha over control even at 100% RDF. Fifty-two demonstration trials on mixed biofertilizer inoculation in pearl millet in farmer's fields (District of Hisar, Bhiwani, Jajjhar, Mahendergarh and Rewari) resulted in an average increase of 5% increase in grain yield and 6% increase in fodder yield at 75% RDN. A higher soybean yield was obtained when using mixed inoculants of *Azospirillum* and *Rhizobium* as compared to inoculations of *Rhizobium* alone. *Azospirillum*, by enhancing the proliferation of root hairs, increased the susceptibility of forage legumes to *Rhizobium* infection. A dual inoculation of *A. brasilense* and VAM fungi increased the root biomass and the absorption of phosphorus by pearl millet, barley yields and the number of colonization sites of VAM fungi in halophytic plants growing in dunes.

Organics have been found to boost the proliferation of *Rhizobium* and enhance nodulation, nitrogen fixation, N and P uptake in legumes and oilseeds. In vertisols of Maharashtra, *Rhizobium* inoculation of groundnut increased the pod yield by 3.9 q/ha while FYM alone @ 5t/ha increased it by 1.5q/ha, combined application of FYM and *Rhizobium* increased it by 7.3 q/ha. Similarly in green gram, the use of *Rhizobium* along with FYM gave 2.8 q/ha additional grain yield respectively over unmanured and uninoculated control. In acid soils (of Orissa), application of micronutrients (molybdenum and cobalt) boosts nodulation, BNF and yield of legumes. In green gram, *Rhizobium* inoculation increased the grain yield (26%). Application of micronutrients along with inoculation further enhanced the grain yield dramatically (78%) over uninoculated control resulting in additional BNF of 24 kg/ha.

In efforts at improving the shelf life of inoculants, survival of *Azotobacter, Azospirillum* and PSB was found to be better (~10 fold) in charcoal based inoculants than lignite based ones at the end of 90 days at HAU, Hisar. For improving the shelf life of *Rhizobium, Bradyrhizobium* and phosphate solubilizing bacteria-*Bacillus* sp., the addition of 2% humic acid to lignite and vermiculite carrier based cultures enhanced the survival of all the bacteria up to 150 days of storage. A new medium for co-culturing *Azospirillum lipoferum, Bacillus* and *Pseudomonas fluorescens* was formulated at TNAU, Coimbatore and staggered inoculation was used to get high titre. In lignite carrier, this co-culture had a population of 10^7-10^8 cfu/g at 6 months in contrast to individual inoculant count of 10^8-10^9 cfu/g. Liquid inoculants of co-culture prepared by addition of 2% PVP supported titre of 10^9 cfu/ml up to six months. Similarly at ANGRAU, Amaravathi, liquid formulations LM2 and LM4 retained maximum population of *Azospirillum,* i.e., 10.7 and 10.64 log cfu/ml after one year.

BIOINOCULANTS USED IN ABIOTIC STRESS MANAGEMENT

Application of plant growth promoting rhizobacteria is one of the best approaches along with conventional breeding in the management of abiotic stresses in crop production. Few reports have been published on PGPR as elicitors of tolerance to abiotic stresses, such as drought, salt and nutrient deficiency or excess. The subject of PGPR-elicited tolerance to heavy metals has been reviewed recently. Yang *et al.* (2009) proposed the term 'induced systemic tolerance' (IST) for PGPR-induced physical and chemical changes in plants that result in enhanced tolerance to abiotic stress. Under stress conditions, the level of plant hormone ethylene is increased that endogenously regulates plant homeostasis and results in reduced root and shoot growth. The most successful strategy for managing the abiotic stresses in plants is lowering the level of ethylene production by utilizing the microbial enzyme ACC deaminase, which cleaves ACC to ammonia and α-ketobutyric acid to establish a sink for ACC and lowering the ethylene level in plants. This can be achieved either through the interaction of ACC deaminase-containing plant growth-promoting bacteria with plant roots or by the development of transgenic plants expressing this enzyme. In either case, ACC deaminase can significantly decrease ACC levels in plants, especially plants subjected to various abiotic stresses, thereby decreasing the amount of stress induced ethylene and subsequent damage to the plant that might occur as a consequence of ethylene.

Drought and Salt Stress

Drought is the most important abiotic factor that adversely affects the crop production in arid and semi-arid areas. Early studies on IST to drought reported that inoculation with the PGPR

Paenibacillus polymyxa enhanced the drought tolerance of *Arabidopsis thaliana*. The mechanisms that have been suggested include reduction of stress ethylene production via ACC deaminase activity and increased expression of the ERD15 (Early Responsive to Dehydration 15) gene. Mayak *et al.* (2004a) isolated *Achromobacter piechaudii* ARV8 that produces ACC deaminase, and conferred IST to drought stress in pepper (*Capsicum annuum* L.) and tomato (*Solanum lycopersicum* L.) plants.

Salt stress has become an ever-increasing threat to food production, irrigation being a major problem of agricultural fields due to gradual salinization. Salt stress has threefold effects: it reduces water potential, causes ion imbalance or disturbance in ion homeostasis and toxicity. Since salt stress involves both osmotic and ionic stress, growth suppression is directly related to total concentration of soluble salts or osmotic potential of soil water. *Achromobacter piechaudii* ARV8 containing ACC deaminase increases the resistance of tomato seedlings to salt. The bacterium reduces the production of ethylene by the seedlings, hence alleviating the suppression of growth and improved water use efficiency. It slightly increased the uptake of phosphorus and potassium, which may contribute in part to activation of processes involved in the alleviation of the effect of salt.

Many studies have demonstrated that inoculation with VAM fungi improves growth of plants under salinity stress conditions. Recently, Rabie (2005) suggested that VAM fungi protected the host plants against the detrimental effects of salt. When mung bean plants were irrigated with different dilution of seawater, VAM plants showed higher growth than non-VAM plants at all levels of irrigation. Mycorrhizae were involved in protection against salt stress, via better access to nutritional status and modification of plant physiology, i.e., osmotic modifications and photosynthesis. To some extent, these VAM fungi have been considered as bio-ameliorators of saline soils. Inoculation with VAM fungi reduced the deleterious effect of salt stress on *Jatropha* seedling growth parameters under salt levels up to 0.5% NaCl (electrical conductivity of 7.2 dS m^{-1}). Inoculation of *Jatropha* seedlings with VAM fungi can promote the establishment of *Jatropha* under NaCl-induced stres. Wang *et al.* (2004) reported that proline accumulation in plants may be a symptom of stress in less salinity-tolerance species and its contribution to osmotic adjustment was apparently negligible as compared with K^+. The proline levels in non-VAM plants with and without NFB were 4.0-and 3.7-fold higher than that of VAM plants at 6.0 dSm^{-1} level of salinity. Although mycorrhizal colonization was reduced with increasing salinity levels, the dependency of faba plants on VAM fungi was increased. It is indicated that symbiotic association between VAM fungus *Glomus clarum* and faba plants was strengthened in saline environment once the association was established. This may be a sign showing the ecological importance of VAM association for plant survival and growth of plants under salinity stress.

Flooding Stress

Deprivation of oxygen to the roots of plants is the main consequence of flooding. Under normal conditions, water dissolves about 230 m mol·m^{-3} oxygen, and hypoxia occurs when the oxygen level falls below 50 m mol·m^{-3}. Within 1 h of flooding, the partial pressure of oxygen declines from 20.8 to 7.9 kPa and further decreases to 1 kPa after 1 d of flooding. Shortly after the onset of flooding, soil microorganisms consume all of the available oxygen, and different toxic compounds begin to accumulate in the soil. Plants respond to flooding with a reduced root permeability, water absorption and mineral uptake; closure of stomata followed by a decrease in photosynthesis; alterations in hormone balance; inhibition of stem and root growth; hypertrophy of lenticels; development of aerenchyma and adventitious roots; epinasty, chlorosis, leaf abscission and premature fruit drop. In flooding, roots release a high amount of ACC into the surrounding soil. The establishment of microbial populations able to break down ACC may be an effective non-invasive approach to ameliorating the damage to plants caused by flooding. In plant growth promoting bacteria, the expression of an ACC deaminase gene, which is increased under anaerobic conditions, helps to lower the oxygen and utilize the ACC that is exuded by plant roots are likely to be selectively enriched. Grichko and Glick (2001) reported that tomato plants that were grown from the seeds bacterized with organisms expressing ACC deaminase such as *Enterobacter cloacae* UW4, *E. cloacae* CAL2, *Pseudomonas putida* ATCC17399/pRKACC or *P. putida* ATCC17399/pRK415 showed a substantial tolerance to flooding stress.

Heavy Metal Stress

When heavy metals are present in excess, they can act as toxicants, reducing the plant life. Among the metals that are most toxic to plant and animal life are those that displace essential metal ions in biological processes. These include cadmium, zinc, mercury, copper, lead and nickel. Nickel is one of the most abundant heavy metal contaminants of the environment due to its release during mining and smelting practices, and it has been the target of many cleanup strategies. Arsenic in contaminated soil affects seed germination, and reduces root length and mass. Arsenite is 4-100 times more toxic than arsenate. In plants, damage from heavy metals occurs due the evolution of active oxygen species, which cause a reduction in chlorophyll and the shutdown of photosynthesis. In addition to this, high metal concentrations in the soil have been shown to cause increased ethylene production, inhibit root and shoot development, reduce CO_2 fixation and limit sugar translocation. Therefore, the best way to prevent plants from becoming chlorotic in the presence of high levels of heavy metals is to provide them with an associated siderophore-producing PGPR that could provide a sufficient amount of iron to the plant. Burd *et al.* (2000) demonstrated that a siderophore over producing mutant of *Kluyvera ascorbata* SUD165 decreases the plant toxicity to three different heavy metals such as nickel, zinc and lead in three different crop plants such as tomato, canola and Indian mustard. ACC deaminase containing plant growth-promoting bacteria can significantly increase the growth of plants in the presence of heavy metals including nickel, lead and zinc by lowering the level of stress-induced ethylene, thus allowing plants to develop longer roots and establish better during early stages of growth.

BIOINOCULANTS USED AS BIOPESTICIDES

Synthetic chemical pesticides had been the widely used approach for reducing the estimated 45% gross crop loss due to pests and diseases, amounting to around Rs. 290 billion per annum. Metchnikoff in 1879 and Krassilnikow in 1888 were the first to document that an entomopathogen, a muscordine fungus, *Metarrhizium anisophilae* could be mass produced and applied as microbial insecticide to control the grain and sugar beet pests. The control of insect pest by bacteria was first attempted by d'Herelle in 1914, approximately 35 years after Pasteur's description of silkworm disease. White and Dutky succeeded in 1940 in demonstrating a control of Japanese beetle by *Bacillus papillae*. The issuing of eight patents between 1960 and 1963 for *Bacillus thuringiensis* led to a revived interest in bacterial insecticides. Biopesticides are gaining importance in Indian agriculture and parallel rural development particularly as a component of the Integrated Pest Management System. The biopesticide market is growing very rapidly. In 2005, biopesticides accounted for about 2.5% of the total pesticide market, which was merely 0.2% during 2000. This share is expected to grow to about 4.2% by 2010 while the market value is estimated to reach more than US$ 1 billion (Source: BCC research). However, the overall growth rate of biopesticides is estimated to be about 10% per annum for the next 5 years. One of the most important factors affecting the efficacy of biopesticides is correct timing of applications. Many of these products are designed to be preventative and won't work once pests are present in large numbers. This is particularly true for many biofungicides, which are based on beneficial microbes that colonize the surfaces of plant roots and act as a barrier to invading plant pathogens. If the pathogen has already invaded the roots prior to application, the biopesticides will not have any impact on it. Timing can also be influenced by the life stage or activity of the pest. Many bioinsecticides (e.g., the Bt products) work best against younger insects and control is greatly reduced when applied against older stages. Biopesticides can be extremely sensitive to environmental conditions such as sunlight, rain, humidity or temperature. The active ingredient in Bt products is sensitive to ultraviolet radiation, and its efficacy may be reduced after prolonged exposure to sunlight. There are several products that are intended for suppression of various plant pathogens in soil. These contain live spores of beneficial microbes the activity of which decreases enormously at low soil temperatures, and thus, their efficacy will be greatly reduced in case these are applied to cool soils.

Bioinoculants Used as Bioinsecticides

The entomopathogenic bacterium *Bacillus thuringiensis* is one of the most promising biological control agent for pest and insect management since many strains are toxic specifically for Lepidopteran and strain *Bacillus thuringiensis* serotype H-14 is highly toxic to Dipterans. Most prominent bacterial biopesticides are insecticides based on various subspecies of *Bacillus thuringiensis* Berliner (*Bt*). These includes *Bacillus thuringiensis kurstaki* with activity against lepidopteran larval species, *Bacillus thuringiensis aizawai* also with activity against lepidopteran larval species, *Bacillus thuringiensis israelensis* with activity against mosquito larvae, black fly and fungus gnats, *Bacillus thuringiensis tenebrionis* with activity against coleopteran adults and larvae, most notably, the Colorado potato beetle *Leptinotarsa decemlineata* (Say), and *Bacillus thuringiensis japonensis* strain buibui with activity against soil inhabiting beetles. *Bacillus thuringiensis* is a widely occurring Gram-positive, spore forming soil bacterium that produces parasporal, proteinaceous, crystal inclusion bodies during sporulation. Upon digestion by the insect, the crystal proteins are solubilized and insect gut proteases convert the original protaxin into a combination of up to four smaller toxins. These hydrolysed toxins bind to the insect midgut cells at high affinity, specific receptor binding sites where they interfere with the potassium ion dependent active amino acid symport mechanism. This disruption causes the formation of large cation selective pores that increases the water permeability of the cell membrane. A large uptake of water causes cell swelling and eventual rupture leading to disintegration of the midgut lining. Different toxins bind to different receptors and with different intensities and this explains the selectivity of different *Bt* strains in different insect species. *Bt* based biological control products contain the endotoxins plus live bacterial cells. The toxin stops feeding and young larvae may starve to death although insects not killed by direct action of the toxin may die from bacterial infection over a longer period.

The insecticidal property of *Bt* is largely a function of the presence of extra-chromosomal plasmids in the cell. These carry genes termed as *cry* genes that code a diverse array of these protein crystalline inclusion bodies that are toxic to insects. The *cry* genes and Cry proteins are grouped into five groups that differ in insecticidal activity or crystal protein size and sequence. *cry*I and *cry*II genes produce proteins that are toxic to lepidopteren larvae, *cry*III gene produce proteins toxic to coleopterans, *cry*IV gene produce proteins toxic to dipteran larvae and *cry*V genes produce proteins toxic to both Lepidoptera and coleopteran. Different endotoxins have different biological spectra and different genes are used in different crops to afford protection from attack by different insects. For example, Monsanto has used *cry*1A(c) genes from *B. thuringiensis* subsp *kurstaki* in cotton and tomatoes and *cry*IIIA genes from *B. thuringiensis* subsp *tenebrionis* in potatoes and Novartis and Mycogen used *cry*IA(b) genes from *B. thuringiensis* subsp *kurstaki* and Monsanto *cry*IIA and *cry*IA(b) genes both from *B. thuringiensis* subsp *kurstaki*, in corn. *Bacillus sphaericus* Neide, closely related species to Bt, has been used to control mosquito larvae notably *Culex* spp, primarily in Europe and Africa. There are several registered *Bacillus sphaericus* products, including Vectolex CG (valent Biosciences). *B. sphaericus* is similar in activity to *B. thuringiensis* subsp *israelensis* (Bti) which is used commercially for control of mosquito larvae and black flies (*Simulium* sp.) primarily in Africa, where black flies are the vector of river blindness disease.

Bioinoculants for Plant Disease Management

Although several genera of rhizobacteria were reported to have antifungal property, *Bacillus* spp. are of great choice as they tolerate extreme heat and desiccation by producing endospores. Antagonistic activity of rhizobacteria towards fungal pathogens is usually related to the production of antifungal compounds and extracellular hydrolytic enzymes. Chitinase and α-1, 3-gluconase are considered to be important hydrolytic enzymes in the lysis of fungal cell walls, as for example, cell walls of *Fusarium oxysporum, Sclerotinia minor*, and *S. rolfsii*. *Bacillus* and related genera also produce peptide antibiotics like bacilopeptins, fusaricidins, iturins, mattacin and different kinds of polymyxins that play a major role in plant disease suppression as well as post-harvest disease management. Antifungal metabolites of *Bacillus* sp. are generally polypeptide and composed of only amino acids, but sometimes contain other residues as in the case of rhizocticin-A which is phosphono-oligopeptide. Antifungal peptides produced by non-ribosomal peptide synthetase (NRPS) of *Bacillus* are reported to have amino acids, which are unique and not commonly found in proteins. Bacillomycin D contains D-amino acid residues in addition to L-amino acid residues while plipastatin B1 contains unusual amino acid residue ornithine. Zwittermicin producing strain *Bacillus cereus* UW85, *B. subtilis* CL27 and *B. pumilus* CL45 were potentially used for the control of *Pythium aphanidermatum*, *Botrytis* sp. and *Alternaria brassicola* respectively. Since the production of antifungal metabolites, extracellular enzymes, and antibiotics appears to be responsible for plant disease suppression by biocontrol bacteria (Table 23.3), it is hypothesized that superior biocontrol activity might be achieved by increasing production levels of these metabolites. Several successful endeavors had been made to enhance the biocontrol potentiality of *Trichoderma* species by exposing the spores to chemical, e.g., ethyl methane sulfonate (EMS) or physical mutagens, e.g., gamma ray. Two mutants (Th50M6 and Th50M11) with enhanced biocontrol activity were developed by exposing the wild type *T. harzianum* conidia to gamma radiation.

Bioinoculants Used as Bioherbicides

Pseudomonas gladioli pv gladioli has been commercialised as biological herbicide by Japan to-bacco as AM301 and Microgen as Camperico for the control of annual meadow grass (*Poa annua* L) in turf. The first mycoherbicide registered and marketed as DeVine was based on the phyto-pathogenic fungus *Phytophthora palmivora* for the control of strangler vine or milkweed vine (*Morrenia odorata*), in citrus orchards. Collego, the second US bioherbicide was based on *Colletotrichum gloeosporioides* f. sp. *aeschynomene* (CGA) was delivered in two packages—one of dried CGA spores in an inert carrier material, the other an inert rehydrating osmoticum for reviving spores before spraying. The components of both packages were added to the desired volume of water immediately before application. BioMal (Philom Bias, Saskatoon, Canada) is another registered mycoherbicide based on the hydrophilic fungus *Colletotrichurn gloeosporioides* f. sp. *rnalvae*. It was delivered as a wettable silica gel powder for control of round leaved mallow (*Malva pusilla*). Granules of several different fungi, such as *C. truncatum* for hemp sesbania control, *F. lateritium* for velvet leaf control, and *F. oxysporurn* for sicklepod control are produced by mixing semolina wheat flour and kaolin clay with fungal propagules contained in a liquid component; either water or residual liquid growth medium. The mixture is kneaded into dough, rolled into thin sheets with a pasta press, and air-dried for 48 h. Sheets are then milled and sieved to obtain uniform-sized granules which are stored at 4°C. These granules, called 'Pesta', provided 90-100% weed control in glasshouse tests. In field tests, 'Pesta' granules containing *C. truncatum* provided 80-85% control of hemp sesbania in 3 years of tests. Various mycoherbicide formulations are listed in Table 23.4.

Table 23.3 List of biofungicides.

Trade name	*Biocontrol organism*	*Crop*	*Target disease*
Bio-Save® 10LP	*Pseudomonas syringae* strain ESC 10	Apples, pears, lemons, oranges, or grapefruit after the fruit is harvested	Ice inducing bacteria and biological decay
Bloomtime Biological™	*Pantoea agglomerans* strain E325	Apples and pears	Fireblight (*Erwinia amylovora*)
Bloomtime Biological™ FD	*Pantoea agglomerans* strain E325	Apples and pears	Fireblight (*Erwinia amylovora*)
Actinovate® AG	*Streptomyces lydicus* WYEC 108	Ornamentals, leafy and fruiting vegetables, fruits, nuts, berries, grapes, cotton and other row	Soilborne pathogens: *Pythium* spp., *Rhizoctonia* spp., *Phytophthora* spp, *Fusarium* spp., *Verticillium* spp.,

Contd.

		crops, citrus, mint, herbs potatoes and other root crops	*Phymatotrichum omnivorum* and other root decay fungi. Foliar pathogens: *Podosphaera* spp., *Botrytis* spp., *Schlerotinia* spp., *Monilinia* spp., *Alternaria* spp., *Peronospora* spp. and other foliar fungi.
Ballad® Plus Biofungicide	*Bacillus pumilus* QST 2808	Soybeans, cereal crops, and potatoes	Rust, powdery mildew, *Cercospora*, and brown spot
Kodiak® Concentrate Biological Fungicide	*Bacillus subtilis* GB03	Cotton, peanuts, soybeans, wheat, barley, peas, and beans	Rhizoctonia, Fusarium, Alternaria, *Aspergillus*, and others that attack the root systems of plants
Serenade® Garden Disease Control Ready to Use	*Bacillus subtilis* strain QST 713 and flowers	Fruits, vegetables,	Bacterial spot, powdery mildew, mildew, rust, gray mold, leaf blight, scab, and more
Serenade® Wettable Powder Biofungicide	*Bacillus subtilis* strain QST 713	Vegetables, fruit, nut, and vine crops	Fire Blight, *Botrytis*, Sour Rot, Rust, *Sclerotinia*, Powdery mildew, Bacterial Spot, and hite Mold
Sonata®	*Bacillus pumilus* QST 2808	Many food and nonfood crops, including trees susceptible to sudden oak death syndrome.	Fungal pests such as molds, mildews, blights, and rusts
Yield Shield® Concentrate Biological Fungicide	*Bacillus pumilus* GB34	Legumes	*Rhizoctonia* and *Fusarium*
Rhapsody®	*Bacillus subtilis* QST708	Turf, ornamentals, bedding plants, tropical plants, seedlings, conifers, fruity and leafy vegetables, and bulbs	Fungal and bacterial diseases; Brown Patch, Anthracnose, and Dollar Spot

Table 23.4 List of bioherbicides.

Microbe	*Formulation*	*Weed host*
Liquid suspension formulations		
Fusarium lateritium	Water + Tween-20 surfactant (0.02%)	Spurred anoda (*Anoda cr/stata*)
Colletotrichum gloeosporioides f. sp. *malvae*	BioMal	Round-leaved mallow (*Malva pusilla*)
Xanthamonas campestris	Camperico	Annual bluegrass (*Poa annua*)
Colletotrichum truncatum	Water + nonoxynol surfactant (0.2%); paraffin wax, mineral oil, soybean oil lecithin; unrefined corn oil	Hemp sesbania (*Sesbania exaltata*)
Alternaria crassa	Water + nonoxynol surfactant (0.4%)	Jimson weed (*Datura stramonium*)

Contd.

Phytophthora palmivora	DeVine (Chlamydospores in water)	Stranglervine (*Morrenia odorata*)
Solid formulations		
Colletotrichum gloeos porioides f. sp. *aeschynornene*	Collego Component-A: dried spores Component-B: rehydrating agent + surfactant	Northern joint vetch (*Aeschynomene virginica*)
Alternaria cassiae	CASST	Sicklepod (*Cassia obtusifolia*)
Colletotrichum truncatum	Fungus-infested wheat gluten/kaolin clay (Pesta)	Hemp sesbania (*Sesbania exaltata*)
Fusarium oxysporum	Fungus-infested wheat gluten/kaolin clay (Pesta)	Sicklepod (*Cassia obtusifolia*)

Solar radiation is one reason for mycoherbicides that perform well in glasshouse trials to fail in the field or exhibit sporadic field efficacy. Exposure to sunlight decreased germination rate and germ tube length of *C. gloeosporioides* conidia isolated from *Polystigma rubrum* subsp. *rubrum*. More recently, UV-A (320-400 nm) photons were found to stimulate appressorium formation, while UV-B (280-320 nm) photons delayed conidium germination in *C. orbiculare* and *Plectosporium alismatis*. As the dose of UV-B increased, these photons deactivated conidia and also delayed germination of the survivors. Studies on UV protection of fungal entomopathogens have indicated that protectants can prolong the viability of conidia. A calcium cross-linked lignin UV barrier produced a tenfold increase in *Beauveria bassiana* germination response time (RT50) from 2.8 to 28.3 h after incubation for 48 h. Ghajar *et al*. (2006a) reported a significant increase in disease development over control levels when *C. orbiculare* was applied with particular UV protectants in leaf disc bioassays. The future of bioherbicides may lie with agents that were once considered too risky. Broad-spectrum bioherbicides such as *Myrothecium verrucaria*, *Sclerotinia sclerotiorum* and others might be made 'safe' by means of appropriate deployment strategies or development of ecologically impaired strains, respectively. Other pathogens with low virulence, but with desirable specificity or epidemiology, might be made more virulent through genetic modification.

CONCLUSION

The use of plant beneficial rhizobacteria as inoculants is a recent area of interest. Inoculants that promote rapid early seedling growth have potential to play an important role in agriculture. In India, an increasing number of systematically developed inoculants are at different stages of commercialization. Our ability to harness soil biological activity through inoculation with specific biological treatments will increase with in-depth studies of microbial ecology and mechanisms of action. Nowadays agrochemical industries are also more sympathetic to the concept of bacterial inoculants than it had been earlier. There is a genuine interest in developing bacterial products that are reliable and which can act as complements to chemicals already in the market. It is relatively easy to isolate a bacterial antagonist to a phytopathogen or to find a bacterium that will increase root development. Most inoculants today are used for legumes and to a lesser extent for cereals. The cost of developing new inoculants may quickly raise the price out of a practical range for agriculture, especially in developing countries. However, there are several high-value speciality markets such as flowers, fresh organic fruits and vegetables, where chemicals are undesirable or become difficult to use because of restrictions. It appears that for legume inoculation with rhizobia, developing inoculants will be the best option for some time to come, since nitrogenase expression in plants is unlikely to occur in the foreseeable future. New environment-friendly, genetically modified microbial inoculants are being produced commercially and used to protect plants from diseases and insects to promote plant growth. These new products are expected to lead to a reduction in the use of biocides and chemical fertilizers. Nevertheless, biological safety issues must be considered prior to the release of these transgenics into the environment. The use of microbial inoculants must take into account the importance of retaining microbial diversity in rhizosphere ecology, and in achieving realistic and effective biotechnological applications. The improvement of molecular biology-based approaches will be fundamental for analysing microbial diversity and community structure, and to predict responses to microbial inoculation or processes in the environment.

FURTHER READINGS

1. Bakshi B.K. (1974) Mycorrhiza and its role in forestry. Forest Research Institute and College, Dehradun, India. Proj. Rep. PL-480.
2. Barker S.J., Stummer B., Gao L., Dispain I., O.'Connor P.J. and Smith S.E. (1998) A mutant in *Lycopersicon esculentum* Mill. with highly reduced VA mycorrhizal colonization: isolation and preliminary characterization. *Plant. J.* **(15):** 791-797.
3. Bashan Y. (1993) Potential use of *Azospirillum* as biofertilizer. *Turrialba.* **(43):** 286-291.
4. Bashan Y. and Holguin G. (1994) Root-to-root travel of the beneficial bacterium *Azospirillum brasilense. Appl. Environ. Microbiol.* **(60):** 2120-2131.
5. Bashan Y. and Holguin G. (1995) Inter-root movement of *Azospirillum brasilense* and subsequent root colonization of crop and weed seedlings growing in soil. *Microbial. Ecology.* **(29):** 269-281.
6. Bashan Y. and Levanony H. (1987) Horizontal and vertical movement of *Azospirillum brasilense* Cd in the soil and along the rhizosphere of wheat and weeds in controlled and field environments. *J. Gen. Microbiol.* **(133):** 3473-3480.
7. Bashan Y. and Levanony H. (1990) Current status of *Azospirillum* inoculation technology: *Azospirillum* as a challenge for agriculture. *Can. J. Microbiol.* **(36):** 591-608.
8. Bashan Y., Puente M. E., Rodriguez-Mendoza M. N., Toledo G, Holguin G, Ferrera-Cerrato R. and Pedrin S. (1995) Survival of *Azospirillum brasilense* in the bulk soil and rhizosphere of 23 soil types. *Appl. Environ. Microbiol.* **(61):** 1938-1945.
9. Beatty P.H. and Jensen S.E. (2002) *Paenibacillus polymyxa* produced fusaricidin type antifungal antibiotics active against *Leptosphaeria maculans*, the causative agent of blackleg disease of canola. *Can. J. Microbiol.* **(48):** 159-169.
10. Belimov A.A., Hontzeas N., Safronova V.I., Demchinskaya S.V., Piluzza G. and Bullitta S. (2005) Cadmium-tolerant plant growth-promoting rhizobacteria associated with the roots of Indian mustard (*Brassica juncea* L. Czern.). *Soil Biol. Biochem.* **(37):** 241-250.
11. Benlloch-Gonzalez, Fournier J., Ramos J. and Benlloch M. (2005) Strategies underlying salt tolerance in halophytes are present in *Cynara cardunculus*. *Plant. Sci.* **(168):** 653-659.
12. Berkum Van and Eardly B. D. (1998) Molecular evolutionary systematic of the Rhizobiaceae. In: *The Rhizobiaceae*. (Eds.) H. Spaink, A. Kondorosi, and P. Hooykaas, Kluwer Academic Pub., Dordrecht, The Netherlands. pp. 1-24.
13. Boyette C.D., Jackson M.A., Bryson C.T., Hoagland R.E., Connick W.J. and Daigle D.J. (2007) *Sesbania exaltata* biocontrol with *Colletotrichum truncatum* microsclerotia formulated in 'Pesta' granules. *Biocontrol.* **(52):** 413-426.

14. Buchanan B.B., Gruissem W. and Jones R.L. (2000) In: *Biochemistry and Molecular Biology of Plants*. Am. Soc. Plant. Physiologists, Rockville, MD U.S.A., pp. 575-588.

15. Burd G I., Dixon D.G and Glick B.R. (1998) A plant growth promoting bacterium that decreases nickel toxicity in seedlings. *Appl. Environ. Microbiol.* **(64)**: 3663-3668.

16. Burd G.I., Dixon D.G and Glick B.R. (2000) Plant growth-promoting bacteria that decrease heavy metal toxicity in plants. *Can. J. Microbiol.* **(46)**: 237-245.

17. Burke D.J., Hamerlynck E.P. and Hahn D. (2003) Interactions between the salt marsh grass season. Spartina patens, arbuscular mycorrhizal fungi and sediment bacteria during the growing. *Soil. Biol. Biochem.* **(35)**: 501-511.

18. Charudattan, (2000) Current status of biological control of weeds. In: Kennedy, G.G and Sutton, T.B. (eds) *Emerging Technologies for Integrated Pest Management: Concepts, Research and Implementation*. APS Press, St Paul, MN, USA, pp. 269-288.

19. Chen W.M., Laevens S., Lee T.M., Coenye T., De Vos P., Mergeay M. and Vandamme P. (2001) *Ralstonia taiwanensis* sp. nov., isolated from root nodules of Mimosa species and sputum of a cystic fibrosis patient. *Int. J. Syst. Evol. Microbiol.* **(51)**: 1729-1735.

20. Connick W.J., Nickle Jr. W.R. and Boyette C.D. (1993) Wheat flour granules containing mycoherbicides and entomogenous nematodes In: Lumsden, R.D. and Vaughn, J.L. (eds) *Pest Management: Biologically Based Technologies*: Proceedings of the 28th BARC Symposium Series. Beltsville, M.D., USA, pp. 238-240.

21. Dave and Patel H.H. (2003) Impact of different carbon and nitrogen sources on phosphate solubilization by *Pseudomonas fluorescens*. *J. Microbiol.* **(43)**: 33-36.

22. Deubel, Gransee A. and Merbach W. (2000) Transformation of organic rhizo-depositions by rhizosphere bacteria and its influence on the availability of tertiary calcium phosphate. *J. Plant. Nutr. Soil. Sci.* **(163)**: 387-392.

23. Diallo, Samb P. and Macauley H. (2001) Water status and stomatal behaviour of cowpea, *Vigna unguiculata* (L) Walp, plants inoculated with two *Glomus* species at low soil moisture levels. *Eur. J. Soil. Biol.* **(37)**: 187-196.

24. El-Katatny M.H., Gudelj M., Robra K.H., Elnaghy M.A. and Gübitz G.M. (2001) Characterization of a chitinase and an endo-â-1,3-glucanase from *Trichoderma harzianum* rifai T24 involved in control of the phytopathogen *Sclerotium rolfsii*. *Appl. Microbiol. Biotechnol.* **(56)**: 137-143.

25. El-Kherbawy M., Angle J.S., Heggo A. and Chaney R.L. (1989) Soil pH, rhizobia and vascular-arbuscular mycorrhizae inoculation effects on growth and heavy metal uptake of alfalfa (*Medicago sativa* L.). *Biol. Fert. Soils.* **(8)**: 61-65.

26. Else M.A., Hall K.C., Arnold G.M., Davies W.J. and Jackson M.B. (1995) Export of abscisic acid, 1-aminocyclopropane-1-carboxylic acid, phosphate, and nitrate from roots to shoots of flooded tomato plants (accounting for effects of xylem sap flow rate on concentration and delivery). *Plant. Physiol.* **(107)**: 377-384.

27. El-Tarabily K.A., Soliman M.H., Nassar A.H., Al-Hassani H.A., Sivasithamparam K., McKenna F. and Hardy G.E. (2000) Biological control of *Sclerotinia minor* using a chitinolytic bacterium and actinomycetes. *Plant. Pathol.* **(49)**: 573-583.

28. Emmert E.A.B. and Handelsman J. (1999) Biocontrol of plant disease: a (Gram) positive perspective. *FEMS. Microbiol. Lett.* **(171)**: 1-9.

29. Fguira L.F., Fotso S., Ameur-Mehdi R.B., Mellouli L. and Laatsch H. (2005) Purification and structure elucidation of antifungal and antibacterial activities of newly isolated *Streptomyces* sp. strain US80. *Res Microbiol.* **(156)**: 341-347.

30. Flowers T.J. (2004) Improving crop salt tolerance. *J. Exp. Bot.* **(55)**: 307-319.

31. Fred E.B., Beldwin I.L. and Mc Coy E. (1932) *Root Nodule Bacteria and Leguminous Plants*. Univ. Wisconsin, Madison, Wisconsin, USA. pp. 142-154.

32. Gerdemann J.W. and Bakshi B.K. (1976) Endogonaceae of India: Two new species. *Trans. Br. Mycol. Soc.* **(66):** 340-343.

33. Ghajar, Holford P., Cother E. and Beattie A. (2006a) Enhancing survival and subsequent infectivity of conidia of potential mycoherbistats using UV protectants. *Biocon Sci. Technol.* **(16):** 451-469.

34. Ghajar, Holford P., Cother E. and Beattie A. (2006b) Effects of ultraviolet radiation, simulated or as natural sunlight, on conidium germination and appressorium formation by fungi with potential as mycoherbistats. *Biocon. Sci. and Technol.* **(16):** 451-469.

35. Glick B.R. (2003) Phytoremediation: synergistic use of plants and bacteria to clean up the environment. *Biotechnol. Adv.* **(21):** 383-393.

36. Glick B.R., Penrose D.M. and Li J. (1998) A model for the lowering of plant ethylene concentrations by plant growth promoting bacteria. *J. Theor. Biol.* **(190):** 63-68.

37. Glick B.R., Todorovic B., Czarny J., Cheng Z., Duan J. and McConkey B. (2007) Promotion of plant growth by bacterial ACC deaminase. *Crit. Rev. Plant. Sci.* **(26):** 227-242.

38. Goenadi, Siswanto H. and Sugiarto Y. (2000) Bioactivation of poorly soluble phosphate rocks with a phosphate solubilizing fungus. *Soil. Sci. Soc. Am. J.* **(64):** 927-932.

39. Goldstein A.H. (1986) Bacterial solubilization of mineral phosphates: historic perspective and future prospects. *Am. J. Altern. Agric.* **(1):** 57-65.

40. Goldstein A.H. (2000) Bioprocessing of rock phosphate ore: essential technical considerations for the development of a successful commercial technology. Alfred University, New York, pp. 1-21.

41. Goren and Siegel S.M. (1976) Mercury induced ethylene production and abscission in citrus and *Coleus* explants. *Plant Physiol.* **(57):** 628-631.

42. Gressel (2002) *Molecular Biology of Weed Control*. Taylor and Francis, New York.

43. Grichko V.P. and Glick B.R. (2001) Amelioration of flooding stress by ACC deaminase-containing plant growth-promoting bacteria. *Plant. Physiol. Biochem.* **(39):** 11-17.

44. Handelsman J. and Stabb E.V. (1996) Biocontrol of soil borne plant pathogens. *Plant Cell.* **(8):** 1855-1869.

45. Hayashi and Murata N. (1998) Genetically engineered enhancement of salt tolerance in higher plants. In: *Stress Response of Photosynthetic Organisms: Molecular Mechanisms and Molecular Regulation.* (Ed.) N. Sato Murata, Elsevier, Amsterdam, pp. 133-148.

46. J.B.P.A.M. Lamarck (1983) *Azolla filiculoides* Lem. *Encycl. Meth. Bot.* **(1):** 343.

47. Jackson M.B. (1985) Ethylene and responses of plants to soil water logging and submergence. *Ann. Rev. Plant. Physiol.* **(36):** 145-174.

48. Jakasaniya M.S. and Trivedi B.S. (2004) Transformation of added phosphorous into inorganic P- fractions in soils of Gujarat. *Madras Agric. J.* **(91):** 163-167.

49. Joo G.J. (2005) Production of an anti-fungal substance for biological control of *Phytophthora capsici* causing *phytophthora* blight in red-peppers by *Streptomyces halstedii*. *Biotechnol. Lett.* **(27):** 201-205.

50. Kajimura Y., Sugiyama M. and Kaneda M. (1995) Bacilopeptins, new cyclic lipopeptide antibiotics from *Bacillus subtilis* FR-2. *J. Antibiot.* **(48):** 1095-1103.

51. Kannaiyan (2000) Use of *Azolla* spores as inoculum in rice field. In: *Biofertilizers-BGA and Azolla*. (Eds) P.K. Singh, D.N. Dhar, S. Pubbi, R. Prasanna and A. Arora, Indian Agriculture Research Institute, New Delhi, pp. 64-82.

52. Kanwer J.S. (1997) Plant nutrient needs, supply, efficiency policy issues: 2000-2025. (eds) Kanwer, J.S and J.C. Katyal, National Academy of Agricultural Sciences, New Delhi, pp-iii-viii

53. Katerji, Hoorn J.W., Hamdy A., Mastrorilli M., Nachit M. and Oweis T. (2005) Salt tolerance analysis of chickpea, faba bean and durum wheat varieties:II. Durum wheat. *Agric. Water. Mangt.* **(72):** 195-207.

54. Klich M.A., Arthur K.S., Lax A.R. and Bland J.M. (1994) Iturin A: a potential new fungicide for stored grains. *Mycopathologia.* **(127)**: 123-127.
55. Kloepper J.W., Lifshitz R. and Zablotowicz R.M. (1989) Free-living bacterial inocula for enhancing crop productivity. *Trends Biotechnol.* **(7)**: 39-43.
56. Kluger M., Loeffler W., Rapp C., Keen A. and Jung G. (1990) Rhizocticin A., an antifungal phosphono-oligopeptide of *Bacillus subtilis* ATCC 6633: biological properties. *Arch. Microbiol.* **(153)**: 276-281.
57. Kozlowski T.T. (1984) Extent, causes, and impacts of flooding. In: *Flooding and Plant Growth*, (ed. T.T. Kozlowski), Academic Press, New York, pp. 1-7.
58. Kramer P.J. and Boyer J.S. (1995) *Water Relations of Plants and Soils*. American Press.
59. Kumar, Sharma S. and Mishra S. (2010) Influence of Arbuscular Mycorrhizal (AM) Fungi and salinity on seedling growth, solute accumulation, and mycorrhizal dependency of *Jatropha curcas* L. *J. Plant Growth Regulation.* **(29)**: 297-306.
60. Leifert, Li H., Chidburee S., Hampson S., Workman S. and Sigee D. (1995) Antibiotic production and biocontrol activity by *Bacillus subtilis* and *Bacillus pumilus* CL45. *J. Appl. Bacteriol.* **(78)**: 97-108.
61. Leland J.E., and Behle R.W. (2005) Coating *Beauveria bassiana* with lignin for protection from solar radiation and effects on pathogenicity to *Lygus lineolaris* (Heteroptera: Miridae). *Biocon Sci. Technol.* **(15)**: 309-320.
62. Malcova, Vosatka M. and Gryndler M. (2003) Effects of inoculation with *Glomus intraradices* on lead uptake by *Zea mays* L. and *Agrostis capillaris L. Appl. Soil. Ecol.* **(23)**: 255-267.
63. Martin N.I., Hu H., Moake M.M., Churey J.J., Whittal R., Worobo R.W. and Vederas J.C. (2003) Isolation, structural characterization, and properties of mattacin (polymyxin M), a cyclic peptide antibiotic produced by *Paenibacillus kobensis* M. *J. Biol. Chem.* **(278)**: 13124-13132.
64. Martinez, J.M., Nunez, Ortiz A. and Cerda A. (1994) Changes in amino acid and organic acid composition in tomato and cucumber plants in relation to salinity and nitrogen nutrition. *J. Plant. Nutr.* **(17)**: 1359-1368.
65. Matsushita, Toyama H., Yamada M. and Adachi O. (2002) Quinoproteins: structure, function, and biotechnological applications. *Appl. Microbiol. Biotechnol.* **(58)**: 13-22.
66. Mattey M. (1992) The production of organic acids. *Rev. Biotechnol.* **(12)**: 87-13.
67. Mayak S., Tirosh T. and Glick B.R. (2004a) Plant growth-promoting bacteria that confer resistance to water stress in tomatoes and peppers. *Plant Sci.* **(166)**: 525-530.
68. Mayak S., Tirosh T. and Glick B.R. (2004b) Plant growth-promoting bacteria that confer resistance in tomato to salt stress. *Plant. Physiol. Biochem.* **(42)**: 565-572.
69. Merguihur A.E., Burity H.A., Tabosa J.N. and Maia F.L. (2002) Salt stress response and proline accumulation in *Brachiaria humidicola. Revista. Argentina de Microbiologia.* **(34)**: 77-82.
70. Michiels K., Vanderleyden J. and Van Gool A. (1989) *Azospirillum*-plant root associations: a review. *Biol. Fert. Soils.* **(8)**: 356-368.
71. Mohamed H.A.L., and Haggag WM. (2006) Biocontrol potential of salinity tolerant mutants of *Trichoderma harzianum* against *Fusarium oxysporum. Brazilian. J. Microbiol.* **(37)**: 181-191.
72. Moore A.W. (1969) *Azolla:* biology and agronomic significance. Bot. Rev. **(35)**: 17-35.
73. Mori, Fani R., Gallori E., Fantappie O. and Bazzicalupo M. (1992) Mutants of *Azospirillum brasilense* altered in the uptake of iron. *Symbiosis.* **(13)**: 115-122.
74. Morton J.B., Bentivenga S.P. and Wheeler W.W. (1993) Germplasm in the international collection of arbuscular and vesicular-arbuscular mycorrhizal fungi (INVAM) and procedures for culture development documentation and storage. *Mycotaxon.* **(48)**: 491-528.
75. Moulin, Munive A., Dreyfus B. and Boivin-Masson C. (2001) Nodulation of legumes by members of the b-subclass of Proteobacteria. *Nature.* **(411)**: 948-950.

76. Mukherjee and Sen S.K. (2006) Purification, characterization and antifungal activity of chitinase from *Streptomyces venezuelae* P10. *Curr. Microbiol.* **(53):** 265-269.

77. Munns R. (2002) Comparative physiology of salt and water stress. Plant Cell Environ. **(20):** 239-250.

78. Nilsen E.T. and Orcutt D.M. (1997) *The Physiology of Plants Under Stress*: Abiotic Factors, John Wiley and Sons Inc., New York, NY, pp. 241-248.

79. Okon Y. and Labandera-Gonzalez C. (1994) Agronomic applications of *Azospirillum*: an evaluation of 20 years worldwide field inoculation. *Soil. Biol. Biochem.* **(26):** 1591-1601.

80. Pascale S.D., Maggio A. and Barbieri G. (2005) Soil salinization affects growth, yield and mineral composition of cauliflower and broccoli. *Eur. J. Agron.* **(23):** 254-264.

81. Perez, Sulbaran M., Ball M.M. and Yarzabal L.A. (2007) Isolation and characterization of mineral phosphate solubilizing bacteria naturally colonizing a limonitic crust in the southeastern Venezuelan region. *Soil Biol. Biochem.* **(39):** 2905-2914.

82. Peypoux F., Besson F., Michel G. and Delcambe L. (1981) Structure of Bacillomycin D., a new antibiotic of the iturins group. *Eur. J. Biochem.* **(118):** 323-327.

83. Plaxton W.C. (2004) Biochemical Adaptations of Phosphate Starved Plants. In: "*Encyclopedia of Plant & Crop Science*". (Ed) R. Goodman, Marcel Dekker, N.Y. pp. 976-980

84. Prasad M.N.V. and Strazalka K. (2000) *Physiology and Biochemistry of Metal Toxicity and Tolerance in Plants*. Kluwer Academic Publishers, Boston, pp. 153-160.

85. Prasanna R. and Kaushik B.D. (1994) Physiological and molecular genetic aspects of nitrogen fixation in non-heterocystous cyanobacteria. *Ind. J. Exp. Biol.* **(32):** 248-251.

86. Prasanna R. and Kaushik B.D. (1996) Nitrogen fixation and *nif* gene organization in branched heterocystous cyanobacteria; variation for the presence of *xis*A. *Folia Microbiol.* **(40):** 176-180.

87. Prinsen E., Costacurta A., Michiels K., Vanderleyden J. and Van Onckelen H. (1993) *Azospirillum brasilense* Indole-3-acetic acid biosynthesis: Evidence for a non-tryptophan dependent pathway. *Mol. Plant. Microbe. Inter.* **(6):** 609-615.

88. Quilambo O.A. (2000). Functioning of peanut (*Arachis hypogaea* L.) under nutrient deficiency and drought stress in relation to symbiotic associations. Ph.D. Thesis. University of Groningen, The Netherlands, Van Denderan B.V. Groningen.

89. Rabie G.H. (2005) Influence of VA-mycorrhizal fungi and kinetin on the response of mung bean plants to irrigation with seawater. *Mycorrhiza.* **(15):** 225-230.

90. Rabie G.H. and Almadini A.M. (2005) Role of bioinoculants in development of salt-tolerance of *Vicia faba* plants under salinity stress. *African. J. of Biotechnol.* **(4):** 210-222.

91. Rao A.V. and Tak R. (2002) Growth of different tree species and their nutrient uptake in limestone mine spoil as influenced by arbuscular mycorrhizal (AM) fungi in India arid zone. J. Arid. Environ. **(51):** 113-119.

92. Rao K.V. B. and Charyulu P. B. B. N. (2005) Evaluation of effect of inoculation of *Azospirillum* on the yield of *Setaria italica* (L.). African *J. Biotechnol.* **(4):** 989-995.

93. Red'Kina T.V. (1990) Fungistatic activity of Bacteria of Genus *Azospirillum.* Agroke' mia' e's Talajtan **(39):** 465-468.

94. Rippka R., Deruelles J., Waterbury J.B., Herdman M. and Stanier R.Y. (1979) Generic assignments, strain histories and properties of pure cultures of cyanobacteria. *J. Gen. Microbiol.* **(111):** 1-61.

95. Salih H.M., Yahya A.I., Abdul-Rahem A.M. and Munam B.H. (1989) Availability of phosphorous in calcareous soil treated with rock phosphate or super phosphate as affected by phosphate dissolving fungi. *Plant Soil.* **(120):** 181-185.

96. Selvakumar G., Kundu S., Joshi P., Nazim S., Gupta A.D., Mishra P.K. and Gupta H.S. (2008) Characterization of a cold tolerant plant growth promoting bacterium *Pantoea dispersa* 1A isolated from a sub-alpine soil in the north western Indian Himalayas. *World. J. Microbiol. Biotechnol.* **(24):** 955-960.

97. Senthilkumar M., Govindasamy V. and Annapurna K. (2007) Role of antibiosis in suppression of charcoal rot disease by soybean endophyte *Paenibacillus* sp. HKA-15. *Curr Microbiol* **(55):** 25-29.

98. Senthilkumar M., Swarnalakshmi K., Govindasamy V., Young-Keun Lee and Annapurna K. (2009) Biocontrol potentials of soybean bacterial endophytes against charcoal rot fungus–*Rhizoctonia bataticola*. *Curr. Microbiol.* **(58):** 288-293.

99. Shanmugasundaram S. and Kannaiyan S. (1994) Studies on the development of *Azolla* hybrid and its biofertilizer value for rice crop. National seminar on *Azolla* and algal biofertilizer for rice. Tamilnadu Agricultural University, Coimbatore, India. P.17

100. Shende S.T. and Apte R. (1982) *Azotobacter* inoculation-A highly remunerative input for agriculture. In: *Biological Nitrogen Fixation*. Proceedings of national symposium held at IARI, New Delhi, by the Food and Agriculture Committee, DAE, Government of India, pp. 532-543.

101. Shetty G., Hetrick D. and Schwat P. (1995) Effects of mycorrhizal fertilizers amendments on Zinc tolerance of plants. *Environ. Pollution.* **(88):** 308-314.

102. Singh C.S. and Subba Rao N.S. (1979) Associative effect of *Azospirillum brasilense* with *Rhizobium japonicum* on nodulation and yield of soybean (*Glycine max*). *Plant Soil.* **(53):** 387-392.

103. Smith K.P., Havey M.J. and Handelsman J. (1993) Suppression of cottony leak of cucumber with *Bacillus cereus* strain UW85. *Plant. Dis.* **(77):** 139-142.

104. Smith R.J. (1986) Biological control of northern joint vetch (*Aeschynomene virginica*) in rice (*Oryza sativa*) and soybeans (*Glycine max*): a researcher's view. *Weed Science.* 34 **(**Suppl. **1):** 17-23.

105. Smith S.E. and Read D.J. (1997) *Mycorrhizal Symbiosis*. 2nd Edition Academic Press, San Diego, California, USA.

106. Stal L.J. and Krumbein W.E. (1985) Nitrogenase activity in the non-heterocystous cyanobacterium *Oscillatoria* sp. grown under alternate light-dark cycle. *Arch. Microbiol.* **(143):** 67-71.

107. St-Arnaud M., Hamel C., Vimard B., Caron M. and Fortin J.A. (1995) Altered growth of *Fusarium oxysporum* f. sp. *Chrysanthemi* in an *in vitro* dual culture system with the vesicular-arbuscular mycorrhizal fungus *Glomus intraradicus* growing on *Daucus carota* transformed roots. *Mycorrhiza* **(5):** 431-438.

108. Stojanovid S., Starovid M. and Matijevh D. (1999) Factors affecting conidial germination of *Colletotrichum gloeosporioides* isolated from *Polystigma rubrum* subsp. *rubrum* stromata. Acta *Phytopathologica et Entomologica Hungarica.* **(34):** 63-73.

109. Subba Rao N.S. (1982) *Biofertilizers in Agriculture and Forestry*. Oxford and IBH Publishing Co., New Delhi, pp. 3

110. Subba Rao N.S., Tilak K.V.B.R. and Singh C.S. (1985a) Effect of combined inoculation of *Azospirillum brasilense* and vesicular-arbuscular mycorrhizae on pearl millet (*Pennisetum americanum*). *Plant. Soil.* **(84):** 283-286.

111. Subba Rao N.S., Tilak K.V.B.R. and Singh C.S. (1985b) Synergistic effect of vesicular-arbuscular mycorrhizae and *Azospirillum brasilense* on the growth of barley in pots. *Soil. Biol. Biochem.* **(17):** 119-121.

112. Sulbaran M., Perez E., Ball M.M., Bahsas A. and Yarzabal L.A. (2008) Characterization of the mineral phosphate solubilizing activity of *Pantoea agglomerans* MMB051 isolated from an iron rich soil in southeastern Venezuela (Bolivar State). *Curr. Microbiol.* **(58):** 378-383.

113. Sundra Rao W.V.B., Mann H.S., Pal N.B. and Mathur R.S. (1963) Bacterial inoculation experiments with special reference to *Azotobacter*. *Indian J. Agric. Sci.* **(33):** 279-290.

114. Tain C.Y., Feng G., Li X.L. and Zhang F.S. (2004) Different effects of arbuscular mycorrhizal fungal isolates from saline or non-saline soil on salinity tolerance of plants. Appl. Soil. Ecol. **(26):** 143-148.

115. Timmusk S. and Wagner G.H. (1999) The plant-growth-promoting rhizobacterium *Paenibacillus polymyxa* induces changes in *Arabidopsis thaliana* gene expression: a possible connection between biotic and abiotic stress responses. *Mol. Plant. Microbe. Interact.* **(12):** 951-959.

116. Tripathi A.K. (2002) Rhizobia of the-subclass of Proteobacteria: a tale of losing the race. *Curr. Sci.* **(82):** 8-9.

117. Tripura, Sashidhar B. and Podile A.R. (2007) Ethyl methane sulfonate mutagenesis-enhanced mineral phosphate solubilization by groundnut associated *Serratia marcescens* GPS-5. *Curr. Microbiol.* **(54):** 79-84.

118. Tsuge K., Ano T. and Shoba M. (1995) Characterization of *Bacillus subtilis* YB8, coproducer of lipopeptides surfactin and plipastatin B1. *J. Gen. Appl. Microbiol.* **(41):** 541-545.

119. Van Assche F. and Clijsters H. (1990) Effect of metals on enzyme activity in plants. *Plant. Cell. Environ.* **(13):** 195-206.

120. Vartapetian B.B. and Jackson M.B. (1997) Plant Adaptations to Anaerobic Stress. *Ann. Bot.* **(79):** 3-20.

121. Vassileva M., Vassilev N., Fenice M. and Federici F. (2001) Immobilized cell technology applied in solubilization of insoluble inorganic (rock) phosphate and P plant acquisition. *Bioresource. Technol.* **(79):** 263-271.

122. Wang S., Wan C., Wang Y., Chen H., Zhou Z., Fu H. and Sosebee E. (2004) The characteristics of Na+, K+ and free proline distribution in several drought- resistant plants of the Alxa Desert, China. *J. Arid Environ.* **(56):** 525-539.

123. Wani S.P. (1990) Inoculation with associative nitrogen fixing bacteria: Role on cereal grain production improvement. Indian *J. Microbiol.* **(30):** 363-393.

124. Weissenhorn, Leyval C. and Berthelin J. (1995) Bioavailability of heavy metals and abundance of arbuscular mycorrhiza in a soil polluted by atmospheric deposition from a smelter. *Biol. Fertil. Soil.* **(19):** 22-28.

125. Will M.E. and Sylvia D.M. (1990) Interaction of rhizosphere bacteria, fertilizer, and vesicular arbuscular mycorrhizal fungi with sea oats. *Appl. Environ. Microbiol.* **(56):** 2073-2079.

126. Wyatt J.T. and Silvey J.K.G. (1969) Nitrogen fixation by *Gloeocapsa*. *Science*. **165:** 908-909.

127. Yahalom E., Okon Y. and Dovrat A. (1987) *Azospirillum* effects on susceptibility to *Rhizobium* nodulation and on nitrogen fixation of several forage legumes. *Can. J. Microbiol.* **(35):** 510-514.

128. Yang J., Kloepper J.W. and Ryu C.M. (2008) Rhizosphere bacteria help plants tolerate abiotic stress. *Trends in Plant. Sci.* **(14):** 1-4.

129. Yano-Melo A.M., Saggin O.J. and Maia C. (2003) Tolerance of mycorrhized banana (*Musa* sp. cv. Pacovan) plantlets to saline stress. *Agric. Ecosystems and Environ.* **(95):** 343-348.

130. Young J.M., Kuykendall L.D., Martinez-Romero E., Kerr A. and Sawada H. (2001) A revision of *Rhizobium* Frank 1889, with an emended description of the genus, and the inclusion of all species of *Agrobacterium* Conn 1942 and *Allorhizobium undicola* de Lajudie *et al.* 1998 as new combinations: *Rhizobium radiobacter, R. rhizogenes, R. rubi, R. undicola* and *R. vitis*. *Int. J. Syst. Bacteriol.* **(51):** 89-103.

131. Youssef B.M. and Aziz N.H. (1999) Influence of gamma-irradiation on the bioconversion of rice straw by *Trichoderma viride* into single cell protein. *Cytobiol.* **(97):** 171-183.

132. Zakharova E., Shcherbakov A., Brudnik V., Skripko N., Bulkhin N. and Ignatov V. (1999) Biosynthesis of indole-3-acetic acid in *Azospirillum brasilense*. Insights from quantum chemistry. *Eur. J. Biochem.* **(259):** 572-6.

133. Zandavalli R.B., Dillenburg L.R. and Paulo V.D. (2004) Growth responses of *Araucaria angustifolia* (Araucariaceae) to inoculation with the mycorrhizal fungus *Glomus clarum*. *Appl. Soil. Ecol.* **(25):** 245-255.

134. Zhuang X., Chen J., Shim H. and Bai Z. (2007) New advances in plant growth-promoting rhizobacteria for bioremediation. *Environ. Int.* **(33):** 406-413.

SECTION C

Biotechnology for Health Applications

CHAPTER 24

Molecular Markers in Animal Health and Production

Over the last two decades advances in molecular genetics have introduced a new generation of molecular markers for the genetic improvement of livestock. This study is focused on the most advanced DNA-based molecular markers which have acted as versatile tools and have found their own position in various fields. Ever since their development, they are constantly being modified to enhance their utility and to bring about automation in the process of genome analysis. The discovery of PCR (Polymerase Chain Reaction) was a milestone in this endeavour and proved to be a unique process that brought about a new class of DNA profiling markers. In this chapter, DNA-based molecular markers developed during the past decades-restriction fragment length polymorphisms (RFLPs), microsatellites (SSRs), amplified fragment length polymorphism (AFLPs), single nucleotide polymorphisms (SNPs) for various applications in the area of animal genome analysis are briefly discussed.

Keywords: Animals molecular markers, Genome analysis, PCR, MAS, QTLs.

INTRODUCTION

All organisms are subject to mutations as a result of normal cellular operations or interactions with the environment, leading to genetic variations (polymorphism). In conjunction with selection and genetic drift, there arises genetic variation within and among individuals, species, and higher order taxonomic groups. For this variation to be useful to geneticists, it must be heritable and discernible to the researchers, whether as a recognizable phenotypic variation or as a genetic mutation distinguishable through molecular techniques. At the DNA level, types of genetic variations include base substitutions, commonly referred to as single nucleotide polymorphisms (SNPs), insertions or deletions of nucleotide sequences (indels) within a locus, inversion of a segment of DNA within a locus, and rearrangement of DNA segments around a locus of interest. Through long evolutionary accumulation, many different instances of each type of mutation should exist in any given specie, and the number and degree of the various types of mutations define the genetic variation within a species. DNA marker technology can be applied to reveal these mutations. Large deletions and insertions (indels) cause shifts in the sizes of DNA fragments produced upon digestion by restriction enzymes, and are among the easiest type of mutations to detect, mainly by electrophoresis of the fragments on an agarose gel; smaller indels require DNA sequencing or more elaborate electrophoretic techniques to determine smaller changes in size. Inversions and rearrangements that involve restriction sites can be easy to detect because they disrupt the ability of a restriction enzyme to cut DNA at a given site and thus can produce relatively large changes in DNA fragment sizes. Point mutations are more difficult to detect because they do not cause changes in fragment sizes.

CONCEPTS

Popular genetic markers include Allozymes, mitochondrial DNA (mtDNA), Restriction Fragment Length Polymorphism (RFLP), Rapid Amplified Polymorphic DNA (RAPD), Amplified Fragment Length Polymorphism (AFLP), Microsatellites, Single Nucleotide Polymorphism (SNP), and Expressed Sequence Tag (EST) markers. Molecular markers are classified into two categories: type I are markers associated with genes of known function, while type II markers are associated with anonymous genomic segments. Under this classification, most RFLP markers are type I markers because they were identified during the analysis of known genes. Likewise, allozyme markers are type I markers because the protein they encode has known function. RAPD markers are type II markers because RAPD bands are amplified from anonymous genomic regions via the polymerase chain reaction (PCR). AFLP markers are type II because they are also amplified from anonymous genomic regions. Microsatellite markers are type II markers unless they are associated with genes of known function. EST markers are type I markers because they represent transcripts of genes. SNP markers are mostly type II markers unless they are developed from expressed sequences (eSNP or cSNP). Indels are becoming more widely used as markers since they are often discovered during genomic or transcriptomic sequencing projects. They can be either type I or type II markers depending on whether they are located in genes. Type I markers have utility in studies of comparative genomics, genome evolution, candidate gene identification, and enhanced communication among laboratories. Due to evolutionary constraints on the genome, many genes and their organization are conserved among species. Comparative genomics deals with the similarity and differences found among genomes. Type I markers serve as a bridge for comparison and transfer of genomic information from a map rich species into a relatively map-poor species. Such inter-specific comparisons can also be made based on type II markers, but the extent to which the comparison can be made is limited to closely related taxa. The requirement for such comparisons lies in sequence conservations. For the most frequently used microsatellite markers, such comparative studies depend on conservation of the flanking sequences used for the design of PCR primers. In contrast, sequence conservation within genes are high, allowing type I markers to serve as anchor points for genomic segments to be compared among species. In general, type II markers such as RAPDs, microsatellites, and AFLPs are considered to be non-coding and therefore selectively neutral. Such markers have found widespread use in population genetic studies whose characterizations of genetic diversity and divergence within and among populations are based on assumptions of Hardy-Weinberg equilibrium and selective neutrality of the markers employed. The usefulness of molecular markers can be measured based on their polymorphic information content (PIC). PIC refers to the value of a marker for detecting polymorphism in a population. PIC depends on the number of detectable alleles and the distribution of their frequencies, and equals 1 minus the sum of the square of all allele frequencies. For instance, the PIC of a microsatellite marker with two alleles of frequency 0.5 each should be $1 - [(0.5)^2 + (0.5)^2] = 0.5$, while PIC for a microsatellite marker of two alleles with allele frequencies of 0.9 and 0.1 is 0.18. Thus, greater the number of alleles, greater the PIC, and for a given number of alleles, the more equal the allele frequencies, greater is the PIC.

PRINCIPLES

In the past years, the developments in understanding the genetic code of animal species have opened the possibility to evolve the genetic evaluation of all species of livestock. Traditionally, the genetic improvement of livestock breeds has been based on phenotypic selection. The past century was characterized by the development of quantitative theory and methodology towards the accurate selection and prediction of genetic response. This resulted in the selection of a number of economically important genetic traits in cattle, sheep, pigs and poultry. The first work on the detection of genome variation in animal livestocks is based on morphological, chromosomal and biochemical markers. Most of the morphological markers are sex limited, age dependent, and significantly influenced by the environment. Biochemical markers show low degree of polymorphism. The various genotypic classes are indistinguishable at the phenotypic level because of the dominance effect of the marker and low genome coverage.

The development of molecular biology during the past three decades created new means for studying livestock genetics and animal breeding. Selection according to genotype has become an important tool in the breeding of farm animals. The molecular markers capable of detecting the genetic variation at the DNA sequence level have removed the above-mentioned limitations of morphological, chromosome and protein markers, but also possess unique genetic properties that make them more useful than other genetic markers. They are numerous and distributed ubiquitously throughout the genome. These markers follow a typical Mendelian inheritance, which usually expresses in a co-dominant fashion, and are often multiallelic giving mean heterozygosity of more than 70 percent. They are noninfluenced by the environmental factors, and generally do not have pleiotropic effects on quantitative trait loci (QTL). Molecular markers, revealing the polymorphism at the DNA level, are now key players in animal genetics. Molecular markers serve as an useful tool for animal identification and genetic distance estimation. Parentage testing using molecular markers yields much higher exclusion probability (> 90%) than the testing with blood groups (70–90%) or other biochemical markers (40–60%). These polymorphisms referred to as molecular markers can be used to build up genetic maps and to evaluate differences between markers in the expression of particular traits that might indicate a direct effect of these differences in terms of genetic determination on the trait. Extensive genetic maps were prepared in the last few decades in a variety of animal species such as cattle, sheep, swine, for marker assisted selection (MAS), QTL segregating analysis and for detection of major genes.

ANIMAL MOLECULAR MARKERS TECHNOLOGY

DNA Based Markers

Various types of molecular markers are utilized to evaluate DNA polymorphism and are generally classified in three major groups:

(1) Hybridization-based DNA markers—Restriction Fragment Length Polymorphisms (RFLPs) and oligonucleotide fingerprinting.

(2) PCR-based DNA markers, which involve *in vitro* amplification of particular DNA sequences or loci with the help of specifically or arbitrarily chosen oligonucleotide sequences (primers) and a thermostable DNA polymerase enzyme—Random Amplified Length Polymorphic DNAs (RAPDs), Simple Sequence Repeats or microsatellites (SSRs), Amplified Length Polymorphism (AFLP).

(3) DNA chip and sequencing-based DNA markers such as Single Nucleotide Polymorphism (SNPs).

Properties of Ideal DNA Markers

The properties of ideal DNA markers are as follows:

- Highly polymorphic nature
- Co-dominant inheritance (determination of homozygous and heterozygous status of diploid organism)
- Frequent occurrence in genome
- Selective neutral behaviour (the DNA sequences of any organism are neutral to environmental conditions or management practices)
- Easy access (availability)
- Easy and fast assay
- High reproducibility
- Easy exchange of data between laboratories

Nowadays the most commonly used molecular markers are RFLP, AFLP, RAPD, SSR, and SNP. These markers differ in genetic information, interpretation and standardization of results, potential for automation and animal genetic improvement. The properties of different molecular markers are listed in Table 24.1.

Table 24.1 Comparison of commonly used genetic markers by Mburu and Hanotte (2005).

Feature	*RFLP*	*SSR*	*RAPD*	*AFLP*	*Isozymes*	*STS/EST*
Origin	Anonymous/ Genic	Anonymous	Anonymous	Anonymous	Genic	Genic
Maximum theoretical number of possible loci in analysis	Limited by the restriction site (nucleotide) polymorphism (tens of thousands)	Limited by the size of genome and number of simple repeats in a genome (tens of thousands)	Limited by the size of genome, and by nucleotide polymorphism (tens of thousands)	Limited by the restriction site (nucleotide) polymorphism (tens of thousands)	Limited by the number of enzyme genes and histochemical enzyme assays available (30-50)	Limited by the number of expressed genes (10,000-30,000)
Dominance	Codominant	Co-dominant	Dominant	Dominant	Co-dominant	Co-dominant
Null alleles	Rare to extremely rare	Occasional to common	Not applicable (presence/ absence type	Not applicable (presence/ absence type	Rare	Rare

Contd.

Feature	RFLP	SSR	RAPD	AFLP	Isozymes	STS/EST
			of detection)	of detection)		
Transferability Across related species	Across genera	Within genus or species	Within species	Within species	Across families and genera	Across related species
Reproducibility	High to very high	Medium to high	Low to medium	Medium to high	Very high	High
Amount of sample required per sample	2-10 mg DNA	10-20 ng DNA	2-10 ng DNA	0.2-1 ìg DNA	Several mg of tissue	10-20 ng DNA
Ease of development	Difficult	Difficult	Easy	Moderate	Moderate	Moderate
Ease of assay	Difficult	Easy to moderate	Easy to moderate	Moderate to difficult	Easy to moderate	Easy to moderate
Automation / multiplexing	Difficult	Possible	Possible	Possible	Difficult	Possible
Genome and QTL mapping potential	Good	Good	Very good	Very good	Limited	Good
Comparative mapping potential	Good	Limited	Very limited	Very limited	Excellent	Good to very good
Candidate gene mapping potential	Limited	Useless	Useless	Useless	Limited	Excellent
Potential for studying adaptive genetic variation	Limited	Limited	Limited	Limited	Good	Limited
Development	Moderate	Expensive	Inexpensive	Moderate	Inexpensive	Expensive
Assay	Moderate	Moderate	Inexpensive	Moderate to expensive	Inexpensive	Moderate
Equipment	Moderate	Moderate to expensive	Moderate	Moderate to expensive	Inexpensive	Moderate to expensive

Allozyme

Allozymes are allelic variants of proteins produced by a single gene locus, and are of interest as markers because polymorphism exists and because they represent protein products of genes and are thus type I markers. Amino acid differences in the polypeptide chains of the different allelic forms of an enzyme reflect changes in the underlying DNA sequence. Depending on the nature of the amino acid changes, the resulting protein products may migrate at different rates (due to charge and size differences) when run through a starch gel subjected to an electrical field. Differences in the presence/absence and relative frequencies of alleles are used to quantify genetic variation and distinguish among genetic units at the levels of populations, species, and higher taxonomic designations.

Mt DNA Markers

Studies of vertebrate species have generally shown that sequence divergence accumulates more rapidly in mitochondrial than nuclear DNA. This has been attributed to a faster mutation rate in mtDNA that may result from a lack of repair mechanism during replication and smaller effective population size due to the strictly maternal inheritance of the haploid mitochondrial genome. Almost the entire mtDNA molecule is transcribed except for the approximately 1-kb control region (D-loop), where replication and transcription of the molecule is initiated. In general, non-coding segments like the D-loop exhibit elevated levels of variation relative to coding sequences such as the cytochrome b gene, presumably due to reduced functional constraints and relaxed selection pressure. Due to its non-Mendelian mode of inheritance, the mtDNA molecule is usually considered as single locus in genetic investigations. In addition, because mtDNA is maternally inherited, the phylogenies and population structures derived from mtDNA data may not reflect those of the nuclear genome due to gender-biased migration or introgression. Species identification and authentication can be done easily using this marker.

RFLP

RFLP markers were regarded as the first shot in the genome revolution, marking the beginning of an entirely different era in the biological sciences. Restriction endonucleases are bacterial enzymes that recognize specific 4, 6, or 8 base pair (bp) nucleotide sequences and cut DNA wherever these sequences are encountered, so that changes in the DNA sequence due to indels, base substitutions, or rearrangements involving the restriction sites can result in the gain, loss, or relocation of a restriction site. Digestion of DNA with restriction enzymes results in fragments whose number and size can vary among individuals, populations, and species. Traditionally, fragments were separated using Southern blot analysis in which genomic DNA is digested, subjected to electrophoresis through an agarose gel, transferred to a membrane, and visualized by hybridization to specific probes. Most recent analyses replace the tedious Southern blot method with techniques based on the polymerase chain reaction (PCR). If flanking sequences are known for a locus, the segment containing the RFLP region is amplified via PCR. If the length polymorphism is caused by a relatively large (> approx. 100 bp depending on the size of the undigested PCR product) deletion or insertion, gel electrophoresis of the PCR products should reveal the size difference. However, if the length polymorphism is caused by base substitution at a restriction site, PCR products must be digested with a restriction enzyme to reveal the RFLP. With the increasing number of 'universal' primers available in the literature, a researcher can target DNA regions that are either relatively conserved or rapidly evolving, depending on the amount of variation observed and the taxonomic level under examination. In addition, PCR products can be digested with restriction enzymes and visualized by simple staining with ethidium bromide due to the increased amount of DNA produced by the PCR method. The major strength of RFLP markers is that they are co-dominant markers, i.e., both alleles in an individual are observed in the analysis. Since the size difference is often large, scoring is relatively easy. The major disadvantage of RFLP is the relatively low level of polymorphism.

RAPD

RAPD procedures were first developed in 1990 using PCR to randomly amplify anonymous segments of nuclear DNA with an identical pair of primers, 8–10 bp in length. Because the primers are short and relatively low annealing temperatures (often 36–40°C) are used, the likelihood of amplifying multiple products is great, with each product (presumably) representing a different locus. Since most of the nuclear genome in vertebrates is non-coding, it is presumed that most of the amplified loci will be selectively neutral. Genetic variation and divergence within and between the taxa of interest are assessed by the presence or absence of each product, which is dictated by changes in the DNA sequence at each locus. RAPD polymorphisms can occur due to base substitutions at the primer binding sites or indels in the regions between the sites. RAPD markers are inherited as Mendelian markers in a dominant fashion and scored as present/absent. In breeding studies, the number of RAPD bands seen in the F1 generation should equal the sum of the bands seen in the parents, assuming parental homozygosity at each locus; polymorphic RAPD then segregates in a 3:1 ratio in F_2 populations. RAPDs have all the advantages of a PCR-based marker, with the added benefit that primers are commercially available and do not require prior knowledge of the target DNA sequence or gene organization. Multilocus amplifications can be separated electrophoretically on agarose gels and stained with ethidium bromide, although higher resolution of bands has been achieved with discontinuous polyacrylamide gel electrophoresis (dPAGE) and silver staining, a somewhat costlier and more labor-intensive method. Other advantages of RAPDs are the ease with which a large number of loci and individuals can be screened. RAPD markers were used for identifying animals with early (precocious) or late (non-precocious) reproductive maturation onset. RAPD assays have been used in animal genetics for identifying polymorphisms that can be used as markers for constructing linkage maps. Polymorphic microsatellite analysis is also a powerful approach for detecting gene–phenotype correlations. However, it demands previous knowledge of the candidate genes and information on the gene sequence for primer design. The RAPD analysis does not require any previous knowledge of the genes related to the trait under study, detecting DNA polymorphisms along the entire genome. The number and intensity of the amplification products and its reproducibility have been often cited as a disadvantage of this method. This has discouraged many investigators from using RAPD. In fact, reliable amplification of scorable RAPD markers requires optimization of the reaction parameters for individual taxa. RAPD analysis can be useful for predicting reproductive maturation onset in animal species.

AFLP

The molecular basis of AFLP polymorphism includes indels between restriction sites and base substitutions at restriction sites. Like RAPDs, it also includes base substitutions at PCR primer binding sites. The unique feature of the technique is the addition of adaptors of known sequence to DNA fragments generated by digestion of whole genomic DNA. This allows for the subsequent

PCR amplification of a subset of the total fragments for ease of separation by gel electrophoresis. Its primary target of genetic variation is the same as RFLP, but instead of analyzing one locus at a time, it allows for the analysis of many loci simultaneously. By using this technique, breed identification markers have been developed in beef cattle.

Microsatellites

Microsatellites, or simple sequence repeats (SSRs), represent a unique type of tandemly repeated genomic sequences, which are abundantly distributed across genomes and demonstrate high levels of allele polymorphism. They are codominant markers of relatively small size, which can be easily amplified with the polymerase chain reaction. The majority of microsatellites (30–67%) found are dinucleotides. In the genome of vertebrates, $(AC)_n$ is the most common dinucleotide motif. It is 2.3-fold more frequent than $(AT)_n$, the second most general type of dinucleotides. Interestingly, in primates, mononucleotide repeats are mostly represented by poly (A/T) tracts, which are the most frequent classes of SSRs. In total, higher order SSR classes (tri-, tetra-, penta-and hexanucluotides) are about 1.5-fold less common in genomic DNA of vertebrates than dinucleotides. Two models (DNA polymerase slippage and unequal recombination) have been suggested to explain microsatellite generation and evolution. The first model involves transient dissociation of the replicating DNA strands with subsequent reassociation. The nonreciprocal recombination (gene conversion) may also play a role in genetic instability of some SSRs, including triplet motifs. Microsatellites consist of multiple copies of tandemly arranged simple sequence repeats (SSRs) that range in size from 1 to 6 base pairs (e.g., ACA or GATA). Microsatellites tend to be evenly distributed in the genome of all chromosomes and all regions of the chromosome. They have been found inside gene coding regions, introns, and in the non-gene sequences. The best known examples of microsatellites within coding regions are those causing genetic diseases in humans, such as the CAG repeats that encode polyglutamine tract, resulting in mental retardation. Most microsatellite loci are relatively small, ranging from a few to a few hundred repeats. The relatively small size of microsatellite loci is important for PCR-facilitated genotyping. Generally speaking, microsatellites containing a larger number of repeats are more polymorphic, though polymorphism has been observed in microsatellites with as few as five repeats. Microsatellite polymorphism is based on size differences due to varying numbers of repeat units contained by alleles at a given locus. Microsatellite mutation rates have been reported as high as 10^{-2} per generation, and are believed to be caused by polymerase slippage during DNA replication, resulting in differences in the number of repeat units. Microsatellites are inherited in a Mendelian fashion as co-dominant markers. This is strength of microsatellite markers in addition to their abundance, even genomic distribution, small locus size, and high polymorphism. However, use of microsatellite markers involves a large amount of upfront investment and effort. Each microsatellite locus has to be identified and its flanking region sequenced for the design of PCR primers. For most efficient marker development, microsatellite-enriched genomic DNA libraries are made. Due to polymerase slippage during replication, small size differences between alleles of a given microsatellite locus (as little as 2 bp in a locus comprised dinucleotide repeats) are possible. Because of this, PCR-amplified microsatellite DNA was traditionally labeled radioactively, separated on a sequencing gel, and then exposed on X-ray film overnight. Significant increases in the number of samples that can be typed in a day have been achieved by using automated fluorescent sequencers coupled with computer imaging systems. The recent advances in genome research have unraveled the genetic basis of heterosis using microsatellite markers in swine. The mapping for growth traits and birth weight by microsatellite markers has indicated that these QTL have important effects on growth traits and birth weight. But the effects of these QTL on some traits could differ between individuals because of the different genotypes of the QTL. The different effects could be attributed to different genotypes of microsatellite markers linked to the QTL. Therefore, a microsatellite locus could act as a significant marker locus when the effect reaches a certain significant level. Although the paternity identification using microsatellite markers in Holstein was well developed in some developed countries, it is worth to establish a new system for a particular dairy cattle population. Chinese yak and different endangered duck breeds were genetically differentiated with excellent characteristics using microsatellite markers. The study helped to better understand the genetic diversity, population structure of yaks and relative distinctiveness of yak genetic resources, and will assist in developing a national plan for conservation and utilization of yaks.

SNPs

Single nucleotide polymorphism (SNP) describes polymorphisms caused by point mutations that give rise to different alleles containing alternative bases at a given nucleotide position within a locus. Such sequence differences due to base substitutions have been well characterized since the beginning of DNA sequencing in 1977, but the ability to genotype SNPs rapidly in large numbers of samples was not possible until the application of gene chip technology in the late 1990s. SNPs are again becoming a focal point in molecular marker development since they are the most abundant polymorphism in any organism, adaptable to automation, and reveal hidden polymorphism not detected with other markers and methods. Theoretically, a SNP within a locus can produce as many as four alleles, each containing one of the four bases at the SNP site: A, T, C, and G. Practically, however, most SNPs are usually restricted to one of the two alleles (most often either the two pyrimidines C/ T or the two purines A/G) and have been regarded as bi-allelic. Obviously, their PIC is not as high as multi-allele microsatellites, but this shortcoming is balanced by their great abundance. SNP markers are inherited as co-dominant markers. Several approaches have been used for SNP discovery including SSCP analysis, heteroduplex analysis, and direct DNA sequencing. DNA sequencing has been the most accurate and most-used approach for SNP discovery. Random shotgun sequencing, amplicon sequencing using PCR, and comparative EST analysis are among the most popular sequencing methods for SNP discovery. SNPs are the most abundant class of genetic markers in the genome. Current estimates place the total number of SNPs in the human population as high as 10 million, and 4 million have already been detected. Many potential differences fixed by selection or genetic drift can be detected only at the level of resolution provided by SNP analysis. Moreover, some SNPs can be associated with particular phenotypes and therefore serve as mapping and diagnostic tools. Most SNPs have only two common alleles, simplifying the genotyping approaches and analysis. Many SNPs, of economically important traits in domestic animals have been identified in recent years.

ESTs

Expressed sequence tags (ESTs) are single-pass sequences generated from random sequencing of cDNA clones. The EST approach is an efficient way to identify genes and analyze their expression by means of expression profiling. It offers a rapid and valuable first look at genes expressed in specific tissue types under specific physiological conditions, or during specific developmental stages. ESTs are useful for the development of cDNA microarrays that allow analysis of differentially expressed genes to be determined in a systematic way, in addition to their great value in genome mapping. For genome mapping, ESTs are most useful for linkage mapping and physical mapping in animal genomics such as those of cattle and swine, where radiation hybrid panels are available for mapping non-polymorphic DNA markers. A radiation panel is composed of lines of hybrid cells, with each hybrid cell containing small fragments of irradiated chromosomes of the species of interest. Typically, the cells from species of interest are radiated to break chromosomes into small fragments. The radiated cells are unable to survive by themselves. However, the radiated cells can be fused with recipient cells to form hybrid cells retaining a short segment of the radiated chromosome. Characterization of the chromosomal break points within many hybrid cell lines would allow linkage and physical mapping of markers and genes.

APPLICATIONS OF ANIMAL MOLECULAR MARKERS TECHNOLOGY

Applications in Animal Health and Production

The development of DNA-based genetic markers has had a revolutionary impact on animal genetics. With DNA markers, it is theoretically possible to observe and exploit genetic variation in the entire genome. The application of DNA markers has allowed progress in genetic variability and inbreeding, parentage assignments, species and strain identification, and the construction of high-resolution linkage maps for different animal species. The advents of DNA marker technology have revolutionized the way animal genetic research is conducted. Broadly defined as the study of genes and their functions, genomics is rapidly impacting many facets of life, from health care and food safety to reproductions and prolificacy.

Improvement of Milk Production Traits

In dairy animals, the primary focus of selection has been to improve milk yield, and significant genetic improvement has been made in cattle using classical quantitative genetics. Milk yield is a polygenic trait and all the genes affecting it are difficult to know, but a few potential candidate genes have been recognized. A candidate gene is selected on the basis of known relationship between physiological or biochemical processes and the traits are tested as putative quantitative trait loci (QTL). It is well established that growth hormone (GH) released from pituitary gland plays an essential role in growth, mammary gland development and lactation process. Genetically improved animals for higher milk yield differed from low producers mainly in their regulation of nutrient utilization, and growth hormone exerts a key control in this process. The variation in milk yield has been reported to be associated with increased levels of GH in dairy cattle. GH gene shares a similar nucleotide sequence containing five exons and four introns in different mammalian species. In small ruminants, exon-4 and exon-5 explained higher diversity and can be correlated with performance data. Molecular marker assisted selection for improvement in milk and meat production in milch animals have been initiated. The alpha-lactalbumin encoding gene is essential for the biosynthesis of lactose in the mammary gland and is a potential quantitative trait locus in dairy animals. It is therefore an interesting candidate gene for MAS studies. Studies have been conducted to detect polymorphism in the full coding region of alpha-lactalbumin at the genetic level and to explore allelic variability of this gene. Jamunapari is the highest milk producer among local Indian goat breeds. PCR-SSCP of all four exons of alpha-lactalbumin (ALA) revealed a total of 9 gel phenotypes of Jamunapari breed of goat. Globally, polymorphism is reported only in exon-3 of ALA gene at position 3E+5 and 3E+7. Genetic evaluation is one of the key issues in dairy breeding, as the increase of genetic progress partially depends on the exact genetic evaluation based on the entire and correct pedigree. Because of the extensive application of artificial insemination in dairy breeding, the increase of mistakes in pedigree has been recorded. For example, the mistakes caused by repetitive insemination; the consequence of this scenario is the reduction of genetic progress.

Improvement of Meat Quality

Much progress in farm animal breeding has been made in the last few decades, but achieving greater understanding in the improvement of meat quality was very slow before molecular markers became an accessible technology with wide applications in breeding schemes. Meat quality is one of the economically important traits in farm animals. From the appearance of the raw material, quality requires analysis and classification of fat content, composition, tenderness, water-holding capacity, color, oxidative stability and uniformity. It is influenced by several factors, such as breed, genotype, feeding, fasting, pre-slaughter handling, stunning, slaughter methods, chilling and storage conditions. In brief, all the factors affecting meat quality can be divided into two aspects on the basis of genetics and management systems. For the genetic basis, the correct selection of breeds or lines is very important because the genetic influence on meat quality is very different among breeds as well as among animals in the same breed. Selective breeding has been carried out in large populations for thousands of years. Such strong selection, especially in recent centuries, has resulted in the accumulation of new mutations with favorable phenotypic effects. These new mutations can provide greater options, especially when molecular technology is used in breeding schemes. Genome research in farm animals progressed rapidly in recent years, moving from linkage maps to genome sequence. The work on farm animal genome sequencing began in the early 1990s, and assists in the understanding of how genomics function in various organisms. In March 2004, the first draft of the chicken genome was released. The chicken genome has a haploid size of 1200 Mb. It is not only a food animal that comprises 41% of the meat produced in the world, but also a model organism for studies of disease and biology. With the chicken genome sequence, especially the genome-wide screening in three chicken breeds yielding a set of 2.8 million SNP markers, chicken breeders will have a framework for investigating polymorphisms of informative quantitative traits to continue the directed evolution of these species. In October 2004, the first draft of the bovine genome sequence was deposited in a free public database. The whole-genome sequencing for pig began in 2005. All this genome information, especially the sequence information, will permit cross-species comparison of the effects of candidate gene allelic polymorphisms on meat quality. Meat quality trait has a multifactorial background and is controlled by an unknown number of quantitative trait loci (QTL). The main goal of genome research in farm animals is to map and characterize trait loci. There are two main strategies to identify trait loci—association tests using candidate genes and genome scans based on linkage mapping DNA markers. The information of the meat quality trait loci can be applied in breeding programs by using marker-assisted selection (MAS). Using different DNA marker technologies, several genes affecting meat quality have been identified. For example, the Halothane gene, the Rendment Napole (RN) gene and insulin-like growth factor-2 (IGF2) gene in pig, the calpastatin and the calpain one gene in bovine, callipyge phenotypes in sheep, etc. Advances in molecular genetics have led to the identification of genes or markers associated with genes that affect the meat quality trait. The molecular basis of meat quality is being revealed by functional genomics approaches. DNA technologies are beginning to change the way by which breeding animals are genetically selected and might soon determine how production animals are managed to better meet the specific market requirements. The technologies themselves have rapidly changed over the past decade, and this has forced changes in understanding by both the research community and livestock industry.

Prolificacy Improvement

Improving the prolificacy of sheep through within-breed selections is a slow process. The incorporation of a major gene for prolificacy into a flock using MAS allows increased selection pressure on the traits leading to increased genetic gain. The major gene has the advantage that it can be introduced into any new breed while retaining the new breed's characteristics. The breeding programs for genetic improvement of meat and wool characteristics as well as disease resistance and fecundity in sheep are now going on in different countries. MAS using FecB (Booroola) gene is warranted to increase litter size in sheep and will be of considerable economic value to mutton producers. FecB gene increases ovulation rate and litter size. Moreover, introgression of FecB gene could improve the fecundities of low prolific flocks.

Tameness and Animal Welfare

The intensive selection procedures for increased production in farm animals causes side-effects on animal behaviour. Modern genetics and genomics offer tools for the study of such side-effects. One of the most prominent examples of classical artificial selection for a behavioural trait is selection for tameness in silver foxes (Vulpes vulpes). Through more than 20 years of selection, lines were developed showing dog-like behaviour towards humans. With the discovery and mapping of polymorphic DNA markers, dense marker maps have been developed for most farm animal species, including cattle, pigs, and chickens. These dense marker maps are essential tools to dissect the underlying genetics of behavioural traits in animals by identifying chromosomal regions affecting polygenic traits, so called Quantitative Trait Loci (QTL), and the causative genes at these loci. Temperament of cattle is important for the safety of the farmer, and may have important bearing for animal welfare. The temperament of an animal can be defined as "an animal's behavioural response to handling by humans". In another study on dairy cattle, temperament was defined as "nervous/aggressive or docile behaviour during milking". The number of QTL for temperament as well as the locations of them differed substantially between the studies. Studies of gene expression patterns and epigenetic modifications caused by stress are likely to be important future instruments in understanding the genomics of animal welfare.

CONCLUSION

The genetic improvement of animals is a fundamental, incessant, and complex process. In recent years many methods have been developed and tested. The genetic polymorphism at the DNA sequence level has provided a large number of markers and revealed potential utility of application in animal breeding. Since the first demonstration of DNA-level polymorphism, known as the Restriction Fragment Length Polymorphism (RFLP), an almost unlimited number of molecular markers have accumulated. The invention of polymerase chain reaction (PCR) in accordance with the constantly increasing DNA sequence data also represents a milestone in this endeavour. The putting into practice of marker-based information for genetic improvement depends on the choice of an appropriate marker system for a given application. Selection of markers for different applications is influenced by certain factors—the degree of polymorphism (PIC), the automation of the analysis, radioisotopes used, reproducibility of the technique, and the cost involved. Presently, the huge development of molecular markers will continue in the near future. It is expected that molecular markers will serve as an underlying tool to geneticists and breeders to create animals as desired and needed by the society.

FURTHER READINGS

1. Allan, M.F. and Smith T.P.L. (2008) Present and future applications of DNA technologies to improve beef production, *Meat Science*. **(80):** 79-85.
2. Alves, B.C.A., Unanian, M.M. Silva, E., Oliveira, M. and Moreira-Filho, C.A.(2005) Use of RAPD markers for identifying Nelore bulls with early reproductive maturation onset, *Animal Reproduction Science*. **(85):** 183-191.
3. Beuzen N.D., Stear M.J., Chang K.C. (2000) Molecular markers and their use in animal breeding. *Vet. J.* **(160):** 42-52.
4. Bishop M.D., Hawkins G.A., Keeler C.L. (1995) Use of DNA markers in animal selection. *Theriogenology.* **(43):** 61-70.
5. Bishop M.D., Kappes S.M., Keele J.W., Stone R.T., Sunden S.L.F. *et al.* (1994) A genetic linkage map for cattle. *Genetics*. **(136):** 619-639.
6. Botstein D, White R.L, Skolnick M., Davis R.W. (1980) Construction of a genetic linkage map in man using restriction fragment length polymorphisms. *Am. J. Hum. Genet.* **(32):** 314-331.
7. Caetano-anolles G., Greshoff P. (1998) *DNA markers. Protocols, Applications, and Overviews*. Wiley-Liss. Inc. p. 364
8. Chambers G.K. and MacAvoy, E.S. (2000) Microsatellites, Consensus and controversy, *Comparative Biochemistry and Physiology part B*. **(126):** 455-476.
9. Chistiakov, D.A. Hellemans, B. and Volckaert F.A.M. (2006) Microsattelites and their genomic distribution, evolution, function and applications:a review with special reference to fish genetics, *Aquaculture*. **(255):** 1-29.
10. Collins D.W., Jukes T.H., (1994) Rates of transition and transversion in coding sequences since the human-rodent divergence. *Genomics.* **(20):** 386-396.

11. Collins F.S., Brooks L.D., Chakravarti A., (1998) A DNA polymorphism discovery resource for research on human genetic variation. *Genome Res.* **(8):** 1229-1231.
12. Cooper D.N., Krawczak M. (1989) Cytosine methylation and the fate of CpG dinucleotides in vertebrate genomes, *Hum. Genet.* **(83):** 181-188.
13. Cornuet J.M., Aulagnier S. Lek S., Franck S., Solignac M. (1996) Classifying individuals among infra-speci_c taxa using microsatellite data and neural networks. *C.R. Acad. Sci.* III **(319):** 1167-1177.
14. Dalvit, C., Marchi, M.D. and cassandro, M. (2007) genetic traceability of livestock products: a review, *Meat Science*. **(77):** 437-449.
15. Dodgson J.B., Cheng H.H., Okimotor R. (1997) DNA marker technology: A revolution in animal genetics. *Poult. Sci.* **(76):** 1108-1114.
16. Drinkwater R.D., Hetzel D.J.S. (1991) Application of molecular biology to understanding genotype-environment interactions in livestock production. In: *Proc. of an International Symposium on Nuclear Techniques in Animal Production and Health*. IAEA, FAO. Vienna, 15-19 April, 1991, 437-452.
17. Erhardt E., Weimann C. (2007) Use of molecular markers for evaluation of genetic diversity and in animal production. *Arch. Latinoam. Prod. Anim.* 15 **(1):** 63-66.
18. Gao, Y., Zhang, R., Hu, X. and Li, N. (2007) Application of genomic technologies to the improvement of meat quality of farm animals. *Meat Science*. **(77):** 36-45.
19. Garcia-mas J., Oliver M., Gomez-paniaguah H., DE vicente M.C. (2000) Comparing AFLP, RAPD and RFLP markers for measuring genetic diversity in melon. *Theor. Appl. Genet.* **(101):** 860-864.
20. Gerber S, Mariette S., Streiff R., Bodeness C., Kremer A. (2000) Comparison of microsatellites and amplified fragment length polymorphism markers for parentage analysis. *Mol. Ecol.* **(9):** 1037-1048.
21. Goldstein D.B., Linares A.R., Cavalli-sforza L.L., Feldman M.W. (1995) An evaluation of genetic distances for use with microsatellite loci. *Genetics.* **(139):** 463-471.
22. Goldstein D.B., Schlotterer C. (1999) *Microsatellites: Evolution and Applications.* Oxford University Press. New York.
23. Guimaraes, Ruane J., Scherf B., Sonnino A., Dargie J. (2007) Marker-assisted selection. Surrent status and future perspectives in srops, livestock, forestry and fish. Food and agriculture organization of the United Nations. Rome. p. 471
24. Gupta, N., Pandey, A., Malik, G. and Gupta, S.C. (2009) Single Nucleotide Polymorphism (SNP) in growth hormone gene of Jakhrana, a prominent milk goat breed in india. *Small Ruminant Research*. **(81):** 35-41.
25. Heaton M.P. (2000) SNP frequency and haplotype diversity in beef cattle cytokine genes. Plant & Animal Genome VIII Conf., January 9-12, 2000. San Diego, CA.
26. Hiendleder S., Thomsen H., Reinsch N., Bennewitz J., Leyhehorn B., Looft C., Xu N., Mededjugorac Djugorac I., Russ I., Kuhn C., Brockmann G.A., Blumel J., Brenig B., Reinhardt F., Reents R., Averdunk G., Schwerin M., Forster M., Kalm E., Erhardt G. (2003) Mapping of QTL for body conformation and behaviour in cattle. *J. of Heredity.* **(94):** 496-506.
27. Hua, G.H. and Yang, L.G. (2009) A review of research progress of Fec B gene in chinese breeds of sheep. *Animal Reproduction Science.* **(116):** 1-9.
28. Jain, A., Gour, D.S., Bisen, P.S., Prashant, Dubey, P.P., Sharma, D.K., Joshi, B.K. and Kumar, D. (2009) Single Nucleotide Polymorphism (SNP) in alpha-lactalbumin gene of Indian jamunapari breed of *Capra hircus*, *Small Ruminant Research*. **(82):** 156-160.
29. Jarne P., Lagoda, P.J.L. (1996) Microsatellites, from molecules to populations and back. *Tree.* **(11):** 424-429.
30. Jensen, P.,Buitenheis, B., Kjaer, J., Zanella, A., Mormede, P. and Pizzari, T. (2008) genetics and genomics of animal behavior and welfare challenges and possibilities. *Applied Animal Behavior Science*. **(113):** 383-403.
31. Jun R., Sheng H., Evens G., Shui A., Jun G., Ke-fei C., Neng-shui D. (2004) AFLP markers for genomic DNA fingerprinting in pigs. *Chinese Journal of Agricultural Biotechnology.* **(1):** 9-12.

32. Liu, Z.J. and Cordes, J.F. (2004) DNA marker technologies and their applications in aquaculture genetics. *Aquaculture*. **(238):** 1-37.
33. Montaldo H.H., Meza-herrera C.A. (1998) Use of molecular markers and major genes in the genetic improvement of livestock. *Journal of Biotechnology.* 1 **(2):** 1-7.
34. Oliver, M., Meehl, M.A., and Lust, G. (1997) Random Amplified Polymorphic DNA (RAPD) sequences as markers for canine genetic studies. *The American Genetic Association*. **(90):** 78-82.
35. Rastogi,G., Dharne, M.S., Walujkar, S., Kumar, A., Patole, M.S. and Shouche, Y.S. (2007) Species identification and authentication of tissue of animal origin using mitochondrial and nuclear markers. *Meat. Science*. **(76):** 666-674.
36. Sasazaki, S., Itoh, K., Arimitsu, S., Imada, T., Takasuga, A., Nagaishi, H., Takano, S., Mannen, H. and Tsuji, S. (2004) Development of breed identification markers derived from AFLP in beef cattle. *Meat Science*. **(67):** 275-280.
37. Sollero, B.P., Paiva, S.R., Faria D.A., Guimaraes, S.E.F., Castro, S.T.R., Egito, A.A., Albuquerque, M.S.M., Piorezan, U., Bertani, G.R. and Mariante, A. Da. S. (2009) Genetic diversity of Barzilian pig breeds evidenced by microsattelite markers. *Livestock Science*. **(123):** 8-15.
38. Spotter, A. and Distl, O. (2006) Genetic approaches to the improvement of fertility traits in the pig. *The Veterinary Journal*. **(172):** 234-247.
39. Su,Y., Long, R., Chen, G., Wu, X., Xie, K. and Wan, J. (2007) Genetic analysis of six endangered local duck population in china-based on microsatellite markers. *Journal of Genetics and Genomics*. 34 **(11):** 1010-1018.
40. Teneva A. (2009) molecular markers in animal genome analysis. *Biotechnology in Animal Husbandry.* 25 **(5-6):** 1267-1284.
41. Tian, F., Sun, D. and Zhang, Y. (2008) Establishment of paternity testing system using microsatellite markers in Chinese Holstein. *Journal of Genetics and Genomics*. **(35):** 279-284.
42. White P.S., Kwok P., Oefner P., Brookes A.J. (2001) 3rd Int. meeting on single nucleotide polymorphism and complex genome analysis: SNP's: 'Some notable progress'. *Eur. J. Hum. Gen.* **(9):** 316-318.
43. Williams J.G.K., Kubelik A.R., Livak K.J., Raflaski J.A., Tingey S.V. (1990) DNA polymorphisms amplified by arbitrary primers are useful as genetic markers. *Nucleic Acids Res.* **(18):** 6531-6535.
44. Young N.D. (1999) A cautiously optimistic vision for marker-assisted breeding. *Mol. Breed.* **(5):** 505-510.
45. Zabeau M., VOS P. (1993) Selective restriction fragment amplification: A general method for DNA fingerprinting. European Patent Application number 92402629.7. Publication number 0534858A1.
46. Zhang, G., Chen, W., Xue, M., Wang, Z., Chang, H., han, X., Liao, X. and Wang, D. (2008) Analysis of genetic diversity and population structure of Chinese yak breeds (Bos grunniens) using microsatellite markers. *Journal of Genetics and Genomics.* **(35):** 233-238.

CHAPTER

25

Embryo Transfer Technology

The embryo transfer technology (ETT) seems to be the technique of choice to increase the number of offspring from excellent parent stock. The non-surgical embryo recovery and transfer into cattle has allowed transfer of this technology from the laboratory to the farm so that increased number of offspring from a superior cow is possible. The ETT in cattle includes techniques like superovulation and breeding of donors, embryo collection and evaluation, selection of recipients and transfer of embryos. This chapter deals with the detailed method and applications of this technology.

Keywords: Embryo transfer technology (ETT), livestock improvement.

INTRODUCTION

Average annual milk production per adult breedable female has grown from 528 kg to 830 kg in cattle and 1041 kg to1355 kg per lactation in buffaloes. During early nineties, it reached to 2141 kg for crossbred cows, 634 kg for Desi and 1355 kg for buffaloes by the end of 2000. Demand for milk and milk products is projected at 7% per annum over the coming two decades, making the total projected demand of milk at 170 million tonnes by 2020 while the projected population size would be about 1500 millions, half of them constituting the urban population. At the current growth rate of 4.5% per annum, milk production will grow to some 140 million tonnes by 2020. The growth target for the milk production enhancement programme should, therefore, be 5-7% per annum to meet the minimum requirement of the teeming millions.

India has a very rich reservoir of genetic diversity and possesses some of the best breeds of cattle and buffaloes in the world. The country's population of 218.8 million cattle accounts for 17% of the total world population of cattle. The best indigenous germplasm of milk, draught and dual purpose animals account for 22-25% of the Indian cattle population, while 7-10% of the cattle population is cross-bred. Most of the indigenous breeds of cattle excel in draught capacity. The native livestock breeds exhibit a distinct superiority in utilizing poor quality feed and are adapted to withstand heat and show better resistance to tropical diseases.

Keeping these things in mind that our own genetic pool is depleting at a faster rate every day, there is an urgent need to conserve, multiply and disseminate the elite indigenous breeds of animals before it becomes too late. To meet these challenges, there are many potent reproductive technologies that can be utilized. Among others, Embryo Transfer Technology (ETT) has emerged as an important tool to improve livestock at faster rate, as in this technique genetic contribution of both the male and female is utilized simultaneously. Although the rate of genetic improvement in dairy cattle may range from 2.5-8.0%, it could be further increased 3-4 times through the ETT, especially in single offspring bearing animals like cow and buffaloes, if dairy herd replacement is selected from top 10% animals. Thus, the application of ETT is highly desirable to produce AI bulls from the best proven bulls and cows. This would be especially worthwhile in improving elite herds, the genetics of which could be spread over a large population using AI. ETT is now commonly used to produce AI sires from proven donor cows. (Although economics at this time would not support the use of embryo transfer technique, but the cattle industry can be benefited by use of bulls produced through a well designed programme.) There are various interdependent steps in embryo transfer technology, which result into birth of calves following *in vivo*/*in vitro* embryo production and transfer to surrogate mother.

CONCEPTS AND PRINCIPLES

It is believed in Indian mythology that Lord Mahavir, the founder of the Jain religion, in 599 BC was born through embryo transfer technology. Devananda was the wife of a priest, in whom the Mahavira was conceived and Trishala, the queen, into whose womb the Mahavira was later transplanted by the horse-headed creature, Harinegameshin. The transfer was deemed necessary because the saint and founders of the religions could only be born of royalty. The concept of transferring a baby from one uterus to another has been a part of human religious thinking for very long time.The technique was perhaps also used for the birth of 100 Kauravas from a single mother during the period of Mahabharat. However, it was Walter Heape who produced live young rabbits by embryo transfer for the 1st time in 1890. He transferred two Angora rabbit embryos into a gestating Belgian doe. It went on to produce a mixed litter of Belgian and Angora bunnies. Embryo transfer in animals reared for their meat began in 1930s using sheep and goat, but it was not until the 1950s that successful embryo transfer was reported in cattle and pigs by Jim Rowson at Cambridge, England. The transplantation of fertilized ova from one variety to another for the purpose of ascertaining whether, the parturition should take place under such circumstances or not was studied critically. He observed for the first time that both the mothers should be in season at about the same time. The necessity for such synchrony could not be firmly established experimentally for another 40 years in rats and for more than 60 years in rabbits . First evidence of interest in embryo transfer beyond the British Isles seems to be at Vienna by Biedl *et al.* (1922) in rabbits during 1911-1913. They made their transfers into the uterus rather than the oviduct, and from 70 experiments achieved only one pregnancy. The late 1020s and 1930s saw the beginning of activities on both sides of the Atlantic that ushered in the notion that embryo transfer could be of practical value to agriculture. In 1940, John Hammond wrote "The economic success of the animal industry depends on the successful production and proper development of the next generation of our farm animals. Experience gained on domestic animals will in future also enable man to control his development more easily. During the last 100 years, great advances have been made in the physical sciences, as witness steam engine, motor car, telephone and wireless. The experiments now proceeding in biological laboratories are beginning to show promise that during the next 100 years equal advances will be made in the control of the animal". Since then many milestones would have been achieved in the development of the embryo transfer technology. Some of the important events are as followings (Table 25.1).

Table 25.1 Milestones in the development of ETT in different species.

Events	*Species*	*Scientist*	*year*
Successful ET	Rabbit	Walter Heape	1890
Successful ET	Rat	J. S. Nicholus	1933
Successful superovulation	Cattle	Casida	1940
Successful ET	Sheep & Goat	B. L. Warwick & R. O. Berry	1949
Successful ET	Pig	A. V. Kvansnickii	1951
Successful ET	Cattle	E. L. Willet	1951
Baby girl in human	Human	Steptoe & Edwards	1979
Calf from frozen embryo	Cattle	Wilmet & Lea Rowson	1973
ET Calf	Buffalo	Morten Drost	1983
Calf born (IVM/IVF)	Buffalo	M. L. Madan	1990
Calf born (frozen embryo)	Buffalo	A. K. Misra	1991
First OPU calf	Buffalo	Shiv Prasad	2008

Embryo transfer is a technique by which embryos are collected from a donor female and transferred to recipient females, which serve as surrogate mothers for the remainder of pregnancy. Embryo transfer techniques have been applied to nearly every species of domestic animal and too many species of wildlife and exotic animals, including humans and non-human primates. Within the past decade, the degree of sophistication of embryo transfer procedures has evolved to permit complete utilization of non-surgical procedures in cow, long term embryo culture and storage with cryopreservation, and, more recently, micromanipulation and many techniques associated with genetic engineering. This is a rapidly developing science with a very short lag-time between discovery and application. The potential applications continue to increase with the development of new technology.

BASIC STEPS IN EMBRYO TRANSFER TECHNOLOGY

Purpose: Embryo transfer is done for a number of purposes, which include the following:

(i) To increase the number of offspring, either male or female, from a genetically superior female.

(ii) To genetically test the bulls for inherited defects. Mating a bull to six or eight of his superovulated daughters will exhibit the recessive genes a bull carries more accurately and in much less time than by testing the population at large.

(iii) To decrease variability in research subjects for the study of the physiology, pathology and immunology of reproduction or other traits.

(iv) For long-term storage of embryos by freezing.

(v) For disease control. Many diseases present in the mother will not be transmitted by the embryo.

(vi) For the treatment of infertility. In general, reproductive traits are less heritable. However, one should consider possible decreases in fertility of subsequent generations before using infertile donors extensively.

(vii) For rapid genetic change within a small population (e.g., from grade to pure-bred herd).

Events in the Entire Process of ETT

ETT involves various interdependent steps in the entire process, which are:

1. Selection of donor and recipient
2. Management of donor and recipient
3. Superovulation/treatment of donor for optimum ova
4. Synchronization of estrous cycles of donor and recipients
5. Breeding of donors
6. Collection of embryo
7. Evaluation of embryo
8. Transfer of embryo
9. Pregnancy following embryo transfer

Selection of donor and recipient

Selection of donor animal should be based on genetic superiority over contemporaries, fertility of the animal and marketability of the calves produced. Animal should have normal reproductive organs, regular cycling, highest milk production record. It should have completed at least one lactation and also should have completed 60 days post partum. The cervix should be negotiable during diestrus, free from diseases and should not be more than 10 years of age. Premature and non-cycling heifers and even calves serve as donor. Studies revealed that even one-year-old buffalo heifers could be successfully superovulated with an average of four ovulation points.

Embryo can be transferred to any recipient of any genetic makeup, provided she has high fertility index, aged between 3-6 years, free from diseases and cervix is negotiable during diestrus phase of estrous cycle.

Management of donor and recipient

Embryo donor/recipient animals should be in positive energy balance, free from worm infestation, and mineral deficiency, vaccinated against tuberculosis, para tuberculosis and Brucellosis etc. Estrus should be detected very critically with the help of teaser bull at every 6-8 hours interval and standing estrus should be recorded.

Superovulation/treatment of donor for optimum ova

The objective of superovulation treatment in the cow is to obtain the maximum number of fertilized and transferable embryos with a high probability of producing pregnancies. Superovulation is the development and ovulation of more than the normal number of follicles within an individual. It is one of the most important steps in embryo transfer programme as it exploits the use of female germ pool and ensures the supply of embryos. Induction of superovulation was reported for the first time by Casida *et al.* (1943). Since then various reports on this aspect have been published. Totey *et al.* (1988) have superovulated 29 Holstein x Sahiwal cattle and found 6.1-6.7, 1.0 -3.0 mean number of corpora lutea, transferable embryos per animal respectively. Further, Totey *et al.* (1989)

have reported 3.90 mean number of transferable embryos. Singla and Madan (1990) found ovulation and embryo recovery upto 6.89 ± 0.99, 3.58 ± 0.98 per donor, respectively. Singla *et al.* (1989) have also studied the superovulatory response during different days of estrous cycle and concluded that superovulatory response, number of embryo recovered and number transferred were better on day 9 of the estrous cycle, compared to days 10, 11, 12 and 13 of the estrous cycle. Presence of dominant follicles before superovulatory treatment may decrease the superovulatory response. The number of corpora lutea (CL) determined by ultrasonography as well as by rectal palpation performed on day 6 of standing estrus was significantly higher, i.e., 11.20 ± 3.70 Vs 3.25 ± 0.75 or 10.40 ± 3.91 Vs 2.25 ± 0.75 in non-dominant follicle group compared to dominant follicle group, respectively. The total number of follicles before the beginning of superovulatory treatment were also high in non-dominant group (22.00±5.95) than dominant (12.5 Vs 1.26) group. More specifically small size follicles (2-3 mm) were in more number in non-dominant group (13.80 Vs 8.00). Superovulatory studies in Ongole cows revealed less number of viable embryos (1.79 ± 0.28). In repeat breeder animal, it was 2.31 ± 1.56, 1.21 ± 0.54 and 0.84 ± 0.60 ovulations, embryo recovery and transferable embryos, respectively.

Superovulatory response was found better in the animals having higher levels of progesterone on the day of initiation of superovulatory treatment compared to those having lower levels of progesterone on the day of initiation of gonadotropin treatment. Further they found that the higher levels of zinc (Zn) and copper (Cu) were also higher in the animals responding well to gonadotropin treatment.

Embryo transfer work at Sabarmati Ashram Gaushala, Bidaj (Gujarat) under DBT project during 1987-1992 had superovulated 528 cattle with total and viable average embryo of 4.8 and 2.3 per cattle with 28 pregnancies after transfer in synchronized recipients. Later on the results improved to 7.1 and 3.7 total and viable embryos per cattle at the Bidaj and resulted into the birth of 94 calves successfully. Extensive work on embryo transfer work was done by National Dairy Development Board (NDDB) as lead agency, under Science and Technology project on cattle herd improvement for increased productivity using embryo transfer technology and supported by National Dairy Research Institute (NDRI), National Institute of Immunology (NII), Central Institute for Research on Buffalo (CIRB) and Indian Veterinary Research Institute (IVRI). One thousand two hundred fifty eight (1258) flushings were done with total and viable recovery of 4.76 and 2.43 embryos /flush. Similar work was done by NDDB under field conditions where 153 flushings were done with 5.45 and 2.59 as total and viable embryos/flush, respectively (NDDB, 1992).

Work on embryo transfer technology at various centers (NDDB, NDRI, IVRI, NII) and under field conditions resulted into 1929 flushings with 8805 (4.58/flush) and 4340 (2.26/flush) total and viable embryo, respectively (NDDB, 1992). Further, the work was continued at NDDB during 1992-1997, which resulted into 1472 flushings with 4630 viable embryos (3.15/flush) (NDDB, 1997).

Effect of various pretreatments (hCG, Estradiol, PMSG, GnRH) to enhance the superovulatory response was also studied. Mean ovulation rate, unovulatory follicles and embryo recovered in Sahiwal pretreated with 250 IU i/m hCG on 9th day of estrous cycle and 2 mg estradiol valerate s/c on 10th day of estrous cycle were 5.4 ± 3.31, 5.00 ± 3.06 and 3.00 ± 2.68. A non-significant increase in the ovulation rate, egg recovery and number of transferable embryos and a significant decrease in the number of unovulated large follicles was observed in the PMSG+GnRH treated group compared to the group given PMSG alone.

Manipulation of dominant follicle by hCG, Estradiol Valerate and GnRH regimen does not yield better superovulatory response as compared to untreated animals. Further, the effect of buserelin acetate on day 8 or 9 of estrous cycle was evaluated and found not beneficial for superovulatory response.

Gonadotropin

In buffalo, though eCG (2000-3000 IU) has been used for superovulation, 21-30 mg PPFE or 600 mg Folltropin (Vetrepharm, Canada) was observed to be more effective. The comparative studies of superovulation with FSH/eCG suggested that FSH (Folltropin) induced better superovulatory response and lead to the recovery of significantly more TE (4.4-4.7 vs 0.7-3.2) and VE (2.3-3.1 vs 0.6-1.2).

Compared to FSH administered twice daily for 4 days, 5 days treatment regimens gave better superovulatory response and embryo recovery in buffaloes. Initial comparison of superovulation of buffaloes with constant/ tapering dosage of FSH administration revealed no significant difference in the ovulation rate or embryo recovery, however, subsequent trials involving large number of buffaloes suggested better superovulatory response and higher yield of embryos with tapering dosage of FSH. Response of buffaloes to superovulation with FSH-P1 (Shering, USA) was observed to be poor than Folltropin, as its first time use with optimum dose resulted in average 6.8 ovulations and recovery of 4.4 TE and 3.1 VE. Later, use of 600 mg NIH-FSH-P1 (1.5 vial of Folltropin) on over 300 buffaloes induced average > 6.0 ovulations and recovery of 2.0 to 2.9 VE on the farm and 6.2 ovulations and 2.8 VE in the field. A trial on repeated superovulations using same superovulatory protocol for the first time on 41 buffaloes lead to an average 8.2 ovulations and recovery of 3.4 VE.

In cattle and buffalo, since the advent of PGF2a, gonadotropins are generally administered during mid cycle when the CL is fully functional and progesterone (P4) concentration is highest, as its level at the time of initiation of superovulation treatment had positive correlation with superovulatory response in buffalo. An attempt to improve CL function and thereby superovulatory response by administration of the GnRH on day 5 of the estrous cycle before superovulation failed to increase the ovulation rate or embryo recovery. Also, attempts to superovulate buffaloes during late (13-15 days) luteal phase did not influence the ovulation rate (Figure 25.1).

Route/Dose of Administration of FSH

Short half life of FSH necessitates its intramuscular (i.m.) administration twice daily for a period of 3 to 5 days, resulting in repeated handling of donor, which is not only stressful but also requires repeated travelling to considerable distances if the donors are located at different places in the rural areas. To overcome this problem, attempts were made to regulate slow absorption of FSH by injecting total dose of FSH as a single dose subcutaneously (s.c). Initially, results following s.c. administration of FSH were similar to multiple i.m. FSH treatment, however, subsequently, s.c. administration of FSH resulted in the poor superovulatory response and embryo recovery. In cows also, multiple i.m. injection regimen seems to have produced better superovulatory response than a single s.c. injection. Intra-vulvo sub-mucosal route (ivsm) was also studied for gonadotropin

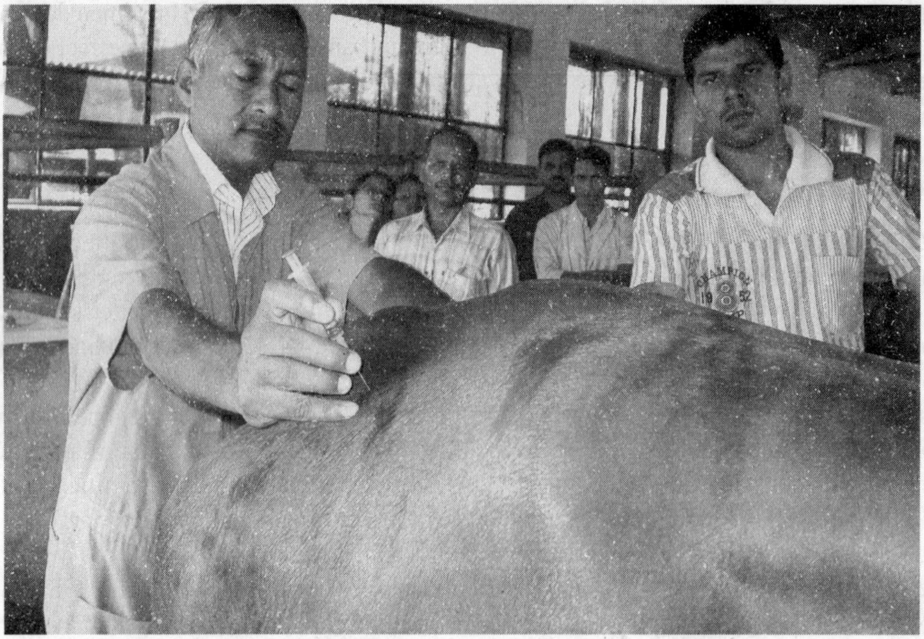

Figure 25.1 Superovulation of donor with gonadotropin.

treatment for superovulation. Mishra and Mishra (1998) reported significantly higher superovulatory response (9.83 ± 1.14 CL) and VE recovery (5.00 ± 0.97) with 50 NIH Super–Ov by using ivsm route compared to i.m. route. Also, half of the dose of Super–Ov by ivsm route resulted in recovery of VE similar to double dose (50 NIH) of Super–Ov by i.m. route (1.66 ± 0.62 vs 1.83 ± 0.70 VE).

Embryo Development/Transport Rate and Day of Nonsurgical Embryo Collection

Knowledge of time of arrival of embryos in the uterus and their subsequent development is necessary to decide the time of collection of embryos of desired stages. One of our studies, in which 30 elite buffaloes were sacrificed, demonstrated that nearly all the embryos reached uterus around day 5.25 after the onset of superovulatory estrus, and most of the early stage (4 cell) embryos developed to 8 to 16-cell/early morula by day 5, morula/compact morula by day 5.5 and blastocysts by day 6. Recovery of 11 hatched blastocysts (of total 184 embryos recovered from 56 buffaloes) following non-surgical embryo collection between Day 6.0 to 6.5 in our earlier study indicated that buffalo embryos develop very fast after reaching the uterus (~ Day 5.25) and hatch (~ Day 6.0-6.5), leaving only about half a day to collect embryos prior to hatching. Thus, the ideal time for the non surgical embryo collection is day 5.5 to 6.0 after the estrus. In this respect, the buffalo seems to differ from superovulated cattle, as in the latter species the ideal time for non surgical embryo collection is Day 7 ± 1 after superovulatory estrus. Embryo development in superovulated buffalo varies considerably and various stages of embryos (8 cells to expanded blastocyst) may be recovered from the same donor buffalo.

Gonadotropin Treatment Protocol

Gonadotropin treatment can be started any day between day 9-14 of the estrous cycle either as single or multiple doses regimen. Experiments over long period on superovulations have concluded that multiple dose regimen is more effective in causing better superovulatory response in cattle and buffaloes (Tables 25.2 and 25.3).

Table 25.2 Superovulatory treatment with FSH-P.

Days of treatment	*Donors*	*Recipients*
– 03	Lutalyse, 25 mg, i/m	Lutalyse, 25 mg, i/m
00	Estrus	Estrus
10	Folltropin, 65 mg, i/m (M)	
	Folltropin, 65 mg, i/m (E)	
11	Folltropin, 55 mg, i/m (M)	Lutalyse, 25 mg, i/m (E)
	Folltropin, 55 mg, i/m (E)	
12	Folltropin, 45 mg, i/m (M)	
	Lutalyse, 25 mg i/m (M)	
	Folltropin, 45 mg, i/m (E)	
13	Folltropin, 35 mg, i/m (M)	–
	Folltropin, 35 mg, i/m (E)	
14	Estrus and AI	Estrus, no breeding

Table 25.3 Superovulatory treatment with FSH-E.

Days of treatment	*Donors*	*Recipients*
– 03	Lutalyse, 25 mg, i/m	Lutalyse, 25 mg, i/m
00	Estrus	Estrus
10	FSH, 7.5 mg, i/m (M)	–
	FSH, 7.5 mg, i/m (E)	
11	FSH, 6.5 mg, i/m (M)	Lutalyse, 25 mg, i/m (E)
	FSH, 6.5 mg, i/m (E).	
12	FSH, 6.0 mg, i/m (M)	–
	Lutalyse, 25 mg i/m (M)	
	FSH, 6.0 mg, i/m (M)	
13	FSH, 5.0 mg, i/m (M)	–
	FSH, 5.0 mg, i/m (E)	
14	Estrus and AI	Estrus, no breeding

Physiology and Endocrinology of the Normal Bovine Estrous Cycle

The endogenous control of the bovine estrous cycle involves the interrelated secretion of a number of hormones from the hypothalamus, anterior pituitary, ovaries and uterus. These include gonadotroplin releasing hormone (GnRH) from the hypothalamus, follicle stimulating hormone (FSH) and luteinizing hormone (LH) from the pituitary gland, estrogen, progesterone and inhibin from the ovary and prostaglandin ($PGF_2\alpha$) from the uterus. The primary timing mechanism of the bovine estrous cycle is the demise of the corpus luteum (CL), which occurs about day 17-18 in the normal cycling, non-pregnant cow. The simplest hypothesis for regression of the CL is that the non-pregnant uterus secretes a luteolytic agent into the uterine venous blood. This material is transferred through a local veno-arterial pathway to the ovarian artery whereby it reaches the ovary and causes luteolysis. $PGF_2\alpha$ has been proposed as the natural luteolytic agent, although definitive proof and details of the mechanism(s) of action are unclear. Regression of the CL results in a rapid fall in serum progesterone concentrations to values less than 1 ng/ml. LH pulse frequency increases and follicular growth is further stimulated. The growth and maturation of the preovulatory follicle results in increasing secretion of estradiol, which causes estrogenic changes in the oviduct and uterus, behavioral estrus, and a preovulatory release of LH. The preovulatory LH peak results in resumption of oocyte meiosis, ovulation 24-32 h later (the LH peak occurs around the onset of estrus) and luteinization of the ovulated follicle to form a secreting corpus hemorrhagicum. Growth and development of the corpus hemorrhagicum into a fully functional CL results in progestational changes in the oviduct and uterus that are conducive to embryonic development and establishment of pregnancy. Should pregnancy not occur, the cycle will begin again with the demise of the CL on about day 17-18 following ovulation.

It has now been shown by ultrasonography that follicles in cattle develop in a wave-like fashion. Bovine estrous cycles are composed of 2 or 3 waves of follicular development. A follicular wave consists of a group of growing antral follicles 3-6 mm in diameter from which a dominant follicle is selected, while the remaining follicles become subordinate and undergo atresia. In both 2- and 3-wave estrous cycles, emergence of the first follicular wave occurs on the day of ovulation (day 0), while the second wave emerges 9 or 10 days after ovulation in 2-wave cycles, and on 8 or 9 days after ovulation in 3-wave cycles, with a third wave emerging on day 15 or 16. Duration of the estrous cycle is approximately 20 days in 2-wave cycles and 23 days in 3-wave cycles. The dominant follicle present at the time of luteolysis will become the ovulatory follicle, and emergence of the next wave is delayed until the ensuing ovulation. The proportion of animals with 2- vs. 3-wave cycles is probably more or less equally distributed. Follicular waves have been reported in heifers before puberty, Adams (1998), and postpartum cows before the first ovulation, Adams (1998). Follicle waves persist in pregnant animals until approximately the last 3 weeks before parturition.

Recruitment of follicular waves and selection of a dominant follicle is based on differential responsiveness to FSH and LH, Adams (1993). Surges in plasma FSH are responsible for eliciting the emergence of a follicular wave. FSH is subsequently suppressed by products of the growing follicles (estradiol and inhibin). In each wave, the follicle that first acquires LH receptors becomes the dominant follicle while subordinates undergo atresia. Suppression of LH as a consequence of progesterone secretion by the CL causes the dominant follicle to eventually cease its metabolic functions and it begins to regress. This leads to FSH release and emergence of a new follicular wave. Luteal regression allows LH pulse frequency to increase. The dominant follicle increases its growth and dramatically higher concentrations of estradiol result in a positive feedback on the hypothalamo-pituitary axis and a surge of LH followed by ovulation.

Estrus synchronization and superovulation are critical components of an embryo transfer program. These techniques involve the manipulation of the basic endocrine patterns outlined above. The key to successful estrus synchronization is obtaining closely synchronized, rapid declines in circulating progesterone to values <1 ng/ml and synchronous growth and ovulation of a viable follicle. It follows, therefore, that $PGF_2\alpha$ is effective only when a fully developed CL is present (days 7-18 of the cycle), and withdrawal of exogenous progesterone is effective only if either natural or induced regression of the CL has occurred. If properly implemented, within the physiological constraints of their mechanism of action, current techniques for estrus synchronization are highly successful. However, variation in ovarian follicular wave dynamics makes it difficult to control the time of estrus and ovulation precisely.

Hormone Profiles in Superovulated Cows

Low progesterone concentrations at the time of initiation of gonadotropin treatment have been shown to be related to a reduced superovulatory response indicating the importance of a functional CL. Progesterone increased within 24 h after treatment with pregnant mare serum/equine chorionic gonadotropin (eCG) or a crude pituitary extract suggesting a luteotrophic action of these gonadotropins. This did not occur with more highly purified pituitary extracts. Normally, the decline in progesterone is rapid after treatment with $PGF_2\alpha$. Levels of progesterone dropped to less than 1 ng/ml of serum within 10-32 h. Ovulation was shown to occur approximately 72 h after $PGF_2\alpha$ treatment in superstimulated cows. At the onset of estrus, progesterone concentrations were lower in superstimulated cows that yielded good quality embryos than in cows that yielded unfertilized ova. A high level of progesterone at the time of estrus may affect LH release and sperm transport and capacitation. After ovulation, the increase in serum progesterone concentration occurred earlier and the slope of the curve was steeper as the number of CL increased in superovulated cattle.

Although embryo transfer technique is widely used around the world, variability in response to the hormonal treatments remains one of the limitations to the widespread application and success of this technology. With a better understanding of ovarian function has come a greater capability of controlling it. Recent protocols, designed to control both luteal and follicular function, permit the initiation of superstimulatory treatments at a self-appointed time and provide the possibilities for superstimulation of cows that have abnormal ovarian function.

Manipulation of the Follicular Wave for Superstimulation

The conventional protocol of initiating ovarian superstimulation during mid-cycle was originally based on anecdotal and experimental information in which a greater superovulatory response was reported when superstimulatory treatments were initiated 8-12 days after estrus. However, none of these early studies evaluated follicular status at the time of initiation of gonadotrophin treatments.

Through information generated by ultrasonography, it is now known that 8-12 days after estrus (equivalent to Days 7-11 after ovulation) would be the approximate time of emergence of the second follicular wave in 2- or 3-wave cycles and a cohort of growing follicles would be present. However, the day of emergence of the second follicular wave differs among individuals and is 1 or 2 days later in two- versus three-wave cycles. In this regard, it has been clearly shown that superovulatory response was higher when superstimulatory treatments were initiated at the time of wave emergence. As little as 1 day asynchrony significantly reduced the superovulatory response compared to initiating treatments on the day of wave emergence.

Based on the duration of the developmental phases of the dominant follicle in two- and three-wave interovulatory intervals, approximately 20% (4 or 5 days) of the estrous cycle is available for initiating treatment at the time of follicular wave emergence. Therefore, 80% of the estrous cycle is not conducive to an optimal superovulatory response. The necessity of waiting until mid-cycle to initiate superstimulatory treatments implies monitoring estrus and an obligatory delay. To obviate these problems, an alternative approach is to initiate superstimulation treatments subsequent to the synchronization of follicular wave emergence. Basically, there are three methods of synchronizing follicle wave emergence for superstimulation.

Methods of Synchronizing Folicle Wave Emergence

Follicle ablation

One approach to the synchronization of follicle wave emergence involves transvaginal ultrasound-guided follicle ablation of all follicles >5 mm, regardless of the stage of estrous cycle. This removes the suppressive effects of follicle products (estradiol and inhibin) on FSH release. As a results, FSH surges and new follicular wave emerges 1 day later. Superstimulatory treatments are then administered, beginning 1 day after ablation and $PGF_2\alpha$ is administered 48 or 72 h later. The timing of estrus was more synchronous when a progestin device was inserted for the period of superstimulation and 2 injections of PGF were administered on the day of progestin removal. Transvaginal ultrasound-guided follicle ablation of all follicles or just the dominant follicle during mid-diestrus, followed in 2 days by superstimulation, also resulted in a higher superovulatory response than cows in which the dominant follicle was not ablated. Conversely, in a retrospective analysis of superovulatory responses of lactating dairy cows, follicle ablation resulted in a significantly higher number of ova/embryos, but a comparable number of transferable embryos than cows superstimulated 7 - 13 days after estrus. In a more recent study, ablation of the 2 largest follicles at random stages of the cycle was as efficacious as ablating all follicles >5 mm in synchronizing follicular wave emergence for superstimulation. However, it is always advised that a progestin device be used during superstimulation.

GnRH

Another method of synchronizing follicular wave emergence for superstimulation could involve the use of GnRH or porcine LH (pLH) to induce ovulation of a dominant follicle followed by emergence of a new follicle wave 2 days later. However, the administration of GnRH or pLH does not always induce ovulation and if ovulation does not occur, follicle wave emergence will not be synchronized. Therefore, the reported asynchrony in follicular wave emergence (range, 3 days before treatment to 5 days after treatment) suggests that GnRH-based approaches may not be feasible for superstimulation. In a study involving 3 different experiments, GnRH or pLH treatments consistently resulted in a lower number of embryos than when follicular wave emergence was synchronized with other methods.

Estradiol and progesterone

Traditionally, estradiol has been administered near the beginning of progestin treatment to induce luteolysis and allow for shortened progestin treatment periods. The mechanism involves suppression of FSH and possibly LH. The initial suppression of FSH and LH results in regression of FSH-

and LH-dependent follicles. Once follicle regression begins and the exogenously administered estradiol is metabolized, FSH surges and a new follicle wave emerges 1 day later. The use of a short acting estradiol-17β in progestin-implanted cows was followed by the emergence of a new wave, approximately 3 to 5 days later, regardless of the stage of follicular growth at the time of treatment. Estradiol-17β is normally injected with 50 to 100 mg of progesterone at the same time as placement of a progestin device. The progesterone prevents an estrogen-induced preovulatory-like LH surge in those animals that do not have a functional CL, and appears to cause regression of LH-dependent follicles.

Therefore, preferred approach for synchronization of follicular wave emergence prior to superstimulation is an injection of 5 mg estradiol-17β + 100 mg progesterone at the time of insertion of progestin releasing device, with FSH beginning 4 days later. Data from experimental and commercial superovulation programs have shown that the superovulatory response of donors given estradiol-17β and progesterone at unknown stages of the estrous cycle was comparable to that of donors superstimulated 8-12 days after observed estrus.

Synchronization of estrous cycles of donor and recipients

Synchrony between the embryo and the uterine endometrium is essential for the establishment of pregnancy and birth. When synchronous condition does not occur, a variety of complications result that include failure of embryo to implant, early embryonic mortality, and retarded embryo growth. All these complications appear to be induced within a week of embryonic development. Progesterone appears to play a causative role in establishing the abnormal growth of the fetus by decelerating or accelerating embryonic development. This may act through increasing the transport of blood born growth factors into the uterine lumen or by stimulating the release of growth factors from the endometrium directly.

Prostaglandin $F_2\alpha$ or its analogues are administered to embryo donor cows at 48-72 hours after gonadotropin treatment initiation. Prostaglandin $F_2\alpha$ causes luteal regression and consequently a marked decrease in serum progesterone, which is necessary to permit the final stage of follicular development, and onset of estrus and ovulation.

It is very important that the donor and the recipient should have come in estrus at almost the same time. The more closely they are synchronized, the better are the chances of conception because the embryo gets almost same environment in the recipient. Synchronization of about half day is better since animals that are thought to be half day asynchronous, may be asynchronous by full day. As far as possible, it is better to choose the recipients, which have shown estrus one day before donor than the one's which have shown estrus one day after.

Methods of Synchronization

Luteolysis by exogenous prostaglandin: Prostaglandins are produced from endometrium and carried to ovaries through utero ovarian vein. The veno constrictive effects of $PGF_2\alpha$ may induce hypoxia, which in turn results into luteolysis. When exogenous prostaglandin is used in cows or buffaloes during 6-16 days of the estrous cycle, the plasma progesterone level rapidly declines to less than 1 ng/ml within 24 hours. Estrus is then usually exhibited within 36 to 72 hours. Recipients synchronized with $PGF_2\alpha$ must be treated 12-24 hours before donor cows because it induces estrus in recipients in 60-72 hours compared to donors' 36-48 hours. Recipients can be synchronized by adopting one of the following ways:

- Prostaglandin is injected @ 25 mg i/m in animals having corpus luteum. Estrus will occur within 2-4 days and majority of them will take about 60 hours.
- Progesterone releasing intravaginal devices are also used for the induction of estrus. The device is inserted into vagina and kept there for 10-11 days and then removed from the vagina. Estrus will occur within 2-4 days.
- Crestar or Synchromate–B ear implants are very successfully used for the induction of estrus in recipients. Silastic capsule (ear implant) is inserted in the outer pinna of the ear and kept there for 9 days and then removed. Most of the recipients will report to estrus within 2-3 days after removal of the ear implant.
- Progesterone administration for long periods also extends the luteal phase of the estrous cycle, and as long as high concentration of the progesterone is maintained, the animal does not exhibit estrus. On withdrawal of progesterone source, the blood level of the progesterone drops down, mimicking the proestrus endocrinological conditions and animal comes into estrus. Nowadays longer duration progesterone therapy (18-21 days) is usually not adopted because of suppression of the fertility at the induced estrus. Shorter duration treatment (8-10 days) can lead to normal fertility. However, short duration treatment is not completely effective in controlling the estrous cycle. If administration begins early in the cycle, the natural CL may outlive the exogenous progesterone treatment and therefore synchronization will not occur. This necessitates the incorporation of a luteolytic agent along with progestogens.

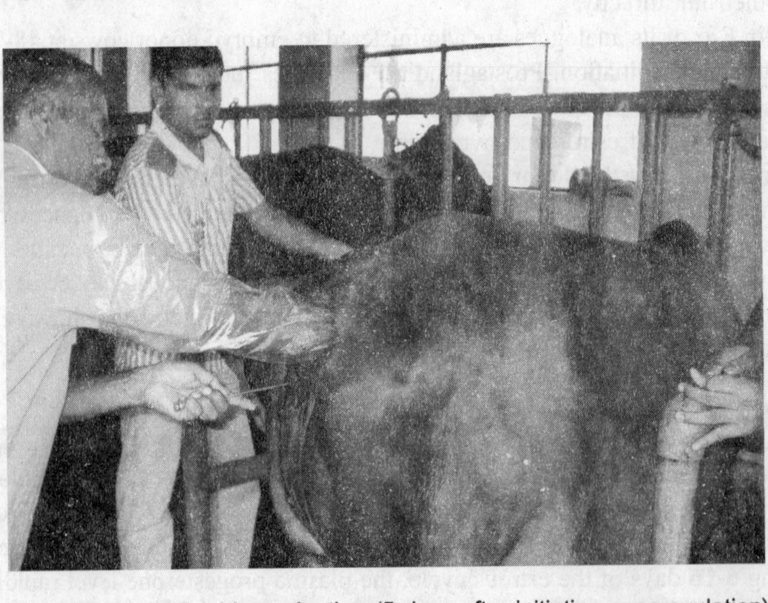

Figure 25.2 Artificial insemination (5 days after initiating superovulation).

Breeding of donors

The donor animals should be watched carefully for external signs of estrus every six hours after 24 hours of $PGF_2\alpha$ injection. The estrus is established on the basis of physical signs of external genitalia, mucus discharge per rectal examination, mounting on other herd mates and by parading of teaser bull. Donor cows are bred three times at 12 hours intervals through artificial insemination using high quality semen, which will cover the protracted period of ovulation (Figure 25.2).

Collection of embryo

Embryos descend into the uterus 4-5 days after estrus and the collection is done between 6-8 days. The donor animals are restrained into cattle crate and prepared for collection. The ovaries are palpated per rectum to estimate the number of CL and unovulated follicles. The estimation of superovulatory response also helps to know the efficiency of flushing. Usually recovery of 50-80% embryos of the total number of CL counted is considered satisfactory. Nowadays embryos are collected by non-surgical method in which catheter along with sanitary sheath is introduced in vagina. On reaching the external os, sheath is broken and catheter is introduced into the cervical canal. Some time cervical dilator may be passed to know the patency of the canal. After negotiating through the cervix and crossing the uterine body, the catheter is first passed into the horn on the

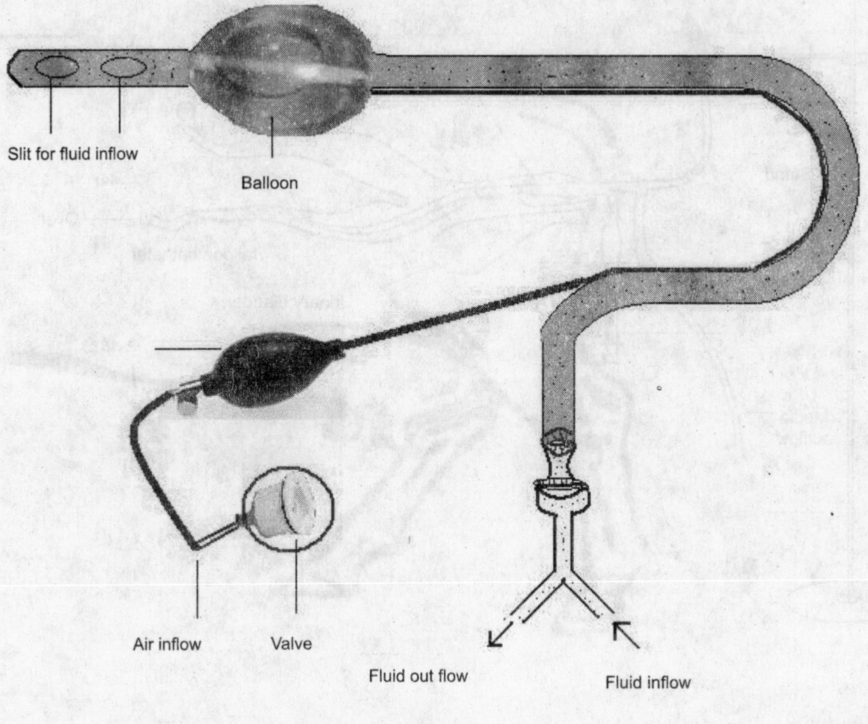

Figure 25.3 Rusch catheter for recovery of embryo.

side of the ovary having a better response. The stylet is unlocked and withdrawn, about 2-3 inches. The rubber catheter is introduced further deep and the process is repeated till the tip of the catheter is positioned about 2 inches from the uterotubal junction. With the help of a syringe, about 12-20 ml of air is infused to inflate the rubber balloon to hold the catheter in the uterine horn after which the stylet is removed (Figure 25.3). Care should be taken while inflating the balloon because over-inflating the balloon will result in the rupture of endometrium. Completely closed tubing system is attached to the catheter with an adapter. The flushing medium is held in one liter capacity bottle and hung above the animal in an inverted position after fixing the tunings to it. The three tubes joined together by the glass Y-junction have tweezer clamp to control the inflow and outflow of the medium into or from the animal. About 10 to 20 ml of medium is passed through the tubings to rinse it and keep it filled and the filter wet. Flushing medium, 20-30 ml, is infused to one horn, then the inflow is cut off and the uterine horn gently massaged to dislodge the embryos from the uterine endometrial folds. Then the outflow tweezer is opened and the flushed medium is collected in the filter by gravity flow. Minimum 1 cm level of medium is left in the filter even after it has been drained out through a filter outflow tube into a separate collection bottle. This is repeated till about 400-500 ml of medium has been used. After one horn is flushed, the balloon is deflated and the

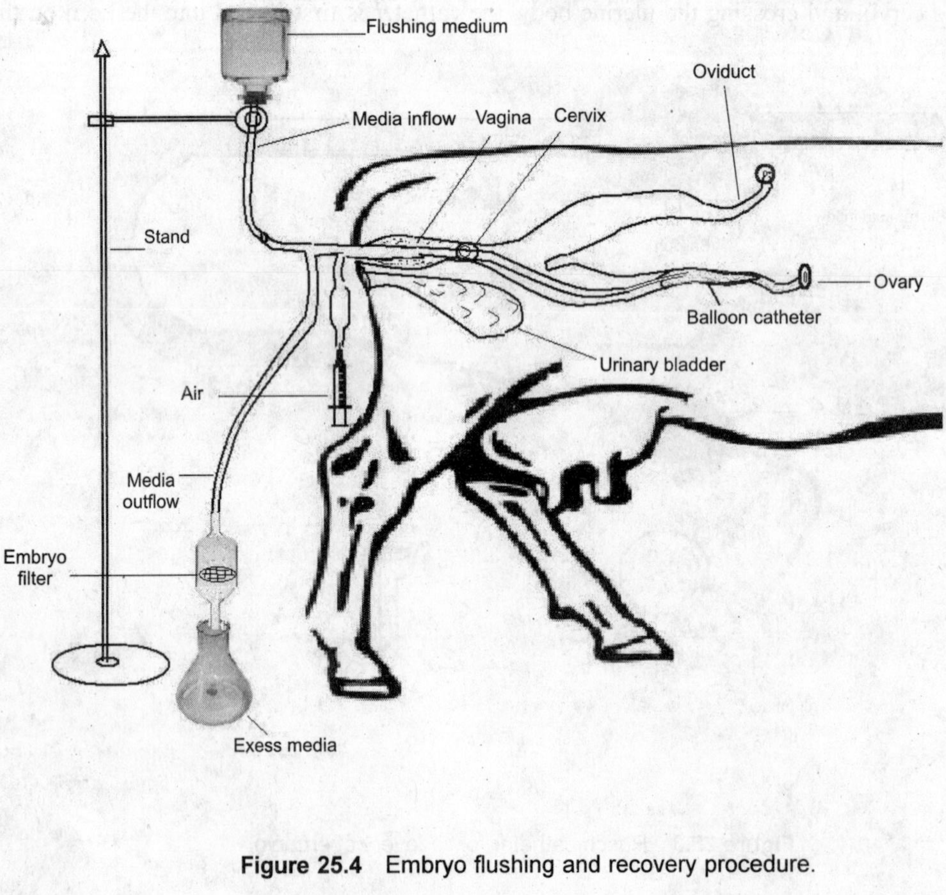

Figure 25.4 Embryo flushing and recovery procedure.

catheter is withdrawn. Flushing is repeated in the other horn. Filter covered with the lid is transferred to the laboratory, taking care that the medium is not exposed to direct sunlight. Although embryos are usually transferred as soon as possible after collection, it is possible to maintain embryos for several hours at room temperature in holding medium. It is also possible to cool bovine embryos in holding medium and to maintain them in the refrigerator for 2-3 days. As a final alternative, embryos may be frozen for use at a later date (Figure 25.4).

Embryos are normally held in the same or a similar medium to that in which they were collected. Media must be buffered to maintain a pH of 7.2 to 7.6 and have an osmolarity around 300 mOs. Dulbecco's PBS or more complex media with Hepes buffer enriched with FCS and antibiotics are normally used in the field. More complex media with a carbonate buffer generally yields superior results for long term culture of bovine embryos.

Evaluation of embryo

After collection of embryos, filter contents are poured into individual Petri dishes for searching of the embryos under steriozoom microscope at magnification 20× (Figure 25.5). Embryo is composed of a cellular mass surrounded by an acellular matrix known as zona pellucida. The area between the embryonic mass and the zona pellucida is known as perivitelline space. The embryonic mass is usually darker than other debris. The bovine embryo is about 160 micron in diameter on day 7 of development, which increases in size and the growth remains synchronus till it reaches 16-cell stages, after which the growth of the embryo becomes asynchronous and individual cell becomes difficult to distinguish. Blastomeres, individual cells of the embryo lose their spherical shape and begin to adhere to one another. Embryos of this stage are termed compact morula and recovered often on day 6.5 to 8 after standing estrus. Later on, blastomere differentiates into two cell types, trophoblast and inner cell mass, and the stage is known as blastocyst. The next developmental stage is expanded blastocyst. The expansion of the blastocyst continues till the mass hatches out of the zona which occurs between day 8-10.

Evaluation of bovine embryos must be done at 50 to 100 × magnification, with the embryo in a small culture dish. It is important to be able to recognize the various stages of development and to compare these with the developmental stage that the embryo should be based on the days from estrus. Often a decision as to whether an embryo is worthy of transfer will depend on the availability of recipients.

Embryos are classified and evaluated by morphological examination at 50 to 100 × magnification according to the Manual of the International Embryo Transfer Society. The overall diameter of the bovine embryo is 150 to 190 μm, including a zona pellucida thickness of 12 to 15 μm. The overall diameter of the embryo remains virtually unchanged from the one-cell stage until blastocyst stage. The best predictor of an embryo's viability is its stage of development relative to what it should be on a given day after ovulation. An ideal embryo is compact and spherical. The blastomeres should be of similar size with even color and texture. The cytoplasm should not be granular or vesiculated. The perivitelline space should be clear and contain no cellular debris. The zona pellucida should be uniform, neither cracked nor collapsed, and should not contain debris on its surface. Embryos of good or excellent quality and at the developmental stages of late morula to blastocyst yield the highest pregnancy rates. It is advisable to select the stage of embryo development for the synchrony of the recipient.

Stages of embryo development

- **Morula:** A mass of at least 16 cells. Individual blastomeres are difficult to discern from one another. The cellular mass of the embryo occupies most of the perivitelline space.
- **Compact Morula:** Individual blastomeres have coalesced, forming a compact mass. The embryo mass occupies 60 to 70% of the perivitelline space.
- **Early Blastocyst:** An embryo that has formed a fluid-filled cavity or blastocoele and gives a general appearance of a signet ring. The embryo occupies 70 to 80% of the perivitelline space. Early in this stage of development, the embryo may appear of questionable quality.
- **Blastocyst:** Pronounced differentiation of the outer trophoblast layer and the darker, more compact inner cell mass is evident. The blastocoele is highly prominent, with the embryo occupying most of the perivitelline space. Visual differentiation between the trophoblast and the inner cell mass is possible at this stage of development.
- **Expanded Blastocyst:** The overall diameter of the embryo increases dramatically, with a concurrent thinning of the zona pellucida to approximately one-third of its original thickness.
- **Hatched Blastocyst:** Embryos recovered at this developmental stage can be undergoing the process of hatching or may have completely shed the zona pellucida. Hatched blastocysts may be spherical with a well defined blastocoele or may be collapsed. Identification of embryos at this stage can be difficult unless it re-expands (Figure 25.6).

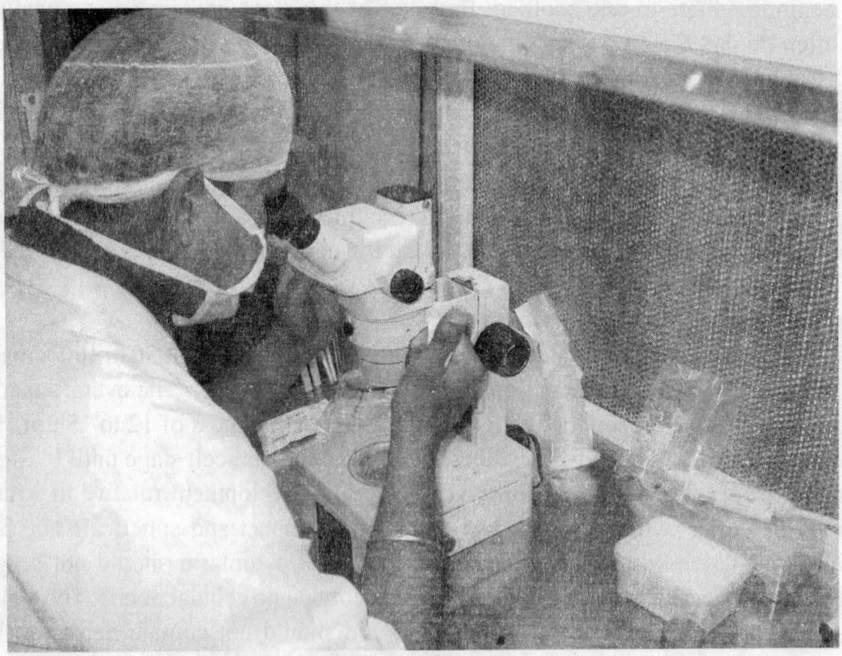

Figure 25.5 Isolation and classification of embryo.

Quality evaluation

- **Excellent:** An ideal embryo, spherical, symmetrical and with cells of uniform size, color and texture.
- **Good:** Small imperfections such as a few extruded blastomeres, irregular shape and a few vesicles.
- **Fair:** Problems that are more definite are seen, including presence of extruded blastomeres, vesiculation, and a few degenerated cells.
- **Poor:** Severe problems, numerous extruded blastomeres, degenerated cells, cells of varying sizes, large and numerous vesicles but an apparently viable embryo mass. These are generally not of transferable quality.

Recommended quality code

The International Embryo Transfer Society (IETS) recommended codes for embryo quality range from "1" to "4" as follows:

- **Code 1:** Excellent or good. Symmetrical and spherical embryo mass with individual blastomeres (cells) that are uniform in size, color and density. This embryo is consistent with its expected stage of development. Irregularities should be relatively minor and at least 85% of the cellular material should be an intact, viable embryo mass. This judgment should be based on the percentage of embryo cells represented by the extruded material in the perivitelline space. The zona pellucida should be smooth and have no concave or flat surfaces that might cause the embryo to adhere to a Petri dish or a straw.
- **Code 2:** Fair. Moderate irregularities in overall shape of the embryo mass or size, color and density of individual cells. At least 50% of the cellular material should be an intact, viable embryo mass.
- **Code 3:** Poor. Major irregularities in shape of the embryo mass or size, color and density of individual cells. At least 25% of the cellular material should be an intact, viable embryo mass.
- **Code 4:** Dead or degenerating. Degenerated embryos, oocytes or 1-cell embryos; non-viable.

Transfer of embryo

Initially, embryo transfers in the cow were done surgically, whereas today most are done using non-surgical methods. Surgical transfers were first done by way of a midline incision, which necessitated the use of general anesthesia and rather elaborate facilities. During the mid to late 1970s, this gave way to a standing flank approach, an approach that was quicker, and because of lesser requirements in facilities made "on farm" embryo transfer possible. More recently, the use of non-surgical embryo transfers has increased the utilization of embryo transfer because of even less elaborate requirements.

Non-surgical embryo transfer techniques utilized the specialized embryo transfer gun. After confirming synchrony of estrus, the recipient is restrained and the rectum is evacuated of feces. At the same time, the presence and side of a functional CL is confirmed. Care is taken to prevent ballooning of the rectum with air. An epidural anesthesia is administered and the vulva is washed with water and dried with a paper towel. The embryo is loaded in 0.25 ml straw between at least two air bubbles and the straw is loaded in the embryo transfer gun. Care must be taken to ensure that the straw engages the sheath tightly so as to avoid leakage. The sheath is coated with sterile, non-toxic obstetrical lubricant and the sheathed gun is passed through the vulvar labia while avoiding contamination. The embryo is placed in the uterine horn epsilateral to ovary bearing the CL by passing the gun through the cervix, very similar to artificial insemination. However, an

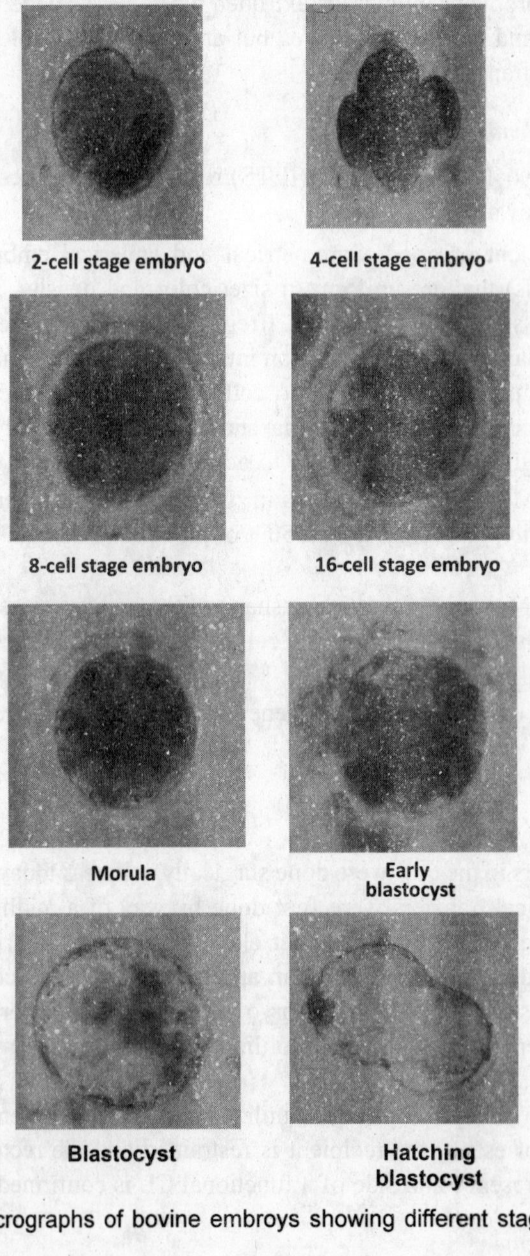

Figure 25.6 Photomicrographs of bovine embryos showing different stages of development.

attempt is usually made to pass the transfer gun at least half-way down the uterine horn. The uterine lumen should be lined-up prior to transfer so as to prevent trauma to the endometrium during passage. The embryo is deposited slowly and firmly while slightly withdrawing the tip of the transfer gun.

Cryopreservation of embryos

Cryopreservation of a living cell constitutes a complex physiochemical process of heat and water transport between the cell and its surrounding medium. There exists an optimum cooling rate for each type of cell. It is dependent on the size of the cell, its surface to volume ratio, permeability to water, and the temperature coefficient of that permeability. Conventional cryopreservation is a slow procedure which exposes the embryo at various phases of freezing to the action of physical, chemical and biological factors. This action can result in the disruption of zona pellucida, cell membrane, and cytoskeleton, ensuing metabolic disturbances. Such cell damage leads to the loss of cell self control and cell death by apoptosis and necrosis. The highest danger for embryonic cell is posed by intracellular ice crystal formation.

The medium that contains the embryos cools below its freezing point without ice crystal formation, a phenomenon referred to as supercooling. Then, at some lower temperature, ice nucleation occurs, followed by a rapid rise in temperature due to the release of latent heat of fusion. To avoid extensive super cooling, ice crystallization is induced in the extracellular medium some 2°C below its freezing point (–4 to –7°C) by seeding the medium with an ice crystal. Water in the cells of the embryo and between the ice crystals outside the embryo does not freeze at this temperature because of solutes lowering its freezing point. During further cooling and enlargement of ice crystals, the solute concentration rises and the embryo responds osmotically by losing water into the extracellular unfrozen medium. Cells are injured during freezing and thawing primarily by solution effects and intracellular ice formation. The latter is especially detrimental when relatively large amounts of large crystals form. To avoid intracellular freezing, embryos must be cooled at 1°C/min or slower. However, very low cooling rates can also damage cells by what has been referred to as the solution effect.

The required thawing rate depends on the freezing regimen used. When embryos are cooled slowly to temperatures between –27 and –40°C and then rapidly to –196°C (liquid nitrogen), thawing must be rapid, e.g., about 200°C/min. Cells treated in this way may contain some intracellular ice, and thawing has to be rapid to prevent injury from the recrystallization of that ice. On the other hand, if embryos are cooled slowly to temperatures below –60°C before transfer to liquid nitrogen, thawing is then normally done slowly at about 20°C/min. Embryos are normally stored in liquid nitrogen at –196°C. The only reactions that occur at –196°C are direct ionizations from background radiation. Consequently, storage times of more than 200 years are unlikely to produce any detectable reduction in survival or cause genetic change in frozen embryos. Glycerol as cryoprotectant in concentrations ranging from 1.0 to 2.0 M is required to ensure embryo survival after freezing. It is thought that cryoprotectants act by reducing the amount of ice present at any temperature during freezing, thereby moderating the changes in solute concentration. Recommended criteria for a cryoprotectant include high solubility, low toxicity at high concentrations, and a low molecular weight both for easier permeation and to exert a maximum colligative effect.

Glycerol has been most often used for the protection of embryos during freezing, but more recently, more permeating cryoprotectants such as ethylene glycol, have been preferred because they can be used with "direct transfer" i.e., transfer into a recipient without prior removal of the cryoprotectant. During the addition and dilution of a permeating cryoprotectant, the cell undergoes osmotic changes resulting in swelling or contraction. Consequently, if the addition or particularly the dilution is carried out inappropriately, the viability of cells can be affected. Glycerol can be added to embryos in a single step, but there is a clear evidence that the rate of glycerol removal is more critical. The standard empirical method was to dilute it by the "step-wise" addition of PBS or to pipette the embryos into decreasing concentrations of glycerol, e.g., 0.25 M steps. However, Leibo and Mazur (1978) suggested a modification in the procedure of cryoprotectant removal by including non-permeable solutes like sucrose into the dilution medium. The sucrose acts as an osmotic counterforce to restrict water movement across the membranes. As the cryoprotectant leaves the embryo, it will shrink in response to the extracellular hypertonic dilution medium. It regains its normal volume at the end of the process when the embryo is placed in normal isotonic culture medium. Using this information, practical methods of quickly removing glycerol from thawed embryos have been devised. As a result, a "one-step straw" was developed so that the embryos could be thawed, and solutions could be mixed within the straw and then transfer to the recipient could be done non-surgically.

The following protocol has been proven successful for the cryopreservation of day 7 bovine embryos in PBS supplemented with 10 to 20% FCS and 1.0 to 1.5 M glycerol. Embryos are pipetted into the freezing medium at room temperature (20°C) and left for 8 to 10 minutes to permit the glycerol to equilibrate within the embryo cells. During this equilibration period, the embryo (s) are transferred in volumes of 0.25 or 0.5 ml of freezing medium into French straws, which are then sealed securely. The samples can be immediately transferred into the freezing chamber at –6 or –7°C and held for 5 min. Ice crystallization (seeding) of the extracellular medium is initiated by touching the outside wall of the straw with a forceps pre-cooled in liquid nitrogen. The samples are held at the seeding temperature for an additional 10 min to allow the crystallization of the medium to progress to equilibrium. Next, embryos are cooled at 0.3 to 0.8°C/min to a temperature between –30 and –40°C, after which they are immersed into liquid nitrogen (-196°C) and stored.

Thawing is carried out by placing the straw into a water bath at a temperature between 20 and 35°C. It has been reported that the incidence of cracked zona pellucida was reduced in an air-thaw or when straws were thawed in air for 10 to 15 seconds prior to being submerged into a 35°C water bath; the thaw rate should be around 200°C/minute. When glycerol is used as the cryoprotectant, it must be removed without causing osmotic damage. The method of choice is the use of sucrose solution between 1.0 M and 0.5 M in a single step for 10 min or 0.3 M sucrose in a 3-step dilution of 5 min each (0.75 M glycerol and 0.3 M sucrose; 0.375 M glycerol and 0.3 M sucrose; 0.3 M sucrose). The embryos are then transferred back into PBS culture medium, washed and evaluated prior to transfer.

The use of highly permeating cryoprotectants such as ethylene glycol has allowed the direct transfer of bovine embryos without the necessity of microscopic examination and cryoprotectant removal. The embryo straw is thawed in a water bath, much like semen, and the contents of the straw are deposited into the uterus of the recipient. There is no need of a microscope or complicated dilution procedures. The cryoprotectant leaves the embryo in the uterus.

Vitrification

Vitrification is a physical process by which a solution is transformed into a stable amorphous glass by rapid cooling, bypassing ice crystal formation while maintaining the properties of liquid in a solidified form. It reduces the equipment and skill required for embryo transfer. Freezing and thawing procedures are time consuming and require the use of biological freezers and a microscope. These steps can be replaced by a relatively simple procedure called vitrification. High concentrations of cryoprotectants are used and the embryo in its cryoprotectant solution is placed directly into liquid nitrogen. Because of the high concentration of cryoprotectants, ice crystals do not form; the frozen solution forms a glass. As ice crystal formation is one of the most damaging processes in freezing, vitrification has much to offer in the cryopreservation of oocytes and IVF embryos.

Procedure of vitrification

Vitrification is done as described by Vajta *et al*. (1998). After removing cotton plugs, 0.25-mL French straws are softened over a hot plate and pulled manually until the inner diameter decreases from 1.7 to approximately 0.8 mm and wall thickness of the central part decreases from approximately 0.15 to 0.07 mm. The straws are then air-cooled and cut at the narrowest point. Before vitrification, the embryos are first incubated in the holding medium (PBS + 10% FCS) supplemented with 7.5% of ethylene glycol and 7.5% dimethyl sulphoxide for 3 min and then transferred into a 20 μL droplet of the holding medium supplemented with 16.5% ethylene glycol, 16.5% dimethyl sulphoxide and 0.5 mol/L sucrose. An approximately 1 to 2μL droplet containing 1-3 embryos are placed in a Petri dish and straws are loaded by the capillary effect to be later submerged into liquid nitrogen. The time between the contact of the embryo with the concentrated cryoprotectant solution and plunging into liquid nitrogen should not exceed 25 sec.

Pregnancy following embryo transfer

Pregnancy following ET in cattle is highly variable and generally, ranges 20 to 50% reported in different studies. In Kankrej breed, transfer of embryos to 27 recipients resulted into 10 (37.0%) pregnancies. However, higher conception rates (72.72%) were reported by Siddiqui *et al.* (2001). Pregnancy following transfer of fresh embryos was reported to be 22.31, 23.93, 23.43, 18.37, and 30.38 at NDDB labs, NDDB field, NDRI, IVRI, NII, respectively, whereas it varied from 15.28-18.05% following transfer of frozen embryos (NDDB 1992). Further work at NDDB resulted into 31 and 18% conception rates following fresh and frozen ET, respectively (NDDB, 1997).

There are limited reports regarding the pregnancy and birth of buffalo calves following ET in India. Initially, the conception rate following ET was reported to be only 10-18%. However, subsequently, following transfer of mostly non-freezable embryos (grade II & III), the pregnancy rate improved significantly to 25-26.4% on the farm and 29.4% in the field. A higher conception rate of 60% was also observed following transfer of only Grade I embryos (Figure 25.7).

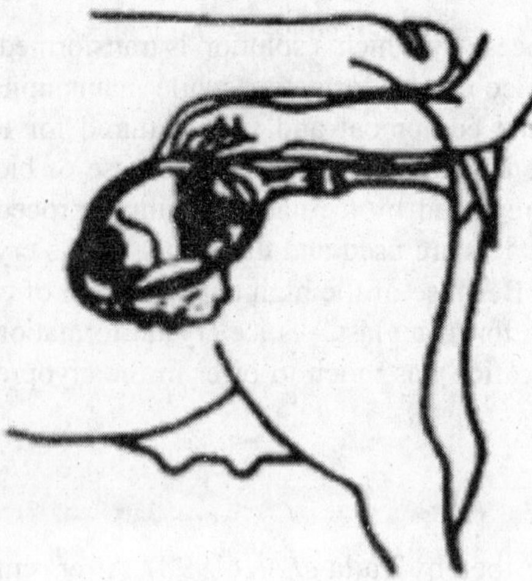

Figure 25.7 Pregnancy diagnosis by palpation through the rectal wall 1 to 3 months after embryo transfer.

In-vitro Embryo Production

Preimplantation embryos can be produced by *in vitro* maturation/*in vitro* fertilization (IVM/IVF) and they are being used in many laboratories worldwide. There has been a great development in biotechnology during the recent years. These new methods enable us to obtain oocytes from the breeding stock. Therefore, these biotechnological methods increase animal productivity and benefit the economy. Viable embryos can be produced from ovarian oocytes collected hours after the death of the animals at the slaughterhouse. By using these techniques, oocytes can be matured and fertilized *in vitro*, stored by freezing and embryos suitable for non-surgical transfer can be produced inexpensively in large numbers. Moreover, IVM/IVF embryos can provide the starting materials for nuclear transfer and other approaches for manipulation of the genome.

The technique of *in vitro* embryo development essentially involves (a) collection of oocytes from slaughterhouse ovaries or from living animals through transvaginal aspiration, (b) *in vitro* maturation of selected oocytes in media containing serum and hormones, *(c) in vitro* fertilization with frozen thawed *in vitro* capacitated spermatozoa (d) *in vitro* culture of embryos in media containing oviduct or cumulus cells upto the morula or blastocyst stage during which they can be either transferred to synchronized recipients or frozen and stored. To date, this technique has given considerable success in both cattle and buffalo, achieving a success rate ranging from 30 – 50% development of preimplantation stage embryo *in vitro*. This technology does not only offer optimization of high-quality dams, but also allows the preservation and rapid multiplication of genetically superior characters by making embryos available for cloning, sexing and nuclear transfer.

Collection of Ovaries

Ovaries are collected from the slaughterhouse soon after the slaughter of the animals, and kept in a sealed container containing physiological saline (0.9% NaC1 with 100 µg/ml Streptomycin and 100 IU/ml Penicillin) at a temperature ranging from 28-33°C. Careful observation of the temperature of the saline is important to maintain the viability of the ovaries during the period of collection. In general, if the time spent from ovary collection to oocyte recovery is short, 30-33°C temperature of the physiological saline is better. However, in cases where the slaughterhouse is distant from the laboratory, a decrease in the temperature is recommended, but the temperature should still be kept above 28°C to maintain the development potential of the oocytes. Prolonging the period of ovary collection may significantly affect the viability of the oocytes for *in vitro* maturation. It is recommended that oocytes should be collected from the ovaries within a 6-hour period. Beyond six hours, development potential is greatly compromised.

Recovery of oocytes

It is necessary to wash the ovaries in fresh, sterile physiological saline (without antibiotics) to further remove any contaminants. Briefly rinsing the ovary in 70% ethyl alcohol is recommended to eliminate surface organisms before the processing begins. The ovaries are dried lightly with sterile paper towels before primary oocytes are recovered from 2-8 mm vesicular follicles. Oocytes are then collected from each ovary by aspiration of follicles using 18 G needle attached to a 10 ml syringe having 1 ml oocytes collection media. The oocyte collection media comprises Dulbecco's phosphate buffered saline with 0.3 % BSA and 50 µg/ml gentamycin. Aspiration medium can be prepared once, stored in a refrigerator and made available for one week's activity. However, it is very important to pre-warm the aspiration medium up to 38°C before use. Alternatively, Medium-199 with Earle's salts, L-glutamine, 25 mM HEPES, supplemented with 3% (v/v) inactivated calf serum (heat-treated at 56°C for 30 min) and trace amounts of antibiotics can also be used.

Visible follicles of 2-8 mm diameter are aspirated in collection medium and contents are gently transferred into 50 m conical tube and allowed to settle down for 10 minutes. Supernatants are removed and bottom contents containing oocytes are poured into 94 × 10 mm Petri dish and searched for oocytes under steriozoom microscope. One of the difficulties associated with the aspiration approach lies in the fact that oocytes may only be retrieved from some 30-60% of the punctured follicles. To minimize this effect, it is necessary to prime the needle and syringe with approximately 0.25-0.5 ml of aspiration medium. This is to provide the initial fluid that helps ensure the retrieval of the follicular contents, especially in collecting the first few oocytes. Oocytes can also be collected by using an ultrasound machine having a trans-vaginal sector transducer of 5/7.5 MHz housed in a modified stainless steel with a needle guide system. The oocytes are collected from each ovary by aspiration of follicles through vaginal wall using 18 gauze (G) disposable needle attached to a special support and vacuum pump that produces a negative pressure of about 45 mm Hg and fluid flow rate of 10-15 ml per minute.

The average recovery of total oocytes per ovary has been reported to vary from 0.7, 1.7 to 2.4. There is a high proportion of oocytes that are atretic or degenerate varying from 40-55 %, and therefore, unusable for *in vitro* maturation. The average recovery of acceptable quality oocytes per ovary further reduced to only 0.4, 0.9 to 1.76. The presene of a corpus luteum further reduces the recovery of total and acceptabile quality oocytes. Although ovary slicing can improve the yield of oocytes, slicing is a more time-consuming process because of the difficulty in searching for oocytes due to the large amount of debris and blood cells in the collection dishes due to the presence of haemorrhagic follicles.

Isolated oocytes are transferred to 35 × 10 mm petri dish washed two to three times in a collection medium and graded as A, B, C or D as per standards set by IETS described earlier in the text. Oocytes with compact multilayered cumulus investment and evenly granulated cytoplasm are selected for *in vitro* maturation. It should be noted, however, that the collected oocytes may have a different appearance. Some are denuded (no cumulus cells attached), some are partly denuded, others have swollen, expanded cumulus cells, while others have deformed ooplasm. These oocytes should not be used, because they lack the potential to undergo normal maturation and will eventually end as degenerating oocytes after *in vitro* fertilization.

In vitro maturation of oocytes

Selected oocytes must be washed four times in a fresh pre-warmed aspiration medium and subjected to a final wash in *in vitro* maturation medium before the *in vitro* maturation droplets are pooled, and also the oocytes must be free from any contaminants. The medium used for *in vitro* maturation of oocytes varies among laboratories. It should be considered that the medium employed in IVM may affect the proportion of oocytes that reach metaphase II and become capable of undergoing fertilization. Usually simple media contains bicarbonate-buffered systems, basic physiological saline with pyruvate, lactate and glucose. The main differences between various types of simple media lie in differences in their ion concentration, and the concentration of the energy sources. The media are generally supplemented with serum or albumin, with trace amounts of antibiotics (penicillin, streptomycin, and gentamicin). Nowadays complex media are used for the maturation of oocytes which contains, in addition to the components of the simple media, amino acids, vitamins, purines and other substances, mainly at levels at which they are found in serum. The most widely used complex media for IVM of cattle and buffalo oocytes is Tissue Culture Medium 199 (TCM-199) with Earle's salt, L-Glutamine and 25 mM HEPES supplemented with 10-20% heat inactivated serum (be it a fetal calf serum, calf serum, steer serum or an estrus cow serum). Other culture media used are Ham's F-10, MEM, IVMD 101, RPMI and Synthetic Bovine Oviductal Fluid medium.

Recently, Nandi *et al.* (2004) observed that the bFF from small follicles had significantly higher potential of developing buffalo oocytes to embryonic stage than from medium or large follicles and cystic follicular fluid was not capable of supporting development of buffalo oocytes. Addition of follicle stimulating hormone (FSH), equine chorionic gonadotropin (eCG), luteinizing hormone (LH) and estradiol either alone or in combination has also been used to induce higher maturation rates. Addition of LH to maturation medium (TCM-199+20% OBS) improved maturation rate from 47 to 77%. Contrarily, however, Madan *et al.* (1994) reported 80% maturation rate in TCM-199+20% OBS without the use of any hormones. On the other hand, Totey *et al.* (1992) reported higher maturation rate (81.7%) in TCM-199 and BES as compared to Ham's F-10 (71.7%). A maturation rate of 70-80% has been achieved by using TCM-199 supplemented with FBS and 5 mg/ml FSH-

P. Additionally, amongst various growth factors such as epidermal growth factor (EGF), EGF plus fibroblast growth factor (FGF), insulin like growth factor II (IGF-II) and vasoactive intestinal peptide (VIP), addition of EGF and IGF II had more beneficial effect on oocyte maturation and subsequent cleavage than FGF or VIP.

Oocyte maturation is commonly considered to be the progression of nuclear maturation from the appearance of the germinal vesicle of the arrested dictyate stage, through meiosis I to metaphase II and extrusion of the first polar body. Extensive redistribution of intracellular organelles occurs, mitochondria migrate to occupy a perinuclear location and the cortical granules migrate outward to lie just beneath the vitelline membrane, development of proteins in the cytoplasm occurs, which regulate meiotic events sperm decondensation, followed by formation of the male pronuclear envelope, initiation of cleavage, completion of cleavage stage embryo development and ability to produce a viable offspring. The development of these regulatory signals can be affected by the duration of *in vitro* maturation period and by the conditions of the *in vitro* maturation culture. Common defects resulting from fertilization of immature oocytes include failure of male pronuclear development and failure to develop to organised blastocyst stage embryo. The latter has been corrected by co-culture *in vitro* co-culture of immature oocytes with granulosa or abundant cumulus cells under stimulation of gonadotrophins and estrogen. Other aspect of the oocytes maturation is the full expansion of the cumulus cells surrounding the oocyte. If cumulus cells are expanded fully, it may enhance sperm capacitation and fertilization rate. A product of cumulus cells stimulated by FSH enhances the motility of bovine spermatozoa. Bovine cumulus cells undergo expansion in response to FSH either *in vitro* or after a small FSH rise accompanying the preovulatory surge of LH *in vivo*. The principal secretory product of FSH stimulated bovine cumulus cells is hyaluronic acid, which forms a mucus matrix between and around cumulus cells. It takes about 24-27 hours in culture to develop from the germinal vesicle stage to metaphase II. This progression is paralleled by progression of cumulus expansion while fertilization is highly temperature dependent, nuclear maturation of bovine oocytes occurs over a temperature range of 35-41°C. Cooling oocytes below 30°C can damage nuclear maturation ability by an apparent disruption of the spindle apparatus.

In vitro fertilization of oocytes

Appropriate preparation of sperm and oocyte is essential for the successful fertilization. Mammalian spermatozoa are not immediately capable of fertilizing oocytes, rather they must undergo a period of preparation, which normally occurs in the female reproductive tract, known as capacitation. Capacitation consists of at least two components, an initial sperm membrane alteration that allows the spermatozoa to undergo the second phase, the fusion of plasma membrane and outer acrosomal membrane. The first phase is referred to as capacitation, while the second phase is referred to as acrosome reaction. In cattle, spermatozoa undergo the acrosome reaction almost exclusively in the ampulla of the oviduct ipsilateral to the side of ovulation and only near and immediately after ovulation.

In vitro, glycosaminoglycans will induce an acrosome reaction or capacitate bovine spermatozoa. Assay of the glycosaminoglycan in bovine and ovine oviduct flushings revealed a high concentration of heparin like material. *In vitro* heparin was shown to be the most potent glycosaminoglycons in its ability to induce the acrosome reaction in bovine epididymal spermatozoa and to capacitate ejaculated bovine spermatozoa. A characteristic of bovine sperm capacitation by heparin is that it is inhibited by 5 mM glucose. Capacitation of bovine spermatozoa by oviduct fluid is also inhibited by glucose. In cows, glucose is present in very low levels in the oviduct, <1 mM, which does not inhibit sperm capacitation by heparin. Capacitation of spermatozoa takes place within the uterus and is accelerated by the exposure of spermatozoa to the uterus and then the oviduct. Capacitation is a reversible phenomenon, which upon completion results in the modification of the sperm membrane surface, causing an efflux of membrane cholesterol that alters the membrane sterol/ phospholipid ratio and results in an influx of Ca^{2+}. The Ca^{2+} activates phospholipase A_2, which catalyzes the synthesis and accumulation of fusogenic lysophospholipids such as lysophosphatidylcholine. In the presence of Ca^{2+} and reduced level of cholesterol, such fusogenic compounds would induce acrosome reaction. The second major event of capacitation is an uptake of Ca^{2+} by spermatozoa. Heparin induces a linear increase in Ca^{2+} uptake during capacitation of bovine spermatozoa that does not occur when spermatozoa are incubated under non-capacitating conditions. It is, however, unknown whether the Ca^{2+} uptake was a result of heparin acting as an ionophore, opening a Ca^{2+} channel in the membrane or the result of membrane changes. Heparin, like glycosaminoglycons, may therefore have direct effect on Ca^{2+} uptake into spermatozoa during capacitation. The third major step in capacitation is the activation of phospholipase A_2 by Ca^{2+} or acrosin. Heparin like glycosaminoglycons may be able to activate phospholipase A_2 through their ability to chelate Zn^{2+}, an inhibitor of phospholipase A_2 or stimulate conversion of proacrocin to acrosin.

In cattle and buffalo, IVF of *in vitro* matured oocytes is usually carried out after 23-24 hours. This is because the peak of oocytes at metaphase II stage is at this period. A 100 μl microdroplets of BO medium containing caffeine, heparin and BSA with 10×10^6 sperm/ml is prepared to accommodate 10 oocytes. This is because 1-oocyte/10 μl is an optimum proportion for successful *in vitro* fertilization of oocyte. Co-culture of sperm-oocyte for *in vitro* fertilization is done in a humidified environment with 5% CO_2 and 38.9°C temperature for 6 to 7 hours. The incubation period was determined by the fact that sperm capacitation inside the female reproductive tract occurred for about 6 hours. Before the *in vitro* matured oocytes are subjected to IVF microdroplets, they are first partially denuded of the surrounding cumulus cells to allow easy penetration of the sperm cells. They are washed twice in pre-warmed IVF medium to maintain the defined component of the IVF medium. Low fertilization rate (19.6%) was recorded when capacitated frozen semen was used in HEPES-TALP medium. Subsequently, this improved to 29.8% by using BO medium. A higher fertilization rate of 78.15% was reported in Murrah buffaloes by Madan *et al.* (1994b). Considerable variations have been reported among different buffalo bulls in terms of the ability of their spermatozoa to fertilize oocytes *in vitro*. Different authors have reported different sperm concentration and sperm oocyte co-incubation period for buffalo IVF. A sperm concentration of 4-5 millions with a co-incubation period of 20-24 h resulted in 60-75% fertilization rate. Some workers observed that 2×10^6 sperm/ml with 20 h sperm-oocyte co-incubation was sufficient for buffalo IVF.

In vitro culture of embryo

In vitro culture of developing embryos on suitable cell lines is an essential step in *in vitro* development of embryo to morula or blastocyst stage, which can be transferred non-surgically. The provision of cell basement support provides the developing zygotes with a comfortable environment, and secretes some growth factors supportive to further development *in vitro*. The most commonly used media for *in vitro* embryo culture are the co-culture of fertilized oocytes with oviduct cells, granulosa cell monolayer, BRL/VERO cell monolayer in defined media. Improvement of the medium and other culture conditions has allowed for full development of the fertilized oocytes, but the great majority of bovine zygotes stop developing within a few cell cycles after initiating cleavage. This developmental block arises in the bovine embryo at the eight-cell-stage and is likely correlated with the cytoplasmic quality of the oocyte. Oocytes harbor all mRNAs and proteins needed to reach the fourth or fifth cell cycle, however, embryos that fail to transcribe their own genome fail to develop further. It is known that cells of the embryo remain alive during the period of blocked development and they cannot be rescued once the block is initiated. In mice, this period of transition from maternal to zygotic control of development is accompanied by the production of a class of proteins known as heat shock proteins. Specifically, heat shock proteins 68 and 70 have been shown to be the first product of the mouse embryonic genome. In mouse embryos, which pass through this critical 2-cell period *in vitro*, heat shock protein 70 returns to a low concentration by the 4-cell stage. Production of heat shock proteins 68 and 70 at this transition period and under *in vitro* culture conditions may reflect the inadequacy of the culture. In spite of the absence of an adequate *in vitro* embryo culture system, embryos have been developed to morula and blastocyst stages.

The efficiency of the embryo development may vary greatly. Totey *et al.* (1992) reported 28% morula/blastocyst development from buffalo oocytes when co-cultured in rabbit oviduct, however, only 8.2% developed oviductal cell monolayer. Madan *et al.* (1994a) and Singh and Dhanda (1997) also reported low blastocyst development (6.10 and 8.10%) from buffalo oocytes co-cultured with cumulus + oviductal cells. On the contrary, Chauhan *et al.* (1997a) recorded a high rate of morula (41%) and blastocyst (31%) development from buffalo oocytes using same co-culture system. Nandi *et al.* (2003) also reported significantly higher embryo development and blastocyst yield in the co-culture system than in defined medium. Using oviductal cell co-culture with mSOF, we observed that on an average 33% (maximum 54%) of the cleaved oocytes became morula and average 7% (maximum 9.4%) became blastocyst and majority hatched during subsequent culture.

Advantages of Embryo Transfer Technology

The embryo transfer technology offers several advantages, which are manifested in its varied applications briefly enumerated below.

- This technology achieves a surprisingly rapid rate of multiplication of animals of the selected superior genotype. In natural course, a single female will produce a single progeny in about one year. But using superovulation and embryo transfer technology, it is feasible to collect around 36 embryos from one female in one year. A single female can be induced to ovulate, on an average, 6 times a year, and in each ovulation cycle about 6 healthy transplantable embryos are obtained. Assuming an average success rate of 50% in the embryo transfer, an average of 18 progeny can be derived from one superior female in one year.

- Each young embryo can be split into 2-4 parts, each of which would develop into a separate progeny. This is called embryo splitting. By combining embryo splitting with superovulation and embryo transfer techniques, the rate of multiplication can be further increased.
- The young embryos can be frozen and stored in liquid nitrogen for up to 10 years or more and used at a subsequent date. The frozen embryos are far easier to transport, and present negligible quarantine problems as compared to the animals themselves. Freezing and storage of young embryos in liquid nitrogen (at –196°C) is known as cryopreservation. The embryos are thawed at a very rapid rate by immersing the ampoule carrying them into a water bath maintained at 0°C.
- Superior course that are unfit to carry the foetus for full term can serve as donors of the young embryos.

Limitations of Embryo Transfer Technology

The embryo transfer technology has some important limitations as follows:

- A high degree of expertise is required for an efficient and successful operation.
- The cost of producing each progeny is several-fold higher than that from natural events.
- The donor females are removed from production for the period they are used as donors of young embryos.

It is therefore necessary to evaluate the gains vis-a-vis the cost of the technology before employing it on a commercial scale. The gains will be attractive in such cases where a relatively rare superior genotype is rapidly multiplied and made available on a commercial scale.

APPLICATIONS OF EMBRYO TRANSFER TECHNOLOGY

This technology achieves a surprisingly rapid rate of multiplication of animals of the selected superior genotype. Some of the important applications are discussed below.

Embryo Transfer and *in vitro* Fertilization in Farm Animals

In recent years, *in vitro* fertilization (IVF) technology in which the fertilization of egg by sperm takes place at artificially maintained optimum conditions has revolutionized the field of animal biotechnology, by the production of more and more animals than that of normal course. IVF was first successfully tried in humans over 25 years ago and this fame goes to "Louise Joy Brown", the first test tube baby born in 1978. Since her birth, thousands of children have been born with the aid of this technology. IVF is the procedure designed to enhance the likelihood of conception in couples for whom other fertility therapies have been unsuccessful or are not possible.

Among farm animals, *in vitro* fertilization has been achieved in the cow, pig and goat; but the number of newborn animals was limited. Lambert *et al.* (1986) produced six calves from a combination of *in vitro* fertilization and incubation in the rabbit oviduct before transfer. Numabe *et al.* (2000) evaluated the difference in birth weight and gestation length between Japanese Black calves obtained from transfer of bovine embryos produced *in vitro* and those developed *in vivo*. The transfer of *in vitro* fertilized embryos is now practicable but the laboratory methods of fertilization still need development. The recent developments in IVP technology in cattle can be adapted to embryo production in small ruminants to overcome limitations exhibited by surgical procedures on preserving the reproductive potential of donors and the efficiency of embryo production. The aim was to assess the current procedures used in cattle for the production of IVP embryos in goats and sheep based on oocytes supplied by laparoscopic aided ovum pick-up (LOPU). Lim *et al.* (2007) developed a defined culture medium that supported improved *in vitro* bovine embryo development and calving rate after embryo transfer (ET). *In vitro*-matured bovine oocytes from abattoir-derived ovaries from Korean native Han Woo cattle were fertilized with frozen-thawed spermatozoa and embryos were cultured in two step culture media.

In vitro fertilization (IVF) is a feasible way to utilize sex-sorted sperm to produce offspring of a predetermined sex in the livestock industry. These technologies (sperm sexing-IVF-vitrification-embryo transfer) provide farmers, as well as the livestock industry, with a valuable option for herd expansion and heifer replacement programmes. In summary, calves were produced using embryos fertilized by sex-sorted sperm *in vitro* and cryopreserved by rapid cooling vitrification.

CONCLUSION AND FUTURE PROSPECTS

Embryo transfer is now accepted as the quickest and the cost efficient method of increasing the rate of genetic improvement within a herd. For beef and dairy operations, it can be a valuable addition to any breeding programme, leading to greater efficiency and profitability. At this point in time scientists are taking embryos and breaking them up into individual cells and making identical animals, this method is called cloning. The cloning aspect is not commercially available yet but should be soon. It really depends on the imagination of the people who are involved with the research. This may lead to farmers taking embryos out of the tank, seven days after examining their own recipients and then transferring the embryo. Embryo transfer offers farmers the chance to (a) produce up to ten or more progeny per year from their best cows, (b) profit from the increased sale of quality genes without losing the bloodlines, (c) extend the productive life of some older cows incapable of carrying another calf by producing further progeny through the use of embryo transfer, (d) conserve the genetics in their herd through the use of embryo freezing for export, domestic sale or future transfers on their own farm, (e) introduce top genes into the farmers' herd, rapidly and economically from other countries. The top cattle in any herd are rarely available for purchase; however the owners are often willing to sell embryos. The importation of new blood stock can be achieved safely and economically through the purchase of embryos from anywhere in the world, once the quarantine regulations have been fulfilled.

Embryo transfer is on the leading edge of biotechnology. There is hardly a distinction made between today's accepted technology and tomorrow's potential developments. The past decade has been witness to a veritable avalanche of technological advances. The lag period between a discovery and its commercial application, while lengthy in many fields, is almost nonexistent in this area.

Undoubtedly within few years we will be commercially sexing embryos, commercially cloning embryos and practising genetic engineering on our domestic livestock. It boggles the mind to contemplate the commercial potential of these innovations.

FURTHER READINGS

1. Alexiev A. Vlahov K. Karaivanov Ch. Kacheva D. Polykhronov O. Petrov M. Nikolov N. Drogoev A. and Radev P. (1988) Embryo transfer in buffaloes in Bulgaria. *Proceedings of the II World Buffalo Congress*, Bulgaria, Vol **(II)**: 591-595.
2. Alkemade S.J. Murphy B.D. Mapletoft R.J. (1993) Superovulation in the cow; Effects of biological activity of gonadotropins. In: *Proc. Ann. Mtg. Am. Embryo Assoc.* Portland, Maine
3. Ambrose J.D. Singla S.K. Jailkhani S. Prakash B.S. and Madan M.L. (1991) Superovulation response in buffaloes (Bubalus bubalis) to different treatment regimens of Folltropin. *Theriogenology.* **(35)**: 181.
4. Ansari M.R. Sharma J.K.P. and Khanna S. (1998) Effect of buserelin on superovulatory response in crossbred cattle treated with PMSG and Folltropin. *Indian Journal of Animal Reproduction.* 19 **(1)**: 10-12.
5. Austin, C.R. (1951) Observation on the penetration of the sperm into the mammalian egg. *Aust. J. Sci. Res.* **(4)**: 581-596.
6. Baguisi, A. Lonergan, P. Overstrom, E. W., Boland, M. P. (1999) Vitrification of bovine embryos: Incidence of necrosis and apoptosis. *Theriogenology.* **(51)**: 62
7. Ball, G.D.. Leibfried, M.L, Lenz, R.W., Ax, R.L., Bavister, B.D. and First , N.L. (1983) Factors affecting successful invitro fertilization of bovine follicular oocytes. *Biol. Reprod.* **(28)**: 717-725.
8. Barnes, F. L. (2000) The effects of the early uterine environment on the subsequent development of embryo and fetus. *Theriogenology.* **(53)**: 649-658.
9. Beal W.E. (1996) Application of knowledge about corpus luteum function in control of estrus and ovulation in cattle. *Theriogenology.* **(45)**: 1399-1411.
10. Beg M.A. Sanwal P.C. and Yadav M.C. (1997) Ovarian response and endocrine changes in buffalo superovulated at midluteal and late luteal stage of the estrous cycle: A preliminary report. *Theriogenology* **(47)**: 423-432.
11. Bergfelt D.R. Bo G.A. Mapletoft RJ *et al.* (1997) Superovulatory response following ablation-induced follicular wave emergence at random stages of the oestrous cycle in cattle. *Anim. Reprod. Sci.* **(49)**: 1-12.
12. Bergfelt D.R. Lightfoot K.C. Adams G.P. (1994) Ovarian dynamics following ultrasound-guided transvaginal follicle ablation in heifers. *Theriogenology.* **(42)**: 895-907.
13. Betteridge K.J. (1981) An historical look at embryo transfer. *J. Reprod. Fert.* **(62)**: 1-13.
14. Betteridge K.J. (2003) A history of farm animal embryo transfer and some associated techniques. *Anim. Reprod. Sci.* **(79)**: 203-244.
15. Bettridge, K.G. Eaglesome, M.D. Randall, G.C.B. and Mitchell, D. (1980) Collection, description and transfer of embryos from cattle 10-16 days after estrus. *J. Reprod. Fertl.* **(59)**: 205-216.
16. Biedl, A., Peters, H. and Hafsttter, R. (1922) Experimentelle studien uber die einnistung und weiterentwichlung des eies im uterus . *Z. Geburtsshilfe Gynak* . **(84)**: 59-130.
17. Bo G.A. Adams G.P. Pierson RA(1995) Exogenous control of follicular wave emergence in cattle. *Theriogenology.* **(43)**: 31-40.
18. Carlson. D., Black, D.L. & Howe, G.R. (1970) Oviduct secretion in the cow. *J. Reprod. Fert.* **(22)**: 549-552.
19. Casida L.E., Meyer R.K., Mcshann W.H. and Wisnicky W. (1943). Effect of pituitary gonadotropins on ovaries and the induction of superfecundity in cattle. *Amer. J. of Veterinary Research.* **(6)**: 76.
20. Casu, B. (1985) Structure and biological activity of heparin: Advances in carbohydrate chem. *Biochem.* **(43)**: 52-143.

21. Chang, M.C. (1951) Fertilizing capacity of spermatozoa deposited into the fallopian tubes. *Nature.* **(168):** 697-698.
22. Chauhan M.S. Singla S.K. Palta P, Manik R.S. Tomar O.S. (1998) IGF-II stimulation of *in-vitro* maturation, in-vitro fertilization and subsequent development of baffalo (Bubalus bubalis) oocytes *in-vitro.* Veterinary Record **(142):** 727-728.
23. Chauhan M.S. Katiyar P.K. Madan M.L. Singla S.K. Manik R.S. (1996) Influence of follicle stimulating hormones on in-vitro maturation and cleavage of buffalo (Bubalus bubalis) oocytes after in-vitro fertilization. *Theriogenology.* **(45):** 243.
24. Chauhan M.S. Palt P. Das S.K. Katiyar P.K. Madan M.L. (1997) Replacement of serum and hormone additives with follicular fluid in IVM media: effects of maturation, fertilization and subsequent development of buffalo oocytes *in vitro. Theriogenology.* **(48):** 461-469.
25. Chauhan M.S. Singla S.K. Palta P. Manik R.S. Madan M.L. (1999) Effect of EGF on cumulus expansion, meiotic maturation and development of buffalo oocytes *in vitro. Veterinary Record.* **(144):** 266-267.
26. Das G.K. Jain G.C. Solanki V.S. and Tripathi V.N. (1996) Efficacy of various collection methods for oocyte retrieval in buffalo. *Theriogenology.* **(46):** 1403-141.
27. Deyo C.D. Colazo M.G. Martinez M.F. (2001).The use of GnRH or LH to synchronize follicular wave emergence for superstimulation in cattle. *Theriogenology.* **(55):** 513
28. Dutt T. Kharche S.D. Ansari M.R. and Taneja V.K. (1995) Superovulation with Folltropin, estrus synchronization / using intra vulvosubmucosal administration of luprostiol and embryo transfer in crossbred cows. *Indian Journal of Animal Sciences.* 65 **(9)**: 990-992.
29. Garcia A. Salaheddine M. (1998) Effects of repeated ultrasound-guided transvaginal follicular aspiration on bovine oocyte recovery and subsequent follicular development. *Theriogenology.* **(50):** 575-585.
30. Gupta P.S.P., Nandi S., Ravindranatha B.M., Sarma P.V.. (2002) In-vitro maturation of buffalo oocytes with epidermal growth factor and fibroblast growth factor. *Indian Journal of Animal Sciences.* **(72):** 20-23.
31. Gupta P.S.P., Nandi S., Ravindranatha B.M., Sarma P.V. (2001) Effect of buffalo follicular fluid alone and in combination with M199 and PMSG on buffalo oocyte maturation. *Asian. Australian Journal of Animal Sciences.* **(14):** 693-696.
32. Guttman, F.M. Guttman, H.A. (1980) Historical note on embryo transfer: 599 BC., with apologies to Drs. Steptoe and Edwards. *Fertil. Steril.* 513-515.
33. Hasler JF, McCauley AD, Schermerhorn EC (1983) Superovulatory responses of Holstein cows. *Theriogenology.* **(19):** 83-99.
34. Herz, Z. Northey, D., Lawyer, M. and First, N.L. (1985) Acrosome reaction of bovine spermatozoa invivo, sites and effects of stages of the estrous cycle. *Biol. Reprod.* **(32):** 1163-1168.
35. Jain G.C. Khanna S. and Chopra S.C. (1992) Efficacy of various superovulatory protocols on superovulation and embryo recovery in buffaloes. In : Seminar on Embryo Transfer and Associated Technologies in Livestock Improvement, Present Status and Future Needs, Indian Veterinary Research Institute, Izatnagar, April 16-17, India.
36. Kasiraj R., Rao M.M., Ranga Reddi N.S. and Misra A.K. (1992) Superovulatory response in buffaloes following single subcutaneous or multiple in 368 tramuscular FSH administration. *Theriogenology.* 37 **(1):** 234.
37. Kasiraj R. Rao M.M. Ranga Reddi N.S., Misra A.K. and Pant H.C. (2000) Superovulation and embryo recovery in Ongole cows using FSH or equine chorionic gonadotropin (ECG). *Indian Journal of Animal Sciences* 70 **(3):** 251-253.
38. Kim H.I., Son D.S., Yeon H. *et al.* (2001) Effect of dominant follicle removal before superstimulation on follicular growth, ovulation and embryo production in Holstein cows. *Theriogenology.* **(55):** 937-945.
39. Kumar, A., Solanki, V..S., Jindal, S.K., Tripathi, V.N., and Jain, G.C. (1997) Oocytes retrieval and histological studies of follicular population in buffaloe ovaries. *Anim. Reprod. Sci.* **(47):** 189-195.
40. Kurup M.P.G. (1988) Present status of embryo transfer in buffalo and future expectations. *Proceedings of the II World Buffalo Congress.* New Delhi. **(II):** 587-590.

41. Kurup, M.P.G. (2000) Milk production in India: perspective 2020. *Indian Dairyman*, **(52):** 25-37.
42. Leibo S.P, Mapletoft R.J. (1998) Direct transfer of cryopreserved cattle embryos in North America. In: *Proc. Ann. Mtg. Am. Embryo. Trans. Assoc.,* San Antonio, TX, 91-98.
43. Leibo SP, Mazur P (1978) Methods for the preservation of mammalian embryos by freezing. In: Daniel JC Jr, ed. *Methods in Mammalian Reproduction.* NY., Academic Press, pp. 179-201.
44. Leibo, S. P. and Loskutoff, N. M. (1993) Cryobiology of *in vitro*-derived bovine embryos. *Theriogenology.* **(39):** 81-94.
45. Macmillan K.L., Thatcher W.W. (1991) Effects of an agonist of gonadotropin-releasing hormone on ovarian follicles in cattle. *Biol Reprod.* **(45):** 883-889.
46. Madan M.L., Chauhan M.S., Singla S.K., Manik R.S.. (1994) Pregnancies established from water buffalo (Bubalus bubalis) blastocysts derived from in-vitro matured in-vitro fertilized oocytes and co-cultured with cumulus and oviductal cells. *Theriogenology.* **(42):** 591-600.
47. Manik R.S., Singla S.K. and Madan M.L. (1996) Embryos recovered and follicular changes monitored using ultrasonography in superovulated Sahiwal cows. *Indian Journal of Animal Production and Management* **(12):** 208-213.
48. Manik R.S. Singla S.K., Chauhan M.S. and Madan M.L. (1992) Superovulatory responses in cattle as influenced by presence or absence of dominant follicle. In: *International Conference on Fertility Regulation,* held at Bombay India. November 5-8. Abstract No. **(29):** p. 296.
49. Mapletoft R.J. (1985) Embryo transfer in the cow: General procedures. *Rev. Sci. Tech. Off. Int. Epiz.* **(4):** 843-858.
50. Mapletoft R.J., Steward K.B., Adams G.P. (2002) Recent advances in the superovulation of cattle. *Reprod. Nutr. Dev.* **(42):** 1-11
51. Martinez M.F., Adams G.P., Bergfelt D. (1999) Effect of LH or GnRH on the dominant follicle of the first follicular wave in heifers. *Anim. Reprod. Sci.* **(57):** 23-33
52. *Massip A.,* Van der zwalmen, P., Scheffen, B., Ectors, F. (1989) Some significant steps in the cryopreservation of mammalian embryos with a note on a vitrification procedure. *Anim. Reprod. Sci.* **(19):** 117-129
53. Matsuoka, K., Sakata, S., Ichino, K., Shimaya, S., Katagihara, T., Suzuki, T. (1995) Ultra-rapidfreezing of *in vitro* produced bovine embryos. *Theriogenology.* **(43):** 274
54. Mishra U.K.and Mishra O.P. (1998) Induction of estrus and multiple ovulation by administration of cloprostenol and super-ov through intra-vulvo submucosal (IVSM) route and embryo transfer in Sahiwal cows. *Indian Journal of Animal Sciences.* 68 **(5):** 450-453.
55. Misra A.K. and Joshi B.V. (1991) Relationship between the synchrony of donor-recipient oestrus in successful pregnancies of embryo transfer in buffalo. *Buffalo Journal.* **(7):** 71-75.
56. Misra A.K. and Pant H.C. (2003) Estrus induction following PGF2a treatment in the superovulated buffalo (Bubalus bubalis). *Theriogenology.* **(59)**:1203-1207.
57. Misra A.K., Chaubal S.A., Kishore G.K., Rajeshwar S., Joshi B.V. and Jaiswal R.S. (1992) Superovulatory response to single subcutaneous injection of folltropin in Holstein and Sahiwal cows. *Theriogenology.* 37 **(1):** 260.
58. Misra A.K., Joshi B.V., Agrawal P.L., Kasiraj R., Sivaiah S, Rangareddy N.S. and Siddiqui M.U. (1990) Multiple ovulation and embryo transfer in Indian buffaloes (Bubalus bubalis). *Theriogenology.* 33 **(5)**:1131-1142.
59. Misra A.K., Kasiraj R., Mutha Rao M., Rangareddy N.S. and Pant H.C. (1999) Embryo Transfer Technology in the Buffalo: Our Experience and Future Prospects. *Bubalus bubalis.* **(IV):** 63-74.
60. Misra A.K., Kasiraj R., Rangareddy N.S., Pant H.C. and Mutha Rao M. (2002) Effect of Gn-RH treatment on superovulatory response and embryo recovery in the buffalo (*Bubalus bubalis*). *Buffalo Journal.* 18 **(3):** 331-338.
61. Misra A.K., Sharma R., Verma P.K. and Yadav S. K. (2004) *In vitro* maturation, fertilization and culture of buffalo oocytes. In 20th Annual convention of ISSAR and National Symposium on Advanced Reproduc-

tive Technologies for management of fertility in livestock, held at College of Veterinary Science & Animal Husbandry, Anjora, Durg, Chhattisgarh. Dec. 14-16, p. 102.

62. Misra A.K. (1993) Superovulation and embryo transfer in buffalo: Progress, problems and future prospects in India, *A Review. Buffalo Journal.* **(1):** 13-24.
63. Misra A.K. (1996) Studies on improving certain aspects of embryo biotechnology in the buffalo. Ph.D. Thesis, CSA University of Agriculture and Technology, Kanpur, India.
64. Moor, R.M. and Gandolfi, F. (1987) Molecular and cellular changes associated with maturation and early development of sheep eggs. *J. Reprod. Fert.* **(34):** 55-69.
65. Moor, R.M., Crosby, I.M. (1985) Temperature induced abnormalities in sheep oocytes during maturation. *J. Reprod. Fert.* **(75):** 467-473.
66. Nandi S., Raghu H.M., Ravindranath B.M., Gupta P.S.P. and Sarma P.V. (2004) *In vitro* development of buffalo oocytes in media-containing fluids from different size class follicles. *Reproduction in Domestic Animals.* **(39):** 33-38.
67. Nandi S., Ravindranath B.M., Gupta P.S.P., Raghu H.M. and Sarma P.V. (2003) Developmental competence and post-thaw survivability of buffalo embryos produced *in vitro*: effect of growth factors in oocyte maturation medium and of embryo culture systems. *Theriogenology.* **(60):** 1621-1631.
68. Nasser L.F., Adams G.P., Bo G.A. (1993) Ovarian superstimulatory response relative to follicular wave emergence in heifers. *Theriogenology.* **(40):** 713-724.
69. NDDB. (1992) Science & Technology Project completion report "Cattle herd improvement for increased productivity using embryo transfer technology" National Dairy Development Board, Anand.
70. NDDB. (1997) Science & Technology Project completion report "Embryo Transfer-Downstream Activities" National Dairy Development Board, Anand.
71. Nicholus, J.S. (1933) Development of transplanted rat eggs. *Proc. .Soc. Exp. Biol. Med.* **(30):** 1111-1113.
72. Palasz AT, Mapletoft RJ (1996) Cryopreservation of mammalian embryos and oocytes: Recent advances. *Biotech. Advan.* **(14):** 127-149
73. Parrish, R.F. Wincek, T.J. and Polakoski, K.L. (1980) Glycosaminoglycons stimulation of the *in vitro* conversion of boar proacrosin to acrosin. *J. Androl.* **(1):** 89-95.
74. Pierson R.A., Ginther O.J. (1987) Follicular populations during the estrous cycle in heifers I. Influence of day. *Anim. Repro. Sci.* **(14):** 165-176.
75. Prasad Shiv (2000). Endocrine and biochemical profile of embryo donor and embryo recipient cattle. Ph.D. thesis. G.B. Pant University of Agriculture and Technology, Pantnagar, U.S. Nagar, Uttarakhand.
76. Prasad Shiv, Maurya S.N. and Misra A.K. (2002) Serum triiodothyronine (T3) and Thyroxine (T4) level in embryo donor and recipient cows. *Indian Journal of Animal Sciences* 72 **(9):** 750-753.
77. Prasad Shiv, Maurya S.N. and Varshney V.P. (2003) Serum progesterone and estradiol 17b concentration in relation to superovulatory response in embryo donor (Sahiwal) and conception rate in embryo recipient (crossbred) cattle. *Indian Journal of Animal Sciences.* 73 **(4):** 353-356.
78. Pursley J.R., Mee M.O., Wiltbank M.C. (1995) Synchronization of ovulation in dairy cows using PGF2á and GnRH. *Theriogenology.* **(44):** 915-923.
79. Raghu H.M., Nandi S., Reddy S.M. (2002) Effect of insulin, transferrin and selenium and epidermal growth factor on development of buffalo oocytes to the blastocyst stage *in vitro* in serum-free, semidefined media. *Veterinary Record.* 151 **(9):** 260-265.
80. Rall W.F., Fahy G.M. (1985) Ice-free cryopreservation of mouse embryos at –196°C by vitrification. *Nature.* **(313):** 573-575.
81. Rao Mutha, Kasiraj R., Reddy K.S.R., Jaiswal R.S., Misra A. K., Ranga Reddy N. S. (1994) A study on repeated superovulation and nonsurgical recovery in buffaloes. In : *Proceedings, 4th World Buffalo Congress,* Sao Paulo, Brazil, Volume **(3):** 498-500.
82. Ravindranatha B.M., Nandi S., Gupta P.S.P., Sarma P.V. 92001a) Comparison of three different media on maturation of buffalo oocytes *in vitro. Indian Journal of Animal Science.* **(71):** 841-843.

83. Ravindranatha B.M., Nandi S., Venkatachalpathy M. and Reddy S.M. (2001b) Conception rates in cows following transfer of vitrified and programmable frozen embryo. *Indian Journal of Dairy and Biosciences.* **(12):** 67-68.
84. Rawat A.K. (2004) Effect of buserelin on superovulatory response & embryo recovery rate in cattle. M.V.Sc. Thesis, G.B.Pant University of Agriculture & Technology, Pantnagar, U.S. Nagar, Uttarakhand, India.
85. Reuben J. Mapletoft (1984) Embryo transfer technology for the enhancement of animal reproduction. Biotechnology. **(2):** 149-160.
86. Rowe R.F., Del Campo M.R., Critser J.K. (1980) Embryo transfer in cattle: Nonsurgical transfer. *Am. J. Vet. Res.* **(41):** 1024-1028.
87. Samad H.A., Khan I.Q., Rehman N.U. and Ahamad N. (1998) The recovery, *in vitro* maturation and fertilization of Nili-Ravi buffalo follicular oocytes. *Asian. Australian. Journal. of Animal. Science.* **(11):** 491-497.
88. Schieve, M. C. (1991) The science and significance of embryo cryopreservation. *J. Zoo and Wildlife Med.* **(22):** 6-22.
89. Seidel G.E. Jr. (1981) Superovulation and embryo transfer in cattle. *Science.* **(211):** 351-358.
90. Seidel G.E. Jr. and Seidel S.M. (1981) The embryo transfer industry, In: *New Technologies in Animal Breeding.* B.G. Brackett, G.E. Seidel, Jr., and S. M. Seidel (eds.), Academic Press, New York. pp. 41-80.
91. Selk, G. Embryo Transfer in Cattle. No. 3158. Cooperative Extension Service , Division of Agriculture , Oklahoma State University
92. Sharma R.K., Siddiqui M.U., Gorani S. and Misra A.K. (2000) Superovulation of German Holstein cows with FSH and PMSG under tropical conditions. *Indian Journal of Animal Reproduction.* 21 **(2):** 98-100.
93. Sharma Utsav (2004) Endocrine manipulation of dominant follicle & its effect on superovulatory response in cattle. Ph.D. Thesis, G.B. Pant University of Agriculture & Technology, Pantnagar, U.S. Nagar, Uttarakhand, India.
94. Shaw D.W., Good T.E. (2000) Recovery rates and embryo quality following dominant follicle ablation in superovulated cattle. *Theriogenology.* **(53):** 1521-1528.
95. Siddique M.U., Sharma, R.K., Misra A.K. and Gorani S. (2001) Superovulatory response, quality of embryos and post superovulatory fertility in repeat breeding Holstein-Friesian heifers. *Indian Veterinary Medical Journal.* 25 **(12):** 322-324.
96. Singh Kamal, Maurya S.N. and Prasad Shiv (2003) Effect of FSH-E and FSH-P administration through single and multiple injections on superovulatory response and embryo recovery rate in cattle. *Indian Journal of Animal Sciences.* 73 **(2):** 136-138.
97. Singh S. and Dhanda O.P. (1997) Rabbit peritoneal fluid as a medium for *in vitro* maturation, fertilization and co-culture of buffalo oocytes. In: *Proc. 5th World Buffalo Congress*. Royal Palace, Caserta, Italy, Oct. 13-16. pp. 800-804.
98. Singla S.K. and Madan M.L. (1990) Response of superovulation in buffaloes (Bubalus bubalis) with SUPER-OV and FSH-P. *Theriogenology* **(33):** 327.
99. Singla S.K., Ambrose J.D. and Madan M.L. (1989) Superovulatory responses to treatment on different dates post estrous using super-OV in dairy cattle. In: proceedings of National Symposium on Applied Reproduction in farm Animals and the VIIIth National Convention of ISSAR, held at Gujrat Agricultural University, Anand, November 10-12. P.1.
100. Sreenan J.M. (1983) Embryo transfer procedure and its use as a research technique. *Vet. Rec.* **(112):** 494-500.
101. Subramaniam A., Devarajan K.P. and Mohanan M. (1990) "On Farm" embryo transfer in crossbred cows under Indian field conditions. *Indian Journal of Animal Reproduction.* 11 **(2):** 114-116.
102. Susko-Parrish, J.L., Parrish, J.J. and Handrow, R.R. (1985) Glucose inhibits the action of heparin by an indirect mechanism. *Biol. Reprod.* 32 **(1):** 80, Abstr.

103. Suzuki, T., Singla, S.K., Sujata, J. and Madan , M.L.(1992) *In vitro* fertilization of water buffalo follicular oocytes and their ability to cleave *in vitro*. *Theriogenology.* **(38):** 1187-1194.

104. Thatcher WW, Drost M, Savio JD (1993) New clinical uses of GnRH and its analogues in cattle. *Anim Reprod Sci.* **(33):** 27-49.

105. Thibault, C. (1977) Are follicular maturation and oocytes maturation independent processes. *J. Reorod. Fert.* **(51):** 1-15.

106. Totey S.M., Singh G.P., Taneja M., Pawshe C.H., Talwar G.P. (1992) *In vitro* maturation, fertilization and development of follicular oocytes from buffalo (Bubalus Bubalis). *Journal of Reproduction and Fertility.* **(95):** 597-607.

107. Totey S.M., Singh Gurpreet and Talwar G.P. (1989) Superovulatory response in lactating Bos indicus x Bos taurus cows primed with FSH-P at the beginning of estrous cycle. *Theriogenology.* 31 **(1):** 268.

108. Totey S.M., Singh Gurpreet, Anand Rajesh, Singh Gurcharan and Talwar G.P. (1988) Embroyo transfer in cattle. *Theriogenology.* 29 **(1):** 319.

109. Vajta, G., Holm, P., Kuwayama J. P., Booth, P. J., Jacobsen, H., Greve, T., Callesen, H. (1998) Open pulled straw (OPS) vitrification: A new way to reduce cryoinjuries of bovine ova and embryos. *Molec. Reprod. Develop.* **(51):** 53-58

110. Verma SK. (2005) Effect of buserelin on superovulation in cattle with reference to the levels of micro-minerals in serum. M.V. Sc. Thesis, G.B. Pant University of Agriculture & Technology, Pantnagar, U.S. Nagar, Uttarakhand, India.

111. Wright J.M. (1981) Non-surgical embryo transfer in cattle embryo-recipient interactions. *Theriogenology.* **(15):** 43-56.

112. Yadav M.C., Misra A.K., Motwani K.T., Rajeshwaran S. and Joshi B.V. (1988) Efficacy of Luprostiol for inducing estrus in superovulated buffaloes. *Proceedings of II World Buffalo Congress*, New Delhi, India, **(II):** 128.

113. Yadav P.S., Hooda O.K., Saini A., Jindal S.K. (2001) *In vitro* cleavage and development of buffalo oocytes with semen from buffalo bulls. *Indian Journal of Animal Sciences.* **(71)**: 752–754.

CHAPTER

26

Stem Cell Technology

Stem cell technology is a rapidly developing field that combines the efforts of cell biologists, geneticists, and clinicians and offers hope of effective treatment for a variety of malignant and non-malignant diseases. Stem cells are defined as pluripotent progenitor cells capable of self-renewal and multilineage differentiation. Stem cells survive well and show stable division in culture, making them ideal targets for *in vitro* manipulation. The ability of stem cells to integrate into the tissue cytoarchitecture under the control of the host microenvironment and developmental cues, makes them ideal for cell replacement therapy. In this chapter, we briefly discuss the basic principles and current research and applications of stem cells.

Keywords: Stem cells, totipotent progenitor cells, embryonic stem cells, self-renewal stem cell therapy.

INTRODUCTION

Stem cells are found in all multicellular organisms. They are characterized by the ability to renew themselves through mitotic cell division and differentiating into a diverse range of specialized cell types. Research in the field of stem cell grew out of findings by Canadian scientists Ernest A. McCulloch and James E. Till in the 1960s. The two broad types of mammalian stem cells are: embryonic stem cells that are isolated from the inner cell mass of blastocysts, and adult stem cells that are found in adult tissues. In a developing embryo, stem cells can differentiate into all of the specialized embryonic tissues. In adult organisms, stem cells and progenitor cells act as a repair system for the body, replenishing specialized cells, but also maintaining the normal turnover of regenerative organs, such as blood, skin, or intestinal tissues.

Stem cells can now be grown and transformed into specialized cells with characteristics consistent with cells of various tissues such as muscles or nerves through cell culture. Highly plastic adult stem cells from a variety of sources, including umbilical cord blood and bone marrow, are routinely used in medical therapies. Embryonic cell lines and embryonic stem cells generated through therapeutic cloning have also been proposed as promising candidates for future therapies. Research on stem cells is advancing knowledge about how an organism develops from a single cell and how healthy cells replace damaged cells in adult organisms. This promising area of science is also leading scientists to investigate the possibility of cell-based therapies to treat diseases, which is often referred to as regenerative or reparative medicine. Study of stem cells is one of the most fascinating areas of biology today. But like many expanding fields of scientific inquiry, research on stem cells raises scientific questions as rapidly as it generates new discoveries.

Scientists discovered ways to obtain or derive stem cells from early mouse embryos more than 30 years ago. After many years of detailed study of the biology of mouse stem cells, in the year 1998 researchers developed the techniques to isolate stem cells from human embryos and grow them in the laboratory. These are called human embryonic stem cells. The embryos used in these studies were obtained from infertility clinics which were produced by *in vitro* fertilization procedures for infertility purposes. When they were no longer needed for transplantation purpose, they were donated for stem cell research, with the consent of the donor. Stem cells are important for living organisms due to many reasons. In the 3- to 5-day-old embryo, called a blastocyst, stem cells in developing tissues give rise to multiple specialized cell types that make-up the heart, lung, skin, and other tissues. In some adult tissues, such as bone marrow, muscle, and brain, discrete populations of adult stem cells generate replacements for cells that are lost through normal wear and tear, injury, or disease. The blastocyst includes three structures: the trophoblast, which is the layer of cells that surrounds the blastocyst; the blastocoel, which is the hollow cavity inside the blastocyst; and the inner cell mass, which is a group of approximately 30 cells at one end of the blastocoel.

It has been hypothesized by scientists that stem cells may, at some point in future, become the basis for treating diseases such as Parkinson's disease, diabetes, and heart disease. Scientists want to study stem cells in the laboratory so that they can learn about their essential properties and what makes them different from specialized cell types. As scientists learn more about stem cells, it may become possible to use the cells not just in cell-based therapies, but also for screening new drugs and toxins and understanding birth defects. However, as mentioned above, human embryonic stem cells have been studied only since 1998. Therefore, in order to develop such treatments, scientists are intensively studying the fundamental properties of stem cells, which include: (1) determining precisely how stem cells remain unspecialized and self-renewing for many years; and (2) identifying the signals that cause stem cells to become specialized cells.

CONCEPTS

A stem is defined as the main stalk of a plant which supports the entire plant. Correspondingly, stem cells are the main trunk from which specialized cells develop and branch out over time by the process of differentiation. Stem cells are the foundation for every organ, tissue and cell in the human body. Stem cells may be able to repair or replace damaged tissue, thereby reversing diseases and injuries such as cancer, diabetes, cardiovascular disease and blood diseases, to name a few. Principally there are two types of stem cells: unlimited stem cells (also known as embryonic stem cells) and limited cells (also known as adult stem cells). The unlimited stem cells are mainly obtained from leftover embryos (2-3 days old) of the fertility clinics with patients' permission that would otherwise be discarded. These embryos are created by the process of *in vitro* fertilization and exist entirely outside the body. Unlimited stem cells can develop into any kind of cell type or tissue in the body. Limited stem cells on the other hand are rare cells that can be found only in some developed organs or tissues. These cells have been successfully used recently in bone marrow (either with bone marrow stem cells or umbilical cord blood stem cells), skin and hair transplants. In 2006, researchers made another breakthrough by identifying conditions that would allow some specialized adult cells to be "reprogrammed" genetically to assume a stem cell-like state. Laboratory studies of stem cells enable scientists to learn about the cells' essential properties and what makes them different from specialized cell types. Scientists are already using stem cells in the laboratory to screen new drugs and develop model systems to study normal growth and identify the causes of birth defects.

PRINCIPLES

Stem cells have two important characteristics that distinguish them from other types of cells. First, they are unspecialized cells that renew themselves for long periods through cell division, sometimes after long periods of inactivity. The second is that under certain physiological or experimental conditions, they can be induced to become cells with special functions such as the beating cells of the heart muscle or the insulin-producing cells of the pancreas. Stem cells have the remarkable potential to develop into many different cell types in the body during early life and growth. In addition, in many tissues they serve as a sort of internal repair system, dividing essentially without limit to replenish other cells as long as the person or animal is still alive. When a stem cell divides, each new cell has the potential either to remain a stem cell or become another type of cell with a more specialized function, such as a muscle cell, a red blood cell, or a brain cell.

STEM CELL TECHNOLOGY

What are Stem Cells?

A stem cell is a cell that can divide for indefinite periods—often throughout the life of an organism. These cells are undifferentiated and lack certain tissue specific markers. These cells remain uncommitted until they receive a signal to develop into a specialized cell.

Unique Properties of Stem Cells

There are some unique properties in the stem cells, which make them different from normal non-stem cells, and so are important. These properties are their proliferation ability, unspecialized nature, differentiation ability, and plasticity.

Proliferation ability: When cells replicate themselves many times, it is called proliferation. Stem cells have long-term self-renewal ability, i.e., stem cells can renew themselves by dividing into the same non-specialized cell type over long periods (many months to years) depending upon the specific type of stem cells.

Unspecialized nature of stem cells: One of the fundamental properties of a stem cell is that it does not have any tissue-specific structures that allow it to perform specialized functions. These cells do not function like their neighboring cells. For example, in blood, these stem cells do not perform oxygen transport (like that of red blood cells), or they do not secrete insulin (like islet cells) in pancreas, which indicates that they do not perform tissue specific functions.

Differentiation ability: The process whereby an undifferentiated embryonic stem cell acquires the features of a specialized cell such as a heart, liver, or muscle cell is called differentiation. After receiving some signal, the undifferentiated stem cells get differentiated into a particular type of cell with specified functions.

Plasticity or transdifferentiation: Stem cells typically generate the cell types of the tissue in which they reside. This is technically known as directed differentiation. For example, a stem cell in the bone marrow normally gives rise to many types of blood cells such as red blood cells, white blood cells and platelets. But it has been found that a blood-forming cell in the bone marrow, which is called a hematopoietic stem cell, bone marrow stromal cells could give rise to the cells of a very different tissue, such as nerve cells in the brain. It has also been proved now that this transdifferentiation also takes place *in vivo*. Researchers have shown that when purified hematopoietic stem cells are injected in the body, cells differentiated into hepatic cells *in vivo*. Stem cells, which are able to differentiate into cell types beyond those of the tissues in which they normally reside, are said to exhibit plasticity or transdifferentiating ability. Examples of such plasticity include blood cells differentiating to neurons; liver cells can be made to produce insulin; and hematopoietic stem cells that can develop into heart muscle.

Difference between Normal Cells and Stem Cells

Normal somatic cells are allowed to divide mitotically up to roughly about 50 times after which they undergo a process called senescence, which means getting old. These will then usually degrade and undergo apoptosis, a term used to define the programmed cell death. In comparison, stem cells have the ability to divide endlessly, which provides the first key difference between stem cells and somatic cells.

Another major difference between stem cells and somatic cells is that when stem cells undergo mitotic division, they give rise to two different kinds of cells. In normal somatic cells, during cell division, a normal cell divides into daughter cells of its own type. But unlike normal cells, stem cells divide into two daughter cells, one of which has characteristics of stem cells, and the other one has potential to differentiate into specialized cells. So stem cells give rise to two different types of cells during mitosis. They mostly give rise to another stem cell, which is important for maintaining the total number of stem cells in the body consistent, and then at the same time stem cells have the ability to give rise to somatic cells. This unique pattern of cell division in stem cells is responsible for their self-renewal properties.

Identification of Stem Cells

Although there is no complete agreement among scientists about identification of stem cells, most tests are based on making sure that stem cells are undifferentiated and capable of self-renewal. Tests are often conducted in the laboratory to check for these properties. One way to identify stem cells in a laboratory, and the standard procedure for testing bone marrow or hematopoietic stem cell (HSC) is by transplanting cells to save an individual without HSCs. If the stem cell produces new blood and immune cells, it demonstrates its potency. Clonogenic assays (a laboratory procedure) can also be employed *in vitro* to test whether single cells can differentiate and self-renew. Researchers may also inspect cells under a microscope to see if they are healthy and undifferentiated or they may examine chromosomes. To test whether human embryonic stem cells are pluripotent, scientists allow the cells to differentiate spontaneously in cell culture, manipulate the cells so that they differentiate to form specific cell types, or inject the cells into an immunosuppressed mouse to test for the formation of a teratoma (a benign tumor containing a mixture of differentiated cells).

Why are Stem Cells Important?

Studying stem cells and their functions is important not only to gain a greater understanding of early human development, including the development of birth defects, but also for our comprehension of medical diseases such as cancer that have their origins in abnormalities of cell division and cell differentiation.

The most exciting potential use of stem cells is "cell therapy," treatment of disease by replacing damaged or dead tissue with stem cells. Earlier people used to employ organ or tissue implantation for replacing the damaged or dead tissues. The major drawback of this system is the limited number of available donors. Apart from this, chance of immune rejection poses a serious threat to this application. Some of the diseases that can be treated with cell therapy include Parkinson's, Alzheimer's, stroke and spinal cord injury; both rheumatoid and osteoarthritis; and heart disease and diabetes. If successful, this regenerative approach would reduce the need for organ and tissue transplants.

Types of Stem Cells

Stem cells can be classified into 3 broad types:

(a) On the basis of differentiation potential
(b) On the basis of differentiated cell type
(c) On the basis of origin

Each of these is further divided into subtypes for a better understanding (Figure 26.1).

(a) On the basis of differentiation potential

On the basis of differentiated cell type, stem cells can be sub-divided into four categories: (i) totipotent stem cells, (ii) pluripotent stem cells, (iii) multipotent stem cells, and (iv) unipotent stem cells.

Totipotent: These stem cells have the potential to become any kind of cell in the body. After an egg is fertilized, it undergoes a series of divisions to become an embryo and later a fetus. The cells that are formed during these first few divisions are totipotent i.e., they can become any cell in the body. Human cells have this capacity only during the first few divisions of a fertilized egg. After 3-4 divisions of totipotent cells, these cells will not be able to differentiate into all types of cells, rather they may undergo specialized cellular differentiation.

Pluripotent: This type of stem cell has the ability to become almost any kind of cells in the body, except the cells of the placenta or other supporting tissues of the uterus. Pluripotent stem cells result after totipotent stem cells undergo the first few divisions. Embryonic stem cells at the blastocyst stage and fetal stem cells are pluripotent. Totipotent and pluripotent cells are essential for the development of an entirely new organism. This is the reason they are found in the early stages of development.

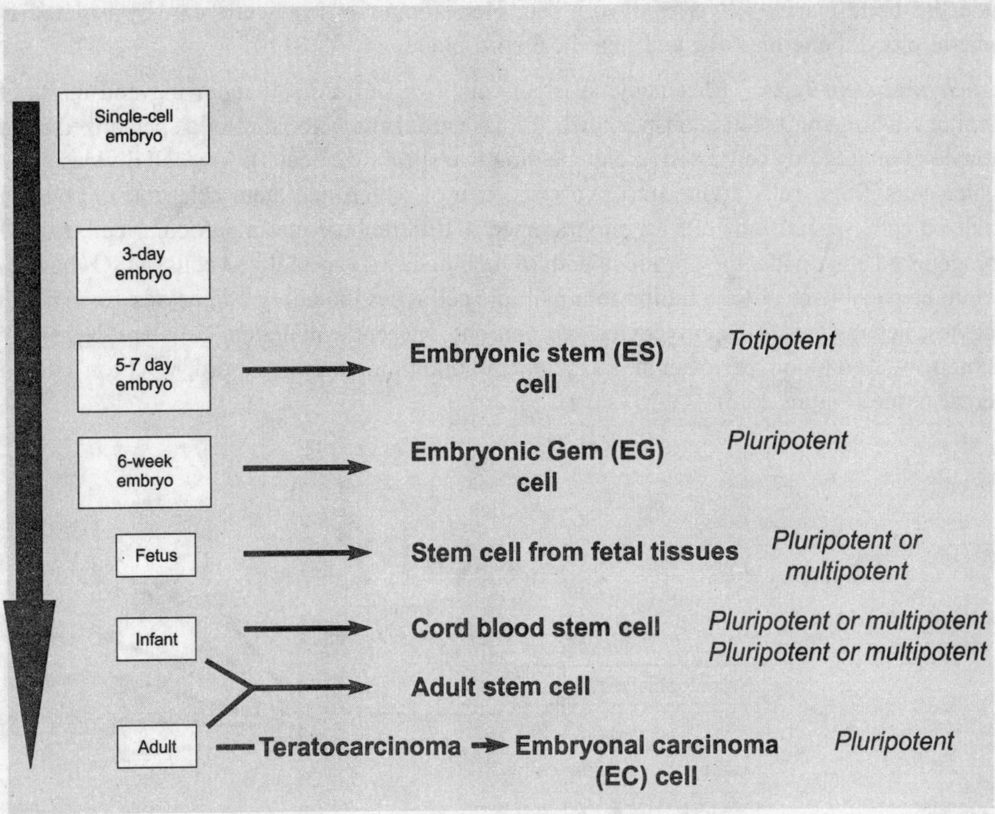

Figure 26.1 Various types of stem cells in human.

Multipotent: These cells can give rise to several other cell types, but those types are limited to mostly cells of the blood, heart, muscle and nerves. These cells function as a repair system for damaged tissue. Adult stem cells are a good example of multipotent stem cells.

Unipotent: A unipotent stem cell refers to a cell that can differentiate along only one lineage. These cells have the capacity to differentiate into only one type of cell or tissue, which is lower in potentiality in terms of differentiation as compared to stem cells that give rise to a broad range of cell types. Although the unipotent adult stem cells in the body's tissues will give rise to only one cell type, they still have the important property of self-renewal that is shared by all stem cells. Skin cells, which are in the epithelium, are one of the most abundant types of unipotent stem cells.

(b) On the basis of differentiated cell type

On that basis of differentiated cell type, stem cells can be sub-divided into two categories: (i) hematopoietic stem cells, and (ii) mesenchymal stem cells.

Hematopoietic stem cells: A stem cell from which all red and white blood cells evolve is called hematopoietic stem cell. The hematopoietic stem cell is derived early in embryogenesis from mesoderm and is deposited in very specific hematopoietic sites within the embryo. These sites include the bone marrow, liver and yolk sac. Hematopoietic stem cells can be isolated from peripheral blood, bone marrow, and umbilical cord blood.

Mesenchymal stem cells: Mesenchymal stem cells (MSCs) are self-renewing and multipotent progenitors (a progenitor cell is unspecialized or has partial characteristics of a specialized cell that is capable of undergoing cell division and yielding two specialized cells). Any cell divides into two daughter cells. Stem cells divide into two cells, one of which is a stem cell, and the other is a specialized cell. Specialized cells are programmed to differentiate into a particular cell. But when the progenitor cells divide, they produce both of their cells into specialized cells. MSCs have been shown to be capable of differentiating into multiple cell types including adipocytes, chondrocytes, osteocytes, hepatocytes, cardiomyocytes and neurons. Mesenchymal stem cells are derived from bone marrow, cord blood, periosteum, fat, skin, amniotic fluid, umbilical cord, Wharton's jelly and placental tissue (Figure 26.2).

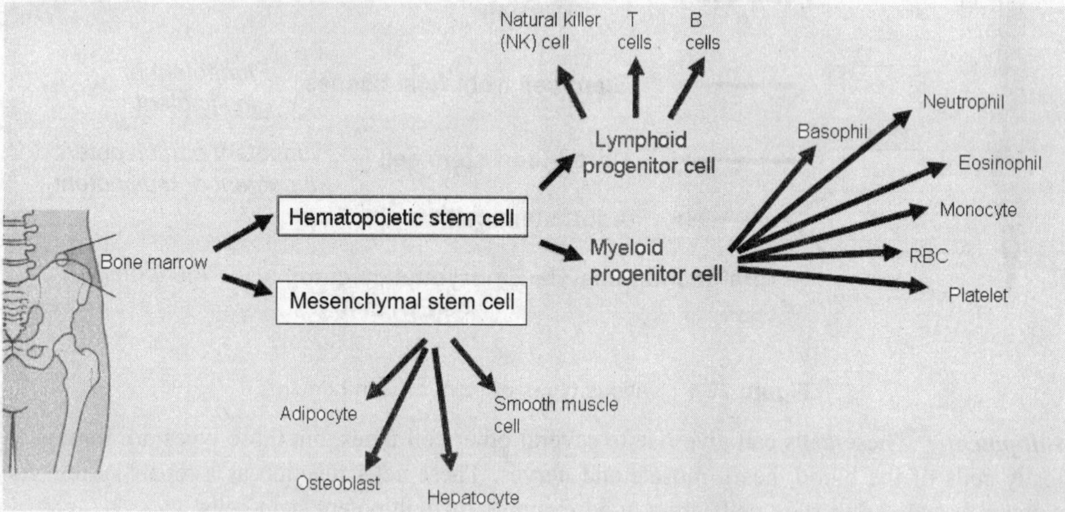

Figure 26.2 Hematopoietic and mesenchymal stem cell differentiation from bone marrow.

(c) On the basis of origin

On the basis of the origin of stem cells, they can be sub-divided into further categories: (i) stem cells from embryo, (ii) stem cells from the fetus, (iii) stem cells from the umbilical cord and cord blood, (iv) and stem cells from the adult.

Embryonic stem cells (ESCs): Embryonic stem cells, as their name suggests, are derived from embryos. An embryonic stem cell is derived from a group of cells called the inner cell mass, which is part of the early (4 to 5 days) embryo called the blastocyst. Once removed from the blastocyst, the cells of the inner cell mass can be cultured as embryonic stem cells. Embryonic stem cells are capable of undergoing an unlimited number of symmetrical divisions without differentiating (long-term self-renewal). They express the transcription factor Oct-4, which maintains ES cells in a proliferative, non-differentiating state. These cells can be induced to continue proliferating or differentiate. Some researchers have shown that they lack the G1 checkpoint in the cell cycle. ES cells spend most of their time in the S phase of the cell cycle, during which they synthesize DNA. Unlike differentiated somatic cells, ES cells do not require any external stimulus to initiate DNA replication. In every somatic cell of a female mammal, one of the two X chromosomes becomes permanently inactivated. However, X chromosome inactivation does not occur in undifferentiated ES cells. One more type of cell, known as embryonic germ cells (EGCs), is also present in the embryo. These cells originate from the primordial germ cells of the gonadal ridge of 5- to 9-week-old fetus. ES cells and EGCs are pluripotent, but they are not identical in all of their characteristics features (Figure 26.3).

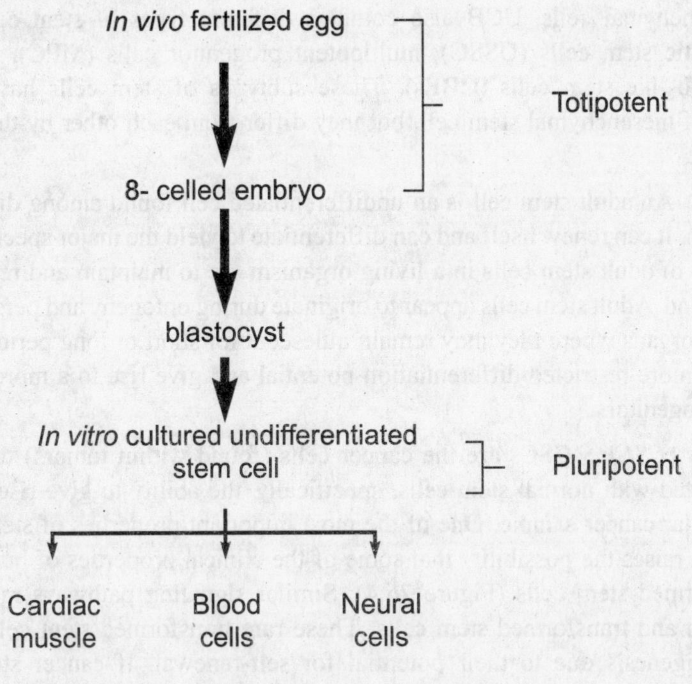

Figure 26.3 Various stages of embryonic stem cells.

Fetal stem cells: After eight weeks of development, the embryo is referred to as fetus. By this time it has developed a human-like form. Fetal stem cells are primitive cell types found in the organs of fetuses. These are responsible for the initial development of all tissues before the birth. They are the earliest cells found in the fetus, which then replicate efficiently and rapidly to create blood, liver, heart tissues, etc. Like that of ESCs, fetal stem cells are also pluripotent.

Umbilical cord (UC) and umbilical cord blood (UCB) stem cells: These cells are in the inter-phase of embryonic and adult stem cells in their characteristic features. They have the proliferation potentiality like that of embryonic stem cells and differentiation capacity like that of an adult stem cell. Umbilical cord transports nutrient and oxygen-rich blood from the placenta to the fetus. After birth the cord is removed from the infant. The UC normally contains two umbilical arteries and one umbilical vein, a main reservoir of UCB. UC is filled with a loose, proteoglycan-rich matrix known as Wharton's jelly (WJ). The main role of this jelly-like material is to prevent the compression, torsion, and bending of the enclosed vessels, which provide bidirectional blood flow between fetal and maternal circulation. Cord derived stem cells are present in both Wharton's jelly and umbilical vein. These stem cells can differentiate into limited types of cells (Multipotent). They can be extracted, cultured, and induced to differentiate into mature cell types such as neurons. Wharton's jelly and umbilical vein are therefore a potential source of adult stem cells.

UCB is the blood remaining in the UC and placenta after birth. It has both hematopoietic and mesenchymal stem cells. Presently the cord blood is used as the most common source of stem cells because it has no ethical concern as with the embryonic stem cells. The frequency of umbilical cord blood hematopoietic stem cells equals or exceeds that of bone marrow. Along with hematopoietic and mesenchymal cells, UCB also contains different types of stem cells, for example unrestricted somatic stem cells (USSC), multipotent progenitor cells (MPC), and cord blood-derived embryonic like stem cells (CBEs). These subtypes of stem cells have differentiation potential as that of mesenchymal stem cell, but they differ from each other by their characteristic surface markers.

Adult stem cells: An adult stem cell is an undifferentiated cell found among differentiated cells in a tissue or organ. It can renew itself and can differentiate to yield the major specialized cell types. The primary roles of adult stem cells in a living organism are to maintain and repair the tissue in which they are found. Adult stem cells appear to originate during ontogeny and persist in specialized niches within the organs where they may remain quiescent for short or long periods of time. They generally show a more restricted differentiation potential and give rise to a more limited number of distinct cell progenitors.

Cancer stem cells (CSC): CSCs are the cancer cells (found within tumors) that possess characteristics associated with normal stem cells, specifically, the ability to give rise to all cell types found in a particular cancer sample. One of the most important properties of stem cells is that of self-renewal. This raises the possibility that some of the clinical properties of human tumors may be due to transformed stem cells (Figure 26.4). Similar signaling pathways may regulate self-renewal in normal and transformed stem cells. These rare transformed stem cells may drive the process of tumorigenesis due to their potential for self-renewal. If cancer stem cells can be prospectively identified and isolated, it should be possible to identify therapies that will selectively target these cells.

Surface Markers

Surface markers are molecules usually found on the plasma membrane of a specific cell type or a limited number of cell types. Stem cells have certain specific surface markers that are absent in non-stem cells. Stem cell markers are given short-hand names based on the molecules that bind

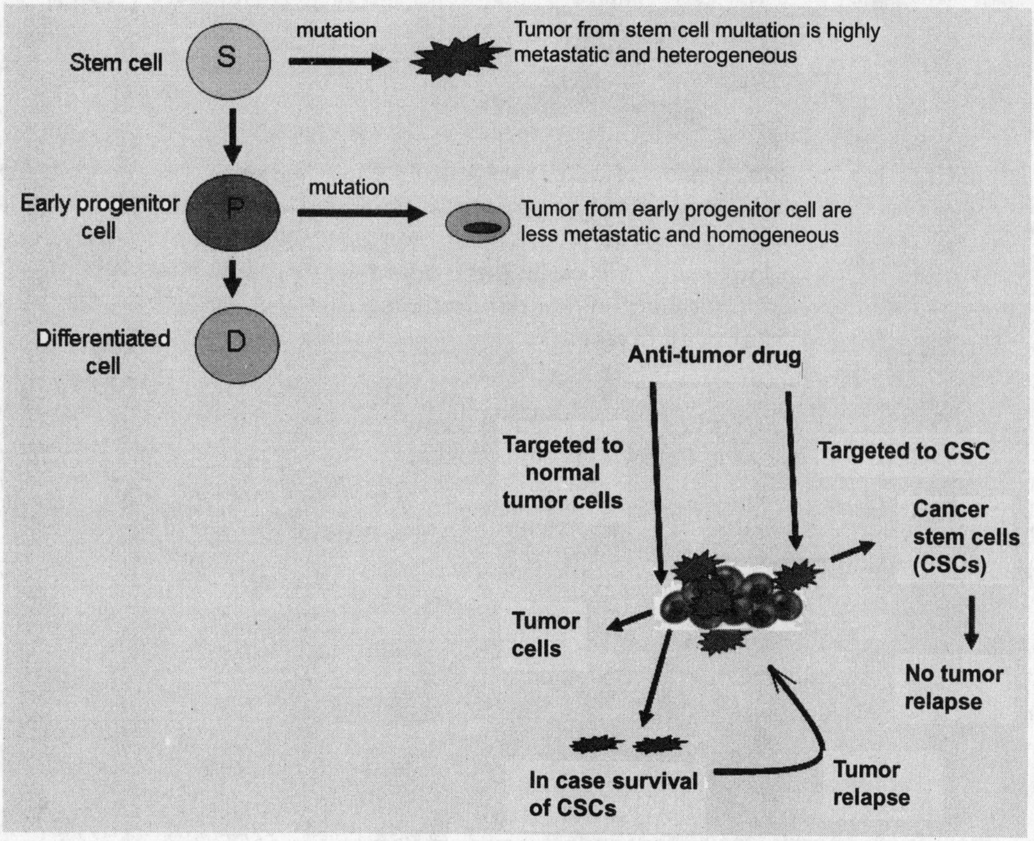

Figure 26.4 Crosstalk between stem cells and developement of cancer.

to the stem cell surface receptors. For example, a cell that has the receptor stem cell antigen–1 on its surface is identified as Sca-1. In many cases, a combination of multiple markers is used to identify a particular stem cell type. Hence, researchers often identify stem cells in shorthand by a combination of marker names reflecting the presence (+) or absence (–) of them. For example, a special type of hematopoietic stem cell from blood and bone marrow called "side population" or "SP" is described as ($CD34^{-}$/low, c-Kit^{+}, Sca-1). Table 26.1 summarizes some of the known cell surface markers from various types of stem cells.

Fluorescence assisted cell sorter (FACS) is used to sort out the rare stem cells from millions of other cells. With this technique, a suspension of tagged cells (i.e., bound to the cell surface specific fluorescent marker) are sent under pressure through an extremely narrow nozzle, i.e., so narrow that only one cell can pass through it at a time. Upon exiting the nozzle, cells then pass, one-by-one, through a light source, usually a laser, and then through an electric field. The fluorescent cells become negatively charged, while non-fluorescent cells become positively charged. The charge difference allows stem cells to be separated from other cells (Figure 26.5).

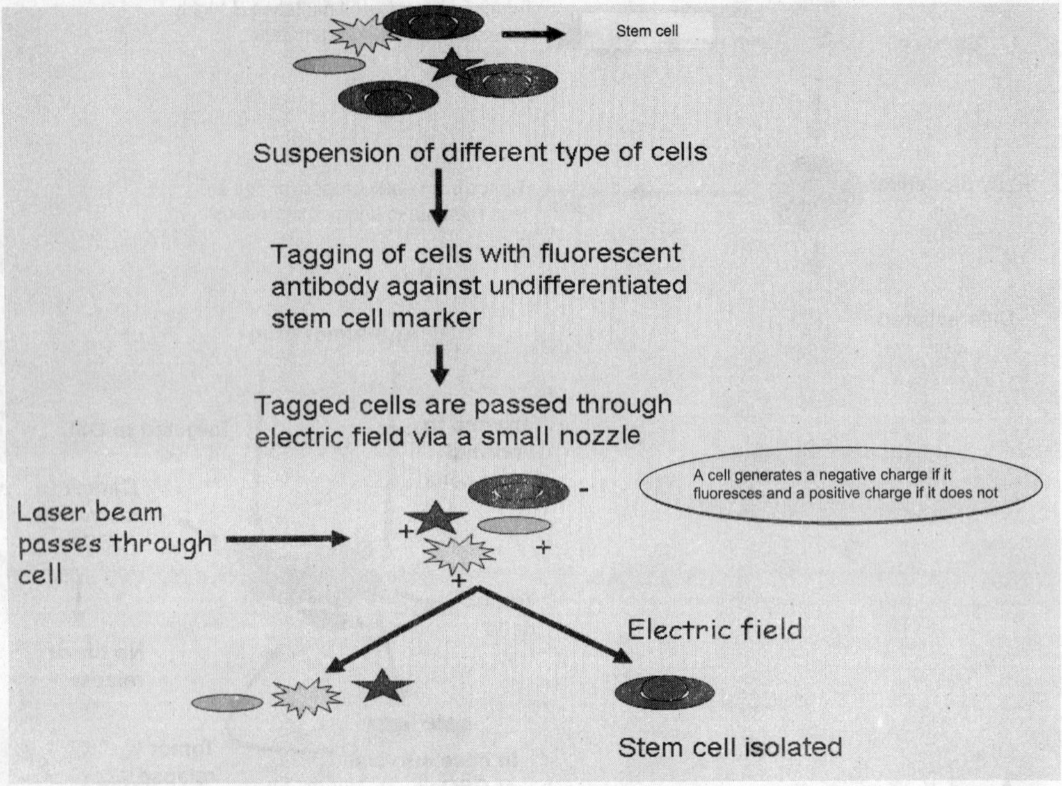

Figure 26.5 Method of separation of stem cells by FACS.

Table 26.1 Some markers commonly used to identify stem cells and characterize differentiated cell types (Source: NIH Appendix E: Stem Cell Markers).

Marker Name	*Cell Type*	*Significance*
Fetal liver kinase-1	Endothelial	Blood vessel Cell-surface receptor protein that identifies endothelial cell progenitor; marker of cell-cell contacts
Smooth muscle cell-specific myosin heavy chain	Smooth muscle	Identifies smooth muscle cells in the wall of blood vessels
Vascular endothelial cell cadherin	Smooth muscle	Identifies smooth muscle cells in the wall of blood vessels
Bone-specific alkaline phosphatase (BAP)	Osteoblast	Bone; enzyme expressed in osteoblast; activity indicates bone formation
Hydroxyapatite	Osteoblast	Mineralized bone matrix that provides structural integrity; marker of bone formation
Osteocalcin (OC)	Osteoblast	Mineral-binding protein uniquely synthesized by osteoblast; marker of bone formation
Bone morphogenetic	Mesenchymal stem	Bone marrow and blood

Contd.

protein receptor (BMPR)	and progenitor cells	Important for the differentiation of committed mesenchymal cell types from mesenchymal stem and progenitor cells; BMPR identifies early mesenchymal lineages (stem and progenitor cells)
CD4 and CD8	White blood cell (WBC)	Cell-surface protein markers specific for mature T lymphocyte (WBC subtype)
CD34	Mesencyhmal stem cell (MSC)	Identifies MSCs, which can differentiate into adipocyte, osteocyte, chondrocyte, and myocyte
CD44	Mesenchymal	A type of cell-adhesion molecule used to identify specific types of mesenchymal cells
c-Kit identifies HSC	HSC, MSC	Cell-surface receptor on bone marrow (BM) cell types that identifies, HSC and MSC; binding by fetal calf serum (FCS) enhances proliferation of ES cells, HSCs, MSCs, and hematopoietic progenitor cells
Stem cell antigen –1 (Sca-1)	HSC, MSC	Cell-surface protein in bone marrow (BM) cell, indicative of HSC and MSC
Adipocyte lipid-binding protein (ALBP)	Adipocyte	Fat; lipid-binding protein located specifically in adipocyte
Albumin	Hepatocyte	Liver; principal protein produced by the liver; indicates functioning of maturing and fully differentiated hepatocytes
CD133	Neural stem cell, HSC	Nervous system; cell-surface protein that identifies neural stem cells, which give rise to neurons and glial cells
Nestin	Neural progenitor	Intermediate filament structural protein expressed in primitive neural tissue
Cytokeratin 19 (CK19)	Pancreatic epithelium	Pancreas; CK19 identifies specific pancreatic epithelial cells that are progenitors for islet cells and ductal cells
Glucagon	Pancreatic islet	Expressed by alpha-islet cell of pancreas
Insulin-promoting factor-1 (PDX-1)	Pancreatic islet	Transcription factor expressed by beta-islet cell of pancreas
Bone morphogenetic protein-4	Mesoderm	Pluripotent stem cells Growth and differentiation factor expressed during early mesoderm formation and differentiation
Alkaline phosphatase	Embryonic stem (ES), embryonal carcinoma (EC)	Elevated expression of this enzyme is associated with undifferentiated pluripotent stem cell (PSC)
Oct-4	ES, EC	Transcription factor unique to PSCs; essential for establishment and maintenance of undifferentiated PSCs

Ethical Issues in Stem Cell Research

The discovery, isolation, and culturing of human embryonic stem cells has been described as one of the most significant breakthroughs in biomedicine of the century. This is because of their ability to self-renew infinitely while retaining a remarkable capacity to differentiate into any form of cell tissue. The culturing of embryonic stem cells holds tremendous potential for the development of new forms of regenerative medicine to treat debilitating or fatal conditions that would otherwise not be curable, but some people oppose embryonic stem cell research on religious grounds. Many

Catholics think that from the moment of conception an embryo is a human being with a soul, and using these embryos is like dismembering a person. And the harvesting of embryonic stem cells results in the destruction of the embryos from which they are harvested. Keeping irony of advantage and harm of embryonic stem cell research, it is finalized that, yes, embryos do have intrinsic moral value but embryos that are surplus to *in vitro* fertilization (IVF) can be used for stem cell isolation. The idea here is that if embryos are definitely not going to be implanted, then 'nothing is lost' by their being used for ES cell research. People also think that stem cell is like a cloning. But these two things are totally different aspects of biological research. A lot of debate is going on in this area. Some countries like United States, United Kingdom, Australia and Switzerland have formulated some laws, and under those regulations only embryonic stem cell research can be done. Under the HFE Act (The Human Fertilization and Embryology Act and Regulations), it is legal to carry out research on human embryos up to 14 days after fertilization in UK. In December 2002, Australia passed two pieces of federal legislation to regulate cloning and embryonic stem cell research. The first, *Prohibition of Human Cloning Act 2002* outlawed any form of human cloning, whether it be to generate tissues (therapeutic cloning) or a new human being (reproductive cloning). The second, *Research Involving Human Embryos Act 2002*, allows researchers to access surplus human embryos under strict conditions. In US, government-funded researchers are not allowed to make stem cells from spare human embryos. But there is no criminal law against it, so researchers in private companies do not have the same constraints as researchers receiving government funding. Whatever the rule, it is critical to undertake stem cell research under strict vigilance to get the benefit out of it but without any misuse.

APPLICATIONS OF STEM CELL TECHNOLOGY

The economic and psychological tolls of chronic, degenerative, and acute diseases in the United States are enormous. It has been estimated that up to 128 million people suffer from such diseases, thus, virtually every citizen is affected directly or indirectly. The total cost of treating diabetes, for example, is approaching $100 billion in the United States alone. With advancement of research, the developmental potential of different kinds of stem cells will be better understood. As of now, although adult stem cells are limited in their potential to differentiate, embryonic germ cells have a great differentiation capacity, and embryonic stem cells are thought to be able to differentiate into almost any tissue. Thus, different types of stem cells could have different applications. Below is a discussion of potential stem cell applications.

Use of Stem Cells in Gene Therapy

Gene therapy involves inserting genes into a person's cells with the aim of providing treatment for a particular disease. At a very simplistic level, gene therapy is the use of a person's own cells to provide a therapeutic effect. In most types of gene therapy, a healthy and normal gene is inserted into a cell or tissue to replace a gene that is abnormal and thus causes disease. There are many reasons why stem cells hold great potential for successful use in gene therapies. Stem cells have the ability to self-renew, which means that the need to provide repeated administrations of gene therapy can be reduced or possibly even eliminated (Figure 26.6).

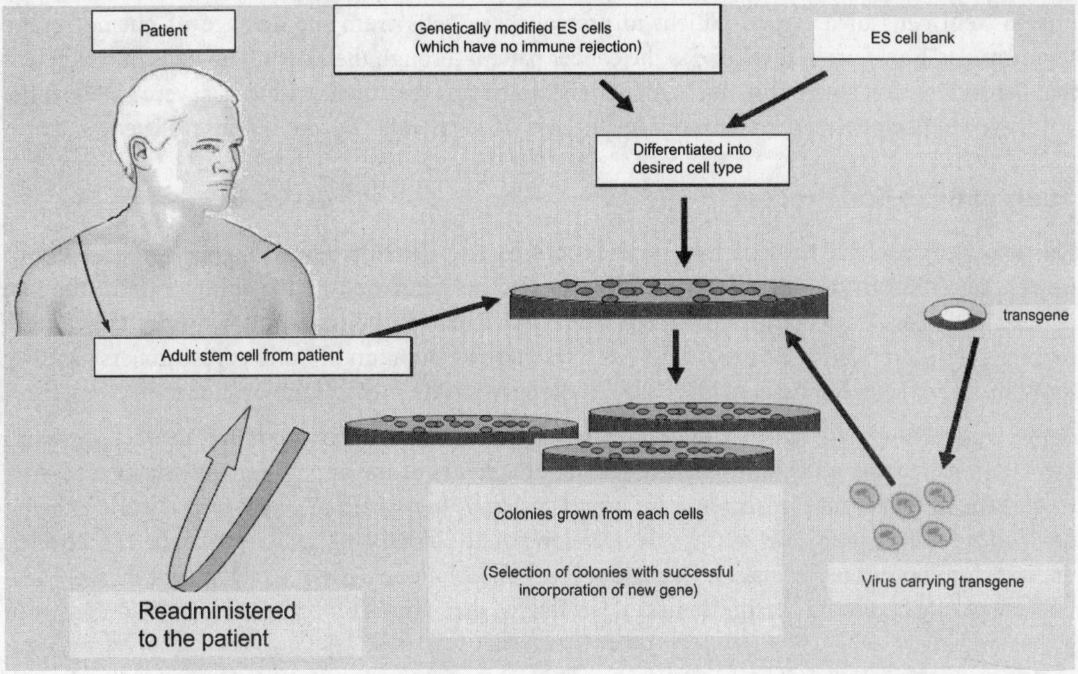

Figure 26.6 Strategies for delivering therapeutic transgenes into patients.

Some breakthroughs in stem cell based gene therapy: The researchers worked with mice breed having poor immunity (thymus of the mice was removed, so that they did not have T-cells, and hence no immune system). Such mice are called nude mice. The mice were injected with blood stem cells (hematopoietic stem cells) that carried a specific gene, which is activated only within a specific mature immune cell called an antigen-presenting cell. The specific gene was tagged with GFP. They were able to monitor the fact that the stem cells ultimately developed into that antigen-presenting cell by measuring the amount of fluorescence in all derivatives of the transplanted cells. Another research group from Jerusalem introduced a gene into the human ESC using lentiviral vector and monitored the expression of the gene in the *in vivo* condition. They found that the modified gene expression continued as the stem cells proliferated and differentiated, demonstrating the technical feasibility of using stem cells for cell therapy.

Cystic fibrosis (CF) is the most common and fatal genetic disorder affecting mainly Caucasians and is characterized by the mutation of *CFTR* gene present on the surface of epithelial cells, including those that line the airways in the lungs. Researchers first isolated the bone marrow stem cells from CF patients and then inserted the corrected *CFTR* gene into the stem cells with the help of Moloney murine leukemia virus vector. After culturing the cells *in vitro* they transplanted the cells back into the patient. The patient showed remarkable recovery by this *ex vivo* gene therapy using stem cell technology.

In another interesting experiment, a group of researchers inserted *MGMT* (O-6-methylguanine-DNA methyltransferase) gene, which is responsible for causing drug resistance, into the hematopoietic stem cells of a cancer patient to protect these cells from the damage of chemotherapy regimens. By transferring this gene to the cancer patient through their own stem cells, it was found that the patient was able to tolerate stronger chemotherapy treatment with less severe side-effects. All these studies provided some basis for the use of stem cells for the purpose of gene therapy.

Study of Biological Process

Our knowledge in the field of biological processes like developmental biology, progression of cancer, target identifications for various disorders etc. is facilitated by the ability to trace the fate of stem cell. This is so because these are the cells, which can be tracked down from their origin to terminal differentiation *in vitro*. This has attracted the attention of various researchers globally to utilize these cells for basic studies as well along with the medical applications.

Some breakthrough in study of biological processes: Researchers are trying to track developmental process of blood and immune system, so that many of the appropriate treatments could be suggested. In this regard, research is in progress across the world and one major work is being done on zebra fish stem cells to trace the development of blood and immune system. The detailed understanding of blood formation (hematopoiesis) and immune system development in zebra fish will eventually be used to design stem cell treatments for various blood or immune disorders even in human beings.

Another group from LA Jolla, California, USA, by utilizing the clues from stem cell research discovered that Wnt signaling pathway is up-regulated in insulin producing cells of pancreases from adults with type 2 diabetes. This fundamental study was possible by observing the developmental pattern of pancreatic cells from ESCs. Studies of these sorts can provide potential new targets for the cure and management of very common metabolic disorder like that of diabetes.

Stem Cells in Drug Discovery

Stem cells are also a valuable source of materials in drug discovery, high-content screening assays, and toxicology studies (Figure 26.7). High-content screening is quantitative study of biological systems at the level of whole living cells. The protein to be studied is tagged with fluorescent protein (e.g. GFP). The expression of that protein is then detected for their spatial (space dependent) and temporal expression (time dependent). The effect of any external drug on the target protein can be monitored by the fluorescence. Stem cells have numerous applications in drug discovery. They are important for understanding differentiation pathways, for identifying factors needed to manipulate cell lineages, for improving screening assays, and for identifying disease targets. In most of the pharmaceutical industries people perform the trials on animal models which many times are not very authentic. Disease models should more faithfully represent the actual human diseases so that underlying mechanisms can be better understood because ultimately we have to use these drugs in human system. Human stem cells can be used for that purpose. Stem cells can be derived from patients with specific diseases and protocols can be established to direct the disease-specific ES cells to become the very types of cells affected in the disease. Such disease-relevant cells should be able to drive more predictive drug discovery and toxicity studies.

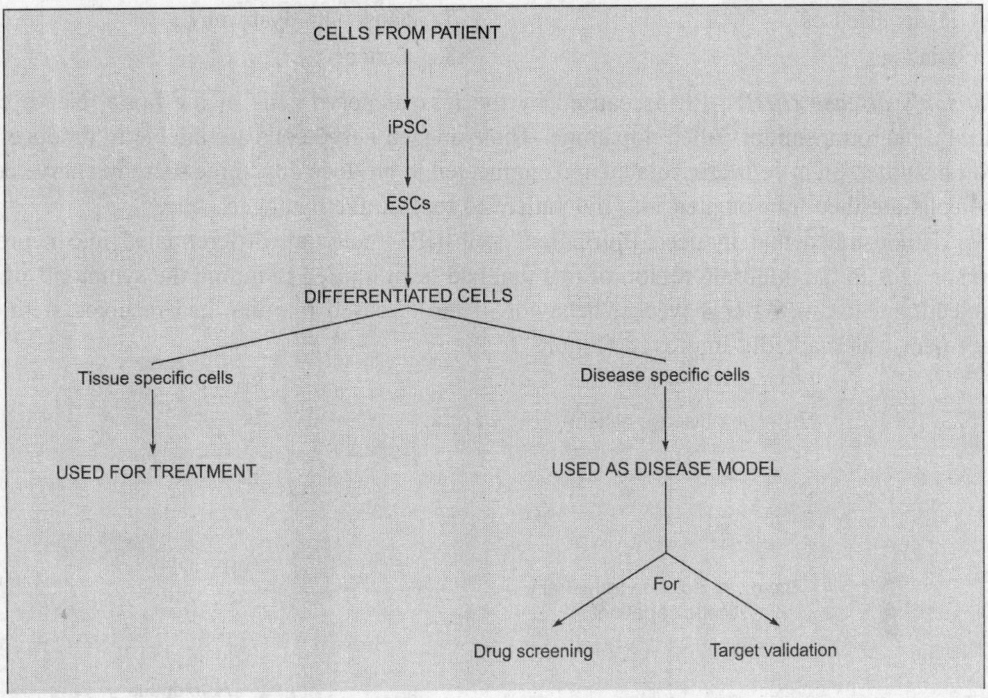

Figure 26.7 Basic scheme for stem cell-based screening assays.

Some breakthrough in drug discovery: Stem cell science (SCS), a company based at USA, provides human nerve stem (NS) cells, which generate physiologically responsive neurons, astrocytes and oligodendrocytes, to pharmaceutical companies for drug screening. This company also provides human multipotent adipose derived stem cells (hMADS). hMADS and their differentiated progeny offer research teams conducting pharmaceutical research a reliable, genetically consistent cellular resource over extended periods. They are an ideal tool for high throughput screens and high content analysis in 96 and 384 well formats.

Stem Cells in Regeneration Therapy

Regenerative medicine helps natural healing processes to work faster, or uses special materials to regrow missing or damaged tissues. Physicians use regenerative medicine to speed up healing, and to help heal injuries that cannot heal on their own. Regenerative therapies have been demonstrated (in trials or the laboratory) to heal broken bones, bad burns, blindness, deafness, heart damage, nerve damage, Parkinson's and other conditions. Because stem cells have self-renewal property and can get converted to bone, muscle, cartilage and other specialized types of cells on providing specific conditions, they have major potential in the field of regeneration therapy. The diseases which can be potentially treated by stem cell therapy include:

1. Parkinson's and Alzheimer's diseases
2. Spinal cord injury
3. Stroke
4. Burns

5. Heart diseases
6. Diabetes
7. Muscular dystrophy
8. Cancer

Parkinson's disease (PD): PD is caused by the loss of nerve cells in the brain. Nerve cells produce a neurotransmitter called dopamine. The damaged nerve cells are unable to produce this neurotransmitter. Stem cells are isolated and engineered to produce dopamine secreting nerve cells. These cells are then transplanted into the patient to replace the damaged cells.

It is demonstrated that induced Pluripotent stem (iPS) cells are differentiated into neuronal precursor cells in the midbrain region of rats that had been injured to mimic the symptoms of PD (by injecting a toxin). After 4 weeks, behavior of the diseased rats that had received stem cell replacement was markedly improved (Figure 26.8).

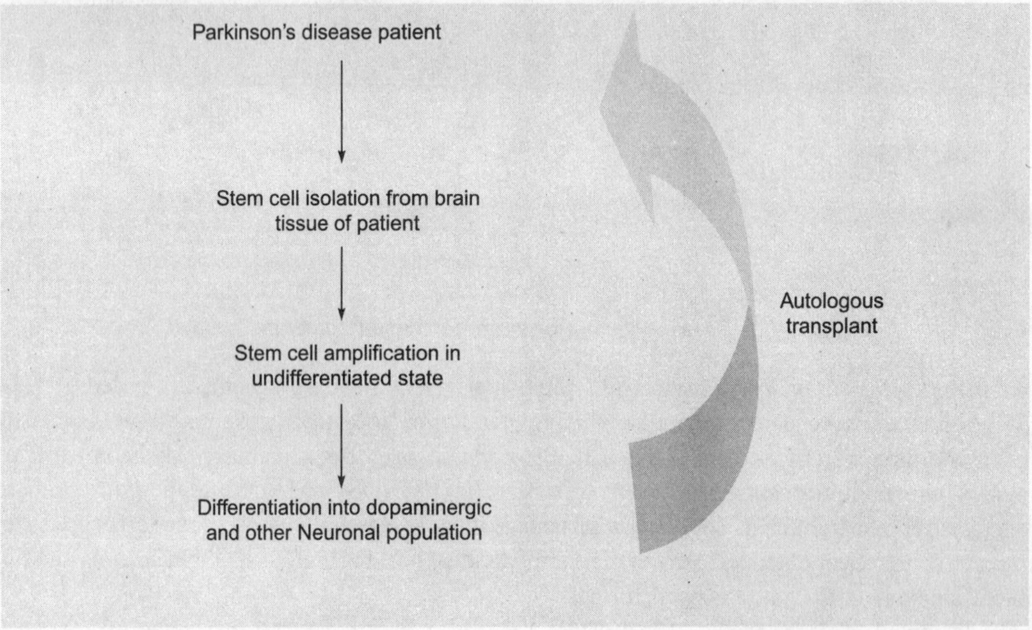

Figure 26.8 A schematic presentation of the cell replacement therapy for Parkinson's disease.

Spinal cord injury: When spinal cord injury occurs, the body creates scar tissue to prevent infection, a mechanism that has little effect on the skin but disastrous on the spinal cord. Scars inhibit nerve-fiber regeneration, creating paralysis. Stem cells may be used to generate new supporting cells that will reform the insulating nerve sheath (myelin) and stimulate re-growth of damaged nerves. When introduced into the spinal cord shortly after injury, stem cells may protect the cells at the injury site from further damage by releasing protective factors. In this regard researchers developed a treatment derived from hESCs to improve mobility in rats with spinal cord injuries. Recently, a similar but preliminary report from a city hospital in Coimbatore, India shows that a 38 years old woman of spinal cord injuries was able to walk after treatment with bone marrow stem cells from the same patient. But all these need further validation and proper methodology based documentation to be really used in therapy.

Stroke: After stroke a gap is created in the brain that can destroy a person's ability to speak and move normally. The most common type of stroke is an ischemic stroke, which involves a blockage of blood (usually in the form of a blood clot) that supplies oxygen to the brain. The other main type of stroke is a hemorrhagic stroke, which involves bleeding in or around the brain. This can be improved by planting immature (stem) cells into the subarachnoid space of the patient via a lumbar puncture. In December 2, 2008, the International Neuroscience Institute (INI), Hannover, announced that the first patient has been treated in the first ever clinical trial for the treatment of stroke with a stem cell product.

Burns: When the skin has been seriously damaged through disease or burns, the body often cannot act fast enough to repair them. Burn victims may die from infection and the loss of plasma. Skin grafts were originally developed as a way to prevent such consequences. Epidermal regenerations obtained with autologous cultured keratinocytes (cultured autografts) can be life-saving for patients suffering from massive full-thickness burn (an injury that extends down to the third layer, subcutaneous tissue, which includes fat, is called a full thickness injury, and formerly known as third degree burn). Adult bone marrow stem cells can be used in constructing artificial skin—marking a leap in healing wounds and burns. Once the artificial skin is attached to the patient and the dermal layer begins to regenerate, stem cells will differentiate into skin cells. Since these cells are self-renewing they will raise the quality of wound healing in terms of recovery and betterment. Few years back a female patient with extensive skin burn (I-II-IIIAB skin burn, total area 40%, area of IIIB degree 30%) was treated using transplantation of allogenic fibroblast-like bone marrow mesenchymal stem cells onto the surface of deep thermal burn. Other than this till date not much has been reported about this mode of therapy.

Heart diseases: Stem cells offer hope to those with heart disease because they might be able to stimulate the growth of new heart-muscle cells. Since the cardiac muscle cells do not replace themselves naturally, those who suffer from a heart attack or from congenital heart disease or from congestive heart failure thus have limited treatment options. On the other hand, while heart transplants potentially could help more patients, limited supply of organs poses a serious limitation to this option. Stem cells can provide some comparatively better modes of therapy, for example, mesenchymal cells can be isolated, cultured and differentiated into cardiomyocites and vascular endothelial cells, which will pump blood to the heart. Recently, a group of Australian scientists made a major breakthrough in the treatment of heart disease when they discovered a method of treating damaged hearts using the patient's own adult stem cells. The new treatment is being developed at the Victor Chang Cardiac Research Institute in Sydney. In the treatment, heart patients were injected with a hormone that causes the release of beneficial stem cells from their bone marrow into the bloodstream. The physical exertion causes the stem cells to travel quickly to their heart and come into action. Upon reaching the heart, the stem cells start creating new blood vessels to restore blood circulation and improve the overall functioning of the heart (Figure 26.9).

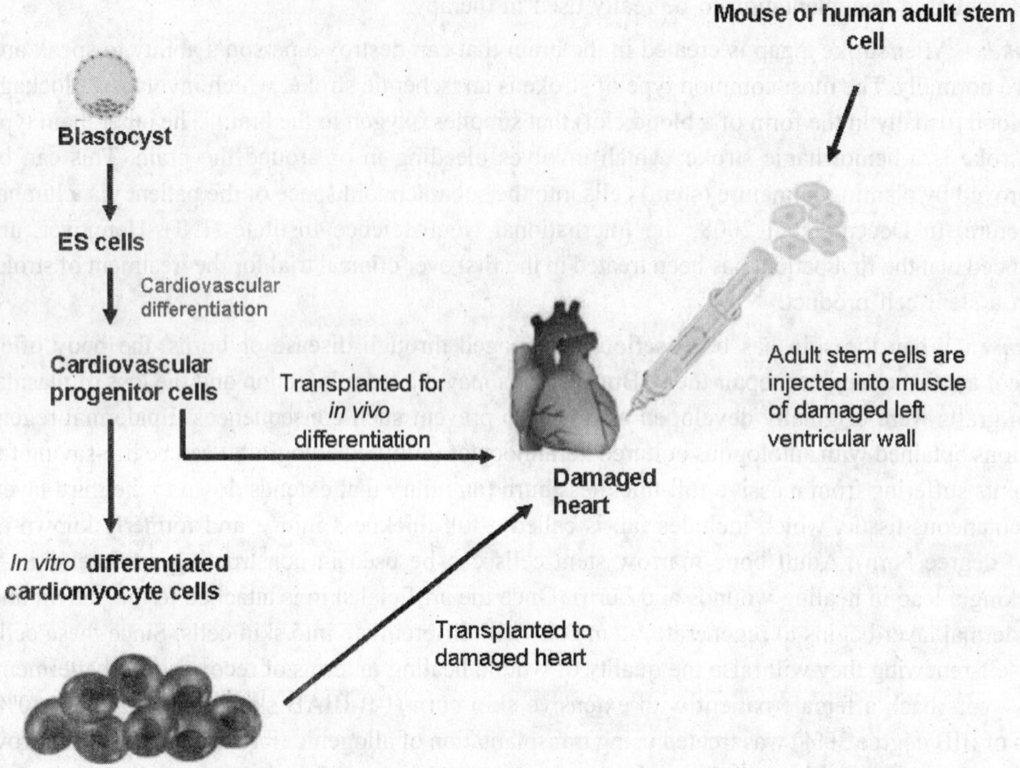

Figure 26.9 Various stages of heart muscle repair with stem cells.

Diabetes: Diabetes is a metabolic disorder in which the utilization of glucose is impaired finally resulting in the high level of glucose in blood. This disease is of two types: type 1, in which the insulin secreting cells of pancreases (islet cells), are destroyed by body's own immune system, and type 2, in which the body becomes insulin tolerant, and cannot use the insulin for glucose metabolism. Both these types of diabetes results in the elevation of blood glucose level in patients. Although there are some drugs available in the market for type 2 diabetes, insulin is the only option for type 1 diabetes which a person has to take throughout his life to maintain glucose level in control. The present-day therapy provides an alternative to it by tissue transplantation to replace the islet cells. However, limited number of donors pose a serious limitation to this method. Hence, now stem cell therapy is the most promising therapy for the diabetes. The mesenchymal stem cells are conditioned to produce insulin secreting cells and then transplanted into the patient's body. A Brazilian study has shown that stem cell transplants in patients with diabetes type 1 may reactivate the pancreas for producing insulin for next 20 months (Figure 26.10).

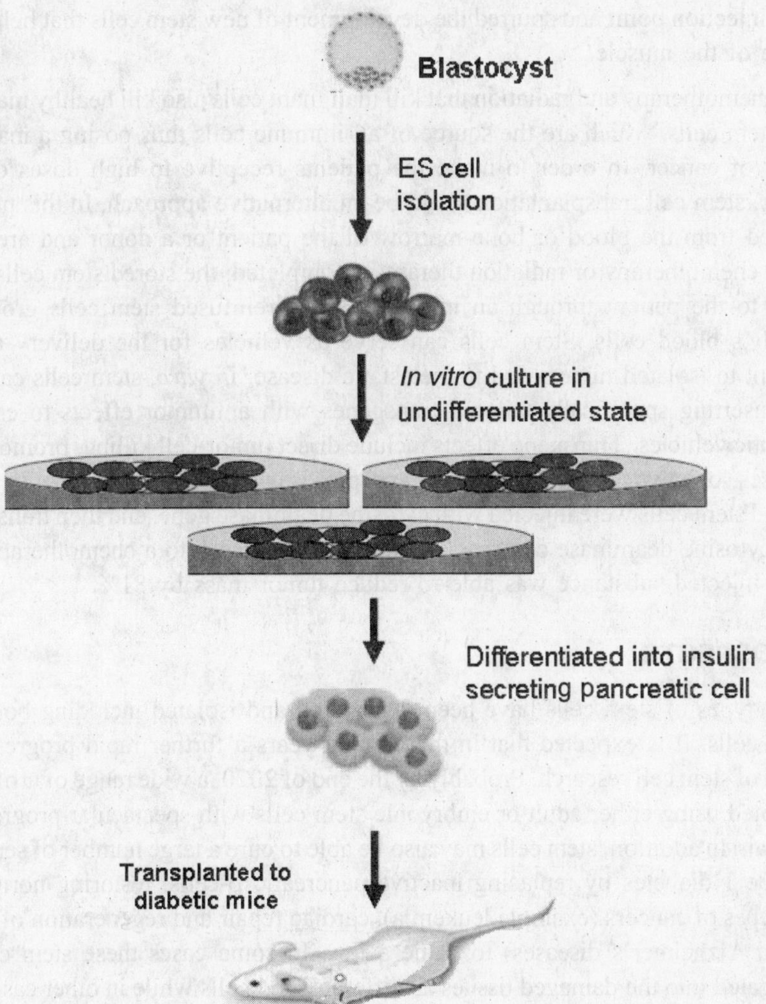

Figure 26.10 Development of insulin-secreting pancreatic-like cells from mouse embryonic stem cells.

Muscular dystrophy: Muscular Dystrophy (MD) is a collection of disorders caused by genetic defects that lead to increasing muscle weakness over time. Although currently there is no cure for this disorder but if stem cells containing normal genes could be delivered to these defective muscles, they could regenerate fully functional muscle fibers. A Harvard research team has developed a new procedure that gave them ready access to a supply of adult muscle stem cells in mice, which they used to counter the effects of Duchenne muscular dystrophy in test animals. They were able to identify muscle stem cells by marker proteins found on the surface of these cells. The cells were harvested and then injected into the muscles of the diseased rodents. The injected stem cells spread from the injection point and spurred the development of new stem cells that helped improve the performance of the muscle.

Cancer: The chemotherapy and radiation that kill malignant cells also kill healthy marrow and its resident blood stem cells, which are the source of all immune cells thus posing a major problem in the treatment of cancer. In order to make the patients receptive to high doses of chemo or radiation therapy, stem cell transplantation could be an alternative approach. In this method, stem cells are removed from the blood or bone marrow of the patient or a donor and are frozen and stored. After the chemotherapy or radiation therapy is completed, the stored stem cells are thawed and given back to the patient through an infusion. These reinfused stem cells grow into (and restore) the body's blood cells. Stem cells can serve as vehicles for the delivery of effective, targeted treatment to isolated tumors and to metastatic disease. *In vitro*, stem cells can readily be engineered by inserting specifically tailored transgenes with antitumor effects to create tumor-seeking therapeutic vehicles. Transgene effects include direct tumor-cell killing, promotion of local immune responses, oncolytic virus production, and pro-drug activation schemes. In another experiment, isolated stem cells were injected with cytosine deaminase gene, and then transplanted into the tumor. The cytosine deaminase converts a non-toxic pro-drug into a chemotherapeutic agent. As a result, the injected substance was able to reduce tumor mass by 81%.

FUTURE PROSPECTS

Till date several types of stem cells have been discovered and isolated including both adult and embryonic stem cells. It is expected that in the coming years a further rapid progress would be made in the field of stem cell research. Probably by the end of 2020, a wide range of artificial tissues would be generated using either adult or embryonic stem cells with spectacular progress in tissue building and repair. In addition, stem cells may also be able to cure a large number of serious human diseases like type 1 diabetes by replacing inactive pancreatic β-cells, restoring normal hearing, curing various types of cancers (example leukemia), cardiac repair and regeneration of neural cells (Parkinson's and Alzheimer's diseases) to name a few. In some cases these stem cells will be actually incorporated into the damaged tissues as differentiated cells while in other cases, they will be temporary assistants in local repair process. Further, we will also see some exciting new pharmaceutical products in the pipeline, which might do the same function without having to remove a single stem cell from the body. These drugs may, for example, activate bone marrow cells and encourage them to migrate to parts of the body where repairs are needed. Along with this, it is expected that a number of biotechnology based companies will emerge working in the fields of regenerative medicines considering its heavy impact in the field of human health improvement. However, the success of all these would be completely dependent on two important issues, first, complete understanding of the basic biology of stem cells and secondly, addressing the ethical issues related to human stem cell research. If these issues are taken care of, in the coming years we will see some breakthrough research on stem cell technology.

CONCLUSION

In recent days stem cells are being exploited in many areas of medical sciences like in gene therapy, studies of biological processes development, in drug discovery and the most extensively in regeneration therapy. But the biggest challenge for stem cell therapy is the immune rejection in which, transplanted cells if not allograft would be treated as foreign cell by the recipient and thus making the ways for immune rejection. Secondly, it was also found that transplantation of fetal and embryonic stem cells in animals can cause tumor. In addition, fetal and embryonic stem cells are extremely unstable and may lead to undifferentiated cell growth and finally causing cancer. But research is in progress to reduce the tendency of stem cells to form cancers.

Studies on human embryonic stem cells may yield information about the complex events that occur during human development. The primary goal of this work is to identify how undifferentiated stem cells become differentiated. Researchers know that turning genes on and off is central to this process. Some of the most serious medical conditions, such as cancer and birth defects, are due to abnormal cell division and differentiation. A better understanding of the genetic and molecular controls of these processes may yield information about how such diseases arise and suggest new strategies for therapy. A significant hurdle to the use of stem cells is that scientists do not yet fully understand the signals that turn specific genes on and off to influence the differentiation of stem cells.

Perhaps the most important potential application of human stem cells is the generation of cells and tissues that could be used for cell-based therapies. Today, donated organs and tissues are often used to replace ailing or destroyed tissue, but the need for transplantable tissues and organs far outweigh the available supply. Stem cells, directed to differentiate into specific cell types, offer the possibility of a renewable source of replacement cells and tissues to treat diseases including Parkinson's and Alzheimer's diseases, spinal cord injury, stroke, burns, heart disease, diabetes, osteoarthritis, and rheumatoid arthritis. To summarize, the promise of stem cell therapies is an exciting one, but significant technical hurdles remain that will only be overcome through years of intensive research.

FURTHER READINGS

1. Barres V., Belluardo N. *et al.* (2003) Transplantation of prodrug-converting neural progenitor cells for brain tumor therapy. *Cancer Gene Therapy.* **(10):** 396-402.
2. Cerletti M., Jurga S. *et al.* (2008) Highly efficient, functional engraftment of skeletal muscle stem cells in dystrophic muscles. *Cell.* 134 **(1):** 37-47.
3. Cui Y., Golob J. *et al.* (2002) Targeting transgene expression to antigen-presenting cells derived from lentivirus-transduced engrafting human hematopoietic stem/progenitor cells. *Blood.* **(99):** 399-408.
4. Daniel R. Marshak, Richard L. Gardner, D. Gottlied (2001) *In: Stem Cell Biology: Introduction to Stem Cell Biology* (eds. Marshak, Gardener, and Gottlied). Cold Spring Harbour Laboratory Press. New York.
5. David T., Phillippe H. *et al.* (2003) The zebrafish as a model organism to study development of the immune system. *Advances in Immunology.* **(18):** 253-330
6. Freshney, I.R., Glyn N. Stacey, Jonathan M. Auerbach. (2007) *Culture of Human Stem Cells.* Wiley. United States of America.

7. Gropp M., Reubinoff B. *et al.* (2006) Lentiviral mediated gene delivery into human embryonic stem cells. *Methods in Enzymology.* **(420):** 64-81.
8. http://neurosurgery.mgh.harvard.edu/oisacson.htm
9. http://www.diabetes.org/ada/c20f.asp
10. http://www.jdfcure.com/JDFINASAisletconfsummary.htm.
11. http://www.mit.edu/afs/athena/user/p/a/pandre/www/Neurology.html.
12. Júlio C., Carlos E. B. *et al.* (2007) Autologous nonmyeloablative hematopoietic stem cell transplantation in newly diagnosed type 1 diabetes mellitus. *JAMA* **(297):** 1568-1576.
13. Keirstead H.S. *et al.* (2005) Human embryonic stem cell derived oligodendrocyte progenitor cell transplants remylinate and restore locomotion after spinal cord injury. *Journal of Neurosciences.* 25 **(19):** 4694-705.
14. Kolls J., Wang G, Bruce A. *et al.* (2005) Adult stem cells from bone marrow stroma differentiate into airway epithelial cells: Potential therapy for cystic fibrosis. *Proceedings of National Academy of Sciences*, **(102):** 186-191
15. Lagasse E., Connors H. *et al.* (2000) Purified hematopoietic stem cells can differentiate into hepatocytes *in vivo*. *Nature Medicine.* **(6):** 1229-1234.
16. Lana R. Skirboll (2000) Stem Cells: Scientific Progress and Future Research Directions: Office of Science Policy.
17. Liu L., Gersonv S., (2006) Targeted modulation of MGMT: Clinical implications. *Clinical Cancer Research.* **(12):** 328-331
18. Paulo A. Fontes and Angus W. Thomson (1999) Stem cell technology. *BMJ.* **(319):** 1-3.
19. Potten C.S. (1997). *In Stem Cells: Tumor Stem Cells* (eds. J. Kummermeher, K-R. Trott). Elsevier. UK.
20. Rasulov M., Vasil'chenkov A *et al.* (2005) First experience in the use of bone marrow mesenchymal stem cells for the treatment of a patient with deep skin burns. *Bulletin of Experimental Biology and Medicine.* **(139):** 141-144(4).
21. Schierle G.S., Hansson O., Leist M., Nicotera P., Widner H. and Brundin P. (1999) Caspase Inhibition Reduces Aptosis and Increases Survival of Nigral Transplants. *Nature Medicine*. **(5):** 97-100.

CHAPTER

27

Animal Transgenic Technology

Animal transgenic technology is a radically new technology for altering the characteristics of animals by directly changing the genetic material. Since DNA contains a universal genetic code for living organisms, it can be transferred between completely unrelated organisms to produce a new/altered organism with particular useful characteristics that would not otherwise be available. In this chapter, we describe the detailed procedure and major applications of animal transgenic technology.

Keywords: Animal transgenic technology, genetically modified animals, somatic cell cloning, nuclear gene transfer, molecular pharming.

INTRODUCTION

There are various definitions of the term transgenic animal. The term transgenic was first used by J.W. Gardon and F. H. Ruddle in 1981. The general definition of transgenic animal is as one carrying recombinant DNA molecules that were introduced by intentional human intervention. Transgenic animal carries and expresses genetic expression not normally found in that species. It can also be defined as an animal, which has received sequences of DNA by artificial means, followed by integration of one or more of the novel sequences into its chromosomal DNA. In another definition, the term transgenic describes organisms that contain in their chromosomes stably integrated copies of genes or gene constructs derived from other species, or not normally found in the host animals. Federation of European Laboratory Animal Associations defines the term transgenic animal as an animal in which there has been a deliberate modification of its genome—the genetic make-up of an organism responsible for inherited characteristics. Transgenic animals contain genetic elements from two different species. Advances in genetic engineering and embryo manipulation technologies made the genetic manipulation of domestic animals possible. It was achieved through the procedures involving the introduction of specific foreign genes into fertilized eggs. It is now possible to generate animals with useful novel properties for dairy, meat, fiber, and biomedical purposes as well as for other human benefits. The first successful transgenic mammal was a mouse. A team led by Richard Palmiter and Ralph Brinster fused elements of a gene (metallothionein) that can be regulated by dietary zinc to a rat growth-hormone gene, and injected it into fertilized mouse embryos. The resulting mice, when fed with extra zinc, grew to be huge (Figure 27.1). This technique paved the way for a wave of genetic analysis using transgenic mice. With the advancement in transgenic technologies, it became possible to apply them for other domestic animals as well as some endangered species (Table 27.1).

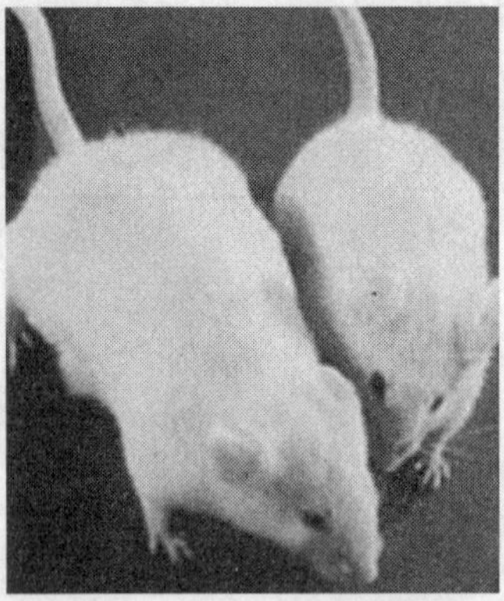

Figure 27.1 A giant mouse grown from an egg injected with rat growth hormone genes weighs nearly twice as much as its normal sibling (left one is transgenic giant mouse) Photo: Ralph Brinster, University of Pennsylvania, School of Veterinary Medicine. (Palmiter *et al.*, 1982).

Table 27.1 Historical background: advances in animal transgenic.

Year	*Events*
1885	August Weismann theorized that genetic information of a cell would diminish as cell went through differentiation
1891	First successful embryo transfer early 1900s *in vitro* embryo culture develops
1894	Hans Dreisch isolated blastomeres from 2- and 4-cell sea urchin embryos and observed their development into small larvae
1901	Hans Spemann split 2-cell newt embryo into two parts, resulting in development of two complete larvae
1902	Hans Spemann split 2-celled salamander embryo and each cell grew to adulthood, providing proof that early embryo cells carry necessary genetic information
1914	Hans Spemann conducted an early nuclear transfer experiment
1951-52	First animal cloning: Robert Briggs and Thomas J. Leing cloned Northern leopard frogs
1961	Mouse embryo aggregation to produce chimeras
1962	John Gurdon announcement: he cloned South African frogs using the nucleus of fully differentiated adult intestinal cells. This was demonstrated that cells' genetic potential does not diminish as the cell became specialized
1963	J.B.S. Haldane coined the term "Clone" in a speech entitled 'Biological Possibilities for the Human Species of the next Ten-Thousand Years'
1966	First report of microinjection of mouse embryos: John B. Gurdon and V Vehlinger grew adult frogs after injecting tadpole intestinal cell nuclei into enucleated oocytes.
1970	Experiments were conducted with embryonal carcinoma cells and teratocarcinoma cells to construct chimeric mice.
1973	Foreign genes function after cell transfection
1974	Development of teratocarcinoma cell transfer
1977	mRNA and DNA transferred to Xenopus eggs
1980	mRNA transferred into mammalian ova
1980-81	Transgenic mice first documented:DNA microinjection first applied to clone mice
1981	Transfer of ES cells derived from mouse embryos
1982	Transgenic mice and a growth hormone phenotype
1983	Tissue specific gene expression in transgenic mice

Contd.

1984	Steene Willadsen cloned a sheep from embryo cells, the first verified example of mammal cloning using a process of nuclear transfer (NT)
1985	Ralph Brinster created the first transgenic livestock: Pigs that produced human growth hormone
1986	Using diffrentiated, one week old embryo cells, Steen Willadsen cloned a cow: Embryonic stem cell mediated gene transfer
1987	Chimeric "knock-out" mice described, Retrovirus mediated: transgenic chicken
1989	Targeted DNA integration & germline chimeric mice, Microinjection for transgenic cattle (Russia), First sperm mediated reports in farm animals
1991	Microinjection for transgenic goats first referred publication
1993	M. Sims and N L First reported the creation of calves by transfer of nuclei from cultured embryonic cells, Germline chimeric mice produced using co-culture
1995	Ian Wilmut and Keith Campbell used differentiated embryo cells to clone two sheep, named Megan and Morag
1996	Dolly the first organism ever to be cloned from adult cells, was born
1997	Scientist at the Roslin institute in Scotland, officially anounced the birth of Dolly (Feb, 1997), Somatic cells from adult sheep used for cloning by nuclear transfer (Dolly), Polly, a poll dorset lamb, cloned from skin cells grown *in vitro* and genetically altered to contain a human gene (July, 1997); Rhesus monkey cloned
1998	Cumulina, the mouse: First clone with "Honolulu method". She was made with the DNA of cumulus cells, which surround developing eggs within the ovaries of female mice, Cloned calves reported
2001	Hosehold pet cloned: CC (carbon copy) the cat was reported, Cloned gaur reported-First endangered species named Noah. It died soon after birth.
2002	Cloned pet (cat) reported named Little Nicky, the birth of five cloned piglets that had a tissue rejection gene ' knocked out' was cloned. They were named Noel, Angel, Star, Joy, and Mary (PPL therapeutics, Near Edinburg)
2003	Prometea: first Horse cloned, Ralph, the rat cloned by Jean-Paul Renard, Dewey: the white tailed deer fawn was cloned
2004	First cloned fruit-flies, First successful cloning of an equine named Idaho Gem
2005	Announcement of a cloned dog named Snuppy by Seoul National University scientists
2009-10	Buffalo calves cloned at NDRI, ICAR named Samrupa, Garima and Shresth by using hand guided cloning techniques.
2010	Creation of first bacterial cell controlled by chemically synthesized genome.

CONCEPTS

Animals are made of billions of cells, all working together. Every cell of the animal has a complete "instruction manual" or genome that is inherited from the parents of the animal as a combination of their genomes. When a cell expresses a gene, a specific protein is produced. Proteins give an individual cell, and therefore the animal, its form and function. Consequently, a gene from one organism can function in another organism. Genes can be altered artificially, so that some characteristics of an animal are changed. When a new gene is put into an animal's genome, it is said to be transgenic. In transgenic animals, transgenes are introduced at the preimplantation embryonic stage of development (prior to birth) and are transmitted through normal Mendelian inheritance, if the introduced genes are expressed in germ cells (sperm or ova), such animals are able to act as "Founder" stock to produce many offspring that carry desirable gene(s). If the germ cells of the founder transmit the transgene stably, then all descendants of this animal are members of a unique transgenic lineage. And if the transgenic animal is fertile, the transgene will be inherited by future progeny. Thus, a transgenic animal, once created, can persist into future generations. Usually animals developing from manipulated cells contain the foreign gene in all somatic cells and the germ line cells if the foreign genes were integrated into the genome of the recipient cell before the first cell division. Integration at a later stage yields genetic mosaics consisting of normal cells with a normal genome and cells with a transgenome. The primary animals developing after gene transfer are always hemizygous because the transgene is not integrated into both copies of a homologous pair of chromosomes. Pure homozygous lines are obtained by crossing of two suitable hemizygous animals (also called founder).

PRINCIPLES

The underlying principle in the production of transgenic animals is the introduction of a foreign gene or genes into an animal. The foreign gene must be transmitted through the germ line, so that every cell, including germ cells, of the animal contains the same modified genetic material. The expression of a transgene requires that the appropriate transcriptional control elements be included in the DNA construct. Expression of some gene might be deleterious or incompatible with proper growth and development of the embryo. Although the basic coding system is the same in all organisms, the fine details of gene control often differ. The basic component of a transgene is the gene to be introduced plus a control sequence (Figure 27.2). All genes are controlled by a special segment of DNA found on the chromosome called a promoter sequence. Promoter is a non-coding DNA sequence that regulates gene expression. These regulatory elements are usually found immediately upstream of the gene, and have critical role in temporal and tissue specific regulation of gene expression, independent of their location and orientation with respect to gene. Signal sequences are short DNA sequences that target protein synthesis into specific intracellular pathways and frequently direct the secretion of the protein from the cell. Secretory signals are usually found directly adjacent to the 5′ end of the gene, and organelle-targeting sequences are found within the 3′ end of the gene or immediately downstream of the 3′ end. These signal sequences are within the reading frame or transcriptional region of the gene, and therefore encode mRNA and short polypeptide products. The 3′ end of the reading frame must also contain a poly-A nucleotide sequence to ensure proper mRNA transcription and translation.

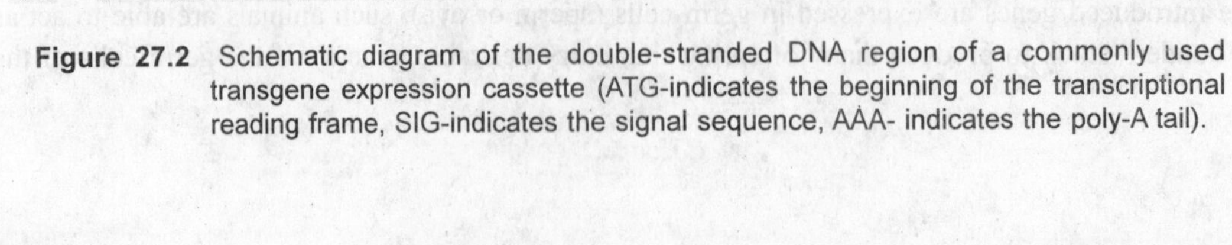

Figure 27.2 Schematic diagram of the double-stranded DNA region of a commonly used transgene expression cassette (ATG-indicates the beginning of the transcriptional reading frame, SIG-indicates the signal sequence, AAA- indicates the poly-A tail).

ANIMAL TRANSGENIC TECHNOLOGY

Gene transfer technology provides the ability to genetically manipulate the cells of higher animals. Gene transfer permits both germ line and somatic cell alterations. Such genetic manipulations are the basis of animal transgenesis. Genetic manipulation of a newly fertilized, single-cell egg (zygote) should in principle result in the development of an organism in which almost all cells contain the identical alteration. Eggs that have undergone cleavage are less than ideal for transgenesis. Where only one cell is transgenically altered, the resulting organism is likely to take the form of a genetic mosaic. Although, mosacism is not always a problem, mosaic transgenics may produce gametes that contain the transgene, allowing the subsequent generation(s) to be fully transgenic. More than one-celled zygotes often reduce the efficiency of transgenesis in comparison with single cell zygote stage eggs. It is also practically not feasible in farm animals because of their relatively longer generation time. A major limitation associated with the egg is that the targeting of transgenes to desired genomic loci is not a practical proposition due to inability in selecting eggs that contain rare targeted integration outcome. Randomly integrated transgenes have got some utility in producing transgenic animals. For example, production of human blood clotting factor VIII in the milk of transgenic sheep.

A number of methods are presently employed for genetic engineering of various animal species. Access to the germline of mammals can be obtained by: (1) direct manipulation (DNA microinjection) of the fertilized egg, followed by its implantation into the uterus; (2) manipulation of the sperm used to generate the zygote; (3) manipulation of early embryonic tissue in place; (4) the use of embryonic stem (ES) cell lines which, after manipulation and selection *ex vivo*, can then be introduced into early embryos, some of whose germline will develop from the ES cells; and (5) manipulation of cultured somatic cells, whose nuclei can be then transferred to enucleated oocytes and thereby provide the genetic information required to produce a whole animal. The last two methods have the advantage of allowing cells containing the modification of interest to be selected prior to undertaking the expensive and lengthy process of generating animals. There are two basic approaches presently in use for inserting DNA into vertebrate germ line cells—transfection and infection with retrovirus vectors. A third approach, transposons-based (mobile genetic elements), has been commonly used for insects and is being explored for germ line modification of vertebrates. Virus mediated transgenesis, the lentiviral technique which was first developed in rodents and later extended to farm animals, is the most successful transgenic method to date in terms, of producing transgenic offspring. It makes use of disarmed retroviral vectors to insert a desirable gene(s) into the host organisms, usually at the single-celled embryo stage. To improve the size limitations of lentiviral vectors, transgene has been placed under the control of long terminal repeats (LTRs). The major drawbacks of this technique are the high embryo lethality, need for specialized containment facilities and limited physical volume of viral particles. There are also lingering concerns about the potential consequences of recombinant events between the viral vector and endogenous retroviruses, leading to the generation of new and more potent pathogenic agents. Transposons are DNA sequences, which contain at least one gene coding for a transposase and motifs located on both ends of the transposons, the role of which is to trigger integration. Foreign gene can be transferred according to animal species. Broadly, three methods are being used for animal transgenesis.

DNA Microinjection

A seminal achievement that paved the way for the transgenic age occurred in 1966 with the description of embryo microinjection. DNA microinjection into the pronuclei of zygote is a classic method of gene transfer in farm animals. Injection is done at the stage of development when mammalian ova have two pronuclei, one from each gamete, which will later fuse to form the diploid nucleus. DNA microinjection generally involves the use of micromanipulators and a microinjection apparatus to inject a solution containing recombinant DNA into embryos (Figure 27.3)

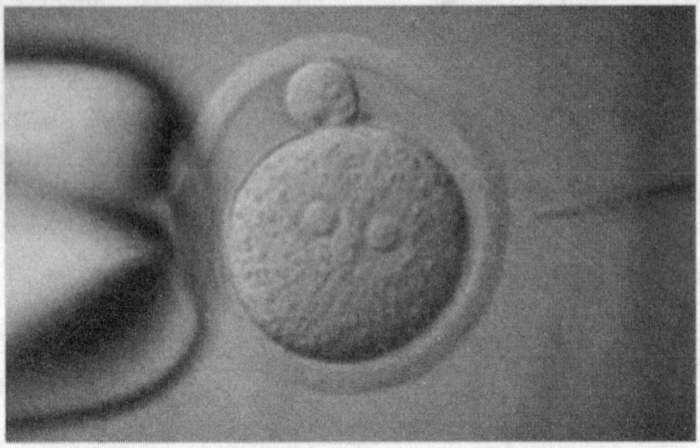

Figure 27.3 DNA microinjection to zygote pronuclei.

Procedure: A finely drawn out glass micropipette loaded with DNA solution is used for the injection. Under the microscope, with the aid of micromanipulators, the egg is held fast and penetrated with the aid of micropipette. The micropipette is guided through the cytoplasm towards one of the egg's pronuclei. Once the tip of the micropipette has entered the pronucleus, around 1-2 picolitre of DNA solution is injected. Some eggs lyse following microinjection, probably due to the physical trauma of being penetrated by the micropipette. Surviving eggs are used for *in vitro* culture and transplantation to surrogate mothers. In this method, embryos are usually recovered from superovulated donor animals. *In vitro* maturation and fertilization of oocyte may be carried out to obtain a sufficient number of zygotes for gene transfer. After this, embryos are transferred to synchronized recipients, which may be done immediately or after in vitro culture. This method has a number of advantages

(i) A high frequency of generating transgenic animals from viable microinjected embryos transferred to recipient females.
(ii) A lack of constraint on the size or type of DNA constructs used.
(iii) The stability of the transgene as it is transmitted from generation to generation.

But this technique allows addition of DNA fragments, which integrate randomly into the genome of the embryo but typically only in a single chromosomal location. Host DNA near the site of integration frequently undergoes various forms of sequence duplication, deletion or rearrangement as a result of transgene incorporation. This random integration of foreign DNA may cause insertional mutation and also has position effects on its expression and/or expression of nearby located genes. Some approaches are available for overcoming/minimizing the position effects. Recombinase enzymes coupled to DNA are reported to increase the efficiency of microinjection. This method of gene transfer can be exploited to insert multiple copies of gene constructs to the genome. When multiple copies are integrated, the transgenes concatenate before the integration event, and as many as few hundred copies of the particular sequence can be incorporated into a single chromosomal location, predominantly as head to tail concatemers. This procedure is particularly suitable for mice because it is easy to collect large numbers of fertilized eggs from a relatively small number of animals. The efficiency of producing transgenic animals by microinjection is 1% for livestock and approximately 3% for mice. For example, Tracy, a transgenic sheep, was produced using this method. Human alpha-1 proteinase inhibitor was produced in her milk.

Sperm Mediated Gene Transfer

Several studies in the last ten years revealed that mammalian spermatozoa can bind exogenous DNA molecules. Studies in mice suggested that plasmid DNA internalized in ejaculated spermatozoa associated with nuclear scaffold is extensively rearranged and undergoes recombination with genomic DNA. Heterologous genome could be incorporated into mammalian spermatozoa and subsequently carried into the ovum during the process of fertilization. The first transgenic mice were obtained by microinjecting SV 40 viral DNA into the blastocoel cavity of embryos, and obtaining between 0.5 and 13 SV 40 genome equivalents per diploid mouse genome, which were identified in various organs. An improvement of this technique was developed in mice, rabbits, sheep and pigs by injecting exogenous DNA into the male pronucleus of zygotes, resulting in germ-line transgenic animals. This pronuclear microinjection technique, an example of passive transgenesis procedure, relies on the injection of a small amount of fluid containing the linearized transgene into the male pronucleus of a zygote, and the repair mechanisms of the zygote nucleus for the insertion of the transgene. In mice, zygote transferred to surrogate mothers results in transgenic animals with random integration of the transgene. Many animals produced by these methods suffer from mosaicism, thus effecting germ line transmission and transgene expression. Furthermore, due to opaque oocyte cytoplasm in bovine and swine, this requires centrifugation of zygote for pronuclei visualization. To overcome the difficulties of male pronuclear microinjection, recently intracytoplasmic sperm injection-mediated transgenesis (ICSI-Tr) has been developed. This technique is also called metaphase II transgenesis. The greatest advantage of this technique is that it allows introduction of very large DNA transgenes (e.g., Yeast artificial chromosomes), with relatively high efficiency into the genome of hosts, as compared to pronuclear injection.

Procedure: Mouse spermatozoa are demembranated either by freeze-thawing or treatment with a detergent such as Triton X-100 or lysolecithin, a natural cellular hydrolysis product of membrane phospholipids. Then sperms are incubated with linear, double-stranded DNA that contains the transgene. The exposed perinuclear theca of the sperm head would interact with the DNA and act as the carrier for the transgene. This sperm-DNA complex is then injected into mature metaphase II oocytes by ICSI, allowing the transgene to be incorporated into the embryonic genome via the DNA repair mechanism. The efficiency of ICSI-Tr is an average of 4.6% of oocyte injected or, 45.5% of animals born, with very little mosaicism demonstrated by such founders. Recently, human decay activating factor (hDAF)-transgenic pig has been generated by sperm-mediated gene transfer. An alternative possibility could be to introduce transgene into the testicular (sperm) stem cells *in vivo*. This would in principle remove the need to collect, manipulate or transfer eggs, thus providing a major streamlining of germ line transgenesis. Preliminary results have been reported in mice where transgene constructs were directly injected into the testis. For example, 60-70% of sperm were reported to carry the transgene following injection of naked DNA into the vas deferens, with a follow up report claiming detection of the transgene in the cells of 7.5% of offspring animals produced following fertilization with the transgene bearing sperm. Lipid associated transgene molecules injected through the testicular capsule demonstrated similar results.

Nuclear Transfer or Cloning

Nuclear transfer (NT) involves the introduction of donor nuclei obtained from either embryonic stem cells, other embryonic cells or differentiated adult cells into enucleated oocytes, thereby reprogramming future development. Reconstructed oocytes are then transferred to a surrogate dam for the remainder of gestation. The advent of NT enabled gene knock out and other gene manipulation experiments in several economically important species. The prospects of germ line transgenesis via NT are very significant. By these methods transgenes can be introduced to donor cells *in vitro*, permitting the production of genetically modified animal. This technique is also suitable to produce gene-targeted transgenic animals. By using this method, first gene-targeted sheep was produced where fetal fibroblasts were transfected with a therapeutic transgene carried by liposomes. Genetic modification in combination with NT is a very powerful technology with many potential biotechnological applications. This technology involves the transfer of a donor nucleus (karyoplast) into the cytoplasm of a zygote or a metaphase II oocyte from which the genetic material has been removed. It is now possible to culture donor cells *in vitro* before using them for nuclear transfer. This method has two implications: first the pool of identical donor cells is available in plenty and second, cultured cell can be transfected before using them for NT. Hence, it provides a new route for the generation of transgenic animals. The donor cells for NT can be harvested from a transgenic animal with the appropriate genetic change, or cultured donor cells can be genetically modified prior to NT. Furthermore, as opposed to DNA microinjection, site specific recombination of gene is possible; therefore the change will be both precise and desired. The donor cell can also be checked to ensure that the appropriate modifications have occurred before time. It will save the efforts and investment in gestating non-modified offspring. This ensures that surrogate mothers are implanted only with genetically modified embryos. By following this method, human factor IX transgenic sheep has been generated using transfected fetal fibroblasts. In fact the establishment of NT using cultured cells is the most important breakthrough in the advancement of transgenic technology. By applying this technique, theoretically it is possible to produce cattle and sheep resistant to bovine spongiformis encephalopathy (BSE) and scrapie, respectively. Gene targeting technology will be useful in inserting any new character or deleting any non-desirable economic traits from farm animals. For example, it will be possible to inactivate milk protein genes such as β-lactoglobulin, which interfere with the cheese-making process and are responsible for allergic responses to milk. Polly, the first transgenic lamb, was produced by NT technology. She was produced from fetal fibroblast cells that were modified by the addition of the human gene coding for blood clotting factor IX.

Somatic cell nuclear transfer (SCNT)

The first live offspring produced from differentiated cell populations was the lamb, Dolly, born in 1995 using cultured embryonic cells as nuclear donors and enucleated unfertilized eggs (metaphase II oocyte, M II) as recipient cytoplasts. Dolly was the first organism ever to be cloned from adult cells (Figure 27.4). Since then, SCNT has been applied successfully to a range of species including cattle, mice, goats, pigs, cats, rabbits, horses, rats, dogs, and ferrets using a range of cell types. The production of animal by SCNT involves multiple steps (Figure 27.5) and each of these may influence the successful outcome. There are numerous variations in the technical steps and applied parameters in SCNT, although all cloning methods are fundamentally similar by achieving the replacement of the oocyte's original nucleus with that from somatic cells.

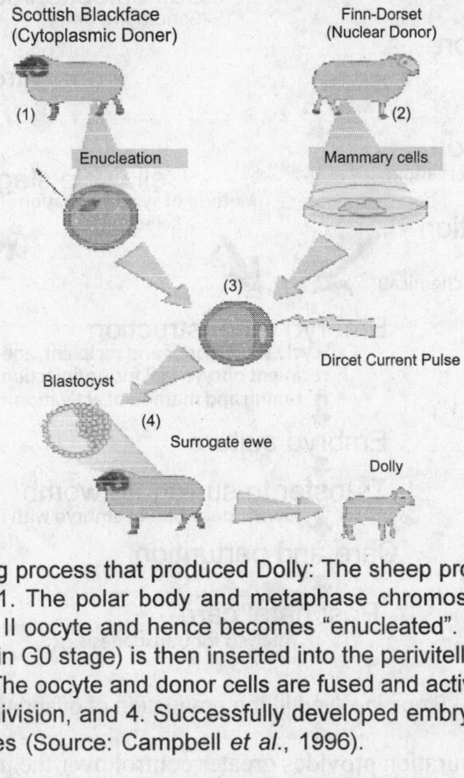

Figure 27.4 The cloning process that produced Dolly: The sheep protocol for nuclear transfer in Rosalin is 1. The polar body and metaphase chromosomes are removed from a metaphase II oocyte and hence becomes "enucleated". 2. A cultured and quiescent donor cell (in G0 stage) is then inserted into the perivitelline space of the enucleated oocyte. 3. The oocyte and donor cells are fused and activated by an electric pulse to begin cell division, and 4. Successfully developed embryos are transferred to surrogate females (Source: Campbell *et al.*, 1996).

Procedure: Three protocols are available based on the presence or absence of the zona pellucida (a coat surrounding the oocyte) during enucleation and reconstruction of the new model embryos.

(i) Conventional zona intact SCNT: This method has been used for a longer time and is still the most popular. It can be used to enucleate oocyte in metaphase II (M II) arrested developmental stage. Genetic material from the recipient oocyte is removed by aspirating the maternal chromosomes and surrounding cytoplasm in a small plasma-membrane envelope in order to obtain cytoplast. This method is very labour-, skill- and technology-intensive due to complicated micromanipulation steps.

(ii) Zona free SCNT: This method is simpler. It uses zona-pellucida free oocytes, which can increase the embryo clones and offspring throughout the production and is also easier to establish in a production environment.

(iii) Zona free *handmade cloning*: This method involves manual sectioning of zona-free oocytes with a microblade, and then the chromatin free portion is fused with another cytoplast to restore the original volume before SCNT. This hand-made cloning is a simple micromanipulation-free cloning technique, and has been applied for the production of cloned embryos and offspring in large livestock species like cows and buffaloes.

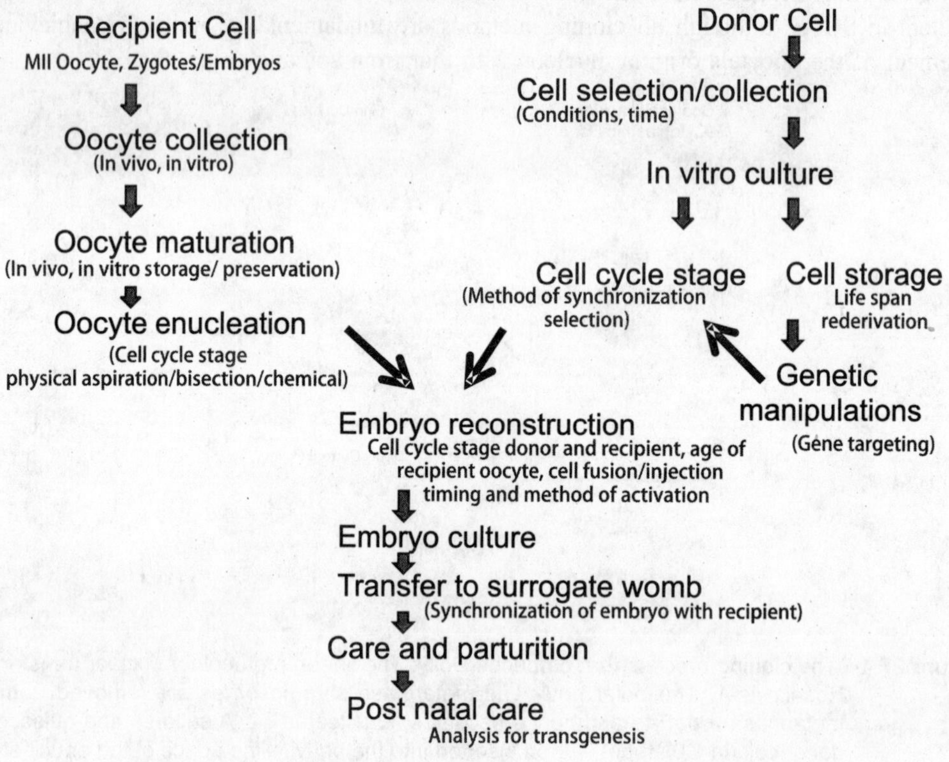

Figure 27.5 Steps involved in the production of offspring by SCNT.

In vitro collection and maturation provides greater control over the maturation process allowing selection of oocytes at defined stages during maturation. In case of porcine, *in vitro* maturation decreases the efficiency of cloning as compared to *in vivo* mature oocytes. To be used as cytoplast recipients for SCNT, the genetic material must be removed from the oocytes. Different enucleation techniques have been developed. It can be performed by mechanical means, chemical means and by some other techniques. Transfer of genetic material from donor cells is done by cell fusion using DC electric pulse. The same pulse may also be used for activation of recipient cytoplast. Now, laser assisted microinjection preceded by laser lyses of the donor cells has also been used. The cell cycle stage of both the donor nucleus and recipient cytoplast at the time of transfer is important whether by fusion or injection and can affect both the efficiency of transfer and subsequent nuclear reprogramming. Efficient artificial activation of reconstructed embryos is critical for development following SCNT. Successful activation has been achieved by a range of treatments (Table 27.2) including electrical stimulation as well as chemicals like strontium in mouse, inomycin, calcium ionophores in cattle and sheep. Inomycin or calcium ionophore combined with 6-dimethyl aminopurine (6-DMAP) or cycloheximide is one of the most widely used activation protocols for reconstructed oocyte after nuclear transfer. After the production of first mammal from cultured embryonic fetal and adult cell lines, numerous studies provided extensive evidence that somatic cell could be used to produce cloned offspring. Subsequently, numerous somatic cell types including mammary epithelial, ovarian cumulus cells, fibroblasts, sertoli cells, lymphocytes, natural killer cells, mature B and T cells, olfactory, neural stem cells, and myoblasts have been used for SCNT. This indicates that different tissues and cells from donors of different ages can be reprogrammed. Culturing somatic cells for prolonged periods is known to alter ploidy, genomic stability and post-translation histone modification. These factors are responsible for reducing cloning efficiency. Contrary to it, somatic cells maintained in culture for prolonged periods or even allowed to senescence have resulted in healthy offspring. Pluripotent cells such as embryonic blastomeres and embryonic stem cells support the development of nuclear transferred embryos at a higher efficiency than somatic cells. Since the production of Dolly in 1996 using SCNT, significant advances have been made in the number of animals cloned and also in understanding the molecular process underlying normal and abnormal development.

Table 27.2 Production of SCNT viable offspring following different activation protocols (Source: Campbell *et al.*, 2007).

Species	*Activation*	*Post-fusion*	*Post-activation treatment*
Cow	Ionophore (5 mM), 4 min	2–4 h	6-DMAP (2 mM), 3 h
	Ionophore (5 mM), 4 min	4–6 h	6-DMAP (2 mM), 4 h
	DC 20 V/mm, 20 ms	-	CHX (10 mg/ml), 5–6 h
Pig	DC 1.5 kV/cm, 100 ms	3–4 h	CB (5 mg/ml), 2 h
	2 x DC 1.5/1.2 kV/cm, 60 ms	-	-
	Ionophore (5 mM), 20 min	2–3 h	6-DMAP (1.9 mM), 3–4 h
Goat	DC 1.4–1.8 kV/cm, 70 ms	-	CB (5 mg/ml), 2 h
	Ionomycin (5 mM), 1 min	30 min	6-DMAP (2 mM), 2 h
	Ionophore (5 mM), 5 min	2–3 h	6-DMAP (2 mM), 2.5–4 h
Sheep	DC 1.25 kV/cm, 80 ms	-	CB (7.5 mg/ml), 1 h
Horse	Ionomycin (5 mM), 4 min	2–3 h	6-DMAP (1 mM), CMX (5 mg/ml), 4 h
Mule	Ionomycin (5 mM), 5 min	2–4 h	CHX (10 mg/ml), 5 h
Rabbit	3 × DC 3.2 kV/cm, 20 ms	1 h	6-DMAP (10 mg/ml), CHX (5 mg/ml), 1 h
Cat	2 × DC1.0 kV/cm, 50 ms	2 h	CHX (10 mg/ml), CB (5 mg/ml), 6-7 h
Dog	Ionophore (10 mM), 4 min	3 h	6-DMAP (1.9 mM), 4 h
Mouse	Sr2+ (10 mM), CB (5 mg/ml), 1–6 h	-	-
Rat	Butyrolactone (150 mM), 2 h	-	MG132 (5 mM) treatment before activation

Abbr: DC: Direct Current electric pulse; Sr: Strontium; DMAP: dimethylaminopurine; CHX: cycloheximide, CB: Cytochalasin B.

Ethical Concerns Regarding Animal Transgenesis

The scientific outlook of right and wrong opinions about transgenic animals is known as ethics of transgenic animals. Environmentalists and medical professionals argue about transgenic animals in different ways and have made the following implications:

(i) Creation of new life-forms: The transfer of genes between 2 species may in course of time affect the genome of the species, leading to some damage to the original genome. Transgenic animals may interact with the environment in a way which is not suitable for the sustainability of safe environment, and produce unexpected outcome. As transgenic animals are best models for human diseases, they are used in the study of progress of diseases. But the fact that changing genomes of animals may lead to reduction in breeding ability and lifespan is not taken care of.

(ii) Increased use of animals: Construction of transgenic animals results in altered phenotypes of the host cell. In transgenic disease models, one model cannot be used for other diseases or even other workers, as it has the selective target gene alone. So the model animals have to be killed. This is an animal wastage.

(iii) Gardon (1997) reported that the genetic and physiological characters in most cases of transgenic animals are different from that what was expected. This is mainly due to unexpected interaction of the desire gene with other genes in the genome.

(iv) Uncontrolled expression of inserted gene may increase the morbidity and mortality, e.g., transgenic animals with inserted growth hormone gene.

APPLICATIONS OF ANIMAL TRANSGENIC TECHNOLOGY

There is a constant expectation for fast improvement of livestock production and human health care products. The advent of DNA recombinant technology and the possibility of gene transfer between organisms of distinct species, or even distinct phylogenic kingdoms, have opened a wide range of possibilities. The recent advances in gene transfer, animal cloning, and assisted reproductive techniques have partly fulfilled the expectation in the field of livestock transgenesis. Some of the recent advances and applications of transgenesis in livestock and their derivative products are discussed. Transgenic animals have become tools for fundamental research in medicine and veterinary science. Application possibilities of transgenic technology in research, medicine, and industry are theoretically almost limitless. However, low level of efficiency is hampering most applications from a technical point of view.

Medical Applications

Transgenic animals became important tools for medical discovery. A number of transgenic animals (mostly mice) have been produced to answer basic research questions like gene regulation, immunology, and developmental biology. Transgenesis and cloning enable domestic animals to be designed to express a certain human illness, and therefore serve as models for study and treatment of human disease. Disease models are animals designed to express certain human diseases either at the genotypic or phenotypic level. They can be used both for further understanding of the disease and initial test on possible treatments. Since the 1980s, a large number of mouse models for human diseases have been developed. These models have limitations due to physiological differences between mice and human beings and also due to the limited life span of mice. Due to the similarity in physiology and size of lungs, small animals like sheep and pigs are an ideal animal model to investigate human respiratory diseases such as cystic fibrosis. Moreover, these animals are relatively inexpensive, breeding and maintenance is well established and their relatively longer life-span may allow diseases to manifest similarly as in human beings. An increasing number of candidate genes are available for establishing possible models of human diseases including neurodegenerative (Parkinson's; Alzhiemer) diseases, skin alterations (psoriasis, epidemolysis bullosa) or, other diseases with known genetic background like certain type of diabetes mellitus, arteriosclerosis and breast cancer. By first knocking out cystic fibrosis gene, to induce the disease, the resulting cloned sheep could be used for drug testing and evaluating new therapies. Cystic fibrosis is caused by a known single gene mutation and, therefore, is a suitable disease for gene targeting investigations. Transgenic monkey model of Huntington's disease has been developed by introducing altered forms of Huntington gene into monkey eggs using a viral vector. The eggs were fertilized and the resulting embryos were introduced into the surrogate mother. This model will be helpful in understanding disease mechanisms and design therapies. Diseases that are not caused by a single gene mutation, but by one of the several genes, or a combination of genes will be more difficult to create as useful animal models. Transgenic animal models have been used to functionally characterize different genes and dissect complex networks of cooperating genes including tissue/organ specific gene regulation and additive polygenic action of genes. A wide variety of oncogenes from viral and cellular sources have been inserted into the germline of mice with subsequent development of neoplasia. These oncomouse act as model animal for various forms of human and animal tumours. Such mice bearing an oncogene targeted for the expression in a specific tissue can reveal how that oncogene influences differentiation and will help to delineate the pathway(s) to malignancy. Transgenic animals are considered to be the powerful models for the investigation of various features of the immune system like studies of the differentiation and tolerance of lymphocytes, cytokines pathways and its pathophysiological consequences, role of different cell surface and major histocompatibility complex (MHC) antigens. The characterization of insertion site of foreign gene sequence in transgenic animals can identify loci that are potentially useful for the genetic analysis of the mammalian genome. In another arena, transgenic pigs are being produced to serve as organ donors for humans. Given its potential for alleviating human diseases due to irreversible tissue or organ failure, and given the acute shortage of human organs for transplant. The development of xenotransplantation as a part of clinical practice promises great benefits in terms of making it possible to dramatically increase supplies of replacement tissues and organs where severe shortages exist today. The field of xenotransplantation covers a great number of procedures, ranging from implantation of single cells to treat Parkinson's disease and tissues, such as pancreatic islets, to treat diabetes; extracorporeal use of intact organs, such as perfusion of patient blood through pig livers to provide short-term support in cases of liver failure; transplantation of whole organs—heart, kidney, liver, and so on. Differences between pigs and humans mean that a normal pig organ, transplanted into a human, would be rejected by the body within a few minutes. This hyperacute rejection (HAR) response occurs because antibodies react with antigenic structures on the surface of the porcine organ and induce HAR by activating the complement cascade. Many articles indicate that the enzyme α-1,3-galactosyltransferase (present on cell surfaces in almost all mammals with the exception of humans, apes and Old World monkeys) is involved in the HAR response. Pigs have been produced that have disrupted genes for the enzyme, thus being unable to express α 1,3-gal sugars on the cell surfaces (so called knock-out pigs). The hope is that an absence of the enzyme in the donor organ will prevent HAR. A similar problem is acute vascular rejection (AVR), which occurs within a few days of transplantation and is thought to be induced by xenoreactive antibodies. Its pathological symptoms are similar to those of HAR. A cellular rejection process occurs within a few days of transplantation. During this process, the blood vessels of the new organ are damaged by T-cells, which invade the intercellular spaces and destroy the organ. In an attempt to prevent hyperacute rejection of pig organs by humans, pigs have been made transgenic for the expression of human complement proteins, which are involved in the regulation of the immune response. The genetic modification of pigs is a requirement for xenotransplantation. Different receptors and antigens of immune system responsible for transplantation failure have been identified, which will be helpful in generating suitable humanized pigs for successful xenotransplantation in future (Table 27.3). However, recipients of xenotransplanted cells, tissues, or organs will be exposed to considerable risk, including the risk of novel infectious disease. The principal concern is that the uniquely close relationship created between xenotransplanted tissue and the host will allow novel opportunities for transmission of infectious disease (e.g., one derived from porcine endogenous retroviruses, or PERVs), and possibly creation of new disease agents in the process like swine flu virus. PERVs are of special concern since the transplant might provide the opportunity for the virus to evolve into a pathogen with the potential for transmission to others.

Table 27.3 Different components responsible for graft rejection (Source: Cascalho and Platt, 2001).

Component	Component mechanism	Target cell	HAR	AVR
1. Complement alternative pathway	Factor H	C3b	+	?
2. Complement regulatory proteins	CD55,CD46,CD57	C3/C$, C3/C4, C2/C9	+	?
3. Natural antibody	Ab.	Galα1,3 Gal	+/-	+
4. Neutrophil	Integrins	-	-	+/-
5. Macrophage	Lectins	Saccharide	-	+/-
6. Platelet	1L-1α	1L1R	-	+/-
7. Thrombin	-	Thrombomodulin,TFP1	-	+/-
8. NK cell	KIR, Lectin, FcR	MHC class I, Gal α 1,3 Gal, Ig Fc	-	+/-

Abb:- KIR:- killer inhibitory receptor, TFP1:- Tissue factor pathway inhibitor, HAR:- hyper acute rejection, AVR:- acute vascular rejection, components thought to initiate HAR or AVR are listed as +, and components for which there is an association but no proof are listed as +/-.

Somatic gene transfer

The first use of gene therapy to treat disease was for adenosine deaminase (ADA) deficiency. This is a disease in which the patients lack the ability to synthesize the ADA enzymes. As a result, a toxic metabolite builds up that poisons the cells of the immune system. The affected children are profoundly immunosuppressed, and if not kept in a specialized environment, they die of infection. The gene therapy trials involve the infection of bone marrow cells from the children with a virus engineered to contain the ADA gene, thereby replacing the missing enzyme. This treatment has caused significant improvement in the immune system of patients. Increasingly, such treatments are being devised and tested for a variety of diseases, including genetic disorders such as cystic fibrosis and muscular dystrophy, cancer, neurological diseases, infectious diseases and transplantation.

Veterinary Applications

Transgenics have shown potential in livestock production systems. The transgenic research in farm animals is mainly focused on production characteristics such as growth performance, increasing feed efficiency, enhancing body composition, lactation performance in bovines, and wool/fibre production in sheep. For example, improving growth in pigs by over expression of growth hormone, IGF-I, or estrogen receptors. The gene for ovine (sheep) growth hormone has been over-expressed in sheep under the control of metallothionein promoter. The transgenic animal showed improved performance in growth, body fat and wool production. In another study, transgenic sheep that over express sheep wool keratin genes have been generated. Over-expression of the type II intermediate filament gene, k2.10 resulted in changed lusture and crimp of the wool. Dairy cattle with altered β–casein and κ-casein ratio and thus improved milk quality. Besides, disease resistance and enhanced immune responsiveness has also been targeted by utilizing transgenic technology the first knock-out mammal, other than a mouse, was cloned by the deletion of the PrP (Prion Protein) gene in ovine fibroblasts before cloning. PrP gene is directly associated with scrapie in sheep, bovine spongiformis encephalopathy (BSE) in cattle and creutzfeld-jacob disease in humans. By knocking out the PrP gene, the resulting prion free livestock should be resistant to diseases such as scrapie and BSE. There are also possibilities to add genes that express proteins that protect animals from bacterial and viral infections. Genetically enhanced cow have been produced, which resist intramammary *Staphylococcus aureus* infection (cause a form of Mastitis). Improvement of reproductive traits of animals like transgenic bulls that produce only female and male offspring would also be feasible by using transgenic technology. In recent years, certain interspecific chimeras have been developed. For example, one interspecific chimera called "GEEP" (Figure 27.6) has been developed from the combination of cells of sheep and goat embryos. These are useful biological models for the study of developmental biology. These interspecific chimeras also provide a model for the study of maternal-foetal incompatibilities. Advances in cloning technology will be helpful in gene pool preservation. Gradual success is being achieved in cloning of endangered and extinct species. For example, argali and banteng resulted in pregnancies, gaur and mouflon pregnancies went on term. A similar approach was used to revive extinct bucardo using cells of cryopreserved skin biopsy and mature oocyte of domestic goats. Spanish ibex was used as surrogate mother. Transgenics in aquaculture has also seen advances in recent years. Different areas like faster growth rate, more efficient feed utilization, freeze resistance, cold and salinity tolerance, improved disease resistance and metabolic modification to improve fish nutritive value are some of the key areas of research. GloFish were the first steps in creating fish that would glow in the presence of certain chemicals, making them useful for detecting pollutants and other environmental contaminants. A gellyfish gene that codes for flourescent protein makes these GloFish glow red, green and yellow. Fish pharming for the production of pharmacologically important proteins was started in recent years. In future, transgenic fish will be able to reduce the amount of mercury or other toxic compounds that fish accumulate from their environment.

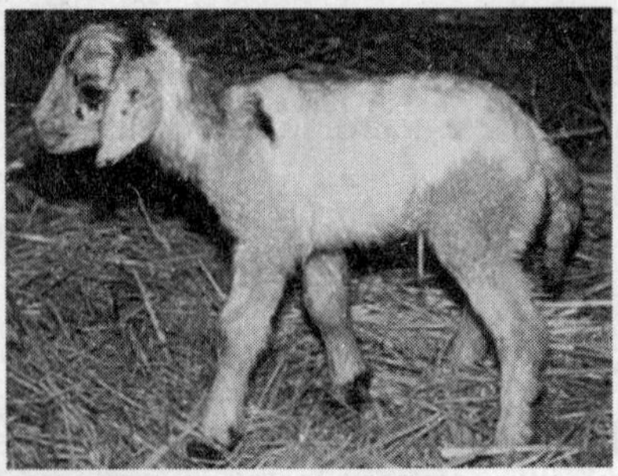

Figure 27.6 Baby GEEP (Source: Fehilli *et al.*, 1984).

"Annie" was the first cow to be cloned with a gene for a veterinary application. She was born in March 2000, a copy of a pure-breed Jersey cow. Now the scientists have started to test her milk for resistance to mastitis, a bacterial disease. Mastitis is often caused by *Staphylococcus aureus*, bacteria that destroy milk-secreting cells in cow's mammary glands. Researchers hope that Annie's mammary glands will secret a protein called lysostaphin that may help her resist attacks from *S. aureus*. They inserted a gene for lysostaphin production obtained from a benign species of *Staphylococcus simulans* that competes with its disease-causing relatives. Antibiotics cure only about 15% of cows infected with *S. aureus*. It is among the most virulent of mastitis-causing pathogens, causing nearly one-third of all infections in cows. If the lysostaphin works, Annie will have an alternative defence bioengineered right inside her cells.

The first reports of transgenic sheep were published by J. P. Simons (1986) of Edinburgh. Two transgenic ewes were produced, each carrying about 10 copies of human antihaemophilic factor IX gene (cDNA) fused with the 10.5 kb BLG (β-lactoglobulin) gene. BLG gene was used because it is necessary for the specific expression of gene in mammary glands. Consequently, the gene had a tissue-specific expression and ewes secreted human factor IX (or alpha 1 antitrypsin) into their milk. This human factor IX is active, even though the expression of the transgene is low. In another report published in 1991, also from Edinburgh, five transgenic sheep were produced (Alan Colman). In all these cases, transgene involved fusion of the Bovine α-lactoglobulin gene promoter fused to the human α_1 antitrypsin (hα_1 AT) gene. Four of these animals were female and one male. In one female, the protein hα_1AT reached a level of 35 g per litre of milk. The protein purified from milk had a biological activity indistinguishable from human plasma-derived antitrypsin. The deficiency of hα_1 AT leads to a lethal diseases, emphysema, which is a common hereditary disorder among Caucasian males of European descent. Hence, any strategy giving high yield of protein economically will be most welcome. In view of this, transgenic sheep with hα_1 AT gene will prove very useful as a bioreactor.

Recombinant DNA technology can also be used to increase the ability of sheep for wool growth. Wool is obtained from Angora, Mohair and Merino sheep. A high class Merino sheep has over 108 hair follicles in the skin, but only 25% of hair follicles possess hairs. This is due to low level of keratin in the cells. Keratin is rich in the sulphur-containing amino acid, cysteine. High level of cystine favours the growth of wool fibres. The following three technologies have been used to develop transgenic sheep for maximum wool production.

(i) Roger, at the University of Adelaide, Australia, isolated the genes coding for serine acetyl transferase (SAT) and O-acyl serine sulphydrase (OAS) from the bacterium *Salmonella typhimurium*. He then fused the two genes and added a promoter to it. The gene construct was introduced into fertilized eggs. The fertilized eggs were allowed to develop into 8-16-celled embryos. The embryos were implanted into a sheep. The sheep delivered a transgenic lamb, which produces dense, long wool fibres.

(ii) In another attempt, Roger introduced genes for isocitrate lyase and malate synthetase of *E. coli* into sheep. These enzymes helped the cells to bypass certain steps in the TCA cycle and helped to synthesize more amino acids. Hence, the transgenic sheep produced more wool.

(iii) R.A. Leng and his co-workers introduced the genes for isocitrate lyase and malate synthetase into rumen bacteria and the sheep were fed with the recombinant bacteria. The bacteria synthesize more amino acids and provide the sheep cells. The sheep skin cells therefore get more amino acids and hence the skin produces dense long wool fibres.

Transgenic goats were successfully produced recently by the groups headed by John Mc Pherson and Karl Ebert in U.S.A. These transgenic goats expressed a heterologous protein (a variant of human tissue-type plasminogen activator = LAtPA) in their milk. This protein is used for dissolving blood cells, i.e., for treatment of coronary thrombosis. A cDNA representing LAtPA was linked with either the murine whey acid promoter (WAP) or a β -casein promoter in an expression vector and used for injecting early embryos obtained surgically from the oviducts of superovulated dairy goats. At this concentration, the dairy goat may become an economically viable bioreactor for human pharmaceuticals (Table 27. 4).

Table 27.4 Transgenic landmarks and reproductive technology in livestock animals (cattle, goats, sheep and swine).

Year	*Important transgenic landmarks*	*Reference*
1985	Transgenic pig and sheep	Hammer *et al.* (1985)
1986	Embryonic cloning by nuclear transfe in sheep	Willadsen (1986)
1991	Transgenic dairy cattle	Krimpenfort *et al.* (1991)
	Transgenic sheep producing altered milk	Wright *et al.* (1991)
1992	Transgenic pigs resistant to viral infection	Muller *et al.* (1992)
1994	Pig expressing inhibitor of human complement system	Fodor *et al.* (1994)
1997	Somatic cloning by nuclear transfer in sheep (Dolly)	Wilmut *et al.* (1997)
	Transgenic livestock production as a model of human disease	Petters *et al.* (1997)
1998	Transgenic cattle produced by nuclear transfer	Cibelli *et al.* (1998)
2000	Transgenic sheep produced by gene targeting	McCreath *et al.* (2000)
2001	"Ecologically correct" transgenic pig	Golovan *et al.* (2001)
2002	Production of biopolymer fibre from transgenic cells	Lazaris *et al.* (2002)
	Calf with human artificial chromosome	Kuroiwa *et al.* (2002)
2003	Transgenic cattle producing altered milk protein compounds	Brophy *et al.* (2003)
	Complete gene inactivation in pigs	Phelphs *et al.* (2003)
2004	Sequential inactivation of 2 bovine genes	Kuroiwa *et al.* (2004)
2005	Transgenic cow resistant to bacterial infection (mastitis)	Wall *et al.* (2005)

Agricultural Applications

By using transgenic technology, it is possible to produce animals that can reduce negative agricultural effects on the environment. The most known of these today is the "EnviroPig": a pig that has the capability to digest plant phytase, leading to less phosphate in the manure from the animal and thus reduces environmental pollution. Pigs have been produced that express the enzymes phytase in their saliva to improve the utilization of feed derived phosphate.

Industrial Applications

The transgenic animal bioreactor industry made a significant stride in recent years. The concept of pharmaceutical pharming where large transgenic mammals are used as bioreactors for protein production is very appealing to the pharmaceutical industry, because it represents a cost-effective alternative to the cell-culture methods and other systems available to produce pharmaceuticals (Table 27.5). Bioreactors are the transgenic animals that have genes which produce human proteins for which genes are inserted into their genome. The production of proteins for treatment of disease is difficult due to their highly complex nature. However, it is now possible to insert a human gene, expressing a medicament, into an animals genome. The goal is to produce pharmaceuticals and nutraceuticals (food with therapeutic value) by exploiting farm animals. Currently mammary gland transgene expression is the preferred option because it allows mass production of large amounts of correctly processed proteins in a temperature-regulated fluid that may be collected daily in a non-invasive fashion. The production of recombinant human proteins in the milk of the transgenic animals presents several advantages over mammalian cell culture system currently being used. Milk is presently most mature systems to produce recombinant proteins from transgenic organism. Theoretically, other possible systems also exist (Table 27.6). Demand of recombinant proteins in large quantities for different therapeutic purpose can be fulfilled by utilizing transgenic technology. The expression levels in the milk of transgenic animals are typically 10-100 folds higher than those in typical mammalian cell culture system. Transgenically produced recombinant proteins have the same amino acid sequences as native human proteins because they are synthesized by the cells of the mammary gland from a recombinant version of the native gene. These recombinant proteins have mammalian glycoprotein pattern and also have appropriate folding, assembly and biological activity of the native molecules. Transgenically produced proteins also avoid the potential risks associated with transmission of different pathogens. Due to high-throughput technology, it guarantees an uninterrupted supply of larger amount needed. Milk also provides a relatively clean "feedstream" consisting of about 87% water, 4% fat, 9% non fat solids. The soluble phase contains the normal milk protein (Casein and whey protein), mineral salts and vitamins. The non-soluble phase contains fat globules, protein aggregates and cells. Recombinant proteins usually accumulate in soluble whey fraction of milk, thereby facilitating their easy recovery. Furthermore, milk does not contain active proteases that can breakdown the protein of interest. Goats, cows, sheep and pigs have been genetically modified and cloned in attempts to produce therapeutic proteins of medical importance (Table 27.7). Atryn is a medicine extracted from the milk of goats whose DNA has been modified by the introduction of a human gene (anti-thrombin gene). Good yield of therapeutic protein is also ensured. Milk from a 2-month-old cloned goat containing the gene for human anti-thrombin III yielded nearly 6g/L when induced to lactate. The gene expressing human coagulation factor IX was introduced into ovine fetal fibroblasts and linked to another gene with a high level of expression in the mammary gland before nuclear transfer. Hence, by linking the gene of interest to milk promoter genes, the protein is expressed in the milk from which it can be harvested economically. Genetically modified cows are used for the production of human therapeutic proteins. Human proteins that have been expressed in cow's milk include human lactoferrin, human α-lactalbumin, human serum albumin, human bile salt stimulated lipase and so on. Hence, large-scale cloning of transgenic livestock has the potential for the production of large quantities of therapeutic proteins (Table 27.8). Transgenic cloned animals can be designed to produce a wide range of medically useful human proteins including insulin for diabetes, interferon for viral infections, and tissue plasminogen factor to dissolve blood clots. This technique has the potential to produce proteins for the treatment of a range of human and animal diseases in near future. The risk of introducing new diseases into humans by animals as disease factories generate a serious need for these biological components to be thoroughly tested before commercialization.

Table 27.5 Comparison of the different systems to produce recombinant pharmaceutical proteins (Source: Houdebine *et al.*, 2009).

Points to consider	*Production systems*					
Bacteria	*Yeast baculovirus*	*Insect cells + cells*	*Animals/ plants*	*Transgenic animal (CHO cells)*	*Transgenic*	
1. Theoretical production level	+++++	+++++	+++	+	+++++	+++++
2. Practical production level	++ (+)	++ (+)	+	+	++	++++
3. Investment cost	+++++	+++++	++	+	++++	+++
4. Production cost	+++++	+++++	++	++	+++++	++++
5. Flexibility	+++++	+++++	++	+	+++++	++++
6. Line conservation	+++++	+++++	+++	+++	+++++	+++++
7. Line stability	+++++	+++++	++++	+++	+++++	+++++
8. Delay for the first production	+++++	+++++	+++	+++++	++++	+++(+)
9. Scaling up	+++++	+++++	++	+	+++++	++++
10. Collection	+++++	+++++	+++++	+++++	+++++	++++
11. Effect on organism	+++ (+)	+++ (+)	+++ (+)	+++ (+)	+++ (+)	+++
12. Post-translational modifications	+	++	+++	++++	+++	++++
13. Glycosylation	+	++	+++	++++	++	++++
14. Stability of product	+++++	+++++	+++	+++	++++	++++
15. Purification	+++	+++	+++	++++	+++	+++
16. Contaminant pathogens	+++++	+++++	+++++	++++	+++++	++++
17. Intellectual property	++++	+++	+++	++	+++	+++
18. Products in the market	++++	+++	+++	+++++	+	+++

Table 27.6 Comparison of the different production systems to produce recombinant pharmaceutical proteins. (Source: Houdebine *et al.*, 2009).

Points to consider	*Production systems*						
	Blood	*Milk*	*Egg white*	*Seminal Plasma*	*Urine*	*Silk gland*	*Drosophila larvae*
1. Theoretical production level	+++++	++++	+++++	+++	++	++	++
2. Practical production level	++	++++	+++ (+)	+	+	++	+
3. Investment cost	+++	+++	+++	+	+	+++	+++
4. Production cost	++++	++++	++++	++	+	+++++	++++
5. Flexibility	+++++	+++++	+++++	++	+	+++++	++++
6. Line conservation	+++++	+++++	+++++	+++++	+++++	+++++	+++++
7. Line stability	+++++	+++++	+++++	+++++	+++++	+++++	+++++
8. Delay for the first production	+++	+++	+++	++	+	++++	++++
9. Scaling up	++++	++++	++++	++	+	++++	+++
10. Collection	+++++	++++	+++++	+++	+++	+++++	+++++
11. Effect on organism	++	+++	+++ (+)	+++ (+)	+++ (+)	++++	++++
12. Post-translational modifications	+++++	++++	+++ (+)	+++ (+)	+++ (+)	++ (+)	++ (+)
13. Glycosylation	++++ (+)	++++	+++	+++ (+)	+++ (+)	++	++
14. Stability of product	+++	++++	++++	+++ (+)	+++ (+)	+++ (+)	+++(+)
15. Purification	++	+++	+++	++ (+)	++ (+)	+++	++ (+)
16. Contaminant pathogens	++	+++	+++	+++	++	++++	++++
17. Intellectual property	++++	+++	+++	+++	+++	+++	+++
18. Products in the market	+	++++	++	+	+	++	+

Table 27.7 Pharmaceutical products derived from transgenic animals (Source: Dunn *et al.*, 2005).

Product	*Use*	*Product development stage*	*Organization*
5G1.1	Rheumatoid arthritis Nephritis	Preclinical	Alexion–GTC Biotherapeutics
α-1 Antitrypsin	Hereditary emphysema Cystic fibrosis	I–T ARC	Bayer–PPL
α-Fetoprotein (rhAFP)	Myasthenia gravis Multiple sclerosis Rheumatoid arthritis	Phase II	Merrimack–GTC
ABX-EGF	Cancer	Phase II	Abgenix–Amgen
ABX-IL8	Rheumatoid	arthritisI–T	Abgenix–GTC
Antithrombin III (ATryn®)	Emboli Thromboses	Phase III Seeking marketing approval	GTC
Bile salt-stimulated lipase	Cystic fibrosis Fat malabsorbtion	I–T	AstraZeneca–PPL

Contd.

Butyrylcholinesterase, BChE (Protexia™)	Biodefense	Preclinical	Nexia
C1 inhibitor	Hereditary angioedema	Phase III	Pharming
Calcitonin	Osteoporosis	I–T	PPL
CD137 agonist	Solid tumors	Preclinical	Mayo Clinic–GTC
CFTR	Ion transport Cystic fibrosis	I–T	GTC
Collagen	Rheumatoid arthritis	Preclinical	Pharming
CTLA4Ig	Rheumatoid arthritis	Preclinical	Bristol-Myers Squibb–GTC
D2E7	Rheumatoid arthritis	Preclinical	Abbott–GTC
Erythropoietin	Anemia	Preclinical	Avigenics
Extracellular superoxide dismutase	Ischemic reperfusion injury	I–T	Pharming
Factor VIII	Hemophilia A	Preclinical	ARC–Pharming
Factor IX	Blood coagulation Hemophilia	Preclinical	GTC PPL ARC–Pharming
Fibrinogen	Tissue sealant development	Preclinical	Pharming
G-CSF	Leukopenia	Preclinical	Avigenics
Glucagon-like peptide-1	Type 2 diabetes	I–T	PPL
Glucosidase	Glycogen storage disease	I–T	Pharming
Glutamic acid decarboxylase	Type 1 diabetes	I–T	GTC–BioSyn
Hemoglobin	Blood substitute development	I–T	Baxter
Human growth hormone	Growth failure Turner's syndrome Cachexia	I–T	GTC
Human serum albumin	Blood pressure Trauma Burn treatment	Preclinical	Fresenius–GTC
Humanized antibodies	Various indications	Phases I, II and III	Medarex
Humanized polyclonal antibodies	Various indications	Preclinical	Hematech Avigenics
huN901	Small-cell lung cancer	Preclinical	ImmunoGen–GTC
Insulin	Diabetes	I–T	GTC
Interferon	Antiviral	Preclinical	Avigenics
Lactoferrin	Immunomodulatory Anti-inflammatory	GRAS filing Phase I	Pharming
Lysozyme	Antimicrobial Immune modulator	I–T	UC-Davis
Merozoite surface protein 1	Malarial vaccine	Preclinical	GTC
PRO542	HIV/AIDS	Preclinical	Progenics–GTC
Prolactin	Enhancement of immunity	I–T	GTC
Protein C	Blood coagulation	I–T	ARC PPL
Remicade®	Crohn's disease Rheumatoid arthritis	Preclinical	Centocor–GTC

Contd.

Rotavirus virus-like particles (VP2,VP6)	Vaccine development	Preclinical	Bioprotein (BPT)
Spider silk (Biosteel™)	Materials development	Preclinical	Nexia
Tissue plasminogen activator	Dissolution of blood clots Heart attacks	I-T	Genzyme
Tissues or organs	Engineered for xenotransplantation	Preclinical	Alexion Bresagen Novartis Mayo Clinic
Tysabri® (formerly Antegren®)	Neurological disorders	Preclinical	Elan–GTC
Xenomouse® (fully human antibodies)	Various indications	Various	Abgenix

Table 27.8 Comparison of the time required to obtain recombinant proteins in different transgenic animal species (Source: Houdebine *et al.*, 2009).

Parameters	*Rabbit*	*Pig*	*Sheep*	*Goat*	*Cow*
1. Gestation time (months)	1	4	5	5	9
2. Age at sexual maturity (months)	5	6	8	8	15
3. Time between gene transfer and first lactation (months)	7	16	18	18	33
4. Number of offspring	8	10	1-2	1-2	1
5. Annual milk yield (liters)	15	300	500	800	8000
6. Recombinant protein per female per year (kg)	0.02	1.5	2.5	4	40

Production of pharmaceuticals and biomolecules

Due to the high cost, the production of transgenic animals such as pig, goat, sheep and cattle must bring an elevated profit in order to be a feasible economical investment. For this reason, the production of high-value pharmaceutical substances, which correspond to a billion-dollar market, is actually the principal and most promising application for animal transgenesis. Despite the lower costs of producing biomolecules in microorganisms, like bacteria and yeast, these organisms do not properly execute several post-translational modifications, such as N-linked glycosylations, authentic O-linked glycosylations, and correct folding in order to produce a wide range of fully active human proteins. Therefore, many human polypeptides must be produced in mammalian cell systems to be recovered with their full activities. However, principally due to the low productive capacity, the price of human biomolecules produced *in vitro* by mammalian cell culture is extremely high. For this reason, many biotechnology companies have been focusing on the production of biopharmaceuticals at high concentrations in transgenic livestock bioreactors. Worldwide those companies are investing great effort in this promising technology. Among them we may mention PPL Therapeutics (UK), GTC Biotherapeutics (USA), Hematech (USA), Genzyme (USA),

ZymoGenetics (USA), Nexia Biotechnologies (Canada), Pharming (Netherlands), BioProtein Technologies (France), Avigenics (USA), Viragen (USA), and TranXenoGen (USA). Pharmaceutical products can be produced in a variety of biological fluids such as milk, urine, saliva, blood and seminal fluid, and their expression can be driven by tissue-specific promoters. Generation of transgenic mice expressing therapeutic heterologous proteins in urine, such as human recombinant erythropoietin (rhEPO) and human alpha I-antitrypsin (alphaIAT), using a uromodulin promoter has been demonstrated recently.

Protein expression into the urine-based system has some advantages, including the expression in both sexes, low contaminant-protein content in urine, and being able to be harvested soon after birth and expressed throughout the life of the transgenic animal. However, the use of this system may be significantly more time and cost consuming than the mammary-gland-based system. Due to its large-scale production, milk is the preferred vehicle to express proteins in transgenic animals. Table 27.9 lists biomolecules expressed in the mammary glands of livestock, which are at an advanced stage of clinical trials, and the respective holders of their commercial rights. The mammary gland can express more than 2g of heterologous recombinant proteins per litre of milk. Based on the assumption average expression levels, daily milk volumes and purification efficiency, 54000 cows would be needed to produce the 100,000 kg of human serum albumin that are required worldwide per year, 4500 ewes would be required for the production of 5000 kg of α antitrypsin, 100 goats for 100 kg of monoclonal antibodies, 75 goats for 75 kg of antithrombin III and sows to produce 2 kg of human clotting factor IX required per year. Therefore, a small herd of transgenic livestock could supply the world demand for pharmaceuticals, which cannot be expressed by other systems such as bacteria or fungi, mainly due to the necessity of complex post translational processing to ensure their proper function. Studies have reported the use of transgenic rabbits as bioreactors, using a rat whey acidic protein (WAP) promoter to produce the human growth hormone (HGH/hgh) in milk.

Table 27.9 Human proteins secreted in the milk of transgenic livestock.

Pharmaceutical	*Bioreactor species*	*Application/ treatment*	*Company*	*Reference*
Antithrombin	Goat	Thrombosis, pulmonary embolism	GTC Biotherapeutics (USA)	Ebert *et al.* (1991) Denman *et al.* (1991)
tPA	Goat	Thrombosis	PPL Therapeutics (UK)	Ebert *et al.* (1994)
α-Antitrypsin	Sheep	Emphysema and cirrhosis	PPL Therapeutics (UK)	Wright *et al.* (1991)
Factor IX	Sheep	Haemophilia b	PPL Therapeutics (UK)	Schnieke *et al.* (1997)
Factor VIII	Sheep	Haemophilia a	PPL Therapeutics (UK)	Paleyanda *et al.* (1997)
Polyclonal antibodies	Gattle	Vaccines	Hematech (USA)	Kuroiwa *et al.* (2004)
Lactoferrin	Cattle	Bactericide	Pharming Group (NED)	Van Berkel *et al.* (2002)

Contd.

Cl inhibitor	Rabbit	Hereditary angioedema	Pharming Group (NED)	Van Boorn *et al.* (2005)
Calcitonin	Rabbit	Osteoporosis and hypercalcaemia	PPL Therapeutics (UK)	McKee *et al.* (1998)

CONCLUSION AND FUTURE PROSPECTS

Since the domestication of first animal humans have been introducing genetic modifications by assisted breeding in a variety of species. Nowadays with the advances of scientific knowledge we can have a better understanding of inheritance mechanisms and make punctual and specific alterations in DNA sequences to meet our requirements. Therefore, discussions on ethics arising with the first GMOs demonstrated the continuity of the human activity in altering the environment, as well as organisms, for our own benefit. Notwithstanding, it does not exempt us from the responsibility for our actions and a recent research field, named biosafety, has been created to manage the ecological impact of GMOs. Regarding individual characteristics of livestock, although we have to consider the low response to artificial selection compared to changes obtained with transgenesis, a continuous application of the former for many generations can introduce huge genetic modifications. Therefore, when an animal is out of a genetic breeding program, in order to insert any genetic modification, the result is an intrinsic loss of the productive ability conferred to their assisted selected counterparts. Moreover, the high cost involved in the transgenic process allows us to obtain only few animals for each genetic modification event. For this reason, a laborious process of reintroduction of those animals in the herd by backcrossing is required. In order to make this process economically feasible, it is essential to have in-depth knowledge about the recent advances in assisted reproduction techniques, such as artificial insemination associated with embryo transfer, or *in vitro* embryo production. Nevertheless, some degree of inbreeding is inevitable, which leads to a loss of genetic variability. Another consequence of the introduction of new characteristics to a livestock product, e.g., milk or meat, is the public perception related to the emergence of new products on the market. The pharmaceutical industry has a history of obtaining products through a variety of microorganisms, plants, animals and human tissue sources. Therefore, the isolation of biopharmaceutical products from milk derived from genetically modified animals does not require significant changes in the production system or market perception by the consumers. However, the prospect of livestock animals with new properties and characteristics would have an enormous impact on the structure of agricultural industry. The benefits of this segmentation can be confirmed by the profitable market of crops in the agriculture sector. But a question remains: is the livestock industry prepared for such changes? This and other questions will be answered as the technical and scientific progress reduces the costs of transgenic livestock and makes it even more feasible and accessible for the production sector.

FURTHER READINGS

1. Baldassarre, H., Wang, B., Kafidi, N., Gauthier, M., Neveu, N., Lapointe, J., Sneek, L., Leduc, M., Duguay, F., Zhou, J.F., Lazaris, A. and Karatzas, C.N. (2003) Production of transgenic goats by pronuclear microinjection of *in vitro* produced zygotes derived from oocytes recovered by laparoscopy. *Theriogenology.* **(59)**: 831-839.

2. Brophy B., Smolenski G., Wheeler T., Wells D., L'Huillier P., Laible G., (2003) Cloned transgenic cattle produce milk with higher levels of beta-casein and kappa-casein. *Nat. Biotechnol.* **(21):** 157-162.
3. Campbell, K.H., Mcwhir, J., Ritchie, W.A., Wilmut, I. (1996) "Sheep cloned by nuclear transfer from a culture cell line". *Nature.* 380 **(6569):** 64-66.
4. Campbell, K.H.S., Fisher, P., Chen, W.C., Choi, I., Kelly, R.D.W., Lee, J.H. and Xhu, J. (2007) Somatic cell nuclear transfer: past, present and future perspectives, *Theriogenology.* **(68S):** S214-S231.
5. Cascalho, M. and Platt, J.L. (2001) The immunological barrier of Xenotransplantation. *Immunity.* **(14):** 437-446.
6. Cibelli J.B., Stice S.L., Golueke P.J., Kane J.J., Jerry J. Blackwell C. *et al.* (1998) Cloned transgenic calves produced from nonquiescent fetal fibroblasts. *Science.* **(280):** 1256-1258.
7. Cournoyer and Caskey (1993) Disruption of the adenosine deaminase (ADA) gene using a dicistronic promoterless construct: Production of an ADA-deficient homozygote ES cell line. *Transgenic Research.***(4):** 247-255.
8. Cowan P. J., Aminian, A., Barlow, H., Brown, A.A., Chen, C.G., Fisicaro, N., Francis, D.M., Goodman, D.J., Han, W., Kurek, M., Nottle, M.B., Pearse, M.J., Salvaris, E., Shinkel, T.A., Sainsbury, G.V., Stewart, A.B. and A'pice, A.J. (2000) Renal xenografts from triple-transgenic pigs are not hyperacutely rejected but cause coagulopathy in non-immunosuppressed baboons. *Transplantation.* **(69):** 2504-2515.
9. Cunningham, E. P. (1999) The application of biotechnologies to enhance animal production in different farming systems, *Livestock Production Science.* **(58):** 1-24.
10. Damak, S., Su, H.Y., Jay, N.P. and Bullock, D.W. (1996) Improved wool production in transgenic sheep expressing insulin-like growth factor 1. *Bio/Technology.* **(14):** 185-188.
11. Denman J., Hayes M., O'Day C., Edmunds T., Bartlett C., Hirani S. *et al.* (1991) Transgenic expression of a variant of human tissue-type plasminogen activator in goat milk: purification and characterization of the recombinant enzyme. *Biotechnology.* (NY). **(9):** 839-843.
12. Dunn, D.A., Kooyman, D.L. and Pinkert C. A. (2005) Transgenic animals and their impact on the drug discovery industry. *Drug Discovery Today.* 10 **(11):** 757-767.
13. Dyck M.K., Lacroix D., Pothier F. and Sirard M.A. (2003) Making recombinant proteins in animals-different systems, different applications. *Trends Biotechnol.* **(21):** 394-399.
14. Ebert K.M., DiTullio P., Barry C.A., Schindler J.E., Ayres S.L., Smith T.E. *et al.* (1994) Induction of human tissue plasminogen activator in the mammary gland of transgenic goats. *Biotechnology.* (NY). **(12):** 699-702.
15. Ebert K.M., Selgrath J.P., DiTullio P., Denman J., Smith T.E., Memon M.A. *et al.* (1991) Transgenic production of a variant of human tissue-type plasminogen activator in goat milk: generation of transgenic goats and analysis of expression. *Biotechnology.* (NY). **(9):** 835-838.
16. Eduardo O. Melo, Aurea M.O. Canavessi, Mauricio M. Franco and Rodolfo Rumpf (2007) Animal transgenesis: state-of-the-art and applications. *J. Appl. Genet.* 48 **(1):** 47-61.
17. Fehilli, C.B., Willadsen, S.M and Tucker, E.M. (1984) Interspecific chimaerism between sheep and goat. *Nature.* **(307):** 634-636.
18. Fishman, J. A. and Patience, C. (2004) Xenotransplantation: infections risk revisited. *American Journal of Transplantation.* **(4):** 1383-1390.
19. Fodor W.L., Williams B.L., Matis L.A., Madri J.A., Rollins S.A., Knight J.W., *et al.* (1994) Expression of a functional human complement inhibitor in a transgenic pig as a model for the prevention of xenogeneic hyperacute organ rejection. *Proc. Natl. Acad. Sci. USA.* **(91):** 11153-11157.
20. Folch, J., Cocero, M. J., Chesne, P., Alabart, J. L., Dominguez, V., Cognie, Y., Roche, A., Fernandez-Arias, A., Marti, J.I., Sanchez, P., Echegoyen, E., Beckers J. F., Sanchez, Bonastre A. and Vignon, X. (2009) First birth of an animal from an extinct subspecies (*Capara pyrenaica pyrenaica)* by cloning. *Theriogenology.* **(71):** 1026-1034.

21. Friedmann T. (1994) Gene therapy for neurological disorders. *TIG* **(10):** 210-214.
22. Gilboa E. and Smith C. (1994) Gene therapy for infectious diseases: The AIDS model (review). *Trends Genet.* **(10):** 139-144.
23. Golovan S.P., Meidinger R.G., Ajakaiye A., Cottrill M., Wiederkehr M.Z., Barney D.J., *et al.* (2001) Pigs expressing salivary phytase produce low-phosphorus manure. *Nat. Biotechnol.* **(19):** 741-745.
24. Gordon, J.W. and Ruddle, F. H. (1981) Integration and stable germ line transmission of genes injected into mouse pronuclei. *Science*. **(214):** 1244-1246.
25. Hammer R.E., Pursel V.G., Rexroad C.E., Jr., Wall R.J., Bolt D.J., Ebert K.M., *et al.* (1985) Production of transgenic rabbits, sheep and pigs by microinjection. *Nature*. **(315):** 680-683.
26. Hong, S.G., Jang, G., Kim, M.K., Oh, H.J., Park, J.E., Kang, J.T., Koo, O.J., Kim, D.Y. and Lee, B.C. (2009) Dogs cloned from fetal fibroblasts by nuclear transfer. *Animal Reproduction Science.* (Article in press).
27. Houdebine, L.M. (2002) The methods to generate transgenic animals and to control transgene expression. *Journal of Biotechnology*. **(98):** 145-160.
28. Houdelbine, L.M. (2009) production of pharmaceutical proteins by transgenic animals. *Comparative Immunology, Microbiology and Infectious Diseases*. **(32):** 107-121.
29. Izsvak, Z., Ivics, Z. and Plasterk, R.H.(2000) Sleeping Beauty, a wide host-range transposon vector for genetic transformation. *Journal of Molecular Biology*. 302 **(1):** 93–102.
30. Kay MA and Woo SLC (1994) Gene therapy for metabolic disorders. *Trends Genet.* **(10):** 253-257.
31. Keefer, C. L. (2004) Production of bioproducts through the use of transgenic animal models. *Animal Reproduction Science*. 82 **(83):** 5-12.
32. Kishigami, S., Wakayama, S., Hosoi, Y., Iritani, A. and Wakayama, T. (2008) Somatic cell nuclear transfer: infinite reproduction of a unique diploid genome. *Experimental Cell Research*. **(314):** 1945-1950.
33. Krimpenfort P., Rademakers A., Eyestone W., van der Schans A., van den Broek S., Kooiman P., *et al.* (1991). Generation of transgenic dairy cattle using *'in vitro'* embryo production. *Biotechnology.* (NY) **(9):** 844-847.
34. Kuroiwa Y., Kasinathan P., Choi Y.J., Naeem R., Tomizuka K., Sullivan E.J. *et al.* (2002). Cloned transchromosomic calves producing human immunoglobulin. *Nat. Biotechnol.* **(20):** 889-894.
35. Kuroiwa Y., Kasinathan P., Matsushita H., Sathiyaselan J., Sullivan E.J., Kakitani M. *et al.* (2004) Sequential targeting of the genes encoding immunoglobulin-mu and prion protein in cattle. *Nat. Genet.* **(36):** 775-780.
36. Larkin D.F., Oral H.B., Ring C.J. *et al.* (1996) Adenovirus-mediated gene delivery to the corneal endothelium. *Transplantation.* **(61):** 363-370.
37. Lavitrano, M., Stoppacciaro, A., Bacci, M. L., Forni, M., Fioretti, D., Pucci, L., Di Stefano, C., Lazzereschi, D., Rughetti, A., Ceretta, S., Zannoni, A., Rahimi, H., Moioli, B., Rossi, M., Nuti, M., Rossi, G., Seren, E., Alfani, D., Cortesini, R. and Frati, L. (1999) Human decay accelerating factor transgenic pigs for xenotransplantation obtained by spermmediated gene transfer. *Transplantation Proceedings*. **(31):** 972-974.
38. Lazaris A., Arcidiacono S., Huang Y., Zhou J.F., Duguay F., Chretien N., *et al.* (2002) Spider silk fibers spun from soluble recombinant silk produced in mammalian cells. *Science.* **(295):** 472-476.
39. Lee, G.S., Kim, H.S., Hyun, S.H., Lee, S.H., Jeon, H.Y., Nam, D.H., Jeong, Y.W., Kim, S., Kim, J.H., Han, J.Y., Ahn, C., Kang, S.K., Lee, B.C. and Hwang, W.S. (2005) Production of transgenic clonedpiglets from genetically transformed fetal fibroblasts selected by green fluorescent protein. *Theriogenology*. **(63):** 973-991.
40. Li, Z., Sun, X., Chen, J., Liu, X., Wisely, S.M., Zhou, Q., Renard, J.P., Leno, G.H. and Engelhardt, J.F. (2006) Cloned ferrets produced by somatic cell nuclear transfer. *Developmental Biology*. **(293):** 439-448.
41. Lipinski D., Jura J., Kalak R., Plawski A., Kala M., Szalata M. *et al.* (2003) Transgenic rabbit producing human growth hormone in milk. *J. Appl. Genet.* **(44):** 165-174.

42. Loi, P., Galli, C. and Ptak, G. (2007) Cloning of endangered mammalian species: any progress? *Trends in Biotechnology*. 25 **(5):** 195-200.

43. Markoulaki, S., Meissner, A. and Jaenisch, R. (2008) Somatic cell nuclear transfer and derivation of embryonic stem cells in the mouse. *Methods*. **(45):** 101-114.

44. McCreath K.J., Howcroft J., Campbell K.H., Colman A., Schnieke A.E., Kind A.J., (2000) Production of gene-targeted sheep by nuclear transfer from cultured somatic cells. *Nature*. **(405):** 1066-1069.

45. McKee C. Gibson A. Dalrymple M., Emslie L. Garner I. and Cottingham I. (1998) Production of biologically active salmon calcitonin in the milk of transgenic rabbits. *Nat. Biotechnol.* **(16):** 647-651.

46. Miller H.I. (2002) As biotech turns 20. *Nat. Rev. Drug. Discov.* **(1):** 1007-1008.

47. Moisyadi, S., Kaminski, J.M. and Yanagimachi, R. (2009) Use of intracytoplsmic sperm injection (ICSI) to generate transgenic animals. *Comparative Immunology. Microbiology and Infectious Diseases*. **(32):** 47-60.

48. Muller M. Brenig B., Winnacker E.L., Brem G., (1992) Transgenic pigs carrying cDNA copies encoding the murine Mx1 protein which confers resistance to influenza virus infection. Gene. **(121):** 263-270.

49. Niemann, H., Halter, R., Carnwath, J.W., Herrmann, D., Lemme, E. and Dieter, P. (1999) Expression of human blood clotting factor VIII in the mammary gland of transgenic sheep. *Transgenic Research*. **(8):** 237-247.

50. Paleyanda R.K. Velander W.H. Lee T.K., Scandella D.H., Gwazdauskas F.C. and Knight JW (1997) Transgenic pigs produce functional human factor VIII in milk. *Nat. Biotechnol.* **(15):** 971-975.

51. Palmiter, R. D. and Brinster, R. L. (1986) Germ-line transformation of mice. *Annual Review Genetics*. **(20):** 465-499.

52. Palmiter, R.D., Brinster, R.L., Hammer, R.E., Trumbauer, M.E., Rosenfeld, M.G., Birnberg, N.C. and Evans, R.M. (1982) Dramatic growth of mice that develop from eggs microinjected with metallothionein-growth hormone fusion genes. *Nature*. **(300):** 611-615.

53. Paterson, L., Desousa, P., Ritchie, W., King, T., and Wilmut, I. (2003) Application of reproductive biotechnology in animals: implications and potential applications of reproductive cloning. *Animal Reproduction Science.* **(79):** 137-143.

54. Petters RM, Alexander CA, Wells KD, Collins EB, Sommer JR, Blanton MR, *et al.* (1997). Genetically engineered large animal model for studying cone photoreceptor survival and degeneration in retinitis pigmentosa. *Nat. Biotechnol.* **(15):** 965-970.

55. Phelps, C.J., koike, C, Vaught, T.D., Boone, J., Wells, K.D., Chen, S.H., Ball, S., Speecht, S.M., Polejaeva, I.A., Monahan, J.A., Jobst, P.M., Sharma, S.B., Lamborn, A.E., Garst, A.S., Moore, M., Demetris, A.J., Rudert, W.A., Bottino, R., Bortera, S., Trucco, M., Starzl, T., Dai, Y. and Ayares, D.L. (2003) Production of 1,3 Galactosyltransferase deficient pigs. *Science*. 299 **(5604):** 411-414.

56. Robl, J.M., Wang, Z., Kainathan, P. and Kuroiwa, Y. (2007) Transgenic animal production and animal biotechnology. *Theriogenology*. **(67):** 127-133.

57. Rockenstein, E., Crews, L. and Masliah, E. (2007) Transgenic animal models of neurodegenerative diseases and their application to treatment development. *Advanced Drug Delivery Reviews*. **(59):** 1093-1102.

58. Roth, T.L., Anderson, G.B., Bon Durant, R.H. and Pahen, R.L. (1989) Survival of sheep x goat hybrid inner cell masses after injection into ovine embryos. *Biological Reproduction*. **(41):** 675-682.

59. Rudolph N.S. (1999) Biopharmaceutical production in transgenic livestock. *Trends Biotechnol.* **(17):** 367-374.

60. Schnieke, A. E., Kind, A. J., Ritchie, W. A., Mycock, K., Scott, A. R., Ritchie, M., Wilmut, I., Colman, A. and Campbell, K. H. S. (1997). Human factor IX transgenic sheep produced by transfer of nuclei from transfected fetal fibroblasts. *Science*. **(278):** 2130-2133.

61. Smith, A. G. (2001) Embryo-derived stem cells: Of mice and men. *Annual Review of Cell and Developmental Biology*. **(17):** 435-462.

62. Smith, K. R. (2002) Gene transfer in higher animals: theoretical considerations and key concepts. *Journal of Biotechnology*. **(99):** 1-22.

63. Vajita, G. and Gjerris, M. (2006) Science and technology of farm animal cloning: state of the art. *Animal Reproduction Science*. **(92):** 211-230.
64. Van Berkel P.H. Welling M.M., Geerts M., Van Veen H.A., Ravensbergen B., Salaheddine M. *et al*. (2002) Large-scale production of recombinant human lactoferrin in the milk of transgenic cows. *Nat. Biotechnol.* **(20):** 484-487.
65. Van Doorn M.B., Burggraaf J. van Dam T. Eerenberg A. Levi M. Hack C.E. *et al*. (2005) A phase I study of recombinant human C1 inhibitor in asymptomatic patients with hereditary angioedema. *J. Allergy Clin.* Immunol. **(116):** 876-883.
66. Velander W.H. Johnson J.L., Page R.L. Russell C.G., Subramanian A. Wilkins T.D. *et al*. (1992) High-level expression of a heterologous protein in the milk of transgenic swine using the cDNA encoding human protein C. *Proc. Natl. Acad. Sci.* (*USA*) **(89):** 12003-12007.
67. Wall R.J., Kerr D.E. and Bondioli K.R. (1997) Transgenic dairy cattle: genetic engineering on a large scale. *J. Dairy Sci.* **(80):** 2213-2224.
68. Wall R.J., Powell A.M., Paape M.J., Kerr D.E. Bannerman D.D. Pursel V.G. (2005) Genetically enhanced cows resist intramammary Staphylococcus aureus infection. *Nat. Biotechnol.* **(23):** 445-451.
69. Wall, R.J., Hyman, P., Kerr, D., Pintado, B. and Wells, K. (1997). Transgenic animal technology. *Journal of Andrology*. 18 **(3):** 236-239.
70. Wall, R.J., Powell, A.M., Paape, M.J., Kerr, D.E., Talbot, N. and Hawk, H.W. (2005) Genetically enhanced cows resist intramammary *Staphylococcus aureus* infection. *Nature Biotechnology*. **(23):** 445-451.
71. Wei, L.N. (1997) Transgenic animals as new approaches in pharmacological studies. *Ann. Rev. Pharmacol. Toxicol.* **(37):** 119-141.
72. Willadsen S.M., (1986). Nuclear transplantation in sheep embryos. *Nature.* **(320):** 63-65.
73. Wilmut, I., Schnieke, A.E., Mcwhir, J., Kind, A.J. and Campbell, K.H. (1997) "Viable offspring derived from fetal and adult mammalian cells. *Nature*. 385 **(6019):** 810-813.
74. Wolf, E., Schernthaner, W., Zakhartchenko, V., Prelle, K., Stojkovic, M. and Brem, G. (2000). Transgenic technology in farm animals- progress and perspectives. *Experimental Physiology*. 85 **(6):** 615-625.
75. Wolf, E., Zakhartchenkov, V. and Brem, G. (1998) Nuclear transfer in mammals: recent developments and future perspectives. *Journal of Biotechnology*. **(65):** 99-110.
76. Wright G. Carver A. Cottom D. Reeves D. Scot A. Simons P. *et al*. (1991) High level expression of active human alpha-1-antitrypsin in the milk of transgenic sheep. *Biotechnology.* (NY). **(9):** 830-834.
77. Zbikowska H.M., Soukhareva N. Behnam R., Chang R., Drews R. Lubon H. *et al*. (2002a) The use of the uromodulin promoter to target production of recombinant proteins into urine of transgenic animals. *Transgenic Res.* **(11):** 425-435.
78. Zbikowska H.M., Soukhareva N., Behnam R. Lubon H. Hammond D. and Soukharev S (2002b) Uromodulin promoter directs high-level expression of biologically active human alpha1-antitrypsin into mouse urine. *Biochem J.* **(365):** 7-11.
79. Zoraqi, G. and Spadafora, C. (1997). Integration of foreign DNA sequences into mouse sperm genome. *DNA and Cell Biology.* **(16):** 291-300.

CHAPTER

28

Liposome Technology

Liposomes are well-recognized delivery vehicles that have been developed to enhance the therapeutic activity of several drugs. The purpose of this chapter is to lay the foundation of basic concepts and practical uses of liposome technology in medical, veterinary, agricultural sciences and industrial application.

Keywords: Liposome technology; bangosomes; unilamellar and multilamellar vesicle; amphipathic compounds, phospholipid vesicles.

INTRODUCTION

A liposome is a tiny bubble (vesicle) made of phospholipids that have a head and a tail. The head is attracted to water, and the tail, which is made of oil (hydrocarbon), is repelled by water. When membrane phospholipids are disrupted, they can reassemble themselves into tiny spheres, smaller than a normal cell, either as bilayers or monolayers, these are liposomes (Figure 28.1). The name liposome is derived from two Greek words 'lipid' meaning fat and 'soma' meaning body. Liposomes are composed of naturally-derived phospholipids with mixed lipid chains (like egg phosphatidylethanolamine, cholesterol, phosphotidylcholine, phosphotidylethanolamine, dipalmitoylphosphatidylcholine, diacetylphosphate, stearylamine, phosphatidic acid, phosphatidylserine, cardiolipin, sphingomyelin, etc.), or pure surfactant components like DOPE (dioleoylphosphatidylethanolamine). Liposomes, usually but not by definition, contain a core of aqueous solution; lipid spheres that contain no aqueous material are called micelles, however, reverse micelles can be made to encompass an aqueous environment.

Liposomes are the smallest artificial vesicles of spherical shape that can be used as drug carriers and are loaded with a great variety of molecules, such as small drug molecules, proteins, nucleotides and even plasmids. Liposomes are extremely versatile and due to the variability of their composition they can be used for a large number of applications. Liposomes are used to deliver certain vaccines, genes, enzymes, or drugs to the body. They are specially effective in treating diseases that affect the phagocytes of the immune system because they tend to accumulate in the phagocytes, which recognize them as foreign invaders. They have also been used experimentally to carry normal genes into a cell in order to replace defective, disease-causing genes. Liposomes are sometimes used in cosmetics because of their moisturizing qualities.

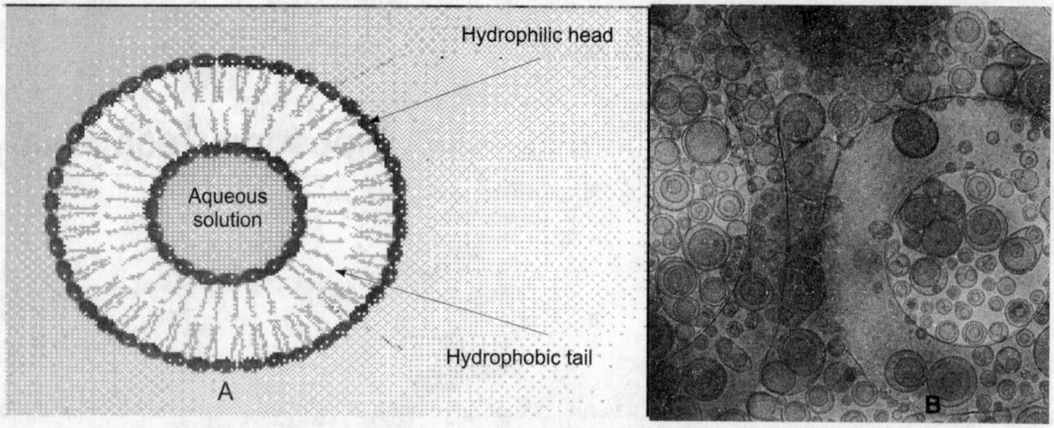

Figure 28.1 A liposome structure B. An electron micrograph of liposomes.

Recent advances in molecular biology, medicine and pharmaceutical technology together have allowed for the development of several new classes of therapeutic modalities, which proved to be a major breakthrough in combating a wide range of genetic, malignant and infectious diseases. The need for effective drug delivery systems is straightforward. For a drug to produce a specific pharmacological response, it must gain access to its specific "Site of action". The last decade has seen the emergence of a great many approaches to the problem of controlled drug delivery, such as polymeric sustained release systems, liposomal drug carriers and antibody drug carriers. Drug targeting is one such pharmaceutical technology that makes a molecule a wonder drug. Drug targeting in simple words means reaching the drug to the site of action and thus achieving the desired response without interactions at other sites. One of the popular experimental approaches to controlled drug delivery has been the use of liposomes, or phospholipid vesicles. In this chapter some of the basic chemical and physical characteristics of liposomes and their applications in various fields of science such as medical, pharmaceutical, veterinary and agricultural are discussed.

CONCEPTS

Liposomes were first produced in England in 1961 by Alec D. Bangham, who was studying phospholipids and blood clotting. It was found that phospholipids combined with water, immediately formed a sphere because one end of each molecule is water-soluble, while the opposite end is water-insoluble. Water-soluble medications added to the water were trapped inside the aggregation of the hydrophobic ends; fat-soluble medications were incorporated into the phospholipid layer. This was the birth of the use of liposomes as model membranes. These liposomes are also sometimes referred to as "Bangosomes", after the name of the discoverer. Liposomes are amphipathic in nature, i.e., part of their structure is water-soluble (hydrophilic or water-loving) and the other part is oil-like (hydrophobic or water-fearing or fat-soluble). Therefore, when added to water, the water-soluble part of the phospholipid interacts with the water and the oil-like part of the molecule avoids the water (Figure 28.2). There are two main concepts of liposomes.

1. Phospholipids dispersed in water can form a variety of structures depending on the molar ratio of lipid to water.
2. At relatively low ratios, the liposomal type structure consisting of aqueous compartments bounded by lipid membranes is the predominant one.

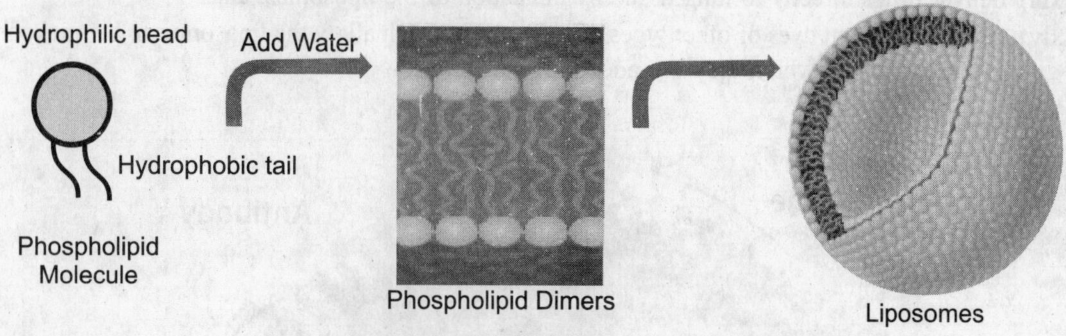

Figure 28.2 Liposome formation.

PRINCIPLES

The most common type of lipid nanoparticle, a liposome, can be thought of as a hollow sphere whose size ranges from 30 nm to 10,000 nm. Liposomes can serve as carriers for all types of molecules including both water-soluble and water-insoluble compounds. Liposomes can be made of a single type of phospholipid or mixtures of different phospholipids. Non-phospholipid components such as cholesterol, fatty acids and other lipid-soluble molecules such as vitamin E are commonly added to liposomes. By varying the type of phospholipid used to make liposomes and/or by attaching certain molecules to the surface of liposomes, they can be engineered to have many useful properties (Figure 28.3). Liposomes, with or without entrapped compounds, can be designed to:

(i) release their contents when they reach a specific temperature;
(ii) release their contents at a specific pH value;
(iii) target certain tissues or cell types by changing the types of lipids in the liposome;
(iv) target tissues, cell types or specific proteins by attaching antibodies to the surface;
(v) avoid certain tissues or cells by attaching complex sugars to the surface;
(vi) evenly distribute fat-soluble (oil-like) compounds such as certain vitamins, antioxidants; antibiotics, flavors, etc., which often cannot be mixed in water-based products including most food;
(vii) fuse with cells, which is important in delivering DNA to a cell;
(viii) serve as model cell membranes making it easier to study specific cellular processes and how certain molecules, such as drugs, interact with cells;
(ix) protect compounds from acidic and enzymatic degradation in the stomach and intestine by using certain molecules to coat the liposome;

(x) protect compounds such as vitamins and antioxidants from premature oxidation for increased shelf-life;
(xi) enhance the intestinal absorption of compounds by coating with certain molecules.
(xii) carry drugs across the nasal mucosa (nasal drug delivery);
(xiii) deliver drugs directly to lung tissue by inhalation of the liposomes; and
(xiv) carry fluorescent dyes or other types of molecules, which allow the liposomes to be tracked in the system to which they are added.

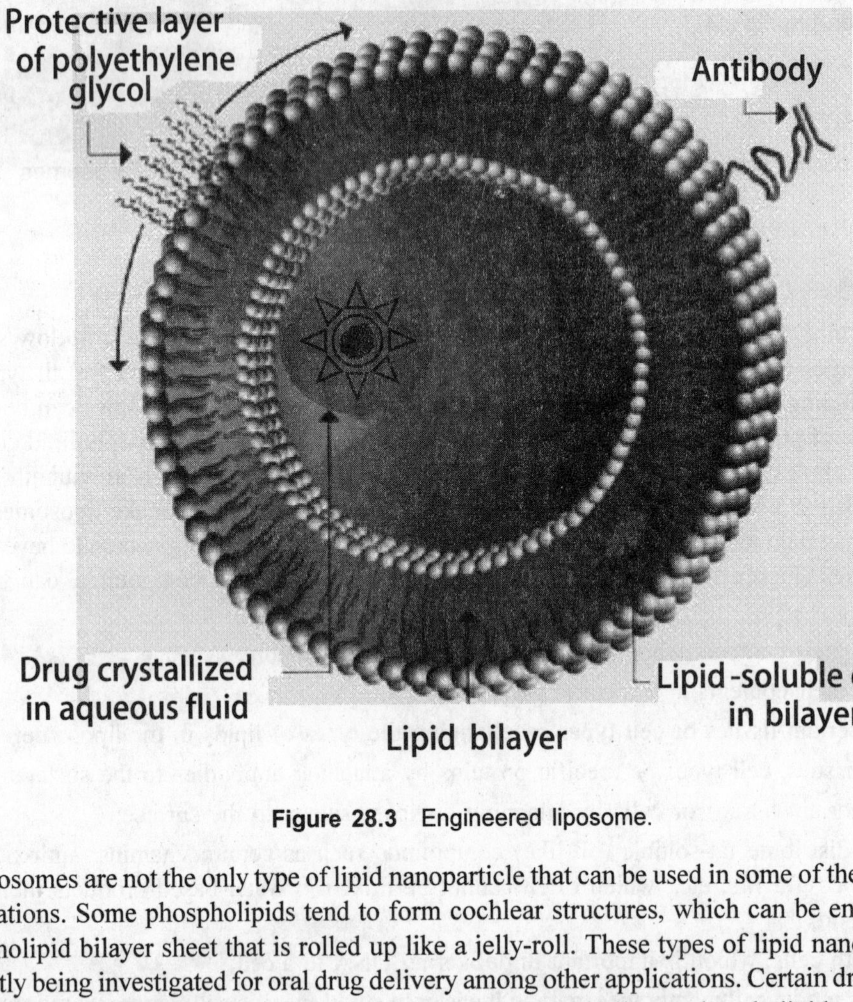

Figure 28.3 Engineered liposome.

Liposomes are not the only type of lipid nanoparticle that can be used in some of the above-listed applications. Some phospholipids tend to form cochlear structures, which can be envisioned as a phospholipid bilayer sheet that is rolled up like a jelly-roll. These types of lipid nanoparticles are currently being investigated for oral drug delivery among other applications. Certain drugs and other molecules, often those which have amphipathic properties similar to phospholipids, form bilayer-like complexes with phospholipids resulting in nanosized particles but usually do not have the capacity to entrap water-soluble compounds. The scientists at Encapsula NanoSciences have experience in all types of lipid nanoparticle systems including the selection of best type of nanoparticle for a particular application.

LIPOSOME TECHNOLOGY

Purpose: The main purpose of liposomes technology includes:

(i) to use a model membrane system in the elucidation of the role of various cell surface molecules, their transport and interaction with various ligands;
(ii) to use as vehicles for delivery of drugs and bio-molecules to a desired site in the living system;
(iii) use as an immunological carrier and an adjuvant; and
(iv) use in immunodiagnosis and genetic engineering.

Types of Liposomes

Liposomes consist of a series of concentric bilayers alternating with aqueous compartments. Based on the number of layers and size of the liposome, they are classified as SUV (small unilamellar vesicle), LUV (large unilamellar vesicle), MLV (multilamellar vesicle) and MVV (multivesicular vesicle) (Table 28.1 and Figure 28.4). The most common preparation is the MLV (multilamellar vesicle), an "onion-like" structure of concentric aqueous and lipid layers. These structures are heterogeneous in size, but range up to several microns in diameter. Sonication can reduce MLVs to SUVs (small unilamellar vesicles), which are single walled vesicles of 200 to 500 Å diameter. It is also possible by various means to construct LUVs (large unilamellar vesicles), where a single large aqueous compartment is bounded by a single bimolecular lipid membrane. These structures are usually about 1 μ in diameter. These vesicles are made by a process of reverse phase evaporation. Typically the thickness of a lipid bilayer membrane is about 50 Å.

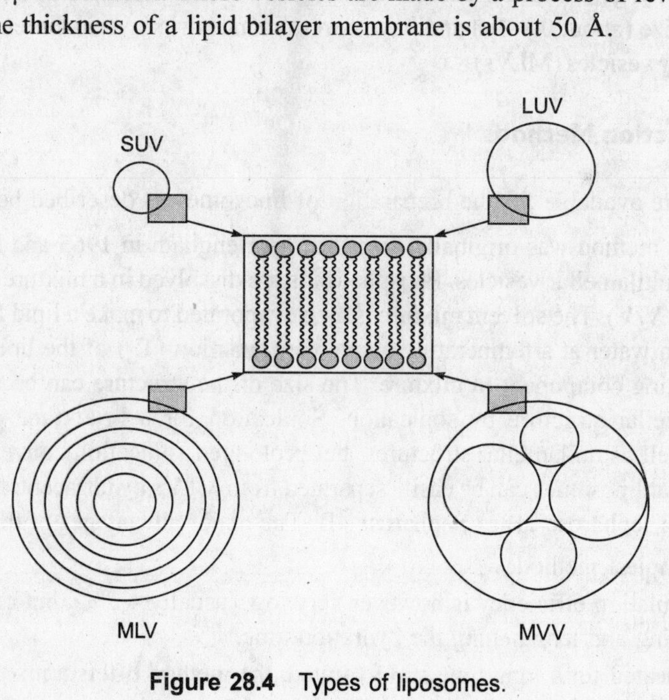

Figure 28.4 Types of liposomes.

Table 28.1 Sizes of liposomes.

Structure	*SUV*	*MLV*	*REV (LUV)*
Size (nm)	20-50	400-3500	200-1000
Capture Volume (il/mg)	0.5	4.1	13.7
Encapsulation	0.5-1.0	5-11	35-65

Small unilamellar vesicles: Small unilamellar vesicles (SUV) consist of a single lipid bilayer having a diameter of 25nm. They may be prepared by exhaustive sonication (solvent dilution technique) of MLVs using a probe or bath type sonicator. Any contaminated MLV can be removed by ultracentrifugation or column chromatography. An alternative method for SUV production involves infection of an ethanolic solution of lipid into an aqueous phase using a fine hypodermic needle. These SUVs are very inefficient in trapping water-soluble compounds.

Large unilamellar vesicles: Large unilamellar vesicles (LUVs) are reformed using acid phospholipids. The preparation requires formation of SUV by sonication and their subsequent fusion into large sheets by the addition of calcium ions. Treatment with EDTA opens out the sheets and LUVs are formed. These vesicles are extremely efficient in terms of trapping water-soluble drug (up to 40-60% entrapment), but seem to be somewhat less stable than other vesicle types.

Multilamellar vesicles: A solution of lipid is dried in an organic solvent. The lipid is then hydrated and dispersed by adding buffer. Aqueous soluble materials are added to the aqueous phase, while lipid-soluble materials are added to the lipid phase. The free and liposome bound drug can then be separated by gel filtration chromatography. The liposomes formed in this manner are heterogeneous in size (about 0.1-3μ) and have several concentric layers of membranes. These are called multilamellar vesicles (MLVs).

Liposome Production Methods

Several methods are available for the preparation of liposomes as described below:

Sonication: This method was originally described by Bengham in 1965 and is usually used for the formation of multilamellar vesicles. Phospholipids are dissolved in a mixture of chloroform and methanol (ratio 2:1 V/V). The solvent mixture is then evaporated to make a lipid film. The lipid film is then dispersed in water at a temperature above the transition (T_C) of the lipid or above the T_C of the highest melting component in mixture. The size of the structure can be further reduced by disrupting the lamellar structure by sonication. Sonication for a brief time gives rise to both multilamellar as well as unilamellar structures, but prolonged sonication converts the former into the later. Unilamellar liposomes can be easily separated from MLVs by ultracentrifugation or column chromatography on sepharose 2B or Sepharose 4B. The major advantages of this method include:

(i) It is the simplest method.

(ii) The encapsulation efficiency is however very low (usually 4-7%), but can be increased by gentle shaking and lengthening the hydration time.

(iii) Unless sonicated for a long time and hydrated, the method offers a mixture of both homogeneous as well as heterogeneous preparation.

Ethanol injection: This method avoids the use of sonicator in preparing liposomes. It involves the injection of a solution of lipid in ethanol, into a buffer. Nearly all vesicles obtained by this method are unilamellar. The major disadvantages are that the lipid dispersion is diluted and the encapsulation efficiency is poor.

Ether infusion: In this method, phospholipids are dissolved in diethyl ether-methanol mixture and are injected into an aqueous solution of the material to be entrapped either at 55- 65°C or under reduced pressure at 0°C. The solvent is then removed by evaporation and large unilamellar vesicles of a mean size between 1500-2500 Å are formed. The method is suitable for macromolecules. The drawbacks are:

(i) Unnecessary exposure of materials to high temperature and organic solvents.
(ii) Low encapsulation efficiency.
(iii) Production of heterogeneous population of liposomes.

Reverse phase evaporation: In this method, the aqueous material is introduced into a mixture of phospholipids and organic solvent. The latter is then removed under reduced pressure. LUV and oligolamellar liposomes are formed. The encapsulation efficiency is very high (up to 65%). The method cannot be applied for entrapment of proteins that get denatured on exposure to organic solvent.

Rehydration-dehydration: This method offers very high entrapment efficiency and can be used for industrial preparation of liposomes. It was developed by Kirby and Gregoriadis in 1984. Initially the liposomes are made by dissolving lipids in organic solvent, removing the solvent under reduced pressure and then dispersing into aqueous phase. The liposome preparation is then freeze-dried and can be stored frozen without any major leakage of entrapped material for more than a year. Whenever desired, the dried lipid can be regenerated into liposomes by adding water. The encapsulation efficiency is achieved when the lipid is fully dehydrated as SUV prior to freeze-drying. The major advantage of this method is that the lipid powder could be stored for a long time and is suitable for diagnostic purposes as it is easy to prepare when desired.

French press: In this method, initially MLVs are made by suspending lipids in aqueous buffer as described in sonication method. Instead of sonication, the dispersion of MLVs are reduced in size by extrusion at high pressure through a French press. When extrusion is done at 20,000 Ibs/in^2 one pass, vesicles with a size range 250-500 Å are formed. Further extrusions may yield more homogeneous preparations of MLV.

Detergent dialysis: Detergent removal method involves the solubilization of unsolicited lipid dispersion with a detergent such as sodium deoxycholate or sodium cholate followed by its removal by gel filtration or dialysis. The major advantage of this method is that liposomes are homogeneous and of the SUV category. However, the complete removal of detergent may not be always possible. It is worth mentioning that the lipid to detergent ratio plays an important role in size of SUV.

Properties of Liposomes

The physical properties of liposomes depend on their chemical composition, thus it is possible to use a variety of different types of saturated or unsaturated phospholipids, to include sterols, fatty acids or a variety of other charged or uncharged amphiphiclic compounds. The physical characteristics of the bilayer membranes of liposomes are also highly dependent on temperature, pH, ionic strength and the presence of divalent cations. In response to temperature changes (or in response to other types of environmental perturbations), bilayer membranes undergo phase transitions, shifting (as the temperature is raised) from a "gel" state in which the fatty acid side chains of the membrane lipid are closely packed and relatively ordered, to a "fluid" state in which the side chains are capable of more rotational motion. This thermotropic phase transition can have major effects on the stability, permeation properties and overall behavior of the lipid vesicles. Discrete phase transitions are observed only in liposomes containing one or a few species of homogeneous phospholipids. Natural lipids, which are mixtures of species containing heterogeneous fatty acyl chains, display broad, and ill defined phase transitions. Cholesterol has a very interesting modulatory effect on the phase transition behavior of bilayers composed of homogeneous phospholipids. This molecule serves as a "fluidity buffer", since below the phase transition cholesterol tends to make the bilayer less ordered, while above the transition it tends to increase the order in the membrane. Thus the presence of cholesterol damps out dramatic phase change behavior of bilayers containing homogeneous phospholipid species.

Incorporation of Drugs in Liposomes

It is clear that polar or hydrophilic drugs will be largely found in the internal aqueous compartments of liposomes, although some degree of binding to the bilayer is also a possibility. By contrast, lipophilic or amphipathic drugs can intercalate into the liposomes membrane, the polar molecule is quickly and completely released as the liposome membrane is breached by sonication while lipophilic drug remains associated with the liposome membrane. For lipophilic drugs, the maximal incorporation into liposomes simply depends on the amount of lipid and the solubility of the drug in the lipid. Drug/lipid molar ratios of 1:10 are usually readily achieved without disrupting bilayer structure. For polar drugs, the entrapment depends on the solubility of the drug in water and the volume of water encapsulated per mass of lipid. This latter parameter can differ substantially among different liposome types. Thus, encapsulation ratios can vary from about 0.5 -1/mol for SUVs to in excess of 15-1/mol for LUVs. One must keep in mind, however, that the encapsulation efficiency is only one of the parameters to be considered in the choice of a liposome type and composition for a particular application. Stability, lack of toxicity or special biochemical characteristics may also be important.

Generally speaking, a variety of drugs are easily incorporated into liposomes. However, it is facing a lot of problems, such as:

(i) Problems of commercial scale formulation of liposomes drugs.

(ii) Amphipathic leak out of the vesicles unless special steps are taken (e.g., charge complexation) to stabilize the drug-liposome association.

Ordinarily, loss or efflux rates of highly polar or highly lipophilic drugs from lipid vesicles tend to be low (less than 1%/hr). Efflux rates of both polar and lipophilic drugs tend to be highest near or at the bilayer phase transition. There may be several obstacles to achieve sufficiently high drug/lipid ratios, narrow size heterogeneity and good chemical stability during prolonged storage. However, the problem of stable incorporation and storage of polar drugs, which reside in the entrapped aqueous compartment, maybe difficult while stable incorporation of lipophilic drugs is less of a problem.

Liposome Cell Interaction

Liposomes can interact with cells via four basic mechanisms namely: a) absorption to the cell surface, b) endocytosis, c) fusion and d) lipid exchange. Although early work suggested that vesicle cell fusion might be important, more recent evidences suggest that for most vesicle compositions and most cell types either absorption or endocytosis are the dominant mechanisms of liposome-cell interaction. Some other mechanisms are as follow:

(i) Solid (i.e., gel state) vesicles tend to adsorb strongly to cell surface, while this is less true for fluid vesicles.

(ii) Cells, which are "professional" phagocytes, such as neutrophils and macrophages tend to engulf and internalize vesicles by an active, energy dependent, actinomycin related phagocytic process.

(iii) Less specialized cells such as fibroblasts tend to internalize vesicles (particularly SUVs) by using the coated pit endocytotic mechanism.

(iv) The presence on the liposome surface of protein or carbohydrate ligands capable of interacting specifically with certain cellular receptors (e.g., Fc-receptor on macrophages) can markedly enchance the rate and extent of cellular uptake of liposomes.

The multiple non-specific mechanisms of liposome cell interaction may pose considerable problems in those cases where more specific interactions are desired.

Targeting of Liposomes

Drug delivery by liposomes has many advantages over simply injecting the drug alone into the bloodstream. First of all, the drug remains concentrated in the liposomes instead of diffusing throughout the body. This means that lower doses can be administered. Since many drugs used in the treatment of diseases such as cancer have toxic side effects to healthy cells as well as the diseased ones, the lower dose means fewer side effects for the patient and lower cost for treatment. Secondly, the liposomes can sometimes be targeted to a tumour or site of disease. Just as biological membranes in a normal cell contain proteins and a variety of other materials, synthetic liposomes can also be manufactured to contain small proteins or carbohydrates that will "lock on" to a specific target molecule when they come in contact with it. Sites of inflammation and some tumours often have specific molecules on their surfaces that are potential targets, including molecules in the liposome that bind these targets that increases the likelihood of the drug reaching the proper area of the body and minimizes uptake by non-target cells. Lastly, the release of the drug at the site is prolonged as the drug slowly releases from the liposome. Since the liposome is composed of lipids like the membrane itself, it can fuse to the membrane and deliver the drug directly inside the cell (Figure 28.5). The direct delivery and prolonged exposure increases the effectiveness of the drug. An attractive but elusive approach in the liposomal drug delivery area has been the notion of coupling antibodies to vesicles so as to target drugs to specific cell populations. While considering the problem of targeting, two important concepts must be kept in mind. First, the specific association of antibody linked vesicles with cells is not a guarantee of effective intracellular delivery of drug molecules from within the vesicle, and secondly, the attainment of specific targeting is much more easily accomplished *in vitro* than *in vivo*, where a variety of processes may frustrate the specific liposome-cell association.

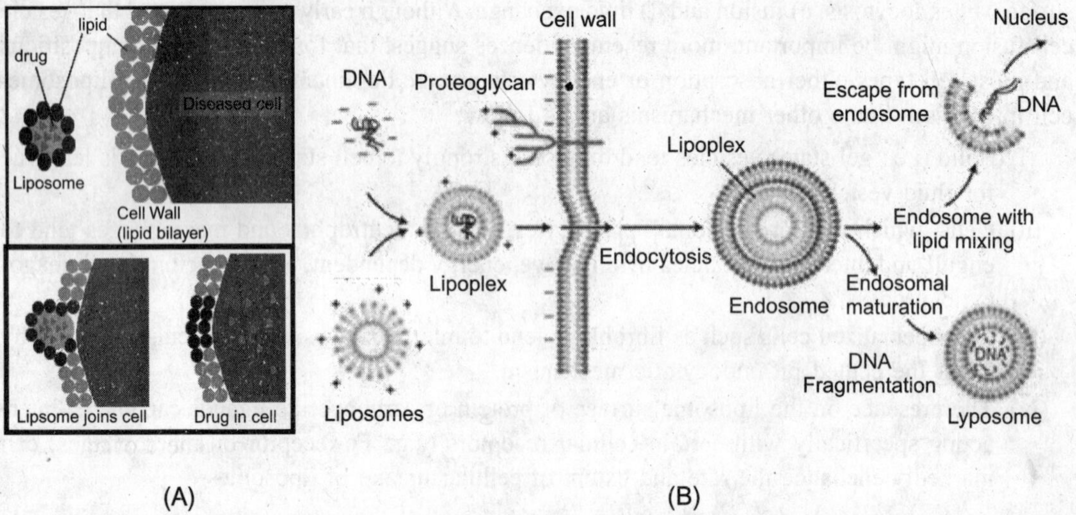

Figure 28.5 Lipoplex-mediated transfection (A) and endocytosis (B).

Some prospects for promoting specific liposome-cell association are:

(i) By simply coating the liposome with antibodies or lectins.

(ii) By coupling of monoclonal antibodies or affinity purified fab fragments to vesicles.

(iii) By incorporation of glycolipid determinants into the liposome membrane so as to promote specific association with lectin-like receptors on cell surfaces.

(iv) By using vesicles coated with an antigen (e.g., myelin basic protein) to specifically manipulate certain aspects of immune function. This model may eventually provide an exciting approach for the specific suppression of a variety of autoimmune or allergic processes by "targeting" vesicles to specific lymphocyte population.

Behaviour of Liposomes *in vivo*

There have been many studies on the *in vivo* fate of liposomes and liposome encapsulated drugs. It has been clear that the primary sites of liposome uptake are the liver and spleen. The liver and spleen are particularly well suited for the clearance of circulating particles since they contain an abundance of phagocytic reticuloendothelial cells and their capillary endothelium is fenestrated there by permitting the egress of comparatively large particles (Figure 28.6).

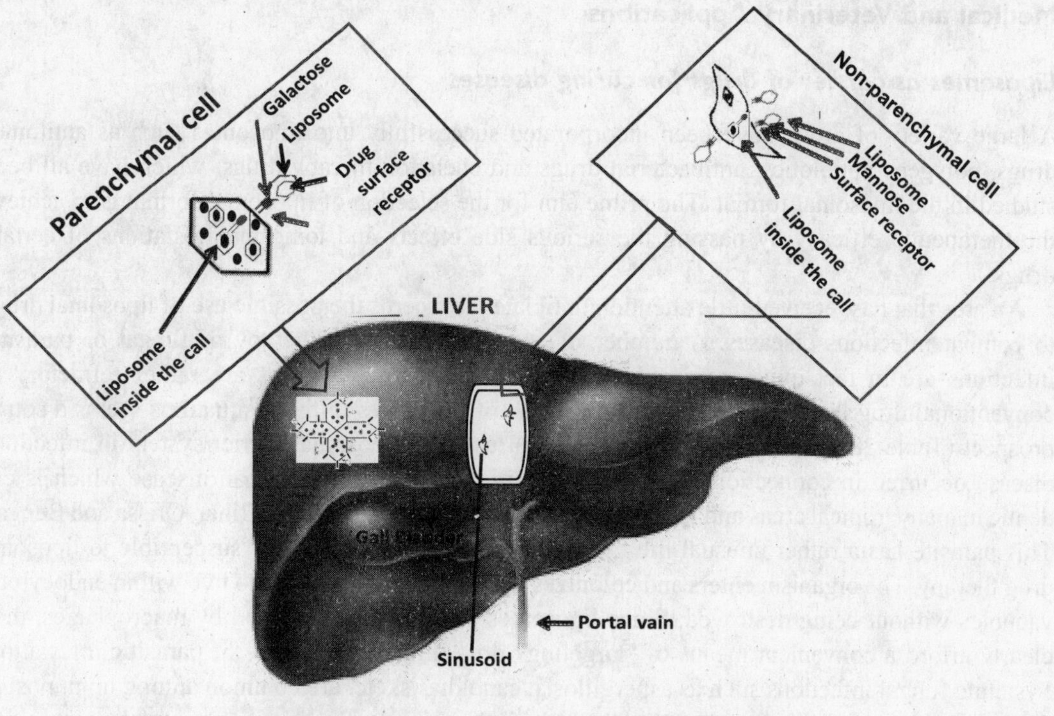

Figure 28.6 Targeting of drug to specific liver-cell types.

A number of studies have explored the role of reticuloendothelial (RE) cells in the clearance of vesicles from the circulation. The behavior of liposomes *in vivo* can be modulated to a considerable degree by altering physical characteristics such as size, surface charge and stability. Early studies of the clearance kinetics of lipid vesicles demonstrated that large vesicles were cleared more rapidly than small ones, and with vesicle populations similar in size, negatively charged liposomes were cleared far more rapidly than neutral or positive ones. Thus, liposomes seem ideally suited as means to deliver drugs to macrophages of the RE system. Despite a number of *in vitro* successes, the problem of antibody-mediated targeting of liposomes *in vivo* is just beginning to be addressed. Clearly, the selective targeting of liposomes *in vivo* will likely remain an elusive goal for sometime to come.

APPLICATIONS OF LIPOSOME TECHNOLOGY

Liposome technology has several potential applications such as gene therapy, cancer therapy, clinical pathogenesis, enzyme replacement therapy, chelation therapy, immunomodulation, thermal transitions of phospholipids, neurobiological applications, leucoyte phagocytosis, botanical research, drug interactions with membranes, bacterial cell wall synthesis, lectin receptor interactions, microvillus formation in cells and many more. Some of the important applications of liposome technology are discussed below.

Medical and Veterinary Applications

Liposomes as carrier of drugs for curing diseases

A large variety of drugs have been incorporated successfully into liposomes such as antitumor drugs, polygene antibiotics, antibacterial drugs and chelation therapy drugs, which have all been studied in the liposomal format. The prime aim for the selection of liposomal format is to achieve the therapeutic efficacy by passing the serious side effects and toxic manifestations of certain drugs.

An area that has received little attention until lately concerns the possible use of liposomal drugs to combat infectious diseases. A number of agents used for the therapy of fungal or parasitic infections are in fact quite toxic, and in some cases these infections are rather refractory to conventional drug therapy. Exploration of the use of liposomes in these situations seems a sound prospect (Table 28.2). The first highly successful use of a liposomal carrier system in infectious disease occurred in connection with leishmaniasis (kala-azar), a protozoan disease which is endemic in many tropical areas and also prevalent in India such as in Assam, Bihar, Orissa and Bengal. This parasite has a rather unusual life cycle, which makes it particularly susceptible to liposome drug therapy. The organism enters and colonizes macrophages, managing to live within endocytotic vacuoles without being destroyed. Since liposomes are avidly internalized by macrophages, they clearly afford a convenient means of "targeting" drug directly to the site of parasitic infestation. Systemic fungal infections such as aspergillosis, candidiasis, etc. are common among immunosuppressed patients suffering from AIDS, tuberculosis, cancer, etc. Such infections can be severe and life threatening to them. Fungizone, a commercial preparation of amphotericin-B (Amp-B) in deoxycholate is the only accepted therapy to treat fungal infections. Amphotericin, which is an antifungal agent, produces serious side effects such as fever, anaphylaxis, nephrotoxicity and abnormalities in pulmonary functions, thus restricting the use of high dosage necessary for the curative effect. The drug being a polyene antibiotic interacts with ergosterol of fungal cell membrane and forms a transmembrane channel leading to the release of vital metabolites, thus causing fungal death and similarly lysis of RBCs simultaneously. Amphotericin is also effective for the treatment of kala-azar. The other important application of the liposomal delivery approach in infectious diseases involves the therapy of systemic fungal infections with polyene antibiotics incorporated into the vesicles. Another very promising example of therapy of an intracellular parasite with liposomal drugs involves the use of liposomal aminoglycosides to treat brucellosis.

Table 28.2 Liposomes as carrier for drugs.

Carrier	*Drug*	*Comments*
Liposomes	Anticancer	Poor tumor accessibility without targeting
Liposomes	Anti-infectious	Excellent penetration to parasites residing in reticuloen dothelial system
Liposomes	Immunomodulators	Exciting possibility of enhancing immune response by encapsulating macrophages activating factor (MAF). Targetting using antibodies and other ligands to specific cell surface receptors.
Liposomes	Chelating agents	Limited accessibility of parenchymal tissue, site of iron storage.

Contd.

Liposomes	Gold products	Potential treatment of rheumatoid arthritis
Liposomes	Amphotericin B	Liposomes generally diminish the generalized cytotoxicity of the antifungal agent
Liposomes	Enzymes	Immunoglobulin-mediated targeting
Liposomes	Interferon	Altered pharmacological properties
Liposomes	Genetic material	Useful for the development of gene delivery both *in vivo* and *in vitro*
Liposomes	Radionucleotide	Diagnostic imaging
Liposomes	Polymerized vesicles	Stabilized time-released carriers

Cancer chemotherapy

Many drugs used in cancer chemotherapy are toxic to normal tissues, particularly bone marrow, kidney, heart and the rapidly dividing cells of the gut lining. Liposomes have their natural ability to target cancer cells. Hence, liposomally carried anti-cancer drugs were hailed as a major new approach to the chemotherapy of cancer. The idea underlying this enthusiasm was that one might be able to "target" the liposomes and their payloads of cytotoxic drugs to tumor cells by manipulating the physical or immunological characteristics of the liposomes injected onto the circulation which must cross the endothelial barrier, and the basement membrane barrier and be effectively taken up by neoplastic cells within the tumour. The endothelial walls of all healthy human blood vessels are encapsulated by endothelial cells that are bound together by tight junctions. These tight junctions stop any large particle in the blood from leaking out of the vessel. Tumour vessels do not contain the same level of seal between cells and are diagnostically leaky. This ability is known as the Enhanced Permeability and Retention (EPR) effect. Liposomes of certain sizes, typically less than 400 nm, can rapidly enter tumour sites from the blood, but are kept in the bloodstream by the endothelial wall in healthy tissue vasculature. Anti-cancer drugs such as Doxorubicin (Doxil) and Daunorubicin (Daunoxome) are currently being marketed in liposome delivery systems. The first objective of Inex's research program is to use a lipid-based drug delivery system, called the Transmembrane Carrier System (TCS) to deliver anticancer drugs more effectively to tumours. Inex is using the anti-cancer drug, vincristine, in liposomes to treat non-Hodgkin's lymphoma and other cancers (Figure 28.7). They are also investigating other key anticancer drugs to see if their

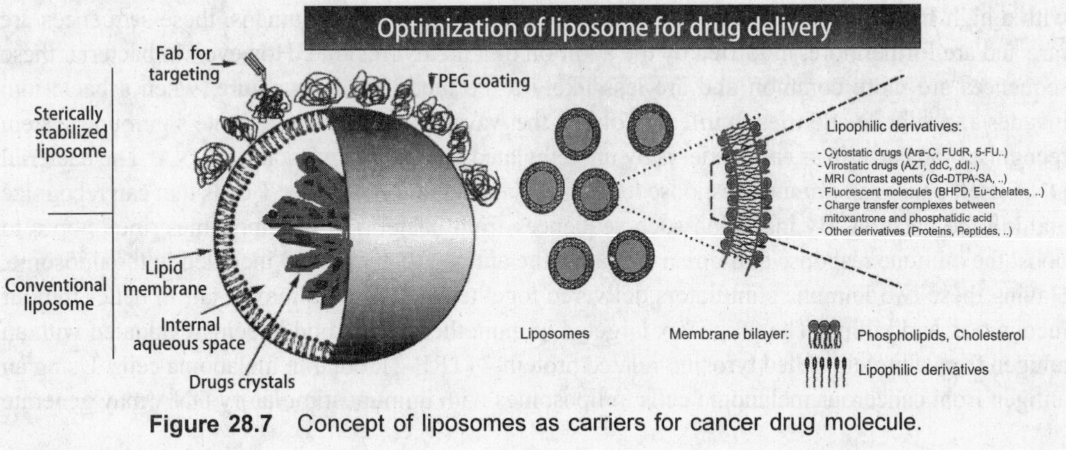

Figure 28.7 Concept of liposomes as carriers for cancer drug molecule.

effectiveness could be improved by encapsulating them in liposomes for more efficient targeting and delivery.

Gene therapy

Gene therapy holds potential for improving the lives of people with genetic diseases by either correcting the defect or using genes to alleviate the symptoms of disease. However, a major obstacle has been targeting the cells that have the defect, while leaving the remainder cells unaltered. Liposomes are one of the method being investigated for use in gene therapy. Liposomes can be induced to fuse with protoplasts using devices like PEG, and therefore have been used for gene transfer. The technique offers several advantages such as protection of DNA/RNA from nuclease digestion; low cell toxicity; stability and storage of nucleic acids due to encapsulation in liposomes; high degree of reproducibility and applicability to a wide range of cell types. The use of liposomes for delivery of gene into cells *in vitro* and *in vivo* and their subsequent expression will help to understand the specific function of a particular gene.

Inex's OligoVax system for targeted immunotherapy uses liposomes containing specific disease markers called antigens, along with an immunostimulatory DNA molecule (Figure 28.8). An antigen is typically a small protein fragment derived from a specific virus, tumour or bacteria. It stimulates the production of immune cells that can specifically attack, kill or neutralize anything they encounter that displays the same antigen. For example, incorporating an antigen from a cancer cell will result in the production of T cells that can kill any diseased cell displaying the same marker on the surface, including those in a primary tumour or metastasis. Similarly, encapsulating a virus antigen (for example, a portion of one of the proteins of the virus' outer coat) will generate immune T cells and antibodies that will recognize whole particles of virus in the body and cells infected with the virus because they will display pieces of viral antigens on their surface for T cell inspection. By incorporating an antigen into the liposome, Inex hopes to guide the immune system to specifically attack the target of interest.

The short piece of DNA also included in the liposome is called an oligonucleotide or "oligo". The oligo can cause immune stimulation in a variety of ways. One method commonly used is to include the so-called Immune Stimulatory Sequences (ISS) or CpG sequences. These are DNA sequences with a high frequency of repeated CG bases. In vertebrates such as humans, these sequences are rare and are furthermore, modified by the addition of a methyl residue. However, in bacteria, these sequences are more common and are less likely to be methylated. In nature, when a bacterium invades a vertebrate and tries to infect it, one of the ways in which the vertebrate's immune system recognises the bacteria as an invader is by unmethylated GG motifs in Bacterial DNA. The bacterial DNA itself causes an immune response leading to the generation of killer T cells that can recognize and kill the bacteria. By including such sequences from bacteria in the liposomes, Inex hopes to boost the immune response and direct it against the antigen that was also included in the liposome. Having these two immune stimulators delivered together by liposome may result in better tumour recognition and killing. The OligoVax targeted immunotherapy method is being evaluated with an antigen from a protein called tyrosine-related protein-2 (TRP-2) found in melanoma cells. Using an antigen from cancerous melanoma cells in liposomes with immunostimulatory DNA may generate enough killer T cells to eliminate the melanoma from the body. The company also plans to develop the immunotherapy program for the treatment of other cancers and infectious diseases.

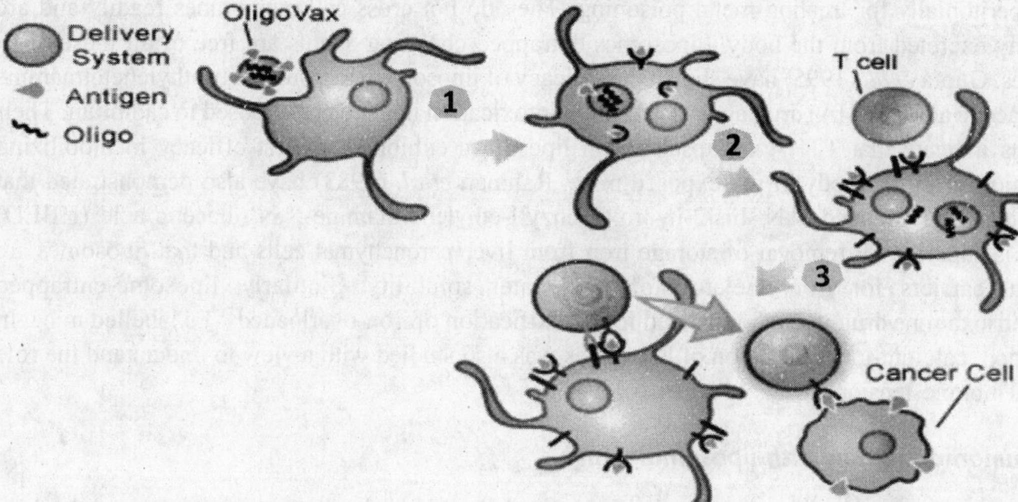

Figure 28.8 An overview of Oligovax. (Image Source: Reproduced from the Inex website). 1. Oligo Vax targets Antigen Presenting Immune cell (APC). 2. Oligo Vax is internalized by the immune cell and the cancer antigen is processed and presented on its surface for recognition by another immune cell called a T cell. The oligo enhance the immune response. 3. T cell binds to antigen complex on the surface of the immune cell and becomes activated. T cell is activated to both kill the cancer cell with the specific antigen and recruit and activate other immune cells to find and kill the cancer kills.

Enzyme replacement theory

Several enzymes can be delivered by liposome for the treatment of genetically inherited storage diseases where the delivery of the missing enzyme to the defective tissue would be of great therapeutic advantage. Cystinosis is an example of a lysosomal storage disease. Cysteamine containing liposomes are effective in mobilizing stored cystine in fibroblast. The feasibility of non-viral gene transfer using liposomes is described for human fetal nigral tissue. This finding might have implications for gene delivery and cell replacement strategies in Parkinson's disease. Lew *et al.* (2002) have performed studies to determine the effects of liposome-mediated adenomatous polyposis coli (APC) gene therapy on intestinal neoplasia *in vivo*. The reduction of intestinal neoplasia by APC gene replacement suggests their role in intestinal tumorigenesis. Luton *et al.* (2004) have also shown that bis (guanidinium)-tren-cholesterol/dioleoylphosphatidylethanolamine (BGTC/DOPE) encapsulated liposomes can mediate gene transfection into the fetal sheep airway epithelium for the treatment of a variety of congenital lung diseases. Similarly, Valencia *et al.* (2006) have shown that 7-Dehydrocholesterol enhances ultraviolet A-induced oxidative stress in keratinocytes. In addition, immobilization of enzymes on liposome significantly decreased entropy and enthalpy of activation of enzyme and made it functionally and thermodynamically more stable and reusable compared to soluble one. Recently, liposome-bound cellulase has been used for the hydrolysis of insoluble cellulose.

Chelation therapy

Chelating agents such as EDTA, DTPA and esferrioxamine are used intravenously and intraperitonially for treating metal poisoning. They do not cross cell membranes readily and are rapidly excreted from the body. Liposomes entrapped chelating agents are free of all these difficulties. Gupta *et al.* (1995) have shown the efficacy of liposome encapsulated triethylenetetraamine hexaacetic acid (TTHA) drug against cadmium intoxication in mice pre-exposed to cadmium. Their results indicate that TTHA encapsulated in liposomes exhibited highest efficacy in mobilizing cadmium from the body of pre-exposed mice. Rahman *et al.* (1983) have also demonstrated that liposome encapsulated N,N'-bis[2-hydroxybenzyl]-ethylene-diamine-N,N'-diacetic acid (HBED) drug is superior for removal of storage iron from liver parenchymal cells and that liposomes are useful carriers for iron chelators of low water solubility. Similarly, liposome-entrapped desferrioxamine drug was administered for detoxification of iron-overloaded ^{59}Fe labelled mice. In addition, calcium-induced fusion of liposomes was also studied with a view to understand the role of membrane tension in this process.

Immunomodulation with liposomal drugs

Macrophages are multicompetent cells that play important roles in several aspects of the host defence system. In particular, macrophages seem to be one of the primary barriers against the growth and metastatic spread of neoplastic cells. Macrophages can be "activated" so as to become cytotoxic to tumor cells. This occurs as a result of exposure to a variety of immunomodulating substances including MAF (a T-celoderived lymphokine) lipopolysaccharide (from gram –ve bacteria) and certain synthetic compounds, muramyl dipeptide being the best known example. Thus, liposomes selectively deliver immunomodulators to macrophages for the purpose of enhancing host defenses against metastases. The other major immunological applications of liposomes are:

(i) As an immunological adjuvant.
(ii) As a carrier for haptens.
(iii) As a carrier of additional immunomodulator.
(iv) As a tool in immunodiagnostics.

The liposome immune lysis assay (LILA) appears to have a potential application in immunodiagnosis in future. This assay system has been exploited to diagnose patients with systematic Lupas Erythematosus (SLE), hemolytic anaemia, Behcet's disease and several other diseases. LILA has certain advantages over the existing assay systems like ELISA and RIA, such as, the assay system is a homogenous one, it does not require the separation of free antigen or antibody from the immune complex, it avoids the use of hazardous chemicals such as radioisotopes and the assay system is very sensitive, almost same to regular EIA or RIA and for detection of some antibodies.

Oral administration of liposome

It has been considered that oral administration of a substance is effective. Thus attempts have been made to administer liposome orally as:

1. Liposome entrapped insulin administered orally could reduce the blood sugar level in diabetic animals.
2. Oral administration in blood coagulation factor *VIII* in liposomes to a hemophillic patient led to a higher rise in blood level.
3. Oral administration of I_gG as passive vaccine.
4. Uptake of orally administered liposomes by the liver suggests an exciting possibility with respect to indigenous ayurvedic drugs.

Industrial Applications

Application of liposomes in cosmetics

The properties of liposomes can also be utilized in the delivery of ingredients in cosmetics. In addition, liposome as a carrier itself offers advantages because lipids are well hydrated and can reduce the dryness of the skin, which is a primary cause for its ageing. Also, liposomes can act as a supply, which acts to replenish lipids and, importantly, linolenic acid. In general, the rules for topical drug applications and delivery of other compounds are less stringent than the ones for prenatal administration, and several hundred cosmetic products are commercially available since Capture (C. Dior) and Niosomes (L'Or´eal) were introduced in 1987. They range from simple liposome pastes, which are used as a replacement for creams, gels, and ointments for do-it-yourself cosmetical products to formulations containing various extracts, moisturizers, antibiotics, and to complex products containing recombinant proteins for wound or sunburn healing. Most of the products are anti-aging skin creams. Unrinsable sunscreens, long lasting perfumes, hair conditioners, after-shave lotions and similar products are also gaining large fractions of the market. Liposomal skin creams already share more than 10% of the over $10 billion market. Table 28.3 shows some of these products. As in the case of topical delivery in medical applications, the workers in the field do not agree on the mechanism of action. Although some claims enhanced permeability of liposomes into the skin, but the others claim that mostly liposomes are a noninteractive, skin-nonirritating, water based matrix (without alcohols, detergents, oils and other non-natural solubilizers) for the active ingredients. In addition to the natural lipids, either phospholipids or 'skin lipids', which contain mostly sphingolipids, ceramides, oleic acid, and cholesterol sulphate, liposomes made from synthetic lipids are also being used. They include mostly liposomes made from non-ionic surfactant lipids, which can be chemically more stable. Some of these liposomes can be made very easily by mixing and homogenizing aqueous solutions with molten surfactants. These liposomes can be more stable than their natural analogues and can be produced easily in large quantities and are very inexpensive.

Table 28.3 Some liposomal cosmetic formulations currently in the market. According to the manufacturers, liposomes may deliver moisture and a novel supply of lipid molecules to skin tissue in a superior fashion to other formulations. In addition they can entrap a variety of active molecules and can therefore be utilized for skin creams, anti-aging creams, after-shave lotion, lipstic, sun screen and make-up.

Product	*Manufacturer*	*Liposomes and key ingredients*
Capture	*Cristian Dior*	*Liposomes in gel with ingredients*
Efect du Soleil	L'Or'eal	Tanning agents in liposomes
Niosomes	Lancome (L'Or'eal)	Glyceropolyether with moisturizers
Nactosomes	Lancome (L'Or'eal	Vitamins
Formule Liposome Gel	Payot (Ferdinand Muehlens)	Thymoxin, hyaluronic acid
Future Perfect Skin Gel	Estee Lauder	TMF, vitamins E, A palmitate, cerebroside, ceramide, phospholipid
Symphatic 2000	Biopharm GmbH	Thymus extract, vitamin A palmitate
Natipide II	Nattermann PL	Liposomal gel for do-it-yourself cosmetics
Flawless finish	Elizabeth Arden	Liquid make-up
Inovita	Pharm/Apotheke	Thymus extract, hyaluronic acid, vitamin E
Eye Perfector	Avon	Soothing cream to reduce eye irritation
Aquasome	LA Nikko Chemical Co.	Liposomes with humectant

Application of liposomes in agro-food industry

The ability of liposomes to solubilize compounds with demanding solubility properties, sequester compounds from potentially harmful milieu, and release incorporated molecules in a sustained and predictable fashion can also be used in the food processing industry. Lipid molecules from fats to polar lipids, are one of the fundamental ingredients in almost any food. For instance, lecithin and some other polar lipids are routinely extracted from nutrients, such as egg yolks or soybeans. Traditionally, polar lipids were used to stabilize water-in-oil and oil-in-water emulsions and creams, or to improve dispersal of various instant powders in water. With the advent of microencapsulation technology, however, liposomes have become an attractive system because they are composed entirely from food acceptable compounds. The sustained release system concept can be used in various fermentation processes in which the encapsulated enzymes can greatly shorten fermentation times and improve the quality of the product. This is due to improved spatial and temporal release of the ingredient(s) as well as their protection in particular phases of the process against chemical degradation. A classical example is cheese-making. The first serious attempts to decrease the fermentation time using cell wall free bacterial extracts were encouraging enough to stimulate efforts to improve enzyme presentation. After preliminary studies in which liposome systems were optimized, the cheese ripening times can be shortened by 30-50%. This means a substantial economic profit knowing that ripening times of some cheeses, such as Cheddar, say, are about one year during which they require well controlled conditions. In addition, due to the better dispersal of the enzymes, the texture of cheeses was even, and bitterness and inconsistent flavour due to the proteolysis of enzymes in the early phase of fermentation was much improved. In addition to improved fermentation, liposomes are being tried in the preservation of cheeses. Addition of nitrates to cheese milk to suppress the growth of spore-forming bacteria is now being questioned due to health concerns and natural alternatives are under study. Lysozyme is effective but quickly gets inactivated due to binding with casein. Liposome encapsulation can both preserve potency and increase effectiveness because liposomes become localized in the water spaces between the casein matrix and fat globules of curd and cheese. This also happens where most of the spoilage organisms are located. These applications of enhancing natural preservatives, including antioxidants such as vitamins E and C, will undoubtedly become very important due to recent dietary trends, which tend to reduce the addition of artificial preservatives and ever larger portion of unsaturated fats in the diet. In other areas of the agro-food industry, liposomes encapsulated biocides have shown superior action due to prolonged presence of the fungicides, herbicides or pesticides at reduced damage to other life forms. Liposome surface can be made sticky so that they remain on the leafs for longer times and do not wash into the ground. In these applications, inexpensive liposomes produced from synthetic lipids are used. The same liposomes are being tried in shellfish farms. These animals are susceptible to many parasitic infections. They are filter feeders and they pump large amounts of water through their body. This seems to offset large dilutions of liposomes in the pool, and the drug molecules as well as some essential nutrients needed in ppm to ppb quantities can be delivered.

Other Biotechnological Applications

Applications of liposomes in bioengineering

Modern genetic engineering and gene recombinant technology is based on the delivery of genetic material, i.e., fragments of DNA, into various cells and microorganisms in order to alter their genetic code and force them to produce particular proteins or polypeptides. Nucleic acids used in gene transfer are large, with molecular weights up to several million Daltons, highly charged and hydrophilic and therefore not easy to transfer across cell membranes. In addition to classical methods, such as direct injection, phosphate precipitation and others, liposomes were tried as transfection vectors. They can deliver the encapsulated or bound nucleic acid into cells predominantly in two ways: the classical approach is to encapsulate the genetic material into liposomes and liposomes act as an endocytosis enhancer, while recently the phosphate or DEAE precipitation was simulated by liposomes. In these cases, the nucleic acid forms a complex with several cationic liposomes and the size of the complex and its adsorption on the cell surface catalyses endocytosis or, possibly, fusion. The third, still unexplored way, would be to use fusogenic liposomes or cause fusion upon adsorption of the liposome on the cell surface. The classical approach used predominantly large unilamellar vesicles made from negatively charged phosphatidylserine in order to prevent interaction with DNA molecules, which may contain up to several thousand negative charges. In some cases, transfection efficiencies were improved several hundred times, and plant protoplast that are very difficult to transfect were successfully altered genetically. In the mid-80s, however, electroporation showed better results and the interest for liposomes markedly diminished. Recently, however, transfection was successfully performed using small unilamellar vesicles made from positively charged lipids. First studies used cationic lipid dioleoyl-propyl-trimethylammonium (DOTMA). Later studies showed better transfection efficiencies by using some of the commercially available cationic lipids. Better transfection efficiencies at reduced toxicity were found by using liposomes containing positively charged cholesterol. Many novel cationic lipids are being synthetised in order to improve transfection, especially *in vivo*. These methods can also be used in gene therapy. The idea is to deliver the nondefective gene into the appropriate cells and hope that they will respond. For instance, patients with cystic fibrosis have a defective gene that encodes the code for a protein critical to the transfer of salts through the cell membrane in the lungs. In recent experiments, upon inhalation of the copies of human gene mixed with liposomes, 70% of the cells lining the lungs of mice incorporated the gene and began using it to make proteins in large amounts. This promises elimination or drastic reduction of the symptoms of the disease if it can be repeated in humans.

Environmental applications

In ecology, liposomes offer improvements in bioreclamation and various monitoring and analytical-diagnostic applications. For instance, it was shown that in an oil spill, the addition of various bacteria with possible nutrients encapsulated in liposomes improves the degradation rates of carbohydrates, which are otherwise very slow. Due to the surfactant action, liposomes also improve the coagulation and sinking of oil spread on the water surface or its cleaning up with floating booms. The Environmental Protection Agency is testing liposomes' ability to deliver nutrients to oil spills to speed up the degradation. Liposomes containing membrane anchored chelators can be used to clean toxic or radioactive metals from solutions. For instance, water contaminated in a nuclear reactor can be purified by the addition of such liposomes, which could be easily precipitated after binding of the toxic ions.

Future Prospects of Liposome Technology

There are only a few of the applications for which liposomes have been used. Reports of new types of liposomes, as well as new uses for liposomes seem to appear almost daily. Further advances in liposome research have been able to allow liposomes to avoid detection by the body's immune system, specifically, the cells of reticuloendothelial system (RES). These liposomes are known as "stealth liposomes", and are constructed with PEG (Polyethylene Glycol) studding the outside of the membrane. The PEG coating, which is inert in the body, allows for longer circulatory life for the drug delivery mechanism. However, research currently seeks to investigate at what amount of PEG coating actually hinders binding of the liposome to the delivery site. In addition to a PEG coating, most stealth liposomes also have some sort of biological species attached as a ligand to the liposome in order to enable binding via a specific expression on the targeted drug delivery site. These targeting ligands could be monoclonal antibodies (making an immunoliposome), vitamins, or specific antigens. Targeted liposomes can target nearly any cell type in the body and deliver drugs that would naturally be systemically delivered. Polymersomes can also be used this way naturally toxic drugs can be much less toxic if delivered only to diseased tissues.

CONCLUSION

Clearly liposome technology is not a panacea for all problems in controlled drug delivery. However, a judicious matching of the characteristic of the liposome technology with particular drugs and particular therapeutic problems can lead to interesting and useful results. This is exemplified by the use of liposomal drugs for treatment of certain infectious diseases and the potential use of liposome-entrapped immunomodulators. Questions remain about the ability to formulate stable, reproducible preparation of liposomal drugs on a pharmaceutical scale. Extremes of aqueous solubility, oil/water partition coefficients, binding, extensive metabolism/degradation of the drug during transit from the point of drug delivery to the target area and narrow therapeutic index are some of the limiting factors of liposome technology. A liposome once designed pays more in terms of its efficacy and safety.

FURTHER READINGS

1. Aichele P., Zinke J., Grode L., Schwendener R.A., Kaufmann S.H.E., and Seiler P., (2003) Macrophages of the splenic marginal zone are essential for trapping of blood-borne particulate antigen but dispensable for induction of specific T cell responses. *J. Immunol.* 171 **(3):** 1148-1155.
2. Alec D. Bangham (1995) Features surrogate cells or trojan horses: The discovery of liposomes. *BioEssays.* 17 **(12):** 1081-1088.
3. Alkhalaf W. Piard J.C., Soda M., Gripon J.C., Desmezeaud M. and Vassal L. (1988) Liposomes as proteinases carriers for the accelerated ripening of St. Paulin type cheese, *J. Food Sci.* **(53):** 1674-1679.
4. Alsarra I.A., Hamed A.Y. and Alanazi F.K. (2008) Acyclovir liposomes for intranasal systemic delivery: development and pharmacokinetics evaluation. *Drug Deliv.* 15 **(5):** 313-321.
5. Alving B.M., Banerji B., Fogler W.E. and Alving C.R. (1987) Lupus anticoagulant activities of murine monoclonal antibodies to liposomal phosphatidylinositol phosphate. *Clin. Exp. Immunol.* **(69):** 403-408.
6. Anne S.U. (2002) Biophysical aspects of using liposomes as delivery vehicles. *Journal of Bioscience* Reports Apr. **(22):** 129-149.
7. Bangham A.D. (2005) Liposomes and the physico-chemical basis of unconsciousness. *FASEB J.* 19 **(13):** 1766-1768.
8. Bauer M., Meyer M., Sautter J., Gasser T., Ueffing M., and Widmer H.R. (2001) Liposome-mediated gene transfer to fetal human ventral mesencephalic explant cultures. *Neurosci Lett.* 308 **(3):** 169-172.
9. Beck-Schimmer B., Rosenberger D.S., Neff S.B., Jamnicki M., Suter D., Fuhrer T., Schwendener R., Booy C., Reyes L., Pasch T., and Schimmer R.C. (2005) Pulmonary aspiration: New therapeutic approaches in the experimental model. *Anesthesiology.* 103 **(3):** 556-566.
10. Bordron A., Dueymes M., Levy Y., Jamin C., Ziporen L., Piette J.C., Shoenfeld Y. and Youinou P. (1998) Anti-endothelial cell antibody binding makes negatively charged phospholipids accessible to antiphospholipid antibodies. *Arthritis Rheum.* **(41):** 1738-1747.
11. Carson D.A., and Raz E. (1997) Oligonucleotide Adjuvants for T Helper 1 (Th1)-specific vaccination. *J Exp. Med.* 186 **(10):** 1621-1622.
12. Carvalheiro M., Jorge J., Eleutério C., Pinhal A.F., Sousa A.C., Morais J.G., and Cruz M.E. (2008) Trifluralin liposomal formulations active against Leishmaniadonovani infections. *Eur. J. Pharm. Biopharm.*. Aug 12 [Epub ahead of print].
13. Chang C.C., Liu D.Z., Lin S.Y., Liang H.J., Hou W.C., Huang W.J., Chang C.H., Ho F.M. and Liang Y.C. (2008) Liposome encapsulation reduces cantharidin toxicity. *Food Chem Toxicol.* Jul 4. [Epub ahead of print].
14. Chanturiya A., Scaria P. and Woodle M.C. (2000) The role of membrane lateral tension in calcium-induced membrane fusion.. *J. Membr. Biol.* 176 **(1):** 67-75.
15. Christopher Kirby and Gregory Gregoriadis (1984) Dehydration-rehydration vesicles: A simple method for high yield drug entrapment in liposomes. *Bio/Technology.* **(2):** 979-984.
16. De Jong W.H. and Borm P.J. (2008) Drug delivery and nanoparticles: applications and hazards. *Int. J. Nanomedicine.* 3 **(2):** 133-149.

17. Di Marzio L., Marianecci C., Cinque B., Nazzarri M., Cimini A.M., Cristiano L., Cifone M.G, Alhaique F. and Carafa M. (2008) pH-sensitive non-phospholipid vesicle and macrophage-like cells: Binding, uptake and endocytotic pathway. *Biochim Biophys Acta*. Aug 12 [Epub ahead of print].
18. Dueymes M., Levy Y., Ziporen L., Jamin C., Piette J.C., Shoenfeld Y., and Youinou P. (1996) Do some antiphospholipid antibodies target endothelial cells? *Ann. Med. Interne* (Paris) 147 Suppl. (1) 22–23.
19. Dutton G. (1993) The promise of liposomes. *Gen. Engin. News*. **(13)**: 6-9.
20. El-Kateb N., Cynober L., Chaumeil J.C., and Dumortier G. (2008) L-cysteine encapsulation in liposomes: Effect of phospholipids nature on entrapment efficiency and stability. *J. Microencapsul.* 25 **(6)**: 399-413.
21. Estruch E.J., Hart S.L., Kinnon C., and Winchester B.G. (2001) Non-viral, integrin-mediated gene transfer into fibroblasts from patients with lysosomal storage diseases. *J. Gene. Med.* **(5)**: 488-97.
22. Ewert K.K., Ahmad A., Bouxsein N.F., Evans H.M., and Safinya C.R. (2008) Non-viral gene delivery with cationic liposome-DNA complexes. *Methods Mol Biol.* **(433)**: 159-175.
23. Felgner P., Gadek T.R., Holm M., Roman R., Wenz M., Northrop J.P., Ringold G., and Danielsen M. (1987) Lipofectin: A highly efficient, lipid mediated DNA transfection procedure. *Proc. Nat. Acad. Sci. USA*. **(84)**: 7413-7417.
24. Finkelstein M.C. and Weissmann G. (1979) Enzyme replacement via liposomes. Variations in lipid compositions determine liposomal integrity in biological fluids. *Biochim. Biophys. Acta*. 587 **(2)**: 202-216.
25. Fraley R.T., Subramani S., Berg P. and Papahadjopoulos D. (1980) Introduction of liposome encapsulated SV40DNA into cells. *J. Biol. Chem.* **(255)**: 10431-10435.
26. Frankenberger, M., Hofmann, B., Emmerich, B., Nerl, C., Schwendener, R.A. and Ziegler-Heitbrock, H.W.L. (1997) Liposomal 1,25 (OH)2 vitamin D3 compounds block proliferation and induce differentiation in myelomonocytic leukemia cells. Br. *J. Haematol.* **(98)**: 186-194..
27. Gao X. and Huang L. (1991) A novel cationic liposome reagent for efficient transfection of mammalian cells. *Biophys. Biochem. Res. Commun.* **(179)**: 280-285.
28. Gatt S., Bercovier J.H. and Barenholz Y. (1991) Use of liposomes to combat oil spills and their potential application to bioreclamation, in: *On Site Bioreclamation*, eds R.E. Hinchee and R.F. Olfenbuttel (Butterworth, Stoneham) pp. 293-312.
29. Gupta S., Behari J.R., Srivastava S., Misra M. and Srivastava R.C. (1995) Efficacy of liposome encapsulated triethylenetetraamine hexaacetic acid (TTHA) against cadmium intoxication: role of lipid composition. *Ind Health*. 33 **(2)**: 83-88.
30. Hippert C., Dubois G, Morin C., Disson O., Ibanes S., Jacquet C., Schwendener R., Antignac C., Kremer E.J. and Kalatzis V. (2008) Gene transfer may be preventive but not curative for a lysosomal transport disorder. *Mol. Ther.* Jun 24. [Epub ahead of print].
31. http://www.inexpharm.com/: Website of Inex Pharmaceuticals Corp.
32. Jean M.M., Gary R.M., Lynn E.S. and Carl R.A. (1999) Oil in water liposomal emulsions: Characterization and potential use in vaccine delivery. *Journal of Pharmaceutical Sciences*. 88 **(2)**: 1332-1339.
33. Jeon B.H., Jang C., Han J., Kataru R.P., Piao L., Jung K., Cha H.J., Schwendener R.A., Jang K.Y., Kim K.S., Alitalo K. and Koh G.Y. (2008) Profound but dysfunctional lymphangiogenesis via vascular endothelial growth factor ligands from CD11b+ macrophages in advanced ovarian cancer. *Cancer Res*. 68 **(4)**: 1100-1109.
34. Kim D.D., Miwa T., Kimura Y., Schwendener R.A., van Lookeren Campagne M. and Song W.C. (2008) Blood Deficiency of DAF and Crry on murine platelets leads to complement-dependent clearance via the macrophage phagocytic receptor CRIg. *Blood*. **(112)**: 1109-1119.
35. Kirby C. (1990) Delivery systems for enzymes. *Chem.* Br. 26 **(9)**: 847-850.
36. Kojima C., Hirano Y., Yuba E., Harada A. and Kono K. (2008) Preparation and characterization of complexes of liposomes with gold nanoparticles. *Colloids Surf. B. Biointerfaces*. Jul 9 [Epub ahead of print].
37. Lasic D.D. (1997) *Liposomes in Gene Delivery*. CRC Press LLC. Boca Raton. FL.

38. Law B.A. and King J.S. (1991) Use of liposomes for proteinase addition to cheddar cheese, *J. Diary Res.* **(52):** 183-188.
39. Lew J.I., Guo Y., Kim R.K., Vargish L., Michelassi F. and Arenas R.B. (2002) Reduction of intestinal neoplasia with adenomatous polyposis coli gene replacement and COX-2 inhibition is additive. *J. Gastrointest. Surg.* **(4):** 563-568.
40. Li C., Yoshimoto M., Fukunaga K. and Nakao K. (2007) Characterization and immobilization of liposome-bound cellulase for hydrolysis of insoluble cellulose. *Bioresour Technol.* 98 **(7):** 1366-1372.
41. Li L., Nie Y., Zhu R., Shi S., Luo K., He B., Yang Y., Yang J. and Gu Z. (2008) Preparation and gene delivery of alkaline amino acids-based cationic liposomes. *Arch Pharm. Res.* 31 **(7):** 924-931.
42. Ludewig, B., Barchiesi, F., Pericin, M., Zinkernagel, R.M., Hengartner, H. and Schwendener, R.A. (2000) In vivo antigen loading and activation of dendritic cells via a liposomal peptide vaccine mediated protective antiviral and antitumor immunity. *Vaccine.* **(19):** 23-32.
43. Lurquin P. (1979) Entrapment of plasmid DNA by liposomes and their interaction with plant protoplasts. *Nucl. Acids Res.* **(6):** 3773-3777.
44. Luton D. Oudrhiri N., de Lagausie P., Aissaoui A., Hauchecorne M., Julia S., Oury J.F., Aigrain Y., Peuchmaur M., Vigneron J.P., Lehn J.M. and Lehn P. (2004) Gene transfection into fetal sheep airways in utero using guanidinium-cholesterol cationic lipids. *J. Gene Med.* **(3):** 328-336.
45. Marty, C., Ballmer-Hofer, K., Neri, D., Klemenz, R., Schott, H. and Schwendener, R.A. (2002) Cytotoxic targeting of F9 teratocarcinoma tumours with anti-ED-B fibronectin scFv antibody modified liposomes. *Br. J. Cancer.* **(87):** 106-112.
46. Meure L.A., Foster N.R. and Dehghani F. (2008) Conventional and dense gas techniques for the production of liposomes: A review. *AAPS Pharm. Sci. Tech.* Jul 3 [Epub ahead of print].
47. Mueller C. and Flotte T.R. (2008) Gene therapy for cystic fibrosis. *Clin. Rev. Allergy. Immunol.* Jul 4. [Epub ahead of print].
48. Nelson D.L. and Cox M.M. (2000) *Lehninger Principles of Biochemistry*, 3rd ed. Worth Publishers: New York.
49. Nicolau C. and Cudd A. (1989) Liposomes as carriers of DNA. *Crit. Rev. Therap. Drug Carr. Systems.* **(6):** 239-271.
50. Pautot S., Barbara J.F. and Weitz D.Z. (2003) Production of unilamellar vesicles using an inverted emulsion. *Journal of Langmuir.* **(19):** 2870-2879.
51. Perrie Y. Gregory (2008) Gregoriadis: Introducing liposomes to drug delivery. *J. Drug. Target.* 16 **(7):** 518-519.
52. Pollock S., Dwek R.A., Burton D.R. and Zitzmann N. (2008) N-Butyldeoxynojirimycin is a broadly effective anti-HIV therapy significantly enhanced by targeted liposome delivery. *AIDS.* Aug 20 [Epub ahead of print].
53. Polo D., Haro I., Alsina M.A. and Reig F. (1997) Physicochemical characterization of Poly (ethylene glycol) coated liposomes loaded with Doxorubicin. *Journal of Langmuir.* **(13):** 3953-3958.
54. Rahman Y.E., Cerny E.A., Lau E.H. and Carnes B.A. (1983) Enhanced iron removal from liver parenchymal cells in experimental iron overload: liposome encapsulation of HBED and phenobarbital administration. *Blood.* 62 **(1):** 209-213.
55. Rahman Y.E. (1979) Potential of the liposomal approach to metal chelation therapy. *Front Biol.* **(48):** 625-652.
56. Rose J.K., Buoncore L. and Whitt M.A. (1991) A new cationic liposome reagent mediating nearly quantitative transfection of animal cells. *Biotechniques.* **(10):** 520-525.
57. Schott, H., Ludwig, P.S., Gansauge, F., Gansauge, S. and Schwendener, R.A. (1997). Synthesis and *in vitro* antitumor activity of 2'-deoxy-5-fluorouridylyl-(3'-5')-2'-deoxy-5-fluoro-N4-octadecylcytidine: A new amphiphilic dinucleoside phosphate. *Liebigs Annalen der Chemie.* 413-417.

58. Schwendener, R.A., Friedl, K., Depenbrock, H., Schott, H. and Hanauske, A.R. (2001) *In vitro* activity of liposomal N4-octadecyl-1-b-D-arabinofuranosyl-cytosine (NOAC), a new lipophilic derivative of 1-b-D-arabinofuranocylcytosine on biopsized clonogenic human tumour cells and haematopoietic precursor cells. *Invest. New Drugs.* **(19):** 203-210.
59. Serikawa T., Kikuchi H., and Oite T. (2008) Enhancement of gene expression efficiency using cationic liposomes on ovarian cancer cells. *Drug Deliv*. Aug 19 [Epub ahead of print].
60. Stribling R., Brunette E., Liggett D., Gaenslar K. and Debs R. (1992) Aerosol gene delivery *in vivo. Proc. Nat. Acad. Sci. USA.* **(89):** 11277-11281.
61. Tahibi A., Sakurai J.D., Mathur R. and Wallach D.F.H. (1991) Novasome vesicles in extended pesticide formulation. *Proc. Symp. Contr. Rel. Bioact. Mat.* **(18):** 231-232.
62. Tiwari S., Goyal A.K., Khatri K., Mishra N. and Vyas S.P. (2008) Gel core liposomes: An advanced carrier for improved vaccine delivery. *J Microencapsul*. **(25):** 1-8.
63. Torchilin V.P. (2006) Multifunctional nanocarriers. *Adv. Drug. Deliv. Rev.* 58 **(14):** 1532-1555.
64. Torchilin V.P. (2008) Antibody-modified liposomes for cancer chemotherapy. *Expert Opin Drug Deliv*. 5 **(9):** 1003-1025.
65. Trabulo S., Mano M., Faneca H., Cardoso A.L., Duarte S., Henriques A., Paiva A., Gomes P., Simões S. and de Lima MC. (2008) S4 (13)-PV cell penetrating peptide and cationic liposomes act synergistically to mediate intracellular delivery of plasmid DNA. *J. Gene Med.* Aug. 27 [Epub ahead of print].
66. Valencia A., Rajadurai A., Carle A.B. and Kochevar I.E. (2006) 7-Dehydrocholesterol enhances ultraviolet A-induced oxidative stress in keratinocytes: roles of NADPH oxidase, mitochondria, and lipid rafts. *Free Radic. Biol. Med.* 41 **(11):** 1704-1718.
67. Van Rooijen N. (2008) Liposomes for targeting of antigens and drugs: immunoadjuvant activity and liposome-mediated depletion of macrophages. *J. Drug. Target.* 16 **(7):** 529-534..
68. Wagner E.J., Krugner-Higby L. and Heath T.D. (2008) Liposome dependent delivery of S-adenosyl Methionine to cells by liposomes: A potential treatment for liver disease. *J. Pharm. Sci*. Jul 18 [Epub ahead of print].
69. Wassef N.M., Roerdink F., Swartz Jr, G.M., Lyon J.A., Berson B..J. and Alving C.R. (1984). Phosphate-binding specificities of monoclonal antibodies against phosphoinositides in liposomes. *Mol. Immunol.* **(21):** 863-868.
70. Young S.P., Baker E. and Huehns E.R. (1979) Liposome entrapped desferrioxamine and iron transporting ionophores: a new approach to iron chelation therapy. *Br. J. Haematol.* 41 **(3):** 357-363.
71. Zeisberger S.M., Odermatt B., Marty C., Zehnder-Fjallman AH, Ballmer-Hofer K. and Schwendener R.A. (2006) Clodronate-liposome-mediated depletion of tumour-associated macrophages: a new and highly effective antiangiogenic therapy approach. *Br. J. Cancer.* 95 **(3):** 272-281.

CHAPTER

29

Vaccine Technology

Prevention of diseases is the most desirable, most convenient and highly effective approach to health; this is achieved by vaccination or immunization using biological preparations called vaccines. A vaccine is a preparation containing a pathogen (disease-producing organism) either in attenuated or inactivated state. This preparation is introduced into an individual to induce adequate antibody production against the pathogen, in particular, so that the individual becomes protected against infection, at a later date, by that pathogen. The introduction of a vaccine in an individual is called vaccination/immunization as it leads to the development of immunity in the vaccinated individuals to the concerned pathogen.

Keywords: Vaccine, vaccination, immunization, vaccinology, variolation.

INTRODUCTION

The publication by Edward Jenner "An Inquiry into the Cause and Effects of Variolae Vaccinae" in 1798 is the first documented evidence for the use of vaccination. In the fifteenth century, Chinese and Turks were using the material from lesions of smallpox infected individuals to infect susceptible persons so that they would develop a mild form of the disease and become resistant. The dried crusts derived from smallpox pustules were either inhaled into the nostrils or inserted into small cuts in the skin (a technique called *variolation*). This was dangerous but much safer than natural exposure to smallpox virus. In 1718, Lady Mary Wortley Montagu, the wife of British ambassador to Constantinpole, observed the positive effects on the native population and had the technique performed on her own children. The method was significantly improved by the English physician Edward Jenner in 1798. He observed that variolation did not "take" in persons who had been previously infected with the pox from the teat of cows. In 1796, Jenner inoculated an eight-year-old boy (James Phipp) with pustular fluid from a milk maid's pox lesion. Within a few days an erythematosus lesion appeared at the inoculation site and then regressed. Six weeks later he challenged the boy with smallpox pustular fluid. A lesion developed but no disease followed. In 1881, Louis Pasteur proposed the term '*vaccination*', honouring Jenner's discovery; the term originating from the Latin word '*vacca*' meaning cow. Pasteur's successful bacterial vaccine for fowl cholera, and the first vaccine ever used, consisted of avirulent cultures of the *Pasteurella multocida* attenuated by prolonged growth on artificial medium. Pasteur also successfully vaccinated against anthrax in 1881. Pasteur's classical vaccine against rabies, developed from infected spinal cord tissue dried at room temperature for 3-14 days, was given in a series of 21-28 inoculations beginning with material dried the longest and progressing through material dried for only 3 days. Even though the last inoculum was virulent enough to cause disease, the earlier inoculations conferred sufficient immunity to protect the recipients. Jenner and Louis Pasteur, through their early vaccination trials, laid the foundation stone of the discipline of *vaccinology*.

The development of vaccines against the various dreaded diseases is one of the most successful achievements. Vaccination is the most economic and efficient way of controlling diseases, and it has become an accepted practice of the preventive medicine. At present vaccination saves countless number of human and animal lives each year throughout the world. Successful vaccination program has led to the regional elimination of diseases like yellow fever, poliomyelitis, and rinderpest. The incidence of diseases such as diphtheria, measles, poliomyelitis and tetanus has declined dramatically. Smallpox, one of the mankind's long lasting and most terrible scourges was eradicated globally in October 1977, nearly two centuries after the discovery of smallpox vaccine by Jenner. A worldwide vaccination program achieved the goal of eradication of this dreaded disease. The Global Rinderpest Eradication Programme was launched in 1994 with a time-bound target to achieve global eradication by the year 2010. The great efforts put into this project have ensured that the whole of the Asian continent is now free of rinderpest. Even then, many diseases pose a serious threat to humans and animals. A crying need remains for vaccines against dreaded diseases like malaria, tuberculosis, AIDS, influenza, etc.

CONCEPTS

A *vaccine* can be defined as the collection of immunological determinants, which when presented to the immune system either as killed or live antigens, provoke protective immune responses.

Immunity to infectious microorganisms can be achieved by active or passive immunization. *Active* immunization can be achieved by natural infection with a microorganism or it can be acquired artificially by administration of a vaccine. Similarly, *passive* immunization can be natural from mother to fetus or artificially acquired by the use of preformed antibodies. Unlike active immunization, passive immunization does not activate the immune system, it generates no memory response and protection provided is transient. Active immunization leads to activation of immune system by proliferation of antigen-reactive T and B cells and formation of memory cells. With a successful vaccination, a subsequent exposure to the pathogenic agent elicits a heightened immune response that successfully eliminates the pathogen or prevents the disease mediated by its product.

Generations of Vaccines

First generation vaccines: Whole microorganism, viral and bacterial vaccines are commonly called first generation vaccines. Viral vaccines consist either of inactivated or killed viruses (i.e., the viruses incapable of multiplying in the body) or attenuated viruses (i.e., live but multiplying at low rates in the body without causing disease symptoms or causing reduced amount of disease). The Salk polio vaccine is an example of the former, while the Sabin oral polio vaccine that of the latter type. Bacterial vaccines are also of similar categories: the whooping cough vaccine has dead cells whereas the tuberculosis vaccine has live, attenuated bacteria. Attenuated organisms provide a higher level of immune response than that obtained by single dose of inactivated organisms. This is due to the reason that attenuated organisms multiply in the body for some time, thus increasing the dose of antigen. This is an advantage of vaccines made with attenuated organisms. But, attenuated organisms may cause health hazards due to this ability of multiplication.

Second-generation vaccine (Cell culture vaccines): The inactivated cell culture vaccines provide better and long lasting immunity compared to conventional nervous tissue vaccines. Although these vaccines are inactivated, they carry unwanted cellular materials and may cause some allergic reactions in vaccinated individuals.

Third generation vaccine (Recombinant and subunit vaccines and synthetic vaccine): Another form of vaccines is the synthetic vaccines, or third generation vaccines. Their preparation is based on the application of recombinant DNA technology. Briefly the whole procedure involves the following:

(i) The immune stimulating antigen must be identified.
(ii) Live cells must be reengineered to produce the antigens.
(iii) The size of the antigens must be increased to promote phagocytosis and immune response. A vaccine of this type was licensed in 1981. This was vaccine for foot and mouth disease. For other vaccines, work is in progress.

Fourth generation vaccine (DNA vaccines): Since the pioneering in early 1990s, DNA vaccines have demonstrated significant advantages over conventional vaccines. Scientists have successfully applied this technique to develop DNA vaccines against infectious pathogens in many different animal models, however, the efficacy of different DNA vaccines has varied widely. With this new technology, recombinant genes encoded by a plasmid expression vector can be delivered and expressed in animal muscle. Based on this technique, a novel type of vaccine, termed nucleic acid vaccine or DNA vaccine with DNA instead of proteins in the vaccine formulation, has been developed.

PRINCIPLES

By the 1970s, it had become apparent that isolated structural components of infectious pathogens were generally immunogenic. Such noninfectious "subunit vaccines" often evoked protective immune responses with fewer undesirable side effects generally associated with inactivated whole agent vaccines. The concept of subunit vaccine, containing only those immunogenic components necessary to elicit a protective response and excluding others unnecessary for immunity, has several attractive features. First and foremost is the element of safety. Subunit vaccines lack infectious material. No infection, either acute, persistent, or latent, can be established in the vaccine/vaccinate, thus substantially reducing complications arising from the vaccination of immunocompromised or pregnant individuals. Extraneous antigens are lacking, reducing or eliminating pyrogenic, allergenic, immunosuppressive, and other undesirable reactogenicity. Subunit vaccines also exhibit considerable stability, potentially allowing for wide distribution and prolonged storage. The composition of a subunit vaccine can be clearly defined, which is a significant advantage in terms of safety considerations and minimization of side effects. Another advantage of the subunit approach is that it allows a ready identification of vaccines/vaccinates. Simple serologic tests can readily distinguish vaccination from infection. Such a vaccine is therefore compatible with, and essential for, disease control and eradication programs. But, these vaccines are not without their shortcomings. Expense is still a major consideration; this is not necessarily the cost of the product itself, but of the research and development cost incurred towards obtaining the same. Also important is the question of efficacy. Non-infectious, non-replicating immunogens are inherently less immunogenic than replicating intact agents. Live vaccines often require only a single inoculation, whereas subunits frequently require multiple administrations before protective immunity is established. They also must incorporate immunostimulants, such as adjuvants to make their efficacy acceptable.

The identification and sequencing of the genes encoding the immunogenic proteins gives a confirmatory evidence of the amino acid sequence present in the immunogenic peptide. Once the amino acid sequence of a particular peptide is known, artificial synthesis of this peptide is possible. Earlier it was believed that most of the antigenic determinants are conformational and not sequential, but subsequent work proved that small linear synthetic peptides react with the intact antigen. These discoveries strengthened the scope of developing the synthetic peptide vaccines. In spite of the manifold advantages of the synthetic peptide vaccines like longer shelf life, accurate composition, and no threat of the presence of live virus, it has been found that synthetic peptides alone have very low immunogenicity even when administered with strong adjuvants. This problem can be overcome by conjugating the synthetic peptides to macromolecular carriers such as proteins, synthetic poly amino acids or liposomes or by incorporating the B and T lymphocyte epitopes and better adjuvants in the peptides. The other disadvantages associated with the synthetic peptide vaccines like short-term immunity and high cost of production restrict their extensive use for vaccination of animals.

Live virus vaccines do have disadvantages, and in many cases some researchers believe that a point of diminishing returns has been reached in regard to new developments. Technologies for biochemical characterization and genetic manipulation of viruses have led to the development of novel mutant and recombinant viruses to be used as genetically modified vaccines (Genetically Engineered Reassortants and Deletion Mutant Vaccines). For example, novel deletion mutants of pseudo rabies virus, derived by genetic engineering, have proven to be nonpathogenic yet effective in protecting swine from wild-type virus challenge. The ability of genetic engineers to manipulate genes allows for the removal of pathogenic genes from infectious agents without destroying their ability to propagate and express immunodominant epitopes. Genes reassorting and deletion techniques are being applied to both viruses and bacteria. Highly attenuated temperature-sensitive mutants of influenza virus or avian strains (that do not replicate efficiently in mammals) are being used with virulent wild-type virus to co-infect cell cultures. Deletion mutants of several bacteria have been engineered and their potential usefulness as vaccines is being explored. Included in these studies are deletion mutants of *Salmonella*, *Shigella* and *Vibrio cholerae*. A mutant strain of *Salmonella* defective in aromatic biosynthesis resulted in the induction of resistance to oral challenge. A hybrid strain of *Salmonella* Typhi/*Shigella sonei* appears to have a potential as a vaccine against both typhoid and dysentery. Using overlapping cosmid clone-based technology, an MDV vIL-8 deletion mutant virus, rMd5 delta vIL-8 was developed, which had attenuated virulence and conferred protection against the challenge. These results confirm the potential of partially attenuated viruses as vaccines against very virulent plus strains and the usefulness of recombinant DNA technology to generate the next generation of Marek's disease virus vaccines.

Besides the possibility of producing recombinant protein immunogens in heterologous hosts, technologies to construct recombinant live viral and bacterial vaccine-delivery vectors carrying foreign immunogens have been developed (vectored vaccines). Compared with proteinaceous subunit vaccines, recombinant live vaccines would potentially be easier and less costly to produce since they do not require extensive purification processes, and they may be able to elicit long-lasting immunity without the need for adjuvants. The attenuated organism serves as a vector, replicating within the host and expressing the gene product of the pathogen. Several viruses have been investigated for their possible use as recombinant vaccines. Herpes viruses, adenoviruses, and poxviruses are the most notable examples of viruses that can serve as vectors for heterologous genes while maintaining full infectivity. Experimental immunizations with infectious virus vectors carrying one or more heterologous genes for immunogenic proteins have been remarkably successful in experimental animal systems. Such immunizations have enabled the presentation of immunogenic proteins to the host immune system in an authentic way, mimicking closely the way antigens are presented in natural infections. Such successes have vaulted infectious virus vectors into consideration as vaccines for humans and animals.

Nucleic acid (NA) vaccination is of recent origin and an effective means of generating an antigen specific immune response by simply inoculating plasmid DNA containing the gene encoding the antigen of interest. Delivery of DNA vaccines requires expression of immunogenic proteins in tissues accessible to the immune system such as muscle or skin or mucous membranes. DNA vaccines have been shown to generate both humoral and cellular immune responses. The major advantage of DNA vaccine is that it is possible to simultaneously introduce plasmids containing genes encoding a wide variety of proteins from different pathogens, from a number of strains of the same pathogen (e.g., influenza virus or HIV) or from different stages of the life cycle of an organism (e.g., parasites). Also it elicits strong and persistent cell mediated and humoral immunity. To further enhance the immune responses by NA vaccines, novel adjuvants like cytokines and immunomodulatory sequence (CpG-cytosine-phosphate-guanosine) are being incorporated along with vaccines. NA vaccines are relatively easy to construct and produce, and considering the post-translational modifications and the presentation of the antigen to the host's immune system, they provide antigen synthesis in the host in a similar way to that which occurs during natural infection. They are also easy to administer, there is no fear of neutralization by maternal antibodies in neonates and there is no requirement of maintenance of cold chain. One drawback of DNA vaccines, which has been extensively discussed, is the potential risk for integration into the host's genome leading to insertional mutation and possible tumorigenesis. This risk could be minimized by using RNA instead of DNA for immunization. Due to the low stability of mRNA, preparation and administration of RNA vaccines are not entirely simple. There is also the possibility of the generation of autoimmune responses, including anti-DNA antibodies or induction of tolerance or the breaking of tolerance to self proteins due to sustained expression of antigen.

Plants provide a very attractive alternative that can be scaled up to a high production system for recombinant proteins. With the availability of excellent plant virus expression vectors, it would not be difficult to express a host of relevant genes encoding immunogenic proteins in plants and hence edible vaccines are rapidly coming within the realm of reality. With the tools of genetic engineering and molecular biology, genes encoding immunogenic proteins of an infectious agent are transferred into the nuclear genome of a plant system via genetic transformation protocols, and these transgenic plants are then capable of producing the desired immunogenic protein subunit vaccines. The production of antigens in genetically engineered plants provides an inexpensive source of edible vaccines and, in turn, increases the value of plants as novel sources of medicinal drugs. This new field of biological science, referred to as molecular "biofarming" has received much attention in the past and promises to become more important in coming years. With advancement of biotechnology, it is possible to use engineered plants to produce vaccines against human or animal diseases, ranging from tooth decay to life threatening infections such as bacterial diarrhea, cholera and AIDS. In perhaps the most far-reaching scenario, it might even be possible to build some vaccine into plants eaten as part of the normal diet. The vaccine, if produced, will be cheaper, easier to administer and free from contamination with animal viruses and cell components, which is always associated with the vaccines manufactured in cultured mammalian cells. There are some limitations to these recombinant antigens produced in plants that should be overcome before this technology can make it to the commercial sector. Among these limitations is the need to achieve high enough yield of the recombinant antigen in the plant tissue, and another limitation is dealing with the presence of plant-specific glycans that might alter the properties of the recombinant protein.

VACCINE TECHNOLOGY

Different Types of Vaccines

The vaccines that are in use in the present time mainly consist of killed vaccines, live attenuated vaccines or subunit vaccines. These types of vaccines have proven to be effective particularly in reducing the clinical manifestation following exposure to virulent field strains of the pathogens. From the experiments of Jenner through the development of live-virus vaccines against yellow fever, poliomyelitis, measles and other diseases, vaccine viruses have been derived empirically, usually by repeated passages in animals, embryonating eggs, or cell cultures. Generally, live-virus vaccines have provided long-lasting protection. Even when immunity levels have fallen with time, natural subclinical reinfections have served as harmless boosters. Inherently, both cell mediated and humoral immunity has usually been stimulated by live-virus vaccines, just as in natural infections. Live vaccines can potentially replicate in the host, but are typically attenuated in their pathogenicity in order not to cause disease. One of the important impediments in the case of live vaccines is to ensure that the organism is attenuated sufficiently not to cause the disease, but still replicate to a sufficient level to induce an appropriate immune response. However, only a limited number of viral diseases can be prevented by live attenuated viral vaccines state and most DNA-containing viruses have the potential to establish persistent (or latent) infection. New viral strains may arise by recombination of the vaccine virus with other viral strains in animal populations; pregnant animals or their offspring may be adversely affected by the vaccine strain. Certain apparently avirulent viral strains can revert to virulence, either by host induced proteolysis or surface proteins of the phenotype, as in the activation of the HN and F0 proteins of influenza virus or by mutations in the genotype, as in the reversion of attenuated oral Sabin poliovirus vaccine.

Killed vaccines are not capable of replication in the host and therefore cannot multiply or revert to pathogenicity, or transmit the disease to another person. Killed vaccines usually function by stimulating the humoral immune response, as well as by priming for immunological memory. The production of such vaccines require large scale culturing of the disease causing microorganisms, which can be associated with both safety risks and problems to achieve cost efficient production. The inactivated vaccines also suffer from the drawback that the protective level of immune response is not generated due to the loss of important antigenic determinants during the process of inactivation. The immunity generated by these vaccines is of shorter duration and thus multiple booster doses are required. Also, the so-called inactivated foot and mouth disease (FMD) viral vaccines are found to be infectious far frequently and cause outbreaks by incompletely inactivated vaccines or due to escape of virus from vaccine manufacturing facilities (Table 29.1).

Table 29.1 Properties, advantages and disadvantages of live vs. non-live vaccines.

	LIVING VERSUS NON-LIVING VACCINES	
	Living	*Non-living*
Preparation	attenuation (not always feasible)	inactivation
Administration	may be natural route (e.g.,oral) may be single dose	injection usually multiple doses
Adjuvant	not required	usually required
Safety	may revert to virulence	pain from injection
Heat lability (for tropical use)	requires cold chain	satisfactory
Cost	low	high
Duration of immunity	usually years	may be long or short
Immune response	IgG, IgA, cell-mediated	mainly IgG, little or no cell-mediated

Subunit vaccines can be (based on) peptides, proteins or polysaccharides that have been shown to contain protective epitopes. Many of the cell-surface carbohydrates of pathogenic bacteria, e.g., *capsular polysaccharides*, are important antigenic determinants for vaccine development. The vaccine for *Streptococcus pneumoniae*, which causes pneumococcal pneumonia and *Neisseria meningitidis*, a common cause of bacterial meningitis, consists of purified capsular polysaccharides. One limitation of polysaccharide vaccines is their inability to activate T_H cells. They activate B cells in a thymus-independent manner, resulting in IgM production but little class switching, no affinity maturation, and little, if any, development of memory cells. One way to involve T_H cells directly in the response to a polysaccharide antigen is to conjugate the antigen to some sort of protein carrier. For example, the vaccine for *Haemophilus influenzae* type b (Hib), the major cause of bacterial meningitis in children less than 5 years of age, consists of type b capsular polysaccharide covalently linked to a protein carrier, tetanus toxoid. The polysaccharide-protein conjugate is considerably more immunogenic than the polysaccharide alone, and since it activates T_H cells, it enables class switching from IgM to IgG. This type of vaccine can also induce memory B cells. Some bacterial pathogens, including those that cause diphtheria and tetanus, produce *exotoxins* that produce many of the disease symptoms that result from infection. Diphtheria and tetanus vaccines are made by purifying the bacterial exotoxin and then inactivating the toxin with formaldehyde to form *toxoid*. Vaccination with toxoid induces anti-toxoid antibodies, which are also capable of binding to the toxin and neutralizing its effects.

These traditional vaccines need improvement for reasons of safety, efficacy and cost effectiveness. Strategies that are currently being applied to the generation of new types of vaccines are:

(i) Recombinant DNA cloning of immunogenic surface protein.
(ii) Chemical synthesis of polypeptide vaccines.
(iii) Construction of recombinant vaccines having guest genes for foreign surface proteins.
(iv) Genetic engineering of non-pathogenic mutant agents.
(v) Production of monoclonal epitopes of the surface proteins of infectious agents.
(vi) Nucleic acid vaccines.

The recent developments in the field of molecular biology and genetic engineering have made a long lasting effect in the field of vaccine production. It has now become possible to design vaccines that no longer have side effects associated with the traditional vaccines. By applying the recombinant DNA technology, production of safe, potent, cost-effective and stable vaccines has become possible. Modern advances in molecular biology and nucleic acid and protein chemistry have contributed to the development of rDNA technology. These advances include:

(i) the elucidation of the structure and functions of bacterial plasmids and viruses;
(ii) the finding that retroviruses possess reverse transcriptase, which permits them to replicate by a recombinant DNA pathway;
(iii) the discovery and isolation of restriction endonucleases that cleave DNA generally where thymine, cytosine, adenine and guanine bases form palindromic sequences on opposite strands;
(iv) the isolation of DNA ligases, S1 nucleases and terminal deoxyribonucleotidyl transferases;
(v) the development of rapid protein and DNA sequencing procedures; and
(vi) the finding that microorganisms such as *E. coli*, *Bacillus subtilis* and yeasts can serve as alternate hosts for chimeric DNA vectors containing guest genes encoding foreign proteins.

Immunogenic components can be isolated directly from pathogenic organisms, e.g., bacterial polysaccharides are often shed during growth and can be enriched from the culture medium. However, the production of subunit vaccines often requires purification of the immunogens from large quantities of the pathogenic organism, which is not without risk and significant cost. Recent advances in immunology and protein engineering have allowed the design and production of recombinant subunit vaccines. Recombinant DNA technology allows controlled production of protein-subunit vaccines in heterologous hosts. Isolation of the genes encoding immunogenic proteins and their expression in heterologous hosts form the basis of recombinant-subunit vaccine development. The problem of obtaining sufficient quantities of the purified toxins to prepare the vaccines has been overcome by cloning the exotoxins genes and then expressing them in easily grown host cells. In this way large quantities of the exotoxin can be produced, purified and subsequently inactivated. A number of genes from the viral, bacterial and protozoan pathogens have been successfully cloned and are being developed as vaccines. The use of gene cloning technologies to bioproduce immunogens provides two additional advantages for vaccine development. The first is the added measure of safety in genes encoding appropriate immunogenic proteins of dangerous or highly pathogenic agents transferred to harmless microbes for safe mass production. Second, they are being considered for exotic and uncultivable pathogens, thus expanding the scope of disease that may be controlled by vaccination.

The DNA encoding the antigenic determinants can be isolated and cloned in bacteria, yeast, insect or mammalian expression systems. *Bacterial expression systems* can express antigens at very high levels and are suitable for expressing vaccine antigens that do not require significant post-translational modifications. *Escherichia coli* is the most commonly used bacterium for production of heterologous proteins, being easy to manipulate, genetically and physiologically well defined, and yielding high expression levels. Other bacteria used are *Salmonella typhimurium*, *Vibrio cholerae* and *Bacillus brevis*. Among the *eukaryotic expression systems*, the baker's yeast *Saccharomyces cerevisiae* is the most commonly used. Yeast cells possess some of the eukaryotic possibilities for post-translationally modifying proteins, e.g., phosphorylation and glycosylation, but since glycosylation differs from that in mammalian cells, it can potentially also be disadvantageous. But, most vaccines requiring eukaryotic post-translational modifications are still being expressed in yeast because of high product yield in yeast and the ease with which yeast can be manipulated and grown. *Baculovirus-based expression system* has been developed for the production of heterologous proteins in cultured insect cells. Advantages of baculovirus over other expression systems are that proteins are expressed at very high levels, and since these cells are eukaryotic, they are able to make many of the post-translational modifications of mammalian cells, even though the glycosylations are not the same as in mammalian systems. *Several mammalian expression systems* for production of recombinant proteins have been developed. The major advantage is that it will post-translationally modify the expressed product with the highest degree of fidelity compared with the other expression systems, and expressed viral proteins will thus be glycosylated in a human-like fashion. Drawbacks of mammalian expression systems are the laborious and time-consuming generation of stable cell lines, the high cultivation costs, and the problems associated with viral and bacterial (e.g., *Mycoplasma*) infections.

Since the synthetic peptide vaccines are safe and lack infectivity, extensive research in this field has led to the development of vaccines against diseases like hepatitis, foot and mouth disease and influenza. A synthetic peptide vaccine developed from two major antigenic sites on capsid protein VP1 induced significant levels of anti-FMDV neutralizing antibodies and protection in guinea pig, swine and cattle. Two peptides derived from highly conserved regions of bovine rotavirus outer capsid proteins (VP7 and VP4) were tried as rotavirus vaccine. With the object of increasing the immunogenicity of the synthetic peptide vaccines, Keyhole Limpet Haemocyanin (KLH), ovalbumin and bovine serum albumin (BSA) have been used for the conjugation of synthetic peptide coding for hepatitis B surface antigen and FMDV. Similarly, the peptides coding for rabies virus glycoprotein when conjucted with KLH elicited better immune response. Research is in progress for chemical synthesis of peptide vaccines for bacterial diseases, for example, diphtheria and cholera. A synthesized hexadecapeptide corresponding to amino acid residues 186-201 of the A chain of diphtheria toxin covalently bound to both synthetic muramyl dipeptide adjuvant and synthetic multichain poly-DL-alanine induced protective anti-toxic immunity in guinea pigs. For cholera, several peptides ranging between 11 and 18 amino acid residues in length corresponding to regions of the 103 amino acid chain of the B subunit of *Vibrio cholerae* have been synthesized and linked either to tetanus toxoid or to multichain poly-DL-alanine. Synthetic peptides derived from predicted loop 2 and loop 5 of outer membrane protein of *Pasteurella multocida* strain X-73 (serotype 1) was tested on chicken. Results showed that synthetic peptide mimicking the predicted loop 2 induced 70% protection in chicken against strain X-73 challenge.

Live viral vaccines have been genetically modified using recombinant DNA technology to attenuate a virus by deleting or altering the virulent gene(s). Temperature sensitive mutant vaccines have been developed for infectious bovine rhinotracheitis, bovine respiratory syncytial disease and bovine viral diarrhea. Genetic engineering has been used to construct deletion mutants by excising a sequence of nucleotides from a gene that is not essential for viral replication but contributes to virulence, such as TK gene in herpes viruses. A deletion mutant has also been prepared for simian immunodeficiency virus and pseudorabies virus. Since such mutants cannot revert to virulence, they are attractive candidates for live viral vaccines. The deletion mutants of the vaccine strains can be used to differentiate the vaccinated animals from the naturally infected ones. The construction of a TK negative pseudorabies vaccine having a deletion in the glycoprotein genes (gI, gIII or gX) enables to distinguish the vaccinated pigs from naturally infected ones based on the ELISA test using the deleted glycoprotein. This approach helps in carrying out the eradication program in parallel to the vaccination program. The overall promise of deletion mutants seems limited, however, especially relative to the promise of insertion mutants.

Vaccinia virus, a member of the pox virus family, is a large double-stranded DNA virus that replicates in the cytoplasm of infected cells. Vaccinia virus has a wide host range, including human, cattle, horses, swine, sheep, goats, mice and monkeys. The vaccinia virus has been widely employed as a vector for the vaccine production. This large, complex virus with a genome of about 200 genes can be engineered to carry several dozens foreign genes without impairing its capacity to infect host cell and replicate, thereby producing the multivalent recombinant vaccines. The vaccinia virus has been successfully used as a vector for developing vaccines against rabies and rinderpest. The rabies glycoprotein gene has been inserted into the thymidine kinase (TK) gene of the vaccinia virus, generating selectable TK negative virus known as VVTGgRAB. It was found safe and effective for fox, raccoon and skunk when used for oral immunization of wild animals. Infectious vaccinia virus recombinants expressing either haemagglutinin or the fusion gene of rinderpest virus, when used to vaccinate cattle, produced neutralizing antibodies against rinderpest virus. In an attempt to produce a multivalent vaccine, the genes from hepatitis B virus, herpes simplex and influenza were expressed in engineered vaccinia virus. The vaccination trials conducted using this vectored vaccine have given promising results. Similarly, the use of vaccinia virus engineered with envelope glycoproteins of the HIV virus is being assessed as a potential vaccine for AIDS. The vectored viral vaccines encoding relevant foreign genes along with immunostimulatory cytokines hold a very promising future.

Two classes of viral vectors may be differentiated. One class comprises *replication-defective* vector viruses that produce infectious progeny only via complementation by specifically transformed (SV40, adenoviruses) or helper-virus super infection (retroviruses). The second class comprises *replication-competent* viruses. Clearly, however, the use of poxviruses, herpesviruses, and adenoviruses as candidate vectors is not without problems. They all have complex *in vivo* replication demands, less-than perfect virulence characteristics, and some undesirable host range traits. They all require further research to define and optimize these characteristics. For example, the persistence of adenoviruses in lymphatic tissues and herpes viruses in neural tissues and the progressive course of vaccinia virus infection in immunocompromised individuals must be studied.

The use of live bacteria as mucosal vaccines has been studied extensively, both against the corresponding disease and also as delivery systems for heterologous diseases. Mucosal vaccines are easy to administer, e.g., by the oral or nasal route, and using bacteria as a delivery vehicle makes the vaccine comparatively inexpensive to produce. The best-studied bacterial delivery systems are based on attenuated *Salmonella* spp. as live vectors expressing heterologous antigens, and numerous studies have been performed for development of oral vaccines against bacterial, viral or parasitic diseases. Live *Salmonella*, being an intracellular pathogen, is generally capable of eliciting cellular immune responses to the antigen delivered—a desired property of the immune responses protecting against viral or parasitic diseases. The possibility of expressing foreign proteins on the surface of bacteria makes live bacterial vectors highly interesting. Surface display of heterologous proteins for the construction of live vectors was first described for Gram-negative bacteria, and more recently systems for surface display on Gram-positive bacteria have also been described. Two basic strategies exist for the generation of bacterial live-delivery vehicles. One type of vehicle is based on colonizing normally pathogenic bacteria, and attenuated or non-pathogenic variants of that bacterium are employed in order to obtain suitable vehicles, e.g., *Salmonella* and mycobacterial strains. A second type of vehicle is based on non-pathogenic commensal or food-grade bacteria, such as *Streptococcus gordonii* and certain staphylococcal or lactococcal strains.

NA vaccines are usually delivered by injection of the plasmid DNA alone, usually into the muscle or skin. The preparation of such a vaccine involves the cloning of the desired target molecule into a plasmid vector, which contains an eukaryotic promoter to enable the gene to be expressed in eukaryotic cells. Such plasmids can also be introduced into the mammalian tissue by a second highly effective method, particle bombardment-mediated gene transfer, whereby plasmid DNA-coated gold particles are accelerated to high velocity to enable their penetration into the target tissue by a device known as gene gun. The direct delivery of genetic material to host cells and the subsequent *in vivo* production of the desired antigen offers the possibility of persistent low-level expression over long periods of time. This results in sustained presentation of the antigen, which overcomes the shortcomings of subunit vaccines where boosting of the immune response is required. Transfected cells then express the antigen encoded on the plasmid resulting in an immune response. Like live or attenuated viruses, DNA vaccines effectively engage both MHC-I and MHC-II pathways allowing for the induction of CD^{8+} and CD^{4+} T cells, whereas antigen present in soluble form, such as recombinant protein, generally induces only antibody response (Figure 29.1).

Like plasmid DNA, naked mRNA encoding immunogenic protein can also be inoculated directly into host to induce immune response against the protein product. RNA expression is short lived, and is thus less effective in inducing an immune response. The preparation and administration of RNA is troublesome because of the low stability of the RNA. RNA vaccination appears attractive in the sense that it would transitorily remain in the host system, hence the possibility of integration and undesirable mutagenic consequences can be avoided.

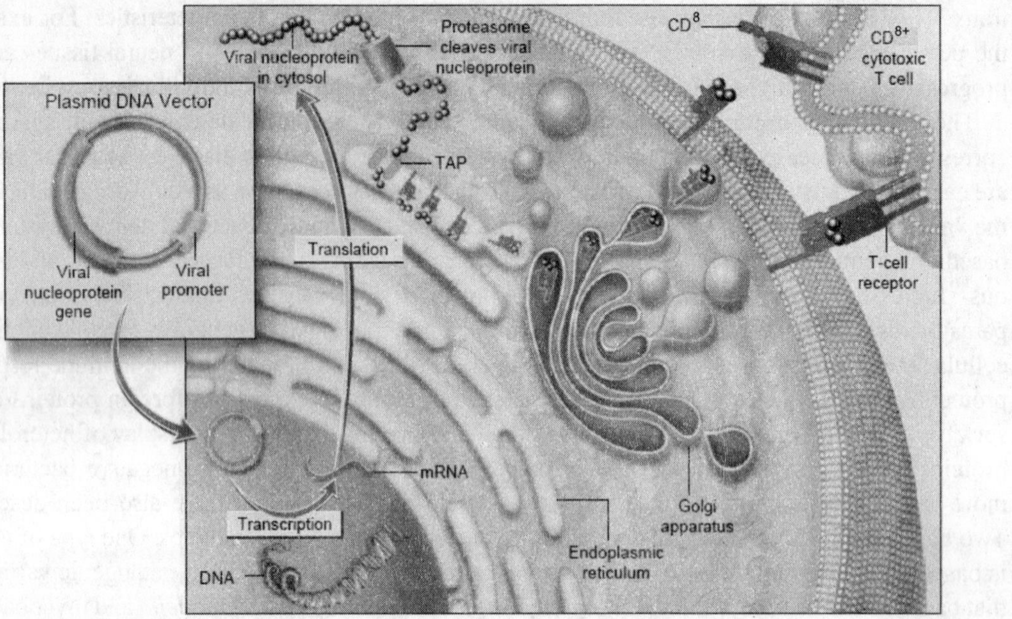

Figure 29.1 Molecular route of a DNA vaccine.

Transgenic plants of tobacco and potato have been produced utilizing the highly active immunogen, the binding subunit of *Escherichia coli* heat labile toxin (LT-B). The plants expressed the foreign peptide, and feeding mice with fresh transgenic potato tubers caused oral immunization thereby demonstrating the feasibility of using transgenic plants as an expression and delivery system for oral vaccines. Similarly, when hepatitis B virus surface protein was expressed in transgenic tobacco, virus specific antibodies were produced by feeding the mice with transgenic tobacco. The cholera toxin B subunit (CTB) against *Vibrio cholerae* was successfully expressed in potato tubers and found to accumulate at high enough levels that induced both mucosal and serum immune responses in mice. The capsid protein of the Norwalk virus was also expressed in potato tubers and found to be immunogenic in test mice as well. Other food crops used for the development of plant-based vaccines include lupine, lettuce, soybean, corn, tomato etc. Plant expression constructs consisted of the universal constitutive cauliflower mosaic virus (CaMV) 35S promoter along with enhancer elements or leader sequences added to the gene of interest to be expressed.

Vaccines of the Future

The vaccines of the future may consist of single viral or bacterial vector containing genes for all required vaccines, the 'one-shot' vaccine. This illustration first appeared in *New Scientist*, London, the weekly review of science and technology (Figure 29.2).

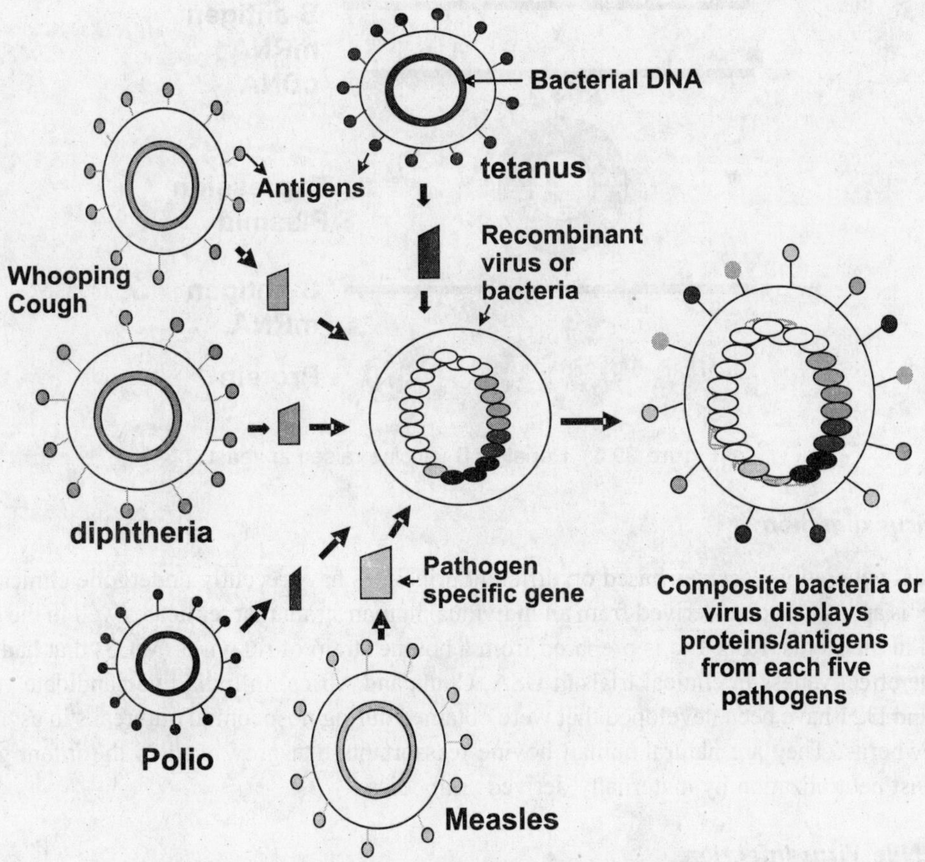

Figure 29.2 The 'one- shot' vaccine.

APPLICATIONS OF VACCINE TECHNOLOGY

Some of the recent developments in the production of new generation vaccines against important diseases are given below.

Medical Applications

Hepatitis B infection

The first recombinant antigen vaccine approved for human use was the hepatitis B vaccine that was developed by cloning the gene for the major surface antigen (HBsAg) of hepatitis B virus in the yeast cells. The expression of the cloned HBsAg antigen facilitated the production of large quantities of recombinant vaccine (Figure 29.3).

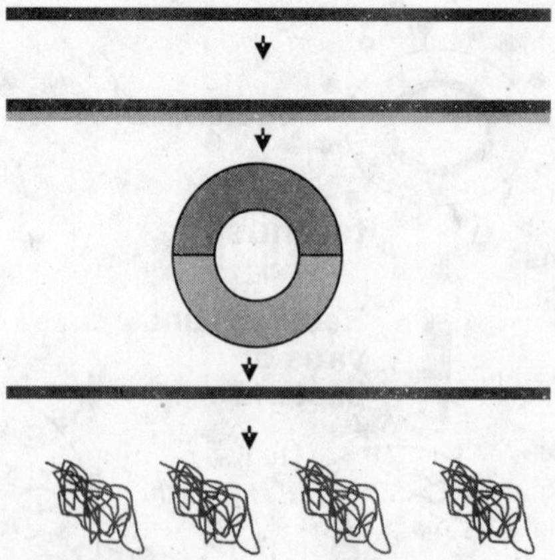

Figure 29.3 Hepatitis B vaccine raised in yeast.

Rotavirus diarrhea

Two next generation vaccines based on different principles have recently undergone clinical trials. Rotarix is an oral vaccine derived from an individual human strain that replicates well in the gut and is shed in the stools. Rota Teq is prepared from a bovine strain of rotavirus (WC3) that had shown variable effectiveness in clinical trials in USA, China and Africa. In India two candidate vaccines 116E and I321 have been developed that were obtained during nosocomial outbreaks in asymptomatic newborns. They are natural human bovine reassortants that grow well in the infant gut, and can resist neutralization by maternally derived antibodies.

West Nile Virus infection

Currently, no WNV vaccine is licensed for use in humans. The experimental vaccine is composed of a small, circular piece of DNA, called DNA plasmid, which contains genes that code for two key surface proteins of the West Nile virus.

Cholera

An indigenous recombinant oral cholera vaccine based on VA 1.3 strain of *Vibrio cholerae* has been found to be safe and provided good vibriocidal antibody response.

Typhoid

Vi polysaccharide conjugate typhoid vaccine using *Salmonella Typhi* outer membrane protein from conjugation has been developed. This Vi conjugate has been shown to be immunogenic in mice.

Japanese Encephalitis

A tissue culture based and inactivated Japanese Encephalitis vaccine has been developed by growing an Indian strain of Japanese Encephalitis Virus (JEV) in Vero cells to high titers and formalin inactivating it. Inactivated virus produced high titers of JEV neutralizing antibodies and challenge experiments in mice indicated that the preparation provided 100 percent protection to the immunized mice against lethal dose of JEV given intracerebrally.

In another approach, a candidate DNA-based JEV vaccine (replication-defective recombinant adenoviruses) is being studied.

Malaria

The vaccine utilizing the recombinant antigens of *Plasmodium falciparum and Plasmodium vivax* is being under study.

Tuberculosis

Efforts have been made to develop novel recombinant DNA-based candidate vaccine and recombinant BCG containing relevant antigens of *Mycobacterium tuberculosis* that are in *E. coli* expression system. The entire DNA candidate antigens were found to elicit specific immune responses in experimental animals. Testing in aerosol challenge models is in progress to select the best candidate for human studies.

Dengue

The existence of multiple but distinct dengue virus serotypes is a major factor that has hindered dengue vaccine development efforts. Available evidence indicates that immunity against an infecting serotype is life-long, whereas cross-protection against other serotypes is transient. Therefore, a safe and effective dengue vaccine should ideally be "tetravalent" or capable of providing solid and long-lasting immunity to all four serotypes. Taking this approach, a tetravalent dengue vaccine candidate is being developed. The strategy is to make non-replicating sub-unit vaccine based on a critical domain of the major dengue structural envelope protein that is involved in the host receptor reception and in the induction of robust protective immunity. Each subunit is being expressed using *Pichia pastoris* as the expression host.

HIV/AIDS

A DNA/MVA based vaccine has been developed for HIV-1, subtype 'C' prevalent in India. The indigenous recombinant DNA/MVA vaccine is constructed from select genetic sequences of HIV and delivered with the help of a plasmid vector in the prime dose and a highly attenuated strain of Vaccinia virus-Modified Vaccinia Ankara (MVA)-as the vector in the booster dose.

Influenza

Flu vaccine is an inactivated vaccine, i.e., it contains killed influenza virus. Two types of influenza vaccines are available: injectable (flu shot) and the nasal spray (FluMist). Both types of influenza vaccine contain three new virus strains *(A/Brisbane/59/2007 (H1N1)-like, A/Brisbane/10/2007(H3N2)-like, and B/Florida/4/2006-like)* that are responsible for the majority of influenza illnesses. FDA approves first U.S. vaccine for humans against the avian influenza virus H5N1. The vaccine could be used to control current H5N1 avian virus which has the capability to efficiently spread from human to human, resulting in the rapid spread of the disease across the globe. Should such an influenza pandemic emerge, the vaccine may provide early protection. The vaccine is obtained from a human strain, which is an inactivated vaccine made from an H5N1 virus isolated in Southeast Asia in 2004.

Anthrax

The efficacy and immunogenicity of a recombinant protective antigen (rPA) against anthrax is being tested in New Zealand white rabbits and Rhesus monkey by pre-exposure and post-exposure prophylactic studies.

Human Papiloma Virus

The work is on expressing L1/L2 proteins of HPV 16/18 as Virus Like Particles (VLPs) and Capsomere Like Particles (CLPs) as possible prophylactic vaccine candidates.

Neurocysticercosis

Two recombinant *Taenia solium* oncosphere antigens, designated TSOL18 and TSOL45-1A, were investigated as vaccines to prevent the transmission of zoonotic diseases, *cysticercosis* through pigs. Both antigens were effective in inducing very high levels of protection (up to 100%) in three independent vaccine trials in pigs against experimental challenge infection with *T. solium* eggs. These two oncosphere antigens provided the basis for the development of a highly effective practical vaccine that could assist in the control and, potentially, the eradication of human neurocysticercosis.

Veterinary Applications

Parvovirus infection

Recombinant subunit vaccine against parvovirus B19 involving the expression of VP1 and VP2 in baculovirus system resulting into synthesis of virus like particles (VLPs) has been shown to be immunogenic and is under clinical trials.

Rabies

A recombinant vaccinia virus expressing the immunizing rabies G glycoprotein was developed. This vaccine was used successfully to protect foxes against rabies. The administration of recombinant rabies vaccine to adult foxes, raccoons and skunks elicited high levels of rabies virus neutralizing antibodies and long-term protection against rabies.

The first combined DNA-based rabies vaccine for the control of rabies in dogs clearly indicates that the combined DNA rabies vaccine provides tremendous boost to the inoculated animals.

West Nile Fever

Centre for Disease Control and Prevention (CDC) has developed the world's first licensed DNA vaccine. The studies showed that the vaccine protected the horses from becoming ill with West Nile virus, with no adverse or major side effects. West Nile virus causes similar disease in horses and humans. Thus, the successful development of this DNA vaccine for horse should enhance the development of human vaccine.

FMD

Foot-and-mouth disease was the first disease against which effective vaccine was produced through gene splicing. The FMD virus genome is a single, positive sense strand of infectious RNA, made of four viral proteins, VPl, VP2, VP3 and VP4. In this virus, the neutralizing immune response appears to be directed primarily against VPl. Studies have shown that the peptide corresponding to residues 141-160 and 200-213 of VP1 are capable of neutralizing FMD virus. A recombinant live vector vaccine was produced by insertion of cDNA encoding the structural proteins (PI) of foot-and-mouth disease virus (FMDV) into a replication-competent human adenovirus type 5 vaccine strain.

The latest technology of the vaccine can replace the ultra filtration method of virus concentration with an alternate technology. It can also replace the imported oil adjuvant with the indigenously developed oil adjuvant. A marker vaccine (Cedivac-FMD) has been developed that does not induce NSP antibodies.

Newcastle disease

Newcastle disease recombinant vaccine had been produced using different virus vectors. The haemagglutinin-neuraminidase (HN) gene and the phosphoprotein (P) gene of Newcastle disease virus (NDV) were inserted into an avian leucosis virus vector. In another study, a cDNA copy of the RNA encoding the fusion (F) protein of NDV was inserted into a fowlpox virus vector.

Infectious bursal disease

A recombinant Newcastle disease virus (NDV) expressing VP2 protein of IBDV was developed. The gene encoding the VP2 protein of the IBDV was inserted into the most 3′-proximal locus of a full-length NDV cDNA for high-level expression. Vaccination with the rLaSotaNP2 generated antibody response against both NDV and IBDV.

Marek's disease

Three glycoproteins (gp 115/110, gp 63 and gp 51) from herpesvirus of turkeys and Marek's disease virus are being targeted for vaccine study.

Blue tongue

VP2 protein of type 10 bluetongue virus induces both neutralizing antibodies and protective immunity in sheep. RNA segment 2, which represents the VP2 neutralizing antigen, has been inserted into an insect baculovirus (Autographa californica, AcNPV). Infection of *Spodoptera frugiperda* cell lines by the recombinant virus produced VP2 protein that was precipitated with BTV-l 0 and to a lesser extent BTV-serotype 11 and 17 virus.

Canine distemper

Vaccinia virus-MVHA and F recombinants were produced and inoculated into dogs.

Colibacillosis

Monoclonal antibody to K99 pilus antigen produced in hybridomas and amplified in mice significantly reduced the severity of scours and the mortality of calves so treated. This product was successfully tested in Canada and has since been approved by the USDA for use in the US.

Pasteurellosis

An edible vaccine against bovine pneumonic pasteurellosis using transgenic white clover expressing a *Mannheimia haemolytica* Al leukotoxin 50 fusion protein Lkt50-GFP has been developed.

Anthrax

Inactivated rabies virus envelope protein was used as a carrier molecule for *Bacillus anthracis* protective antigen (PA).

Ectoparasitic infections

First recombinant vaccine against *Boophilus* ectoparasite tick has been commercialized utilizing recombinant Bm 86 antigen.

Others

R&D efforts are being initiated for several other vaccines such as recombinant DNA based vaccines for filarial, pneumococcal, bovine tuberculosis, brucellosis and duck plague.

Agricultural Applications

Transgenic plants for edible vaccines

Genes for peptide epitopes of pathogens can be used for the production of vaccines against a variety of human and animal diseases. This concept of vaccine production in transgenic plants was introduced in 1992. In the year 1995, a biopharmaceutical company, Prosigene, from Texas (USA) conducted clinical trials, where pigs, fed with an edible maize vaccine, were found protected against the transmissible gastroenteritis virus (TGEV). The company has also obtained patents on this and other edible vaccines produced in transgenic crops. Such vaccines, whenever successful, will provide a technology for the production and delivery of inexpensive vaccines, especially in the developing world. This technology will also be cheaper than the expensive recombinant cell cuture-based expression systems.

A mucosal immune response is necessary particularly for combating infections due to bacteria/viruses invading epithelial membrane. Mucosal immune system involves the production of secretory IgA (S-IgA) at mucosal surfaces such as gut and respiratory epithelia. Such a response is more easily achieved by oral vaccine rather than by parenteral (administered elsewhere than in alimentary canal) antigen delivery system. Particulate antigens rather than subunit or soluble antigens have been shown to be effective oral immunogens. The subunit vaccines, whenever used, require larger amounts of antigens and will be expensive if produced in recombinant cell culture expression system, which will need fermentation technology. In contrast to this, transgenic plants can be made to express the antigens in particulate form in the edible tissue, which can then be used as food, thus providing an inexpensive oral vaccine production and delivery system.

Factors affecting choice of transgenic plants for vaccines

While using transgenic plants for vaccines, several factors need to be taken into consideration:

(i) It should stimulate a mucosal immune response and therefore diarrheal diseases were the first target for oral vaccine through transgenic plants.

(ii) Antigen should assemble into ordered structures such as virus-like particles (VLP), which are resistant to digestion and reach the gut associated lymphoid tissue (GALT), which is used as foreign antigen for production of antibodies.

(ii) Plant system should be such that it may be used as food/feed, although tobacco was initially used, it is not suitable. Potato and banana were subsequently used/suggested, with an expression system, where antigen is produced or stored in the tuber in potato and in the fruit of banana. Alfalfa, coarse grain crops and beans can also be used for animal vaccines.

Transgenic tobacco, potato and banana as edible vaccines

Several examples of successful production of prospective edible vaccines through transgenic plants are listed in the Table 29.2. It may be seen that in majority of cases, transgenic tobacco plants were used, although other plants like potato, cowpea and blackeyed bean were also used. In some of these cases, the oral immunogenicity was tested in mice and positive results were obtained and recovery of antibodies was possible. It is hoped that eventually transgenic banana will be the fruit of choice to be used as edible vaccine, because banana is grown extensively throughout the world and can be consumed raw without any modification or processing of the edible part. The diseases that will be targeted for the production of edible banana vaccines may initially include measles, polio, diphtheria, yellow fever, viral diarrhea and hepatitis B, which will be successfully produced and used in the developing countries.

Table 29.2 The production of vaccines in transgenic plants.

Applications	*Plant*	*Protein*
Hepatitis B	Tobacco	Recombinant HBsAg
	Tobacco	Murine hepatitis epitope
Dental caries	Tobacco	*Streptococcus mutans* surface protein SpaA
Autoimmune diabetes	Potato	*Vibrio cholerae* toxin B subunit-human insulin fusion
	Potato	Glutamic acid decarboxylase
Cholera and *E.coli* diarrhea	Tobacco/potato	*E.coli* heat-labile enterotoxin LT-B
Cholera (oral vaccine)	Potato	*V.cholerae* toxin CtoxA and CtoxB subunits
Mucosal vaccines not requiring adjuvants	Cowpear	D2 peptide of fibronectin binding protein B of *Staphylococcus aureus*

Transgenic as edible vaccines for hepatitis B

An important target for vaccines is hepatitis B, a virus causing chronic liver disease. Serum derived antigens were initially used for immunization against this disease, but due to a variety of safety concerns against this vaccine, recombinant vaccines were developed in yeast. These recombinant vaccines also failed due to high expense and lack of facilities at several places for their production.

Therefore, in 1990s and in the year 2000, transgenic tobacco and potato were produced, which expressed hepatitis B surface antigen (HbsAg).

In the year 2002, transgenic carrot plants were also produced at Giessen University in Germany, which have the potenital as an edible vaccine against hepatitis B. In future, HbsAg may also be produced in banana, which can be eaten raw. Thus, it is hoped that the transgenic plants, without any treatment of edible parts that are ingested, will provide edible vaccines against hepatitis B in developing countries. It has already been shown that transgenic potato expressing HbsAg, when orally administered to mice, can elicit humoral immune responses.

Future Prospects of Vaccine Technology

Research in vaccine technology continues on many fronts to provide safe, efficacious, and affordable vaccine products. Many at-risk individuals living in the Third World and endemic areas do not have ready access to health care, so compliance to the multidose regimens required to achieve full protection may be difficult. Also, cold chains may not exist for those vaccine preparations that must be kept refrigerated to maintain proper levels of potency. Improvements in the thermal stability of vaccine preparations is advantageous. One approach to improve coverage that is being adopted by many vaccine manufacturers is to combine antigens into single preparation so that immunity to two or more diseases can be achieved with a single injection. Timerelease polymeric preparations are also being explored even for monovalent preparations to achieve repeated antigenic stimulation of the immune system without the need for multiple injections. Other research initiatives seek to eliminate the need for needles for delivery of vaccines through the use of oral vaccines, aerosolizers for inhalation, or needleless devices that use compressed gases at high pressure to deliver transdermal doses of vaccine preparations. A fairly recent development in vaccine technology may offer several advantages over more conventional preparations in terms of manufacturing ease, potency, and flexibility in terms of delivery systems and disease targets. Observations in the early 1990s that plasmid DNA-encoding antigenic proteins can elicit an immune response when injected directly into animals have sparked intensive research and tremendous excitement as well as concern over long term safety. With DNA vaccines, the coding region for a specific antigenic protein is incorporated into plasmids that are amplified in a host bacterial strain, such as *Escherichia coli*, and then purified. The bacterial hosts for the coding plasmids are easily scaleable, and generic purification schemes may be possible because the product would always be plasmid DNA. After injection, the naked plasmid DNA yields protein expression in its native conformation to which both humoral and cell-mediated antibody responses are mounted. The DNA constructs can be customized to coexpress both the coding region for the antigen as well as an immune modulator to enhance the immune response or increase its specificity. The tremendous amount of research in the past few years has led to progress in the development of vaccines against disease targets associated with bacterial, viral, and parasitic infections and provides hope for combating autoimmune and inflammatory diseases as well as cancer.

CONCLUSION

Vaccines are crucial for maintaining public health. They are safe, cost-effective, and an efficient way to prevent sickness and death from infectious diseases. Vaccines have led to some of the greatest public health triumphs ever, including the eradication of naturally occurring smallpox from the globe and the near-eradication of polio. In recent years, researchers have increased their understanding of the immune system and how it fights off harmful microbes. Scientists working on vaccines also have advanced technology to draw on, including recombinant DNA technology and the ability to "read" and analyze the genomes of disease-causing organisms. This new knowledge and technology promises to usher in a renaissance in the already vital field of vaccinology. Scientists are hard at work creating improved vaccines, designing new vaccine strategies, and identifying new vaccine candidates to prevent diseases for which no vaccines currently exist.

FURTHER READINGS

1. Alving, C.R., Detrick B., Richards R.L., Lewis M.G., Shafferman, A. and Eddy, G.A. (1993) Novel Adjuvant Strategies for Experimental Malaria and AIDS Vaccines. *Ann. N.Y. Acad. Sci.* **(690):** 265-275.
2. Babiuk L. A., Babiuk S. L. and Baca-Estrada M. E. (2002). Novel vaccine strategies. *Advances in Virus Research* **(58):** 29-79.
3. Bonn D. and Bradbury J. (1998) The warts and all approach to tackling cervical cancer *The Lancet.* 351 **(9105):** 810.
4. Canales M., Enriquez A., Ramos E., Cabrera D., Dandie H., Soto A., Falcón V., Rodriguez M., and De la Fuente J. (1997) Large-scale production in Pichia pastoris of the recombinant vaccine Gavac against cattle tick. *Vaccine.* 15 **(4):** 414-422.
5. De Kruif, P. (1954) P. *Microbe Hunters*, Harcourt Brace Jovanovich, New York.
6. Elelman, R. (1997) Adjuvents for the future. In: Leving MM, Woodrow G.C., Kaper, J.B. and Cobon G.S. eds., *New Generation Vaccines.* **(2):** 173-192.
7. Elliott, A.Y. (1990) in A.S. Lubiniecki ed. *Large-scale Mammalian Cell Culture Technology*, Dekker, New York, pp. 207-216.
8. Eskola J. and Käyhty H. (1998) Early immunization with conjugate vaccines. *Vaccine.* 16 **(14-15):** 1433-1438.
9. Excler J.L. (1998) Potentials and limitations of protein vaccines in infants. *Vaccine.* 16 **(14/15):** 1439-1443.
10. Gizurarson S. (1996) Optimal delivery of vaccines. Clinical pharmacokinetical considerations. *Clin. Pharmacokinet.* **(30):** 1-16.
11. Hansson M., Nygren P. and Stahl S. (2000). Design and production of recombinant subunit vaccines. *Biotechnology and Applied Biochemistry.* **(32):** 95-107.
12. Hayflick L., Moorhead P.S. (1961) The serial cultivation of human diploid cell strains. *Exp. Cell Res.* **(25):** 585-621.
13. Hayflick, L. (1989) History of cell substrates used for human biologicals. *Dev. Biol. Stand.* **(70):** 11-26.
14. Hayflick, L. Plotkin S., and Stevenson R.E. (1987) History of the acceptance of human diploid cell strains as substrates for human virus vaccine manufacture. *Dev. Biol. Stand.* **(68):** 9-17.
15. Hilleman, M. and W.W. Ellis ed., (1993) *Hepatitis B Vaccines in Clinical Practice*, Dekker, New York, pp. 17-39.
16. Hinman A.R. (1998) Global Progress in Infectious Disease Control. *Vaccine.* 16 **(11/12):** 1116-1121.
17. Ho, S.V. Ladisch M.R., Willson R.C., Painton C.-d.C., Builder S.E. eds., (1989), *Protein Purification from Molecular Mechanisms to Large-scale Processes*, American Chemical Society Press, pp. 14-34.
18. Keeling M. J., Woolhouse M. E. J., May R. M., Davies G. and Grenfell B. T. (2003). Modelling vaccination strategies against foot and mouth disease. *Nature.* **(42):** 136-142.
19. Kistner O., Barrett P.N., Mundt W., Reiter M., Schober-Bendixen S. and Dorner. F. (1998) Development of a mamalian cell (Vero) derived candidate influenza virus vaccine. *Vaccine.* 16 **(9-10):** 960-968.

20. Korban S. S., Krasnyanski S. F. and Buetow D. E. (2002). Foods as production and delivery vehicles for human vaccines. *Journal of the American College of Nutrition.* 21 **(3):** 212-217.
21. Leclerc C. (2003). New approaches in vaccine development. *Comparative Immunology, Microbiology & Infectious Diseases.* **(26):** 329-341.
22. Lee C.J., Banks S.D. and Li J.P. (1991) Virulence, immunity, and vaccine related to *Streptococcus pneumoniae*. *Crit. Rev. Microbiol.* 18 **(2):** 89-114 .
23. Leitner W. W., Ying H. and Restifo N. P. (2000). DNA and RNA-based vaccines: principles, progress and *prospects. Vaccine.* **(18):** 765-777.
24. Lightfoot E.N., in Ladisch M.R., Willson R.C., Painton C.-d.C., Builder S.E. eds. (1989), Protein *Purification from Molecular Mechanisms to Large-scale Processes*, American Chemical Society Press, pp. 35-51.
25. Marchetti M., Rossi M., Giannelli V., Giuliani M.M., Pizza M., Censini S., Covacci A., Massari P., Pagliaccia C., Manetti R., Telford J.L., Douce G., Dougan G., Rappuoli R. and Ghiara P. (1998) Protection against *Helicobacte pylori* infection in mice by intragastric vaccination with *H. pylori* antigens is achieved using a non-toxic mutant of *E. coli* heat-labile enterotoxine (LT) as adjuvant. *Vaccine.* 16 **(1):** 33-37
26. Marsano L.S., West D.J., Chan I., Hesley T.M., Cox J., Hackworth V. and Greenberg R.N. (1998) A two-dose hepatitis B vaccine regimen: proof of priming and memory responses in young adults. *Vaccine.* 16 **(6):** 624–629
27. Maynard J.E., Kane M.A. and Hadler S.C. (1989) Global control of hepatitis B through vaccinations: role of hepatitis B vaccine in the Expanded Programme on Immunization. *Rev. Infect. Dis.* **(2):** S574-S578.
28. Prasad G. and Minakshi (1997). Trends in antiviral vaccines. *Indian Journal of Microbiology.* **(37):** 165-176.
29. Relyveld E.H., (1986) Preparation and use of calcium phosphate adsorbed vaccines. *Dev. Biol. Stand.* **(65):** 131-136.
30. Relyveld E.H., Bizzini B. and Gupta R.K. (1998) Rational approaches to reduce adverse reactions in man to vaccines containing tetanus and diphtheria toxoids. *Vaccine.* 16 **(9-10):** 1016-1023.
31. Robbins J.B. Schneerson R. (1990) Polysaccharide-protein conjugates: a new generation of vaccines. *J. Infect. Dis.* 161 **(5):** 821-832.
32. Scarselli M., Giuliani M. M., Adu-Bobie J., Pizza M. and Rappuoli R. (2005). The impact of genomics on vaccine design. *Trends in Biotechnology.* 23 **(20):** 84-91.
33. Shapiro C.N. and Margolis H.S. (1990) Hepatitis B epidemiology and prevention. *Epidemiol. Rev.* **(12):** 221-227.
34. Spier, R.E. (1997). The 3rd European Conference on Vaccinology: Building lifelong immunity,: Berlin. *Vaccine.* **(15):** 1163-1164.
35. Tindle R.W. (1997) Immunomanipulative strategies for the control of human papillomavirus associated cervical disease. *Immunol. Res.* 16 **(4):** 387-400.
36. Tiollais P., Buendia MA. (1991) Hepatitis B virus. *Sci. Am.*, 264 **(4):** 116-123.
37. Vogel F.R. (1995) Immunologic adjuvants for modern vaccine formulations. *Ann. N.Y. Acad. Sci.* **(754):** 153-160.
38. Vos A, Muller T., Schuster P., Schluter H. and Neubert A. (2000). Oral vaccination of foxes against rabies with SAD B19 in Europe, 1983-1998: a review. *Veterinary Bulletin.* **(70):** 1-5.
39. *Weekly Epidemiological Record: WHO* **(70):** 221-228 (1995).
40. West D.J., Calandra G.B. (1996) Vaccine induced immunologic memory for hepatitis B surface antigen: implications for policy on booster vaccination. *Vaccine* 14 **(11):** 1019-1027
41. Wiebe M.E. and May L.H., in Lubiniecki A.S. ed. (1990), *Large-Scale Mammalian Cell Culture Technology*. Dekker, New York, pp. 147-160.
42. Willson R.C. and Ladisch M.R., in Ladisch M.R., Willson R.C., Painton C-d.C., Builder S.E. eds. (1989) *Protein Purification from Molecular Mechanisms to Large-Scale Processes*, AChS Press, pp. 1-13.
43. Zuckerman A.J. (1990) Vaccines against hepatitis A and B. *Baillieres Clin. Gastroenterol.* **(4):** 775-788.

CHAPTER 30

Synthetic Biological Technology

Engineering of new biological components, organisms and redesigning the existing ones comprises the newly emerging field of "Synthetic Biology". It brings biology parallel to engineering with requirement for standardized components and defined functions. Initially tools of synthetic biology were used for understanding of complex cellular mechanisms by building of simple synthetic models.

In recent years, advances in key technologies like fast and error-free *de novo* DNA synthesis, high-throughput DNA sequencing and advances in computer algorithm for building synthetic genes have contributed immensely to this field. The basic building blocks of synthetic biology are called "bio bricks" and a library of standardized biological components is maintained in Massachusetts Institute of Technology, USA. Since 2004, an annual International Genetically Engineered Machine Contest is being held, where a number of amazing cellular devices built by the synthetic biologists are displayed. Using "synthetic genomics", a synthetic species of bacteria, *Mycoplasma laboratorium* was recently created. Even though the field is nascent, it has found practical applications in human medicine, veterinary medicine, agriculture and industry. The most notable applications are artificial synthesis of antimalarial drug artemisinin and in renewable energy production and environmental decontamination. Since it has the potential to create new life with unpredictable behavior, extreme caution and ethics are needed to be adopted for its use.

Keywords: Synthetic biology, bio bricks, biofuel; metabolic pathway.

INTRODUCTION

Synthetic biology is a newly emerging exciting field of science. The name "Synthetic Biology" was coined by a Polish geneticist, Waclaw Szybalski in 1974. A few years later, Barbara Hobom used the term to describe genetically engineered bacteria. Interest in this field is driven by diverse groups of scientists like biologists, chemists, engineers and rewriters. The tools provide biologists with means for testing current understanding of biological systems. The engineers can finally use biology as any other technology. It excites rewriters to prove that the genes encoding biological systems can be rewritten.

Till recently, genetic and biochemical manipulations were used to study different genetic pathways in cells. Answer to many biological questions depends on how interaction among genes and proteins forming genetic circuits gives rise to specific cellular function. These questions can probably be answered using the tools of newly emerging field of synthetic biology. With the help of modern technologies, one can construct and analyze synthetic genetic circuits based on their natural counterparts. Such synthetic circuits can be used as simple *in vivo* models to understand the relations between structure and functions of a genetic circuit. To elaborate it further, usually biologists work out the working of different phenomena in cells by gradually breaking and reassembling them. A very common example usually given by pioneers of synthetic biology is the working of the circadian clock (day and night cycle) in Drosophila. The genes and proteins involved have been isolated using different genetic and biochemical methods. Even then the mechanisms have not been completely worked out and many fundamental questions remain difficult to answer. To answer all these questions, one can design and build new circuits using similar genes and proteins and study their dynamics in the organism, as was recently done for yeast regulatory networks. In fact, several simple genetic clocks have been constructed in bacteria. Even though they are not as perfect, they provide a synthetic approach to understanding of genetic circuits.

Definition: The most widely accepted definition of synthetic biology is: Synthetic biology involves engineering of new biological components and organisms and the redesigning of the existing ones.

CONCEPTS AND PRINCIPLES

In many cases, knowledge about the functioning of various pathways in living cells is not sufficient to explain the total happenings inside a cell. As elaborated by Sprinzak *et al.* (2005), there may be several reasons for lack of complete understanding:

(i) Several interactions in the pathways may be missed.

(ii) Certain interactions that are not actively involved in the pathways *in vivo* are thought to be involved, i.e., may be one of the proteins is actually not expressed under the relevant conditions.

(iii) Incomplete understanding of the rules regulating proteins and gene interaction inside the living cells, e.g., *in vivo* values of kinetic parameters such as affinities, binding and degradation rates, etc. are not yet fully worked out.

(iv) Intracellular environment is intrinsically 'noisy', i.e., so many different reactions are always occurring simultaneously. Small copy numbers of molecular species limit the predictability of biochemical reactions in real living cells.

(v) These factors make interpretations and conclusions drawn from different reactions, completely or slightly erroneous.

Reconstructive (Synthetic) Approach

On the other hand, a reconstructive (synthetic) approach to genetic circuits may avoid the above-mentioned problems. Here genetic circuits are synthesized from scratch out of well characterized components such as genes, proteins, regulatory sequences etc. and introduced into the living cells (bacteria etc.), and their dynamics in living cells are observed. As again elaborated by Sprinzak et al., there are several advantages of this approach.

- New circuits or pathways for a particular function can be built from the current understanding and tested. It may be possible that the newly designed circuit can be tested in living cells without interfering other cellular functions.
- For carrying out one function, many different circuits may be built and compared.

Therefore, synthetic genetic circuits can function as physical models of natural genetic circuits, e.g., understanding of protein interaction will facilitate design of synthetic interacting proteins. In fact, novel functionality could be obtained by recombining protein modules as in case of polydactyl zinc finger DNA binding proteins. Using tools of synthetic biology, some degree of functional re-programming has also been achieved in the level of protein-protein interactions in case of signaling proteins. Recent technologies of molecular biology such as chemical synthesis of DNA molecules in the laboratory and recombinant DNA techniques have made synthetic pathway or circuit reconstruction possible. This field has benefited greatly from further advances in faster and longer DNA synthesis and rapid sequencing of DNA.

SYNTHETIC BIOLOGICAL TECHNOLOGY

The components used in synthetic biology: In order to build synthetic circuits, the required genetic components should be (1) well characterized, (2) modular (functions similarly in different systems) and (3) act independently of other cellular processes.

Frequently Used Components

Early synthetic biology experiments focused on the components used for transcription regulation in living cells, because they were relatively well understood and easy to configure. For example, repressors were used to create feedback loops in *E coli*; use of one repressor to understand noise suppression in cells, use of two repressors to understand bio-stability and use of three repressors to understand oscillation, etc.

However, many pathways in nature are controlled in non-transcriptional manner. For example, working of Cyanobacterial circadian clock is controlled by protein phosphorylation. So other interaction mechanisms such as protein modification, regulated degradation etc., are to be properly understood and models prepared for their use in synthetic biology.

Small molecules such as hormones and metabolites have also been used in synthetic biology. Fung *et al.* (2005) reported a creation of a synthetic "metabolator". In their synthetic circuit, transcriptional control of metabolic enzymes was used to create oscillation between 2 metabolic pools, Acetyl CoA verses Acetyl phosphate and acetate. This principle was later used to produce amorha 4, 11, diene, a precursor of artemisinin, an antimalarial drug. Using synthetic biology, metabolic enzymes from plants, yeasts and *E. coli* were arranged in synthetic pathways for this purpose.

After at least thirteen years of trial, Palsson's group has recently reported a genome scale reconstruction of *E. coli* metabolic network. Synthetic metabolic pathway construction has the potential to enable synthesis of medically important components and may also shed light on the fundamental issues of pathway design. In recent times, protein engineering and advances in synthetic biology has expanded the technologies available to metabolic engineers, so that multi-genic changes rather than single pathway manipulations could be achieved in cells.

Other small diffusible molecules, which are naturally used for communications between cells, have also been used in synthetic biology. One of the small molecules, AHL (acryl homoserine lactone), a signaling molecule present in diverse bacteria, was used to generate a simple multicellular patterning system in *E. coli*. In this model, mixed population of modified *E. coli* strains were placed in a Petri dish. The sender strains placed in the centre of a Petri dish produced AHL that diffused away. A second set of receiver strains contained a synthetic transcriptional circuit that combined positive and negative responses to AHL, thereby served as a ring of band pass detector. Band pass detector strains responded to specific ranges of AHL either positively or negatively using synthetic detector circuit components. Depending on the concentration gradient of AHL present in the Petri dish, fluorescent output gene was expressed only in bacteria within a specific range of distance from the centre producing colour in a ring form. They included two different detector strains (green and red) to be turned on at specific distances from the source, therefore concentric ring pattern of the gene expression appeared in red and green. Recently, Balagadde created an *E. coli* predator-prey ecosystem using complex synthetic circuits. Here, two populations of *E. coli* were created from a single strain by introduction of complex synthetic circuits. When placed together, they could influence each other population density using interconnected quorum sensing modules.

Recently, RNA molecules have also been used in synthetic biology and a vast amount of work is going on in the field of micro RNAs—the *trans*-acting RNA molecules (micro RNAs). As predicted by Sprinzak, these have potential for use in synthetic biology as they are versatile and use sequence based targeting mechanism. Synthetic variants of miRNAs have been used to understand micro RNA function in cells. Synthetic mi RNAs has also been used to understand their role in interferon modulation in viral infections.

Key Technologies for Synthetic Biology

Several technologies hold the key for future growth in synthetic biology; sequencing and fabrication of DNA in large scale, and availability of quality standardized biological parts. Availability of standardized methods and components in biological engineering will make design libraries of compatible parts available and outsourcing possible.

For fast and error-free synthesis of long pieces of DNA, scientists are nowadays using microarray technology to do parallel synthesis of large amount of DNA simultaneously. Selection oligos or naturally occurring enzymes are being used for rapid error correction. Releasable parallel synthesis and error correction makes it possible to assemble long relatively error free DNA constructs rapidly and cheaply. Recently, a Quantum behaved Particle Swarm Optimization (QPSO) algorithm has been developed for optimizing the codon usage in synthetic genes, which will make synthetic gene production easier. In recent years, advances in rapid and high throughput DNA sequencing techniques have become available, which will be of great help for synthetic biologists.

Library of Biological Components

A group of scientists at the Massachusetts Institute of Technology, USA have developed/and developing a library of biological components similar to the libraries available to chip designers. The registry of standard biological parts should facilitate a wide range of biological building projects. So far the registry contains more than 1000 individual components called Bio Bricks.

Bio Bricks

Bio Brick standard biological components are DNA sequences with defined structure and function. The term "Bio Brick" was introduced By Tom Knight, Drew Endy and Christopher Voigt. Each Bio Brick consists of DNA sequences, usually held in a circular plasmid, with flanking regions containing known restriction sites, which enables it to be joined with others and make bigger structures. The term "Brick" brings the parallel with engineering. The three basic types of Bio Bricks are (i) Parts: (building blocks encoding basic biological function), (ii) Devices: (collection of parts implementing some defined function), (iii) Systems: (performing higher level tasks). The working group at MIT has also defined a standard for signal transduction in synthetic biology, polymerase per second "POPS" akin to the current in a wire connecting two electronic components.

Example of a Bio Brick

In 2000, the first basic biological circuit elements, i.e., a ring oscillator and a toggle switch was built. In the synthetic ring oscillator, the basic circuit consisted of a plasmid containing 3 genes *tet R, LacI and λcI*, encoding proteins Tet R, LacI and λcI respectively. Lac I protein binds to *tel R* promoter, λcl protein binds to *LacI* promoter, and tet R protein binds to *λCI* promoter. These proteins binding to the promoters block polymerase from binding and inhibit gene transcription. So, manufacture of 3 proteins remains in an oscillatory cycle (Figure 30.1). When one of the protein products in this cycle was also linked to a gene for making green fluorescent protein and the entire circuit was inserted in bacteria, oscillation of this device could be observed as the bacteria blinked on and off like holiday lights. Latest versions of genetic toggle switches are being used to programme bacteria to detect cellular DNA damage and then report their findings by arranging themselves into bio-films.

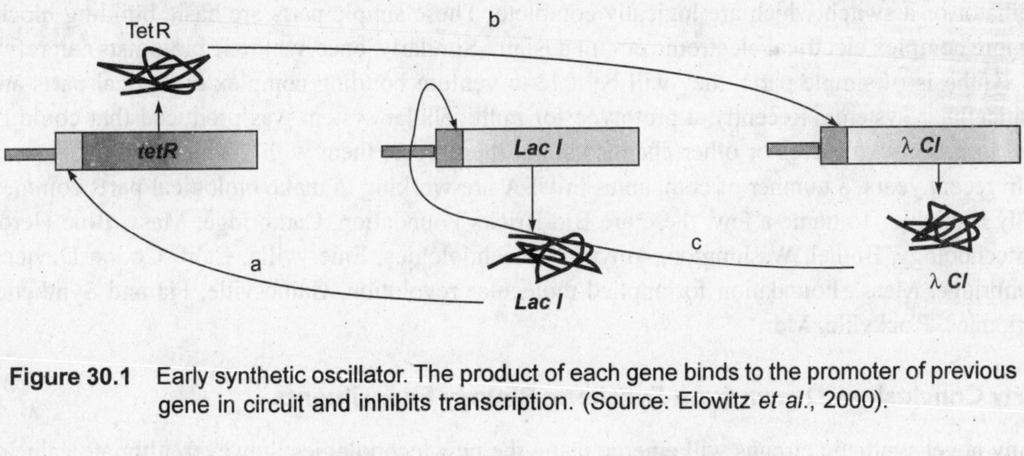

Figure 30.1 Early synthetic oscillator. The product of each gene binds to the promoter of previous gene in circuit and inhibits transcription. (Source: Elowitz *et al.*, 2000).

International Genetically Engineered Machines: (IGEM) Contest

The first course in Bio Fab engineering with biological parts was offered by MIT in 2003. An annual competition is being held from 2004 onwards, in which university students participate in the International Genetically Engineered Machine (IGEM) contest. The main goals of IGEM program, as stated in their site are: (a) to enable the systematic engineering of biology; (b) to promote open and transparent development of tools for synthetic biology, and (c) to help to build a society that constructively applies tools of synthetic biology (IGEM publicity page: 2007). From 5 participating teams in 2006, the competition grew to 34 teams with 400 students in 2006. Some of the projects in 2006 included: (1) creation of images and dynamic patterns using engineered bacteria; (2) engineering bacteria for controlled movement; (3) programming bacterial cells to create computational logic devices; (4) demonstration of engineered bacteria to detect important environmental chemicals (arsenic, hydrogen or metals); (5) programming the differentiation of mouse stem cells; (6) engineering bacteria to produce new scents like banana etc. and (7) modification of human cell lines to resist sepsis. Over the years, the contest has generated a number of amazing cellular devices, including bio-films that can record and display a photograph, as well as programmed cells that are able to sense and respond like switches to small molecular inputs such as caffeine. The most amazing synthetically built device demonstrated was smart bacteria that "photograph" a light pattern as a high – definition chemical image. In this system, synthetic sensor kinases were introduced inside *E. coli* cells. As a result *E. coli* behaved as a biological photographic film. Projection of a pattern of light onto the lawn of engineered *E. coli* produced high (up to 100 mega pixel per square inch) chemical image. This system may have potential applications like bacterial microlithography and in the study of multicellular signaling networks. The students participating in IGEM contest may represent the first generation of biological engineers. Until now biotechnology has been characterized by self-contained teams working to develop single purpose applications such as drug compounds. Much of the future of biological technology will require many different groups to contribute to subsystems.

Parallel with Engineering

The synthetic biological circuits are very similar in function to the early engineering circuits, like oscillator or a switch which are logically complete. These simple parts are basic building blocks of more complex electrical/electronic circuit design. Similarly, once synthetic biologists can refine the synthesis of simple parts, they will be able to venture building complex biological parts and multicellular systems. Recently, a prototype for multicellular system was produced that could be used to detect explosives or other chemicals and then report them with visible signal.

In recent years, a number of companies in USA are working to make biological parts commercially available. To name a few, these are Bio-Bricks Foundation, Cambridge, Mass, Blue Heron Biotechnology, Bothel, Washington, Amyris Biotechnologies, Emeryville, Calif, Codon Devices, Cambridge, Mass., Foundation for applied molecular revolution, Gainesville, Fla and Synthetics Genomics, Rockville, Md.

Early Conclusions Drawn from Synthetic Biology Experiments

Many novel synthetic circuits will emerge using the new technologies; however, ultimate value of this field will depend on what general principles it reveals after the use of synthetic circuits in living cells. According to Springzak and Elowitz, the early pioneers of synthetic biology, so far several important lessons have emerged from early results. The intracellular environment is too complex. Most mathematical models are based on laboratory experiments in test tubes, which are very different from real living cells.

Intracellular environment is variable. Many cellular molecules exist in low copy numbers. Therefore, stochastic effects or intrinsic noise (the effect of other biochemical reactions occurring simultaneously) can be significant. It makes the real effect of a particular biochemical reactions occurring inside a cell become partly unpredictable, therefore difficult to model. Moreover the cells are surrounded by other cells and they differ from one another in many ways. The events in which one cell affects the neighboring cell in some ways is called, 'extrinsic noise'. There is also interplay between these 2 types of noises. Some events in one cellular component such as transcription factor production may contribute to extrinsic noise in other cellular components, e.g., effect on its target genes. Synthetic biology is instrumental in probing both types of noises and revealing the strong effect they have on function of genetic circuits. It has become evident that extrinsic component of the noise makes a dominant contribution to the total noise.

Usually synthetic biologists rearrange modular elements to create novel circuits. Moreover combinational libraries of many possible circuits can be used for building a specific circuit. Recently, Guet created a synthetic circuit slot machine in which each of the 3 transcriptional regulatory genes could be controlled by one of the 5 possible promoters. The resulting library was screened for response to 2 different chemical inputs that interacted with 2 of the repressors. A surprisingly large fraction of the combinations worked and produced effects. In some cases the same circuit architecture produced different functions, whereas in some others, the same function was encoded by circuits with different architecture. So it was possible to obtain rich functional diversity from relatively small number of components.

Technical Challenges Faced by Synthetic Biologists

Constructing a functional synthetic biological machine requires assembling diverse genetic elements and getting them to work together. In general, combining disparate components requires the tuning of different biochemical parameters such as affinities and rate constants, which is often difficult to implement in biological circuits. Scientists are working on these aspects. Now several approaches are being used for this:

- Use of tunable element such as transcription factors derived from known elements. This allows external control over some parameters.
- One can screen libraries of mutated components to find out which component works better.
- Using robust designs that are insensitive to unknown or variable parameters.

A related challenge is computational modeling of genetic circuits. Modeling is essential both for analysis of natural system and also for design of synthetic ones. Ultimately it would be desirable to have computer aided design tools for synthetic biology as is being done in other fields of engineering.

APPLICATIONS OF SYNTHETIC BIOLOGICAL TECHNOLOGY

The main goals of these synthetic circuit paradigm or synthetic biology are to better understand the natural circuits by building minimal replica circuits; observing their dynamics *in vivo* and comparing them to one another and to their natural counterparts. In recent years, reconstruction of metabolic networks of *E. coli* has reached the genome scale. These constructed networks are being utilized for purposes of metabolic engineering, model directed discoveries, interpretation of phenotypic screens, analysis of network properties and studies of evolutionary processes.

As was elegantly described by Benner *et al*. (2005), work in this field is going on with the aims of:

(i) chemical synthesis of a large repertoire of genetic components;
(ii) to develop DNA polymerase for better handling artificial genetic systems;
(iii) to incorporate artificial genetic systems in experimental evolutionary processes;
(iv) to use synthetic biology in chemical evolution in artificial environments; and
(v) to use synthetic biology in diagnostics, detection and genotyping systems.

In this context, "Synthetic Genomics", a nascent field of synthetic biology has emerged. In this naturally occurring genes in their life form are not used. Rather it uses custom designed nucleotide base pairs for making the parts. Using this approach, a planned partially synthetic species of a bacterium, *Mycoplasma laboratorium* was being synthesized in J Craig Ventor Institute, USA. In this effort, also called the "Minimal Genome Project", genes were systematically removed from *Mycoplasma genitalium* to build *Mycoplasma laboratorium*, with minimal set of genes that can sustain life.

Synthetic biology can be and has been used to learn about fidelity in signal transduction. Park *et al*. (2003) used a synthetic approach to study how signal fidelity is maintained within pathways that share components. The study was done in yeast cells, where both the mating pheromone and osmolarity stress response pathways are signaled through mitogen activated protein kinase (MAP Kinases) ste11; yet there are no cross responses. They built synthetic components of the 2 pathways and rewired them differently from nature. They could demonstrate that by rewiring, pheromones induced osmoregulatory responses and vice versa. So it was concluded that the proximity of the components was more important for signal transduction and there are simple ways in which signal transduction pathways can evolve.

Synthetic biology can be used to discover which other natural circuit designs are possible given realistic biological components, and which of these operate reliably *in vivo*. This can be achieved by building and characterizing a variety of alternative circuit designs in living cells. Non-natural (synthetic) designs may prove useful for biotechnology applications. The most intriguing problem is how a synthetic circuit operates in the context of a complete organism.

The potential applications of synthetic biology, as discussed in MIT Synthetic Biology working group brain storming session in 2003, were very promising (Open Wet Ware). However, since the field is nascent, the potential benefits/ products are not yet fully actualized. It holds great promises for medical sciences, veterinary sciences, agricultural sciences and industry, in general. The various fields in which research is going on and some amount of progress that has been achieved are as follows.

Medical Applications

Cancer therapy: The broad categories of applications in health sciences are exploring new ways of combating disease by rapid early diagnosis using multiplexing approach for infections and cancer. Studies using synthetic biology are going on for programming bacteria or viruses to identify malignant cells and deliver therapeutic agents. As recently reviewed by Cattaneo *et al*. (2008), viruses can be converted into oncolytic vectors with the use of synthetic biology. They can be used for cancer cell targeting by incorporating cancer cell specificity. For cancer therapy, they can be armed with cancer pro-drug convertases and cytokines. Coating them with polymers or different envelopes or capsid proteins will make these evade host immune response.

Synthesis of specific enzymes for gene therapy: Synthetic biology has great potential for gene therapy, especially for delivery, using the above approach. The most shining example of use of synthetic biology in medicine is the artificial synthesis of anti-malarial wonder drug, artemisinin (C-15 sees quiterpene). The sweet worm plant (normally found in Northern China) produces too little of artemisinin, making it expensive and unaffordable in Africa and Asia. In the plants, artemisinin is synthesized using a total of nine genes in mevalonate pathway. Each gene is approximately 1500 bp long. One group of researchers at Lawrence Berkeley National Laboratories, Physical Bio Sciences Division and Chemical Engineering Department of University of California at Berkeley, USA are trying for last several years to copy all these genes and insert them into *E. coli* to mass produce the drug. They have been able to redesign the key subsets of the gene and produce an artemisinin precursor called amorphadiene; yield being 1,00,000 times greater than in plants. Further increase in yield to the point of making the drug widely available would require re-engineering of entire artemisinin pathway, and the scientists working on it and are almost there.

Pathogen destruction: Synthetic biology approach is also being uesd to understand DDT and other insecticide resistance in mosquitoes. Scientists are also using synthetic biology to produce anti-cancer drugs, which were highly effective but limited in supply due to tricky natural sources—isoprenoids like Eluntherobin having natural sources as marine coral, or Taxol having natural sources as a plant. Efforts are being made to produce analogues of other anti-cancer drugs like epothilones using synthetic biology. Synthetic biology holds a great potential for the synthesis of compounds for pathogen destruction, mostly multidrug resistant bacteria. Bio-films are crucial in pathogenesis of many infections, especially device related infections and are usually associated with tenacious resistance to antimicrobials. With the aid of synthetic biology, an engineered bacteriophage expressing biofilm degrading enzymes during infections has been developed, which will be very helpful in combating infections in which biofilms play an important role.

Anti-HIV drugs: Synthetic biology approach is being used to synthesize newer anti-HIV drugs. It has also provided newer hopes for HIV vaccine with artificial antigens. It has also been helpful in the design and synthesis of HIV proteins: Type 1 proteases of HIV could be synthesized using synthetic biology and this will be helpful in understanding pathogenesis. Using synthetic biology approach, SARS virus and new flu virus (Avian influenza virus) were characterized in record time. Protein based vaccine could be designed against them in record time.

Synthetic catalytic scavengers: Artificial antioxidants have been demonstrated to extend cellular life in *C. elegans* and have shown some promise in mice. They act like other antioxidants.

Veterinary Applications

Majority of the applications of synthetic biology in human health can be potentially applied to animal health. Multiplexing approach can use synthetic biology for rapid cancer and disease diagnosis in animals similar to human diseases.

Synthetic biology approach is being used for the development of vaccines against different animal diseases like anthrax, psittacosis etc and fish diseases. In fact an oral vaccine is being developed for fish using potato tubers for vaccine production and delivery using synthetic biology. This vaccine includes gut adhesion molecule and a viral peptide. The gut adhesion molecule mediates binding to and uptake in gut, viral protein acting as antigen and evoking immune response. This can be given as standard dietary feed pellet.

The environmental pollutants like Endocrine Disrupting Chemicals (EDC) present in pesticides, household cleaning agent surfactants, etc., which are present in municipal and industrial effluents, sewage plants, etc. and are going to water bodies affect fertility in fish and other aquatic creatures. Using synthetic biology approach (Vg gene induction in aquatic invertebrates and fish), the presence of these substances in water bodies can be assessed. For experimental purposes, three-dimensional extracellular matrix substrates have been developed for animal cell culture.

Agricultural Applications

A synthetic biology approach is being used for augmenting the defense pathways in plants to control pests, diseases and weeds. For example, in near future it will be possible to develop insect resistant transgenic maize expressing protease inhibitors. Moreover, newer classes of agricultural fungicides are being developed with the aid of synthetic biology.

Synthetic biology approach is being used to improve the grass land soil by addition of synthetic sheep urine. Genetically modified Rhizobia have been released into the fields to contribute to nodulation. Moreover, application of synthetic biology will be helpful in increasing food safety, nutrition and development of the product in the gradients. Natural raspberry ketones have been produced in enngineered bacteria.

Industrial Applications

As reviewed recently by R Patnaik from Du Pont Central Research and Developenment Laboratory, USA, synthetic biology has found many applications in industry for various purposes especially for development of "green technologies", moreover the primary metabolic pathways of many industrial organisms has been engineered in the laboratory. To elaborate a few applications:

Renewable bio-fuel using synthetic biology

Synthetic biology will be helpful in converting cheap renewable resources into energy rich molecules, production of inexpensive drugs including antimicrobials, and decontamination of polluted sites using engineered bacteria. Production of biofuels is the greatest dream of synthetic biologists. LS9, Inc, a San Francisco based company, is specializing in the development of renewable biofuels using synthetic biology. A number of US based companies, Amyris Biotechnologies, Codexis, Gevo, Mascoma and SunEthanol are trying to convert non-food biomass into fuel. Most of them are designing microbes that will digest crop in a refinery.

Cheap, high yield hydrogen production

For a long time scientists have realized that conversion of organics in waste water into hydrogen gas can do both waste reduction and renewable energy production. Hydrogen is already being tested as an important alternative to fossil fuel. In nature, green algae and cyanobacteria can split water using photosynthesis to produce molecular hydrogen. Using synthetic biology, the relevant components of the bacteria can be synthesized and used for hydrogen production. European Union funded Bio Modular H2 project is working towards this end. In an experiment, a synthetic pathway consisting of 13 enzymes derived from 5 different organisms including *Bacillus subtilis* has been developed to produce H_2 from cellulose.

Decontamination of environment

There is a possibility of using synthetic alternatives of metabolic and genetic control mechanism of microorganisms capable of biodegradation, to be put into use, especially for more efficient biodegradation of hazardous environmental contaminants like heavy metals.

Biofuel production from corns

Using synthetic biology approach efforts are being made to produce more ethanol from corn, and even from leaves and stalks. The US based company, Agrivida, is trying to insert a gene that will make an enzyme, which gets activated once the corn is heated to $60^{\circ}C$ and attacks cell wall making more ethanol. Phospholipase A(2) plays an important role in the production of lysophospholipids. Till date, they were made from bovine or porcine pancreas. Recently, using a synthetic biology approach, they have been produced in genetically engineered *E. coli*.

Synthesis of enzymes from scratch

David Baker and his team from University of Washington has recently created eight enzymes from scratch using synthetic biology to catalyse two reactions for Kemp elimination for which no natural enzymes existed. Moreover, enzymes like proteinase K could be synthesized using synthetic biology, which will make it cheap and easily available.

Future Prospects of Synthetic Biology Technology

One concern while building synthetic genetic circuits is the effects they might have on endogenous cellular functions. Ideally one would like the circuit to operate independently of the rest of the cells, but the limits to such independence remain unclear. Over the last few years, there is a global concern about the danger of synthetic biology becoming a double-edged sword because of its ability to create new life with the possibility that the creators will not be able to predict its exact behavior. This can potentially harm environment, humankind, and society (bio-weapons), and may have effects on natural evolution in many possible ways. The main concerns are about the new types of microbes (bacteria, viruses etc) created in the laboratory for which treatment will be difficult to find. Once synthetic life will be created, its impact will be permanent. The ethical, legal and practical issues arising from this will be numerous, and proper evaluation of these needs to be done before its creation. Therefore, in every meeting of synthetic biologists from 2004 onwards, the scientists discussed about the biological risks, safety, security and public understanding of this new science and tried to formulate a moral code of conduct for themselves.

Advances Towards Creation of Synthetic Life

The most exciting and recent advance in synthetic biology technology towards creation of a synthetic life came in May 2010. Researchers at J Craig Ventor Institute in Rockville, Maryland, USA led by Dr J Craig Ventor published the successful transplantation of fully functional complete synthetic genome (1.1 Mb) of *Mycoplasma mycoides* into *Mycoplasma capricoloum* cell. The progeny bacterial cells formed typical *Mycoplasma mycoides* colonies, that contains only synthetic genome identified by the introduced "water mark" DNA sequences and further verified by proteomic analysis. This feat was achieved after more than 10 years of work by 20 scientists and with an estimated $40 million cost.

Two landmark developments in the field made this possible: i.) Synthesis and assembly of full 538 kb *Mycoplasma genitalium* genome based on sequence data by the same group and ii.) Successful replacement of one bacterial genome by another. Latigue *et al.* cloned the full *Mycoplasma mycoides* genome into a yeast centromeric plasmid and transplanted it to a *Mycoplasma capricoloum* cell.

The synthetic genome of *Mycoplasma mycoides*. (1.1 Mb size) was created in steps. First, the researchers synthesized 1078 cassettes of 1080 bp each with 80 bp overlaps. Groups of these were recombined in yeast, to produce 109 assemblies of 10 kb each. The process was repeated with the 10 kb products to produce 11 assemblies of 100 kb each. The process was repeated to produce a single chromosome which was introduced in to *Mycoplasma capricoloum* cell. During synthesis, several short nucleotide sequences were introduced into the synthetic genome as "water mark" sequences to differentiate it from natural genome.

This remarkable work demonstrated conclusively that a functional bacterial genome could be reconstituted from an *in silico* copy based entirely on genome sequence data. Even though real applications and possible misuses will take time to come, this remains undoubtedly the most important achievement of synthetic biology technology till date.

CONCLUSION

There are no dotted lines inside the cells isolating circuits from one another. The ultimate test for this synthetic approach is to delete defective natural circuits and replace them with synthetic counterparts within organisms. This will require synthetic circuits to interface with rest of the cells. However, the most optimistic synthetic biologist would expect such circuits to be less functional than their natural counterparts.

The futurologists like Ian Pearson predict that, as simple viruses are now being synthesized in the laboratory by taking their genetic code from data base and reconstruction in laboratory, in the next few years the living bacteria from scratch may be created using tools of synthetic biology.

The nascent field of synthetic biology may learn lessons from synthetic chemists of earlier century to apply analytical and rational approaches in building novel biological systems.

FURTHER READINGS

1. Altmann K.H., Memmert K. (2008) Epothilones as lead structures for new anticancer drugs—pharmacology, fermentation, and structure-activity-relationships. *Prog. Drug. Res.* 66; **(273):** 275-334.
2. Alves R., Savageau M.A. (2000) Extending the method of mathematically controlled comparison to include numerical comparisons. *Bioinformatics.* 16; **(9):** 786-98.
3. Anderson J.C., Clarke E.J., Arkin A.P., Voigt C.A. (2006) Environmentally controlled invasion of cancer cells by engineered bacteria. *J. Mol. Biol.* 27; 355 **(4):** 619-27.
4. Baker D. (2008) Making the paper: David Baker: *Nature:* 453; 8 (7192):xii (e publication)
5. Baker D., Church G., Collins J., Endy D., Jacobson J., Keasling J., Modrich P., Smolke C., Weiss R (2006) Engineering life: building a fab for biology. *Sci. Am.* 294 **(6):** 44-51.
6. Balagaddé F.K., Song H., Ozaki J., Collins C.H., Barnet M., Arnold F.H., Quake S.R., You L. (2008) A synthetic *Escherichia coli* predator-prey ecosystem. *Mol. Syst. Biol.* **(4):** 187.
7. Basu S., Gerchman Y., Collins C.H., Arnold F.H., Weiss R. (2005) A synthetic multicellular system for programmed pattern formation. *Nature.* 28; 434 **(7037):** 1130-4.
8. Basu S., Mehreja R., Thiberge S., Chen M.T., Weiss R. (2004) Spatiotemporal control of gene expression with pulse-generating networks. *Proc. Natl. Acad. Sci. U S A.* 101 **(17):** 6355-60.
9. Becskei A., Serrano L. (2000) Engineering stability in gene networks by autoregulation. *Nature.* 405 **(6786):** 590-3.
10. Beekwilder J., van der Meer I.M., Sibbesen O., Broekgaarden M., Qvist I., Mikkelsen J.D., Hall R.D. (2007) Microbial production of natural raspberry ketone. *Biotechnol J.* 2 **(10):** 1270-9.
11. Belshe R.B. (2007) Translational research on vaccines: influenza as an example. *Clin. Pharmacol. Ther.* 82 **(6):** 745-9.
12. Benner S.A., Sismour A.M. (2005) Synthetic biology. *Nat. Rev. Genet.* 6 **(7):** 533-43.
13. Blancafort P., Segal D.J., Barbas C.F. (2004) Designing transcription factor architectures for drug discovery. *Mol. Pharmacol.* 66 **(6):** 1361-71.
14. Cai Y., Sun J., Wang J., Ding Y., Tian N., Liao X., Xu W. (2008) Optimizing the codon usage of synthetic gene with QPSO algorithm. *J. Theor. Biol.* 254 **(1):** 123-127.
15. Cattaneo R., Miest T., Shashkova E.V., Barry M.A. (2008) Reprogrammed viruses as cancer therapeutics: targeted, armed and shielded. *Nat. Rev. Microbiol.* 6 **(7):** 529-40.
16. Cello J., Paul A.V., Wimmer E. (2002) Chemical synthesis of poliovirus cDNA: generation of infectious virus in the absence of natural template. *Science.* 297 **(5583):** 1016-8.
17. Chang M.C., Keasling J.D. (2006) Production of isoprenoid pharmaceuticals by engineered microbes. *Nat. Chem. Biol.* 2 **(12):** 674-81.
18. Church G. (2005) Let us go forth and safely multiply. *Nature.* 438 **(7067):** 423.
19. Church GM (2006) Genomes for all. *Sci. Am.* 294 **(1):** 46-54.
20. Companjen A.R., Florack D.E., Bastiaans J.H., Matos C.I., Bosch D., Rombout J.H. (2005) Development of a cost-effective oral vaccination method against viral disease in fish. *Dev Biol.* (Basel). **(121):** 143-50.
21. Companjen A.R., Florack D.E., Slootweg T., Borst J.W., Rombout J.H. (2006) Improved uptake of plant-derived LTB-linked proteins in carp gut and induction of specific humoral immune responses upon in feed delivery. *Fish Shellfish Immunol.* 21 **(3):** 251-60.
22. Corich V., Giacomini A., Vendramin E., Vian P., Carlot M., Concheri G., Polone E., Casella S., Nuti M.P., Squartini A. (2007) Long term evaluation of field-released genetically modified rhizobia. *Environ. Biosafety Res.* **6 (3):** 167-81.

23. Dueber J.E., Yeh B.J., Chak K., Lim W.A. (2003) Reprogramming control of an allosteric signaling switch through modular recombination. *Science.* 301 **(5641):** 1904-8.
24. Editorial: *Nature:* (2004) Futures of artificial life: 431 **(7009):** 613
25. Elowitz M.B., Leibler S. (2000) A synthetic oscillatory network of transcriptional regulators. *Nature.* 403 **(6767):** 335-8.
26. Endy D. (2005) Foundations for engineering biology. *Nature*. 438 **(7067):** 449-53.
27. Expert Review on Vaccines: (2007) Artificial antigens for HIV vaccine design: Expert. *Rev. Vaccines:* 6 **(3):** 301
28. Feist AM, Palsson B.O. (2008) The growing scope of applications of genome-scale metabolic reconstructions using *Escherichia coli. Nat. Biotechnol.* 26 **(6):** 659-67.
29. Ford L.P., Cheng A. (2008) Using synthetic precursor and inhibitor miRNAs to understand miRNA function. *Methods. Mol. Biol.* **(419):** 289-301.
30. Forster A.C., Church G.M. (2006) Towards synthesis of a minimal cell. *Mol. Syst. Biol.* **(2):** 45.
31. Fung E., Wong W.W., Suen J.K., Bulter T., Lee S.G., Liao J.C. (2005) A synthetic gene-metabolic oscillator. *Nature.* 435 **(7038):** 118-22.
32. Gaertner H., Offord R., Botti P., Kuenzi G., Hartley O. (2008) Semisynthetc analogues of PSC-RANTES, a potent anti-HIV protein. *Bioconjug. Chem.* 19 **(2):** 480-489.
33. Gardner T.S., Cantor C.R., Collins J.J. (2000) Construction of a genetic toggle switch in *Escherichia coli. Nature.* 403 **(6767):** 339-42.
34. George D., Ferry N., Back E.J., Gatehouse A.M. (2008) Characterisation of midgut digestive proteases from the maize stem borer Busseola fusca. *Pest. Manag. Sci.* Jun. 6 (e publication)
35. Gibbs WW (2004) Synthetic life. *Sci. Am.* 290 **(5):** 74-81.
36. Gibson D.G., Benders G.A., Andrews-Pfannkoch C., Denisova E.A., Baden-Tillson H., Zaveri J., Stockwell T.B., Brownley A., Thomas D.W., Algire M.A., Merryman C., Young L., Noskov V.N., Glass J.I., Venter J.C., Hutchison CA 3rd, Smith HO (2008) Complete chemical synthesis, assembly, and cloning of a Mycoplasma genitalium genome. *Science*. 319 **(5867):** 1215-20.
37. Gibson D. G., Glass J.I., Lartigue C., Noskov V.N., Chuang R.Y., Algire M.A., Benders G.A., Mantague M.G., Ma L., Moodie M.M., Merryman C., Vashee S., Krishnakumar R., Assad-Garcia N., Andrew-Pfannkoch C., Denisova E.A., Young L., Qi Z.Q., Sequall-Shapiro T.H., Calvey C.H., Parmar PP, Hutchison CA3rd, Smith HO, Ventor JC. Creation of a bacterial cell controlled by chemically synthesized genome. *Science.* (2010) 329 (5987): 5256, Epub May 20th May 2010 (doi; 10.1126. *Science* 1190719)
38. Gibson D. G., Benders G.A., Andrew-Pfannkoch C., Denisova E.A., Baden-Tillson H., Zaveri J., Stockwell T.B., Brownely A., Thomas D.W., Algire M.A., Merryman C., Young L., Noskov V.N., Glass J.I., Ventor J.C., Hutchison CA3rd, Smith HQ. (2008) Complete chemical synthesis, assembly and cloning of *Mycoplasma genitalium* genome. *Science.* **(319):** 1215-1220.
39. Ginkel S.V., Sung S., Lay J.J. (2001) Biohydrogen production as a function of pH and substrate concentration. *Environ Sci. Technol.* 35 **(24):** 4726-30.
40. Graveley B.R. (2008) Molecular biology: power sequencing. *Nature*. 453 **(7199):** 1197-8.
41. Guet C.C., Elowitz M.B., Hsing W., Leibler S (2002) Combinatorial synthesis of genetic networks. *Science*. 296 **(5572):** 1466-70.
42. Hale V., Keasling J.D., Renninger N., Diagana T.T. (2007) Microbially derived artemisinin: a biotechnology solution to the global problem of access to affordable antimalarial drugs. *Am. J. Trop. Med. Hyg.* 77 (6 Suppl.): 198-202.
43. Hardin P.E. (2005) The circadian timekeeping system of Drosophila. *Curr. Biol.* 15 **(17):** R714-22.
44. Heinemann M., Panke S. (2006) Synthetic biology—putting engineering into biology. *Bioinformatics*. 22 **(22):** 2790-9.
45. Hobom B. (1980) Gene surgery: on the threshold of synthetic biology. *Med. Klin.* 75 **(24):** 834-41.

46. Hsu C.W., Juan H.F., Huang H.C. (2008) Characterization of micro RNA-regulated protein-protein interaction network. *Proteomics*. **(10):** 1975-9.

47. htpp://wwwTimes online.co.uk/tol/news/environment/article4133668.ece,2008,Scientists find bug that eat waste and excrete petrol.) Scientists find bug that eat waste and excrete petrol, Times June 14th.

48. Huang W., Zhao P.L., Liu C.L., Chen Q., Liu Z.M., Yang G.F. (2007) Design, synthesis, and fungicidal activities of new strobilurin derivatives. *J. Agric. Food. Chem.* 55 **(8):** 3004-10.

49. IGEM publicity page: (http:// igem2007.com)

50. Jiang L., Althoff E.A., Clemente F.R., Doyle L., Röthlisberger D., Zanghellini A., Gallaher J.L., Betker J.L., Tanaka F., Barbas CF 3rd, Hilvert D, Houk KN, Stoddard BL, Baker D (2008) De novo computational design of retro-aldol enzymes. *Science*. 319 **(5868):** 1387-91.

51. Johnson E.C., Malito E., Shen Y., Rich D., Tang W.J., Kent S.B., (2007) Modular total chemical synthesis of a human immuno deficiency virus type 1 protease. *J. Am. Chem. Soc.* 129 **(37):** 11480- 11490

52. Kaern M., Blake W.J., Collins J.J. (2005) Stochasticity in gene expression: from theories to phenotypes. *Nat. Rev. Genet.* 6 **(6):** 451-64.

53. Kaern M., William J. Blake, and J.J. Collins (2003) The engineering of gene regulatory networks. *Ann. Rev. Biomed. Eng.* **(5):** 179- 206

54. Keasling J.D. (2008) Synthetic biology for synthetic chemistry. *ACS Chem. Biol.* 3 **(1):** 64-76.

55. Kern A., Tilley E., Hunter I.S., Legisa M., Glieder A. (2007) Engineering primary metabolic pathways of industrial micro- organisms. *J. Biotechnol.* 129 **(1):** 6-29

56. Knight T. (2003) Idem potent Vector Design for standard assembly of Biobricks. MIT Synthetic Biology Working Group. http://hdl.handle.net/1721.1/21168.

57. Latrigue C. V. ashee S., Algire M.A., Chuang R.Y., Benders G.A., Ma L., Noskov V.N., Denisova E.A., Gibson D.G., Assad-Garcia N., Alperovich N., Thomas D.W., Merryman C., Hutchison CA3rd, Smith H.Q., Ventor J.C., Glass J.I. (2009) Creating bacterial cells from genomes that have been cloned and engineered in yeast. *Science*. **(325):** 1693-1696

58. Lee D.Y., Yun C., Cho A., Hou B.K., Park S., Lee S.Y. (2006) WebCell: a web-based environment for kinetic modeling and dynamic simulation of cellular networks. *Bioinformatics*. 22 **(9):** 1150-1.

59. Lemerle C., Di Ventura B., Serrano L. (2005) Space as the final frontier in stochastic simulations of biological systems. *FEBS Lett.* 579 **(8):** 1789-94.

60. Levskaya A., Chevalier A.A., Tabor J.J., Simpson Z.B., Lavery L.A., Levy M., Davidson E.A., Scouras A., Ellington A.D., Marcotte E.M., Voigt C.A. (2005) Synthetic biology: engineering *Escherichia coli* to see light. *Nature*. 438 **(7067):** 441-2.

61. Liao J., Warmuth M.K., Govindarajan S., Ness J.E., Wang R.P., Gustafsson C., Minshull J. (2007) Engineering proteinase K using machine learning and synthetic genes. *BMC Biotechnol.* **(7):** 16.

62. Lu T.K., Collins J.J. (2007) Dispersing biofilms with engineered enzymatic bacteriophage. *Proc. Natl. Acad. Sci. U S A*. 104 **(27):** 11197-202.

63. Luo Ruoyu, Liao Sha, Zeng Shaoqun, Li YiXue, Luo Q.M. (2006) Flux Explorer: A general platform for modeling and analyses of metabolic networks based on stoichiometry *Chin. Sci. Bull.* 51 **(6):** 689-696.

64. Markert Y., Mansfeld J., Schierhorn A,. Rücknagel K.P., Ulbrich-Hofmann R. (2007) Production of synthetically created phospholipase A(2) variants with industrial impact. *Biotechnol. Bioeng.* Sep. 1; 98 **(1):** 48-59.

65. Martin V.J., Pitera D.J., Withers S.T., Newman J.D., Keasling J.D. (2003) Engineering a mevalonate pathway in Escherichia coli for production of terpenoids. *Nat Biotechnol.* 21 **(7):** 796-802.

66. Matozzo V., Gagné F., Marin M.G., Ricciardi F., Blaise C. (2008) Vitellogenin as a biomarker of exposure to estrogenic compounds in aquatic invertebrates: A review. *Environ Int*. 34 **(4):** 531-45.

67. Nair V., Uchil V., Chi G., Dans L., Cox A., Seo B. (2007) Biologically validated HIV integrase inhibitors with nucleobase scaffolds: structure, synthesis, chemical biology, molecular modeling and antiviral activity. *Nucleosides Nucleotides Nucleic Acids*.: 26 **(6-7):** 665-668.

68. Nakajima M., Imai K., Ito H., Nishiwaki T., Murayama Y., Iwasaki H., Oyama T., Kondo T. (2005) Reconstitution of circadian oscillation of cyanobacterial KaiC phosphorylation *in vitro*. *Science*. 308 **(5720):** 414-5.
69. Nitschke M., Pastore G.M. (2006) Production and properties of a surfactant obtained from *Bacillus subtilis* grown on cassava waste water. *Bioresour. Technol.* 97 **(2):** 336- 341.
70. Park S.H., Zarrinpar A., Lim W.A. (2003) Rewiring MAP kinase pathways using alternative scaffold assembly mechanisms. *Science.* 299 **(5609):** 1061-4.
71. Patnaik R. (2008) Engineering complex phenotypes in industrial strains. *Biotechnol Prog*. 24 **(1):** 38-47.
72. Pearson I. (2008) The future of life. Creating natural, artificial, synthetic and virtual organisms EMBO reports 9, S1, S75-S77.
73. Pedersen I.M., Guofeng Cheng, Stefan Wieland, Stefano Volinia, Carlo M. Croce, Francis V. Chisari & Michae David (2007) Interferon modulation of cellular microRNAs as an antiviral mechanism. *Nature*. 449 **(7164):** 919-922.
74. Price N.D., Reed J.L., Palsson B.O. (2004) Genome-scale models of microbial cells: evaluating the consequences of constraints.*Nat. Rev. Microbiol.* 2 **(11):** 886-97.
75. Rajesh R., Gunasekaran K., Muthukumaravel S., Balaraman K., Jambulingam P. (2007) *In silico* analysis of voltage- gated sodium channel in relation to DDT resistance in vector musquitoes. *In. Silico. Biol.* 7 **(4-5):** 413- 421.
76. Reed J.L., Palsson B.O. (2003) Thirteen years of building constraint-based in silico models of *Escherichia coli*. *J. Bacteriol.* 185 **(9):** 2692-9.
77. Reid A.J. It is alive (GENOME WATCH). *Natutre. Rev. Microbiol*. 2010.8(Jul): 468 The above paragraph is to be inserted as last but one paragraph (just before conclusion) in page no. 12 of the article "Synthetic biological technology", Chapter 30. The 4 references are for this paragraph.
78. Ro D. K., Paradise E.M., Quellet M., Fisher K.J., Newman K.L., Ndungu J.M., Ho K.A., Eachus R.A., Ham T.S., Kirby J., Chang M.C., Withers S.T., Shiba Y., Saprong R., Keasling J.D. (2006) Production of the anti malarial drug precursor artemisinic acid in engineered yeast. *Nature:* 440 **(7086):** 940-943).
79. Rooney D., Kennedy N., Deering L., Gleeson D., Clipson N. (2006) Effect of sheep urine deposition on the bacterial community structure in an acidic upland grassland soil. *Appl. Environ. Microbiol.* 72 **(11):** 7231-7.
80. Rosenfeld N., Alon U. (2003) Response delays and the structure of transcription networks. *J. Mol. Biol.* 13; 329 **(4):** 645-54.
81. Rosenfeld N., Elowitz M.B., Alon U. (2002) Negative autoregulation speeds the response times of transcription networks. *J. Mol. Biol.* 323 **(5):** 785-93.
82. Röthlisberger D., Khersonsky O., Wollacott A.M., Jiang L., DeChancie J., Betker J., Gallaher J.L., Althoff E.A., Zanghellini A., Dym O., Albeck S., Houk K.N., Tawfik D.S., Baker D. (2008) Kemp elimination catalysts by computational enzyme design. *Nature.* 453 **(7192):** 190-5.
83. Sathaliyawala T., Rao M., Maclean D.M., Birx D.L., Alving C.R., Rao B.V. (2006) Assembly of human immunodeficiency virus (HIV) antigens on bacteriophage T4: a novel *in vitro* approach to construct multi component HIV vaccines: *J. Virol.* 80 **(15):** 7688-7698.
84. Shivachandra S.B., Li Q, Peachman K.K., Matyas G.R., Leppla S.H., Alving C.R., Rao M., Rao V.B. (2007) Multi component anthrax toxin display and delivery using bacteriophage T4. *Vaccine:* 25 **(7):** 1225-1235.
85. Sprinzak D., Elowitz M.B. (2005) Reconstruction of genetic circuits. *Nature*. 438 **(7067):** 443-8.
86. Szybalski W. (1974) *In vivo* and *in vitro* initiation of transcription. P405 In: Kohn A. and Shatkay A. (eds). *Contol of Gene Expression.* pp. 23-*24 and Discussion* pp. 404-405. (Szybalski's concept of Synthetic Biology) 411-412, 415-417, New York: Plenum Press.

87. Tan D. .X., Manchester L.C., Terron M.P., Flores L.J., Reiter R.J. (2007) One molecule, many derivatives: a never ending interaction of melatonin with reactive oxygen and nitrogen species. *J. Pineal. Res.*: 42 **(1):** 28-42.

88. Tian J., Gong H., Sheng N., Zhou X., Gulari E., Gao X., Church G. (2004) Accurate multiplex gene synthesis from programmable DNA microchips. *Nature.* 432 **(7020):** 1050-4.

89. Tyo K.E., Alper H.S., Stephanopoulos GN (2007) Expanding the metabolic engineering toolbox: more options to engineer cells. *Trends Biotechnol.* 25 **(3):** 132-7.

90. Voytik-Harbin SL (2001) Three-dimensional extracellular matrix substrates for cell culture. *Methods Cell Biol.* **(63):** 561-81.

91. Wong D., Robertson G. (2004) Applying combinatorial chemistry and biology to food research. *J. Agric. Food. Chem.* 52 **(24):** 7187-98.

92. Yeh B.J., Lim W.A. (2007) Synthetic biology: lessons from the history of synthetic organic chemistry. *Nat. Chem. Biol.* 3 **(9):** 521-5.

93. Yokobayashi Y., Weiss R., Arnold F.H. (2002) Directed evolution of a genetic circuit. *Proc. Natl. Acad. Sci. U S A.* 99 **(26):** 16587-91.

94. Zhang M.Q., Wilkinson B. (2007) Drug discovery beyond the 'rule-of-five'. *Curr. Opin. Biotechnol.* 18 **(6):** 478-88.

95. Zhou J., Qiu C., Cao X.A., Lin G. (2007) Construction and immunogenicity of recombinant adenovirus expressing the major outer membrane protein (MOMP) of Chlamydophila psittaci in chicks. *Vaccine.* 25 **(34):** 6367-72.

96. Zhu J., Zhang B., Smith E.N., Drees B., Brem R.B., Kruglyak L., Bumgarner R.E., Schadt E.E. (2008) Integrating large-scale functional genomic data to dissect the complexity of yeast regulatory networks. *Nat. Genet.* 40 **(7):** 854-61.

CHAPTER

31

Bioengineering

Bioengineering is an interdisciplinary science which uses the principles of engineering to address the problems in biology and medicine. It thus leads to the development of innovative biologics, materials, processes, implant devices for the prevention, treatment and diagnosis of incurable diseases. Bioengineering has shown applications in medicine, agriculture and industry. Applicability of bioengineering to medicine has led to the development of new areas in medical sciences like regenerative medicine and tissue engineering. Concepts of tissue engineering are being applied for the restoration of damaged tissues and organs like skin, cornea, bone, cartilage, heart, CNS, etc. Bioengineering has been applied in agriculture for increasing the productivity and decreasing soil erosion by using superabsorbent polymers. It has the applicability in industry for the production of therapeutic proteins and purified cell population. Bioengineering being a multidisciplinary area educates a student in diverse fields so that they can gain technical expertise in biology and medicine simultaneously and contribute effectively in the development and improvement of health care solutions. This unique field encompasses bio-instrumentation, bio-materials, bio-mechanics, medical imaging, genetic engineering, orthopedic surgery cellular and tissue engineering. Bioengineering acts as a trendsetter in establishing a symbiotic relationship between the classical sciences like engineering, medicine, biology and physics with a goal to develop the overall health care facilities. With such a contribution to the society bioengineering tends to be a very important area both in terms of its applicability and in career development.

Keywords: Bioengineering, tissue engineering, regenerative medicine, medical devices, biomaterials, agriculture, industry.

INTRODUCTION

"Bioengineering" or "biological engineering" or "biotechnological engineering" is an emerging area which applies the principles of engineering to address the challenges in the fields like biology and medicine. Bioengineering has shown its applications in all the fields of life sciences and medicine like molecular biology, biochemistry, microbiology, immunology, neuroscience, regenerative medicine, etc. The word bioengineering was coined by British scientist and broadcaster Heinz Wolff in 1954. The term "bioengineering" was then used to describe an activity which was designed to make huge advances in technology applicable to biological science during the Second World War. Bioengineering can be differentiated from its originating sciences like pure biology and classical engineering. This differentiation can be qualified by the following relevant definitions: (a) "Bioengineering is the optimization of the performance of a task or set of tasks performed by a biological system through the application of engineering designing process". (b) According to the NIH definition of bioengineering "it integrates physical, chemical, mathematical science and engineering to study biology, medicine, behaviour and health. It further develops innovative biologics, materials, processes, implants, devices, and other informatics approaches for the prevention, diagnosis and treatment of some incurable diseases for improving the overall health of the society". Although there exists a very feeble boundary between bioengineering and biomedical engineering, bioengineering is broader in its application and at the same time it is restricted mainly to biological field unlike biomedical engineering where non-biological field do come under this terminology. Some opined that Biological Engineering (like biotechnology) has a broader base which spans molecular methods (tends to emphasize the use of biological substances—applying engineering principles to molecular biology, biochemistry, microbiology, pharmacology, protein chemistry, cytology, immunology, neurobiology and neuroscience, cellular and tissue based methods (including devices and sensors), whole organisms (plants, animals), and up increasing length scales to ecosystems. So biological engineers use the principles of basic biology and tools of classical engineering to create novel and economically beneficial products. Apart from using the conventional scientific areas, bioengineers also utilize the knowledge and expertise from other pure and applied sciences like, biomechanics, bioinformatics, bioreactor design, surface science and polymer science for devising new technologies. Bioengineers tend to either mimic biological systems to create medically valuable products or modify and control biological systems so that they can replace or sustain the chemical and mechanical processes. Bioengineering has originally emerged from other areas of sciences which is schematically depicted in Figure 31.1.

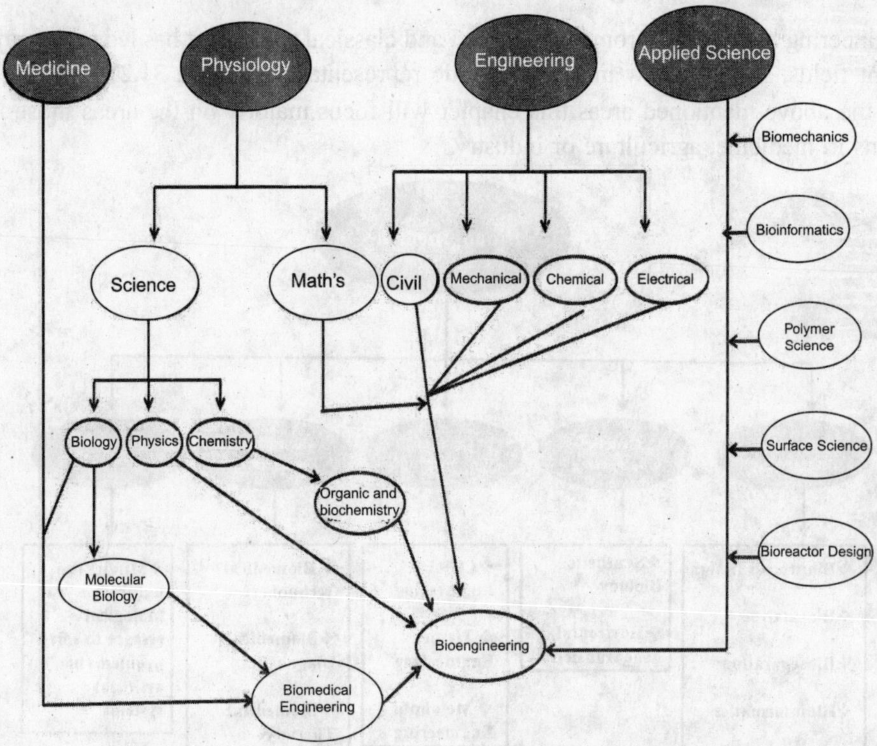

Figure 31.1 Schematic showing the emergence of bioengineering from different basic and applied fields of science.

CONCEPTS AND PRINCIPLES

Bioengineering is the application of the principles of engineering and natural sciences to tissues, cells and molecules. It utilizes the concept of "biomimesis" which means that it mimics the natural biological essence which is the chief factor in the phenomenon of healing and in the restoration of lost natural substances. Closely related to this is biotechnology, which deals with the implementation of biological knowledge in industrial, agricultural and medicinal processes. Applications from both fields are widely used in other applied areas like medical science, natural sciences and in engineering. Bioengineering is a field of biotechnology where biology is manipulated for benefits of humankind. It simply implies that life is basically a machine which takes in fuel and performs work by applying principles of physics and analytical chemistry. Life can be modified in a way able to perform certain special functions.

Bioengineering integrates physical, chemical, or mathematical sciences and engineering principles for the study of biology, medicine, behavior, or health. It advances fundamental concepts, creates knowledge for the molecular to the organ systems levels, and develops innovative biologics, materials, processes, implants, devices, and informatics approaches for the prevention, diagnosis, and treatment of disease, for patient rehabilitation, and for improving health.

Main Fields of Bioengineering

As bioengineering has evolved from both applied and classical sciences it has led to the emergence of different fields, shown below in the schematic representation (Figure 31.2).

Out of the above-mentioned areas this chapter will focus majorly on the areas those have the applications in medicine, agriculture or industry.

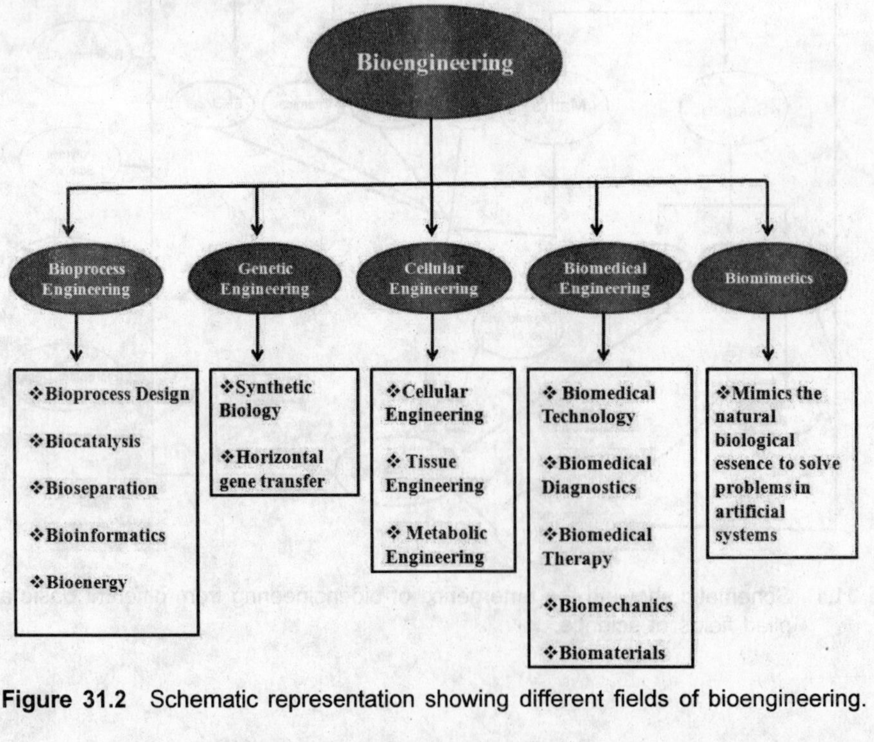

Figure 31.2 Schematic representation showing different fields of bioengineering.

APPLICATIONS OF BIOENGINEERING

Live cells have evolved over several billion years since the beginning of life into highly specialized units secreting bioactive molecules coded by DNA chains that have been selected during evolution while exposed to environments with limited resources. By using combinatorial bioengineering approach it is possible to attain an entirely new level of biotechnological research.

Medical Applications

In recent times the field of medicine has been revolutionised by the development of bioengineering area. Bioengineering applies its concepts to the medical field for the development of novel treatment strategies. Applications of bioengineering to medical sciences are discussed as follows:

Tissue engineering: Tissue engineering is a developing multifaceted area which has shown its applicability in the repair or replacement of damaged tissue or organ. The advances in tissue engineering can be credited to the significant advances in cell, molecular biology and biomaterials. According to Langer and Vancati (1993), Tissue Engineering can be defined as *"an interdisciplinary field that applies the principles of engineering and life sciences towards the development of biological substitutes that restore, maintain, or improve tissue function or a whole organ"*. Major aim of tissue engineering is to surpass the limitations of conventional repair strategies like organ transplantation and biomaterial implantation. It produces artificial immunotolerant organ and tissue substitutes those can be implanted in the patient, so this approach can be used as a permanent solution to damaged organs and thus avoiding the expensive treatments. One of the principle methods behind tissue engineering involves growing the relevant human or animal cells *in vitro* into the required three-dimensional (3D) organ or tissue. Such 3D tissue mimics are formed by seeding the appropriate cell type onto porous matrices, known as scaffolds. Scaffolds are generally fabricated from natural or synthetic polymers, so seeded cells attach and colonize the available surface in the 3D scaffold. Langer and his group have done pioneering work in the area of scaffold design that provide the fundamentals for tissue engineering As scaffold acts as a substrate for the cell adherence it is an important component of tissue engineering. Other important components are growth factors or bioactive components. Figure 31.3 is the schematic representation of components of tissue engineering.

Scaffold being the crucial component of tissue engineering should possess desirable properties which are listed as follows: (a) entire scaffold be fabricated as an extensive network of pores for the proper and uniform cell migration and efficient diffusion of nutrients to the deeper areas of scaffold together with the removal of wastes, (b) should possess interconnected pores which can favour the integration of scaffold with the host tissue following the vascularisation, (c) should have an easy fabrication process in various desirable formats, (d) should be fabricated from the materials those are biocompatible and bioresorbable, (e) should possess a suitable surface chemistry which can favour the cell attachment and proliferation, and (f) should possess a good mechanical strength. Keeping in mind all the necessary properties many materials have been synthesised and fabricated into scaffolds. Scaffold materials commonly used include: ceramics (hydroxyapatite and tricalcium phosphate) used in bone tissue engineering, aliphatic polyesters such as polyglycolic acid (PGA), polylactic acid (PLLA), their copolymers (e.g., PLGA) and polycaprolactone (PCL) are the most commonly used polymers for tissue engineering scaffold applications as in soluble stitches. Naturally derived protein or carbohydrate polymers like agarose, gelatin, chitosan, alginate, collagen, etc. have been used as scaffolds in various tissue engineering applications. The most popular natural polymer used for tissue engineering scaffolds is collagen.

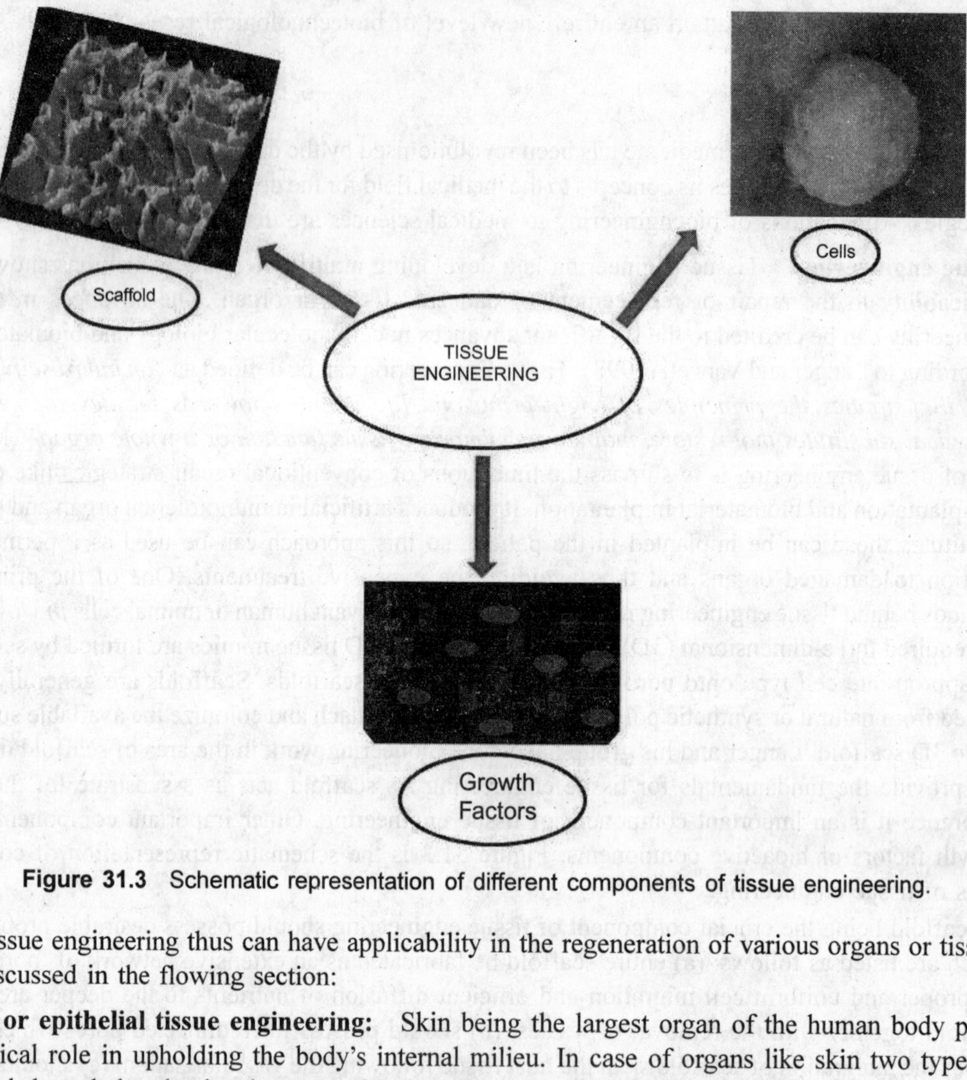

Figure 31.3 Schematic representation of different components of tissue engineering.

Tissue engineering thus can have applicability in the regeneration of various organs or tissues as discussed in the flowing section:

Skin or epithelial tissue engineering: Skin being the largest organ of the human body plays a critical role in upholding the body's internal milieu. In case of organs like skin two types of wounds have led to the development of various tissues engineered skin substitutes, on one side are the burn wounds and on the other side are the chronic wounds. In both the cases deep open wounds or third degree burn sites are prone to secondary bacterial infections which can be fatal to the patient. Tissue engineering has emerged as an interdisciplinary science for the development of ideal skin substitutes for the full thickness and deep wounds. Primary goal of any skin substitute is the restoration of the skin functions which minimizes the protein and fluid loss thus avoiding the infection. An ideal skin replacement should allow the rapid healing together with the restoration of skin layers like dermis and epidermis; should be ready to use; and most importantly should not carry the risk of transmission of disease or infectious agents. Different types of skin substitutes are available in market and few of them are listed in Table 31.1. These skin substitutes vary in complexity, in presence or absence of cultured skin cells in the desired polymeric graft.

Table 31.1 List of the commercially available bioengineered skin substitutes.

Skin Substitutes (Commercial name)	*Dermal Component*	*Epidermal Component*	*Medical Usage*
Allo Derm	Allogenic acelluair dermis	None	In repair of soft tissue defects etc.
Apligraft	Collagen gel with allogenic fibroblast	Allogenic keratinocytes	In burn wounds, chronic foot ulcers etc.
Biobrane	Nylon mesh coated with collagen	Semipermeable silicon membrane	In partial thickness burn wounds
Dermagraft	Polyglactin mesh scaffold with allogeneic fibroblast	None	In diabetic foot ulcers
Epicel	None	Autologous keratinocyte sheet	In burn wounds
Epidex	None	Autologous keratinocytes with silicon membrane support	In chronic leg ulcers
Integra	Collagen and Chondroitin-6 -sulfate matrix	Silicon polymer coating	In burn wounds
OrCel	Collagen sponge with allogeneic fibroblast	Allogenic keratinocytes	In epidermolysis bullosa
SureDerm	Allogenic acellular human dermis	None	In repair of soft tissue defects
TranCell	None	Autologous keratinocytes on acrylic acid polymer	In burn wounds

Further ongoing research focuses on the fabrication of the novel scaffolds for skin tissue engineering. In this direction, scaffolds composed of nano- and micro-diameter fibers have been used as they mimic the morphology and architecture of skin. Composite scaffolds made from natural polymers like collagen-chitosan in combination with fibrin has shown application in the construction of tissue engineered skin. Different research groups have investigated different methods to develop full thickness skin equivalents using different dermal substitutes based on biological materials, e.g, collagen and fibrin or synthetic materials like PLA and PLGA. To further enhance the mechanical stability of the synthesised scaffolds, recently scaffolds fabricated by using a mixture of collagen and agarose has shown potential in skin tissue engineering. Stem cells particularly mesenchymal stem cells (MSCs) are proving useful in burn treatments.

Artificial blood: Red cell substitutes are being developed for use in blood replacement therapies, either for perioperative haemodilution or for resuscitation from haemorrhagic blood loss. Unlikely true blood, artificial blood is designed for the sole purpose of transporting oxygen and carbon dioxide throughout the body. The ideal artificial blood product has the following characteristics; it must be safe to use and compatible within the human body with different blood types. It must be able to transport oxygen throughout the body and release it where it is needed and lastly it must be shelf stable. It should be used as an alternative and/or supplement to homologous and autologous transfusion, or in combination with the use of erythropoietin. Artificial blood can be produced in different ways using synthetic production, chemical isolation, or recombinant biochemical technology. Depending on the type of artificial blood that is made, various raw materials are used. The two significantly different products, i.e., perfluorocarbons (PFC) and hemoglobin-based products are under development as blood substitutes. They differ primarily in the way that they carry oxygen and have been used for perfusional protection of organs. Hemoglobin molecules and perfluorochemicals used can reach to blocked capillary beds, while increasing the drug sensitivity of the peripheral tissues by oxygenation. Hemoglobin-based products use either isolated hemoglobin or synthetically produced hemoglobin reconstituted in an artificial blood formula. These agents have the oxygen carrying solution which can be used in culture media of the tissues and bacteria (aerobes); in chemical examination such as an indicator for oxygen sensor, and a standard solution for oxygen calibrator; and in some kinds of bioreactor. If the oxygen affinity of the artificial red cells can be controlled, they can also be used as an oxygen absorbent agent paradoxically. PFC products involve a polymerization reaction. PFC is chemically inert compound consisting of fluorine substituted hydrocarbons. Unlike Hb based substitutes, PFCs have the following advantages: 1) they do not react with oxygen or other gases; 2) increase the oxygen solubility in the plasma compartment; 3) the dissolved oxygen is not subject to the effects of temperature, pH, 2,3-DPG, etc. (thus the oxygen dissociation curve is linear); and 4) facilitate effortless transfer of oxygen from red cells to the tissue. The final goal of any transfusion service is to create a transfusion system with no side effects and with more effective medical care. Although current system of homologues blood is working well with low cost, acceptable efficacy and relatively less side effects.

Corneal bioengineering: Human corneal endothelium acts as a permeable barrier with a high metabolic activity. It also functions in the maintenance of corneal transparency by regulating the stromal hydration utilizing ATPase pumps. Due to the limited *in vivo* regeneration capacity of corneal endothelium the only repair strategy left out is the corneal transplantation which has the associated limitations like the imitated donor availability, risk of disease transfer, etc. With the emergence of bioengineering/tissue engineering, novel scaffolds or cell carriers are being developed for the transplantation. Corneal endothelial cells (CEC) or human donor-derived corneal endothelial cells can be cultured and expanded *in vitro*. Such expanded cells can be then seeded onto a biological or synthetic (polymethylmethacrylate) graft material to replace the damaged cornea. Several graft materials both biological and synthetic have been used as scaffolds for the corneal transplantation. Such materials include human amniotic membrane, collagen sheets, cross-linked gelatin films, etc. But such materials can also have some disadvantages like, less mechanical strength which makes the handling difficult and can have poor integration with the host tissue. To avoid some of these disadvantages recently some research groups are using decellularized human corneal stromas cultured with CEC's. Such neo-corneas are showing potential to be used as high quality corneal tissue for transplantation.

Bone tissue engineering: Bone is a complex and highly vascularised tissue that provides internal support for higher vertebrates. It further functions as a mineral reservoir and can withstand heavy loads. Bone is subjected to injuries during accidents or chronic diseases. Current treatments are based on the approaches like autologous bone grafts, allografts or metallic or ceramic implants. Autologous bone grafts have a disadvantage of donor site morbidity, while allografts carry the risk of pathogen transfer. Alternative treatments like metallic or ceramic implants exhibit poor integration capacity with the host tissue and less tensile strength. With such limitations there is a need of novel materials for bone regeneration and a possible solution can be tissue engineering. Naturally derived matrices made from hyaluronic acid, chitosan, collagen, fibrinogen, etc. have been used in bone tissue engineering. But the disadvantage with the use of these matrices is that they are difficult to sterilize and can also elicit immune response in the host. Synthetic polymers like poly(α-hydroxy acid), polypropylene fumarate, poly ethyleneglycol, etc. have an advantage that they can be fabricated with desired paramaters, but they degrade into toxic components. Wide range of bioactive inorganic materials is showing potential in bone tissue engineering, e.g., bioactive glass, hydroxyapatite, porous coralline, tricalcium phosphate, etc. Composites made from inorganic and organic materials have shown additional advantages in case of bone tissue engineering. Such composites combine the toughness of polymeric part and compressive strength of inorganic component. The combination generates a bioactive material with good mechanical strength and desired degradation profile suitable for bone tissue engineering. Examples of these composites include hydroxyapatite/poly([epsilon]-caprolactone), poly(lactide-co-glycolide) (PLGA) and PLGA/Bioglass, poly(propylene fumarate)/ poly(DL-lactic-co-glycolic acid), poly(L-lactide)/bioactive glass, etc. Further combination of biomaterials and cell therapy has shown applications in bone tissue engineering. Type of cells for this application varies from primary osteoblasts to bone mesenchymal stem cells. Further work is being focused on enhancing the bio-functionality of the scaffold by the incorporation of osteinductive cues which can enhance osteoblast proliferation on these scaffolds. Recently supermacroporous cryogels synthesised at sub-zero temperature have shown applications in bone tissue engineering by supporting the growth and proliferation of human osteoblast cell lines. Kumar and his group has recently fabricated organic/inorganic composite cryogel scaffolds of polyvinyl alcohol–tetraethylorthosilicate–alginate–calcium oxide (PTAC) for the growth and proliferation of human osteoblast cell lines which is shown by scanning electron micrographs in Figure 31.4.

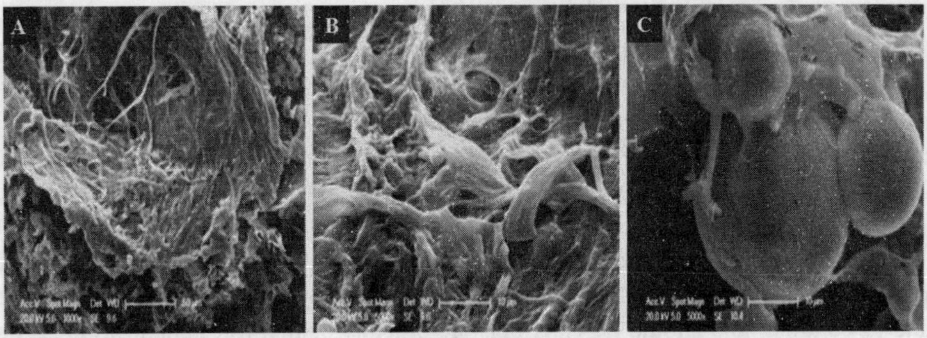

Figure 31.4 Scanning electron micrographic analysis of polyvinyl alcohol–tetraethylorthosilicate–alginate–calcium oxide (PTAC) cryogels (A and B); human osteoblasts growing on the cryogel surface with the synthesis of extracellular matrix (ECM) (C); calcium phosphate deposits on the surface of PTAC cryogels. (Source: Mishra and Kumar, 2010).

Cartilage tissue engineering: Articular cartilage is an avascular and aneural tissue which lines the surface of joints and ensures the frictionless movement of the knee. The unique property of articular cartilage is its high mechanical durability which enables it to bear the high loads during the normal activities. Cartilage is composed of cells called chondrocytes which makes up to 2-5% of the volume and rest (95-98%) is the extracellular matrix (ECM). Two major components of ECM are collagen and glycosaminoglycans (GAG), these components of cartilage are responsible for the tissue's material strength. Cartilage is subjected to degradation either due to injuries or damage due to congenital abnormalities. Due to the limited self-repair capacity of the cartilage the damages can progressively lead to osteoarthritis. The available treatment strategies like autologous chondrocyte transplantation, mosiacplasty or marrow stimulation techniques have the associated limitation. Recently tissue engineering has emerged as a novel approach which has shown potential for the treatment of damaged cartilage. Scaffolds fabricated from natural and synthetic polymers are being used in cartilage tissue engineering. Examples of natural polymers include agarose, alginate, chitosan, collagen, fibrin, hyaluronan, etc. and synthetic polymers are poly (α-hydroxy ester), polylactic acid (PLA), polyglycolic acid (PGA) and their copolymers, etc. An ideal scaffold for cartilage tissue engineering should possess following important properties; high mechanical strength, large and interconnected pores for proper cell migration and integration with the native host tissue. Together with the three-dimensional scaffolds injectables are also being considered for the cartilage tissue engineering to avoid the need of surgical intervention. Naturally derived polysaccharide gel, alginate has successfully shown to support chondrocyte proliferation and retention of phenotype. The other concern is the source of cells to be used for the cartilage tissue engineering, although primary chondrocytes are still used but the limitations like donor site morbidity, and loss of phenotype has brought the mesenchymal stem cells (MSC's) to the forefront of such applications. Research is being further focused on the generation of the neo-cartilage on the surface of cryogels with similar characteristics to the native cartilage and thus be used as a sealant for damaged cartilage. Kumar *et al.* (2010) has recently fabricated cryogel matrices from natural polymers like gelatin, chitosan, alginate and agarose which have shown applications in cartilage tissue engineering by supporting the growth and proliferation of primary goat chondrocytes as shown in Figure 31.5.

Cardiac tissue engineering: Heart failure is the leading cause of death worldwide particularly in industrialised countries accounting for 40% of all deaths. Myocardial infarction which leads to the massive cell loss due to ischemia leads to the impaired cardiac functions permanently. As myocardial tissue lacks intrinsic regeneration capacity, heart transplantation is the ultimate solution to the end stage heart failure. Due to the lack of organ donors and complications associated with the immune suppression treatments there is demand for the new strategies to regenerate the injured heart. Tissue engineering has emerged as an interdisciplinary field and has sown application in cardiac tissue engineering. Scaffold constructed for myocardial tissue engineering should be flexible, able to contract, and should be electrophysiologically stable. Substantial progress has been made in the areas of biopolymers, cell material interactions and bio-mimetic culture devices. Three dimensional tissue constructs, those express characteristics similar to native cardiac tissue have been engineered using fetal or neonatal rat cardiac myocytes on collagen. Similar studies have been performed with other natural polymers like, collagen fibers, fibrous polyglycolic acid scaffolds or

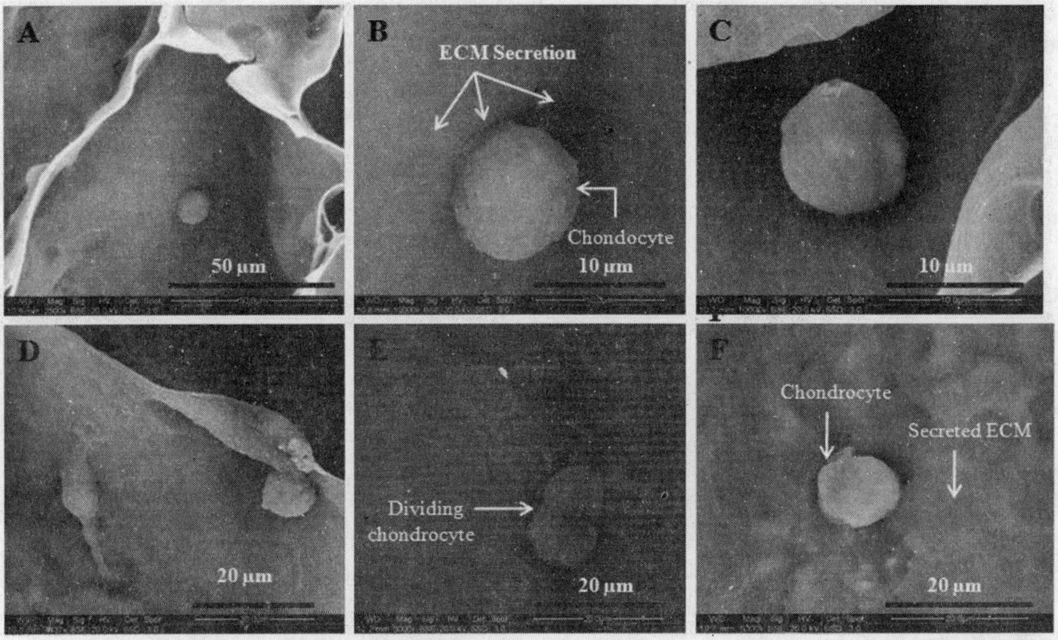

Figure 31.5 Scanning electron microscopic images showing growth and proliferation of primary goat chondrocytes on the surface of cryogel matrices (Source: Bhat *et al.*, 2010).

porous collagen scaffolds. Synthetic and biodegradable polymers used in cardiac tissue engineering include poly(lactide-co-glycolide) (PLGA), polycaprolactone (PCL), poly(glycerol–sebacate) (PGS), poly(trimethylene carbonate–co-lactide) (PTMCLA), polyurethane, etc. Cell sheet engineering which is scaffold free tissue engineering combines several monolayer cell sheets to form thick 3D tissue has shown promisin g results when implanted at the site of infracted myocardium.

Neural tissue engineering: Adult central nervous system (CNS) which is comprised brain and spinal cord is largely in-capable of self repair or regeneration after the injury. Currently grafting is done to repair any injury to CNS. Grafts can be either autograft or allograft. But grafting techniques have the major limitations like multiple surgeries, lack of donor tissue and chances of immune rejection. Due to the limitations with the existing treatment regimes tissue engineering has been utilized to repair CNS injuries. Studies have shown that ECM proteins like laminin, fibronectin, and collagen have shown promising results when used for the nerve repair applications. Other natural polymers those have shown application in nerve regeneration are hyaluronic acid, fibrinogen, fibrin gels, alginate, agarose etc. Research is in progress to explore the utility of synthetic materials for nerve repair applications. Some of these synthetic polymers have already shown applications in nerve regeneration and examples include PGA, PLA, PLGA, etc. Additionally other synthetic materials those are under investigation for their applications in CNS repair include poly (lactides), poly (2-hydroxyethyl methacrylate) (pHEMA), PLGA, and poly (ethylene glycol) glue. Recently poly (epsilon caprolactone) nanowire surfaces have been synthesised and have shown applications in regeneration of spinal injuries. The concept discussed in different areas of tissue engineering is represented schematically in Figure 31.6.

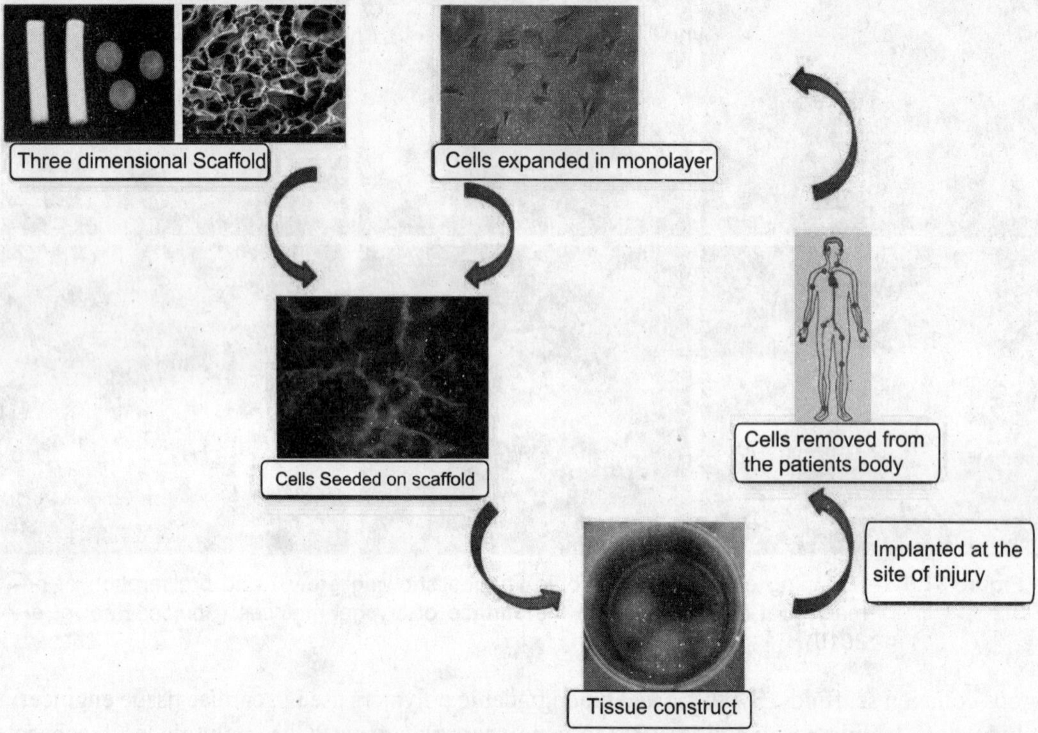

Figure 31.6 Schematic representation of tissue engineering. Cells are removed from the patient and expanded in monolayer, expanded cells are then cultured on three-dimensional scaffold and the resulting tissue construct is implanted in patient at the site of injury.

Extracorporeal devices: These devices are used to process the patient's blood outside the body before it is returned to the circulation. Examples of these devices include gas and heat exchangers, dialysers, apheresis devices, bioartificial liver, etc. All these devices are designed to optimise the flux of material between body fluids and other fluids separated from each other by a membrane. The application of these extracorporeal devices in bioengineering are:

(i) Gas exchangers are required during open heart surgeries. Their role is to supplement cardiovascular functions when they are severely impaired. They function both to oxygenate the blood and also to remove carbon dioxide.

(ii) Heat exchangers are used during certain surgeries to reduce the body temperature which subsequently reduces the metabolic rate. This is achieved by passing the blood through the tube surrounded by coolant.

(iii) Dialysers are used for patients suffering from end stage renal failure. They remove excess fluids and wastes from the body.

(iv) Apheresis units are used to remove pathological agents from the patients or are used to collect useful materials from a healthy donor. Technique uses either ultracentrifugation or continuous centrifugation.

(v) Bioartficial liver devices are used to support the patients suffering with acute liver failure. These devices either use hepatocytes in bioreactor which provides both exchange and synthetic functions or uses non-living components which remove toxins accumulated due to liver failure. These devices are used to assist the patient till transplantation.

Breast Implant: In 1963, the quality of the artificial implants was revolutionized by the introduction of the silicone gel-filled implant. Breast implantation is one such example which has been used for about four decades for both reconstructive and aesthetic purposes. There are two primary types of breast implants; saline-filled and silicone-gel-filled implants. Saline implants have a silicone elastomer shell filled with sterile saline liquid. Silicone gel implants have a silicone shell filled with a viscous silicone gel. Silicone gel breast implants has certain drawbacks with it, it may rupture and cause local symptoms, but do not cause systemic health hazard for patients who have undergone augmentation mammaplasty or postmastectomy reconstruction. Cohesive silicone gel implant has been introduced to reduce the above-mentioned disadvantages. The best advantage of this implant is that it maintains both its shape and integrity if it ruptures.

Cell sheet engineering: As discussed earlier in the tissue engineering approach a mature tissue engineered construct is implanted at the site of injury and with time as the scaffold degrades the space is filled by the ECM secreted by the native cells. But the deposited ECM often results in the fibrosis which is a pathological condition. Further under some situations properties of the scaffold may not be desirable to the tissue, for example, opaque scaffolds may not be suitable for ophthalmological applications. To answer this limitation of the 3D tissue engineering, few research groups have proposed the concept of "cell sheet engineering". It is a novel tissue engineering methodology which constructs the 3D functional tissue by layering 2D sheets over each other without the use of 3D matrices. To remove such cell sheets an interesting approach involves grafting of temperature sensitive polymer poly(*N*-isopropylacrylamide) (PNIPAAm) to the normal tissue culture polystyrene dishes (TCPs) covalently by using electron beam. Such surface being hydrophobic, cells attach and proliferate at physiological temperature, i.e., 37 °C. By reducing the temperature below 32 °C surface changes reversibly to hydrophilic to which cells cannot attach. Such surface changes allow the cultured cell sheet to get detached from the grafted surface. Cardiomyocyte sheets cultured on such grafted surfaces have been used for the constriction of myocardial tissue. Cell sheets made on such temperature responsive culture dishes have shown applications in other biomedical applications like ocular surface regeneration, periodontal regeneration, bladder augmentation and cardiac patches. In this direction Kumar and his group has developed fructose/glucose sensitive cell sheets for the application in tissue engineering. In this process phenylboronate containing terpolymer was synthesised using dimethylaminoethyl methacrylate (DMAEMA) as amine provider. Amino group of DMAEMA acts lewis base and donates a pair of electron boron of vinyl phenyl boronic acid (VPBA) which becomes tetrahedral. This structure synthesised with amine stabilizes the phenylboronate moieties and form a complex gel with PVA at a pH of 7.4. Monosaccharide's like fructose and glucose have high affinity towards phenylboroate in comparison to PVA. Addition of such sugars competitively displaces PVA from the complex causing the dissolution of the gel. Such phenylboronate terpolymer/PVA hydrogels were then used as cell culture substrate. Cell sheets were removed from the treated dishes by the addition of fructose or glucose. The nano- or microparticles synthesised from such hydogel systems have the applicability as glucose sensitive delivery systems in diabetic patients. Such system can also be used for the fabrication of cryogel scaffolds with controlled degradation regulated by the addition of fructose which can be an alternative to the non-degradable synthetic tissue engineering scaffolds.

Drug delivery: The ability to deliver therapeutic agents to a patient in a pulsatile or staggered release profile remains an important challenge in medicine over the last two decades. Extremely sophisticated and potent drugs cannot be effectively delivered using current drug delivery techniques (e.g., pills and injections). There are a number of mechanisms that can provide controlled release of drugs, including transdermal patches, implants, bioadhesive systems and microencapsulation. Transdermal delivery is an attractive alternative, but it is limited by the extremely low permeability of skin. Together with drugs, growth factors like vascular endothelial growth factor (VEGF), basic fibroblast growth factor (bFGF) stimulates the vascularisation of the tissue *in vivo*, which play an important role in regenerative medicine. Similarly members of bone morphogenetic proteins (BMP's) enhance the bone formation. So delivery of drug is equally important as the delivery of growth factors. The mechanism by which drug is delivered can be classified into three major mechanisms discussed as follows:

(i) Diffusion: It is a thermodynamically driven process and has a well understood kinetics.
(ii) Erosion: It is defined as sum of all the processes those lead to the mass loss from a drug delivery device. Materials can either dissolve in an aqueous environment or in case of lipophilic polymers, materials can degrade into water soluble oligomers that allow the initiation of matrix erosion releasing the drug.
(iii) Swelling: This phenomenon increases the polymer chain mobility due to uptake of water which reduces the glass transition temperature of the polymer. Due to increase in flexibility by enhanced diffusibility release rate of the drug is enhanced.

Strategies to deliver the growth factor or drug to a tissue are diverse, but some of them are discussed here:

Use of classical controlled delivery vehicles: This approach uses the vehicles developed for the parenteral application of the drug, e.g., implants (e.g., monolithic system), microspheres (particulate system) and injectable gels (gel like system). First delivery system made from polymeric materials were monolithic matrices. These matrices can be easily synthesised either by solvent casting or injection molding techniques. Such matrices provide an excellent control over the release of drug. In case of degradable systems there are more variables those can be adjusted for control over the release rate. One example is PLA/PLGA system where degradation rate is influenced by the crystalinity, copolymer composition and molecular weight which in turn influences the release rate. Disadvantage with these delivery vehicles is that they may not allow for a homogenous distribution of the drug in tissue, resulting in undesirable concentration gradients. Particulate system uses microparticles and advantage with this system is that the particles can be evenly distributed either in the tissue by injection or in cell suspension which avoids the formation of a drug gradient. Particulate systems have been used for the delivery of nerve growth factors for the treatment of neurodegenerative diseases. Natural polymers like collagen and gelatin have emerged as promising materials for the fabrication of microparticles. Gel like systems have excellent properties and have shown applications in tissue engineering and bioengineering. A system made up of a block copolymer that consists of poly (ethylene oxide) (PEO), poly (L-lactic acid) and urethane units has exhibited sol gel transition at 37 °C which subsequently released dextran incorporated in the system.

Drug delivery via cell carriers: This approach uses cells as delivery vehicles. This is done by genetically altering a portion of the cell or all of them for the production of specific protein or drug molecule.

Biomimetic systems: This approach involves the attachment of drug or growth factor to the surface of material. These systems have exhibited application in drug delivery and medicine for the treatment of diseases.

Hydrogels as drug delivery systems: Hydrogels are emerging as boon to bioengineering which is very efficient in delivering drugs in a controllable manner. Hydrogels have been used extensively in the development of the smart drug delivery systems. Hydrogels can protect the drug from hostile environments like the presence of enzymes and low pH in the stomach and intend to deliver drug at predetermined rates for predefined periods of time. A hydrogel is a network of hydrophilic polymers that can swell in water and hold a large amount of water while maintaining its structure. A three-dimensional network is formed by cross-linking polymer chains. Cross-linking can be provided by covalent bonds, hydrogen bonding, van der Waals interactions, or physical entanglements. Hydrogels contain 'sensor' properties that can undergo reversible volume phase transitions or gel–sol phase transitions upon only minute changes in the environmental conditions. Many physical (temperature, electric fields, solvent composition, light, pressure, sound and magnetic fields) and chemical stimuli (pH, ions and specific molecular recognition events) have been applied to induce various responses of the smart hydrogel systems. Environment-sensitive hydrogels are also called 'intelligent' or 'smart' hydrogels. They are classified on the basis of stimuli perceived, i.e., temperature sensitive hydrogels, pH-sensitive hydrogels, glucose-sensitive hydrogels, electric signal-sensitive hydrogels, light-sensitive hydrogels, etc. This environment-sensitive property is dependent on the type of polymer used to prepare hydrogels. Some of them are shown in Table 31.2.

Table 31.2 Responsive polymers for hydrogel synthesis.

S. No.	*Type of hydrogel*	*Polymer used*
1	Temperature sensitive	poly(N-isopropylacrylamide) (PNIPAAm), Poly(N,N-diethylacrylamide (PDEAAm), Copolymers of NIPAAm & butyl methacrylate (BMA), copolymers made of poly (ethylene oxide) (PEO) and poly(propylene oxide) (PPO), etc.
2	Glucose sensitive	porous filter grafted with polyanions, e.g. poly (methacrylic acid co-butyl methacrylate) and immobilized glucose oxidase, Concanavalin A (Con A)
3	Light-sensitive	leuco derivative molecule like bis(4-di methylamino) phenylmethyl leucocyanide, tri trisodium salt of copper chlorophyllin to poly(N-iso propylacrylamide)
4	pH sensitive	Pendant acidic (e.g., carboxylic and sulfonic acids) or basic (e.g., ammonium salts) groups, Poly(acrylic acid) (PAA), poly (diethylaminoethyl methacrylate) (PDEAEM)

High water content of most of the hydrogels aid in relatively rapid release of drug from the matrix for the extended period of time. In addition to the entrapment of drugs, liposomes can also be entrapped in hydrogels for example liposome entrapped in poly (hydroxyethyl methacrylate) hydrogels mimicking contact lenses can regulate the release of anti-glaucoma drug for up to 8 days. Microparticles entrapped within a hydrogel, i.e., microgels have shown applications in drug delivery. For example gelatin microparticles entrapped in thermal-gelling poly(ethylene glycol fumrate) matrix delivered TGF-α and has shown application in cartilage tissue engineering. Surfactant stabilized microemulsion droplets, surfactant micelles and polymeric micelles can also be entrapped in hydrogel network for a prolonged drug or growth factor release. Hoffman and coworkers have conjugated temperature, pH and light sensitive polymers at specific sites on recognition proteins near the active site. On exposure of polymer to specific stimuli its phase separates and in case of site specific conjugates its active site is blocked. Further the reverse of the same stimuli restores the protein activity. This principle is applied to affinity separation and enzyme processes. In a same way light sensitive polymers have been conjugated to specific site on enzyme like endogluconase (or cellulose). Such enzyme can be turned on or off by altering the supply of visible or UV light. So hydorgels exhibit applications in both drug delivery and tissue engineering.

Preparation of hydrogels: Hydrogels can be prepared from monomers, prepolymers or existing hydrophilic polymers. Hydrogels are synthesized by the following different approaches:

(i) **Synthesis of hydrogels from monomers:** Hydrophilic network structures are formed by the copolymerization of hydrophilic monomers and polyfunctional comonomers, which act as crosslinkers. Most commonly used monomers and copolymer are hydrophilic meth-acrylates, meth-acrylamides and 2-hydroxyethyl methacrylate (HEMA) and ethyleneglycol dimethacrylate (EGDMA), respectively. Polymerization of vinyl monomers is most frequently initiated via radical initiators (peroxides, azo-compounds). Radicals are generated by heating, by the use of a redox initiator (e.g., ammonium persulfate + N,N'-tetramethyl ethylene diamine, TEMED) or a photoinitiator. An alternative way to initiate the radical polymerization process is by high energy irradiation. Figure 31.7 shows the hydrogel synthesis from monomers, prepolymer or existing hydrophilic polymers.

1

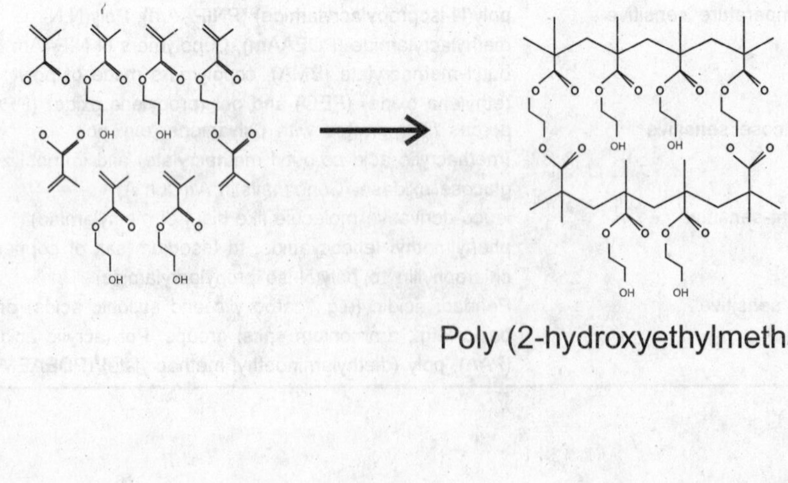

Poly (2-hydroxyethylmethacrylate)

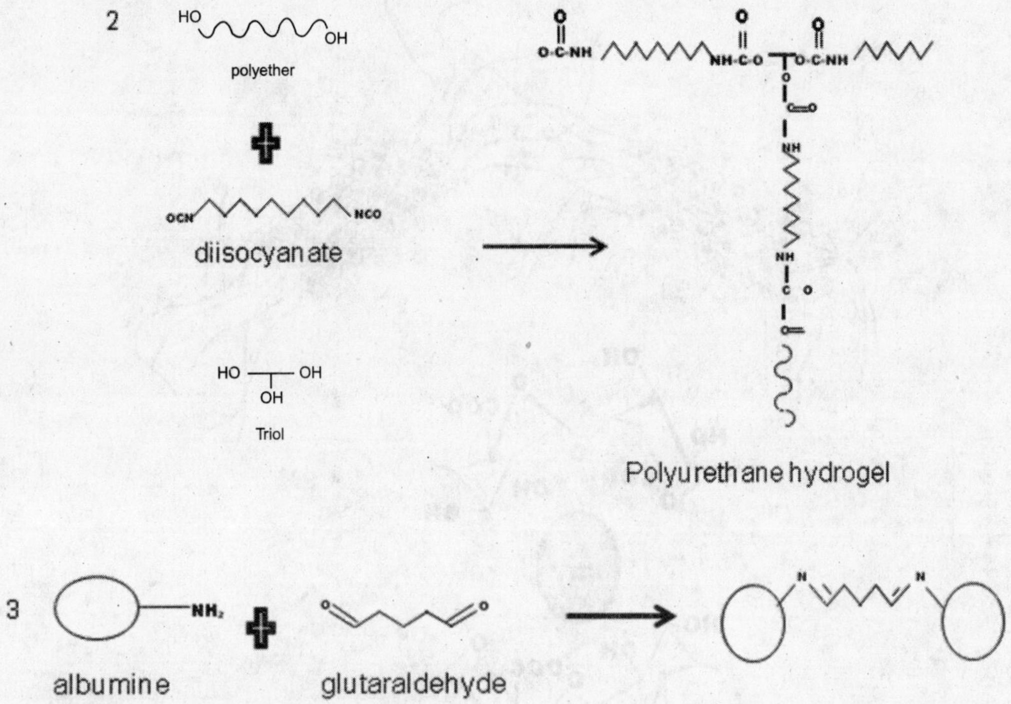

Figure 31.7 Preparation methods of hydrogels: starting from monomers (1), prepolymers (2) or existing hydrophilic polymers (3).

(ii) **Synthesis of hydrogels from prepolymers:** Hydrogels have been prepared by crosslinkage of low molecular weight hydrophilic polymers or oligomers. Example of such kind of linkage is the reaction of α,ω-hydroxyl poly (ethylene glycol) with a diïsocyanate in the presence of a triol as crosslinker. This reaction leads to the formation of crosslinked hydrophilic polyurethanes. Hydroxyl end groups of poly(ethylene glycol) are converted into meth-acrylate to be used as crosslinker via radical polymerization which is an alternative approach.

(iii) **Synthesis of hydrogels from polymers:** Chemical crosslinkage of hydrophilic polymers also results in the formation of a hydrogel. Example of these includes proteins crosslinked with formaldehyde, gluteraldehyde or a polyaldehyde, preparation of stationary phases for gel filtration chromatography, like, Sephadex crosslinked with epichlorohydrin. Ionic polymers can be crosslinked by the addition of di- or tri-valent counterions, e.g., gelation of sodium alginate by addition of Ca^{2+}-ions (Figure 31.8).

These physically crosslinked hydrogels have a sol-gel transition temperature. Chemical crosslinkage are used to form permanent crosslinkage, e.g., gelatin-based hydrogels (Figure 31.9) used for preparing material for wound dressing.

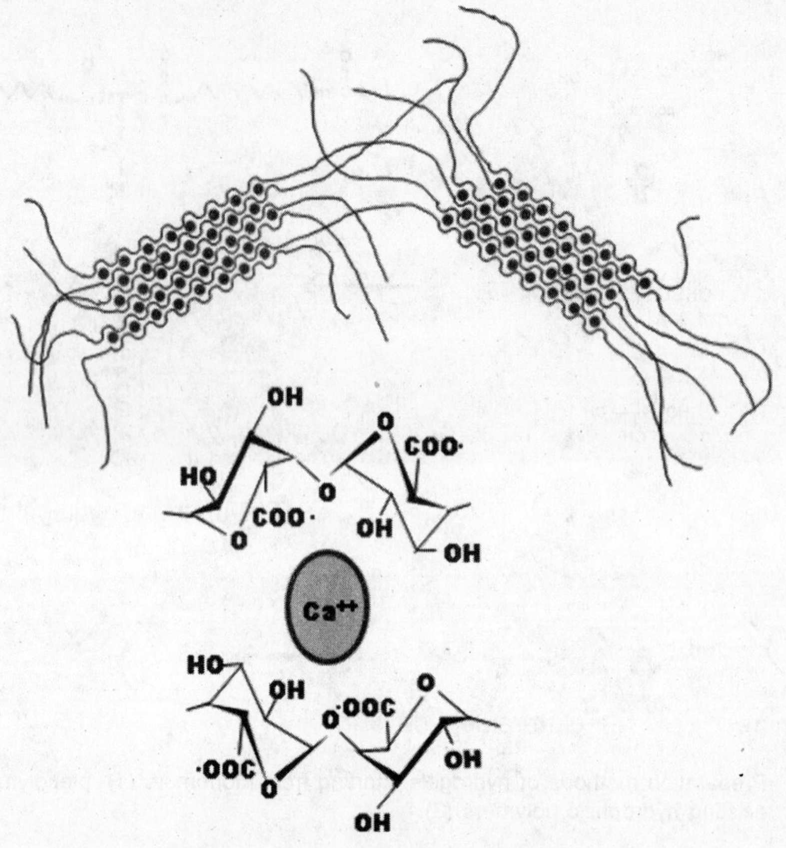

Figure 31.8 Gelation of sodium alginate by addition of Ca^{2+} -ions.

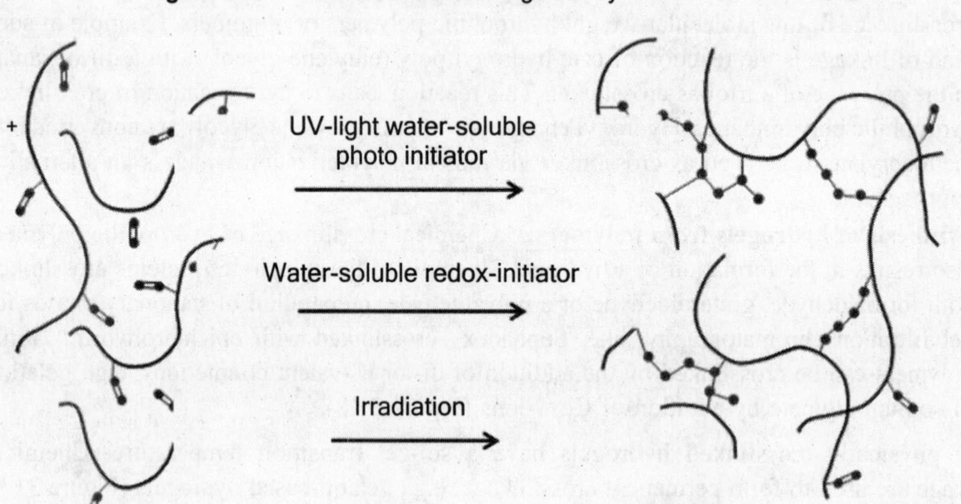

Figure 31.9 Chemical modification of gelatin with methacrylate side groups.

Microfabrication technique, another way to deliver drugs is used to make arrays of microneedles which are long enough to cross the permeability barrier but short enough to stimulate nerves. Microfabrication technology has also created a new class of controlled release of drugs based on programmable devices. These devices are important and efficient due to their small size, potential for integration with microelectronics and their ability to store and release chemicals on demand. The device was fabricated by the sequential processing of a silicon wafer using microelectronic processing techniques including UV photolithography, chemical vapour deposition, electron beam evaporation and reactive ion etching. One step ahead to this technology are certain biodegradable polymeric microchips which has been built that do not require electric power sources or micro-processors. Bioadhesive drug delivery is nowadays most accepted method for delivering the drugs for specific targeting as it intensifies the contact with mucosal epithelial barrier and thus increasing the drug concentration gradient.

Agricultural Applications

Utilization of water resources and fertilizer nutrients is very important as they are the external limiting factors affecting production of agriculture. The most widely and commonly used macro-nutrients are nitrogen (N), phosphorous (P) and potassium (K) or NPK fertilizers. They are used in large quantity than a plant can assimilate, leading to leaching and surface and groundwater contamination. Transport of P from agricultural soils to surface waters has led to eutrophication in freshwater and estuaries. Nitrogen and P accumulation in fresh or brackishwater can over-stimulate the growth of algae creating conditions that interfere with the health and diversity of indigenous plant and animal population. Nitrates and nitrites are implicated in many fatal physiological disorders such as methemoglobinemia in babies, oral cancer, and cancer of the colon, rectum, gastrointestinal cancers, and other health issues.

One possible way to improve nutrients use efficiently while reducing the environmental hazards is by using slow-release fertilizers. These slow release fertilizers have many advantages, such as decreasing fertilizer loss rate, supplying nutrients sustainably, lowering application frequency and minimizing potential negative effects associated with over dosage. These slow release fertilizers include coated fertilizers, i.e., physically prepared by coating fertilizer granules with various materials. Release of fertilizer depends on the soil moisture. Superabsorbent polymers (SAPs) have come up as novel polymers which have shown applications in agriculture, disposable diapers, hygienic napkins and drug delivery systems. SAPs are the functional polymers with an ability to absorb large amounts of water so also known as "miniature water reservoirs". Earlier agricultural water absorbents were made from biopolymers through grafting of hydrophilic monomers onto natural polymers like starch. Such natural superabsorbents are gradually replaced by synthetic absorbents and acrylamide is a major component in that. Such gel forming or superabsorbent polymers act as soil conditioners and were developed for the sustenance of plants in drought prone soil. Major advantages of SAP in agriculture are as follows;

(i) it reduces death rate of plants:

(ii) it increases the water availability in soil enabling the plants to survive even under water stress; and

(iii) it prevents erosion and water runoff.

Increased industrialization has led to the degradation of agricultural land which has severely affected the productivity, so ecological restoration of such land is a major challenge for mankind. Such lands can be restored by the application of SAPs. As SAPs are hydrophilic and have carboxylic groups they can act as artificial humus, which enables them to bind cations and water which helps in the restoration of the degraded land. Polymers used for the construction of SAP with an application in agriculture are polyelectrolyte gels often composed of acrylamide (AM), acrylic acid (AA) and potassium acrylate (KA). All these polymers when crosslinked, i.e., polyacrylamide (PAM), polyacrylic acid (PAA) and potassium polyacrylate (PAAK) have shown potential in agriculture. For example PAM/PAAK co-polymer possesses porous structure and has fast swelling capacity. Such gels are studied for water retention properties of sandy soils. These polymers can be made in the form of nano-composite carbohydrate graft copolymer, to yield particles those are nano-composite superabsorbent containing fertilizer. These nano-fertilizers have unique features like the ultra high absorption, the increase of 20% to 200% in production, the increase of 3.5 times in photosynthesis, and an increase of 70% in the leave's surface area. Nano fertilizers are absolutely environmentally sustainable due to their organic base. In addition to the enhancing potential of the agricultural productivity research has shown that SAPs can increase the nodulation of actinorhizal plants. Use of SAP for ornamental plants like *Cipressus arizonica* has recently been studied which indicates its application in horticultural applications. SAP hydrogels have also been investigated for artificial cultivation of edible food products like mushrooms. SAPs influence the mycelial growth and sporophore production of edible mushrooms. SAPs can also be used in agriculture to aid the germination and seedling establishment.

The widespread usage of agrochemicals to enhance the productivity has led to contamination of groundwater which is affecting the human health and environment severely. Solution to this problem is the slow release formulations in which active materials are released at a slow and constant rate over a long duration of time. In this regard an ideal fertilizer should be able to provide essential nutrients with good water holding capacity and should be eco-friendly. SAP hydrogels can be designed as controlled release system by favoring the uptake of some vital nutrient elements and delaying their further dissolution. So plant can have access to these nutrients for longer duration and thus wastage of fertilizer is also avoided. Urea is majorly used as a fertilizer in various agricultural practices. Approximately 40-70% of the applied urea is lost in the environment leading to environmental pollution. In these situations slow release techniques are applied to enhance the efficiency of the fertilizer and also to reduce the environmental pollution. Fertilizers can be loaded onto the hydrogel by immersing the polymer in fertilizer solution which further leads to the slow release of the fertilizer. For example, for the slow release of nitrogen fertilizer SAP system has been prepared by solution polymerization of AA and maleic anhydride in presence of urea. Further to improve the slow release of fertilizer the product was surface cross-linked with trihydroxymethyl propane glycoidol ether. A similar type of controlled release system for NPK (nitrogen, phosphorous and potassium) fertilizers have been constructed by Liang and co-workers. It has a core/shell structure which has water retention capacity. Its core is made from formaldehyde and polyphosphate fertilizer and shell is made from poly (AA-co-AM)/kaolin SAP composite. Such SAPs are shown in the schematic representation (Figure 31.10).

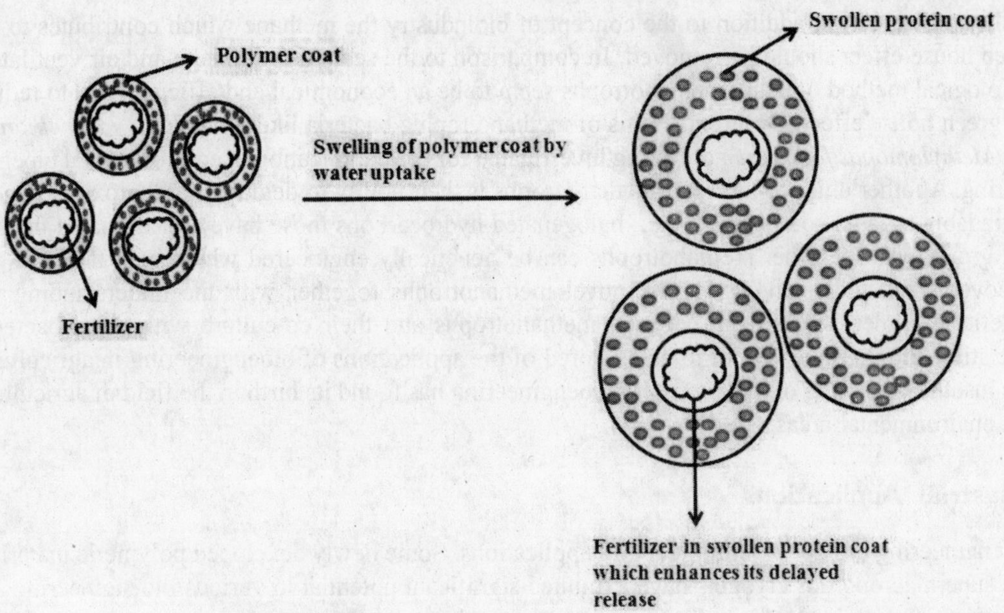

Figure 31.10 A typical NPK controlled system for the delayed release of the fertilizer based on the concept of SAP.

Recently a new type of chitosan coated NPK systems have been prepared, these systems possess a three-layer structure, i.e., core which possesses NPK fertilizer, inner coating made from chitosan and outer coating made from poly (AA-co-AM) SAP hydrogel. Similarly, nanoencapsulated pesticides are also prepared which are highly efficient and minimize the damage to the environment. The smaller quantities of the pesticides are used effectively over a given period of time interval. It also enables them to resist the severe environmental processes, i.e., leaching, evaporation and photolytic, hydrolytic and microbial degradation.

Bioengineering has also helped to solve the global issues like enviornmental pollution and shortages of food, feed, phytomass (plant biomass) and natural resources including fossil fuels and usable water aroused as a result of population explosion. With an increase in population, consumption of food and fuels and also the amount of CO_2 release has raised as a result of which global warming has occurred. Methane is the most significant contributor of the greenhouse effect after CO_2. Methane in atmosphere is contributed by different sources like landfills and coal mines. There is an urgent need to increase our phytomass and microorganisms so that we can decrease the CO_2 present in the environment. To minimize these problems, bioengineering concepts have been applied to develop the bioindustry. In bioengineering, the global and local flows of energy, mass/ materials and information and last but not the least the organic and inorganic metabolisms of plants, animals, microorganisms and humans are analyzed. One of the examples of bioengineering and bioindustry is transplant production, also known as closed production system. This is very essential in developing a production system with minimum use of resources and minimum enviornmental pollution by using artificial lighting for producing billions of quality transplants. In this production system the by-products are recycled to minimize the release environmental pollutants and improve the productivity of the system. This closed transplant system has resulted in higher yield and better quality of harvest. In addition to the concept of bioindustry the methane which contributes to the green house effect should be removed. In comparison to the seam gas drainage and air ventilation a biological method of using methanotrophs seem to be an economical and efficient way to reduce the green house effect. Different strains of methanotrophic bacteria like *Methylomonas methanica* and *Methylomonas fodinarum* are being investigated for their application in environmental bioengineering. Another unique feature of methanotrophs is their ability to degrade highly toxic and non-degradable organic compounds, e.g., halogenated hydrocarbons those have contaminated the soil and groundwater. Further methanotrophs can be genetically engineered which may facilitate the discovery and understanding of the novel methanotrophs together with the understanding the benefits of synergistic effects between methanotrophs and their co-culture with other bacteria. One still believes there is a lot to be explored of the applications of bioengineering in agriculture. It is just the beginning of the era where bioengineering has found its birth in the field of agriculture and environmental areas.

Industrial Applications

Bioengineering has got several industrial applications. Some newly developed polymeric materials like supermacroporous cryogels have exhibited significant potential in various bioengineering applications. Cryogels are the gel matrices synthesised at sub-zero temperature and typically have interconnected pores allowing unhindered diffusion of solutes of practically any size, as well as mass transport of nanoparticles. This unique structure of cryogels, in combination with their osmotic, chemical and mechanical stability, makes them attractive matrices for chromatography of biological nanoparticles and cells. It has also been utilized in a number of processes like cell separation, tissue engineering (as discussed earlier), bioreactor for therapeutic protein production and extracorporeal devices. Different cryogel matrices synthesised from natural and synthetic polymers, e.g., polyacrylamide-chitosan (PAAC), poly (N-isopropylacrylamide)-chitosan polyacrylonitrile (PAN) have been analysed for the growth of different hybridoma cell lines and for the production of therapeutic proteins like monoclonal antibodies. Synthetic polymer, polyacrylamide (pAAM) cryogel matrices have shown their potential to support the proliferation of cell lines like HT 1080 (human fibrosarcoma) and HCT116 (human colon cancer) for the production of urokinase. The potential of cryogels for the separation of stem cell from umbilical cord blood is explored recently using the affinity cryogel matrices made from the synthetic polymers like polyacrylamide and polydimethylacrylamide. Thus, polymeric cryogels have an immense role in the production of industrially important products like therapeutic proteins, purified cell population, etc.

CONCLUSION AND FUTURE PROSPECTS

This chapter introduces students and researchers from academia and industry to the emerging area of bioengineering and its applications to medicine, agriculture and industry. In the area of regenerative medicine bioengineering has led to the development of new technologies and devices which has and in future will be used to combat incurable diseases. Apart from this bioengineering in drug delivery has developed newer ways for the delivery of bioactive molecules and drugs to the target site which has provided an intelligent approach in drug delivery. Applications of bioengineering to agriculture have increased the productivity and soil fertility. So this chapter can be concluded with anticipation that bioengineering has an immense potential and can be utilized in other areas also.

Such developments which will lead to betterment of human health and overall standards of living and also help the areas of agriculture research.

FURTHER READINGS

1. Aubrecht, J., Manivasakam, P., and Schiestl, R.H., (1996) Controlled gene expression in mammalian cells via a regulatory cascade involving the tetracycline transactivator and the lac repressor. *Gene*. **(172):** 227-231.
2. Ayse, B.C., Scott, G., Jeffery, O.H., and Michael, M. (2007) *Tissue Enginneirng* applications-bone. In: Tissue Engineering. Fisher, J.P., Mikos, A.G., and Bronzino, J.D. (eds) CRC Press NY. pp. (21-1 to 21-22).
3. Bechara, S.L., Judson, A., and Popat, K.C. (2010) Template synthesized poly (epsilon-caprolactone) nanowire surfaces for neural tissue engineering. *Biomaterials.* **(31):** 3492-3501.
4. Berthhod, F., and Damour, O (1997) *In vitro* reconstituted skin models for wound coverage and deep burns. *British Journal of Dermatology*. **(136):** 809-816.
5. Bhat, S., Tripathi, A., and Kumar, A. (2010) Supermacroprous chitosan-agarose-gelatin cryogels: *in vitro* characterization and *in vivo* assessment for cartilage tissue engineering. *Journal of Royal Society Interface*. **(8):** 540-554.
6. Boorsma, M., Nieba, L., Koller, D., Bachmann, M.F., Bailey, J.E., and Renner, W.A. (2000) A temperature-regulated replicon- based DNA expression system. *Nature Biotechnology*. **(18):** 429-432.
7. Butler, D.L., Goldstein, S.A., and Guilak, F. (2000) Functional tissue engineering: the role of biomechanics. *Journal of Biomechanical Engineering.* **(122):** 570-576.
8. Carpentier, B., and Ash, S.R. (2007) Sorbent-based artificial liver devices: principles of operation, chemical effects and clinical results. *Expert Review of Medical Devices.* **(4):** 839-861.
9. Choi, J.S., Williams, J.K., Greven, M., Walter, K.A., Laber, P.W., Khang, G., and Soker, S. (2010) Bioengineering endothelialized neo-corneas using donor-derived corneal endothelial cells and decellularized corneal stroma. *Biomaterials.* **(31):** 6738-6745.
10. Cuello, J.C. (2005) 'Engineering to biology' and 'biology to engineering': The bidirectional connection between engineering and biology in biological engineering design. *International Journal of Engineering Education*. **(21):** 1-7.
11. Currie, L.J., Sharpe, J.R. and Martin, R. (2001) The use of fibrin glue in skin grafts and tissue-engineered skin replacements: a review. *Plastic and Reconstructive Surgery.* **(108):** 1713-1726.
12. D'haeseleer, P., Liang, S., and Somogyi, R. (2000) Genetic network inference: from co-expression clustering to reverse engineering. *Bioinformatics*. **(16):** 707-726.
13. Doillon, C.J., Watsky, M.A., Hakim, M., Wang, J., Munger, R., Laycock, N., Osborne, R., and Griffith, M. (2003) A collagen-based scaffold for a tissue engineered human cornea: physical and physiological properties. *The International Journal of Artificial Organs.* **(26):** 764-773.
14. Encyclopaedia Britannica, (1994) 15th ed., Encyclopaedia Britannica, Inc., Chicago, IL
15. Eschenhagen, T., Fink, C., Remmers, U., Scholz, H., Wattchow, J., Weil, J., Zimmermann, W., Dohmen, H.H, Schafer, H., Bishopric, N., Wakatsuki, T., and Elson, E.L. (1997) Three-dimensional reconstitution of embryonic cardiomyocytes in a collagen matrix: a new heart muscle model system. *The Federation of American Societies for Eeperimental Biology Journal.* **(11):** 683-694.
16. Gallico, G.G. (1990) Biological skin substitutes. *Clinics in Plastic Surgery.* **(17):** 519-526.
17. Gaspar, A., Moldovan, L., Constantin, D., Stanciuc, A.M., Sarbu Boeti, P.M., and Efrimescu, I.C. (2011) Collagen-based scaffolds for skin tissue engineering. *Journal of Medicine and Life*. **4**: 172-177.
18. Goorha, Y.K., Deb, P., Chatterjee, T., Dhot, P.S. and Prasad, R.S. (2003) Artifical blood. *Medical Journal Armed Force India.* **(59):** 45-50.
19. Han, C., Zhang, L., Sun, J., Shi, H., Zhou, J., and Gao, C. (2010) Application of collagen-chitosan/fibrin glue asymmetric scaffolds in skin tissue engineering. *Journal of Zhejiang University Science.* **(11):** 524-530.

20. Hidaka, C., Ibarra, C., Hannafin, J.A., Torzilli, P.A., Quitoriano, M., Jen, S.S., Warren, R.F., and Crystal, R.G. (2002) Formation of vascularized meniscal tissue by combining gene therapy with tissue engineering. *Tissue Engineering*. **(8):** 93-105.
21. Hoare, T.R., and Kohane, D.S. (2008) Hydrogels in drug delivery: progress and challenges. *Polymer.* **(49):** 1993-2007.
22. http://en.wikipedia.org/wiki/Biological_engineering
23. http://www.becon.nih.gov/ bioengineering_definition.htm
24. http://www.heinzwolff.co.uk/
25. Hutmacher, D.W. (2001) Scaffold design and fabrication technologies for engineering tissues-state-of-the-art and future perspectives. *Journal of Biomaterial Science*-Polymer Edition. **(12):** 107-124.
26. Ishino, Y., Sano, Y., Nakamura, T., Connon, C.J., Rigby, H., Fullwood, N.J., and Kinoshita, S. (2004) Amniotic membrane as a carrier for cultivated human corneal endothelial cell transplantation. *Investigative Ophthalmology and Visual Science.* **(45):** 800-806.
27. Joyce, N.C. (2003) Proliferative capacity of the corneal endothelium. *Progress in Retinal and Eye Research.* **(22):** 359-389.
28. Jumblatt, M.M., Maurice, D.M., and Schwartz, B.D. (1980) A gelatin membrane substrate for the transplantation of tissue cultured cells. *Transplantation.* **(29):** 498-499.
29. Kamihira, M., and Kumar, A. (2007) Development of separation technique for stem cells, In: *Cell Separation: Fundamentals, Analytical and Preparative Methods,* Kumar, A., Galaev, I.Y. and Mattiasson, B. (volume eds) Springer-Verlag Berlin Heidelberg. pp. 173-193.
30. Kumar, A., and Srivastava, A. (2010) Cell separation using cryogel-based affinity chromatography. *Nature Protocols.* **(5):** 1737-1747.
31. Kumar, A., Galaev, I.Y., and Mattiasson, B. (2008) Smart polymers in affinity precepatation of proteins, In: *Smart Polymers: Applications in Biotechnology and Biomedicine,* Galaev, I.Y. and Mattiason, B. (eds) CRC Press, NY, pp. 401-436.
32. Kumar, 'A., Jain, E., and Srivastava, A. (2010) Macroporous polymeric scaffolds for tissue engineering applications, In: *Macroporous Polymers: Production Properties and Biotechnological/ Biomedical Applications,* Mattiasson, B., Kumar, A., and Galaev, I.Y. (eds) CRC Press, NY. pp. 405-466.
33. Kumar, A., Srivastava, A., and Jain, E. (2009) Biomaterial applications, In: *Advanced Biomaterials: Fundamentals, Processing and Applicatins,* Basu, B., Katti, D.S., and Kumar, A. (eds); John Wiley & Sons, Inc., *Hoboken, New Jersey.* pp. 535-550.
34. Langer, R. and Peppas, N.A. (2003) Advances in biomaterials, drug delivery and bionanotechnology. *Bioengineering Food and Natural Products.* **(49):** 2990-3006.
35. Langer, R., and Vacanti, J.P. (1993) Tissue engineering. *Science*. **(260):** 920-926.
36. Lee, D.Y., Ahn, H.T. and Cho, K.H. (2000) A new skin equivalent model: dermal substrate that combines de-epidermized dermis with fibroblast-populated collagen matrix. *Journal of Dermatological Science.* **(23):** 132-137.
37. Lee, L.K., and Roth, C.M. (2003) Antisense technology in molecular and cellular bioengineering. *Current Opinion in Biotechnology.* **(14):** 505-511.
38. Lever, M.J. (2005) Cardiovascular assistance system, In: Artificial Exchange Systems in Biomaterials: Artificial Organs and Tissue Engineering, Hench, L.L., and Jones, J.R. (eds) CRC Press NY, pp.179-190.
39. Lu, W., Zhang, Y.J., and Jin, Y. (2009) Potential of stem cells for skin regeneration following burns. *Expert Review of Dermatology.* **(4):** 97-99.
40. Mishra, R., and Kumar, A. (2010) Inorganic/organic biocomposite cryogels for regeneration of bone tissue. *Journal of Biomaterial Science Polymer Edition.* (DOI:10.1163/092050610X534230).
41. Oh, S., Oh, N., Appleford M. and Ong, J.L. (2006) Bioceramics for tissue engineering applications- Review. *American Journal of Biochemistry and Biotechnology.* **(2):** 49-56.

42. Patrick, C.W., Mikos, A.G., and McIntire, L.V. (1998) Prospects of tissue engineering. In: *Frontiers in Tissue Engineering*. Patrick, C.W., Mikos, A.G., and McIntire, L.V. (eds.) Elsevier Science Ltd, Oxford. pp. 3-11.
43. Qiu, Y., and Park, K. (2001) Enviornment- sensitive hydrogels for drug delivery. *Advanced Drug Delivery Review.* **(53):** 321-339.
44. Riley, M.R. (2007) Introducing journal of biological engineering. *Journal of Biological Engineering.* **(1):** 1-3.
45. Sachlos, E., and Czernuszka, J.T. (2003) Making tissue engineering scaffolds work. Review on the application of solid freeform fabrication technology to the production of tissue engineering scaffolds. *European Cells and Materials,* **(5):** 29-40.
46. Salgado, A.J., Coutinho, O.P., and Reis, R.L. (2004) Bone tissue engineering: State of the art and future trends. *Macromolecular Bioscience.* **(4):** 743-765.
47. Schmidt, C.E., and Leach, J.B. (2003) Neural tissue engineering: Strategies for repair and regeneration. *Annual Reviews of Biomedical Engineering.* **(5):** 293-347.
48. Sekiya, S., Shimizu, T., Yamato, M., Kikuchi, A. and Okano, T. (2006) Bioengineered cardiac cell sheet grafts have intrinsic angiogenic potential. *Biochemical and Biophysical Research Communications.* **(341):** 573-582.
49. Shay, J.W., and Wright, W.E. (2000) The use of telomerized cells for tissue engineering. *Nature Biotechnology.* **(18):** 22-23.
50. Shea, L.D., Smiley, E., Bonadio, J., and Mooney, D.J. (1999) DNA delivery from polymer matrices for tissue engineering. *Nature Biotechnology.* **(17):** 551-554.
51. Shibasaki, S., Tanaka, A., and Ueda, M. (2003) Development of combinatorial bioengineering using yeast cell surface display-order-made design of cell and protein for bio-monitoring. *Biosensors and Bioelectronics,* **(19):** 123-130.
52. Stosich, M.S., Moioli, E.K., Wu, J.K., Lee, C.H., Rohde, C., Yoursef, A.M., Ascherman, J., Diraddo, R., Marion, N.W., and Mao, J.J. (2009) Bioengineering strategies to generate vascularized soft tissue grafts with sustained shape. Methods. **(47):** 116-121.
53. Tao, S.L. and Desai, T.A. (2003) Microfabricated drug delivery system: from particles to pores. *Advanced Drug Delivery Reviews.* **(55):** 315-328.
54. Tuan, R.S., Boland, G., and Tuli, R. (2003) Adult mesenchymal stem cells and cell-based tissue engineering. *Arthritis Research and Therapy* **(5):** 32-45.
55. Tuli, R., Li, W., and Tuan, R.S. (2003) Current state of cartilage tissue engineering. *Arthritis Research and Therapy.* **(5):** 235-238.
56. Venkatesh, S., Byrne, M.E., Peppas, N.A., and Hilt, J.Z. (2005) Applications of biomimetic systems in drug delivery. *Expert Opinion on Drug Delivery.* **(2):** 1085-1096.
57. Weber, W., and Fussenegger, M. (2002) Artificial mammalian gene regulation networks-novel approaches for gene therapy and bioengineering. *Journal of Biotechnology.* **(98):** 161-187.
58. Zele, D.V., and Heymans. O. (2004) Breast implants. A review. *Acta Chirurgica Belgica.* **(104):** 158-165.
59. Zhu, C., and Joyce, N.C. (2004) Proliferative response of corneal endothelial cells from young and older donors. Investigative *Ophthalmology and Visual Science.* **(45):** 1743-1751.
60. Zimmermann, W.H., Fink, C., Kralisch, D., Remmers, U., Weil, J., and Eschenhagen, T. (2000) Three-dimensional engineered heart tissue from neonatal rat cardiac myocytes. *Biotechnology and Bioengineering.* **(68):** 106-114.
61. Zimmermann, W.H., Schneiderbanger, K., Schubert, P., Didié, M., Münzel, F., Heubach, J.F., Kostin, S., Neuhuber, W.L., and Eschenhagen. T. (2002) Tissue engineering of a differentiated cardiac muscle construct. *Circulation Research.* **(90):** 223-230.
62. Zohuriaan-Mehr, N.J., Omidian, H., Doroudiani, S. and Kabiri, K. (2010) Advances in non-hygenic applications of Superabsorbent hydrogels. *Journal of Material Science.* **(45):** 5711-5735.

SECTION D

Biotechnology for Industrial Applications

CHAPTER

32

Immobilized Biocatalyst Technology

Immobilization of enzymes, cells, and organelles has found vast analytical, technological, and medical applications. The purposes of this chapter are to lay the foundation of basic concepts and practical uses of immobilized biocatalyst technology in analytical, clinical and therapeutic and industrial applications.

Keywords: Immobilized biocatalyst technology; carrier binding; cross-linking; enzyme immobilization method; immobilized enzyme; water-insoluble enzyme, trapped enzyme, fixed enzyme, and matrix-supported enzyme.

INTRODUCTION

An immobilized biocatalyst is an enzyme which is attached to an inert, insoluble material that can provide increased resistance to changes in conditions such as pH or temperature. It also allows enzymes to be held in place throughout the reaction, following which they are easily separated from the products and may be used again. It is a far more efficient process and is widely used in industry for enzyme catalyzed reactions. Immobilized enzymes are very important for commercial purpose as they possess many benefits to the expenses and processes of the reaction:

(i) **Convenience:** Minuscule amounts of protein dissolve in the reaction, so workup can be much easier. Upon completion, reaction mixtures typically contain only solvent and reaction products.

(ii) **Economical:** The immobilized enzyme is easily removed from the reaction, making it easy to recycle the biocatalyst.

(iii) **Stability:** Immobilized enzymes typically have greater thermal and operational stability than the soluble form of the enzyme.

Supports employed range from different variants of natural and synthetic polymers via polyelectrolytic complexes; biocompatible supports and erythrocytes to glass, graphite, brick-dust and magnetic particles; silicon wafer; and carriers responding to light, temperature, and electric and magnetic fields. Selection of support material and method of immobilization is made by weighing the various characteristics and required features of the enzyme/cell application against the properties/limitations/characteristics of the support. All principal binding methods including adsorption, covalent attachment, multipoint attachment, gel entrapment, cross linking, immobilization based on bioselective interactions, chelation, co-immobilization, reversible immobilization, photochemistry and electrochemistry-based immobilization have their relative merits and drawbacks. Therefore, a number of practical aspects should be considered before embarking on experimental work to ensure that the final immobilized enzyme and/or cell preparation is fit for the planned purpose or application and will operate at optimum effectiveness. This chapter deals with the review of available methods of enzyme immobilization and provides some background to assist in choice evaluation for support and method of immobilization for medical, veterinary, agricultural sciences and industrial application.

CONCEPTS

The use of immobilized cells is not a new idea. Since the early 18th century, they have been used in the production of vinegar and for disposal of sewage effluent. In both instances a microbial film is formed naturally and is held in place by a combination of microbial produced exopolysachharides ('slime') and physical forces with microbial support. Since growth of the organisms occurs, enzyme decay is not a problem. There is also a continual release of aggregates of microorganisms ('flocks').

In 1916, Nelson and Griffin found that an enzyme in water-insoluble form showed catalytic activity. They reported that invertase extracted from yeast was adsorbed on charcoal, and the adsorbed enzyme showed the same activity as native enzyme. In 1948, Sumner found that urease from jack bean became water-insoluble on standing in 30% alcohol and sodium chloride for 1 to 2 days at room temperature and that the water-insoluble urease was active. Thus, it has been known for a long time that enzymes in water-insoluble form show catalytic activity. However, the first attempt to immobilize an enzyme to improve its properties for a particular application was not made until 1953, when Grubhofer and Schleith immobilized enzymes such as carboxypeptidase, diastase, pepsin, and ribonucleases by using diazotized polyaminopolystyrene resin. On the other hand, before this (1949), immobilization of physiologically active protein was carried out by Micheel and Ewers. Further, in 1951, Campbell *et al.* prepared immobilized antigen by binding albumin to diazotized p-aminobenzylcellulose. Subsequently, a number of reports on the preparation and application of immobilized antigens and antibodies appeared.

In the 1960s, many papers appeared; in particular, Professor Katchalski-Katzir and his co-workers at the Weizmann Institute of Science, Israel, carried out extensive studies on new immobilization techniques and the enzymatic, physical, and chemical properties of immobilized enzymes. In 1969, Chibata *et al.* at Tanabe Seiyaku Co., Ltd., in Japan succeeded in the industrialization of a continuous process for the optical resolution of D- & L- amino acids using immobilized aminoacylase. This was the first industrial application of immobilized enzymes in the world.

In 1971, the first Enzyme Engineering Conference was held at Henniker, New Hampshire, and the predominant theme of this conference was immobilized enzymes. A definition and classification of immobilized enzymes was proposed at the conference. After that, different methods of enzyme immobilization were developed in the 1970s and 1990s. Up to now, more than 5000 publications and patents have been published on enzyme immobilization techniques. Several hundred enzymes have been immobilized in different forms and approximately a dozen immobilized enzymes, e.g., penicillin G, acylase, lipases, proteases, invertase, etc. have been used as catalysts in various large-scale processes.

In conclusion, general concepts of immobilized biocatalyst technology are:

(i) Enzyme immobilization is the confinement of enzyme molecule in a distinct phase or attachment to some solid support.

(ii) The distinct phase allows exchange from the bulk phase in which substrate effecter or inhibitor molecules are dispersed.

PRINCIPLES

Principles of immobilized biocatalyst technology can be defined as "enzymes physically confined or localized in a certain defined region of space with retention of their catalytic activities and which can be used repeatedly and continuously." Accordingly, enzymes modified to a water-insoluble form by suitable techniques satisfy this definition of immobilized enzymes. In addition, when an enzyme reaction using a substrate of high molecular weight is carried out in a reactor equipped with a semipermeable ultrafiltration membrane without leakage of the enzyme from the reactor, this can also be considered a kind of immobilized enzyme system. The term immobilized enzyme was recommended at the First Enzyme Engineering Conference in 1971. Before that time, various terms such as water-insoluble enzyme, trapped enzyme, fixed enzyme, and matrix-supported enzyme were used.

Free amino and carboxyl groups, the sulfhydryl group of cystein, the imidazole group of histidine, phenolic groups, and hydroxyl groups of serine and threonine may be considered functional groups involved in enzyme immobilization. For immobilization of an enzyme, it is necessary that the functional groups in the active center should not be involved in the reaction leading to immobilization of the enzyme. Further, because the tertiary structure of enzyme protein is maintained by relatively weak binding forces, such as hydrogen, hydrophobic, and ionic bonds, it is necessary to carry out the immobilization reaction under mild conditions.

The nature of the immobilized enzyme preparation depends upon the character of the enzyme phase. The enzyme phase is usually insoluble in water and is often a high molecular weight hydrophilic polymer. The attachment of the enzyme may be achieved by various means. The enzyme can be covalently bonded to, adsorbed onto or physically entrapped within the solid support or matrix. Chemical coupling of enzymes with reactive supports is currently the most frequently used method of enzyme immobilization. Chemical coupling techniques are reactions occurring between an enzyme and a support. These phases may be both organic and inorganic. The most extensively used organic enzyme phase in immobilization is insoluble polymer matrix such as cellulose, polyacrylamide collagen, gelatin, sugar, alginate, carrageenan and polystyrene. The polymer, however, may be in the form of a particulate powder in sheet form as a membrane. A variety of inorganic phase materials have been used for immobilizing enzymes. These include alumina, bentonite, charcoal, glass, hydroxyapetite, nickel oxide silica, titana and zirconia. The inorganic materials may be porous or non-porous. Porous inorganic materials have large surface areas than non-porous ones.

IMMOBILIZED BIOCATALYST TECHNOLOGY

Purpose: It is quite pertinent in an immobilized enzyme system because:

(i) The immobilization enzyme system is stable than the existing system.
(ii) The immobilization enzyme system is efficient biocatalyst than the existing system.
(iii) The immobilized enzyme processes is reusable.

Immobilization Methods

In recent years, several techniques for immobilizing both enzymes and whole cells have been devised that can be classified into three basic categories as follows.

Carrier binding method

It is the binding of enzymes to water-insoluble carriers such as polysaccharide derivatives, synthetic polymers and porous glass etc. The carrier-binding method is the oldest immobilization method for enzymes, and many papers have been published on this method. When enzymes are immobilized in this way, care is required regarding the selection of carriers as well as in binding techniques. The carrier-binding method can be further divided into three categories according to the binding mode of the enzyme, i.e., physical adsorption, ionic binding, and covalent binding.

Physical binding: The oldest technique of enzyme immobilization involves simple adsorption. Enzymes or whole cells adhere loosely (without chemical bonding) to the surface of a support material (polymer matrix). A variety of adsorbents have been used; the binding forces may be ionic, hydrophobic, hydrogen bonds or van der Waals interaction. Cells immobilized in this way have a tendency to autolyse and activity is often partially or totally lost. Sometimes such adsorbed agents wash away, but some last a surprisingly long time.

Ionic binding: Immobilization of enzymes by the ionic binding method can be achieved simply under mild conditions. Accordingly, in this case, preparations having relatively high activity are obtained. However, the binding forces between enzyme and carrier are weak in comparison with those in the covalent binding methods. Therefore, leakage of the enzyme from the carrier may occur after changes in the ionic strength, pH of the substrate or product solution. This type of immobilized enzyme can be regenerated when the enzyme activity decreases after prolonged operation. Thus, the ionic-binding method is advantageous in comparison with the covalent-binding method, particularly when expensive carriers or enzymes are used.

Covalent binding: Immobilization by covalent binding to activated polymers is probably the most extensively used method, although often tedious. The enzyme may even be covalently bonded onto itself forming an insoluble, but active, polymeric enzyme. For isolated enzymes, chemical bonding between the enzyme molecule and the surface of the support material achieves a much firmer hold and results in a stable biocatalyst preparation capable of extended service. Immobilization of enzymes by covalent binding is carried out under relatively severe conditions in comparison with those of physical adsorption or ionic binding. Thus, in the former cases, conformational change of the enzyme structure and partial destruction of the active center may occur. Accordingly, unless immobilization of an enzyme by covalent binding is carried out under well controlled conditions, immobilized enzyme having high activity cannot be obtained. However, the binding forces between the enzyme and carrier are strong and the enzyme cannot be easily lost from carriers even in the presence of substrates or salts at high concentrations. However, when the activity of enzymes immobilized by covalent binding decreases on long term operation, regeneration is impossible.

Cross-linking method

The immobilization of enzymes is performed by the formation of intermolecular cross-linkages between the enzyme molecules by means of bifunctional or multifunctional reagents such as glutaraldehyde, bisdiazobenzidine and hexamethylene diisocyanate, etc. Immobilization of enzymes by cross-linking is carried out under relatively severe conditions like covalent binding in comparison with those of physical adsorption or ionic binding. The cross-linking method is based on the formation of chemical bonds, but water-insoluble carriers are not used in this method.

Entrapping method

The entrapping method is based on incorporating enzymes into the lattice of a polymer matrix or enclosing enzymes in semipermeable membrane or polymeric membrane, such as collagen, gelatin cellulose triacetate polyacrylamide, and κ-carrageenan, etc. and it can be classified into the lattice and microcapsule types. This technique reduces the rate of reaction because substrate, nutrient and product molecules must all diffuse through the solid matrix structure. A compensating advantage, however, is that living cells can be firmly retained, without damage. The entrapment of an enzyme molecule can be achieved in one of the three ways:

(i) Inclusion within the matrix of a highly cross-linked polymer.
(ii) Separation from bulk phase by a semipermeable microcapsule.
(iii) Dissolution indistinct non-aqueous phase.

The membrane is semipermeable, i.e., relatively small substrates and product molecules can pass readily through the encapsulating membrane but the larger enzyme molecules and the still larger structure of a complete cell cannot escape. This method differs from the covalent binding and cross-linking method in that the enzyme itself does not bind to the gel matrix or membrane. Thus, this method may have wide applicability. However, if a chemical polymerization reaction is used for entrapping, relatively severe conditions are required and loss of enzyme activity occurs in some cases. Therefore, it is necessary to select the most suitable conditions for the immobilization of various enzymes. A major disadvantage of the entrapping method is that its application is limited to small molecular substrate and product molecules; the entrapped enzyme shows little or no activity toward macromolecular substrates. It should be readily recognized that no single immobilization technique and no single support system are ideal for all enzymes. Figure 32.1 depicts various forms of immobilized enzymes.

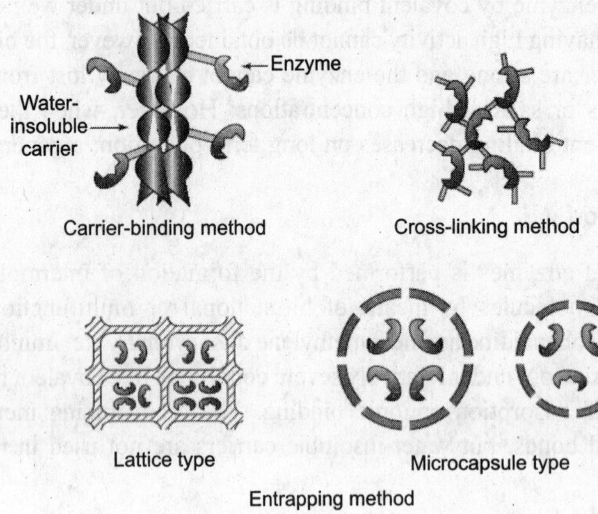

Figure 32.1 Schematic diagram of immobilized enzymes.

Each method of immobilization has its own advantages and disadvantages, which are compared in Table 32.1. As evident, no method is perfect and the selection of method is often dictated by the enzyme to be immobilized and its intended application.

Table 32.1 Preparation and characteristics of immobilized enzyme.

	Carrler-binding method				
Characterstic	*Physical adsorption*	*Ionic binding*	*Covalent binding*	*Cross-linking method*	*Entrapping method*
Preparation	Easy	Easy	Difficult	Difficult	Difficult
Enzyme activity	Low	High	High	Moderate	High
Substrate specificity	Unchangeable	Unchangeable	Changeable	Changeable	Unchangeable
Binding force	Weak	Moderate	Strong	Strong	Strong
Regeneration	Possible	Possible	Impossible	Impossible	Impossible
General applicability	Low	Moderate	Moderate	Low	High
Cost of immobilization	Low	Low	High	Moderate	Low

Kinetics of Immobilized Enzyme

The kinetic behavior of a bound enzyme can differ significantly from that of the same enzyme in free solution. The properties of an enzyme can be modified by suitable choice of the immobilization protocol whereas the same method may have appreciably different effects on different enzymes. These changes may be due to conformational alterations within the enzyme due to the immobilization procedure or the presence and nature of the immobilization support. Immobilization can greatly affect the stability of an enzyme. Additional stabilization is derived by preventing the enzyme molecules from interacting with each other and the protection that immobilization exerts towards proteolytic and microbiological attack. This latter effect is due to a combination of diffusional difficulties and the camouflage to enzymic attack produced by the structural alterations. In order to achieve maximum stabilization of the enzymes, the surfaces of the enzyme and support should be complementary with the formation of many unstrained covalent or non-covalent interactions. Often, however, this factor must be balanced against others, such as the cost of the process, the need for a specific support material and it should be ensured that the substrates are not sterically hindered from diffusing to the active site of the immobilized enzyme in order to react at a sufficient rate. The kinetic constants (e.g., K_m, V_{max}) of enzymes may be altered by the process of immobilization due to internal structural changes and restricted access to the active site. Thus, the intrinsic specificity ($k./K_m$) of such enzymes may be changed relative to the soluble enzyme. An example of this involves trypsin where the freely soluble enzyme hydrolyses fifteen peptide bonds in the protein, pepsinogen, but the immobilized enzyme hydrolyses only ten. The apparent value of these kinetic parameters, when determined experimentally, may differ from the intrinsic values. This may be due to changes in the properties of the solution in the immediate vicinity of the immobilized enzyme or the effects of molecular diffusion within the local environment (Figure 32.2).

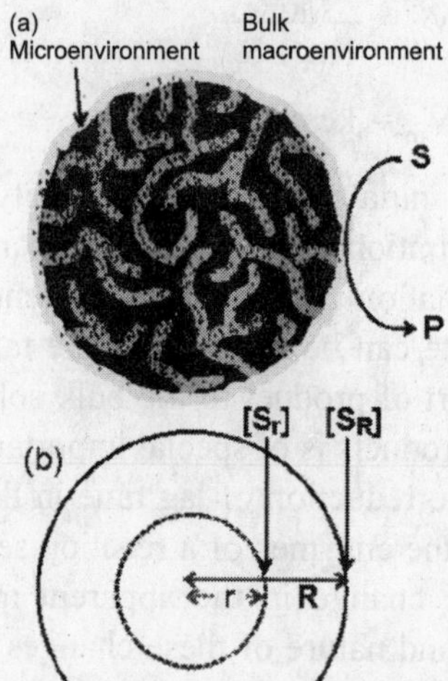

Figure 32.2 A schematic cross-section of an immobilized enzyme particle (a) shows the macro-environment and micro-environment. Triangular dots represent the enzyme molecules. The microenvironment consists of the internal solution plus that part of the surrounding solution which is influenced by the surface characteristics of the immobilized enzyme. Partitioning of substances will occur between these two environments (Source: Goldstein, 1972).

The following depicts the effect of substrate and product diffusion in a heterogeneous enzyme system.

Soluble enzyme:

$$E + S \xrightarrow[km]{} ES \xrightarrow{kcat} E + P$$

Fixed enzyme:

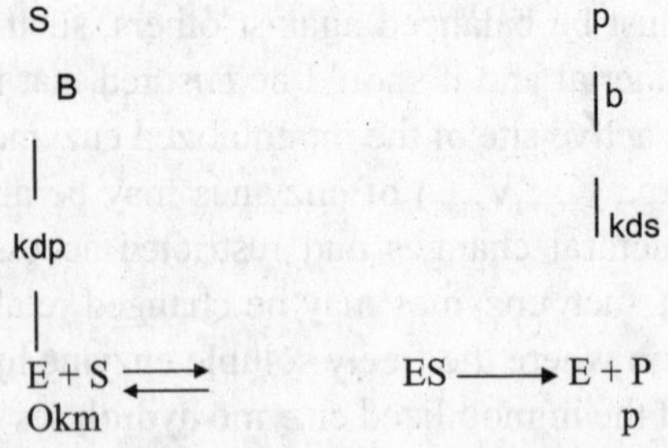

(1)

The subscript b and p represent bulk solution and the enzyme vicinity, respectively. The rate constant kds governs the enzyme, and kdp governs the diffusion product into the bulk phase. The constants Km and kcat occur in the Michaelis-Menten equation.

$$V_o = \frac{V_m \, S_o}{K_m + S_o} \tag{2}$$

$$V_m = kcat \quad E_o$$

The terms are defined as: V_o, initial velocity; V_m, velocity at S K_m; S_o, initial substrate concentration; E_o, total enzyme concentration of the E_o complex: and K_m, the Michaelis constant which, in the simplest case, is a dissociation constant. It is evident from Eqs. 1 and 2 that the reaction rate catalyzed by a fixed enzyme can be affected by the rate of transport of the substrate to the enzyme, and the rate of transport of product to the bulk solution. In fixed multienzyme systems, the diffusion of substrates and products is of special importance since the effects may be amplified along the reaction sequence. The reduction of lag time in the appearance of the ultimate product is the principal effect of fixing the enzymes of a reaction sequence in close proximity. Immobilization often causes a dramatic change in the apparent measured parameters of the enzyme-catalyzed reaction. The degree and nature of these changes will depend not only on the immobilization method used but also on the enzyme reaction.

Choice of Immobilization Method

The art of enzyme immobilization lies in knowing which method to choose. Choice is governed by a number of factors some of which will not be apparent until the procedure is tried. For successful immobilization, therefore, the following factors should, if possible, be considered:

1. The operational stability of the immobilized catalyst i.e., the enzyme must be stable under the conditions required for reaction.
2. The reagents should preferably react with chemical groups other than those present at active site.
3. The cost of the immobilized catalyst should be minimum.

4. For high activity and yield of immobilized catalyst, following considerations should be made:
   (i) If possible, cross-linking reagents should react preferentially with chemical groups other than those at active site.
   (ii) If the above condition cannot be met (as is usually the case), the cross-linking reagent should be as large as possible to prevent it from penetrating the active site. A polymer such as 'activated' cellulose is thus preferable to a small bifunctional reagent (e.g., glutaraldehyde).
   (iii) Where feasible, the active site of the enzyme should be protected in the same way. This may be achieved in sulphydryl enzymes by first reacting the enzyme with glutathione or cystine and then reactivating it once it is immobilized. Certain enzymes, for example, papain, may be immobilized in the inactivated state, for other enzymes blocking the active site can sometimes be successfully achieved by incorporating maturating concentrations of substrate in the reaction mixture.
   (iv) The washing procedure used to remove the uncross linked enzyme from the preparation must not adversely effect the enzyme. Cellulose polymers will usually strongly adsorb the enzyme such that high ionic strength solutions are required to wash the immobilized enzymes. Thus, the use of cellulose as a support material for a polymeric enzyme is sometimes not advised, as the process of washing may cause the enzyme to associate.
   (v) If the enzyme, once immobilized, is to be used as a high efficiency catalyst in some chemical reaction, consideration must be given to the nature of the reaction before choosing the immobilization method.
5. The regenerability of the catalyst must be there.
6. The mechanical stability and physical form of the support material must be considered.
7. The cost of the appropriate reactor configuration must also be considered. The mechanical properties of certain particulate immobilized enzyme preparations make them unsuitable for use in large scale reactor system. Others, however, may be specifically designed for use in a reactor.

Initially, the choice of method is empirical, but subsequently the process must be thoroughly analyzed, tested, and considered on its merits.

The choice between immobilized cells and immobilized enzymes

There is rather no difficulty in choosing between cells or enzymes for immobilization. If the enzyme with the desired activity is secreted from the cell, then clearly it is the enzyme, which should be immobilized. With protein engineering, it is even possible to combine several enzymic activities in a single protein molecule. If the activity of the enzyme is dependent on its spatial arrangement in the cell membrane, then clearly it is the cell, which should be immobilized. Immobilized cells may be more useful in this respect, because if the cell membrane remains intact during the immobilization step, the coenzymes are retained as all the enzymes are necessary for recycling them. However, if the cell membrane does not remain intact, then diffusion of the substrate and product across it may be rate limiting.

In recent years, the practice of using non-growing whole or lysed microbial cells, rather than purified enzymes, is gaining popularity, and it is therefore pertinent to enquire the relative advantages of these two types of catalyst. Throughout the following discussion, it must be remembered that the overriding consideration is usually one of cost. One theoretical advantage in the use of the immobilized purified enzyme, as opposed to the immobilized cell, is that it is possible to obtain higher loadings of catalyst. The maximum activity per gram of solid of an immobilized enzyme preparation is often 10 times that of a preparation of immobilized cells from which the enzyme was obtained, although 'activation' of immobilized cells (e.g., lysis) can provide activity loading nearly as great as that of an immobilized purified enzyme.

The following considerations should be met in choosing the two systems:

(i) More often there is little to choose between the two systems, and the overriding factor is the cost. In this context, it is not the cost immobilization but sum of the capital and recurrent costs associated with initiating and running the process.

(ii) Of particular importance is the retention of activity on immobilization and the operational half-life.

(iii) To date the commercially developed immobilized systems are the ones in which the catalyst has no requirement for a co-factor.

The commonest co-factors are NAD/NADP and ATP, and their cost is such that it is not economically feasible to add them continuously with the substrate. The only practical preposition is to recycle the co-factors. This can be done in enzyme factors, but usually two substrates must be added and two products are obtained, only one of which is required. In addition, the co-factors must also be immobilized or they will be lost from the system and such immobilized co-factors tend to have a short half-life.

Operational Stability of Immobilized Cell and Enzyme Reactors

A number of factors can affect the operational stability of immobilized cell and enzyme reactors. These are:

Purity of the substance

Impurities may affect the operational stability because of two reasons:

(i) They can accumulate during prolonged factor operation and either foul the reactor bed or, worse still, irreversibly inactivate the catalyst.

(ii) These impurities can act as substrate for the growth of microbial contaminants. The growth of contaminants can be minimized by the use, wherever possible, of high temperatures and pH values and high substrate concentrations.

Gas exchange

A different problem is gas exchange. In some immobilized cell systems, the viability of the cells has to be maintained, which can be achieved by providing a supply of oxygen. This can best be achieved by using a fluidized bed. In such a system, the beads of immobilized cells are kept in suspension by the introduction of air into the bottom of the reactor. Cells can be prevented from leaving the reaction in the effluent stream.

Generation of heat

A factor, which can preclude the use of immobilized biocatalysts, is the generation of heat. It is not easy to design reactors for immobilized cells and enzymes which efficiently remove the heat produced by an exothermic reaction. Thus, the heat generated in the middle of an aggregate of immobilized catalyst may be sufficient to inactivate the enzyme. Since the heat produced will be proportional to the substrate concentration, one solution is to reduce the concentration of the substrate in the feed solution. However, this will reduce the concentration of the product in the reactor effluent, making product recovery more difficult and expensive and the process may not be economic. Thus, before embarking on demonstration of a large-scale reactor, it is advisable to check the thermodynamics of the reaction in a calorimeter.

The Economic Argument for Immobilized Biocatalyst Technology

An important factor determining the use of enzymes in a technological process is their expense. Several hundred enzymes are commercially available at prices of about £1 mg^{-1}, although some are much cheaper and many are much more expensive. As enzymes are catalytic molecules, they are not directly used up by the processes in which they are used. Their high initial cost, therefore, should only be incidental to their use. However due to denaturation, they do lose activity with time. If possible, they should be stabilized against denaturation and utilized in an efficient manner. When they are used in a soluble form, they retain some activity after the reaction, which cannot be economically recovered for re-use and is generally wasted. This activity residue remains to contaminate the product and its removal may involve extra purification costs. In order to eliminate this wastage and give an improved productivity, simple and economic methods must be used which enable the separation of the enzyme from the reaction product. The easiest way of achieving this is by separating the enzyme and product during the reaction using a two-phase system; one phase containing the enzyme and the other phase containing the product. The enzyme is imprisoned within its phase allowing its re-use or continuous use but preventing it from contaminating the product. Other molecules, including the reactants, are able to move freely between the two phases. This is known as immobilization and may be achieved by fixing the enzyme to, or within, some other material. Immobilization of enzymes often incurs an additional expense and is only undertaken if there is a sound economic or process advantage in the use of the immobilized rather than free (soluble) enzymes. The most important benefit derived from immobilization is the easy separation of the enzyme from the products of the catalyzed reaction. This prevents the enzyme from contaminating the product, minimizing downstream processing costs and possible effluent handling problems, particularly if the enzyme is noticeably toxic or antigenic. It also allows continuous processes to be practicable, with a considerable saving in enzyme, labor and overhead costs.

APPLICATIONS OF IMMOBILIZED BIOCATALYST TECHNOLOGY

The practical applications of immobilized enzymes can be divided into three main categories.

(1) **Analytical Applications:** Analytical applications of immobilized enzymes may be divided into two areas, the enzyme electrode and automated analyzers. Enzyme electrodes are probes capable of generating an electrical potential as a result of a reaction catalyzed by an immobilized enzyme, which is used to replace soluble enzyme in an existing automatic analyzer system.

(2) **Industrial Applications:** Any industrial process is ultimately concerned with producing a product of the highest possible quality for the lowest possible price. Immobilized catalysts are used for the commercial production of a number of chemicals. Among these the best example of the commercial realization of immobilized biocatalyst technology is the production of high-fructose corn syrup (HFCS), low calorie sweeteners and certain antibiotic intermediates.

(3) **Medical and Therapeutic Applications:** Enzyme may be employed as a therapeutic agent, either to replace enzymes that are missing because of genetic or other malfunctions in the individual or as agents for the specific degradation of unwanted metabolites in the diseased individual. Recent decade has seen more applications in organic synthesis, especially exploring chirality and enantio selecting of lipases.

Medical and Therapeutic Applications

Many of the basic functions of the human body are based on enzymatic reactions carried out in intracellular environments. Despite the basic importance of enzymes in body functions, enzyme therapy has not yet played an important role in the field of medicine. The reason for this is that most enzymes administered into the body present a number of problems except for a few digestive enzymes that can be administered orally and one or two enzymes, which might be useful for external wound debridement by local application. The main problem in enzyme therapy using enzymes extracted from cells are instability and short duration of action in the body because the enzyme is rapidly removed as a foreign protein, the possible allergic reaction, toxic contamination from the cell extract and development of immunological reaction and the production of antibodies to inactivate subsequently injected enzymes.

Can immobilized enzymes help to solve these problems? The questions of stability and duration of action may be solved by any of the immobilized enzymes described, since many of the enzymes become much more stable when immobilized (Table 32.2). However, no immobilized enzymes can solve the problems of recognition as a foreign protein, the production of allergic reaction, the production of antibodies with repeated injection, and enzyme inactivation by antibodies. Thus, enzymes immobilized by covalent binding are not completely prevented from coming into direct contact with external antibodies or leucocytes. Enzymes prepared by molecular entrapment are prevented from coming into direct contact with the external environment. Enzyme immobilization by microencapsulation may be the most appropriate approach for administrative enzymes, since it gives the enzyme an intracellular environment even after administration into the body. The enclosing membrane prevents the enzyme from coming in contact with external antibodies (leucocytes) and loading out to cause immunological and allergic toxic reaction.

Table 32.2 Pilot scale production by immobilized enzymes and whole cells.

Enzyme or whole cells	*Carrier*	*Method of Immobilization*	*Application*
Aminoacylase	DEAE-Sephadex	Adsorption	Preparation of L-amino acids from a rac DL-amino acid mixture
Xylose isomerase (glucose isomerase)	Duolite A 7 (ceramic beads) Amberlite IRA 904 exchange resin	Adsorption Adsorption	Preparation of fructose glucose mixture
E.coli containing asparate ammonia-lyase	*Polyacrylamide*	Entrapment	Preparation of L-*aspartate*
Pseudomonas putida containing arginine deaminase	Polyacrylamide	Entrapment	Preparation of citrulline
Ahcromobacter liquidum containing histidine ammonialyase	Polyacrylamide	Entrapment	Preparation of uraconic acid
E. coli containing pencillin amidase	Polyacrylamide, cellulose	Entrapment	Preparation of 6-acid aminopenicillanic acid
Brevibacterium ammoniagenes containing fumarate hydratase	Polyacrylamide	Entrapment	Preparation of malate and fumarate
Lactase (β-galactosidase)	Silica particles	Adsorption	Preparation of lactose-free milk

The most important therapeutic uses of immobilized biocatalyst are as fellow:

Enzyme replacement for hereditary enzyme defects

There are many diseases that are characterized by the absence of a particular enzyme because of genetic or tissue malfunction. Hereditary enzyme defects may result in an accumulation of substrates to toxic level or the deficiency of essential products. Although the solution to this problem exists, but not useful because of the earlier mentioned problems of enzyme administration. However, feasibility of using immobilized enzyme to correct inborn errors of metabolism has been determined. Examples of genetically derived enzyme deficiency include the broad classification of lysosomal storage diseases, where a lysosomal enzyme is absent and its substrate will accumulate within the cell, often with disastrous results and also diseases such as favlem where an enzyme involved in a metabolic pathway, in this case glucose-6-phosphate dehydrogenase of RBC, is absent. Tissue malfunction, particularly of the liver and kidney may result in the accumulation of toxic waste materials, for example, urea, within the body. These toxic waste materials can be eliminated from the body by use of immobilized enzymes.

Although the majority of enzyme replacements involve simple hydrolytic or oxidase reactions. Certain enzyme deficiency diseases involve dehydrogenases or kinases. In these cases, NAD/ NADH or ADP/ATP regeneration systems must be included with the replacement enzyme because coenzymes are not generally available in the extracellular compartment. For example, the inherited galactokinase deficiency disease may be treated (experimentally) by injection of galactokinase co-encapsulated with an ATP regenerating system of ATP/ADP and pyruvate kinase.

Suppression of substrate dependent tumor using enzyme therapy

Enzyme therapy differs from enzyme replacement in that the enzyme to be added to the body is not one that is normally found within the body (or is present but not pathologically diminished in quantity), the rationale behind the addition of such an enzyme is to alter the normal environmental conditions in the body in order to control a diseased state. The best example of this is the use of L-asparginase, which can suppress the growth of certain asparagine dependent tumors, e.g., treatment of certain leukaemias. Normal cells have the ability to synthesize asparagine, but certain leukaemic cells do not have this ability and they cannot grow without an extraneous supply from the blood.

Sufficient asparginase for clinical trail could only be obtained from bacterial sources. However, parentally injected bacterial L-asparaginase is removed rapidly as foreign protein. Furthermore, antibodies produced as a result of repeated injections cause even more rapid removal and inactivation of injected L-asparagines, making the treatment ineffective. The first animate using immobilized asparagines to suppress asparagine-dependent tomora were reported in 1969. In these studies, the asparaginase was immobilized by microencapsulation and then injected interperitoneally into mice. The addition of immobilized asparaglase to the blood or contiguous satracellular compartment reduces the blood asparagines concentration to a minimal level and leukaemic cells die from asparagines starvation. The asparagines must be immobilized in a biodegradable form, e.g., by inclusion in a Tiposome or polylactic acid capsule. Administration can be either intravenous or intraperitoneal.

Management of lactose intolerance

Lactose intolerance is particularly widespread among the inhabitants of the third world. It is due to the deficiency of lactose enzyme. The clinical result of milk consumption by such people is severe gastrointestinal upset, diarrhea, flatulence, and abdominal pain. It is not clear whether the deficiency of lactase is a genetic abnormality. Thus, another good reason for the development of an immobilized lactase system lies in the inability of many individuals to metabolize lactose, because they lack the lactase enzyme. The objective then is to able to remove, cheaply, the lactose from milk without affecting its nutritional or physical characteristics. The most obvious method would be a one-step process based upon an immobilized lactase preparation by which virtually complete food, lactose-free milk is obtained. It is most suitable for the persons suffering from lactose intolerance.

Industrial Applications

Enzyme reactors: An enzyme reactor consists of a vessel or a series of vessels used to perform a desired conversion by enzymic means. A number of important types of such reactors are shown diagrammatically in Figure 32.3. There are several important factors that determine the choice of reactor for a particular process. In general, the choice depends on the cost of a predetermined productivity within the product's specifications. This must be inclusive of the costs associated with substrate(s), downstream processing, labor, depreciation, overheads and process development, in addition to the more obvious costs concerned with building and running the enzyme reactor. Other contributing factors are the form of the enzyme of choice (i.e., free or immobilized), the kinetics of the reaction and the chemical and physical properties of an immobilization support including whether it is particulate, membranous or fibrous, and its density, compressibility, robustness, particle size and regenerability. Attention must also be paid to the scale of operation, the possible need for pH and temperature control, the supply and removal of gases and the stability of the enzyme, substrate and product. These factors will be discussed in more detail with respect to the different types of reactor. A batch reactor is one in which the entire product is removed, as rapidly as is practically possible, after a fixed time. Generally this means that the enzyme and substrate molecules have identical residence time within the reactor, although in some circumstances there may be a need for further addition of enzyme and/or substrate (i.e., fed-batch operation). The

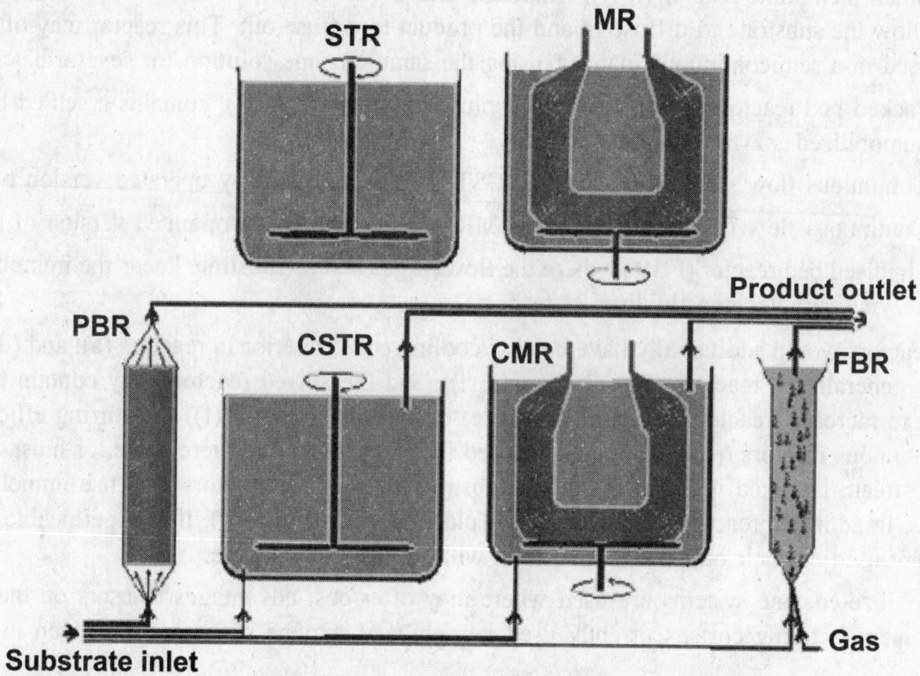

Figure 32.3 Diagrams of various important enzyme reactor types.

operating costs of batch reactors are higher than continuous processes due to the necessity for the reactors to be emptied and refilled both regularly and often. This procedure is not only expensive in itself but means that there are considerable periods when such reactors are not productive; it also makes uneven demands on both labor and services. Batch reactors generally consist of a tank containing a stirrer (stirred tank reactor, STR). The tank is normally fitted with fixed baffles that improve the stirring efficiency. STRs can be used for processes involving non-immobilized enzymes if the consequences of these contaminating the product are not severe. Batch reactors also suffer from pronounced batch-to-batch variations, as the reaction conditions change with time, and may be difficult to scale-up due to the changing power requirements for efficient fixing. They do, however, have a number of advantageous features. Primary amongst these is their simplicity, both in use and in process development. For this reason they are preferred for small-scale production of highly priced products, especially where the same equipment is to be used for a number of different conversions. They offer a closely controllable environment that is useful for slow reactions, where the composition may be accurately monitored and conditions (e.g., temperature, pH, coenzyme concentrations) varied throughout the reaction. They are also of use when continuous operation of a process proves to be difficult due to the viscous or intractable nature of the reaction mix. Different reactor types include:

(i) Stirred tank batch reactor (STR), which contains all the enzymes and substrates until the conversion is complete;

(ii) Batch membrane reactor (MR), where the enzyme is held within membrane tubes, which allow the substrate to diffuse in and the product to diffuse out. This reactor may often be used in a semicontinuous manner, using the same enzyme solution for several batches;

(iii) Packed bed reactor (PBR), also called plug-flow reactor (PFR), contains a settled bed of immobilized enzyme particles;

(iv) Continuous flow stirred tank reactor (CSTR), is a continuously operated version of (a);

(v) Continuous flow membrane reactor (CMR), is a continuously operated version of (b);

(vi) Fluidised bed reactor (FBR), where the flow of gas and/or substrate keeps the immobilized enzyme particles in a fluidised state.

All reactors would additionally have heating/cooling coils (interior in reactors (a), and (d), and exterior, generally, in reactors (b), (c), (e) and (f)), and the stirred reactors may contain baffles in order to increase (reactors (a), (b), (d) and (e) or decrease (reactor (f)) the stirring efficiency. The continuous reactors ((c)-(f)) may all be used in a recycle mode where some, or most, of the product stream is mixed with the incoming substrate stream. All reactors may use immobilized enzymes. In addition, reactors (a), (b) and (e) (plus reactors (d) and (f), if semipermeable membranes are used on their outlets) may be used with the soluble enzyme.

Immobilize-enzyme systems are used where they offer cost advantages to users on the basis of total manufacturing costs. Currently used immobilized-enzyme processes are given in Table 32.3.

Table 32.3 Some of the more important industrial uses of immobilized enzymes.

Enzyme	CE number	Product
Aminoacylase	3.5.1.14	L-Amino acids
Aspartate ammonia-lyase	4.3.1.1	L-Aspartic acid
Aspartate 4-decarboxylase	4.1.1.12	L-Alanine
Cyanidase	3.5.5.x	Formic acid (from waste cyanide)
Glucosmylase	3.2.1.3	D-Glucose
Glucose isomerase	5.3.1.5	High-fructose corn syrup
Histidine ammonia-lyase	4.3.1.3	Urocanic acid
Hydantoinasea	3.5.2.2	D-and L-amino acids
Invertase	3.2.1.26	Invert sugar
Lactase	3.2.1.23	Lactose-free milk and whey
Lipase	3.1.1.3	Cocoa butter substitutes
Nitrile hydratase	4.2.1.x	Acrylamide
Penicillin amidases	3.5.1.11	Penicillins
Raffinase	3.2.1.22	Raffinose-free solutions
Thermolysin	3.2.24.4	Aspartame

Analytical Applications

Biosensors

A biosensor is an analytical device that converts a biological response into an electrical signal (Figure 32.4). The term 'biosensor' is often used to cover sensor devices used in order to determine the concentration of substances and other parameters of biological interest even where they do not utilize a biological system directly. Enzymes are the biologically responsive material, but it should be recognized that other biological systems may be utilized by biosensors, for example, whole cell metabolism, ligand binding and the antibody-antigen reaction. Research and development in biosensor is wide and multidisciplinary, spanning biochemistry, bioreactor science, physical chemistry, electrochemistry, electronics and software engineering. Most of this current endeavor concerns potentiometric and amperometric biosensors and colorimetric paper enzyme strips. However, all the main transducer types are likely to be thoroughly examined, for use in biosensors, over the next few years.

The biological response of the biosensor is determined by the biocatalytic membrane which accomplishes the conversion of reactant to product. Immobilized enzymes possess a number of advantageous features which makes them particularly applicable for use in such systems. They may be re-used, which ensures that the same catalytic activity is present for a series of analyses. This is an important factor in securing reproducible results and avoids the pitfalls associated with the replicate pipetting of free enzyme otherwise necessary in analytical protocols. Many enzymes are intrinsically stabilized by the immobilization process, but even where this does not occur, there is usually considerable apparent stabilization. It is normal to use an excess of the enzyme within the immobilized sensor system. This gives a catalytic redundancy (i.e., $h << 1$), which is sufficient to ensure an increase in the apparent stabilization of the immobilized enzyme. Even where there is some inactivation of the immobilized enzyme over a period of time, this inactivation is usually steady and predictable. Any activity decay is easily incorporated into an analytical scheme by regularly interpolating standards between the analyses of unknown samples. For these reasons, many such immobilized enzyme systems are re-usable up to 10,000 times over a period of several months. Clearly, this results in a considerable saving in terms of the enzymes' cost relative to the analytical usage of free soluble enzymes. When the reaction, occurring at the immobilized enzyme membrane of a biosensor, is limited by the rate of external diffusion, the reaction process will possess a number of valuable analytical assets. Control of biosensor response by the external diffusion of the analyte can be encouraged by the use of permeable membranes between the enzyme and the bulk solution.

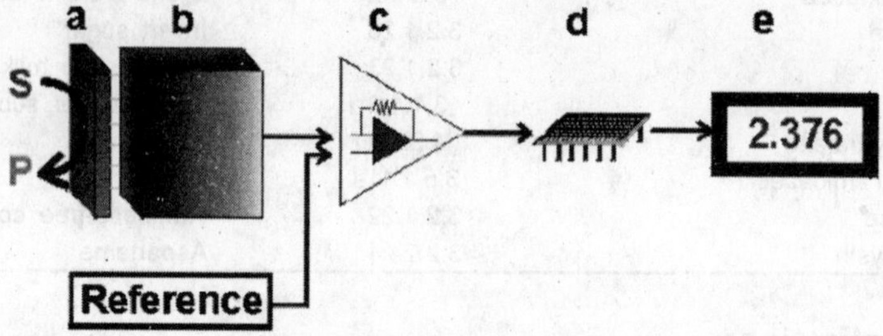

Figure 32.4 Schematic diagram showing the main components of a biosensor. The biocatalyst (a) converts the substrate to product. This reaction is determined by the transducer (b) which converts it into an electrical signal. The output from the transducer is amplified (c), processed (d) and displayed (e).

Production of antibiotics

Benzylpenicillins and phenoxymethylpenicillins (penicillins G and V, respectively) are produced by fermentation and are the basic precursors of a wide range of semi-synthetic antibiotics, e.g., ampicillin. The amide link may be hydrolyzed conventionally, but the conditions necessary for its specific hydrolysis, whilst causing no hydrolysis of the intrinsically more labile but pharmacologically essential β-lactam ring, are difficult to attain. Such specific hydrolysis may be simply achieved by use of penicillin amidases (also called penicillin acylases). Different enzyme preparations are generally used for the hydrolysis of the penicillins G and V, pencillin-V-amidase being much more specific than pencillin-G-amidase. Penicillin amidase may be obtained from *E. coli* and has been immobilized on a number of supports including cyanogen bromide-activated Sephadex G200. It represents one of the earliest successful processes involving immobilized enzymes and is generally used in batch or semicontinuous STR processes (40,000 Ukg-1penicillin G, 35°C, pH 7.8, 2 h) where it may be reused over 100 times. It has also been used in PBRs, where it has an active life of over 100 days, producing about two tonnes of 6-aminopenicillanic acid kg-1of immobilized enzyme.

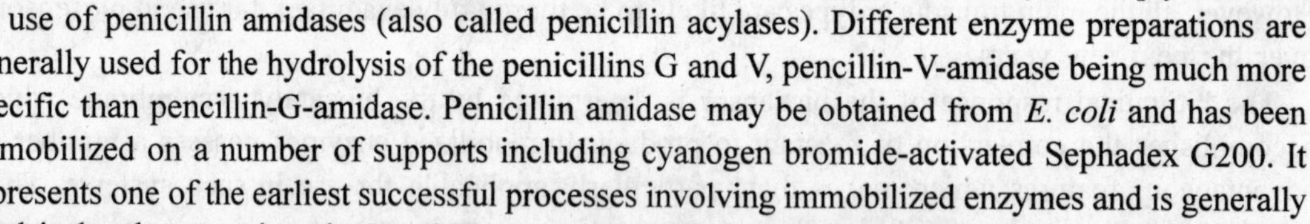

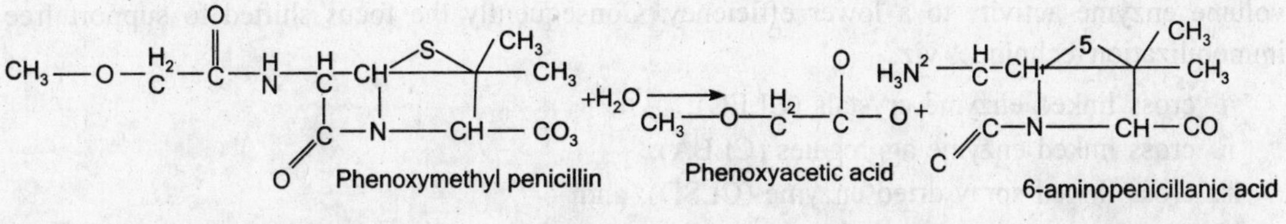

The penicillin-G-amidases may be used 'in reverse' to synthesize penicillin and cephalosporin antibiotics by non-equilibrium kinetically controlled reactions. Ampicillin has been produced by the use of penicillin-G-amidase immobilized by adsorption to DEAE -cellulose in a packed bed column:

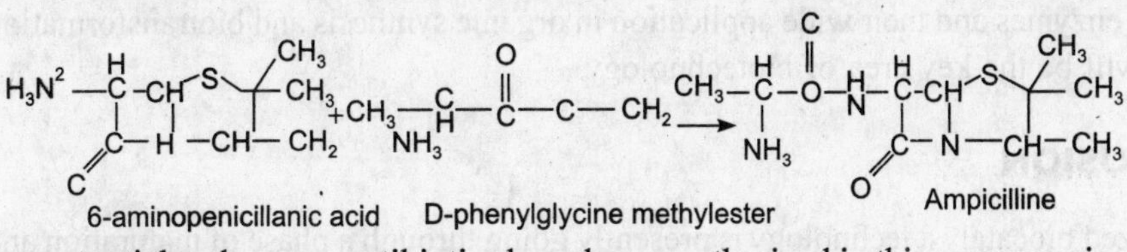

Many other potential and proven antibiotics have been synthesized in this manner using a variety of synthetic β-lactams and activated carboxylic acids.

Recent Advances in Immobilized Biocatalyst Technology

A number of possibilities now exist for the construction of artificial enzymes. These are generally synthetic polymers or oligomers with enzyme-like activities, often called synzymes that can be immobilized on solid support. They must possess two structural entities, a substrate-binding site and a catalytically effective site. It has been found that producing the facility for substrate binding is relatively straightforward, but catalytic sites are somewhat more difficult. Both sites may be designed separately, but it appears that if the synzyme has a binding site for the reaction transition state, this often achieves both functions. Synzymes generally obey the saturation Michaelis-Menten kinetics. For one-substrate reaction, the reaction sequence is given by:

$$\text{synzyme} + \text{S} \rightleftharpoons (\text{synzme-S complex}) \rightarrow \text{synzyme} + \text{P}$$

Some synzymes are simply derivatised proteins, although covalently immobilized enzymes are not considered here. An example is the derivatisation of myoglobin, the oxygen carrier in muscle, by attaching $(Ru(NH_3)_5^{3+}$ to three surface histidine residues. This converts it from an oxygen carrier to an oxidase, oxidising ascorbic acid whilst reducing molecular oxygen. The synzyme is almost as effective as natural ascorbate oxidases.

FUTURE PROSPECTS

In recent years, several techniques for immobilizing both enzymes and whole cells have been devised. Even since their initial development, the possibility of the use of immobilized enzyme as practical re-usable catalysts has been recognized and an enormous quantity of research has been carried out in this area. However, continual promises, the "golden egg" are yet to be laid. Of late advances have been made in the development of support/carrier free enzymes. Support constitutes large non-catalytic mass in immobilized enzyme system, thereby drastically reducing per unit volume enzyme activity to a lower efficiency. Consequently the focus shifted to support free immobilization techniques viz.

i. cross linked enzyme crystals (CLEC);
ii. cross linked enzyme aggregates (CLEA);
iii. cross linked spray dried enzyme (CLSD); and
iv. protein coated microcrystals (PCMC)

These emerging techniques have been very successful in obtaining very efficient and remarkable stable derivatives. In case of hydrolases, it is believed that rational design of CLEA of various industrial enzymes and their wide application in organic synthesis and biotransformation of pharma middles will be the key area of biotechnology.

CONCLUSION

Immobilized biocatalyst technology is presently going through a phase of maturation and evolution. The maturation is shown by the development of the theory concerning how enzymes function and how this is related to their primary structure through the formation and configuration of their three-dimensional structure. The evolution is shown by the ever broadening range of enzymic applications. There still remains much room for the development of useful processes and materials based on this hard-won understanding. Immobilized enzymes will clearly be used more widely in the future and this will be reflected in the number of enzymes available on an industrial (and research) scale, the variety of reactions catalyzed and the range of environmental conditions under which they will operate. Established immobilized enzymes will be put to new uses; and novel enzymes, discovered within their biological niches or produced by design using enzyme engineering will be used to catalyze hitherto unexploited reactions. This is just the beginning of the immobilized biocatalyst technology era.

FURTHER READINGS

1. Baret, J. L. (1987) Large-scale production and application of immobilized lactase. *Methods in Enzymology.* **(136):** 411-423.
2. Barker, S.A. (1982) New approaches to enzyme stabilization. In: *Topics in Enzyme and Fermentation Biotechnology*, Vol. 6, ed. A. Wiseman. Ellis Horwood Ltd., Chichester, UK, pp. 68-78.
3. Bicker staff, G.F. (1997) *Immobilization of Enzymes and Cells*. Humana Press Inc., New York.
4. Bodálo, A., Gómez, J.L., Gómez, E., Bastida, J., Iborra, J.L. and Manjón, A. (1986). Analysis of diffusion effects on immobilized enzymes on porous supports with reversible Michaelis-Menten kinetics. Enzyme and Microbial Technology **(8):** 433-438.
5. Buchholz, K., Kasche, V, and Bornscheuer, U. T. (2005) *Biocatalysts and Enzyme Technology*. Marcel-Dekkar, New York.
6. Campbell D.H., L ıescher E., and Lerman L.S. (1951) *Proc. Nat. Acad. Sci.* **(37):** 575-581.
7. Cao, L, and Schmed, R.D. (2006) *Carried Baus Immobilized Enzyme: Principles Application and Design*. Wiley-VCH, Weiuheim.
8. Cheetham, P.S.J. (1987) Screening for novel biocatalysts. *Enzyme and Microbial Technology.* **(9):** 194-213.
9. Chibata I, Tosa T, Sato T, Mori T, and Matuo Y (1972) *Proc. of the 4th Int. Fermentation Symp.: Fermentation Technology Today,* p. 383-389.

10. Cornish-Bowden, A. (1976) *Principles. of Enzyme. Kinetics.* Butterworth., London.
11. Daniels, M. J. (1986) Immobilized enzymes in carbohydrate food processing. In: *Biotechnology in the Food Industry*, Pinner: Online Publications, pp. 29-35.
12. Daniels, M. J. (1987) Industrial operation of immobilised enzymes. Methods in Enzymology, **(136):** 356-370.
13. Engasser, J-M. and Coulet, P.R. (1977) Comparison of intrinsic stabilities of free and bound enzymes by graphical removal of diffusional effects. *Biochimica et Biophysica Acta.* **(485):** 29-36.
14. Engasser, J-M. and Horvath, C. (1976) Diffusion and kinetics with immobilised enzymes. *In: Applied Biochemistry and Bioengineering*, Vol. 1 *Immobilised Enzyme Principles*. ed. L. B. Wingard.
15. Gekas, V. and Lopez-Leiva M. (1985) Hydrolysis of lactose: a literature review. *Process Biochemistry.* **(20):** 2-12.
16. Goldstein, L. (1972) Microenvironmental effects on enzyme catalysis. A kinetic study of polyanionic and polycationic derivatives of chymotrypsin. *Biochemistry.* **(11):** 4072-4084.
17. Gordon F. Bickerstaff ed. "Immobilization of Enzymes and Cells" (1997) Humana Press. N.J.
18. Grubhofer N., Schleith L. (1953) Modified ionexchange resins as specific adsorbent. *Naturwissenschaften* **(40):** 508.
19. Guilbault, G.G. and de Olivera Neto, G. (1985) Immobilized enzyme electrodes. In *USES451 Immobilized Cells and Enzymes: A Practical Approach* ed. J.Woodward, Oxford: IRL Press Ltd., pp. 55-74.
20. Guisan Jose M. *et al.* (2007) Improvement of enzyme activity, selectivity and stability via immobilization techniques". *Enzyme and Microbial Technology.* 40 **(6):** 1451-1463.
21. Guisan, J. M. (2006). *Immobilized of Enzyme and Cells*, Humana Press Inc. New York.
22. Hall, EAH. (1986) The developing biosensor arena. *Enzyme and Microbial Technology.* **(8):** 651-657.
23. Howaldt, M. W., Kulbe, K. D. & Chmiel, H. (1986) Choice of reactor to minimise enzyme requirement. 1. Mathematical model for one –substrate Michaelis-Menten type kinetics in continuous reactors. *Enzyme and Microbial Technology.* **(8):** 627- 631.
24. Jensen, V. J. and Rugh, S. (1987) Industrial-scale production and application of immobilized glucose isomerase. *Methods in Enzymology.* **(136):** 356-370.
25. Katchalski-Katzir, E. and Goldstein L. (1983) Guidelines for the characterization of immobilized biocatalysts. *Enzyme and Microbial Technology.* **(5):** 304-307.
26. Kennedy, J.F. and Cabral, J.M.S. (1987) Enzyme immobilisation. In: *Biotechnology*, Vol. 7a, *Enzyme Technology*, ed. J.F. Kennedy, Weinheim: VCH Verlagsgesellschaft mbH, pp. 347-404.
27. Klyosov, A. A. (1986) Enzymic conversion of cellulosic materials to sugar and alcohol: the technology and its implications. *Applied Biochemistry and Biotechnology.* **(12):** 249-300.
28. Kricka, L.J. and Thorpe, G.H.G. (1986) Immobilized enzymes in analysis. *Trends in Biotechnology.* **(4):** 253-258.
29. Lerner, R. A. and Tramontano, A. (1987) Antibodies as enzymes. *Trends in Biochemical Sciences.* **(12):** 427-430.
30. Lingiu Cao. (2005) Immobilized enzymes: science or art?. *Current Opinion in Chemical Biology.* 9 **(2):** 217-226.
31. Lowe, C.R. (1984) Biosensors. *Trends in Biotechnology.* **(2):** 59-64.
32. Manson, M.-A. and Mosbach, K. (1987) Immobilized active coenzymes. *Methods in Enzymology.* **(136):** 3-9.
33. Martinek, K., Klibanov, A.M., Goldmacher, V.S. and Berezin, I.V. (1977a) The principles of enzyme stabilization 1. Increase in thermostability of enzymes covalently bound to a complementary surface of a polymer support in a multipoint fashion. *Biochimica et Biophysica Acta.* **(485):** 1-12.
34. Martinek, K., Klibanov, A.M., Goldmacher, V.S., Tchernysheva, A.V., Mozhaev, V.V., Berezin, I.V. and Glotov, B.O. (1977b) The principles of enzyme stabilization 2. Increase in the thermostability of enzymes

as a result of multipoint noncovalent interaction with a polymeric support. *Biochimica et Biophysica Acta.* **(485):** 13-28.

35. Micheel F. and Ewers J. (1949) Makromol. *Chem.* **(3):** 200-209.
36. Mosbach, K. (1987) Immobilized enzymes and cells, *Methods Enzyme* Vol. 135, Academic Press, NY.
37. Nelson J.M. and Griffin E.G. (1916) *J. Am. Chem. Soc.* **(38):** 1109-1115.
38. Pike, V. W. (1987) Synthetic enzymes. In: *Biotechnology*, Vol. 7a *Enzyme Technology*, ed. J.F. Kennedy, Weinheim: VCH Verlagsgesellschaft mbH, pp. 465-485.
39. Gupta Sanjay Mohan, Gupta Supriya and Kumar Anil (2009) Development of bed reactor using brick-dust immobilized CM-Cellulase from seeds of cowpea (*Vigna sinensis* L.). *J. Plant Bioch. & Biotech.* 18 **(1):** 113-116.
40. Sheldon, R. A. (2007) Crosslinked enzyme agqregalies *Biochem. Soc. Trans.* **(35):** 1583- 1587.
41. Soda, K. and Yonaha, K. (1987) Application of free enzymes in pharmaceutical and chemical industries. In: Biotechnology, Vol. 7a *Enzyme Technology*, ed. J.F. Kennedy, Weinheim: VCH Verlagsgesellschaft mbH. pp. 605-52.
42. Sumner J.B. (1948) Denaturation of Urease Without Inactivation. *Science.* **(108):** 410-413.
43. Turner, A.P.F. (1987) Biosensors: Principles and potential. In: *Chemical. Aspects of Food. Enzymes,* ed. A.T. Andrews, London: Royal Society of Chemistry, pp. 259-270,
44. Turner, A.P.F., Karube, I. and Wilson, G.S. eds. (1987) *Biosensors: Fundamentals and Applications*, Oxford University Press. Oxford, U.K.
45. Vieth, W. R., Venkatasubramanian, K., Constantinides, A. and Davidson, B. (1976) Design and analysis of immobilized-enzyme flow reactors. In: *Applied Biochemistry and Bioengineering*, Vol. I *Immobilized Enzyme Principles*, ed. L. B. Wingard & E. Katchalski -Katzir, Academic Press. London, pp. 221-327.
46. Wingard LB (1972) Jr. ed., *Enzyme Engineering*, Wiley, New York.
47. Woodward, J. (1985) Immobilized enzymes: Adsorption and covalent coupling. In: *Immobilized Cells and Enzymes: A Practical Approach*, ed. J. Woodward, Oxford:IRL Press Ltd., pp. 3-17.
48. Zaborsky O.R. (1973) *Immobilized Enzymes*, Chemical Rubber Co. Press, Ohio.

CHAPTER

33 Bioprocess Technology

Bioprocess technology makes use of microbial, animal and plant cells and components of cells such as enzymes to manufacture new products and destroy harmful wastes. Application areas commonly associated with bioprocess technology include the production of biofuels, ethanol, amino acids and other organic acids, antibiotics, design and operation of fermentation systems, development of food processing systems, application and testing of product separation technologies, design of instrumentation to monitor and control biological processes, and many more. The purpose of this chapter is to lay the foundation of basic concepts and practical uses of bioprocess technology in agriculture, medical, veterinary and industrial applications.

Keywords: Bioprocess technology; bioreactor; downstream processing; batch processing; metabolites.

INTRODUCTION

Bioprocess technology works at the frontiers of biological and engineering sciences to *"Bring Engineering To Life"* through the conversion of biological materials into other forms needed by mankind. Bioprocess technology is a specialization of Chemical Engineering or of Agricultural Engineering. It deals with the design and development of equipment and processes for the manufacturing of products such as food, feed, pharmaceuticals, nutraceuticals, chemicals, and polymers and paper from biological materials. Application areas commonly associated with bioprocess technology include the production of biofuels, design and operation of fermentation systems, development of food processing systems, application and testing of product separation technologies, design of instrumentation to monitor and control biological processes, and many more. Like other engineering disciplines, bioprocess engineers are trained in the application of engineering sciences and problem solving techniques. What separates them from other engineers is their understanding of how every engineering field relates to living materials.

Bioprocess development for biopharmaceuticals involves all aspects of generating a safe, effective, and stable product. It begins with the biological system, continues with product isolation and purification, and finishes when the product is placed in a stable, efficacious, and convenient form. The product is initially derived either directly or indirectly from a living organism. Thus, process development starts with the development of the biological system. It is usually a living organism that expresses the desired protein; but it might be an enzyme for protein modification or an antibody for immuno-affinity purification. rDNA and hybridoma technology allows the biological system to be optimized for maximal formation of the product, for facilitation of downstream processing, for high product quality, and for improved interaction with the production equipment (Figure 33.1). In this phase of bioprocess engineering, many disciplines must be applied, including molecular biology, genetics, biochemistry, analytical chemistry, and bioprocess engineering. Thus, engineers become full partners with experts trained in the bioscience disciplines in developing and scaling up manufacturing technology for biopharmaceuticals. As the task of process development proceeds through isolation, purification, and formulation, multidisciplinary approaches continue to be advantageous. Bioprocess engineers combine their skills with those of biochemists and analytical biochemists to develop the optimal process. The multidisciplinary task of bioprocess engineering is usually applied to developing processes for the production of biopharmaceutical products, but it can also be applied to the discovery of new products. For example, automated screening methods that use purified cell receptors can be developed. More efficient methods for producing and isolating families of precisely modified proteins can be devised, and the technology required to produce protein pharmaceuticals efficiently with mammalian cells can be applied to develop cell-based assays to screen for product activity or toxicity.

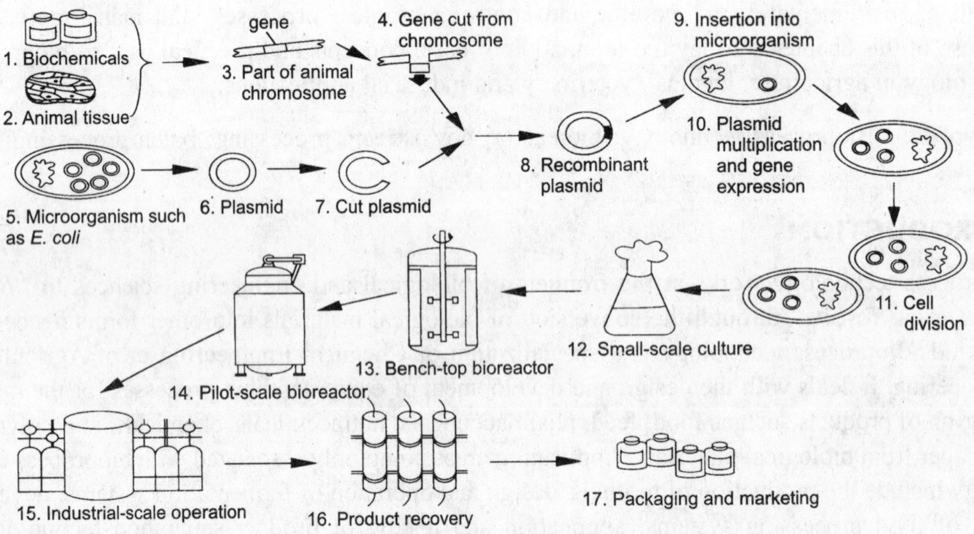

Figure 33.1 Steps in the development of a complete bioprocess for commercial manufacture of a new recombinant-DNA-derived product.

The bioprocessing of renewable and nonrenewable resources requires the application of multiple disciplines in a cross-disciplinary approach. As in the case of biopharmaceuticals, products are derived either directly or indirectly from living organisms. Unlike those in the biopharmaceutical sector, however, bioprocess engineers dealing with renewable and nonrenewable resources are involved with high processing volumes and often design and operate large installations. The processes themselves must still be reliable, robust, and cost-effective. The goal is to generate products from renewable resources or to produce microbial and other biocatalysts for use in processing renewable or nonrenewable resources to obtain value-added products. Economies of scale and scalable equipment are important, if not critical, process characteristics. This sector of the biotechnology industry also produces specialty products (enzymes, amino acids, organic acids, and animal-health products) for which the processing technology and regulatory issues are similar to those associated with high-volume biopharmaceutical products, but the ratio of market price to processing cost can be much lower. Production efficiency, as well as product quality, is paramount. A key function of bioprocess engineering is the design, operation, and improvement of manufacturing technology to yield bioproducts at high volume and acceptable costs. Success will require bioprocess engineers to become partners with molecular biologists and geneticists, biochemists, carbohydrate chemists, wood chemists, food scientists, analytical chemists, and microbial physiologists. With the rapid growth of biologically based technologies, bioprocess engineers are uniquely qualified to solve the problems of today and tomorrow. The demand for bioprocess engineers continues to grow. They provide a bridge between the research laboratory and the economic, large-scale implementation of biotechnologies and food production systems.

CONCEPTS

Bioprocess technology evolved as a means of producing food, beverages, and medicines. More than 8,000 years ago, it was used to make leavened bread. Some 5,000 years ago, moldy soybean curd was used to treat skin infections in China. The malting of barley and fermentation of beer was used in Egypt in 2500 BC. Louis Pasteur proved in 1857 that yeast is a living cell that ferments sugar to alcohol; in 1877, he showed that some bacteria kill anthrax bacilli. In 1923, Banting and Best showed that insulin from animals could be used to treat people suffering from diabetes. In 1928, Alexander Fleming showed that growing colonies of Penicillium notatum inhibit Staphylococcus cultures. Beginning in 1939, Florey and Chain rediscovered that Fleming's Penicillium could lyse bacteria, but the yield of penicillin was small; in addition, the penicillin it did produce was unstable. They realized that producing penicillin on a large scale would require isolation and purification procedures that minimized product loss. Early bioprocess engineers found solutions to this problem when researchers in the U.S. Department of Agriculture (USDA) laboratory in Peoria, Illinois, discovered that mold on a cantaloupe (P. chrysogenum) could be grown in large tanks in submerged cultures. During World War II, government incentives encouraged several pharmaceutical companies to develop cost-effective manufacturing processes for penicillin. Chemical engineers, industrial chemists, and microbiologists quickly devised methods of countercurrent extraction, crystallization, and lyophilization to recover penicillin in an active and stable form and established the viability of submerged fermentations. The benefits of biotechnology might be an anomaly if it were not for engineering, specifically bioprocess technology, the discipline that puts biotechnology to work. To quote Louis Pasteur, bioprocess engineering is to biotechnology "as the fruit is to the tree." Neither can exist without the other. The realization of the benefits of penicillin required the development of methods of transforming microbial growth on the surface of a moldy cantaloupe to cultures grown in large stirred tanks fed by sterile air. It took engineers to design the tanks, impellers, pumps, compressors, columns, pipes, and valves that have made biotechnology products available to large numbers of people. The lifesaving benefits of insulin required engineering for the extraction and purification of insulin from cow and pig pancreas, and later, the large-scale propagation of bacteria engineered to make human insulin, as well as methods of recovery, refolding, and purification to obtain an active molecule. Biochemical manufacturing and bioseparations have made it possible to purify products derived from biotechnology on a large scale.

PRINCIPLES

The basic principles of bioprocess technology are based on understanding of the microorganisms or biocatalysts involved. This ensures:

(i) consistent product quality and product safety, regardless of scale;
(ii) addressing environmental consequences of the manufacture and use of the products; and
(iii) continually improving and developing processes in response to the competitive pressures generated by consumer markets.

The engineering operations that cut across those requirements include the development of bioreactor technology, the processing of impure dilute product streams into purified and concentrated form, and the ability to apply engineering economics in decision-making processes during the design, development, operation, and improvement of bioprocess facilities. That requires engineers who can solve engineering problems on the basis of an understanding of the biochemistry and genetics of living organisms. A sustained policy is needed to foster development of a fundamental knowledge base for the manufacture of a broad spectrum of bioproducts and the training of bioprocess engineers who will grow with the growing industry.

BIOPROCESS TECHNOLOGY

Purpose: Bioprocess technology has been used for the following purposes:

(i) In the formation of complex molecular structure such as antibiotics and proteins where there is no practical alternative.
(ii) In the exclusive production of one specific form of an isomeric compound.
(iii) Because micro-organisms may efficiently execute many sequential reactions.
(iv) Because bioconversions may give high yields.

Requirements for Bioprocessing

Raw materials

Current bioprocess technology uses an extremely limited range of raw materials just a few agricultural commodities in many of the existing industrial bioprocesses. The need for raw materials for bioprocesses, however, could become a major factor in commodity grain markets if bioprocesses find a place in large scale fuel or chemical production.

Biocatalysts

The substances that actually cause chemical changes in bioprocesses are the enzymes produced by a living cell. Biological transformation of the substrate involves several sequential and interrelated chemical reactions, each catalyzed by a separate enzyme, however whole cells (e.g., microorganisms such as bacteria, yeast or fungi) are used as biocatalysts. Bioprocesses used for the synthesis of complex molecular structures (e.g., antibiotics or proteins such as insulin) require entire system of enzymes. Sometimes animal cells and tissues are employed for vaccine production and related activities but the catalytic capabilities of plant cells except for some algae, have not yet been employed commercially. Biocatalysts generally exhibit great sensitivity to changes in temperature, pH and even concentrations of certain nutrients or metal ions. The success of a bioprocess depends on the extent to which these factors are controlled in the medium where interaction between biocatalyst and substrate take place. Biocatalysts that can withstand high temperatures and high pressure may also be useful industrially. Wider availability of thermo tolerant biocatalysts is important for all industries using bioprocesses. The advantages of thermo tolerance include:

(i) Reduced susceptibility to contamination
(ii) easier removal of conversions
(iii) more complex and rapid conversions
(iv) easier recovery of volatile products

Water

Water is the dominant component of the medium for virtually all current bioprocesses and is needed in many of the ancillary services such as heating, cooling, cleaning and rinsing. Clean water of consistent composition is therefore required in large quantities from reliable permanent sources. When assessing the suitability of a water supply it is important to consider pH, dissolved salts and effluent contamination. Products must usually be purified from the dilute aqueous solution. The environment is closely controlled and this necessity markedly influences their design.

Supply of Nutrients

The medium must provide for the nutritional needs of living cells in addition to establishing a suitable environment. A primary requirement is a source of carbon. In addition to supplying the energy needed for metabolism and protein synthesis, carbon sources contribute structural elements required for the formation of complex compounds. Other important nutrients required by living cells are nitrogen and phosphorus which are sometimes oxygen; nitrogen and phosphorus are incorporated into structural and functional molecules of a cell and may also become part of product molecules. A number of other nutrients such as vitamins and metal ions, though required only in very small amounts, are nevertheless essential.

On a large scale the normally used sources of nutrients to create a medium which will meet as many as possible of the following criteria:

(i) It should produce the maximum yield of product or biomass per gram of substrate used.
(ii) It should produce the maximum concentration of product or biomass.
(iii) It should permit the maximum rate of product formation.
(iv) There should be the minimum yield of undesired products.
(v) It should be of a consistent quality and be readily available throughout the year.
(vi) It should cause minimal problems during media making and sterilization.
(vii) It should cause minimal problems in other aspects of the production process particularly aeration and agitation, extraction, purification and waste treatment.

Energy sources

Energy for growth comes from either the oxidation of medium components or from light. Most industrial microorganisms are chemo-organotrophs, therefore, the commonest source of energy will be the carbon source such as carbohydrates, lipids and proteins. Some microorganisms can also use hydrocarbons or methanol as carbon and energy sources.

Carbon source

The main product of a bioprocess will often determine the choice of carbon source, particularly if the product results from the direct dissimilation of it. It is now recognized that the rate at which the carbon source is metabolized can often influence the formation of biomass or production of primary or secondary metabolites. Fast growth due to high concentrations of rapidly metabolized sugars is often associated with low productivity of secondary metabolites. The purity of the carbon source may also affect the choice of substrate. The method of media preparation, particularly sterilization, may affect the suitability of carbohydrates for individual bioprocesses. It is often best to sterilize sugars separately because they may react with ammonium ions and amino acids to form black nitrogen containing compounds which will partially inhibit the growth of many microorganisms.

In the most common practice carbohydrates are used as the carbon source in microbial fermentation processes. The most widely available carbohydrate is starch obtained from maize grain. It is also obtained from other cereals, potatoes and cassava. Maize and other cereals may also be used directly in a partially ground state, e.g., maize chips.

Barley grains may be partially germinated and heat treated to give the material known as malt, which contains a variety of sugars besides starch. Malt is the main substrate for brewing beer and lager in many countries. Malt extracts may also be prepared from malted grain.

Sucrose is obtained from sugar cane and sugar beet. It is commonly used in fermentation media in a very impure form as beet or cane molasses which are the residues left after crystallization of sugar solutions in sugar refining. Molasses is used in the production of high-volume flow-value products such as ethanol, SCP, organic and amino acids and some microbial gums. Molasses or sucrose also may be used for production of higher value/low-bulk products such as antibiotics, special enzymes, vaccines and fine chemicals.

Nitrogen sources

Most industrially used microorganisms can utilize inorganic or organic sources of nitrogen. Inorganic nitrogen may be supplied as ammonia gas, ammonium salts or nitrates.

Organic nitrogen may be supplied as amino acid, protein or urea. In many instances growth will be faster with a supply of organic nitrogen, and a few microorganisms have an absolute requirement for amino acids. However, amino acids are more commonly added as complex organic nitrogen sources which are non-homogeneous, cheaper and readily available. Other proteinaceous nitrogen compounds serving as sources of amino acids include corn-steep liquor, soya meal, peanut meal, cotton-seed meal and yeast extract.

Supply of Oxygen

Since most of the microorganisms currently used by industry perform their conversions aerobically. The fundamental problem in supplying sufficient oxygen is oxygen's low solubility. Solubility of oxygen decreases as the concentration of dissolved solutes increases. However, solubility of oxygen in the growth medium can be increased by:

(i) Increasing oxygen pressure of the gas phase by increasing reactor pressure.
(ii) Using oxygen rich gas for aeration.
(iii) Changing in process design and operation.

For small-scale culture, e.g., less than 1L, it is possible to supply adequate amounts of oxygen by growing the microbe in an Erlenmeyer flask which is agitated constantly, provided that the volume of growth medium does not exceed 10-20% of the flask volume. For large-scale culture and/or high cell densities the oxygen demand of the culture can be met by blowing air through the culture.

At laboratory-scale cultures may be aerated by means of the *shake-flask technique* where the culture is grown in a conical flask shaken on a platform contained in a controlled environment of the chamber.

At Pilot- and industrial-scale fermentations broth or culture is aerated by *stirred or agitation method.*

Some bioreactors or fermenters are so designed that adequate supply of oxygen is obtained without agitation and such bioreactors or fermenters are called *bubble columns and air-lift fermenter.*

Bartholomew *et al.* (1950) represented the transfer of oxygen from air to the cell, during fermentation, as occurring in a number of steps:

(i) The transfer of oxygen from an air bubble into solution.
(ii) The transfer of the dissolved oxygen through the fermentation medium to the microbial cell.
(iii) The uptake of the dissolved oxygen by the cell.

The individual steps involved in oxygen transfer from a gas bubble to the reaction site inside the individual cell are given bellow: (Figure 33.2)

1. Diffusion of oxygen from the bulk gas to the gas liquid interface.
2. Transport across the gas liquid interface.
3. Diffusion of oxygen through a relatively stagnant liquid region adjacent to the gs bubble i.e. from the gas-liquid interface to the well-mixed bulk liquid.
4. Transport of oxygen through the well-mixed liquid to a relatively unmixed liquid region surrounding of the cells.
5. Diffusion through the stagnant region surrounding the cells.
6. Transport from the liquid to the pellet cell aggregate etc.
7. Diffusion transport of oxygen into the pellet etc.
8. Transport across the cell envelope.
9. Transport from the cell envelope to the intracellular reaction site, e.g., the mitochondria.

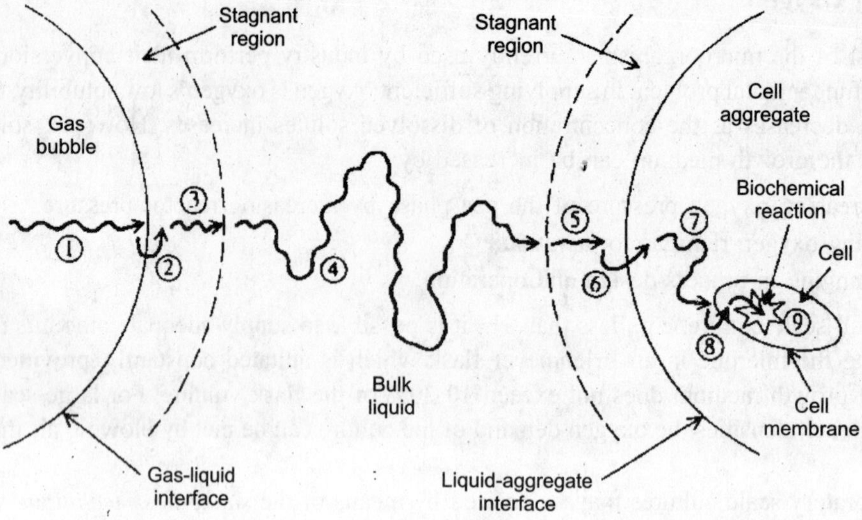

Figure 33.2 The individual steps involved in oxygen transfer from a gas bubble to the reaction site inside the individual cell.

Pure Culture and Sterilization

Most of the products of bioprocesses are formed through the action of a single biocatalyst, either a microorganism or an enzyme. If foreign organisms contaminate the process system, they may disrupt its operation in a variety of ways. They can directly inhibit or interfere with the biocatalyst, whether it is a single enzyme or a complete cell and they may even destroy the biocatalyst completely. Alternatively, contaminating organisms may leave the catalyst unaffected but modify or destroy the product. Also, there substances are difficult to separate from the primary product. In the manufacture of pharmaceutical products, the risk of toxic impurities is of particular concern. To avoid or minimize contamination, most current bioprocess technologies employ pure culture techniques. The medium and its container are sterilized and a pure culture consisting of a population of a particular species is introduced. In order to avoid subsequent contamination, all materials entering the system, including the large amounts of air required for aerobic processes, are sterilized. The apparatus must be designed and operated so that the opportunities for invasion by unwanted organisms are minimized.

Bioprocessing Modes (Batch ver. Continuous Operation)

A bioprocess may, in principle, use any of the operating modes employed by conventional chemical technology. These modes range from batch processing to continuous steady state processing which include – batch processing, semi-batch processing, fed-batch processing continuous steady-state processing.

Batch Processing

In batch processing the reaction vessel (e.g., fermenter) is filled with the medium containing substrate, sterilized, inoculated (or added biocatalyst) and the bioconversion is allowed to proceed. It takes time ranging from a few hours to several days. During this time, nutrients as well as substrates, agents for pH control and air are supplied and product gases are removed from the reaction vessel. When conversion is complete, the reaction vessel is emptied and cleaned and prepared for a fresh run. Simultaneously, the purification process begins. In some instances, this turnover time between the batches can be prolonged.

A semi-batch processing ***allows either input or output of mass, but not both.***

A fed-batch processing ***allows input of material to the system but not output.***

Continuous Steady-state Processing

In this process raw materials are supplied to the vessel at a rate volumetrically equal to that at which product and spent medium are withdrawn. The possibility of the long runs (i.e. several weeks duration) is the potential advantage offered by continuous processing over batch processing which leads to significantly higher productivity, greater ease of product recovery through the reuse of contaminating biocatalyst and lower cost due to reuse of biocatalyst. The extent of increase in productivity will depend on the ratio of processing time and turnover time: the smaller the ratio, the more advantageous is continuous operation. A second advantage is that the growth rate of the cells which is required for optimal product formation can be maintained.

Continuous culture is ideally suited for the production of biomass or simple metabolites or simple metabolites such as ethanol where synthesis is proportional to cell density. It is not suitable for the production of other metabolites such as amino acids and antibiotics where synthesis is not associated with growth. The most widespread use of continuous culture is in the effluent disposal industry where waste organic materials (substrate) are converted into microbial cells (biomass). Batch operation currently dominates specially in chemical and pharmaceutical bioprocesses and is likely to continue to do so in the near future. In addition to technical limitations on continuous processing, other considerations have led manufacturers to choose the batch mode. Batch processing is often used because it offers the operational flexibility needed when a large number of products are manufactured, each at fairly low production levels. Each process unit, more or less standard in design, can easily rapidly be switched from one product line to another. The simplest approach to the implementation of a continuous processing system is to modify a batch reactor so that fresh substrate and nutrients can continually be added while a product stream is removed. Furthermore, a switch from batch to continuous processing is expensive. This arrangement has also one serious drawback: the biocatalyst leaves the reactor continuously with the outlet stream and must be separated from the product. Several techniques, all of which involve fixing the biocatalyst in some manner, have been developed to avoid the biocatalyst's escape with the reaction mixture and allowed its repeated use. The development of techniques for the immobilization of continuous bioprocesses, although still not widely employed for large scale bioprocess, the biocatalyst immobilization techniques now available (discussed in Chapter 32) offer a diversity of new opportunities for more effective bio-processing. Increased use of genetically manipulated biocatalysts could affect the design and operation of bioconversion units. Harvey Blanch points out:

"One of the difficulties which arise from the insertion of foreign DNA into the organism is reversion. This can be minimized by placing the cell in an environment in which cellular replication is minimized, while cellular activity such as the production of enzymes and products is maintained at high levels."

Achieving the dual objective of minimal growth and maximum conversion activity requires restrictive nutrient supplies and high cell densities. Immobilized biocatalysts could be used to achieve these objectives.

Novel Reactor Designs in Bioprocess Monitoring

The main function of a bioreactor is to provide a controlled environment for the growth of microorganisms or animal cells, to obtain a desired product. As a result of the growing need for efficient and cost effective means of producing large quantities of important biological compounds from living cells and enzymes, novel bioreactor types and the modes in which they are operated have been developed. Currently bioreactors are used for small to large-scale production of many different compounds from plant, microbial and animal cells as well as from isolated enzyme systems.

In choosing a bioreactor type and mode of operation, a biotechnology company usually balances medium costs, downstream processing costs and technological advantages.

During the designing and constructing a bioreactor following points must be considered (Figure 33.3):

1. The vessel should be capable of being operated aseptically for a number of days and should be reliable in long-term operation and meet the requirements of containment regulations.
2. Adequate aeration and agitation should be provided to meet the metabolic requirements of the microorganism. However, the mixing should not cause damage to the organism.
3. Power consumption should be as low as possible.
4. A system of temperature control should be provided.
5. A system of pH control should be provided.
6. Sampling facilities should be provided.
7. Evaporation losses from the fermenter should not be excessive.
8. The vessel should be designed to require the minimal use of labor in operation, harvesting, cleaning and maintenance.
9. Ideally the vessel should be suitable for a range of processes, but this may be restricted because of containment regulations.
10. The vessel should be constructed to ensure smooth internal surfaces, using welds instead of flange joints whenever possible.
11. The vessel should be of similar geometry to both smaller and larger vessels in the pilot plant or plant to facilitate scale-up.
12. The cheapest materials which enable satisfactory results to be achieved should be used.
13. There should be adequate service provisions for individual plants.

The first two points are probably the most critical. It's obvious from the above points that the design of a bioreactor will involve co-operation between experts in microbiology, biochemistry, chemical engineering, mechanical engineering and costing.

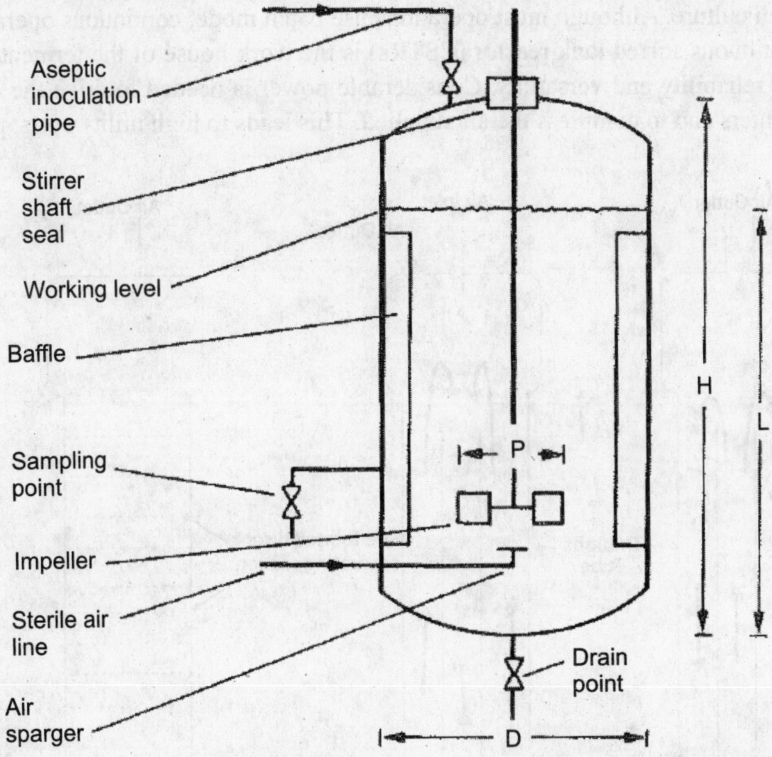

Figure 33.3 Diagram of a bioreactor.

Types of bioreactors: There are two types of bioreactors: 1) conventional bioreactors 2) and membrane bioreactors (Figure 33.4).

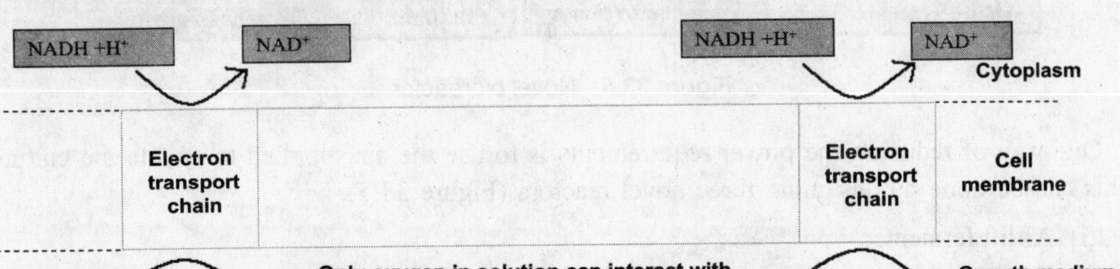

Figure 33.4 Membrane bioreactor.

Conventional Bioreactors

Conventional bioreactors have been used almost universally for fermentation in food, beverage and drug industries. Because of their widespread use and operator familiarity, they have also been adapted for cell culture. Although most operations use batch mode, continuous operations are also used. The continuous stirred tank reactor (CSTRs) is the work house of the fermentation industry because of its reliability and versatility. Considerable power is needed to drive the agitators used in large fermenters and to compress the air supplied. This leads to high utility costs, principally for electricity.

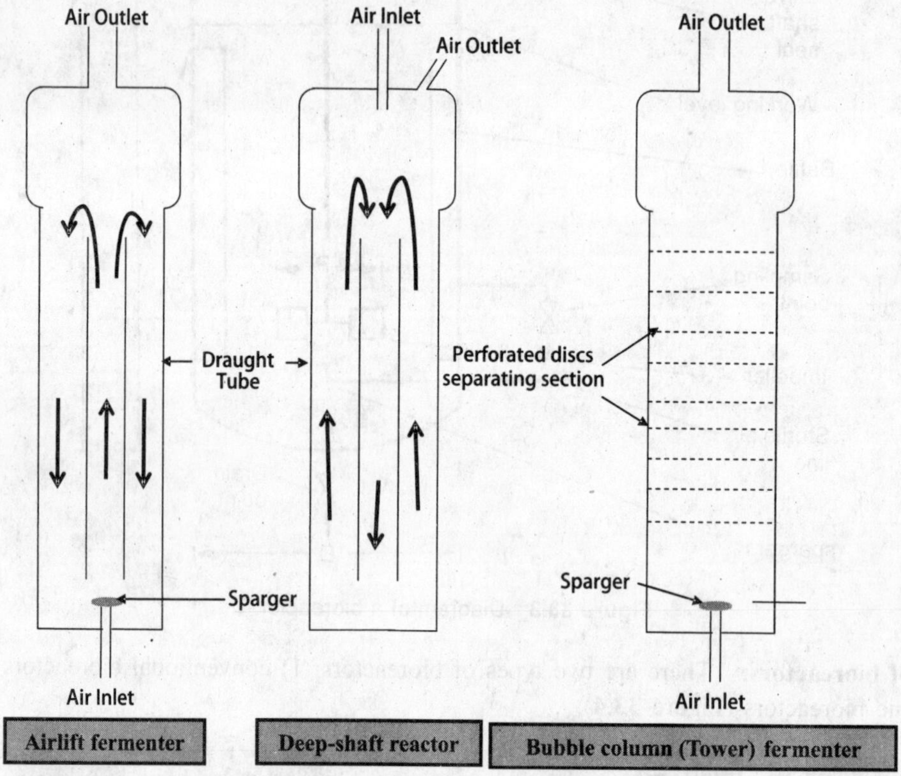

Figure 33.5 Novel bioreactor.

One way of reducing the power requirements is to use the air supplied to agitate the culture. This can be done by designing three novel reactors (Figure 33.5).

(i) Airlift fermenter.

(ii) Deep-shaft reactor.

(iii) Bubble column (tower) fermenter.

In an airlift fermenter, the air is introduced at high velocity at the bottom of the vessel. The use of a draught tube enables the liquid to circulate with considerable turbulence. For efficient oxygen transfer it is necessary for the fermenter to have a height to diameter ratio (10:1- 40:1) that is much greater than with a conventional stirred tank reactor (1:1 – 4:1).

As a gas bubble ascends a column of liquid, the hydrostatic pressure on it decreases and the volume of the bubble increases. Since there now is a decrease in the surface area to volume ratio there is a decrease in the rate of oxygen transfer from the gas phase to the bulk liquid. Furthermore, in a well agitated fermenter over 50% of the oxygen supplied is utilized. Thus, as the bubble ascends the column, the partial pressure of oxygen within it will decrease and this too will decrease the rate of oxygen transfer to the liquid.

A novel reactor design which overcomes these disadvantages is the deep-shaft reactor. Here the air is introduced at high velocity at the top of the reactor and forces the liquid downwards. Although oxygen is utilized during the downward passage the bubble size will diminish because of the hydrostatic pressure and should give rise to a more uniform oxygen transfer rate.

Both the airlift fermenter and the deep-shaft reactor can be operated continuously. The entire vessel contents are essentially homogeneous, both spatially and temporally. By contrast, in a bubble column reactor, which is a variant of the airlift fomenter, the contents of the vessel are not homogeneous. Since there is no mixing, the medium moves through the fermenter as a 'plug' and its composition varies spatially. By dividing the fermenter into sections it is possible to vary the physiochemical environment at will e.g. pH 7.0 at temperature 30°C in one section and pH 40°C in another section.

Membrane Bioreactors

Membrane bioreactors, which simulate the *in vivo* capillary tissue environment by retaining the biological catalyst (cell or enzymes) behind a barrier, have proven to be quite successful in both design goals (as discussed earlier). Membrane systems provide a very mild method of immobilizing cells and enzymes composed with technique requiring chemical attachment. Other advantages include their high surface to volume ratios (important for substrate delivery and waste removal) and their ability to isolate the cells/enzymes from shearing and contamination. With recycle, membrane systems can often achieve higher product concentrations, yields and productivities than batch reactors. These reactors retain the cells in a stable environment with a continuous supply of nutrients, substrates and cofactors while simultaneously removing metabolic wastes. In this manner, cells can be maintained in a state of low or non-proliferating state for long periods of time while still producing the desired products.

Typical system configurations are the hollow fiber and the plate and frame (flat sheet membrane reactors have been used successfully for entrapped culture of microbial, plant mammalian cells. Entrapment of selected cells/ enzymes in spiral wound modules is only beginning to be explored. These membrane systems can also act as integrated production and separation devices.

Despite the advantages of using membrane bioreactors with or without perfusion for culturing cells and producing large amount of products, these systems do have limitations. One of the proclaimed disadvantages of membrane systems is the potential for concentration polarization and fouling which can severely diminish the trans-membrane and nutrient transport.

Fouling can usually be avoided by using hydrophilic membranes with low surface charge density which has the effect of minimizing adsorption on the pore walls and surfaces of the membrane. Concentration polarization can be minimized by the use of high flow rates through the lumen space which increases the wall shear rate and by using the highly porous membrane which lowers the protein refraction coefficient. Another disadvantage is the existence of diffusional limitations. Since in many systems transport of nutrients and by-products relies primarily on diffusion, cells further from the membrane surface may be subjected to low substrate and high waste concentrations leading to cell stagnation and a possible decrease in viability.

Other concerns with the use of hollow fiber bioreactors are the need to maintain aseptic operation and the need to sterilize the bioreactor prior to each run. The use of steam and harsh chemicals often degrades the membranes and the plotting materials such as polyurethane and epoxy that hold and seal the fibers in the cartridge. Several approaches have been used to solve this problem. Porous polypropylene and porous modified glass have been used as auto-cleavable membrane materials. Cold sterilization techniques such as ethylene oxide and radiation have been successfully used. Some companies offer pre-sterilized and disposable, semi- or fully autoclavable hollow fiber cartridges.

The membranes used in reactors must be chosen carefully from the many available types. When a membrane is used to act as a preamble barrier between cells and the cell-free culture medium which carries both nutrients and products, it must be hydrophilic to allow for adequate transport across the membrane. In other reactors where gases and /or organic solutions are used, a combination of hydrophilic and hydrophobic membranes may be more appropriate. The pore size (MWCO) must be chosen to allow the proper selectivity and mechanical strength should be adequate to withstand operational pressures. Ultra filtration (MWCO form 10^3 to 10^6) or micro porous (0.01- 10 μm pore size) membranes are typically used for immobilizing cells in reactors. Micro porous membranes will retain cells yet allowed passage of product molecules while ultra filtration membrane may retain some product molecule in the cell space, increasing its concentration with time. Table 33.1 lists some of the types of membrane and module as well as the catalysts which have been used in bioreactors (Figure 33.6).

Table 33.1 Membrane materials used in bioreactors.

Membrane material	*Catalyst*	*Module* [a]
Acrylic copolymer	SV3T3 cells	HF
Cellulose acetate	Hepatome cells BHK and L929 cells hybridomas	HF
Mixed cellulose esters	B. Cells	HF
Polyacrylonitrile	SV 3T3 Cells	HF
Polyamide	Glucose oxidose	HF
Polypropylene	L. delpreuckii	HF
	S. cerevisiae	HF
	N. tabacum	HS
	S. aureofaciens	HF
	E. coli	HF
Polysulfone	SV3T3 cells	HF
	S. cerevisiae	HF
	D. corota	HF
	Hybridomas	HF
	Fibroblasts	HF
	H. henricii	HF
Hydrophilic PVDF	Hybridomas	FS
Teflon	Hybridomas	HH

a HF. hollow fiber; FS, flat sheet

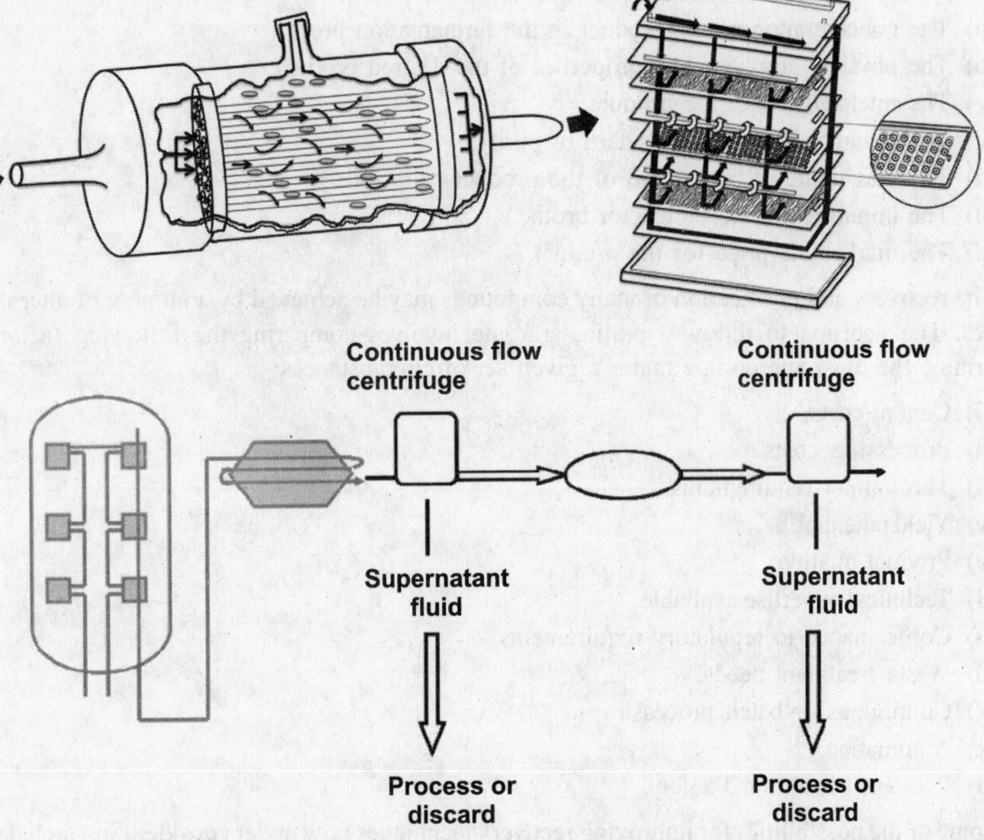

Figure 33.6 Various types of bioreactors.

Downstream Processing (Separation and Purification of Products)

The bioprocesses also release a variety of unwanted metabolites associated with useful products. Separation and purification of useful products from these other associated unwanted metabolites is also needed and is sometimes described as 'downstream processing'. Separation and purification techniques used in bioprocesses are the aspect of bioprocess engineering and needs of attention, especially for the production of novel products such as proteins. Once fermentation is complete, it is necessary to recover the desired and product. At a minimum this will involve separation of the cells from the fermentation both but also may include purification of metabolites with or without cell disruption. Such operations are referred to as downstream processing. Research is need to find highly selective recovery techniques that leave as little residual product as possible in the medium and thus lessen the labor intensity associated with downstream processing.

The choice of recovery process is based on the following criteria:

(i) The intracellular or extracellular location of the product.
(ii) The concentration of the product in the fermentation broth.
(iii) The physical and chemical properties of the desired product.
(iv) The intended use of the product.
(v) The minimal acceptable standard of purity.
(vi) The magnitude of bio-hazard of the product or broth.
(vii) The impurities in the bioreactor broth.
(viii) The marketable price for the product.

The recovery and purification of many compounds may be achieved by a number of alternative routes. The decision to follow a particular route involves comparing the following factors to determine the most appropriate under a given set of circumstances:

(i) Capital costs.
(ii) Processing costs.
(iii) Throughput requirements.
(iv) Yield potential.
(v) Product quality.
(vi) Technical expertise available.
(vii) Conformance to regulatory requirements.
(viii) Waste treatment needs.
(ix) Continuous or batch processing.
(x) Automation.
(xi) Personnel health and safety.

Some of the possibilities for improving recovery techniques now under consideration include the following:

1. Some cells rapidly settle out of suspension once aeration and agitation of the fermented broth cease and the setting may be assisted by the addition of flocculating agents. Many of these flocculating agents are polyelectrolyte's which neutralize the charge on the microbial cell surface and keeps cells in suspension by electrostatic repulsion. Where cells settling occur, or can be induced to occur, the cell removal becomes easy and inexpensive for the fermentation broth and can be decanted or filtered off.
2. Where cell settling does not occur, cell removal can be effected by centrifugation.
3. An alternative to centrifugation is ultra filtration. Membranes and other filtration systems such as porous metals offer many advantages, and considerable experience in other areas of chemical technology is already available. Some U.S. companies such as Millipore, Amicon and Needeopor are making advances in this area. The term ultra filtration describes processes in which particles significantly greater in size than the solvent are retained when the solution is forced through a membrane of very fine pore size, usually less than 0.5 µm.

4. The clarified fermentation liquor will contain microbial metabolites and extracellular enzymes and many methods are available for their recovery including continuous chromatography, ion exchange chromatography, high performance liquid chromatography, precipitation and solvent extraction. The use of ion exchange resins is particularly desirable since they can be used for concentration as well as having capacity and being cheap and reusable.
5. Electrophoretic methods, especially continuous flow can separate proteins, peptides and nucleic acids on the basis of their electrical charge. The advantage of this separation method over some others is that it can run continuously and can effectively separate molecules in large sample volumes.
6. Immobilized monoclonal antibodies are being used as purification agents for protein products (see in hybridoma technology). This technique best suits large molecular weight and high value added products such as proteins.

If the desired product is retained within the cell then cell disruption will be necessary to affect its release. Although many methods of cell disruption and used in the laboratory, most of them cannot be used on a large scale. Two methods which are suitable for large scale use are high pressure homogenization and the use of high speed bead mills. After cell disruption the cell debris needs to be removed. For the removal of intact cells the most widely used methods are centrifugation and ultra filtration.

Advantages of Bioprocessing

Bioprocesses may offer the following advantages over conventional chemical processes:

(i) Milder reaction conditions (temperature, pressure and pH).
(ii) Use of renewable (biomass) resources as raw materials for organic chemical manufacture, providing both carbon skeletons and the energy required for synthesis;
(iii) Less hazardous operation and reduced environment impart.
(iv) Greater specificity of catalytic reaction.
(v) Less expensive or more readily available raw materials
(vi) Requires less complex manufacturing facilities and smaller capital investments.
(vii) Improved process efficiencies (e.g., higher, yields, reduced energy consumption) and
(viii) The use of recombinant-DNA-technology to develop new processes.

Disadvantages of Bioprocessing

Some of the conceivable disadvantages of bioprocesses on the other hand, the following:

(i) The generation of complex product mixtures requiring extensive separation and purification especially when using complex substrates as raw materials (e.g., lignocelluloses)
(ii) Problems arising from the relatively dilute aqueous environments in which bioprocesses function (e.g., the problem of low reactant concentrations and hence, low reaction rates.)
(iii) The susceptibility of most bioprocess system to contamination by foreign organisms, and in some cases, the need to contain the primary organism so as not to contaminate the surrounding.

(iv) An inherent variability of biological processes due to such factors as genetic instability and raw material variability.

(v) For recombinant DNA systems, the need to contain the organisms and sterilize the waste streams, an energy intensive process.

Solutions to some of these problems through the use of biotechnology may make bioprocesses more competitive with conventional chemical synthesis.

APPLICATIONS OF BIOPROCESS TECHNOLOGY

Bioprocess technology has several implications in medical, veterinary, agricultural sciences and industrial applications such as in production of cell matter (biomass itself) (e.g., banks yeast, single cell protein); production of cell components (e.g., enzymes nucleic acids); production of metabolites (chemical products of metabolic activity) including both primary metabolites (e.g., ethanol, lactic acid) and secondary metabolites (e.g., antibiotics); catalysis of specific, single-substrate conversion (e.g., glucose to fructose, penicillin to 6-aminopencillanic acid and; catalysis of multiple-substrate conversions e.g., biological waste treatment; production of microbial insecticide and many more. Some of the important applications are discussed.

Medical Applications

In medical sciences bioprocess technology has several applications such as production of bacterial vaccines (e.g., for cholera, whooping cough, plague, typhoid, paratyphoid fever and typhus fever); production of the diversity of commercially useful low molecular weight compound produced by microorganism such as antibacterial agent, antifungal agent, anti-heliminthic agent, pharmacologically active agents (e.g., ergot alkaloids (vasoconstrictor), cyclosporine (immuno-suppressor drug), mevinolin (cholesterol reduction) vitamins, amino acids, therapeutically useful steroids, etc.); Production of some human proteins with therapeutic potential using recombinant microorganisms (e.g., the proteins include interferons, human growth hormone, insulin, etc.) and many more.

Gene-Based Pharmaceuticals and Gene Therapy

New classes of products are being tested for use in humans and animals, all sharing genes as common targets. Products based on antisense technology directed toward neutralizing messenger RNA are probably being pursued most vigorously; gene therapy through permanent alteration of chromosomes might hold the greatest potential for treatment of diseases like cancer and for correction of genetic disease. The products depend either on classes of compounds that are related to nucleic acids (oligonucleotides and oligonucleotide analogues), on cells that have been genetically altered, of on viruses that bear appropriate nucleic acids. For the large-scale production of nucleotides and nucleotide analogues, new molecular techniques must be developed. There are now no procedures for making substantial quantities of these types of materials in high purity and with appropriate chirality's. Basic chemical and biochemical techniques must be developed for their preparation; new techniques (probably based on high-pressure chromatography) will be required for large-scale purification, and biological methods might be required for preparation of precursors and perhaps for formation of bonds. For genetically modified cells and viruses, the usual techniques for mammalian-cell culture and molecular biology will be required, as will additional measures for safety and for economical, patient-specific production.

Biopharmaceuticals and Biopesticides from Insect Cell-Baculovirus System

Insect cells from moths can be cultivated in a manner similar to (but not identical with) the manner in which mammalian cells can. Unlike mammalian cells, insect cells are naturally continuous cell lines. They can be adapted easily to growth in serum-free media. The unique biphasic life cycle of the baculovirus, which readily infects cultured insect cells, makes it an ideal vector for expression of foreign genes. The baculovirus contains a late promoter that is very strong perhaps the strongest eukaryotic promoter known. Consequently, the insect cell baculovirus expression can be used to produce very high levels of protein (up to 40% of total protein) in a non-transformed host cell (i.e., noncancerous) with a vector that is non-pathogenic to vertebrate animals. Those features of high expression levels and increased safety distinguish this system from the commonly used mammalian expression systems. However, the high expression levels are not typically obtained with secreted, glycosylated proteins. Although insect cells have most of the post-translational machinery of mammalian cells, proteins produced in the baculovirus system are not processed in precisely the same way as in mammalian hosts. Currently, the insect cell-baculovirus system is widely used to produce research quantities of proteins in many industrial laboratories. It is a convenient system for gene expression, and most proteins are produced in the correctly folded conformation. One product, a coat protein from HIV (the virus responsible for AIDS) produced from the baculovirus system, is in Phase II clinical trials and could be produced commercially within 5 years. Other commercial developments of the baculovirus system will depend on bioprocess research to increase expression levels of secreted glycosylated proteins. The baculovirus itself has been approved for use as a pesticide. Genetic modifications to the virus to increase its effectiveness (e.g., speed of killing) are being tested. Large-scale production of such a biopesticide with cell culture will present unprecedented challenges for large-scale, inexpensive animal-cell reactor designs.

Cells, Organs, and Biomaterials

Production of human skin is already a commercial business in the United States; clonal production of lymphocytes is in an early stage of development. With the enormous advances in the biology of differentiation and development, a clear target for the future is large-scale production of cells (initially) and intact organs (later) for use in therapy and organ replacement. Bioprocess engineering will be required to develop new types of reactors and to delineate biological mechanisms that affect growth and maintenance of the cells and differentiated state of these cells. Although lymphocytes in culture can be prepared now, economical production still requires substantial improvement of existing techniques. The technology for production of organs will be much more complex. The rapid increase in knowledge concerning the role of growth factors, cytokines, and other molecules important in cellular communication, coupled with the realization that the three-dimensional matrix in which tissue cells grow is crucial in maintaining cell phenotype, has opened up the possibility of cultivation of viable functioning organ structures. The first applications, already well under way, are in bone marrow cultures and tissues for cosmetic reconstruction. With the increasing concern about the safety of blood products, the ability to culture specific types of blood cells might be crucial for treatment of many diseases and wounds and for surgical procedures. There are serious engineering challenges in developing a system for successful large-scale cultures. Important problems remain in understanding the role of mass transfer, protein matrix for cell attachment and growth, and medium formulation, particularly the proper combination of growth factors required to optimize production of specific cell types. Cosmetic applications include cartilage and artificial skin. Great strides in the latter field in the last decade have resulted in many applications, from burn treatment to reconstruction after surgical procedures, such as breast-cancer removal. But there is need for much improvement even here. Longer-range opportunities include hepatic, pancreatic, and kidney cell cultures. A complex three-dimensional substrate is required to maintain cell differentiation and organ function. Again, many engineering problems must be solved. Providing new vasculature for substrate delivery and product removal is vital. Most organ cells have a polarity that is required for proper function. The overall basic biology of the complex systems required to direct and control differentiating cells is not now understood, and it is impractical to specify in any detail the types of reactors that will be required in the future, other than to say that they will be much more complex and interactive than those now used. With an aging population, there is increasing interest in biologically compatible materials for replacement of organs, joints, and ligaments and for related applications. Collagen, biologically derived polyesters, hyaluronic acid, and other materials have all shown attractive properties in some applications. New biological materials (for example, spider silk or protein adhesives from barnacle and mussel) might be usable for such applications as sutures and bioadhesives. They are "specialties," rather than true pharmaceuticals, even if they are used in human health-care applications. Thus, the economics of production are more important for them than for conventional drugs, and the process aspects of their production are critical.

Veterinary Applications

Transgenic animals

Transgenic animals are being developed for a wide variety of applications, and bioprocess engineering will play a role in the use of these animals in several ways. If transgenic animals are used as factories for production of biological substances (e.g., as protein in milk), bioprocess engineering will be required to develop appropriate techniques for isolation and purification of the desired products. More important in the short term is that transgenic animals might provide test beds for proving the safety of new pharmaceutical entities and for accelerating their passage through the regulatory process. Bioprocess engineering can play an important role in controlling the testing technologies, perhaps in maintaining transgenic tissues and organs, and in coupling the testing available for use in transgenic animals with the development of processes that are acceptable and robust from a regulatory viewpoint.

Agricultural Applications

Agricultural chemicals and food

Bioprocess engineering in agriculture sciences involves the application of biocatalysts (living cells or their components) to produce useful and value-added products, and it offers opportunities to design and produce new or improved agricultural and food products and their manufacturing processes. This will likely have a great impact on the U.S. food-processing industry, which has estimated annual sales of $255 billion. In our increasingly health-conscious society, genetically engineered microorganisms and specialty enzymes will find increased use in improving the nutritional, flavoring, and storage characteristics and safety of food products. Products under development range from genetically improved strains of freeze-resistant yeast used in frozen bakery products to phage-resistant dairy (yogurt) starter cultures. Chymosin, a product of recombinant *E. coli*, is already used in the milk-clotting step of cheese manufacture, and a recombinant maltogenic amylase is being used as an anti-staling agent. Enzyme-based immunoassays could develop into a widely used method for detecting pesticides in foods at parts-per-billion concentrations. Challenges that must be addressed include the economics of production and regulatory issues. The most important applications of bioprocess-engineering research and development related to agriculture and food involve production of agricultural chemicals for control of animal and plant diseases, growth-stimulating agents for improved yield, and biological insecticides and herbicides; increasing bioprocess efficiencies for fermented foods, natural food additives, food enzymes as processing aids, and separation and purification of the products; use of plant-cell culture systems to produce secondary metabolites or chemical substances of economic importance; and efficient use of renewable biomass resources for production of liquid fuel and chemical feedstock and efficient treatment and management of agricultural wastes and wastes from food-processing industries.

Plant-cell culture

The commercial potential of plant-cell tissue culture has not yet been fully recognized and is underexploited. Plant-cell tissue culture has two primary products: plant tissue for efficient micropropagation of plants and the use of plant-tissue culture to produce specialty chemicals. Plant-cell, -tissue, and-organ cultures can be used in processes analogous to traditional fermentation processes for producing chemicals. Although less than 5% of the world's plants have even been identified taxonomically, from among the known plants over 20,000 chemicals are produced—about 4 times as many as from all microorganisms. Very few of the chemicals in pure or semipure form have been tested for their pharmacological activity for other uses. The enzymatic systems in plants can be used to generate completely new compounds when supplied with analogues of natural substrates; thus, plants contain underused biochemical diversity. Even the limited use of this vast biochemical potential has had important impacts on mankind; in western countries, about one-fourth of all medicines are derived from compounds extracted from plants. Other plant products are used as flavors, fragrances, or pesticides. Plant-cell tissue culture to produce chemicals commercially has been exploited in Japan, although regulatory approval for medicinal uses has proved difficult and commercial production is restricted to food uses and pigment production. In

Japan, a government-sponsored consortium of universities and corporations was recently developed to establish a foundation for plant-cell culture exploitation (i.e., a precompetitive research thrust). In the United States, plant-cell tissue is not being exploited for chemical production, although at least two companies are actively developing processes for the production of the chemotherapeutic agent taxol. The major technical barriers to the commercial exploitation of plant-cell tissue culture are low growth rates and relatively low product yields. To mitigate those problems, research is needed in subjects as diverse as bioreactor strategies to maintain high-density cultures and enable large-scale production of chemicals through organ cultures and a mechanistic understanding of the role of elicitors in activating pathways for secondary metabolites that could lead to higher productivities of compounds with therapeutic value.

Plants and seeds

Basic research in plant molecular biology has allowed the clonal production of plants through the process of somatic embryogenesis, in which somatic cells develop through the stages of embryogenesis to yield whole plants without gamete fusion. Somatic embryos have been induced from a variety of plant tissues, and this system is commercially attractive for the high-volume multiplication of genetically improved embryos in culture. The clonal embryos are synthetic "seeds" that can be delivered to commercial growers. For many applications, somatic embryos have powerful advantages over conventional clonal propagation methods and other *in vitro* regeneration systems for mass propagation. One advantage is the very high multiplication rates. Depending on the plant species, virtually unlimited numbers of embryos can be generated from a single explant. A second advantage is that, for many species, growth and tissue development of somatic embryos can be carried out in a liquid medium. That fact gives somatic embryogenesis the potential to be combined with engineering technology to create large-scale culture systems. The development of such engineering technology is the limiting step in commercialization. The use of submerged liquid culture for the efficient mass production of embryos, artificial seeds, or plant propagates is a promising industrial technique now used in Israel and other countries. For crop and forest plants, micropropagation on solid medium is too expensive. The use of bioreactors, which reduces labor costs greatly, will probably be necessary for mass production of crop and forest plants generated by genetic engineering or nontraditional breeding methods. The key engineering problem in such systems is the control of environmental conditions necessary for development of organized tissues from unorganized, minimally differentiated tissues. Fundamental studies on the interaction of concentration gradients with cellular developmental processes are required.

Transgenic plants

Transgenic plants are capable of generating specialty chemicals or other bioproducts. Special bioprocessing capabilities will then also need to be developed for extracting, concentrating, and purifying such products from plant tissue. This sector of bioprocess engineering might also be important to the prospects of expanding crops or developing new varieties that are rich in fermentable carbohydrates, which are readily used as feedstocks for large-scale manufacturing of specialty and industrial chemicals. Transgenic tobacco plants have been developed to produce monoclonal antibodies identical in function with the original mouse antibody. Other proteins produced in plants are human serum albumin and enkephalins. Processes to recover and purify proteins from plant-cell extracts will be needed if such systems are commercialized.

Industrial Applications

New catalysts

New types of catalysts based on biological systems are being developed. Among them are catalytic antibodies (abzymes) and catalytic nucleic acids (ribozymes). Those types of materials can, in principle, be used both in specialty-chemical production and in human therapy. Although the techniques required for preparing abzymes will be the same as those used in other kinds of monoclonal-antibody manufacture, production of ribozymes (initially for applications in human health) will require an entire new array of manufacturing, purification, and production technologies; there are no large-scale methods for preparation, isolation, and purification of high-molecular-weight nucleic acids.

Microbial metabolites

The metabolites produced during the trophophase of culture are referred to as primary metabolites and include amino acids, nucleotides, proteins, nucleic acids, lipids and carbohydrates, and the by-products of energy-yielding metabolism are ethanol, acetone and butanol. Some of the commercially important primary metabolites are given in Table 33.2.

Table 33.2 Some commercially important microbial primary metabolites.

Primary metabolite	*Producing microbe*	*Commercial signification/application*
Ethanol	*Saccharomyces cerevisiae*	Production of alcohol
Acetone, butanol	*Clostridium acetobutyricum*	Solvents
Lysine	*Corynebacterium glutamicum*	Feed supplement
Glutamic acid	*Corynebacterium glutamicum*	Flavour enhancement
Polysaccharides	*Xanthomonas* spp.	Food industry, enhanced oil recover

The metabolites produced during the idiophase are referred to as the secondary metabolites. Secondary metabolites are synthesized from the intermediates and end-products of primary metabolism. Few of the secondary metabolites include antibiotics (penicillin. cephalosporin, tetracyclines, streptomycin and griseofulvin), anti-tumour agents (actinomycin), anticancer agents (krestin and bestatin) and immunosuppresant (cyclosporin A). The production of microbial metabolites may be achieved in continuous, as well as in batch systems. The secondary metabolites are produced by slow-growing organisms in continuous cultures.

Microbial enzymes

Microbial enzymes are most widely used in the food and beverage industries and to a lesser extent in clinical and analytical laboratories and as protease detergents in washing powders. The most economical and convenient method of producing these enzymes is by microbial fermentation. Bacillus stearothermophilus produces amylases as secondary metabolites, but most other microbes produce enzymes as primary metabolites, during exponential growth. The major commercial utilization of microbial enzymes is in the food and beverage industries, in pharmaceutical textile and leather industries, in analytical processes as well as in detergent and dairy industry. Most enzymes are synthesized in the logarithmic phase of the batch culture and may, therefore, be considered primary metabolites. However, some, for example, amylases of Bacillus stearothemophilus are produced by idiophase, type cultures and may be considered equivalent to secondary metabolites. Enzymes may be produced from animals and plants as well as microbial sources, but the production by microbial fermentation is the most economical and convenient method. For example, microbial rennin is being used instead of calf rennin and proteases used in detergents are produced by microbes. It is now possible to engineer microbial cells to produce animal or plant enzymes. Most of the enzymes in industrial use are extracellular proteins produced by *Aspergillus* sp. or Bacillus sp. and include α-amylase, β-glucanase, cellulase, dextranase, lactase, lipase, pectinase, proteases and others. The extent of purification required for most of these enzymes is minimal, and they can be produced in tonnes without serious problems. Some of the important microbial enzymes, their source and applications are described in Table 33.3.

Table 33.3 Some important microbial enzymes and their applications.

Source (genus)	*Enzymes*	*Reaction*	*Application*
Bacillus	α-Amylase	Starch hydrolysis	Converts starch to glucose or dextran in food industry
	Proteases	Protein digestion	Help laundering
Escherichia	Penicillin Acylase	Benzoyl cleavage	Production of 6-APA
	L-Asparaginase	Removal of L-asparagine involved in tumour growth	Leukaemia/cancer treatment
Aspergillus	Amyloglucosidase	Dextrin hydrolysis	Glucose production
	β-Galactosidase	Lactose hydrolysis	Lactose hydrolysis in milk or whey
	Aminoacylase	Hydrolysis of acylated L-amino acids	Resolution of racemic mixtures
	Glucose oxidase	Oxidation of glucose	Glucose detection in blood
Streptomyces	Glucose isomerase	Conversion of glucose of fructose	Production of high fructose syrups
Several marine bacteria	Luciferase	Bioluminescence	Assay for ATP
Several bacteria and cyanobacteria	Nucleases (restriction endonucleases)	Hydrolysis of phosphodiester bonds in nucleic acids	Genetic engineering

Fermented Foods

Thousands of kinds fermented foods are being produced industrially in Japan, Korea, China and other oriental countries. Miso, shoyu, ontjam, khimchi, beet, tempeh and fermented fish and meat are good examples. Fermentation often makes the food more nutritious, more digestible, safer, or having better flavour. It also tends to preserve the food, increasing its shelf life and lowering the need for refrigeration. Fermentation can be applied to all kinds of foods. Eight classes of fermented food may be recognized, viz., beverages, cereal products, diary products, fish products, fruit and vegetable products, legumes, meat products and starchy products. Of these, dairy products, cereal products and beverages are the most common. Beer is produced from cereal grains which have been malted, dried and ground into fine powder. The powder is washed in warm water. Fermentation of the washed powder is mediated either by bottom yeast (e.g., *Saccharomyces uvarum*) or by a top-yeast (*S. cerevisiae*). The final product (beer) has up to about 8% alcohol. Grapes can be directly fermented by yeasts to wine. Wine is made by distillation of the alcoholic broth formed by fermentation of grape juice (Table 33.4).

Table 33.4 Industrial chemicals produced by fermentation.

Chemicals	*Microbial source*	*Some uses*
Formic acid	Aspergillus	Textile dyeing, leather treatment, electroplating, rubber manufacture
Ethanol	Saccharomyces	Industrial solvent, intermediate for vinegar, esters and ethers; beverages
Oxalic acid	Aspergillus	Printing, dying, bleaching; cleaner; reducing agent
Glycerol	Saccharomyces, Dunaliella	Solvent; Plasticizer, sweetener, manufactures of explosives; printing, cosmetics; soaps
Propylene glycol	Bacillus	Antifreeze solvents; synthetic resin manufacture; mould inhibitor
Acetone	Clostridium	Industrial solvent; intermediate for several organic chemicals
Malonic acid	penicillium	Manufacture of barbiturates
Lactic acid	Lactobacillus, Streptococcus	Food acidulant; dyeing; intermediate for lactates; leather treatment
Acrylic acid	Bacillus	Industrial intermediate for plastics
Butanol	Clostridium	Industrial solvents; intermediate for several organic chemicals
Methylethyketone	Chlamydomonas	Industrial solvent; intermediate for explosives and synthetic resins
Succinic acid	Rhizopus	Manufacture of lacquers
Tartaric acid	Acetobacter	Acidulant, tanning, printing, esters for lacquers
Itaconic acid	Aspergillus	Textile and paper manufacture

Other Biotechnological Applications

Nontraditional organisms

Many unusual chemicals or enzymes with unique properties come from organisms that are difficult to culture effectively. In particular, marine microbes (especially algae) and extremophiles (primarily the archaebacteria) present important, but long-range opportunities. Bioprocess engineers have already demonstrated the ability to design devices and protocols to culture microbes from deep-sea vents and undoubtedly have the skills necessary to develop techniques for other difficult-to-culture organisms.

Energy and renewable resources

A broad range of technical opportunities might require large-scale engineering. For example, if biologically produced materials (surfactants and viscosifiers) are used in enhanced oil recovery and in transportation of heavy crudes and coal slurries; appropriate biological manufacturing facilities must be developed. Particularly for those purposes, the ability to produce materials economically on-site from local raw materials might be important and might require development of completely new technology. Although ideas for desulfurization of coal and liquid hydrocarbons seem, at present, to be improbable, the development of materials from biological processes to aid in transportation and burning of coal, for example, seems plausible. The largest-volume process that bioprocess engineering might be called on to address would be consumption of carbon dioxide (CO_2) from combustion. If it is necessary to reduce CO_2 emissions from stationary sources substantially to ameliorate the greenhouse effect, a plausible approach would be to couple CO_2 release with growth of a CO_2-requiring organism (either photosynthetic or non-photosynthetic). The scale of any facility that would be used in this type of application would be enormous and would require innovative engineering to minimize costs. In addition to those large-scale processes, there are plausible uses for biological catalysts on a smaller scale in a number of fields related to energy production and bioprocessing. For example, fuel cells based on enzymatic catalysis would provide an attractive method of using ethanol and perhaps other biologically derived fuels with high thermodynamic efficiency in an environmentally acceptable way. A range of chemicals can, of course, in principle be produced from renewable resources. The process for production of acrylamide from acrylonitrile has re-emphasized the practicality of large-volume production of some types of commodity chemicals with enzymatic catalysis. If energy costs continue to go up, if petroleum feedstocks become more expensive or more erratic in supply, and if processes based on conventional non-biological catalytic systems become unacceptable from an environmental point of view, biological processing might be able to overcome what is usually an intrinsic economic disadvantage. In that event, bioprocess engineering will be called on to provide reactors and control systems appropriate for the production of commodity products (chemicals and fuels) with tight environmental and economic constraints. Bioprocess engineering is an essential component for addressing those challenges. Fundamental understanding of the changes that occur in pre-treated cellulose to make it more reactive and identification of inexpensive approaches to the engineering of large-scale processes are first steps in producing a reactive substrate. Improvement of both the rate and the extent of xylose fermentation to ethanol require an understanding of microbial physiology and of the optimal control of fermentation conditions to maximize productivity and yield. The fractionation of solutes from water is a challenge common to most fermentation, where the product is present at less than 10% concentration and is less volatile than water. Identification of sorbents, for example, that remove the solutes from the water could be an important first step in improving the process.

The environment

Many environmental problems will require bioprocess engineering. Some are discussed elsewhere in this report. Here we mention that, in addition to the types of problems commonly considered (minimization of manufacturing waste, treatment of municipal waste, environmentally friendly manufacturing), new classes of problems might arise from the concept of "life-cycle environmental responsibility." That idea is being actively considered in various European countries for such products as automobiles. The manufacturer would be responsible for its product throughout its life cycle, including its ultimate disposal. If that responsibility becomes a reality in any of the major markets, it will be necessary to develop new classes of processes for final disposal of components. The need for biodegradable polymers, for example, coupled with efficient biodegradation systems for disposing of manufactured components, would become a reality. Large volume and low cost in operation would be essential. Because there are virtually no counterparts for them at present, there is no experience to guide future development; these types of engineering and process problems would be truly novel. The removal and oxidation of organic gases from contaminated air by microorganisms fixed in beds of soil, compost, or other solid materials might gain expanded acceptance as a process by which air is cleaned through biological means. Bio-filtration has already enjoyed industrial success in Europe and Japan. Nonetheless, significant bioprocess engineering challenges remain in the use of organisms to remove gas-phase organic chemicals. These include gas-solid contacting, maintaining stable microbial populations, and predicting performance for scale-up purposes.

Space

The unique problems presented by the manned exploration and colonization of space pose major and important challenges for bioprocess engineering. Space biology—the behavior of living systems in a zero-gravity (and perhaps high radiation) environment is just beginning to be investigated. The long-term influence of the space environment on cellular development remains to be determined. In principle, however, a plausible (from an economic point of view) application of processing in space would be to produce new cell lines. If it is possible to carry out manipulations of genetic materials or cell types in space that cannot be conducted on earth and if the modifications of cell behavior or germ-line composition that result from the manipulations can be preserved on return to earth, very high value could, in principle, be achieved. Because cells can be propagated and relatively small volumes of starting material (genetically altered cells) can be converted into large numbers of product cells after return to earth, the very high cost of manipulations in space would have a smaller effect on the overall cost of genetic manipulation of cell lines than of products that are sold by weight. The development of reactor systems and assay systems that are appropriate for use in space thus represents an important investment in this speculative field. Reduced gravity (Moon and Mars) and microgravity (space station) would present some unique opportunities for the study of complex biological systems. One new interest is in the possible use of a microgravity environment to produce three-dimensional differentiated tissue structures in the fluid phase without a solid support. That could lead to a new tool for tissue engineering and the study of cell differentiation and developmental biology. Limitations in the knowledge of how cell suspensions and cell-to-cell communication affect the growth of such biomaterials might be quickly overcome once experiments are carried out on a space platform in low earth orbit. The objective would be research on manufacturing technologies, rather than manufacturing itself. Specific objectives include developing and testing experimental models for testing mammalian cell and tissue properties and for providing the necessary nutrients, bio-modifiers, gases, and control. Important studies in developmental biology should be possible, including the generation of high-order tissue morphology of primary cells and ultimately perhaps complete organ generation. Once developed, the necessary techniques could be brought back to earth for manufacture. Bioprocess engineering is an element of all phases of such a project, from the design and implementation of orbiting bioprocess laboratory experiments to the implementation of the results for manufacturing processes on earth. The problem of development of life-support systems for humans and other organisms in space is separate and highly important (if specialized). The engineering of even conventional equipment for the space environment presents a unique set of problems. If the National Aeronautics and Space Administration (NASA) continues with its long-term goal of manned exploration of space, a major component of the reduction of space biology to engineering systems appropriate for life support of astronauts on long voyages will require the development of a specialized, light-weight, gravity-insensitive set of operations for handling and maintaining the appropriate environments for biological systems in space. The number of appropriately trained bioprocess engineers required for that effort would be substantial. NASA supports relatively small programs in space biotechnology through the Microgravity Science and Applications Division (MSAD) and the Life Sciences Division. One field in which the lack of density gradient-driven convection could be important is protein nucleation and crystallization. Several active research projects are supported by MSAD (NASA, 1991). Another potential use of microgravity is in separation of large biological molecules (such as chromosomes) or cells (such as lymphocyte subpopulations), in which again gravity-induced sedimentation and density-gradient-driven convection could destroy separation ability. This committee feels that space manufacturing of biological products for use on earth will not be fiscally feasible in the near future. For example, improvements in earth-based crystallization and separation systems and rapid developments in three-dimensional matrices for tissue engineering will make space-manufactured biomaterials too expensive. The space environment does provide a laboratory for interesting experiments in developmental biology and physiology, which should be pursued. Integration of those experiments into the space stations or the Moon-and Mars-based modules will require substantial collaboration between bioprocess engineers and basic biological scientists. That is particularly true because changes in local mass transport and fluid mechanics can often have important biological consequences on cell growth and structure formation, which must be separated from any effects of microgravity alone.

FUTURE PROSPECTS

Bioprocess engineering is concerned with translating biological science into biologically based manufacturing. To be prepared for the biological manufacturing systems of the future, it is important to identify the fields of science and technology that have reached or will soon reach early prototypes and to begin to develop engineering systems to deal with them. The lead time in development of any new technology is long. Biological science is so prolific that any present list of future developments of technology must be incomplete. It is, however, straightforward to identify subjects in which new engineering techniques must be developed now, if the technologies are to be available when they are needed in large-scale manufacturing 5-15 years from now.

CONCLUSION

The challenge of bioprocess engineering lies in identifying the needs of the industry and promoting technology transfer and training of engineers who will fit the wide range of markets, activities, and products that are being encompassed by biotechnology and bioprocess-engineering developments. The synthesis and innovation to develop the enabling technologies for industry to exploit the potential of modern biology and chemistry fully is a significant part of this challenge. The vignettes in this chapter illustrate how bioprocessing technology facilitates amplification of existing microbial products, application of new manufacturing techniques for existing products, and the production of proteins derived from mammalian systems that would otherwise not be available in sufficient quantities for practical use as therapeutic agents. Challenges that bioprocess engineering faces include specialty-equipment design that meets regulatory, biological, and economic constraints; integration of manufacturing processes into environmentally acceptable and economically feasible process concepts; and rapid purification and monitoring of purification processes to obtain high quality, high purity, and consistent output. Improvements in the design of bioreactors and in conditions for cultivating microorganisms and obtaining products are also needed. Both solid-substrate and submerged fermentations present major opportunities for bio-manufacturing and improvement through bioprocess engineering. Novel bioreactor designs, membrane-separation technologies, and processing aids could all improve the economics of producing specialty bioproducts. The challenges and opportunities of bioprocessing technology for the manufacture of specialty bioproducts are similar to those related to biopharmaceuticals, except for the special hazards of pathogens and the specialty-product emphasis on economics of production—the lower the value of the product, the more intense the economic focus.

FURTHER READINGS

1. Aiba, S., Humphrey A.E. and Millis N.F. (1973) *Biochemical Engineering*, 2nd ed. Academic Press, New York.
2. Antrim, R. L., Colilla W. and Schnyder B. J. (1979) Glucose isomerase production of high fructose syrups. In: *Applied Biochemistry and Bioengineering,* Vol. 2, L. B. Wingard, Jr., E. Katchalski-Katzir, and L. Goldstein, eds. Academic. Press, New York, pp. 97-156.
3. Atkinson, B., and Mavituna, F. (1983) *Biochemical Engineering and Biotechnology Handbook*, The Nature Press, N.Y., U.S.A. pp. 581-669.
4. Avgerinos, G. C., and Wang. D.I.C. (1983) Selective solvent delignification for fermentation enhancement. *Biotechnol. Bioeng.* **(25):** 67-83.
5. Baret, J. L. (1987) Large-scale production and application of immobilized lactase. *Methods in Enzymology.* **(136):** 411-423.
6. Brodelius, P. (1978) Industrial applications of immobilized biocatalysts. *Adv. in Biochem. Eng.* **(10):** 1-23.
7. Brodelius, P. (1983) Production of biochemicals with immobilized plant cells. Possibilities and problems. *Annals N.Y. Acad. Sciences*. **(413):** 383-393.
8. Bungay, H. (1992) Product opportunities for biomass refining. *Enzyme Microb. Technol.* **(14):** 501-507.
9. Calabresi, P., McCarthy, K.L., Dexter, D.L., Cummins, F.J., and Rotman, B. (1981) Monoclonal antibody production in artificial capillary cultures. *Proc. Amer. Assoc. Cancer Res.* **(22):** 362.
10. Chance, R E., Kroef E.P. and Hoffmann J.A. (1981) Chemical, physical, and biologic properties of recombinant human insulin in insulin. In: *Growth Hormone, and Recombinant Technology,* edited by J.L. Gueriguian. Raven Press. New York, pp. 71-85.

11. Decker Eva L. and Reski Ralf (2008) Current achievements in the production of complex biopharmaceuticals with moss bioreactor. *Bioprocess and Biosystems Engineering.* **(31):** 3-9.
12. Feder, J. and Tolbert, W.R. (1983) The large-scale cultivation of mammalian cells. *Amer. Sci.* **(248):** 36-43.
13. Glacken, M.W., Fleischaker, R.J., and Sinskey, A.J. (1983) Large scale production of mammalian cells and their products: engineering principles and barriers to scale-up. *Annals N.Y. Acad. Sciences*. **(413):** 355-372.
14. Glaser, V., and Dutton G. (1992) Food processors seek to adapt bioproducts for large-scale manufacturing. *GEN* 12 **(2)**:6–8.
15. Gong, C.-S., Chen L.-F., Flickinger M. C., Chiang L. C. and Tsao G. T. (1981) Production of ethanol from D-xylose using D-xylose isomerase and yeasts. *Appl. Environ. Microbiol.* 41 **(2)**: 430-436.
16. Hiatt, A., Cafferkey R. and Bowdish K. (1989) Production of antibodies in transgenic plants. *Nature.* **(342):** 76-78.
17. Ingram, L. (1992) Genetic engineering of novel bacteria for the conversion of plant polysaccharides into ethanol. In: *Harnessing Biotechnology for the 21st Century*, M. Ladisch and A. Bose, eds. American Chemical Society, Washington, D.C. pp. 507-509.
18. Jain, M. K., Datta R. and Zeikus J. G. (1989) High value organic acids fermentation—Emerging products and processes. In: *Bioprocess Engineering*. T.K. Ghose, ed. Horwood, London, pp. 367-389.
19. Kirk, T. K., and Chang H.-M. eds. (1990) *Biotechnology in Pulp and Paper Manufacture:Applications and Fundamental Investigations*. Butterworth-Heinemann. Boston: pp. 696
20. Kleid, D.G. (1983) Using genetically engineered bacteria for vaccine production. *Annals N.Y. Acad. Sciences*. **(413):** 23-30.
21. Konig, B., Seewald, C., and Schugerl, K. (1981) Process engineering investigations of penicillin production. *Europ. J. Microbiol. Biotechnol*. **(12):** 205-211.
22. Ladisch, M. R., and Svarczkopf J. A. (1991) Ethanol production and the cost of fermentable sugars from biomass. *Bioresour. Technol.* **(36):** 83-95.
23. Ladisch, M. R., and Dyck K. (1979) Dehydration of ethanol: New approach gives positive energy balance. *Science.* **(205):** 898-900.
24. Ladisch, M. R., Ladisch C. M. and Tsao G. T. (1978) Cellulose to sugars: New path gives quantitative yield. *Science.* **(201):** 743-745.
25. Ladisch, M.R. (2002) Bioprocess Engineering (Biotechnology). In: Vol. 1 of *Scientific Encyclopedia*, 9th ed. Van Nostrand, New York, pp. 434-459.
26. Luckow, V. A. (1990) Cloning and expression of heterologous genes in insect cells with baculovirus vectors. In: *Recombinant DNA Technology and Applications*, C. Ho, A. Prokop, and R. Bajpai, eds. McGraw-Hill Book Company, New York.
27. Lynd, L. R., Cushman J. H., Nichols R. J. and Wyman C. E. (1991) Fuel ethanol from cellulosic biomass. *Science.* **(251):** 1318-1323.
28. Maiorella, B. L., Blanch H. W. and Wilke C. R. (1984) Economic evaluation of ethanol fermentation processes. *Biotechnol. Bioeng.* **(26):** 1003–1025.
29. Margaritis, A. and Wallace, J.B. (1982) The use of immobilized cells of *Zymomonas mobilis* in a novel fluidized bioreactor to produce ethanol. *Biotech. Bioeng. Symp*. **(12):** 147-159.
30. Marshall, R. O., and Kooi E. R. (1957) Enzymatic conversion of D-glucose to D-fructose. *Science* **(125):** 648-649.
31. Moore, G.E., Hasenpusch, P., Gerner, R.E., and Burns, A.A. (1968) A pilot plant for mammalian cell culture. *Biotech. Bioeng*. **(10):** 625-640.
32. Pitcher, W.H. (1978) Design and operation of immobilized enzyme reactors. *Adv. Biochem. Eng.* **(10):** 75-129.
33. Prenosil, J.E. and Pedersen, H. (1983) Immobilized plant cell reactors. *Enzyme Microb. Technol.* **(5):** 323-332.

34. Prouty, W.F. (1991) Production-Scale Purification Processes. In: *Drug Biotechnology Regulation.* 13, edited by Y.-Y.H. Chen and J.L. Gueriguian. New York, pp. 221-262

35. Scott, C.D. and Hancher, C.W. (1976) Use of a tapered fluidized bed as a continuous bioreactor. *Biotech. Bioeng*. **(18):** 1393-1403.

36. Shuler, M. L., and Kargi F. (1991) *Bioprocess Engineering: Basic Concepts*. Prentice Hall, Englewood Cliffs, N.J., p. 448

37. Shuler, M. L., Cho T., Wickham T., Ogonah O., Kool M., Hammer D. A., Granados R. R. and Wood H. A. (1990) Bioreactor development for production of viral pesticides or heterologous proteins in insect cell cultures. *Ann. NY Acad. Sci.* **(589):** 399-422.

38. Veliky, I.A. and Jones, A. (1982) Bioconversion of gitoxigenin by immobilized plant cells in a column bioreactor. *Biotech. Lett*. **(3):** 551.

39. Wang, D.I.C., Avgerinos G. C., Biocic I., Wang S.-D. and Fang H.-Y. (1983) Ethanol from cellulosic biomass—Direct conversion using a mixed culture of *Clostridium thermosac-charolyticum*. *Philos. Trans. R. Soc. London B* **(300):** 323-333.

40. Watson, J. S., and Scott C. D. (1988) The Impact of Bioprocessing on Enhanced Oil Recovery. Oak Ridge National Laboratory Report ORNL/TM-10676. Oak Ridge, Tenn.: Oak Ridge National Laboratory.

SECTION E

Biotechnology for Environmental Applications

CHAPTER

34

Metagenomics Technology

Metagenomics is the study of metagenomes, *genetic* material recovered directly from *environmental* samples. The broad field may also be referred to as environmental genomics, ecogenomics or community genomics. Traditional *microbiology* and microbial *genome sequencing* rely upon cultivated *clonal cultures*. This relatively new field of *genetic* research enables studies of organisms that are not easily cultured in a laboratory as well as studies of organisms in their natural environment. Early environmental gene sequencing relied on cloning specific genes (often the *16S rRNA* gene) to produce a profile of diversity in a natural sample. Such work revealed that the vast majority of *microbial biodiversity* had been missed by cultivation-based methods. Recent studies use "shotgun" *Sanger sequencing* or massively parallel *pyrosequencing* to get (mostly) unbiased samples of all genes from all members of sampled communities.

Keywords: Metagenomics, environmental genomics, unculturable microorganisms, DNA libraries, novel bioproducts.

INTRODUCTION

In the past two decades, molecular biology has changed the face of agriculture, medicine and most other disciplines, primarily in the area of genomics and relatively new offshoot areas of functional genomics, proteomics, transcriptomics, metabolomics and metagenomics. The word "metagenomics" i.e., direct extraction of genetic material from environmental samples was coined to capture the notion for analysis of a collection of similar but not identical items, as in a meta analysis. Microbiology has long relied on diverse methods for analysis and metagenomics can provide the tools to balance the abundance of knowledge attained from culturing with an understanding of the uncultured majority of microbial life. In recent years, phylogenetic diversity of environments such as ocean surfaces, deep sea vents, hot springs, soil, animal rumen and gut, human oral cavity and intestine have been described and many new lineages were classified based on their molecular signatures. Facts are available to prove that metagenomes are rich resource for the discovery of even novel natural products like enzymes and drugs etc. Metagenomic technology has been successful at all scales. It has been used to study single gene for example cellulase, antibiotic synthesis, organisms and bacterial communities. Moreover, recently it has been used to understand microflora in the gut environment.

The science of metagenomics only a few years old will therefore make it possible to investigate microbes in their natural environments and the complex communities in which they normally live. It will bring about a transformation in biology, medicine, ecology, and biotechnology that may be as profound as that initiated by the invention of the microscope.

CONCEPTS

The term "metagenomics" was first used by Jo Handelsman and others at the University of Wisconsin, Department of Plant Pathology and first appeared in publication in 1998. The term metagenome referred to the idea that a collection of genes sequenced from the environment could be analyzed in a way analogous to the study of a single genome. The exploding interest in environmental genetics along with the buzzword like nature of the term, has resulted in the broader use of metagenomics to describe any sequencing of genetic material from environmental (i.e., uncultured) samples even work that focuses on one organism or gene. Recently, Kevin Chen and Lior Pachter (researchers at the University of California, Berkeley) defined metagenomics as "the application of modern genomics techniques to the study of communities of microbial organisms directly in their natural environments, bypassing the need for isolation and lab cultivation of individual species." Conventional sequencing begins with a culture of identical cells as a source of DNA. However, early metagenomic studies revealed that there are probably large groups of micro-organisms in many environments that cannot be cultured and thus cannot be sequenced. These early studies focused on 16S ribosomal RNA sequences which are relatively short, often conserved within a species and generally different between species. Many 16S rRNA sequences have been found which do not belong to any known cultured species indicating that there are numerous non-isolated organisms.

Early molecular work in the field was conducted by Norman R. Pace and colleagues, who used PCR to explore the diversity of ribosomal RNA sequences. The insights gained from these break-through studies led Pace to propose the idea of cloning DNA directly from environmental samples as early as 1985. This led to the first report of isolating and cloning bulk DNA from an environ-mental sample which was published by Pace and colleagues in 1991, while Pace was in the Department of Biology at Indiana University. Considerable efforts ensured that these were not PCR false positives and supported the existence of a complex community of unexplored species. Although this methodology was limited to exploring highly conserved, non-protein coding genes, it did support early microbial morphology-based observations that diversity was far more complex than was known by culturing methods.

Soon after that, Healy reported the metagenomic isolation of functional genes from "zoo librar-ies" constructed from a complex culture of environmental organisms grown in the laboratory on dried grasses in 1995. After leaving the Pace laboratory Ed DeLong continued in the field and published work, which has largely laid the groundwork for environmental phylogenies based on signature 16S rRNA sequences, beginning with his group's construction of libraries from marine samples.

PRINCIPLES

Microbes are essential for every part of life on Earth. Every process in this biological world is directly or indirectly dependent on microbes. All plants and animals have closely linked microbial communities that make necessary nutrients, metals and vitamins available to their hosts. Moreover, fermentation and other natural processes substitute additive value to many foods that are staples of the human diet. Further, microbes play a crucial role in biodegradation and bioremediation of toxins and non-toxic wastes, an essential part of environmental management.

Discovery of microscope made microbes visible to us, but with the help of microscope we can see only culturable bacteria and still a large variety of microbes are invisible. There are ~ 1.9×10^6 species of microorganisms but less than 10^5 species of bacteria and fungi are documented. In the case of bacteria, a small fraction form observable colonies on culture media and there is no clear-cut evidence that cultivable bacterial portion play a significant role in their environment because enrichment cultures are for those adapted to grow in media and selective for fast growing microbes. Studies reveal that 99% microbes are unculturable in laboratory conditions, showing the bias of cultivation based technologies. According to information present in literature, one of the important reasons for bacterial unculturability is the prerequisite for cellular signals from organisms in co-culture. Therefore, to unreveal the complete microbial community an approach should be there that provides an easy way to explore these invisible magicians. The concept of cloning DNA directly from environmental samples was proposed by Norman R. Pace in 1991 wherein a phage vector was reported for such cloning. Modification by Delong group in direct DNA cloning from seawater provided the landmark for this field. After these initiative steps, lots of other groups used this idea for the exploration of unculturable microbial flora. Various new modifications and methodologies have been developed to find out the unseen prokaryotic diversity of many different environments.

METAGENOMICS TECHNOLOGY

Extraction of Metagenomic DNA and Library Construction

The basic steps for the construction of a metagenomic library are described in Figure 34.1. The first step is the extraction of highly pure, large size DNA/RNA from environment, which is necessary for high cloning efficiency. Several methods have been developed to isolate the large size DNA. The extraction of DNA from soil is more problematic than any other resource. Challenges associated with soil DNA metagenomics are responsible for the slow development of this technology in complex soil matrix. Factors that complicate soil DNA extraction are the pH of soil and soil-DNA interaction. DNA is degraded under acidic conditions. Soil contains several components such as montmorillonite, kaolinite, and quartz, which bind with DNA and create complexity during the extraction. In acidic soil it becomes more difficult because clay-DNA binding increases in acidic pH. However, reports are also available for successful isolation of inhibitor free-metagenomic DNA. e.g., DNA from acidic volcanic soil, humic acid removal from crude soil DNA.

After the extraction of metagenomic DNA, the next critical step is its cloning in a suitable vector. The choice of the vector depends on the size of insert DNA. BAC cloning is well suited for large size insert. However, cosmid library can also be prepared for the same purpose. Schmitz *et al.* (2008) recently developed a rapid DNA library construction method for metagenomic screening which utilizes linker amplification with topoisomerase cloning and allows for inducible transcription in *Escherichia coli*. This technique is suited for functional screening, as it rapidly generates expression libraries with gene-sized inserts. These libraries are referred to as expressible LASLs (E-LASLs). Several other terminologies have also been used for metagenomic library, such as environmental DNA libraries; zoolibraries; eDNA libraries; whole genomes treasures; community genome; soil DNA libraries; whole genome shotgun sequencing, etc.

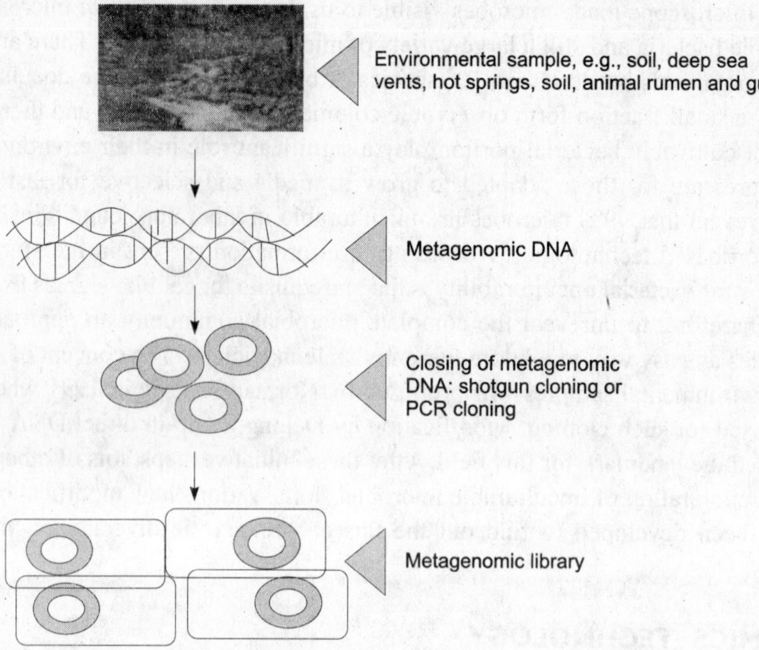

Figure 34.1 Basic steps for the construction of metagenomic library.

Approaches and Techniques of Metagenomics

Two different analyses have been used to obtain information from metagenomic libraries: a function-driven approach in which metagenomic libraries are initially screened for an expressed trait and a sequence-driven approach, in which libraries are initially screened for particular DNA sequences (Figure 34.2).

The potential of discovery from metagenomics is dependent on the advancement of methods that are central to library construction and analysis. For sequence-based approaches, the speed and cost of nucleotide sequencing will be a barrier of rapidly diminishing significance as sequencing technology continues to improve. Moreover sequence-based assignment of function will also benefit from advances in the detection of homology which will increasingly rely on the tertiary structures of predicted proteins rather than simply on primary sequence. Advances that will facilitate the management and analysis of large libraries include bioinformatics tools to analyze vast sequence databases and reassemble multiple genomes rapidly, affordable gene chips for library profiling to readily distinguish clones that are expressing genes from those clones that are silent. On the other hand, functional approach will require more innovation in method development. Most important among these are strategies to improve heterologous gene expression and approaches for efficient screening of large libraries.

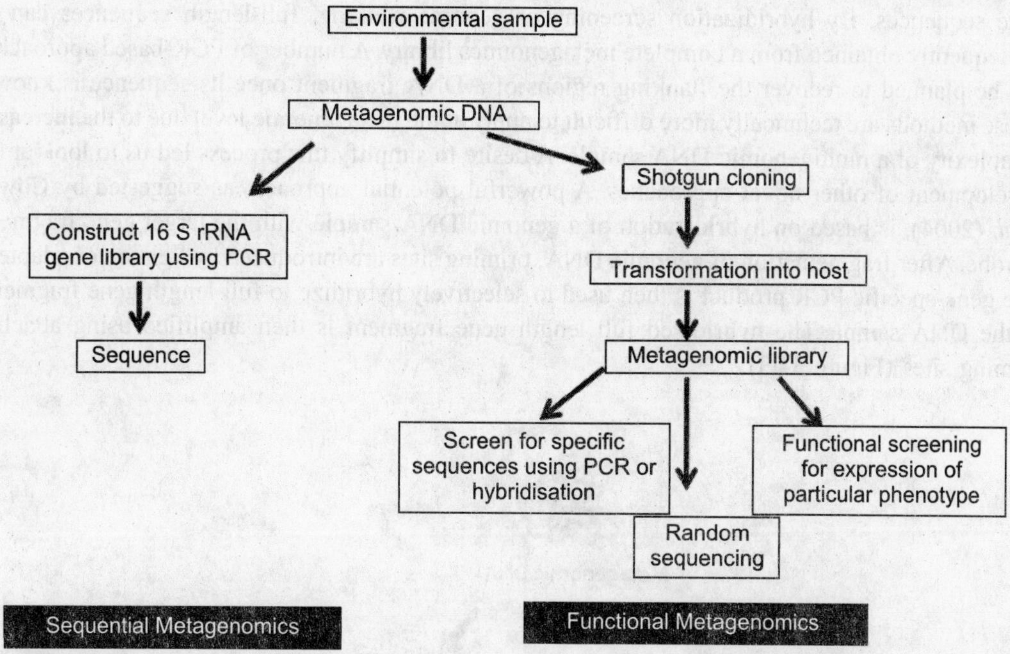

Figure 34.2 Two different metagenomic approaches: sequenced-based and function based.

The study of nucleic acids extracted directly from the environmental samples provides information on the structural composition of microbial communities as well as the presence or absenceof functional genes independent from traditional cultivation techniques. If RNA is used, the expression of certain genes in response to certain environmental stimuli can be studied. The growing database of partial or complete microbial sequences is essential for the development of tools such as primers or probes. Many of the common methods of cultivation independent microbiology are based on PCR. The modern PCR technology provides a sight of microbial diversity that was not distorted by the culturing bias, and revealed that the uncultured majority is highly diverse and contains members that diverge deeply from the readily culturable minority. Further, nucleic acid probes with fluorescent labels that facilitate visualization of single cells *in situ* led to a recrudescence of microscopy as a central tool of microbiology and microbial phylogeny, however, traditional microscopy provides little phylogenetic information and fluorescent antibody studies require prior knowledge and culturing of an organism or one closely related to it to raise antibodies. Phylogenetic strains require only a rRNA sequence, which can be derived from an environmental sample without culturing. Phylogenetic strains corroborated evidence from PCR-based studies but provided quantitative information as well, because the findings are based on direct observation that is not subjected to the skewing of organism abundance potentially observed with PCR. The amplified PCR product can be used for preparing clone libraries and a range of microbial community fingerprinting techniques.

On another front, PCR amplification methods, which have been used successfully to identify families of homologous genes, suffer from the limitation that the primary PCR generates only partial gene sequences. By hybridization screening or genome walking, full-length sequences can be subsequently obtained from a complete metagenomics library. A number of PCR-based approaches can be planned to recover the flanking regions of a DNA fragment once its sequence is known. These methods are technically more difficult to apply at the metagenomic level due to the increased complexity of a multigenomic DNA sample. A desire to simplify this process led us to look at the development of other novel approaches. A powerful potential approach, as suggested by Cowan *et al.* (2004), is based on hybridization of a genomic DNA sample with the target gene fragment, a probe. After fragmentation of genomic DNA, priming sites are introduced by ligation of adapters. The gene-specific PCR product is then used to selectively hybridize to full-length gene fragments in the DNA sample.The hybridized full length gene fragment is then amplified using attached priming sites (Figure 34.3).

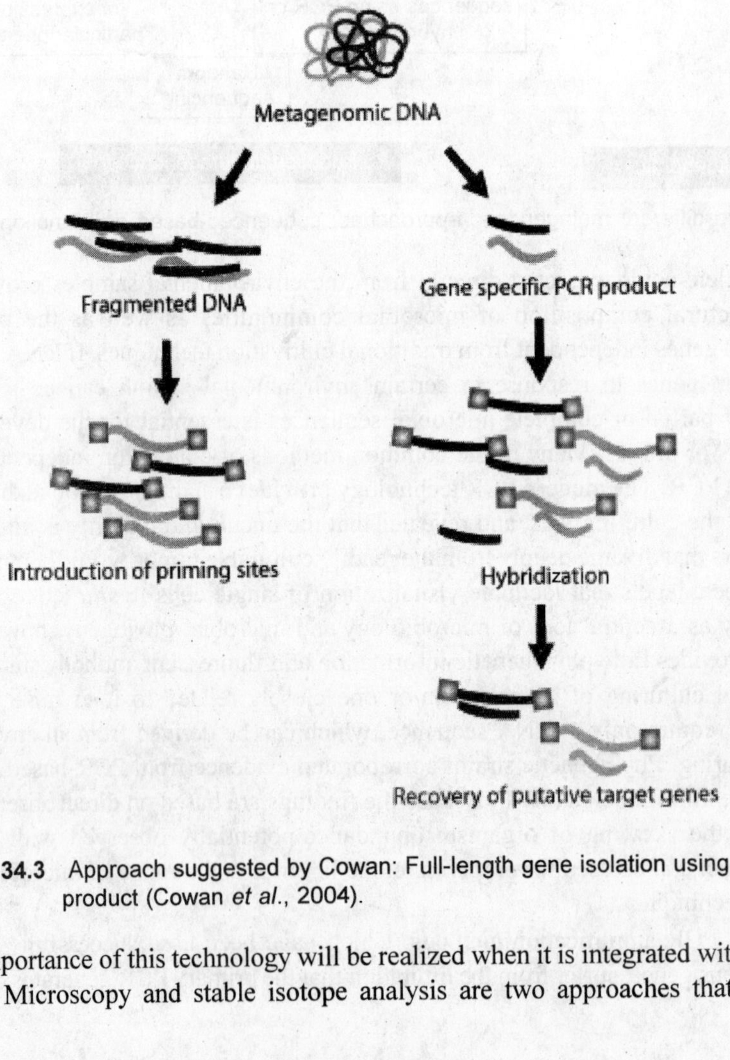

Figure 34.3 Approach suggested by Cowan: Full-length gene isolation using gene specific PCR product (Cowan *et al.*, 2004).

The importance of this technology will be realized when it is integrated with classical ecological methods. Microscopy and stable isotope analysis are two approaches that will be particularly informative when linked to metagenomics. It is used to visualize microbes that have ribosomal RNA, which hybridizes with fluorescently labeled probe most often directed toward the 16S rRNA gene. Nowadays other modified form of FISH like RING-FISH and FISH-MAR are routinely used in microbial ecology. Nevertheless, the use of stable isotopes to understand cycling of elements in microbial communities presents a singular opportunity in metagenomics. Libraries with labeled metagenomic DNA to enrich genes associated with active species can be constructed. Scientists use various advanced techniques during their metagenomic studies, which are summarized in Table 34.1.

Table 34.1 Few advanced techniques used to screen different environmental metagenomes.

Techniques used	*Aim of Metagenomic study*	*References*
Most-probable-number PCR and immunofluorescence	Assessment of the fate of *Mycobacterium* chlorophenolicum strain PCP-1 in different soils.	van Elsas *et al.*, 1997
Competitive PCR and RT-PCR	Metabolic Activity of the Bacterial Community.	Ka *et al.*, 2001
Microarray	Metagenomic Profiling.	Sebat *et al.*, 2003
Real time	1) Direct quantification of fungal DNA from soil.	Filion *et al.*, 2003
	2) Quantitative analyses of nitrogen cycling genes.	Wallenstein *et al.*, 2005
Metagenomic DNA shuffling	Development of metagenomic DNA shuffling for the construction of a xenobiotic gene.	Boubakri *et al.*, 2006
DNA-stable isotope probing	Identification of 2,4-dichloro-phenoxyacetic acid-degrading soil microorganisms.	Cupples & Sims, 2007
ni H PCR-DGGE	Diazotrophic community in rice.	Wartiainen *et al.*, 2008

Exploiting microbial activities or metabolic pathways successfully via a metagenomic approach requires a large number of crucial steps. Firstly, the selected environment must contain the gene(s) of interest. Secondly, the DNA extraction and cloning methods must allow for the capture of intact genes or operons. Next, the target genes must be detectable, either genetically or phenotypically. Lastly, after the detection of potential target activities it must be possible to modify their expression into viable production schemes. Prediction of success rate can be modeled depending on the nature of the target genes and the proportional abundance of the microorganisms harbouring them.

Myriad environments on Earth have not been studied with culture-independent methods other than PCR-based 16S rRNA gene analysis and they invite further analysis. Culture-independent molecular microbial diversity studies not only revealed the vast unexplored bacterial diversity, but also helped in the development of techniques suitable for isolation of high purity microbial community DNA (metagenome) from various environmental samples.

Although metagenomics has the potential to generate tremendous amounts of sequence information, this information needs the involvement of bioinformatics interpretation. Bioinformatics challenges are encountered at several steps of metagenome analyses, namely: (1) sequence assembly, (2) sequence annotation and (3) broader use and analysis of metagenomic sequence information. Of course, the recovered sequence information is made available via public databases, but this is often in a less useful form than the original datasets. Opening up metagenomic datasets for interrogation by a broader group of researchers, whose interests span a greater breadth of microbial functions, seems to be a relatively easy step that could greatly increase the understanding gleaned from large-scale metagenomics initiatives.

APPLICATIONS OF METAGENOMIC TECHNOLOGY

Scratching the secrets of earth's microbial communities via metagenomics will reveal solutions to heap challenges in medicine, agriculture, biotechnology and many others areas. Novel antibiotics, vitamins, proteins involved in antibiotic resistance and pollutant degradation have already been discovered by researchers using functional screening of metagenomic libraries. Beyond this sequence based analysis have further shaped the fundamental biological concepts. Better knowledge on community's sequence helps to determine the complete genome of an individual microbial species and the genome of the community as a whole which can offer insights about population ecology and evolution.

Medical Applications

Probing in microbial communities that inhabit on and in the human body can lead to new strategy for diagnosing, treating, and perhaps preventing diseases. Microbes residing in the human gut perform functions such as detoxifying potentially harmful chemicals in the food we eat, help in extracting nutrients and calories from otherwise stodgy components of our diets and making indispensable vitamins and amino acids. Metagenomics of human microbiome can help can us to gain a deeper understanding of both the beneficial and harmful microbial communities, which may lead to more valuable guidelines in nutrition, strategies for preventing pathogen invasion and diagnosing complex diseases such as cancer, immune disorders, obesity, drug discovery and preventive medicine.

Metagenomics of microbial world also offers astonishing range of biologically active chemicals. Traditional antibiotic screening for the molecules that inhibit bacterial growth have led to the discovery of antibiotics in metagenomic libraries. However, detection of antibiotic-producing clones at a low frequency (approx. one producer per 10^4 clones) hinders their discovery. Some of the antibiotics discovered so far are mentioned in Figure 34.4 with their chemical structures.

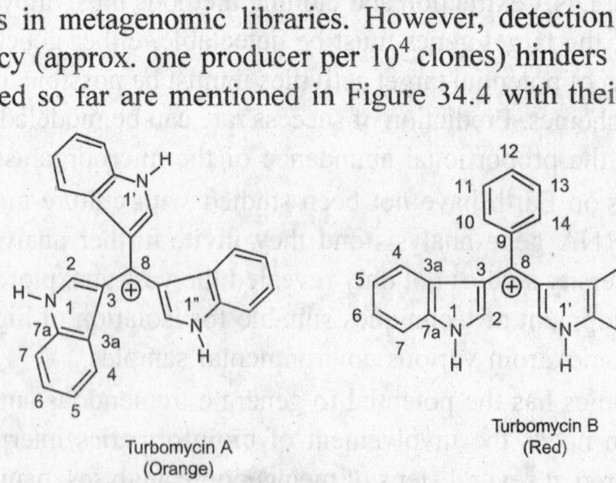

Turbomycin from the libraries of Gillespies *et al.*, 2000.

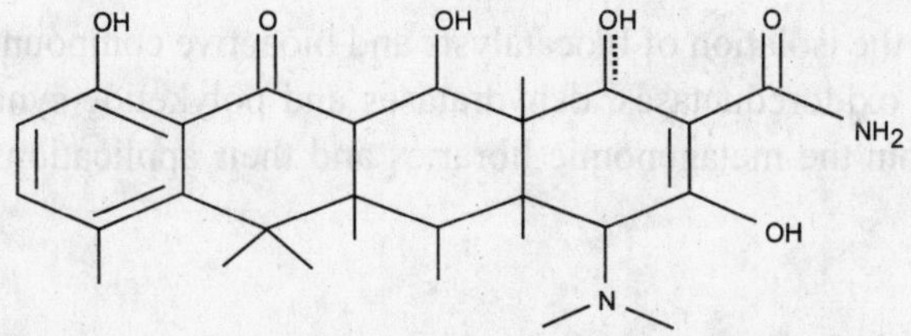

Tetracycline from the libraries of Toree *et al.*, 2003

Figure 34.4 Antibiotics developed through metagenomic libraries.

Metagenomic and antimicrobial drug discovery

Presently there is an urgent need for novel drugs of desirable clinical utility due to growing incidence of antibiotic resistance among microbial pathogens. Microorganisms continue to evolve and adapt at a remarkable rate, therefore they have developed resistance to every class of antibiotic currently in clinical use. Furthermore, an escalating number of bacteria have acquainted multiple resistance systems for avoiding and/or reducing the action of an antibiotic. Therefore, it is the need of this hour to develop novel antimicrobial agents possessing new mechanisms of action. Function-driven metagenomic analysis is initiated through identification of clones that express a desired trait (antibacterium), followed by characterization of the active clones by sequence and biochemical analysis. This approach quickly identifies clones that have potential application in medicine or industry. The only constraint of the approach is that it requires expression of the function of interest in the host cell and clustering of all gene required for the function.

Moreover, metagenomics analysis of soil is challenging because soil is a very complex environment containing diverse organisms in a dynamic matrix with vast potential. Discovery of metabolic networks and small molecules from the cultured microorganisms in soil has been unparalleled in any other environment and therefore it is likely that the potential for discovery from the uncultured community is similarly enormous. As most of the uncultured life forms in soil appear to be new species and many represent new genera, there is much to learn about the functioning of soil microbial communities and these communities have already yielded new enzymes and antibiotics. Technical advances in DNA recovery, gene expression and functional analysis will enhance the rate of discovery and make possible productive prospecting of soil for the medicinal, agriculture and industrial chemicals.

Biotechnology

The knowledge of DNA and biochemical fingerprints of microbial communities are mind-boggling. In biodefence and microbial forensics, the study helps to monitor pathogens, generate more effective vaccines and therapeutics against bioterror agents, and reform attacks that entailed microorganisms. Metagenomics helps to study the products of cellular processes viz. proteins and metabolites and in identifying the genes and metabolic pathways. Metagenomic libraries are the key to find out the genes coding for the functions like antibiotic resistance, cold tolerance, nitrogen fixation, and metal resistance etc. The application of construction and screening of metagenomic libraries has resulted in the isolation of biocatalysts and bioactive compounds of industrial interest, e.g., amylases, lipases, oxidoreductases, dehydratases and polyketide synthases etc. Some of the enzymes discovered from the metagenomic libraries and their applications are (Table 34.2) summarized below.

Table 34.2 Novel biocatalysts retrieved from metagenomics libraries.

Source	*Enzymes discovered*	*Functions*	*Applications*	*References*
Soil	Lipases/esterases	Biocatalyst	Baking, laundry detergents	Yun *et al.*, 2006
Deep-Sea Sediments	New alkaline esterases EM2L8	Biocatalyst	Food industry	Jung *et al.*, 2007
Soils and compost	Lipases Phosphatases	Biocatalyst Removes phosphate group from its substrate	Enzyme modified cheese	Lammle *et al.*, 2007
Marine sample	Chitinases	Digestive enzymes that break down glycosidic bonds in chitin.	Used in agriculture to control pathogens	Cottrell *et al.*, 1999
Agricultural/ river valley soil	4-hydroxy butyrate dehydrogenases	-	-	Henne *et. al.*, 1999
Soil sample	Polyketide synthase	Synthesis of polyketides.	Antibiotic production	Seow *et al.*, 1997
Laboratory enrichment cultures	β-agarases Cellulases Amylases	Cleave the β-D-1,4) linkages of agar. Degrade cellulose fibers to glucose. Hydrolyses chemical bonds between glucose molecules in starch.	Food and Feed additives as a solidifying agent Food processing in coffee, textile, Pulp and paper industries, detergents. Corn syrup and in baking processes.	Voget *et al.*, 2003
Endosymbiont of *Riftia pachyptila*	Histidine protein kinase RuBisco	Signal transduction Enzyme used in calvin cycle		Hughes *et al.*, 1997 Robinson *et al.*, 1998

Agricultural Applications

Metagenomics plays a vital role in agriculture. The microbial communities in the soil are responsible for the healthy plants and thus make direct impact on the yield. The manipulation by selecting ideal combination of the microbes and crops will help to increase the yield parameter. The Biological Nitrogen Fixation (BNF) is an important source of nitrogen and helps to reduce the use of chemical nitrogen fertilizer. The capacity for nitrogen fixation is unique to certain groups within the domains of bacteria and archaea. The *nifH* gene encoding the iron protein subunit of nitrogenase is highly conserved among all diazotrophs and the phylogeny based on *nifH* genes has been shown largely to resemble the 16S rRNA phylogeny. During the last few years, successful amplification of the *nifH* gene have been achieved by polymerase chain reaction (PCR) to examine the diazotroph communities in various soil habitats.

Challenges and limitations in metagenomics analysis

Although metagenomic libraries have yielded interesting information about biological systems, there are many barriers. Many genes are derived from organisms that are phylogenetically distant from *E. coli* or another culturable species, which is used as host to the library, and thus functional analysis will not detect these genes.

In addition to the large number of species currently estimated at 10^4 or more per g of soil, there is likely microheterogeneity among genomes within a species. Recent work on *Cenarchaeum symbiosum,* a species that forms an intimate associate with a sponge, showed substantial variation among genomes within a local population of the bacterium. Therefore, layers of complexity may make it impossible to reconstruct a genome, as is possible in simpler communities, but association of genes, their functions and genomic organization with particular taxa will be a fruitful area of endeavor in soil metagenomics.

Future prospects of metagenomics technology

Metagenomic analysis depends on technical innovations that will provide improved access to DNA, heterologous gene expression and DNA sequence analysis. To access DNA from a wider range of organisms, we need methods that facilitate aggressive bacterial cell lysis while protecting integrity of the DNA. We need strategies to increase representation of rare members of the community by removing the DNA from the abundant organisms. This might involve antibodies that remove certain bacterial cell genomes after lysis, although the latter will be challenging because of the conservation among all bacterial genomes. Gene expression can be enhanced by transferring clones to a variety of organisms that represent a range of G+C content, preferred codon usage, and protein secretion strategies. This requires shuttle vectors that replicate in *E. coli* and a host cell with gene expression machinery that differs substantially from that of *E. coli*, such as *Bacillus* (a low G+C Gram-positive) or *Streptomyces* (a high G+C Gram-positive). Highly sensitive detectors and small volume assays that maintain high local concentration of products from a clone will likely increase the rate of finding active clones and will be the most appropriate approach.

Our on-going efforts

To explore the unculturable microbial diversity of Uttarakhand Himalayan region, efforts are underway at different fronts: one is direct quantification of bacterial rRNA gene to know the bacterial load on soil, and the other is isolation of functional genes like bacterial cold shock genes (*csp*) and *nifH* gene etc. The metagenomic Csp library was constructed from the temperate and glacier soils. Homology search of cloned sequence revealed their identity with the *Csp* genes of *Pseudomonas fluorescens, Psychrobacter cryohalolentis K5* and *Shewanella* sp.MR-4. Further, analysis of amino acid sequence of Csp recombinants revealed the sequence similarity with several cold stress induced proteins like rbfA, IF2, DEAD-boxhelicase, cold acclimation proteins (EFTs) and temperature induced proteins (SRP1/TIP1). This study highlights the prevalence of *Csp* gene(s) from cold Himalayan environments, which can be explored for tailored made crop as per the need of that region in future.

Besides, a 16s rRNA gene library was constructed and sequenced from metagenome isolated from six places i.e., Pantnagar (29.00 N, 243.8 mts), Chamoli (30. 51°N, 79.4°E, 1300mts), Ranichauri (78°30'E, 30°15'N, 1600 mts), Pithoragarh (80°2' E, 29° 47'N, 1967 mts), Badrinath (30.44°N, 79°E, 3110mts) and Mana Glacier (30.44°N, 79°E, 3, 133m) of Uttarakhand. More than 30 finally selected clones were sequenced and analyzed. Most of the clones show homology with free living species like *Nostoc sp.* symbiotic: *Azorhizobium, Mesorhizobium* nitrogen fixing and others related to nitrogen fixation process *Nitrobacter* sp., *Nitrosococcus* etc. community like. It would be interesting to further screen them completely in view of their 100% exploitation.

CONCLUSION AND FUTURE PROSPECTS

Microbes run the world. It is that simple. Although we cannot usually see them, microbes are essential for every part of human life—indeed all life on Earth. Every process in the biosphere is touched by the seemingly endless capacity of microbes to transform the world around them. The chemical cycles that convert the key elements of life—carbon, nitrogen, oxygen, and sulfur—into biologically accessible forms are largely directed by and dependent on microbes. All plants and animals have closely associated microbial communities that make necessary nutrients, metals and vitamins available to their hosts. Through fermentation and other natural processes, microbes create or add value to many foods that are staples of the human diet. We depend on microbes to remediate toxins in the environment—both the ones that are produced naturally and the ones that are the by-products of human activities, such as oil and chemical spills. The microbes associated with the human body in the intestine and mouth enable us to extract energy from food that we could not digest without them and protect us against disease-causing agents.

These functions are conducted within complex communities—intricate, balanced, and integrated entities that adapt swiftly and flexibly to environmental change. But historically, the study of microbes has focused on single species in pure culture, so understanding of these complex communities lags behind understanding of their individual members. We know enough, however, to confirm that microbes, as communities, are key players in maintaining environmental stability.

FURTHER READINGS

1. Aardema B.W., Lorenz M.G., Krumbein W.E. (1983) Protection of sediment-adsorbed transforming DNA against enzymatic inactivation. *Appl. Environ. Microbiol.* **(46):** 417.
2. Amann, R.I., Ludwig, W., Schleifer, K.H., (1995) Phylogenetic identification and *in situ* detection of individual microbial cells without cultivation. *Microbiol. Rev.* **(59):** 143-169.
3. Bell, P.J.L., Sunna, A., Gibbs, M. D., Curach, N. C., Nevalainen, H. and Bergquist, P. L. (2002) Prospecting for novel lipase genes using PCR. *Microbiology*. **(148):** 2283-2291.
4. Berry Andrew E., Claudia Chiocchini Tina Selby, lMargherita Sosio, Elizabeth M.H. (2003) Wellington Isolation of high molecular weight DNA from soil for cloning into BAC vectors. *FEMS Microbiology Letters.* (223) 15-20.
5. Bertrand He´le‘ne, Franck Poly, T., Van Tran Vana, B., Nathalie Lombarda, Renaud Nalinb,Timothy M. Vogela, Pascal Simonet (2005) High molecular weight DNA recovery from soils prerequisite for biotechnological metagenomic library construction. *Journal of Microbiological Methods.* **(62):** 1-11.
6. Boubakri Hasna, Mélanie Beuf, Pascal Simonet, Timothy M. Vogel (2006) Development of metagenomic DNA shuttling for the construction of a xenobiotic gene. *Gene.* **(375):** 87–94.

7. Bu¨ rgmann, H., Widmer, F., Sigler, W.V. and Zeyer, J. (2004) Newmolecular screening tools for analysis of free-living diazotrophs in soil. *Appl. Environ. Microbiol.* **(70):** 240-247.
8. Bull A.T., Goodfellow M. and Slater J.H. (1992) Biodiversity as asource of innovation in biotechnology. *Annu. Rev. Microbiol.* **(l46):** 219.
9. Cottrell, M. T., Moore J. A. and Kirchman D. L. (1999) Chitinases from uncultured marine microorganisms. *Appl. Environ. Microbiol.* **(65):** 2553-2557.
10. Cowan D.A., Arslanoglu A., Burton S.G., Baker G.C., Cameron R.A., Smith J.J. and Meyer Q. (2004) Metagenomics, gene discovery and the ideal biocatalyst. Biochemical Society Transactions. Volume 32, part 2.
11. Cupples, M. and Gerald K. Sims (2007) Identification of *in situ* 2,4-dichlorophenoxyacetic acid-degrading soil microorganisms using DNA-stable isotope probing. *Soil Biology & Biochemistry.* **(39):** 232-238.
12. Daniel R. (2004) The soil metagenome – a rich resource for the discovery of novel natural products *Current Opinion in Biotechnology.* **(15):** 199-204.
13. Daniel, R. (2005) The metagenomics of soil. *Nat. Rev. Microbiol.,* **(3):** 470-478.
14. Desai Chirayu, Datta Madamwar (2006) Extraction of inhibitor-free metagenomic DNA from polluted sediments, compatible with molecular diversity analysis using adsorption and ion-exchange treatments. *Bioresource Technology.* **(98):** 761-768
15. Diaz-Torres, M. L., McNab, R., Spratt, D. A., Villedieu, A., Hunt, N., Wilson, M., and Mullany P. (2003) Novel tetracycline resistance determinant from the oral metagenome. *Antimicrob. Agents Chemother*. **(47):** 1430-1432.
16. Dong Dexian, An Yan, Haiming Liu, Xuehong Zhang, Yuquan Xu (2006) Removal of humic substances from soil DNA using aluminium sulfate *Journal of Microbiological Methods*. **(66):** 217-222.
17. Filion, M., Arnaudb, M. S., Suha, H., Harea, J. (2003) Direct quantification of fungal DNA from soil substrate using real-time PCR. *J. Microbiol. Meth.* **(53):** 67-76.
18. Gabor, E.M., Alkema, W.B., Janssen, D.B., (2004) Quantifying the accessibility of the metagenome by random expression cloning techniques. *Environ. Microbiol.* **(6):** 879–886.
19. Garrett R. H., Grisham C. N. (1995) in *Biochemistry*. (Saunders College Publishing: USA. p. 213
20. Gillespie, D.E., Brady, S.F., Bettermann, A.D., Cianciotto, N.P., Liles, M.R., Rondon, M.R., Clardy, J., Goodman, R.M., and Handelsmann J. (2002) Isolation of antibiotics turbomycin A and turbomycin B from a metagenomic library of soil microbial DNA. *Appl. Environ. Microbiol*. **(68):** 4301-4306.
21. Green R.D., Qureshi M.A., Long J.A., Burfening P.J., Hamernik D.L. (2007) Identifying the future needs for long-term USDA efforts in agricultural animal genomics. *Int. J. Biol Sci.* 3 **(3):** 185-91.
22. Hammond, P.M. (1995) Described and estimated species numbers:an objective assessment of current knowledge. In: Microbial 5 diversity and ecosystem function: proceedings of the IUBS/IUMS workshop, Egham, UK: University Press, Cambridge, UK, p. 2.
23. Handelsman, J. (2004) Metagenomics: application of genomics to uncultured microorganisms. *Microbiology and Molecular Biology Reviews.* **(68):** 669-685.
24. Handelsman, J. (1998) Molecular biological access to the chemistry of unknown soil microbes: a new frontier for natural products. *Chem. Biol.* **(5):** R245-R249.
25. Handelsman, Jo. (2004) Soil - the metagenomics approach. *In: Microbial Diversity and Bioprospecting.* (eds). Alan T. Bull. ASM Press, Washington, D.C., pp. 109-119.
26. Henne, A., Daniel R., Schmitz R.A., and Gottschalk G. (1999) Construction of environmental DNA libraries in *Escherichia coli* and screening for the presence of genes conferring utilization of 4-hydroxybutyrate. *Appl. Environ. Microbiol.* **(65):** 3901-3907.
27. Henneberger, Ruth M., A. B. Malcolm, R. Walter, A.B.C. and Anitori Roberto P. (2006) Extraction of DNA from acidic, hydrothermally modified volcanic soils. *Environ. Chem*. **(3):** 100-104.
28. Hughes, D.S., Felbeck H., and Stein J.L. (1997) A histidine protein kinase homolog from the endosymbiont of the hydrothermal vent tubeworm *Riftia pachyptila. Appl. Environ. Microbiol.* **(63):** 3494-3498.

29. Ka J.O., Yu Z., Mohn W.W. (2001) Monitoring the size and metabolic activity of the bacterial community during biostimulation of fuel-contaminated soil using competitive PCR and RT-PCR. *Microb. Ecol.* **(42):** 267-273.
30. Kaeberlein, T., Lewis. K. and Epstein, S.S., (2002) Isolating 'Uncultivable' microorganisms in pure culture by a simulated natural environment. *Science.* **(296):** 1127-1129.
31. Khanna M., Stotzky G. (1992) Transformation of *Bacillus subtilis* by DNA bound on montmorillonite and effect of DNase on the transforming ability of bound DNA. *Appl. Environ. Microbiol.* **(58):** 1930.
32. Kowalchuk George A., G.C.L. Arjen Speksnijder, Zhang Kun, Goodman Robert M. and Johannes A. van Veen (2007) Finding the Needles in the Metagenome Haystack Microbial Ecology DOI: 10.1007/s00248-006-9201-2
33. Lammle, K., Zipper, H., Breuer, M., Hauer, B., Buta, C., Brunner, H., and Rupp. S. (2007) Identification of novel enzymes with different hydrolytic activities by metagenome expression cloning. *J. Biotechnol.* **(127):** 575-592
34. Morita H., Kuwahara T., Oshima K., Sasamoto H., Itoh K., Hattori M., Hayashi T. & Takami H. (2007) An improved DNA isolation method for metagenomic analysis of the microbial flora of the human instetine. *Microbes Environ.* 22 **(3):** 214-222.
35. Morris D.D., Reeves R.A., Gibbs, M.D., Saul, D.J. and Bergquist, P.L. (1995) Correction of the beta-mannanase domain of the celC pseudogene from Caldocellulosiruptor sacchorolyticus and activity of the gene product on kraft pulp. *Appl. Environ. Microbiol.* 61 **(6):** 2262-2269.
36. Ochman, H., Jose Ayala, F. and Hartl, D.L. (1993) Use of polymerase chain reaction to amplify segments outside boundaries of known sequences. *Methods Enzymol.* **(218):** 309-321.
37. Park H-J, Jeong Ho Jeon, Sung Gyun Kang, Jung-Hyun Lee, Sung-A Lee, Hyung-Kwoun Kima. (2007) Functional expression and refolding of new alkaline esterase, EM2L8 from deep-sea sediment metagenome. *Protein Expression and Purification.* **(52):** 340-347.
38. Pettit R.K. (2004) Soil DNA libraries for anticancer drug discovery. *Cancer Chemother Pharmacol.* **(54):** 1-6.
39. Pietramellara G., Dal Canto L., Vettori C., Gallori E., Nannipieri P. (1997) Effects of air drying and wetting cycles on the transforming ability of DNA bound on clay minerals. *Soil Biol. Biochem.* **(29):** 55-61.
40. Poly Franck, Lucile Jocteur Monrozier, René Bally (2001) Improvement in the RFLP procedure for studying the diversity of *nifH* genesin communities of nitrogen fixers in soil. *Res. Microbiol.* **(152):** 95-103.
41. Raymond, J., Siefert, J.L., Staples, C.R., Blankenship, R.E., (2004) The natural history of nitrogen fixation. *Mol. Biol. Evol.* **(21):** 541-554.
42. Riesenfeld, C.S., Schloss, P.D. and Handelsman J. (2004) Metagenomics: Genomic analyses of microbial communities. *Annu. Rev. Genet.* **(38):** 525-529.
43. Robinson, J. J., Stein J. L. and Cavanaugh C. M. (1998) Cloning and sequencing of a form II ribulose-1, 5-biphosphate carboxylase/oxygenase from the bacterial symbiont of the hydrothermal vent tubeworm *Riftia pachyptila. J. Bacteriol.* **(180):** 1596-1599.
44. Rondon, M. R. (2000) Cloning the soil metagenome: a strategy for accessing the genetic and functional diversity of uncultured microorganisms. *Appl. Environ. Microbiol.* **(66):** 2541-2547.
45. Schleper, C., DeLong E.F., Preston C.M., Feldman R.A., Wu K.Y. and Swanson R.V. (1998). Genomic analysis reveals chromosomal variation in natural populations of the uncultured psychrophilic archaeon Cenarchaeum symbiosum. *J. Bacterial.* 180 **(19):** 5003-5009.
46. Sebat, J.L. (2003) Metagenomic profiling: Microarray analysis of an environmental genomic library. *Applied and Environmental Microbiology.* **(69):** 4927-34.
47. Seow, K. T., Meurer G., Gerlitz M., Wendt-Pienkowski E., Hutchinson C. R. and Davies J. (1997) A study of iterative type II polyketide synthases, using bacterial genes cloned from soil DNA: a means to access and use genes from uncultured microorganisms. *J. Bacteriol.* **(179):** 7360-7368.

48. Stein J.L.; Marsh T.L. wu K.Y., Shizuya H, Delong E.F. (1996) Characterisation of uncultivated prokaryotes :isolation and analysis of a 40 kilobase-pair genome fragment front a planktonic marine archaeon. *J. Bacteriol.* **(178):** 591-599.
49. Torsvik, V. and Ovreas, L. (2002) Microbial diversity and function in soil: from genes to ecosystems. *Curr. Opin. Microbiol.* **(5):** 240-245.
50. Tyson, G. W. (2004) Community structure and metabolism through reconstruction of microbial genomes from the environment. *Nature*. (428), 37-43.
51. Van Elsas J.D., MaÈntynen V., Wolters A.C. (1997) Soil DNA extraction and assessment of the fate of Mycobacterium chlorophenolicum strain PCP-1 in different soils by 16S ribosomal RNA gene sequence based most-probable-number PCR and immunofluorescence. *Biol. Fertil. Soils.* **(24):** 188-195.
52. Voget, S., Leggewie, C., Uesbeck, A., Raasch, C., Jaeger, K.-E. and Streit W.R. (2003) Prospecting for novel biocatalysts in soil metagenome. *Appl. Environ. Microbiol.* **(69):** 6235-6242.
53. Voget, S., Steele H.L., Streit W.R. (2006) Characterization of a metagenome-derived halotolerant cellulase. *Journal of Biotechnology.* **(126):** 26-36.
54. Wakelin, S.A., Colloff, M.J., Harvey, P.R., Marshner, P., Gregg, A.L., Roger, S.L., (2007) The effect of stubble retention and nitrogen application on soil microbial community structure and functional gene abundance under irrigated maize. *FEMS Microbiol. Ecol.* (59), 661-670.
55. Wallenstein Matthew D., Vilgalys Rytas J. (2005) Quantitative analyses of nitrogen in soils. *Pedobiologia.* **(49):** 665-672.
56. Wang P. and Dick W.A. (2004) Microbial and genetic diversity in soil environments. *Journal of Crop Improvement.* **(12):** 249-287
57. Wartiainen Ingvild, Eriksson Torsten, Zheng Weiwen, Rasmussen Ulla (2008) Variation in the active diazotrophic community in rice paddy—nifH PCR-DGGE analysis of rhizosphere and bulk soil. *Appl. Soil Ecol.,* doi:10.1016/ j.apsoil.2007.11.008
58. Yeager, C.M., Kornosky, J.L., Housman, D.C., Grote, E.E., Belnap, J., Kuske, C.R., (2004) Diazotrophic community structure and function in two successional stages of biological soil crust from the Colorado plateau and Chihuahuan desert. *Appl. Environ. Microbiol.* **(70):** 973-983.
59. Yun-Jung Kim, Gi-Sub Choi, Seung-Bum Kim, Gee-Sun Yoon, Yong-Sung Kim, and Yeon-Woo Ryu. (2006) Screening and characterization of a novel esterase from a metagenomic library. *Protein Expression and Purification.* **(45):** 315-323.
60. Zehr J.P., MacReynolds L.A. (1989) Use of degenerate oligonucleotides for amplification of the nifH gene from the marine Cyanobacterium Trichodesmium thiebautii, *Appl. Environ. Microbiol.* **(55):** 2526-2552.
61. Zhang, L., Hurek, T., Reinhold-Hurek, B., (2006) A nifH-based oligonucleotide microarray for functional diagnostics of nitrogen-fixing microorganisms. *Microbial. Ecol.* **(53):** 456-470.
62. Zhou J., Thompson D.K., Tiedje M.J. (2004) Microbial Functional Genomics, pp. 21-40.

CHAPTER

35

Bioremediation Technology

Bioremediation technology deals with the removal or detoxification of man-made, partially or wholly non-biodegradable xenobiotic compounds by using microorganisms, plants and fungi or their enzymes for solving tremendous pollution and health hazard problems. The goal of bioremediation should be clarified from the points of view of human health, protection of the global environmental and preservation of biodiversity. In this chapter we described the detailed procedures and applications of bioremediation technology in various fields.

Keywords: Bioremediation technology, xenobiotics, detoxification, bioaugmentation, biostimulation.

INTRODUCTION

Enormous quantities of organic and inorganic compounds are released into the environment each year as a result of human activities. In some cases these releases are deliberate and well regulated (e.g., industrial emissions), while in other cases they are accidental (e.g., chemical or oil spills). Detoxification of the contaminated sites by conventional chemical or physical methods is expensive and time consuming. Bioremediation is a combination of two words, "bio", means living and "remediate" means to solve a problem or to bring the sites and affairs into the original state, and "bio-remediate" means to use biological organisms to solve an environmental problem such as contaminated soil or groundwater through technological innovations.

Bioremediation technologies can be generally classified as *in situ* or *ex situ. In situ* bioremediation involves treating the contaminated material at the site, while *ex situ* involves the removal of the contaminated material to be treated elsewhere. Some examples of bioremediation technologies are bioventing, landfarming, bioreactor, bioaugmentation, rhizofiltration, and biostimulation. However, not all contaminants are easily treated by bioremediation using microorganisms. For example, heavy metals such as cadmium and lead are not readily absorbed or captured by organisms. The assimilation of metals such as mercury into the food chain may worsen matters. Phytoremediation is useful in these circumstances, because natural plants or transgenic plants are able to bioaccumulate these toxins in their above-ground parts, which are then harvested for removal. The heavy metals in the harvested biomass may be further concentrated by incineration or even recycled for industrial use. A wide range of bioremediation strategies is being developed to treat contaminated soils. In bioremediation, microorganisms transform hazardous chemical compounds to non-hazardous end products, however, in phytoremediation, plants are used for this purpose. Two basic methods are available for obtaining the microorganisms to initiate the bioremediation:

(i) Bioaugumentation—In this mehod, adapted and genetically coded toxicants degrading microorganisms are added.

(ii) Biostimulation—This involves the injection of necessary nutrients to stimulate the growth of the indigenous microorganisms.

The effectiveness of bioremediation is mainly influenced by the degradability and the toxicity of the chemical compounds. Based on this, the chemical may be divided into degradable and nontoxic, degradable and toxic, nondegradable and toxic and nondegradable and nontoxic chemical compounds. The main goal of bioremediation can be fulfilled by enhancing the rate and extent of biodegradation of the pollutants, utilizing or developing microorganism. Selecting the most appropriate strategy to treat a specific site can be guided by considering three basic principles: the amenability of the pollutant to biological transformation to less toxic products (biochemistry); the accessibility of the contaminant to microorganisms (bioavailability); and the opportunity for optimization of biological activity (bioactivity). Bioremediation is the use of biological treatment systems to destroy or reduce the concentrations of hazardous wastes from a contaminated site. Such systems have numerous applications, including clean up of ground water, soil, lagoons, sludges and process waste-streams. At present, there are three commonly used methods of carrying out *in situ* bioremediation of contaminated soil and groundwater. The first is to inoculate the subsurface environment with non-indigenous, contaminant-degrading bacteria, together with a balanced nutrient formulation. The second is to periodically introduce a hydrogen peroxide/nutrient formulation to the subsurface environment. The rationale behind this approach is that the subsurface environment already contains microorganisms adapted to the contaminant, but it is deficient in both nutrients and oxygen, which would enable the indigenous microorganisms to metabolize the contaminants to the end products—carbon dioxide and water. By supplying these growth-limiting factors, the indigenous microbes can then mineralize the contaminants. The third method is bioreactor-based. Whereas the first two methods are considered relatively passive means of bioremediation, the third method flushes contaminants from the soil so that they can be recovered and treated in the above-ground bioreactor, into which a continuous supply of nutrients, oxygen and microorganisms is introduced. Variations or combinations of these three basic technologies provide a range of *in situ* bioremediation methods.

CONCEPTS

Bioremediation is defined as the process whereby organic wastes are biologically degraded under controlled conditions to an innocuous state, or to levels below concentration limits established by regulatory authorities. Bioremediation process involves detoxification, where the waste is made less toxic, and mineralization, where the waste material is converted into inorganic compounds such as carbon dioxide, water and methane. According to Dr. Ting, bioremediation processes may be classified into two main categories: *in situ* and *ex-situ*. Bioremediation can often be carried out on site, without causing a major disruption of normal activities. This also eliminates the need to transport quantities of waste off site and the potential threats to human health and the environment that can arise during transportation. Bioremediation is an option that offers the possibility to destroy or render harmless various contaminants using natural biological activity. As such, it uses relatively low-cost, low-technology techniques, which generally have a high public acceptance and can often be carried out on site. Factors such as site conditions, indigenous microorganism population, and the type, quantity, and toxicity of contaminant chemicals present determine the bioremediation technology most suitable for a specific site. Bioremediation can be applied to an environmental problem in a variety of ways. There are five general approaches to bioremediation: above-ground reactors, solid phase treatment, composting, landfarming, and *in situ* treatment. Bioremediation can prove less expensive than other technologies that are used for clean-up of hazardous waste. The economics of bioremediation are almost always significantly more favorable than other techniques. The primary reason is that there is no need for the hauling and expensive disposal costs of contaminated soils. It is estimated that bioremediation costs 1/3 to 1/2 that of incineration, and for complex mixtures of waste, bioremediation typically offers savings of 60-90% over landfill-disposal costs. The estimated cost of biotreatment of biodegradable contaminants in soil range between 40 and 100$ per cubic yard, as compared with cost as high as 250-800 $ per cubic yard for incineration and 150-250$ per cubic yard for landfilling. The current technology based land remediation market is worth in the region of 120-130 £ million. Technologies such as soil washing, bioremediation and other extractive methods have developed to a stage where they are both commercially viable and compete head-to-head with excavate and landfill options.

PRINCIPLES

The key players in bioremediation are bacteria—microscopic organisms that live virtually everywhere. Microorganisms are ideally suited to the task of contaminant destruction because they possess enzymes that allow them to use environmental contaminants as food, and they are so small that they are able to contact contaminants easily. *In situ* bioremediation can be regarded as an extension of the purpose that microorganisms have served in nature for billions of years: the breakdown of complex human, animal, and plant wastes so that life can continue from one generation to the next. Without the activity of microorganisms, the earth would literally be buried in wastes, and the nutrients necessary for the continuation of life would be locked up in detritus.

Whether microorganisms will be successful in destroying man-made contaminants in the subsurface depends on three factors: the type of organisms, the type of contaminants, and the geological and chemical conditions at the contaminated site. This chapter explains how these three factors influence the outcome of a subsurface bioremediation project. It reviews how microorganisms destroy contaminants and what types of organisms play a role in *in situ* bioremediation. Then, it evaluates which contaminants are most susceptible to bioremediation in the subsurface and describes the types of sites where bioremediation is most likely to succeed.

BIOREMEDIATION TECHNOLOGY

Role of Microbes in Bioremediation

The goal of bioremediation is to stimulate microorganisms with nutrients and other chemicals that will enable them to destroy the contaminants. The bioremediation systems in operation today rely on microorganisms native to the contaminated sites, encouraging them to work by supplying them with the optimum levels of nutrients and other chemicals essential for their metabolism. Thus, today's bioremediation systems are limited by the capabilities of the native microbes. However, researchers are currently investigating ways to augment contaminated sites with nonnative microbes—including genetically engineered microorganisms—specially suited to degrading the contaminants of concern at particular sites. It is possible that this process, known as bioaugmentation, could expand the range of possibilities for future bioremediation systems. Regardless of whether the microbes are native or newly introduced to the site, an understanding of how they destroy contaminants is critical to understanding bioremediation. The types of microbial processes that will be employed in the cleanup dictate what nutritional supplements the bioremediation system must supply. Furthermore, the by-products of microbial processes can provide indicators that bioremediation is successful.

In microbial bioremediation, living microorganisms are used to convert complex toxic compounds into harmless by-products of cellular metabolism such as CO_2 and H_2O. However, in phytoremediation, plants are used to remove contamination from the soil and water. In a non-polluted environment, microorganisms are constantly at work, utilizing toxic compounds, however, most of them die at contaminated sites. Few of them, due to their inherent genetic material, grow, survive and degrade the chemicals. The successful use of microorganisms in bioremediation depends on the development of a basic understanding of the genetics of a broad spectrum of microorganisms and biotechnological innovations. Pure, mixed, enriched and genetically engineered microorganisms have been used for the degradation of these compounds. Routes of degradation of the major natural compounds have been well established. The entire spectrum of microbial degradation is related to the breakdown of xenobiotic chemicals, which are non-degradable and recalcitrant. A large number of microorganisms have been isolated in recent years that are able to degrade compounds previously considered to be non-degradable. This suggests that, under the selective pressure of environmental pollution, a microbial capacity for the degradation of recalcitrant xenobiotics is developing that might be harnessed for pollutant removal by biotechnological processes. Nevertheless, the fact that many pollutants persist in the environment emphasizes the current inadequacy of this catabolic capacity to deal with such pollutants.

Degradation by fungi: The process of natural bioremediation of persistent compounds involves a range of microorganisms. Most fungi are robust and generally more tolerant to high concentration of polluting chemicals than bacteria. A variety of fungi have been used for the degradation of pollutants in the environment. The contaminants present in water and soil from industrial and agriculture activities are degraded and utilized by fungi. But the use of fungi for degradation of industrial pollutants such as chlorophenols, nitrophenols and polyaromatic hydrocarbons is limited. In spite of the toxicity of the effluent and presence of chlorophenols, the microbial flora of tannery liquid wastes is relatively rich, with the *Aspergillus niger* group predominant. Sixteen species of fungi belonging to 6 genera, and 2 yeasts belonging to one genus were isolated from tannery effluent. The extracellular enzymes and cell mass from the pregrown *Phanerochaete chrysosporium* cultures were used for the degradation of pentachlorophenol (PCP). The lignin degrading fungi *Phanerochaete chrysosporium, P. sordida, Trametes hirusta*, and *Ceriporiopsis subvermispora* were evaluated for their ability to decrease the concentration of pentachlorophenol.

Degradation by bacteria: These bacteria can be separated into aerobic types, which require oxygen to live, and anaerobic, which can live without oxygen. Aerobic bioremediation is usually preferred because it degrades pollutants 10 to 100 times faster than anaerobic bioremediation. Facultative types can thrive under both aerobic and anaerobic conditions. Certain bacteria belonging to the *Bacillus* and *Pseudomonas* species have these desirable characteristics. They consume organic waste thousands of times faster than the types of bacteria that are naturally present in the waste. Bacteria, *Arthobacteria, Flavobacterium, Pseudomonads* and *Sphingomonas* have been isolated and applied for the degradation of chlorinated phenol and other toxic organic compounds. A number of bacteria viz., *Pseudomonas, Flavobacterium, Xanthomonas, Nocardia, Aeromonas* and *Arthrobacterium* are known to utilize lignocellulosic components of the bleached plant effluent containing lignosulphonics and chlorinated phenols. One particularly promising mechanism for the detoxification of PCDDs and PCDFs is microbial reductive dechlorination. So far only a limited number of phylogenetically diverse anaerobic bacteria have been found that couple the reductive dehalogenation of chlorinated compounds with the substitution of chlorine for a hydrogen atom to energy conservation and growth in a process called dehalorespiration. Microbial dechlorination of PCDDs occurs in sediments and anaerobic mixed cultures from sediments, but the responsible organisms have not yet been identified or isolated. Here we show the presence of a Dehalococcoides species in four dioxin-dechlorinating enrichment cultures from freshwater sediment highly contaminated with PCDDs and PCDFs. Various microbial cultures capable of aerobic PCB biodegradation have been isolated. Up to 85% degradation of Arochlors 1248 and 1242 has been shown. The more highly chlorinated 1254 and 1260 Arochlors have not shown significant aerobic biodegradation in the laboratory or in the field. Anaerobic degradation by dechlorination reactions is widespread a even for the 1254 and 1260 Arochlors.

Bioremediation Processes and Technologies

Bioremediation techniques are divided into three categories: *in situ*, *ex situ* solid, and *ex situ* slurry. *in situ* techniques (Figure 35.1), the soil and associated groundwater is treated in place without excavation, while it is excavated prior to treatment with *ex situ* applications. The potential applications of biotechnology can be applied in terms of the contaminated matrix, degrading organisms of the contaminants, the type of reactor technology used and the types of compounds present. The anaerobic and aerobic treatment methods applied for reducing the pollution load have been proved successful up to some extent. Pump-and-treat systems, which are applied to saturated-zone remediation, involve the removal, treatment and return of associated water from a contaminated soil zone. The returned water is supplemented with nutrients and saturated with oxygen. Percolation consists of applying water, containing nutrients and possibly a microbial inoculum, to the surface of a contaminated area and allowing it to filter into the soil and mix with the groundwater, if present. Bioventing supplies air to an unsaturated soil zone through the installation of a well(s) connected to associated pumps and blowers, which draw a vacuum on the soil. Air sparging involves the injection of air into the saturated zone of a contaminated soil.

Ex situ solid-phase techniques consist of soil treatment units, compost piles and engineered biopiles. Soil treatment units consist of soil contained and tilled (to supply oxygen) with application of water, nutrients and possibly microbial inocula. Compost piles consist of soil supplemented with composting material (i.e., wood chips, straw, manure, rice hulls, etc.) to improve its physical handling properties and water and air-holding capacities. Compost piles require periodic mixing to provide oxygen to the soil. Biopiles are piles of contaminated soil that contain piping to provide air and water. *Ex situ* solid applications involve the addition of water, nutrients and sometimes cultured indigenous microbes or inocula. They are often conducted on lined pads to ensure that there is no contamination of the underlying soil. *Ex situ* slurry techniques involve the creation and maintenance of soil-water slurry as the bioremediation medium. The slurry can be maintained in either a bioreactor or a pond or lagoon. Adequate mixing and aeration are key design requirements for slurry systems. Nutrients and, perhaps, inocula may be added to the slurry.

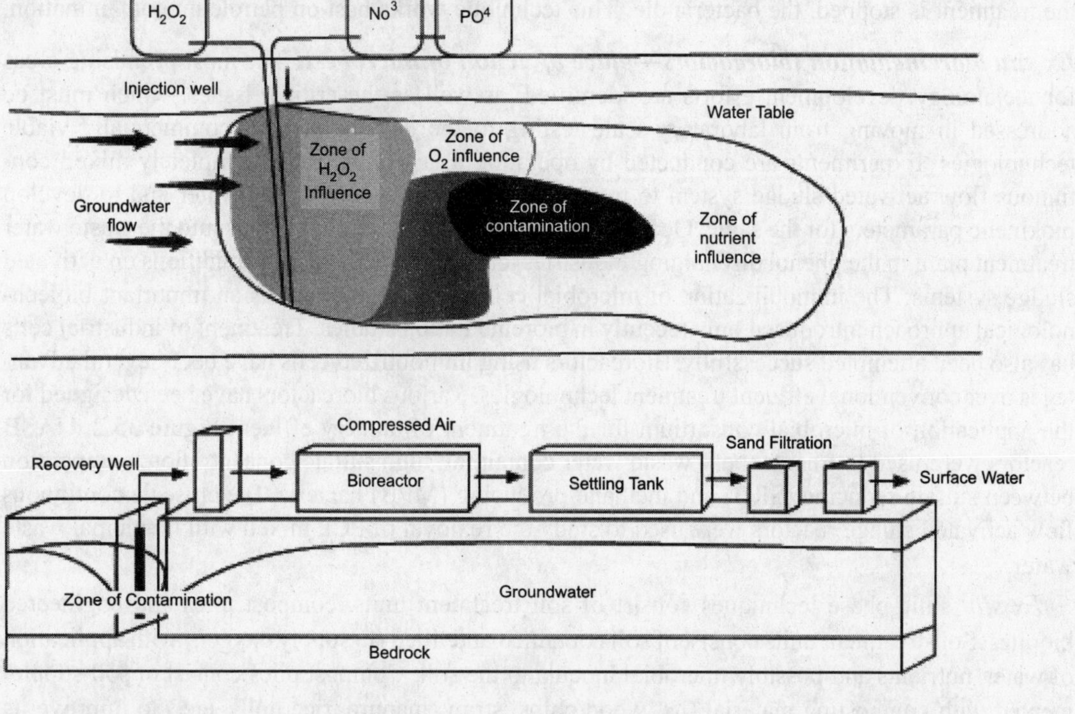

Figure 35.1 *In situ* bioremediation processes of bioaugmentation and biostimulation.

Monitoring the Efficacy of Bioremediation

The general acceptance of bioremediation technology as an environmentally sound and economic treatment for hazardous waste requires the demonstration of its efficacy, reliability and predictability, as well as its advantages over conventional treatments. An effective monitoring design includes protocols for treatment-specific, representative sampling, control and monitoring. These should take into account abiotic and biotic pollutant fate processes in all relevant process compartments. A number of well-established and novel chemical and molecular biological monitoring techniques and parameters are available.

Bioremediation research is generally conducted at one of the three scales: laboratory, pilot scale, or field trial. To help ensure that results achieved at the first two scales can be translated to the field, the research program should be conceived as a continuum, with investigators working at each scale involved throughout the research conceptualization and planning process. The aim is to translate research findings from the laboratory into viable technologies for remediation in the field. Mechanisms of bioremediation include bioaugmentation in which microbes and nutrients are added to the contaminated site or biostimulation in which nutrients and enzymes are added to supplement the intrinsic microbes. In the injection method, bacteria and nutrients are injected directly into the contaminated aquifer, or nutrients and enzymes, often referred to as 'fertilizer', that stimulate the activity of the bacteria are added. In soil remediation, usually nutrients and enzymes are added to stimulate the natural soil bacteria, though sometimes both nutrients and bacteria are added. When the treatment is stopped, the bacteria die. This technique works best on petroleum contamination.

Ex situ bioremediation (bioreactors—place of action of microbes): The most promising areas for technology development efforts are identified, as well as the critical issues, which must be addressed in moving from laboratory-scale testing to the development of commercially viable technologies. Experiments are conducted by operating a laboratory scale completely mixed continuous flow activated sludge system to treat settled chrome tannery waste water and to develop biokinetic parameters for the same. Occasionally a large amount of phenol gets into the waste water treatment plant in the phenol discharging industries, creating shock-loading conditions on activated sludge systems. The immobilization of microbial cells on solid supports is an important biotechnological approach introduced only recently in bioremediation studies. Treatment of industrial cells has also been attempted successfully. Bioreactors using immobilized cells have been several advantages over conventional effluent treatment technologies. Various bioreactors have been designed for the application of microbial consortium for the treatment of tannery effluent Figure 35.2. UASB reactors were used to treat tannery waste water containing high sulfate concentration, competition between sulfate-reducing (SRB) and methane-producing (MPB) bacteria. Bench scale continuous flow activated sludge reactors were used to study the removal of PCP mixed with municipal waste water.

Ex situ solid-phase techniques consist of soil treatment units, compost piles and engineered biopiles. Soil-treatment units consist of soil contained and tilled (to supply oxygen) with application of water, nutrients and possibly microbial inocula to the soil. Compost piles consist of soil supplemented with composting material (i.e. wood chips, straw, manure, rice hulls, etc.) to improve its physical handling properties and its water- and air-holding capacities.

Flavobacterium cells are immobilized on polyurethane and the degradation activity of cells is studied in semi-continuous batch reactor. The ability of *Arthrobacter* cells to degrade PCP in mineral salt medium was evaluated for immobilized, non-immobilized and co-immobilized cells. The immobilized cells were encapsulated in alginate. A microbial consortium able to degrade PCP in contaminated soil was used in a fed batch bioreactor. The microorganism in the biofilm employs natural biological processes to efficiently degrade complex chemical process and can remediate high volume of waste more cheaply than other available clean up procedures.

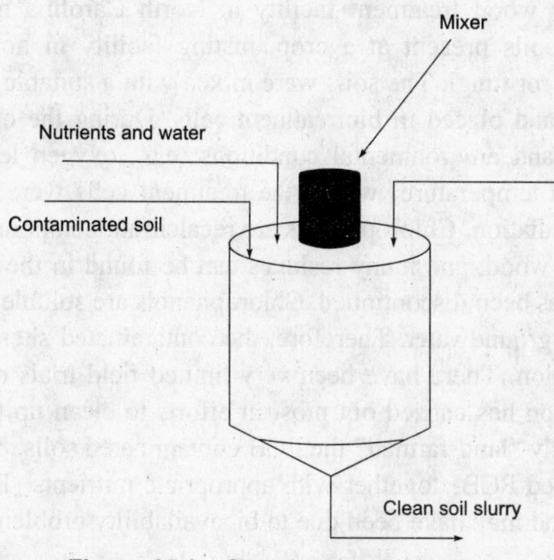

Figure 35.2 One chamber bioreactor.

In situ bioremediation: With *in situ* techniques, the soil and associated groundwater is treated in place without excavation, while it is excavated prior to treatment with *ex situ* applications. Pump-and-treat systems, which are applied to saturated-zone remediation, involve the removal, treatment and return of associated water from a contaminated soil zone. The returned water is supplemented with nutrients and saturated with oxygen. Percolation consists of applying water, containing nutrients and possibly a microbial inoculum, to the surface of a contaminated area and allowing it to filter into the soil and mix with the groundwater, if present. Bioventing supplies air to an unsaturated soil zone through the installation of a well(s) connected to associated pumps and blowers that draw a vacuum on the soil. Air sparging involves the injection of air into the saturated zone of the contaminated soil.

It has long been recognized that microorganisms have distinct and unique roles in the detoxification of polluted soil environments and in recent years, this process has been termed bioremediation or bioreclamation. The role of microorganisms and their limitations for bioremediation must be better understood, so that they can be utilized more efficiently. Application of the principles of microbial ecology will improve methodology. The enhancement of microbial degradation as a means of bringing about the *in situ* clean-up of contaminated soils has spurred much research. The rhizosphere, in particular, is an area of increased microbial activity that may enhance transformation and degradation of pollutants. The most common methods to stimulate degradation rates include supplying inorganic nutrients and oxygen, but the addition of degradative microbial inocula or enzymes as well as the use of plants should also be considered. Approximately 750 tons of soil, which had been contaminated by a wood preservative, was bioremediated in North Carolina using white rot fungi. Primary contaminants of concern at the site included pentachlorophenol and lindane. The field degradation of polychlorinated dibenzo-p-dioxins and dibenzo furans in soil at a former wood treatment facility in North Carolina has been demonstrated. Toxaphene-contaminated soils present at a crop dusting facility in northern California were bioremediated using white rot fungi. The soils were mixed with a suitable substrate that had been inoculated with the fungi and placed in biotreatment cells. During the operation of the project, toxaphene concentrations and environmental conditions (e.g., oxygen levels, moisture content, carbon dioxide levels, and temperature) within the treatment cells were monitored to track the progress of fungal bioremediation. Chlorophenols are recalcitrant compounds that have been used for decades to impregnate wood, and many residues can be found in the environment long after the use of chlorophenols has been discontinued. Chlorophenols are soluble in water and may leach from contaminated soil to groundwater. Therefore, the contaminated sites must be cleaned up to prevent further contamination. There have been very limited field trials of PCB bioremediation. General Electric Corporation has carried out most in efforts to clean up their own contaminated sites. One, in 1987, basically "land-farmed" the PCB contaminated soils. They tilled the soils and added bacteria that degraded PCBs together with appropriate nutrients. This was less than laboratory results had shown and may have been due to bioavailability problems with the PCBs in the field (Figure 35.3).

Measuring Bioremediation in the Field

Many microorganisms have been isolated that are capable of remarkable enzymatic transformations of traditionally recalcitrant harmful compounds. Bioremediation of contaminated sites and waste treatment in activated sludge bioreactors relies on microbial communities to transform and remediate undesirable industrial wastes. Only a subset of the microorganisms in an ecological system will be crucial for driving the desired chemical transformation. Therefore, it is important to understand the dynamics of this active community and to develop ways of detecting its presence and measure its activity.

In situ physical/chemical treatment

Air sparging: This is injection of gas (usually air or oxygen) under pressure into well(s) installed within the saturated zone to volatilize contaminants dissolved in groundwater, present as non-aqueous phase liquid, or sorbed to the soil matrix. This technique is most applicable for volatile organic contaminants in relatively moderate to high permeability geologic materials.

Blast-enhanced fracturing: A technique used at sites with fractured bedrock formations to improve the rate and predictability of recovery of contaminated groundwater by creating "fracture trenches" or highly fractured areas through detonation of explosives in boreholes (shotholes). Blast-enhanced fracturing is distinguished from hydraulic or pneumatic fracturing in that the latter technologies do not involve explosives, are generally conducted in the overburden, and are performed within individual boreholes.

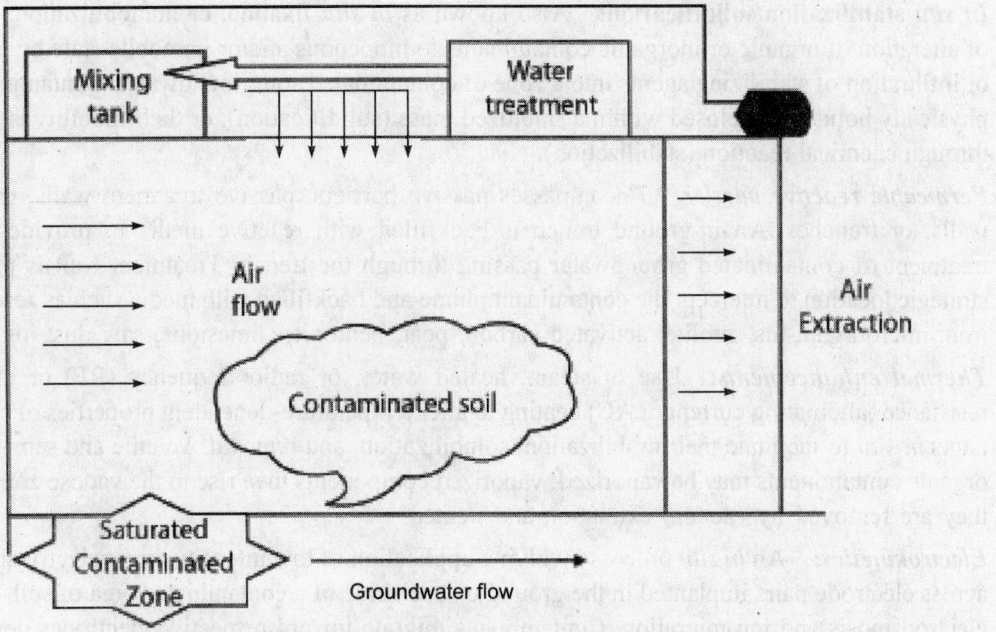

Figure 35.3 *In situ* bioremediation of contaminated site.

Directional wells: Encompasses horizontal wells, trenched or directly drilled wells installed at any non-vertical inclination for purposes of groundwater monitoring or remediation. This technology can be used in the application of various remediation techniques such as groundwater and/or non-aqueous phase liquid extraction, air sparging, soil vapor extraction, *in situ* bioremediation, *in situ* flushing, permeable reactive barriers, hydraulic and pneumatic fracturing, etc.

Ground water recirculation well: Encompasses *in situ* vacuum, vapor, or air stripping, in-well vapor stripping, in-well aeration, and vertical circulation wells. Creation of groundwater circulation "cell" through injection of air or inert gas into a zone of contaminated groundwater through center of double cased stripping well, which is designed with upper and lower double screened intervals.

Hydraulic and pneumatic fracturing: Techniques to create enhanced fracture networks to increase soil permeability to liquids and vapors and accelerate contaminant removal. Especially useful for vapor extraction, biodegradation and thermal treatments. Hydraulic fracturing involves injection of high pressure water into the bottom of a borehole to cut a notch; a slurry of water, sand and thick gel is pumped at high pressure into the borehole to propagate the fracture from the initial notch.

In situ flushing: Also known as injection/recirculation or *in situ* soil washing. General injection or infiltration of a solution into a zone of contaminated soil/groundwater, followed by downgradient extraction of groundwater and elutriate (flushing solution mixed with the contaminants) and above-ground treatment and/or re-injection. Solutions may consist of surfactants, cosolvents, acids, bases, solvents, or plain water.

***In situ* stabilization/solidification:** Also known as *in situ* fixation, or immobilization. Process of alteration of organic or inorganic contaminants to innocuous and/or immobile state by injection or infiltration of stabilizing agents into a zone of contaminated soil/groundwater. Contaminants are physically bound or enclosed within a stabilized mass (solidification), or their mobility is reduced through chemical reaction (stabilization).

Permeable reactive barrier: Encompasses passive barriers, passive treatment walls, treatment walls, or trenches. An in-ground trench is backfilled with reactive media to provide passive treatment of contaminated groundwater passing through the trench. Treatment wall is placed at strategic location to intercept the contaminant plume and backfilled with media such as zero-valent iron, microorganisms, zeolite, activated carbon, peat, bentonite, limestone, saw dust, or other.

***Thermal enhancements*:** Use of steam, heated water, or radio frequency (RF) or electrical resistance (alternating current or AC) heating to alter temperature-dependent properties of contaminants *in situ* to facilitate their mobilization, solubilization, and removal. Volatile and semi-volatile organic contaminants may be vaporized; vaporized components then rise to the vadose zone where they are removed by vacuum extraction and treated.

Electrokinetics: An *in situ* process involving application of low intensity direct electrical current across electrode pairs implanted in the ground on each side of a contaminated area of soil, causing electroosmosis and ion migration. Contaminants migrate toward respective electrodes depending upon their charge. Process may be enhanced through the use of surfactants or reagents to increase contaminant removal rates at the electrodes. Process separates and extracts heavy metals, radionuclides, and organic contaminants from saturated or unsaturated soils, sludges, and sediments.

Biological treatment

Bioslurping: Use of vacuum-enhanced pumping to recover light, non-aqueous phase liquid (LNAPL) and initiate vadose zone remediation through bioventing. In bioventing, air is drawn through the impacted vadose zone via extraction wells equipped with low vacuum to promote biodegradation of organic compounds.

Intrinsic bioremediation: Natural, non-enhanced microbial degradation of organic constituents by which complex organic compounds are broken down to simpler, usually less toxic compounds through aerobic or anaerobic processes.

Monitored natural attenuation: Encompasses intrinsic bioremediation. Reliance on a variety of physical, chemical, or biological processes (within the context of a carefully controlled and monitored site clean-up approach), under favorable conditions, act without human intervention to reduce the mass, toxicity, mobility, volume, or concentration of contaminants in soil or groundwater.

Biocolloid formation: Solid materials containing the basic elements produced by bacterial transformation assume a discrete particle and are refered as biocolloids. Biological colloid is the negative charge that is usually present on the particle surface and forms the electric double layer surrounding the colloid particles. The biocolloid system may be appropriate in remediation of groundwaters and flowing surface water. The basic requirements would be the addition of bacteria and metabolism in the presence of the metal followed by recovery of the biocolloids. Biocolloid methods can be used for the treatment of contaminated groundwater *in situ* in recovery of metals.

Phytoremediation

Phytoremediation, the use of plants for environmental restoration, is an emerging cleanup technology to exploit plant potential to remediate soil and water contaminated with a variety of compounds. Several technological subsets have been proposed. Phytoextraction is the use of higher plants to remove inorganic contaminants accumulants, primarily metals, from polluted soil. In this approach, plants capable of accumulating high levels of metals are grown in contaminated soil. At maturity, metal-enriched above-ground biomass is harvested and a fraction of soil metal contamination removed. Plants have a natural propensity to take up metals. Some metals such as Cu, Co, Fe, Mo, Mn, Ni, and Zn are essential mineral nutrients. Others, however, such as Cd and Pb, have no known physiological activity. Perhaps not surprisingly, phytoremediation as an environmental cleanup technology, was initially proposed for the remediation of metal-contaminated soil. The general use of plants to remediate environmental media *in situ* includes rhizofiltration (absorption, concentration, and precipitation of heavy metals by plant roots), phytoextraction (extraction and accumulation of contaminants in harvestable plant tissues such as roots and shoots), phytotransformation (degradation of complex organic molecules to simple molecules, which are incorporated into plant tissues), phytostimulation or plant-assisted bioremediation (stimulation of microbial and fungal degradation by release of exudates/enzymes into the root zone), and phytostabilization (absorption and precipitation of contaminants, principally metals, by plants). A wide range of organic and inorganic contaminants; most appropriate for sites where large volumes of groundwater with relatively low concentrations of contaminants must be remediated to strict standards. It is most effective where groundwater is within ten feet of the ground surface, and soil contamination is within three feet of the ground surface.

Waste

An agricultural establishment produces many types of wastes in its daily operations. It is important that these wastes are identified and managed properly to protect oneself, co-workers, and others in the community, as well as the environment. As a waste generator, we are responsible for all wastes generated at our site, including both hazardous and non-hazardous wastes.

Biological waste: These processes produce significant quantities of toxic or hazardous by-products. To the extent that these plastics can be displaced by products made from cleaner, biological sources, the wastes associated with current plastic production can be minimized. Additionally municipal solid waste streams contain significant amounts of paper, food wastes, scrap wood, yard wastes, etc. (biological materials). These waste streams are potential feedstocks for creating plastics. By diverting biological wastes from the municipal solid waste stream, these materials become valuable products with productive reuse.

Solid waste: Solid waste means any garbage or refuse; sludge from a wastewater treatment plant, water supply treatment plant, or air pollution control facility; and other discarded material, including solid, liquid, semi-solid, or contaminated gaseous material resulting from industrial, commercial, mining, and agricultural operations, and from community activities.

Hazardous waste: A waste may be considered hazardous if it is ignitable (i.e., burns readily), corrosive, or reactive (e.g., explosive). Waste may also be considered hazardous if it contains certain amounts of toxic chemicals. In addition to these characteristic wastes, EPA has also developed a list of more than 500 specific hazardous wastes. Hazardous waste takes many physical forms and may be solid, semi-solid, or even liquid. Acute hazardous wastes contain dangerous chemicals that could pose a threat to human health and the environment even when properly managed. These wastes are fatal to humans and animals even in low doses.

Universal waste: The universal waste rule is designed to reduce the amount of hazardous waste items in the municipal solid waste (MSW) stream, encourage recycling and proper disposal of certain common hazardous wastes, and reduce the regulatory burden on businesses that generate these wastes. Universal wastes include:

(i) **Batteries** such as nickel-cadmium (Ni-Cd) and small sealed lead-acid batteries, which are found in many common items in the business and home setting, including electronic equipment, mobile telephones, portable computers, and emergency backup lighting.
(ii) **Agricultural** pesticides that have been recalled or banned from use, are obsolete, have become damaged, or are no longer needed due to changes in cropping patterns or other factors. They are often stored for long periods of time in sheds or barns.
(iii) **Thermostats**, which can contain as much as 3 grams of liquid mercury and are located in almost any building, including commercial, industrial, agricultural, community, and household buildings.

Hazardous Waste Management

Hazardous waste is everywhere. It comes from paints, motor oil, hair spray, household cleaners, automotive chemicals, and all kinds of toxic medical, industrial and military products. Most industrial processes—from which come cosmetics and pharmaceuticals, computers and garden pesticides—generate wastes that the EPA, acting under the Resource Conservation Recovery Act (RCRA), says can harm human health or the environment if not properly managed. As a waste-disposal technology, incineration has been around for about 5,00,000 years—an interesting technology. The high-temperature incineration is the best available technology for disposing of most hazardous wastes. Hazardous waste goes into an incinerator, comes out as potentially harmful air emissions, although these emissions are strictly controlled, and as ash that's treated to meet EPA standards, and then disposed of in an authorized landfill. The hazardous site remediation process consists of four steps:

(i) The preliminary assessment—It involves identification of any conditions at a site that pose an imminent threat to human health and the environment.
(ii) Selection and implementation of appropriate interim remedial measures—It addresses any imminent hazards that may exist at a site.
(iii) Site investigation and remediation technology feasibility study—In this stage, nature and extent of contamination are defined, and potential final remedial methods are identified and evaluated.

(iv) Selection of final remedial methods—Selection processes are taken into account based on the results of the site investigation including effectiveness of different remedial methods and cost associated with the methods.

Risk assessment is an integral part of the remedy selection process at hazardous waste sites. A quantitative risk assessment includes hazards evaluation, exposure assessment and risk characterization. Hazards are evaluated by sampling and analysis of soil, water and other environmental media at contaminated sites. Once the chemical of concern at a site is identified, available toxicity data is collected and evaluated to ascertain the nature of health effects associated with exposure to chemicals. Different methodologies are used to characterize dose response relationship. Exposure assessment is characterized by identification of major exposure pathways, exposure concentrations and exposure scenarios, and finally the risk is characterized.

The potential hazards have long term and short term effects on overall ecosystem, depending upon the type of contaminants, their chemical species and spatial distribution, the concentration, and the hydrological characteristics of the soil media. Several treatment options are available for the removal of toxic compounds in the environment (Figure 35.4).

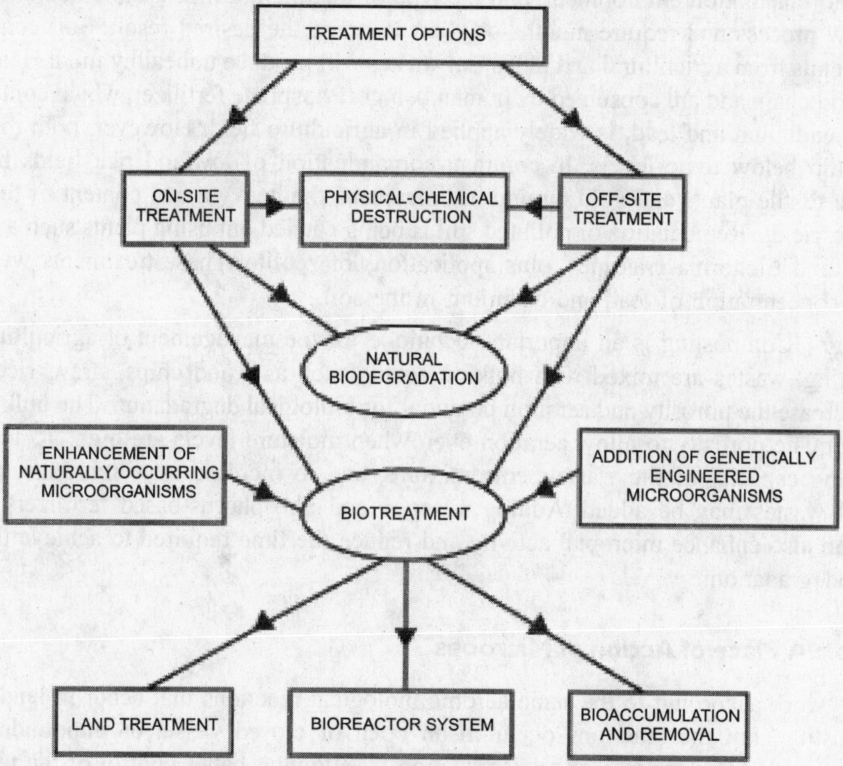

Figure 35.4 *In vivo* and *in vitro* design strategies.

A variety of strategies for designing new or improved catalysts for bioremediation have been developed over recent years. The simplest strategy is improving the biodegradative performance of a consortium (a mixed bacterial culture) through the addition of a 'specialist' organism; in this case, a consortium is designed. Consortia that exhibit novel catabolic activities can also be obtained by sustained selective pressure in, for example, a chemostat. Here, although it is not possible to talk about design in the sense of the deliberate combination of known genetic elements to achieve a desired phenotype, the design of the selection system results in the desired phenotype.

Agriculture Waste and its Management

The agricultural industry has a large waste stream. Animal manure and food wastes contain nutrients that are more valuable to reuse than to landfill. Anaerobic digestion and composting are two bioremediation methods that stabilize the waste product, kill pathogens, and produce a nutrient-rich usable product. Some advantages of biological treatment of agriculture wastes are: it is relatively environmentally benign; generates few emissions; wastes are converted into products; and it requires minimal, if any, transportation. Sometimes, bioremediation is used as an interim treatment or disposal step, which reduces the overall level of hydrocarbon contamination prior to final disposal. Bioremediation can create a drier, more stable material for landfilling, thereby reducing the potential to generate leachate. Depending on the composition of the hydrocarbon components, the bioremediation environment, and the type of treatment utilized, bioremediation may be a fairly slow process and require months or years to reach the desired result. Soil contaminated by heavy metals from agricultural and industrial wastes will produce unhealthy food. Heavy metals enter the food chain and are consumed by human beings. Phosphate fertilizer, which contains small amounts of cadmium and lead, is widely applied in agriculture field. However, both these heavy metals remain below toxic levels. In contrast, contamination of lowland rice fields by sewage sludge from textile plants and gold mining has increased the heavy metal content of the soil and reduced rice yields. Remediation of polluted soil is being carried out using plants such as Vetiveria zizanioides and Eichornia crassipes, plus applications of zeolite. These treatments were able to reduce the concentration of lead and cadmium in the soil.

Composting: Composting is an important technique for the management of agriculture wastes. In composting, wastes are mixed with bulking agents such as wood chips, straw, rice hulls, or husks to increase the porosity and aeration potential for biological degradation. The bulking agents provide adequate porosity to allow aeration even when moisture levels are high. To increase the water-holding capacity of the waste-media mixture, and to increase trace nutrients, manure or agricultural wastes may be added. Adding nitrogen and phosphorus-based fertilizers and trace minerals can also enhance microbial activity and reduce the time required to achieve the desired level of biodegradation.

Bioreactor: A Place of Action of Microbes

Bioreactors work according to the same aerobic biological reactions that occur in land treatment and composting, but the reactions occur in an open or closed vessel or impoundment. This environment accelerates the rate of biodegradation by allowing better control of the temperature and other conditions that affect the biodegradation rate. Bioreactor processes are typically operated as a batch or semi-continuous process. In a bioreactor, nutrients are added to slurry of water and waste, and air sparging or intensive mechanical mixing of the reactor contents provides oxygen. This mechanical mixing results in significant contact between microorganisms and the waste components being degraded. To accelerate system start-up, introduction of microbes capable of degrading the organic constituents of the waste may be useful, although some companies have not had favorable experience with designer bugs. Many of the additives used for bioreactors are common agricultural products and plant or animal wastes. In tank-based bioreactors, operating conditions (temperature, nutrient concentration, pH, oxygen transport and mixing) can be monitored and controlled easily. Optimized biological processes ensure the best rate of biodegradation and allow for reduced space requirements relative to land-based biological treatment processes. However, capital, operation and maintenance costs for bioreactors are high relative to other forms of biological treatment (Figure 35.5).

Vermiculture: Vermiculture is the process of using worms to decompose organic waste into a material capable of supplying necessary nutrients to help sustain plant growth. For several years, worms have been used to convert organic waste into organic fertilizer. Recently, the process has been tested and found successful in treating certain synthetic-based drilling wastes.

Industrial effluent: Industrial waste consists of both organic and inorganic substances. Organic wastes include pesticide residues, solvents and cleaning fluids, dissolved residue from fruit and vegetables, and lignin from pulp and paper to name a few. Effluents can also contain inorganic wastes such as brine salts and metals. The Clean Water Act has standards for the permitted release of a limited amount of contaminants into waterways. This is an incentive for industry to pre-treat their water by neutralizing the chemically active components, recycling, dilution or extraction and collection for proper disposal. More than 200,000 sources of waste water are regulated by the National Pollutant Discharge Elimination System (NPDES) permit program. Industries that use large amounts of water in their processes include chemical manufacturers, steel plants, metal processers, textile manufacturers, and the following:

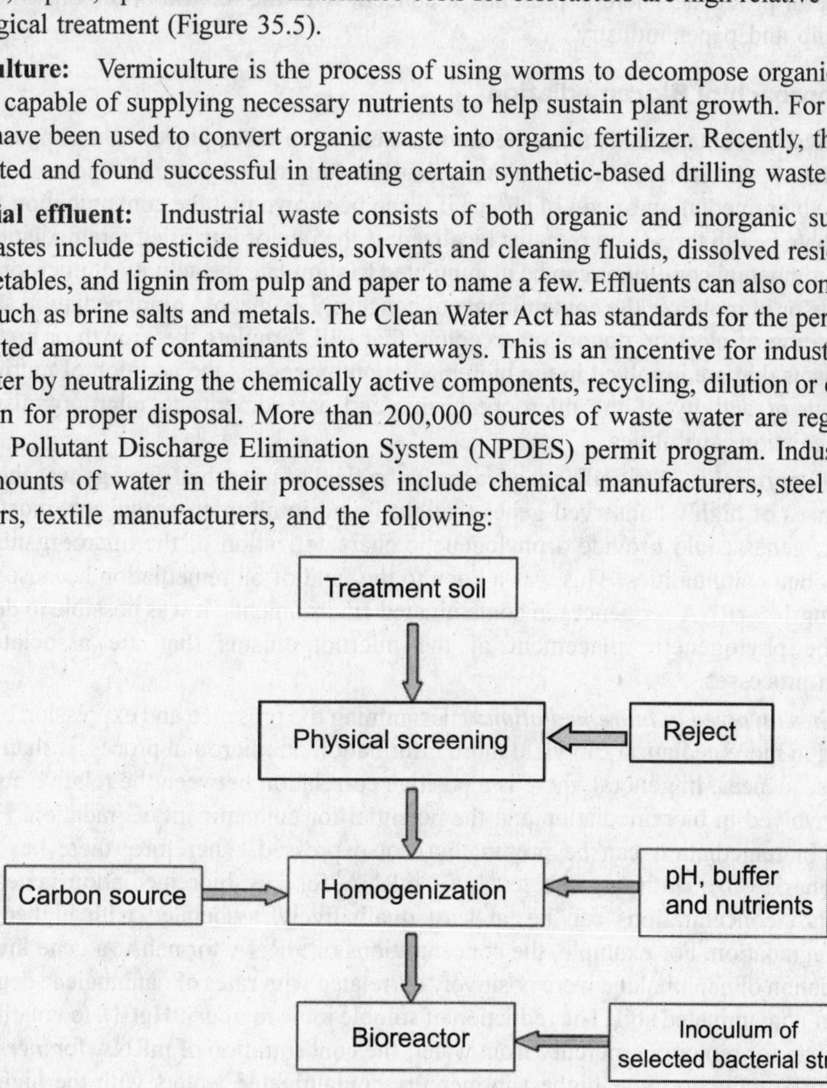

Figure 35.5 Treatment strategies in bioreactor.

Agriculture: Run-off from crops contains pesticides, fertilizer, and sediment. Run-off from animal production facilities contains bacteria, organic matter, nitrates, and phosphates.

Fruit and vegetable processing: Waste water contains high concentrations of dissolved organic matter and may be highly alkaline from the use of lye. Most of this water is now recycled.

Petroleum refining: Oil is mixed with water in the refining process to remove salts and other impurities. It is then separated and collected. Most of this water is now recycled.

Pulp and paper: The use of bisulfate and sulfurous acid or sulfur dioxide in the pulping process yields waste sulfite liquor containing various wood by-products. This can be reduced or recycled into various useful products. There is presently a concern over the release of dioxins into waterways by the pulp and paper industry.

Molecular Approach of Bioremediation

Microbial removal of contaminants from the environment often takes place without human intervention. This has been termed intrinsic bioremediation. Relying on intrinsic bioremediation is increasingly the bioremediation option of choice if it can be shown that the contamination does not pose an immediate health threat and remains localized. If the rate of intrinsic bioremediation is too slow, then environmental conditions can be manipulated to stimulate the activity of microorganisms that can degrade or immobilize the contaminants of concern. Engineered bioremediation strategies include the addition of electron donors or acceptors that will stimulate the growth or metabolism of microorganisms that are involved in the bioremediation processes; the addition of nutrients that limit the growth or activity of the microorganisms; and amendments to microorganisms with desired bioremediation capabilities.

The 16S rRNA approach: A significant advance in the field of microbial ecology was the finding that the sequences of highly conserved genes that are found in all microorganisms, most notably the 16S rRNA, genes could provide a phylogenetic characterization of the microorganisms that comprise microbial communities. This was a boon to the field of bioremediation because it meant that by analysing 16S rRNA sequences in contaminated environments, it was possible to determine definitively the phylogenetic placement of the microorganisms that are associated with bioremediation processes.

Analysis of genes involved in bioremediation: Examining the presence and expression of the key genes involved in bioremediation can yield more information on microbial processes than analysis of 16S rRNA sequences. In general, there is a positive correlation between the relative abundance of the genes involved in bioremediation and the potential for contaminant degradation. However, the genes for bioremediation can be present but not expressed. Therefore, there has been an increased emphasis on quantifying the levels of mRNA for key bioremediation genes. Often, increased mRNA concentrations can be, at least qualitatively, associated with higher rates of contaminant degradation. For example, the concentrations of mRNA for nahA, a gene involved in aerobic degradation of naphthalene were positively correlated with rates of naphthalene degradation in hydrocarbon-contaminated soil. The reduction of soluble ionic mercury, Hg(II), to volatile Hg(0), is one mechanism for removing mercury from water; the concentration of mRNA for *merA*, a gene involved in Hg(II) reduction was highest in mercury contaminated waters with the highest rates of Hg(II) reduction. However, the concentration of *merA* was not always proportional to the rate of Hg(II) reduction, illustrating that factors other than gene transcription can control the rates of bioremediation processes. Highly sensitive methods that can detect mRNA for key bioremediation genes in single cells are now available. This technique, coupled with 16S rRNA probing of the same environmental samples, could provide data on which phylogenetic groups of organisms express the genes of interest.

Cells isolated from the environment provide the opportunity for in-depth physiological analysis as well as information on gene composition that can be used for the analysis of mRNA and proteins that are extracted directly from the environment. Genomic DNA extracted from the environment furnishes data on the genetic potential of as-yet-uncultured organisms. mRNA and proteins extracted from the environment provide information on gene expression under different environmental conditions. Analysis and comparison of pure cultures and mixed communities yields data for the development of models of microbial function in the environment.

The application of genomics: Although the molecular techniques have outlined to improve our understanding of bioremediation, investigations in this field are on the cusp of a new era, which promises for the first time to provide a global insight into the metabolic potential and activity of microorganisms living in contaminated environments. This is the 'genomics era' of bioremediation. With the application of genome-enabled techniques to study not only pure cultures, but also environmental samples, it will be possible to develop the models that are needed to model microbial activity predicatively under various bioremediation strategies (Figure 35.6).

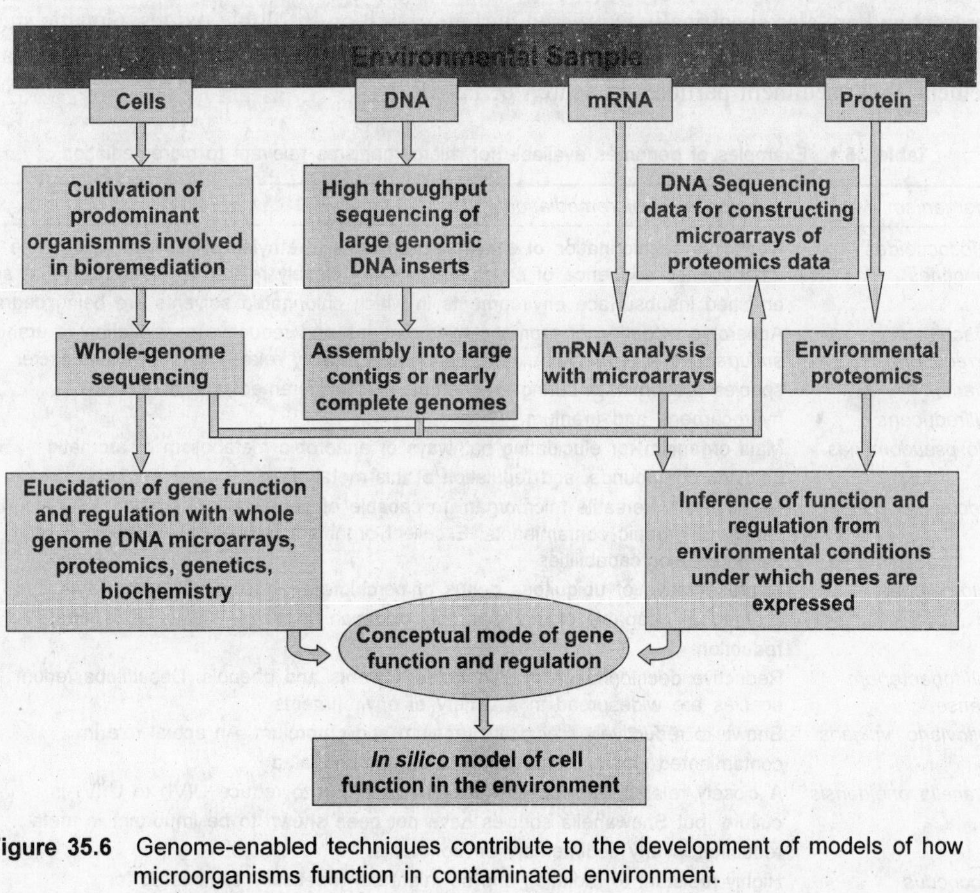

Figure 35.6 Genome-enabled techniques contribute to the development of models of how microorganisms function in contaminated environment.

The application of genomics to bioremediation initially revolutionized the study of pure cultures, which serve as models for important bioremediation processes. Complete, or nearly complete, genome sequences are now available for several organisms that are important in bioremediation (Table 35.1). Whole-genome sequencing is especially helpful in promoting the understanding of bioremediation-relevant microorganisms,whose physiology has not previously been studied in detail. For example, as noted earlier, molecular analyses have indicated that *Geobacter* species are important in the bioremediation of organic and metal contaminants in subsurface environments. The sequencing of several genomes of microorganisms of the genus *Geobacter*, as well as closely related organisms, has significantly altered the concept of how *Geobacter* species function in contaminated subsurface environments. For instance, before the sequencing of the *Geobacter* genomes, *Geobacter* species were thought to be non-motile, but genes encoding flagella were subsequently discovered in the *Geobacter* genomes. Further investigations revealed that *Geobacter metallireducens* specifically produces flagella only when the organism is growing on insoluble Fe(III) or Mn(IV) oxides (Figure 35.7). Genes for chemotaxis were also evident in the *Geobacter* genomes, and experimental investigations have revealed that *G. metallireducens* has a novel chemotaxis to Fe(II),which could help guide it to Fe(III) oxides under anaerobic conditions. Pili genes are present and are also specifically expressed during growth on insoluble oxides. Genetic studies have indicated that the role of the pili is to aid in attachment to Fe(III) oxides, as well as facilitating movement along sediment particles in search of Fe(III).

Table 35.1 Examples of genomes available for microorganisms relevant to bioremediation.

Microorganism	*Relevance to bioremediation*
Dehalococcoides ethanogenes	Reductive dechlorination of chlorinated solvents to ethylene. The 16S rRNA gene ethanogenes sequence of *D. ethanogenes* is closely related to sequences that are enriched insubsurface environments in which chlorinated solvents are being degraded
Geobacter sulfurreducens *Geobacter metallireducens*	Anaerobic oxidation of aromatic hydrocarbons and reductive precipitation of uranium. *sulfurreducens,* 16S rRNA gene sequences closely related to known Geobacter species predominate during eranaerobic *in situ* bioremediation of aromatic hydrocarbons and uranium.
Rhodo pseudomonas	Main organism for elucidating pathways of anaerobic metabolism of aromatic palustris compounds, and regulation of this metabolism.
Pseudomonas putida	Metabolically versatile microorganism capable of aerobically degrading a wide variety of organic contaminants. Excellent organism for genetic engineering of bioremediation capabilities
Dechloromonas	Representative of ubiquitous genus of perchlorate-reducing microorganisms and *aromatica* capable of the anaerobic oxidation of benzene coupled to nitrate reduction.
Desulfitobacterium hafniense	Reductive dechlorination of chlorinated solvents and phenols. Desulfitobacterium species are widespread in a variety of environments
Desulfovibrio vulgaris	Shown to reductively precipitate uranium and chromium. An actual role in contaminated environments is yet to be demonstrated
Shewanella oneidensis	A closely related Shewanella species was found to reduce U(VI) to U(IV) in culture, but Shewanella species have not been shown to be important in metal reduction in any sedimentary environments
Deinococcus	Highly resistant to radiation and so might be genetically engineered for *radioactive* bioremediation of highly environments radiodurans

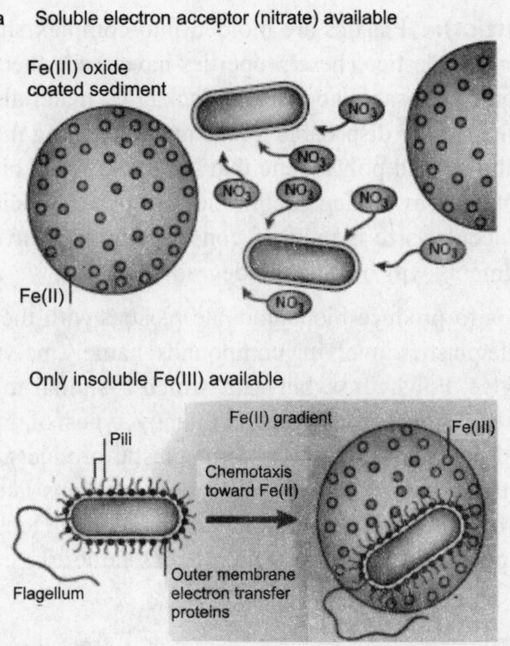

Figure 35.7 Genome-derived model for physiological differences in *Geobacter* during growth on soluble electron acceptors or insoluble Fe(III) oxide.

This energy-efficient mechanism for locating and reducing Fe(III) oxides in *Geobacter* species contrasts with the strategies for Fe(III) reduction in other well studied organisms, such as *Shewanella* and *Geothrix* species. These other organisms release Fe(III) chelators, which solubilize Fe(III) from Fe(III) oxides, and electron shuttling compounds, which accept electrons from the cell surface and then reduce Fe(III) oxides. These strategies make it possible for *Shewanella* and *Geothrix* species to reduce Fe(III) without directly contacting the Fe(III) oxide.

APPLICATIONS OF BIOREMEDIATION TECHNOLOGY

Industrial Applications

Xenobiotics are synthetic (man-made) organic compounds that are foreign to existing biological system. They possess such molecular structures and chemical bond-sequences that are not recognized by microbial degradative enzymes. Many of the xenobiotics are toxic to living system and their accumulation in aquatic and terrestrial habitats often results in serious ecological consequences including major killing of indigenous biota. The dispersal or accidental spillage of these compounds has created serious environmental pollution problems, particularly when their degradation by microbial activities fails to remove these pollutants quickly enough to prevent environmental damage. Sewage treatment and water purification systems are usually unable to remove them if they enter municipal water supply and, therefore, they result in potential human health hazard. Although there are varieties of xenobiotic pollutions, some major ones that are practically proving hazardous are synthetic polymers (plastics), pesticides, petroleum pollutants, laundry detergents, cellulosic wastes from various industries, etc.

Synthetic polymers (plastics): Plastics are molded into complex shapes, have high chemical resistance, and are more or less elastic. These properties have made them popular in the manufacture of garments, durable and disposable goods, and packaging materials. It is estimated that over 90% of the plastic materials, mainly disposable goods and packaging materials, consist mainly of polyethylene, polyvinyl chloride and polystyrene that appear to resist biodegradation indefinitely. Resistance of these constituents to biodegradation seems to be associated with their excessive molecular size. If their molecular size is reduced considerably in short polymer chain fragments e.g., by pyrolysis, the fragments will become biodegradable.

The second alternative is to produce biodegradable plastics with the help of microorganisms. Production of biodegradable plastics involving compounds, namely, polyhydroxybutyrate (PHB) is a recent biotechnology device. Polyhydroxybutyrate, which is similar to synthetic polyesters used in the textile industry, is the storage compound of many types of bacteria (e.g., *Alcaligenes eutrophus*). The compound can be processed to form plastic products. PHB is used in surgical sutures, as the threads of this compound inserted during operations later dissolve once their job is over. However, polyhydroxybutyrate is now being manufactured in tons and should soon become a large scale commercial product to compete with plastics now used.

Pesticides

Most of the organic pesticides used are extensively biodegraded (or mineralized) within the time of one growing season or less as a result of biochemical processes alone or in combination with purely chemical reactions. But, a simple change in the substituent of a pesticide may make it "recalcitrant" or nonbiodegradable. The chemical structures of some biodegradable and recalcitrant pesticides are given in Figure 35.8 (A, B). The herbicide 2, 4-D is biodegraded within months (approximately 3 months), but 2, 4, 5-T (2, 4, 5-trichlorophenoxy acetic acid), which differs only by an additional chlorine substitution in the meta-position, persists for years (approximately 2-3 years). The insecticide, methoxychlor is less persistent than DDT [1, 1, 1-trichloro-bis-(p-chorophenyl) ethane] because the para-methoxy groups are subject to dealkylation and the para-chloro substitution renders DDT with great biological and chemical stability. In some cases, one portion of the pesticide molecule is susceptible to degradation while the other is recalcitrant. Microbial acylamidases attack herbicide propanil and cleave its propionate moiety (aliphatic portion), which is subsequently mineralized. A portion of the released 3, 4-dichloroaniline (DCA) is acted upon by microbial oxidases and peroxidases resulting in highly persistent residues such as TCAB (3, 3' 4, 4'-tetrachloroazobenzene) and related compounds (Figure 35.8 C).

Genetic engineering may help to degrade the recalcitrant pesticides by combining various plasmids in a bacterium. For convenience, microorganisms harbouring a variety of plasmids encoding degradation of various aromatic compounds were incubated with 2, 4, 5-T, and after 8-10 months, microbes capable of growing on 2,4, 5-T as a sole carbon source were isolated. Almost certainly a plasmid has evolved by recruitment of genes from other plasmids. This is a very exciting observation. Nevertheless, in future, such a plasmid should be constructed *in vitro*.

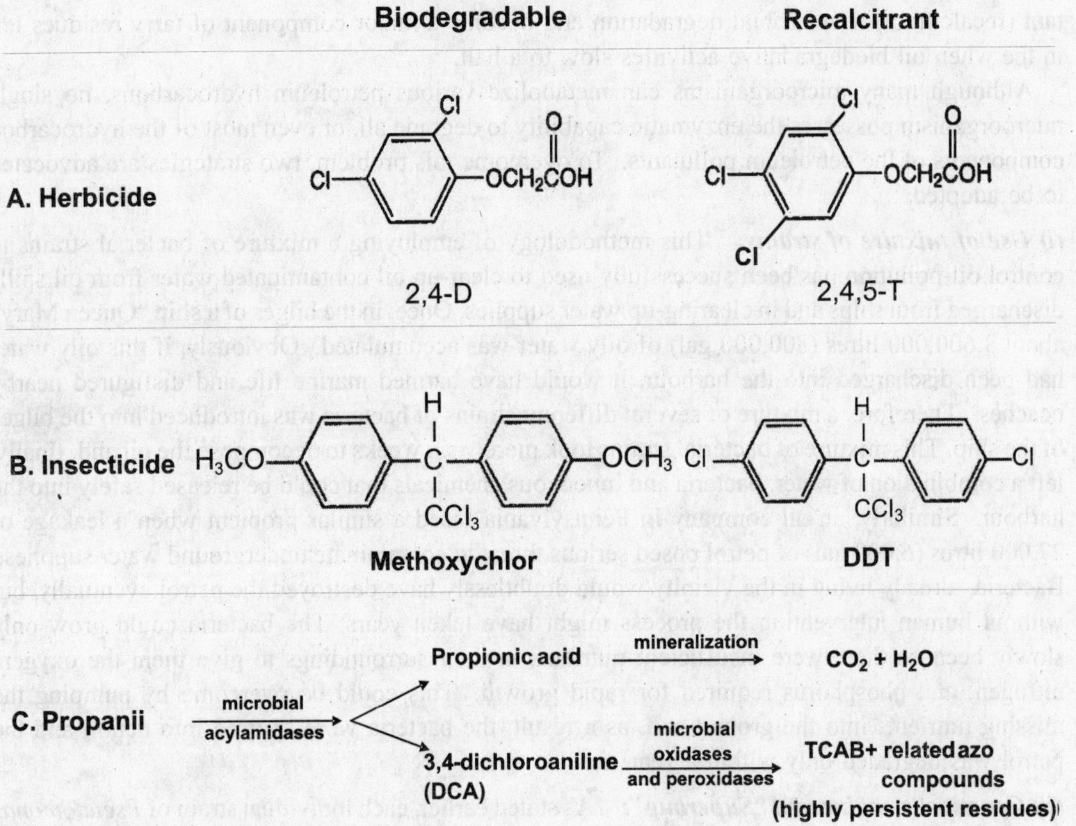

Figure 35.8 (A) Biodegradable (2, 4-D) and recalcitrant (2, 4, 5-T) herbicides. (B) Biodegradable (methoxychlor) and recalcitrant (DDT) insecticides and (C) Biodegradation pathway for propanil herbicide.

Petroleum pollutants

Over 10 millions metric tons of petroleum pollutants (oil pollutants) enter the marine environment each year as a result of accidental spillages and disposal of oily wastes. In addition to killing birds, shellfish, fish and other invertebrate animals, these petroleum pollutants pose more subtle effects on marine life. Their even very low concentration may disrupt the "chemoreception" of some marine organisms and, as a result, such marine organisms may be eliminated because their feeding and mating responses largely depend upon chemoreception. Another problem that disturbs people is the possibility that condensed polynuclear components of petroleum many move up marine food-chains and accumulate in fish and shellfish that we eat. Petroleum is a complex mixture composed of hundreds of individual components, and the challenge for microorganisms to degrade all of the components of a petroleum pollutant is immense. Although most of the petroleum components are biodegradable either most rapidly or slowly, the polynuclear aromatic components are most resistant (recalcitrant) to microbial degradation and become a major component of tarry residues left in the when oil biodegradative activities slow to a halt.

Although many microorganisms can metabolize various petroleum hydrocarbons, no single microorganism possesses the enzymatic capability to degrade all, or even most of the hydrocarbon components of the petroleum pollutants. To overcome this problem, two strategies are advocated to be adopted.

(i) Use of mixture of strains: This methodology of employing a mixture of bacterial strains to control oil-pollution has been successfully used to clear-up oil contaminated water from oil spills discharged from ships and in clearing-up water supplies. Once, in the bilges of a ship "Queen Mary" about 3,600,000 litres (800,000 gal) of oily water was accumulated. Obviously, if this oily water had been discharged into the harbour, it would have harmed marine life and disfigured nearby beaches. Therefore, a mixture of several different strains of bacteria was introduced into the bilges of the ship. This mixture of bacterial strains took merely six weeks to decompose the oil and, finally, left a combination of water, bacteria and innocuous chemicals that could be released safely into the harbour. Similarly, an oil company in Pennsylvania faced a similar problem when a leakage of 27,000 litres (6,000 gal) of petrol posed serious threat to contaminate underground water supplies. Bacteria, already living in the vicinity would doubtlessly have destroyed the petrol eventually, but without human intervention the process might have taken years. The bacteria could grow only slowly because there were insufficient nutrients in their surroundings to give them the oxygen, nitrogen, and phosphorus required for rapid growth. This could be overcome by pumping the missing nutrients into the ground and, as a result, the bacteria were spurred into action and the petrol was degraded only within a year.

(ii) Genetically engineered "Superbug": As stated earlier, each individual strain of *Pseudomonas* can utilize only one or a few of the many different types of hydrocarbons present in oil. This means, no single strain of *Pseudomonas* can consume all varieties of hydrocarbons constituting oil because the same does not contain all the genes that code the enzymes, which attack the hydrocarbon varieties. Genetic engineering has come forward to make it possible. Ananda Chakrabarty (1979), an India born American scientist, created a single such strain of *Pseudomonas* that would be able to contain all the genes responsible for oil consumption and thus mop up all the types of hydrocarbon in the oil. This unique bacterial strain, the product of genetic engineering, is called a "superbug". This superbug was created by introducing plasmids from different strains of *Pseudomonas* into a single cell. Oil consists of a variety of hydrocarbons, the main being xylenes, naphthalenes, octanes and camphors. Certain strains of *Pseudomonas putida* can consume each of these hydrocarbons, but no single strain found in nature can consume all four types. The genes that enable these strains to feed on hydrocarbons are found on four types of plasmids, referred to as XYL, NAH, OCT, and CAM. By introducing all four sets of genes into a single cell, a superbug was created that could consume all the four hydrocarbons present in oil. Since the CAM and OCT plasmids cannot coexist inside the same cell, the relevant genes from each plasmid are first joined into a single plasmid. Figure 35.9 illustrates this whole act of creating a superbug diagrammatically.

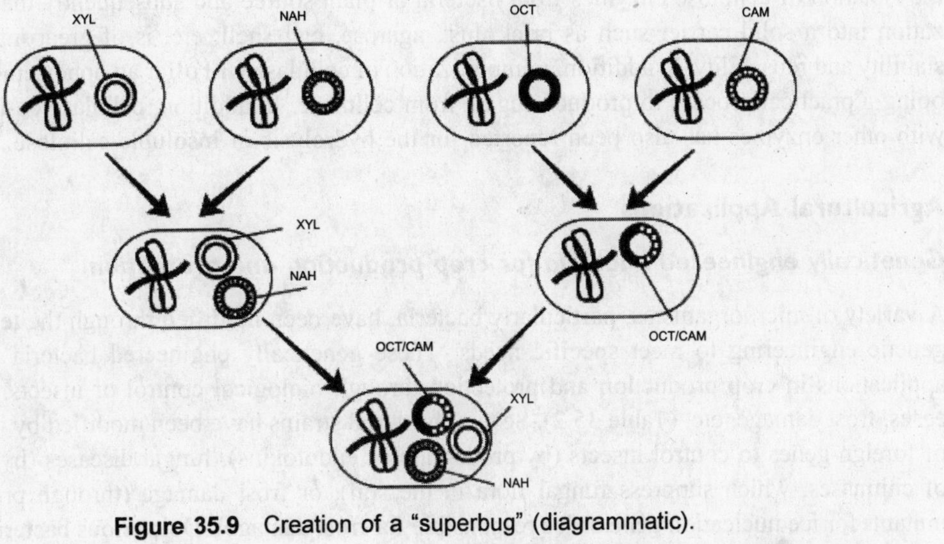

Figure 35.9 Creation of a "superbug" (diagrammatic).

The theme behind the creation of a superbug using genetic engineering in laboratory was to mix them with straw and dry them. The superbug laden straw could then be stored and, when needed, could be scattered over the oil spills. The straw, when at work, would first soak up the oil and then the superbug would break it down into harmless, non-polluting materials. However, the usefulness of Chakravarty's superbug under field conditions has yet to be proved.

Laundry detergents

Laundry detergents normally contain alkyl benzyl sulfonate (ABS) as a major component. The alkyl portion of ABS molecule is branched (nonlinear) and proves to be recalcitrant, and causes extensive foaming in water bodies. If the branching design of alkyl portion is changed to linear design, the alkyl benzyl sulphonate turns to be more easily biodegradable. Detergent industries of many advanced countries have switched from nonlinear to linear ABS to overcome the problem. The ABS story is particularly important because it is the first instance in which a synthetic compound's structure is altered to avoid recalcitrance.

Cellulosic wastes

Annually, great amounts of cellulosic wastes, which could be measured in many billions of tons, are produced worldwide as residues from fabric, paper and pulp, syrup, ethanol, food processing industries causing serious pollution to the environment. In order to remove, reduce or ameliorate these potential polluting materials by using microorganisms or their enzymes is a real challenge to the environment. Nevertheless, no practical process has still been reported for the enzymatic hydrolysis of cellulosic waste. The main reason for this is the high cost of cellulose degrading enzymes such as cellulose, which has low specific activity in soluble form and is also susceptible to inactivation and difficult to recycle. How to maintain the cellulase activity is one of the most practical problems for an efficient enzymatic hydrolysis of cellulosic waste. It can be achieved by the isolation of cellulose enzymes from bacteria or plant source and subsequently their immobilization into a solid carrier such as brick dust, agarose, egg shell, etc. is of great interest for its stability and reusability. In addition, immobilization of cellulase will offer an opportunity for developing a practical process to produce sugars from cellulose. In addition, cellulase co-immobilized with other enzymes has also been reported for the hydrolysis of insoluble cellulose.

Agricultural Applications

Genetically engineered bacteria for crop production and protection

A variety of microorganisms, particularly bacteria, have been modified through the techniques of genetic engineering to meet specific needs. These genetically engineered bacteria have found applications in crop production and protection through biological control of insects, fungal diseases, frost damage, etc. (Table 35.2). Several bacterial strains have been modified by introduction of foreign genes to control insects (by production of endotoxins), fungal diseases (by production of chitinases, which suppress fungal flora in the soil), or frost damage (through production of mutants for ice nucleation gene or ice responsible for frost damage). Deleterious bacteria and fungi or their effects have been controlled in some cases by using a variety of approaches, which include the following:

(i) production of avirulent mutant of the pathogen and releasing it to compete with the virulent strains;
(ii) production of antibiotic producing strains of plant associated bacteria to control pathogen through antibiotic production; or
(iii) production of bacterial strains that will degrade the toxin produced by the pathogen.

There are also other positive measures, where the N_2 fixing efficiency of Rhizobia can be enhanced by transfer of useful *nif* genes and other related genes involved in nodulation, nitrogenase activity and other related functions. Some examples of these genetically engineered bacteria responsible for increase in crop production and protection are given in Table 35.2.

Table 35.2 Genetically engineered bacteria in crop production and protection.

Bacterium	*Altered trait*	*Possible use*
1. *Clavibacter xyli*	Transfer of *B.thuringiensis* delta endotoxin gene	Control of corn ear worm
2. *Pseudomonas fluorescens*	Transfer of *Serratia marcescens* chitinase gene	Control of fungal disease
3. *P.fluorescens, syringae*	Delection of 'ice' gene	Control of frost damage
4. *P. fluorescens*	Addition of lac ZY	Assessment of movement of bacteria for biological control ('take all disease' of wheat)
5. *A. radiobacter*	Delection of 'tra' gene of Agrocin 84 plasmid	Biological control of crown gall
6. *Rhizobium melilotii*	Additional copies of '*nif*' gene	Increased efficiency of N_2 fixation

Limitations of Bioremediation Technology

The bioremediation technology appears to be limited to soils contaminated with non-halogenated and certain halogenated organic compounds. The technology may become technically or economically infeasible when dealing with soils with excessively high contaminant concentrations. The developers claim that the technology would probably not treat soils contaminated with polychlorinated biphenyls (PCBs) or highly halogenated organics. In addition, high levels of heavy metals, soil pH ~2, and excessive amounts of buried debris may limit the rate at which biodegradation proceeds. Furthermore, the *in situ* application of the technology is limited to the depth to which the soil can be physically tilled. *Ex situ* applications of the technology may be limited by community acceptance of the inherent hazards (e.g., noise, dust, etc.) associated with excavation activities. Of course, a number of natural physical and chemical factors may affect the activity and longevity of contaminant-degrading microorganisms in general. The bioremediation technology addresses many of these factors directly (i.e., moisture content, soil particle size distribution, clay content, nutrient limitations, and oxygen limitations). In addition, some factors (i.e., temperature) are indirectly addressed by implementation of the bioremediation technology. For instance, a cover (i.e., greenhouse) used for moisture control also adds inherent heat value.

CONCLUSION

The application of genome-enabled techniques to the study of bioremediation is clearly in its infancy. There are many technical issues that will need to be addressed before some of the more novel approaches, such as environmental genome sequencing and arrays, or *in silico* modeling of multi-species consortia, can be routinely employed in this field. However, for bioremediation to advance as a science, there is a strong need for the comprehensive understanding of physiological properties that genome-enabled approaches can provide. The ultimate goal of such studies is the coupling of models of microbial growth and metabolism in contaminated environments with existing geochemical and hydrological models to predict accurately the microbial assisted natural attenuation of contaminants or the likely outcome of engineered strategies to accelerate bioremediation.

FURTHER READINGS

1. Derek R. Lovley. (2003) Cleaning up with genomics: applying molecular biology to bioremediation. *Nature Reviews.* **(1)**: 35-43.
2. Derek R. Lovley (1995) Bioremediation of organic and metal contaminants with dissimilatory metal reduction. *J. of Ind. Microbiol. and Biotechnol..* **(14)**: 85-93.
3. Fetzner, S and Lingens, F. (1994) Bacterial dehalogenases: biochemistry, genetics, and biotechnological applications. *Microbiological. Reviews,* 641-685.
4. Gupta Sanjay Mohan, Gupta Supriya and Kumar Anil (2009) Development of Bed Reactor Using Brick Dust Immobilized CM-Cellulase from Seeds of Cowpea (*Vigna sinensis* L). *J. Plant Biochemistry & Biotechnology.* 18 **(1)**: 113-116.
5. Jaroslav Drobník. (1999) Genetically modified organisms (GMO) in bioremediation and legislation. *International Biodeterioration & Biodegredation,* **(44)**: 3-6.

6. Juan L. Ramos, Asuncibn Delgado, Estrella Duque, Maria-Dolores Fandila, Matilde Gil, Ali Haidour, Gloria Lucchesi, Carmen Michan, Rafael Salto. (1997) Biodegradation of nitroaromatics by microbes. *Bioremediation Protocols.* **(2)**: 187-200.
7. Karube I., Tanaka S., Shirai T. and Suzuki S. (1977) Hydrolysis of cellulose in a cellulase-bead fluidized bed reactor. *Biotechnol. Bioeng.* **(19)**: 1183-1191.
8. Leahy, J. G. and Colwell, R. R. (1990) Microbial degradation of hydrocarbons in the environment. *Microbiol Rev.* 54 **(3)**: 305-315
9. Lee Y. J., Kim B. K., Lee B. H., Jo K. I., Lee N. K., Chung C. H., Lee Y. C and Lee J. W. (2008) Purification and characterization of cellulase produced by *Bacillus amyoliquefaciens* DL-3 utilizing rice hull. *Biorcsour. Technol.* 99 **(2)**: 378-386.
10. Lovley D.R. (2003) Cleaning up with genomics: applying molecular biology to bioremediation. *Nat. Rev. Microbiol.* **(1)**: 35-44.
11. Michael Moldowan, Dahl, J., Mark, Jeremy A., McCaffrey Smith, Fetzer William J., John C. (1995). Application of biological marker technology to bioremediation of refinery byproducts. *EnergyFuels.* 9 **(1)**: 155-162.
12. Moran-Mirabal J.M., Santhanam N., Corgie S.C., and Craighead H.G. (2008) Immobilization of cellulose fibrils on solid substrates for cellulase-binding studies through quantitative fluorescence microscopy. *Biotechnol Bioeng.* **(101)**: 1129-1141.
13. Nevin, K. P. & Lovley, D. R. (2002) Mechanisms for accessing insoluble Fe(III) oxide during dissimilatory Fe(III) reduction by *Geothrix fermentans. Appl. Environ. Microbiol.* **(68)**: 2294-2299.
14. Nierman, W. C. & Nelson, K. E. (2002). Genomics for applied microbiology. *Adv. Appl. Microbiol.* **(51)**: 201-245.
15. Oremland, R.S., Lonergan, D.J., Culbertson, C.W and Lovley, D.R.(1996) Microbial degradation of hydrochlorofluorocarbons (CHCl2F and CHCl2CF3) in soils and sediments. *Appl. Environ. Microbiol.* **(62)**: 1818-1821,
16. Parekh, S.R. 2004. *The GMO Handbook: Genetically Modified Animals, Microbes, and Plants in Biotechnology.* Humana Press, Michigan.
17. Satinder, K. Brar, Verma M., Surampalli Y., Misra K., Tyagi R. D., Meunier N. and Blais J. F. (2006). Bioremediation of hazardous wastes—A review. *Pract. Periodical* of Haz., *Toxic, and Radioactive Waste Mgmt.* Vol. 10, Issue 2, pp. 59-72.
18. Saul L. and Neidleman, Allen. (1964) *Advances in Applied Microbiology.* Academic Press.
19. Schneegurt, M. A. & Kulpa, C. F. Jr (1998) The application of molecular techniques in environmental biotechnology for monitoring microbial systems. *Biotechnol. Appl. Biochem.* **(27)**: 73-79.
20. Sohel D., Aparna S. and Munishwar N.G. (2007) A multipurpose immobilized biocatalyst with pectinase, xylanase and cellulase activities. *Chemistry Central Journal.* **(1)**: 16.
21. Spormann, A. M. & Widdel, F. (2000) Metabolism of alkylbenzenes, alkanes, and other hydrocarbons in anaerobic bacteria. *Biodegradation.* **(11)**: 85-105.
22. Stroud J., Paton G. I., Semple K. T. (2007) Microbe-aliphatic hydrocarbon interactions in soil: implications for biodegradation and bioremediation. Polymicrobial Communities. Symposium, Edimburgh., Vol. 102, pp. 1239-1253 .
23. Todd A. Anderson, Joel R. Coats. (2004) Enhanced microbial degradation of pesticides. *Encyclopedia of Pest Management*, pp. 205-225.
24. Warren, J., Lyman, Patrick J. Reidy., Benjamin S.(1992) *Mobility and Degradation of Organic Contaminants in Subsurface*, CRC Press.
25. Yi-Li Huang, Qing-Biao Li, Xu Deng, Ying-Hua Lu, Xin-Kai Liao, Ming-Yuan Hong and Yan Wang.(2005) Aerobic and anaerobic biodegradation of polyethylene glycols using sludge microbes. *Process Biochemistry.* Vol. 40, Issue 1, pp. 207-211.

Glossary

AB SoLid system has been adopted by Applied Biosystems to develop the sequencers. In this method, library of adaptor flanked DNA fragments is constructed by emulsion PCR.

Abzymes The use of antibodies as enzymes is described as Abzymes.

Acquired immunity is another term for adaptive immunity.

Activated sludge process Aerobic sewage treatment process using aerobic microorganisms present in sewage sludge to break down organic matter in sewage.

Activator is a protein that stimulates the expression of a gene, typically by acting at a promoter to stimulate RNA polymerase. In eukaryotes, the sequence to which it binds in the promoter is called a response element.

Active site is the restricted part of an enzyme to which a substrate binds.

Active transport is an energy-consuming process that moves molecules against an electrochemical gradient. Energy for the movement is provided by hydrolysis of ATR.

Adaptive immunity is the response mediated by lymphocytes that are activated by their specific interaction with antigen. The adaptive immune response develops over several days as lymphocytes with antigen-specific receptors are stimulated to proliferate and become effector cells. It is responsible for immunological memory.

Adaptor any synthetic single- or double-stranded oligodeoxynucleotide useful in recombinant DNA technology for joining two incompatible cohesive ends of restriction fragments.

Addiction system is a survival mechanism used by plasmids. The mechanism kills the bacterium upon loss of the plasmid.

Aerated pile Microbial composition of organic waste matter where the wastes are heaped in piles and forced aeration supplies oxygen.

Affinity chromatography a general chromatographic method that may, in principle, be used to isolate either of the components of a reversibly reacting chemical system provided that one component can be coupled to an insoluble matrix through a covalent linkage.

Agglutination-Test is that in which visible clumping or aggregation of cells or particles takes place due to the reaction of surface-bound antigens of such cells or particles with homologous antibodies.

Agrobacterium a genus of Gram-negative aerobic rod-shaped soil bacteria. Most strains can initiate formation of galls in plants. A feature of the infection of plants by *Agrobacterium* species is that the bacterium can subvert the host plant tissue to produce amino acids known as opines, which the bacterium can use as an energy, carbon, and nitrogen source. Transformation by *Agrobacterium tumefaciens* has been shown to be due to large plasmids (140 -235 kb). These are known as tumour-inducing or Ti plasmids, and they have been exploited in the production of transgenic plants.

Allele *or* **allelomorph** any of the forms of the same gene that occur at the same locus on a homologous chromosome but differ in base sequence. Two or more alleles are said to be allelic or allelomorphic to each other, and if more than two alleles exist in a population, the locus is said to show multiple allelism.

Allele Specific PCR This method differentiates the sequences solely on the basis of their ability to bind to an oligo primer.

Allelic exclusion describes the expression in any particular lymphocyte of only one allele coding for the expressed immunoglobulin. This is caused by feedback from the first immunoglobulin allele to be expressed that prevents activation of a copy on the other chromosome.

Allosteric regulation describes the ability of a protein to change its conformation (and therefore activity) at one site as the result of binding a small molecule to a second site located elsewhere on the protein.

Amperometric sensitivity biosensor can detect electroactive species present in biological test samples.

Amphipathic structures have two surfaces, one hydrophilic and one hydrophobic. Lipids are amphipathic; and some protein regions may form amphipathic helices, with one charged face and one neutral face.

Amplified Fragment Length Polymorphism (AFLP) is a technique based on the detection of genomic restriction fragments by PCR amplification and can be used for DNA of any origin or complexity.

Anaerobic digestion A microbial fermentation of organic matter to methane and CO_2 which occurs in near absence of air; a sewage treatment process.

Anchored PCR utilized only one primer instead of two.

Aneuploid set of chromosomes differs from the usual diploid constitution by loss or duplication of chromosomes or chromosomal segments.

Animal Transgenic Technology deal with the production of transgenic animals that depends upon the success of a series of several complex technical experimental manipulations.

Annealing of DNA describes the renaturation of a duplex structure from single strands that were obtained by denaturing duplex DNA.

Annie was the first cow to be cloned with a gene for a vetnary application.

Antibiotic A specific type of chemical substance that is used to fight microbial infections, usually in humans or animals. Most antibiotics are produced by microorganisms. Semi-synthetic antibiotics are natural antibiotics that have been modified chemically.

Antibody A protein produced by the immune system on exposure to a specific antigen, characterized by specific reactivity with its complementary antigen.

Antigen A molecule introduced into an organism and recognized as a foreign material, resulting in the elicitation of antibody production (immune response) directed specifically against the foreign molecule.

Antisense gene codes for an (antisense) RNA that has a complementary sequence to an RNA that is its target. Genes in which the mirror image of the normal nucleotide base sequences is inserted, preventing expression of the natural genes.

Antisense refers to short DNA or RNA sequences, termed oligonucleotides, which are designed to be complementary to a specific gene sequence.

Antisense Technology are a suite of techniques that together, form a very powerful weapon for studying gene function and discovering new and more specific treatments of diseases in humans, animals and plants.

Antitoxin any antibody to a toxin of a (micro) organism that neutralizes the toxin both *in vitro* and *in vivo*.

Apoenzyme the protein part of an enzyme that forms a catalytically active enzyme (holoenzyme) when combined with an activator, a coenzyme, or a prosthetic group. It determines the specificity of the catalytic system.

Apoptosis (programmed cell death) is the capacity of a cell to respond to a stimulus by initiating a pathway that leads to its death by a characteristic set of reactions.

Arbitrarily primed PCR is based on the amplification of genomic DNA with a single primer selected from an arbitrary nucleotide sequence.

ARS (autonomous replication sequence) is an origin for replication in yeast. The common feature among different *ARS* sequences is a conserved 11 bp sequence called the A-domain.

Ascites Liquid accumulation in the peritoneal cavity, widely used as a method for propagating hybridoma cells for monoclonal antibody formation.

Ascites-route Technology provides an alternative for MAbs production commercially.

Asymmetric PCR In this method the addition of one primer is vast excess over the other primer during the PCR, results in the generation of an excess of one amplified strand relative to the other.

Atmospheric pressure chemical ionization (APCI) technique is advantageous for analysis of nonpolar and neutral molecules that are thermally stable such as lipids and is tolerant to higher buffer concentrations.

Atmospheric pressure photoionization (APPI) directly photoionizes metabolites and therefore can ionize compounds that cannot be ionized as effectively using other atmospheric pressure techniques such as less polar metabolites.

Atomic force microscopy (AFM) imaging is a unique direct visualization technique that is used to characterize mechanism involved in DNA-protein recognition and DNA-protein complex formation in different conditions (air and liquids).

Attenuation describes the regulation of bacterial operons by controlling termination of transcription at a site located before the first structural gene. An **attenuator** is a terminator sequence at which attenuation occurs.

Autogenous control describes the action of a gene product that either inhibits (negative autogenous control) or activates (positive autogenous control) expression of the gene coding for it.

Autoimmune disease is a pathological condition in which the immune response is directed to self antigen.

Autoradiograph *or* **autoradiogram** the image produced by autoradiography. Autoradiography is a method by which radioactive material can be localized in, e.g., a tissue, cell, a cell part, or molecule, or in a chromatogram or electrophoretogram. The sample containing a radioactive substance is put in direct contact with a thick layer of specially prepared photographic emulsion. The radiation emitted in the decay of the radionuclide(s) activates individual silver halide grains in the emulsion rendering them susceptible to conversion to metallic silver grains by a photographic developer. After fixation the silver grains may be located either visually or by microscopy.

Autotroph *or* **lithotroph** any organism that requires only simple inorganic substances to fulfill its nutritional requirements and for which gaseous or dissolved carbon dioxide is the sole source of carbon for the synthesis of cellular constituents.

Auxotroph any strain of microorganism (alga, bacterium, or fungus) that differs from the wild-type by requiring a supply of one or more growth factors.

Avirulent mutants of a bacterium or virus have lost the capacity to infect a host productively, that is, to make more bacterium or virus.

B

B cell memory is responsible for rapid antibody production during a secondary immune response and subsequent responses. Memory B cells produce antibodies of higher affinity than native B cells.

Backcross (also known as a testcross) describes a genetic cross in which a hybrid strain is crossed to one of its two parental strains.

Bacterial artificial chromosome (BAC) is a synthetic DNA molecule that contains the sequences needed for replication and segregation in bacteria. This is used in genomic cloning to amplify sequences typically 100-200 kb long. They are usually derived from derived from the naturally-occurring F factor episome.

Bacteriophage A virus that multiplies in bacteria.

Batch processing In batch processing the reaction vessel (e.g. fermenter) is filled with the medium containing substrate, sterilized, inoculated (or added biocatalyst) and the bioconversion allowed to proceed.

Bayesian inference In order to model the uncertainty in the complex model, a statistical approach known as Baysian inference is used.

Bayesian mapping methodology has become popular in QTL mapping because of the availability of simulation based MCMC algorithms.

Bio Brick standard biological components are DNA sequences with defined structure and function. Each Bio Brick consist of DNA sequences, usually held in a circular plasmid, with flanking regions containing known restriction sites, which enables it to be joined with others and make bigger structures.

Bio-affinity sensors have wide versatility because of the use of radiolabelled, enzyme-labelled or fluorescein-labelled substances or the optical systems employing bioluminescence or chemiluminescence.

Biocatalysts The substances that actually cause chemical changes in bioprocesses are the enzymes produced by a living cell.

Bioengineering is the application of engineering principles to address challenges in the fields of biology and medicine.

Bio-fertilizers are live formulations of agriculturally beneficial bacteria and fungi, which on application to seed, root or soil can fix atmospheric nitrogen or solubilise phosphorus and oxidize sulphur in the soil by their biological activity and help to improve the soil health.

Bioinformatics and *in silico* Technology It occupies a unique niche amongst the sciences, lying at intersectional of biology, genetics, biochemistry, computer science, mathematics, statistics and numerous other allied fields.

Bioinoculant Technology deals with the prospect of improving agriculture by inoculation with bio-fertilizers, bio-pesticides and organic decomposers.

Biological oxygen demand (BOD) The oxygen used in meeting the metabolic needs of aerobic organisms in water containing organic compounds.

Biomass All organic matter that derives from the photosynthetic conversion of solar energy.

Bioprocess Engineering is the sub-discipline within biotechnology that is responsible for translating the discoveries of life science with practical products, processes, or systems that can serve the needs of society.

Bioreactor (fermenter) Containment system for fermentation purposes.

Bioremediation technology: Bioremediation is a process which relies on microorganisms to break down and detoxify organic chemicals such as hydrocarbons and some oreganochlorines.

Biosensor An electronic device that uses biological molecules to detect specific compounds.**Biosensor Technology** deals with the use of an analytical device mat converts a biological response into an electrical signal.

Blotting *or* **blot transfer** a technique useful for identifying similar macromolecules, e.g. sets of DNA or RNA fragments, or mixtures of intact proteins, that are separable by gel electrophoresis. The separated components are then transferred from the gel to a sheet of an appropriate medium while preserving their two-dimensional relationships. The original version of the technique, used for DNA fragments and often referred to as Southern blotting, has been extensively developed and adapted for other applications, e.g. dot hybridization (or dot blotting), colony hybridization, electrophoretic transfer, Northern blotting, and Western blotting.

Blue Biotechnology Term used to describe the marine and aquatic applications of biotechnology.

Bovine somatotropin Growth hormone that can be produced by recombinant DNA technology and used to increase the milk yield by cows.

Ca-DNA co-precipitation (or calcium phosphate co-precipitation) In this method, DNA is mixed with $CaCl_2$ solution and isotonic phosphate buffer to form a DNA-calcium phosphate co-precipitate (also called Ca-DNA coprecipitate).

Callus a mass of relatively unspecialized tissue that develops at wound sites in plants, forming a protective covering. Callus cells are used in tissue culture as the starting material for the propagation of plant clones.

Capsid is the external protein coat of a virus particle.

Carcinogen is a chemical that increases the frequency with which cells are converted to a cancerous condition.

Caspases comprise a family of proteases some of whose members are involved in apoptosis (programmed cell death).

cDNA is a single-stranded DNA complementary to an RNA, synthesized from it by reverse transcription *in vitro.* The cell cycle is the set of stages through which a cell progresses from one division to the next.

cDNA library a collection of cloned recombinant cDNA, usually in bacteria or yeast. The clones represent cDNAs prepared from all the mRNAs in any particular species or organ.

Cell Designer is a modelling tool of biochemical networks with graphical user interface.

Cell fusion the formation of a single hybrid cell containing the nuclei and cytoplasms from different cells. It may be induced by treatment of a mixed cell population with certain fusogens (e.g. killed Sendai virus or polyethylene glycol). It is an important step in the technique of forming hybridoma cells for the production of monoclonal antibodies.

Cell line a population of cells cultured *in vitro* those are descended through one or more generations (and possibly Sub-cultures) from a single primary culture. The cells of such a population share common characteristics.

Central dogma describes the basic nature of genetic information: sequences of nucleic acid can be perpetuated and interconverted by replication, transcription, and reverse transcription, but translation from nucleic acid to protein is unidirectional, because nucleic acid sequences cannot be retrieved from protein sequences.

Chemical proofreading describes a proofreading mechanism in which the correction event occurs after addition of an incorrect subunit to a polymeric chain, by reversing the addition reaction.

Chloroplast DNA (ctDNA) is an independent genome (usually circular) found in a plant chloroplast.

Chloroplast Transformation Today chloroplast transformation has become an important technique in plant biotechnology and is effectively used for obtaining transgenic plants.

Chromatin immunoprecipitation (CHIP) is a powerful tool to identify there *in vivo* interaction of a specific protein at particular region in the chromatin.

Chromosomal microarray Microarray-based genomic copy-number analysis is now a commonly ordered clinical genetic test for patients and is defined under various names.

Chromosome is a discrete unit of the genome carrying many genes. Each chromosome consists of a very long molecule of duplex DNA and an approximately equal mass of proteins. It is visible as a morphological entity only during cell division.

Chymosin An enzyme used to clot milk, which is used in the manufacture of cheese.

Cisgenesis Plant transformation using its own genetic material or gene(s) from species with which it can intercross or able to breed conventionally (cisgenes) has gained much significance. This process is known as cisgenesis or intragenesis.

Cistron a unit of DNA sequences that code for a single polypeptide or protein. It may be a smaller unit than the gene, which contains the unit of DNA determining a single character. Whether or not a cistron is the same as a gene can be determined by the *cis-trans* complementation test, hence the name cistron *(cis* means 'on this side').

Clonal selection theory proposed that each lymphocyte expresses single antigen receptor specificity and that only those lymphocytes that bind to a given antigen are stimulated to proliferate and to function in eliminating that antigen. Thus, the antigen "selects" the lymphocytes to be activated. Clonal selection is now an established principle in immunology. The cloverleaf describes the structure of tRNA drawn in two dimensions, forming four distinct arm-loops.

Clone A collection of genetically identical cells or organisms derived from a common ancestor; all members of the clone have identical genetic composition.

Clone contig approach The "clone-by-clone" strategy involves the constructions of genomic DNA libraries in suitable vectors such as PAC (P1 derived Artificial Chromosome) and BAC (Bacterial Artificial Chromosome), which can clone up to 150 kb of DNA fragment.

Cloning in gene technology, making many copies of a fragment of an organism's genome, after it has been spliced into a bacterial plasmid or lambda phage, or by polymerase chain reaction.

Cloning vector *or* **cloning vehicle** the DNA of any transmissible agent (e.g. plasmid or virus) into which a segment of foreign DNA can be spliced in order to introduce the foreign DNA into cells of the agent's normal host and promote its replication and transcription therein. (1) Plasmid vectors contain (i) an origin of replication, (ii) an antibiotic resistance gene, (iii) often, a 'polylinker' containing several different restriction enzyme recognition sites and a second marker gene.

Co-activators are factors required for transcription that do not bind DNA but are required for (DNA-binding) activators to interact with the basal transcription factors.

Coding region is a part of the gene that represents a protein sequence. The coding strand (sense strand) of DNA has the same sequence as the mRNA and is related to the protein sequence that it represents by the genetic code.

Cofactor is a small inorganic component (often a metal ion) that is required for the proper structure or function of an enzyme.

Complete dominance is the state in which the phenotype is the same when the dominant allele is homozygous or heterozygous.

Computational Biology Conceptualizing biology in terms of molecules and than applying informatics techniques to understand and organize the information associated with these molecules, on a large scale.

Conjugation is a process in which two cells come in contact and exchange genetic material. In bacteria, DNA is transferred from a donor to a recipient cell. In protozoa, DNA passes from each cell to the other.

Constant regions (C regions) of immunoglobulins are coded by C gene segments and are the parts of the chain that vary least. Those of heavy chains identify the type of immunoglobulin.

Constitutive genes are expressed following interaction between a promoter and RNA polymerase without additional regulation. *Also known as* housekeeping genes, they are expressed in virtually all cells since they are essential for the cell's activity.

Continuous fermentation A fermentation process that can run for long periods, in which raw materials are supplied and products and microorganisms are removed continuously.

Co-operativity in protein binding describes an effect in which binding of the first protein enhances binding of a second protein (or another copy of the same protein).

Copasi is a software application for simulation and analysis of biochemical networks and their dynamics.

Copy number the number of copies of any gene or plasmid in a given cell.

Co-repressor is a small molecule that triggers repression of transcription by binding to a regulator protein.

Cosmid a hybrid cloning vector used for cloning DNA. Cosmids are derived from plasmids but also contain cos sites from phage lambda. ***cos*** site the cohesive ends (sticky ends) of certain phage DNA molecules.

Co-transduction the transduction of two or more identifiable genes in a single event, probably because the transduced element contains more than one genetic locus.

Co-translational translocation describes the movement of a protein across a membrane as the protein is being synthesized. The term is usually restricted to cases in which the ribosome binds to the channel. This form of translocation may be restricted to the endoplasmic reticulum.

Crown gall disease is a tumor that can be induced in many plants by infection with the bacterium *Agrobacterium tumefaciens*.

Cryptic satellite is a satellite DNA sequence not identified as such by a separate peak on a density gradient; that is, it remains present in main-band DNA.

Cybrid a plant derived from a cell containing the nucleus from one species and the cytoplasm from another species.

Cytokinin *or* phytokinin any of a group of plant hormones that have a stimulatory effect on the division of plant cells and a retarding effect on leaf senescence. They are purine derivatives.

Cytomer is a relational database on organs, tissues, cell types, physiological systems and developmental stages, presently focusing on the human system.

Cytoplasmic inheritance is a property of genes located in mitochondria or chloroplasts.

Cytoscope is a project dedicated to building open-source network visualization and analysis software.

D

DDRT-PCR is used to amplify and display many cDNAs derived from the mRNAs of a given cell or tissue type.

Degeneracy the existence of two or more synonyms specifying a particular item or function. One such is the genetic code, wherein a specific amino acid may be encoded by two or more nucleotide triplets, or codons present in a nucleic acid or polynucleotide.

Degenerate PCR is used to amplify (fish out) conserved sequences of a gene or genes from the genome of an organism and to get the nucleotide sequence after having sequenced some amino acids from a protein of interest.

Denaturation of protein describes its conversion from the physiological conformation to some other (inactive) conformation.

Denitrification the reduction of nitrate ions to oxides of nitrogen or molecular nitrogen (N_2), carried out by certain aerobic soil bacteria, especially in the absence of sufficient oxygen under waterlogged conditions.

Density gradient is used to separate macromolecules on the basis of differences in their density. It is prepared from a heavy soluble compound such as CsCl.

Deoxyribonucleic acid (DNA) is a nucleic acid molecule consisting of long chains of polymerized (deoxyribo) nucleotides. In double-stranded DNA the two strands are held together by hydrogen bonds between complementary nucleotide base pairs.

Dephosphorylation the process of removing one or more phosphoric (ester or anhydride) residues from a molecule.

Derivatization involves chemically modifying a compound to produce a new compound which is volatile and hence suitable for analysis using a GC.

Desorption electrospray ionization (DESI) technique has been proved to work for polar and non-polar organic and biological compounds and enables *in situ* analysis of biological tissues.

Diabetes is a metabolic disorder in which the utilization of glucose is impaired finally resulting in the high level of glucose in blood.

Dideoxy method *or* **dideoxy (nucleotide)** sequencing analysis *an alternative name for* chain-termination method (for sequencing DNA molecules).

Direct analysis in real time (DART) This technique uses an atmospheric-pressure ion source that permits analysis of gases, liquids, solids, or materials on surfaces in open air at ground potential under ambient conditions.

Direct infusion mass spectrometry (DIMS) This type of analysis can be helpful with metabolites that are challenging to measure by gas chromatography-mass spectrophotometry (GC-MS) and can increase the throughput of the analysis.

Divergence is the percent difference in nucleotide sequence between two related DNA sequences or in amino acid sequences between two proteins.

Diversity Array Technology (DArT) - Relies on hybridization to previously defined clones; Needs a small amount of very high quality DNA; Can be mechanized and you get many loci per run; Do not have multiple alleles (dominant); Require much discovery and optimization for each species before use; Require special equipment to visualize; generally better to outsource.

DNA amplification restricted transcription translation (DARTT) has been used to describe the PCR-based amplification of protein encoding genes and truncations coupled to the rapid analysis of protein functions following transcription and translation of the encoded protein.

DNA fingerprinting analyzes the differences between individuals of the fragments generated by using restriction enzymes to cleave regions that contain short repeated sequences. Because these are unique to every individual, the presence of a particular subset in any two individuals can be used to define their common inheritance (e.g. a parent-child relationship).

DNA foot printing has been used to identify exact region in DNA which interacts with the protein binding factors.

DNA helicase an enzyme that catalyses unwinding of the DNA double helix during DNA replication and repair. It requires ATP.

DNA ligase makes a bond between an adjacent 3'-OH and 5'-phosphate end where there is a nick in one strand of duplex DNA.

DNA polymerase is an enzyme that synthesizes a daughter strand(s) of DNA (under direction from a DNA template). Any particular enzyme may be involved in repair or replication (or both).

DNA probes Isolated single DNA strands used to detect the presence of the complementary (opposite) strands, and used as very sensitive biological detectors.

DNA protein interactional technology DNA proteins interactions are fundamental to the existence of life forms, providing the key to the genetic plan as well as mechanisms for its maintenance and evolution.

DNA replicase is a DNA-synthesizing enzyme required specifically for replication.

DNA topoisomerase is an enzyme that changes the number of times the two strands in a closed DNA molecule cross each other. It does this by cutting the DNA, passing DNA through the break, and resealing the DNA.

DNAases are enzymes that attack bonds in DNA. The initial association of a translating ribosome with the translocation channel in the membrane of the ER is called docking.

Dosage compensation describes mechanisms employed to compensate for the discrepancy between the presence of two X chromosomes in one sex but only one X chromosome in the other sex.

Dotplots method is basically based on the graphical representation of the alignment between the given two sequences.

Down regulation a decrease in response of a cell to a hormone brought about either by a decrease in receptor number or by the uncoupling of an effector component.

Downstream processing Separation and purification of product(s) from a fermentation process.

DRTF A database of rice transcription factors.

Edman degradation In this method the phosphoprotein is radiolabelled with ^{32}P by in vivo or in vitro methods and then digested with protease to produce the peptides which are purified by HPLC.

Edman Sequencing One of the earliest methods used for protein identification was sequencing by Edman degradation to obtain N-terminal amino acid sequences.

Electrochemical Biosensors are mainly used for the detection of hybridized DNA, DNA-binding drugs, glucose concentration etc.

Electronic-PCR (ePCR) has been successfully utilized for conducting electronic PCR without the use of PCR machine or PCR reaction mixtures.

Electrophoresis the phenomenon of the movement of ions (including macromolecular ions) or charged particles or ions through a fluid under the influence of an electric field applied to the fluid. A number of different media have been used as the fluid support, including paper, cellulose acetate, starch gel, and polycrylamide gel.

Electroporate to create momentary pores in the membranes of living cells, without loss of their viability, by exposing them to a sequence of brief electrical pulses of high field strength. The reversible breakdown of the cell membranes thus caused enables treated cells to take up exogenous material (e.g. drugs or foreign DNA).

Electrospray ionization In ESI, liquid sample flows from a microcapillary tube into the orifice of the mass spectrometer, where a potential difference between the capillary and the inlet results in the generation of fine charged droplets.

ELISA is based on, as the name suggests, enzyme-linked antibodies adsorbed on some solid surface.

Embryo transfer Implementation of embryos from donor animals or generated by *in vitro* fertilization into the uteri of recipient animals.

Embryogenesis cells belonging to normal (vegetative) cells of a plant, or protoplasts derived from such cells, can sometimes be induced to divide and differentiate into the parts of a new embryo. This process involves transfers through appropriate culture media.

Embryonic stem cells (ESCs) as their name suggests, are derived from embryos.

EMSA or gel shift assay experiment includes incubating a^{32}p-end labelled DNA with a protein or protein mixture in an incubating buffer wherein the DNA binding proteins binds to the DNA upon electrophoressing, the mobility of protein bound DNA is retarded and is detected as a separate higher order band in the autoradiogram.

End labeling describes the addition of a radioactively labeled group to one end (5' or 3') of a DNA strand.

Endocytosis describes the process by which material at the surface of the cell is internalized. The process involves the formation of a membranous vesicle.

EndoNet is a database on intercellular signalling paths as they are exerted by e.g., hormones to constitute the endocrine network of the human body.

Endonucleases cleave bonds within a nucleic acid chain; they may be specific for RNA or for single-stranded or double stranded DNA.

Endotoxin is a toxin that is present on the surface of Gram negative bacteria (as opposed to exotoxins, which are secreted). LPS is an example of an endotoxin.

Enzyme bioreactor A reactor in which a chemical conversion reaction is catalyzed by an enzyme.

Enzyme turnover is the process through which the enzyme returns to its original shape, enabling the enzyme to catalyze another reaction.

Enzyme-linked immunosorbent assay *abbr.:* ELISA; a form of quantitative immunoassay based on the use of antibodies (or antigens) that are linked to an insoluble carrier surface, which is then used to 'capture' the relevant antigen (or antibody) in the test solution. The antigen-antibody complex is then detected by measuring the activity of an appropriate enzyme that had previously been covalently attached to the antigen (or antibody).

Epigenetic changes influence the phenotype without altering the genotype. They consist of changes in the properties of a cell that are inherited but that do not represent a change in genetic information.

Episome a genetic element that is sometimes found in cells, especially those of bacteria, and that can replicate either when integrated into or independently of the host chromosome.

Epitope is the portion of an antigen that is recognized by the antigen receptor on lymphocytes. It is also called an antigenic determinant.

ESTs are single pass sequences of cloned mRNAs (cDNA clone taken from a cDNA library).

Exocytosis is the process of secreting proteins from a cell into the medium, by the fusion of the secretory vesicle with the plasma membrane.

Exon is any segment of an interrupted gene that is represented in the mature RNA product.

Exonucleases cleave nucleotides one at a time from the end of a polynucleotide chain; they may be specific for either the 5' or 3' endofDNAorRNA.

Expressed sequence tag (EST) is a short sequence of DNA taken from a cDNA copy of an mRNA. The EST is complementary to the mRNA and can be used to identify genes corresponding to the mRNA.

Expression vector is generally a plasmid that is used to introduce and express a specific gene into a target cell.

Extrachromosomal genome in a bacterium is a self-replicating set of genes that is not part of the bacterial chromosome. In many cases, the genes are necessary for bacterial growth under certain environmental conditions.

Extractive Electro-spray Ionization (EESI) is a method for the ionization of analytes in complex matrices. The technique was established for the direct analysis of vaporized samples such as breath for clinical diagnosis.

Feedback inhibition describes the ability of a small molecule product of a metabolic pathway to inhibit the activity of an enzyme that catalyzes an earlier step in the pathway.

Feedback repression an inhibitory feedback system in which the accumulation of a substance produced in a metabolic pathway represses the synthesis of an enzyme that is required at an earlier stage of the pathway.

Fermentation The process by which microorganisms turn raw materials such as glucose into products such as alcohol.

Flanking marker (DNA) a DNA marker on either side of a locus; a DNA sequence on either side of a gene.

Fluidised bed reactor (FBR) where the flow of gas and/or substrate keeps the immobilized enzyme particles in a fluidised state.

Fluorescence immunoassay *or* fluorescent immunoassay *or* fluoroimmunoassay *abbr.:* FIA; a method of assaying very small amounts of material that is similar in principle to radioimmunoassay but uses a fluorescent rather than a radioactive label for the antigen.

Fluorescence *in situ* hybridization *abbr.:* FISH; a procedure that involves the use of DNA probes to locate in tissue section specific regions of DNA in the chromosomes.

Fluorescence the emission of light of a different wavelength to light that has been absorbed.

Fluorescene resonance energy transfer (FRET) is a technique by which protein-protein interaction can be studied in vivo.

Fluxome The complete set of all fluxes through the different biochemical reactions that are involved in the interconversion of metabolites.

Foot printing is a technique for identifying the site on DNA bound by some protein by virtue of the protection of bonds in this region against attack by nucleases.

Fourier transform infrared spectroscopy (FT-IR) primarily measures vibrations of functional groups and highly polar bonds.

Frame shift mutations arise by deletions or insertions that are not a multiple of 3 bp; they change the frame in which triplets are translated into protein.

Functional genomics The knowledge of complete genome sequences has led to the development of functional genomics, which studies gene expression pattern and gene functions.

Fusion protein an expression product resulting from the fusion of two genes. Such a protein may be produced, e.g., in recombinant DNA expression studies or, naturally, in certain viral oncogenes in which the oncogene is fused to *gag.* Their production sometimes results from the need to place a cloned eukaryotic gene under the control of a bacterial promoter for expression in a bacterial system; sequences of the bacterial system are then frequently expressed linked to the eukaryotic protein.

Gas Chromatography (GC) is the oldest form of automated separation. It uses a carrier gas as a mobile gas phase and a stationary liquid or polymer phase within a column.

Geiger counter *or* Geiger-Muller counter a device for detecting and measuring ionizing radiation (alpha or beta particles or gamma-ray photons).

GenBank a large database of protein and nucleic-acid sequences.

Gene are segment of DNA sequence that are both transcribed into mRNA and stable RNA (e.g. rRNA, tRNA) that can be translated into polypeptides (structural genes) and those that function as regulators of the expression of the other two types (regulator genes).

Gene expression the process by which the information carried by a gene or genes becomes manifest as the phenotype. It involves transcription of the gene into complementary RNA sequences and, for structural genes, subsequent translation of mRNA into polypeptide chains and their assembly into the ultimate protein products. Gene expression is tightly regulated by promoters, enhancers, and transcription factors.

Gene frequency a measure of the proportion of an allele in a given population, equal to the number of loci at which a given allele occurs, divided by the total number of loci at which it could occur.

Gene library *or* **cloned library** *or* **gene bank** *or* **shotgun collection** a random collection of DNA fragments cloned in a vector, and which may include all the genetic information of a particular species. It may be prepared from a variety of sources, including an extract of mRNA, in contrast to a genomic library which is prepared from genomic DNA.

Gene pool the sum of the genetic information in the reproductive members of a population of sexually reproducing organisms.

Gene transfer The use of genetic or physical manipulations to introduce foreign genes into host cells to achieve desired characteristics in progeny.

Genetic code all the regularities in nucleotide sequence according to which genetic information for the sequences of all the polypeptides synthesized by transcription and translation is encoded in DNA (or RNA in some viruses). A sequence of three nucleotide residues (a codon) is required to code for one amino-acid residue, and since there are four different kinds of base in nucleic acids (apart from minor constituents), 43 i.e. 64 different nucleotide triplets can exist.

Genetic drift any change with time in gene frequency in a population. It may be either directed, steady drift, or undirected, random drift.

Genetic engineering Technologies, including DNA technologies, used to isolate genes from an organism, manipulate them in the laboratory, and insert them into another cell system.

Genetic map any diagram showing the linear order of, and the relative distances between, mutable sites on a chromosome as deduced from genetic recombination experiments.

genetic perturbations with the ultimate goal to identify discriminating metabolites.

Genome Annotation Generation of long contiguous sequence is of no use unless it is annotated for the presence of coding sequences or genes. Genome annotation is the process of integrating biological information to genomic sequences.

Genome is the complete set of sequences in the genetic material of an organism. It includes the sequence of each chromosome plus any DNA in organelles.

Genomics Technology Genomics is the study of the genomes of organisms.

Genomics The term coined by T.H. Roderick in 1987, refers to the study of genome which is entire complement of chromosomal and extrachromosomal genes present in an organism.

Genotype the total genetic constitution of an organism. It comprises the genetic information carried both in the chromosomes and extrachromosomally.

Glycomics The neoglycolipids can be probed with proteins of known carbohydrate binding specificity to confirm identification of predicted protein–oligosaccharide interactions.

Green Biotechnology is biotechnology applied to agricultural processes.

Hapten is a small molecule that acts as an antigen when conjugated to a protein.

HeliScope In this technology, the DNA fragments are sequenced without clonal amplification.

Helper T cell is a T lymphocyte that activates macrophages and stimulates B cell proliferation and antibody production. Helper T cells usually express cell surface CD4 but not CD8.

Helper virus provides functions absent from a defective virus, enabling the latter to complete the infective cycle during a mixed infection.

Hematopoietic stem cells A stem cell from which all red and white blood cells evolve, is called as hematopoietic stem cells

Heterochromatin describes regions of the genome that are highly condensed, are not transcribed, and are late-replicating. Heterochromatin is divided into two types, which are called constitutive and facultative.

Heteroduplex DNA (hybrid DNA) is generated by base pairing between complementary single strands derived from the different parental duplex molecules; it occurs during genetic recombination.

Highly repetitive DNA (simple sequence DNA) is the first component to reassociate and is equated with satellite DNA.

High-pressure liquid chromatography a technique of column chromatography that is rapid and provides high resolution. It can be used with the various modes of liquid chromatography, the liquid being forced at high pressure, normally up to 420 kg cm^{-2} (6000 psi); through the column (which is usually of stainless steel) and thence through a detector into a fraction collector.

Histone acetyltransferase (HAT) enzymes modify histones by addition of acetyl groups; some transcriptional coactivators have HAT activity.

Homologous recombination (generalized recombination) involves a reciprocal exchange of sequences of DNA, e.g. between two chromosomes that carry the same genetic loci.

Hot spot any site at which mutations are observed with an unusually high frequency.

Housekeeping genes (constitutive genes) are those (theoretically) expressed in all cells because they provide basic functions needed for sustenance of all cell types.

HPLC is a form of chromatography that separates compounds dissolved in solution. The instrument consists of a reservoir of mobile phase, a pump, an injector, a separation column and a detector.

Humoral response is an immune response that is mediated primarily by antibodies. It is defined as immunity that can be transferred from one organism to another by serum antibody.

Hybrid cell any cell containing the nuclei and cytoplasms from differing cells, formed artificially by cell fusion.

Hybridization describes the pairing of complementary RNA and DNA strands to give an RNA-DNA hybrid.

Hybridoma A unique fused cell which produces quantities of a specific antibody, and reproduces endlessly.

Hybridroma Technology for production of monoclonal antibodies by hybridoma cells.

Hypermutation describes the introduction of somatic mutations in a rearranged immunoglobulin gene. The mutations can change the sequence of the corresponding antibody, especially in its antigen- binding site.

Hypersensitive site is a short region of chromatin detected by its extreme sensitivity to cleavage by DNAase I and other nucleases; it comprises an area from which nucleosomes are excluded.

IAPs are inhibitors of apoptosis. They function by antagonizing the actions of caspases.

Illumina genome analyzer This is commonly referred as "the Solexa" technology for sequencing. In this method DNA fragments are ligated with specific adaptor fragments and amplified in vitro by the method known as bridge PCR.

Immobilized biocatalyst technology can be defined as "enzymes physically confined or localized in a certain defined region of space with retention of their catalytic activities, and which can be used reputedly and continuously".

Immobilized enzyme An enzyme which is physically defined or localized in a defined region, enabling it to be re-used in a continuous process.

Immobilized metal affinity chromatography (IMAC) is based upon the electrostatic interaction of negatively charged phosphate group with a positively charged metal ion which is immobilized on the resin beads.

Immune response is an organism's reaction, mediated by components of the immune system, to an antigen.

Immunity in phages refers to the ability of a prophage to prevent another phage of the same type from infecting a cell. It results from the synthesis of phage repressor by the prophage genome.

Immunofluorescenc The fluorescent-antibody technique (immunofluorescence) is often used to identify unknown antigen.

Immunosensors Biosensors may be used in conjunction with enzyme – linked immunosorbent assays (ELISA).

***In Planta* Transformation** Thus recently *in planta* transformation systems have been developed in which DNA is introduced either by *Agrobacterium* or by direct transfer methods into intact plants, with no need for plant regeneration under tissue culture conditions.

In *situ* hybridization a technique of hybridization analysis in which chromosomes *in situ* are used as the target for hybridization with radioactive or fluorescent putative complementary DNA or RNA.

***In vitro* fertilization (IVF) Technology** In this method the fertilization of egg by sperm takes place at artificially maintained optimum conditions has revolutionized the field of animal biotechnology, by the production of more and more animals than that of normal course.

In vitro *Latin (of any biological process, reaction, or experiment)* occurring or made to occur outside an organism, e.g. in extracts or cultures; literally it means 'in glass'.

In vivo *Latin (of any biological process, reaction, or experiment)* occurring or made to occur within a living organism; literally it means 'in life'.

Incomplete dominance is a state in which the heterozygote has a phenotype in between that of each of the homozygotes.

Induced mutations result from the action of a mutagen. The mutagen may act directly on the bases in DNA or it may act indirectly to trigger a pathway that leads to a change in DNA sequence.

Inducer is a small molecule that triggers gene transcription by binding to a regulator protein.

Induction of prophage describes its entry into the lytic (infective) cycle as a result of destruction of the lysogenic repressor, which leads to excision of free phage DNA from the bacterial chromosome.

Innate immunity is the rapid response mediated by cells with non varying (germline-encoded) receptors that recognize pathogen. The cells of the innate immune response act to eliminate the pathogen and initiate the adaptive immune response.

Integration of viral or another DNA sequence describes its insertion into a host genome as a region covalently linked on either side to the host sequences.

Inter Simple Sequence Repeat markers (ISSR) In this technique, reported by Zietkiewicz *et al.* (1994), primers based on microsatellites are utilized to amplify inter-SSR DNA sequences.

Interactome The complete set of interactions between different components within the cell. These interactions include protein-protein interactions, protein-DNA interaction, protein-metabolite interactions as well as other possible interactions.

Intron (intervening sequence) is a segment of DNA that is transcribed, but removed from within the transcript by splicing together the sequences (exons) on either side of it.

Inverses PCR In this technique, the amplification of those DNA sequence takes place, which are away from the primers, and not those, which are flanked by the primers.

Ion-Sensitive Biosensors These are semiconductor FETs having an ion-sensitive surface. The surface electrical potential changes when the ions and the semiconductor interact.

Isoschizomers are restriction enzymes that cleave the same DNA sequence but are affected differently by its state of methylation.

Isotope-coded affinity tag labelling This method relies on the labelling of protein samples from two different sources with two chemically identical reagents that differ only in mass as a result of isotope composition.

Karyotype the visual appearance of the set of chromosomes of a typical somatic eukaryotic cell of a given species, individual, or cell strain.

Kinetic proofreading describes a proofreading mechanism that depends on incorrect events proceeding more slowly than correct events, so that incorrect events are reversed before a subunit is added to a polymeric chain.

Kirromycin is an antibiotic that inhibits protein synthesis by acting on EF-Tu.

Laser diode thermal desorption (LDTD) source contains an infrared diode laser with an X-Y moveable stage capable of holding one 96-well plate.

Leaky mutations leave some residual function, either because the mutant protein is partially active (in the case of a missense mutation), or because a small amount of wild-type protein is made (in the case of a nonsense mutation).

Library is a set of cloned fragments together representing the entire genome (genomic library) or all the expressed genes (cDNA library).

Ligand is an extracellular molecule that binds to the receptor on the plasma membrane of a cell, thereby effecting a change in the cytoplasm.

Ligase enzyme An enzyme used by genetic engineers to join cut ends of DNA strands.

Linkage describes the tendency of genes to be inherited together as a result of their location on the same chromosome; measured by percent recombination between loci.

Linker any small synthetic single-chain oligodeoxynucleotide that is six or more residues long and has a self-complementary base sequence. When self-annealed it forms a stable duplex with blunt ends and containing a restriction site.

Lipofection are closed, self-sealing, solvent-filled vesicles bound by a single bilayer and possess many properties similar to those of biological membranes. This use of liposomes as a transformation or transfection system is called lipofection.

Liposome Technology uses well recognized liposomes as delivery vehicles that have been developed to enhance the therapeutic activity of several drugs.

Liquid Chromatography (LC) is an analytical chromatographic technique used for separating molecules or ions dissolved in a solvent.

Loop is a single-stranded region at the end of a hairpin in RNA (or single-stranded DNA); it corresponds to the sequence between inverted repeats in duplex DNA.

Loss-of-function mutation inactivates a gene. It is recessive.

Luxury genes are those coding for specialized functions synthesized (usually) in large amounts in particular cell types.

Lysis describes the death of bacteria at the end of a phage infective cycle when they burst open to release the progeny of an infecting phage (because phage enzymes disrupt the bacterium's cytoplasmic membrane or cell wall). The same term also applies to eukaryotic cells; for example, when infected cells are attacked by the immune system. Lysogeny describes the ability of a phage to survive in a bacterium as a stable prophage component of the bacterial genome.

Major histocompatibility complex (MHC) is a chromosomal region containing genes that are involved in the immune response. The genes encode proteins for antigen presentation, cytokines, and complement proteins. The MHC is highly polymorphic.

MALDI is a very fast and sensitive technique, implemented on small, relatively inexpensive instruments that do not require extensive expertise in mass spectrometry.

MAP kinase (MAPK) is a Ser/Thr protein kinase named for its original identification as a mitogen-activated kinase. There is a large group of cytosolic Thr/Ser protein kinases that form several signaling pathways. The name reflects their original isolation as mitogen-activated protein kinases.

Marker assisted backcrossing (MAB) is the process of using the results of DNA tests to assist in the selection of individuals to become the parents in the next generation of a genetic improvement program.

Marker assisted recurrent selection (MARS) It involves crossing in selected individuals at each cycle of crossing and selection.

Marker assisted selection Technology is a complementary technology for use in conjunction with more established conventional methods of genetic section for plant and animal improvement.

Marker gene any gene of known function and known location on a chromosome.

Mass Spectrometry (MS) provides protein structural information like peptide masses or amino acid sequences which can be used to identify the protein by nucleotide and protein databases searching. A mass spectrometer separates proteins and other analytes according to their mass-to-charge (m/z) ratio.

Maternal inheritance describes the preferential survival in the progeny of genetic markers provided by one parent.

Memory cell is a lymphocyte that has been stimulated during the primary immune response to antigen and that is rapidly activated upon subsequent exposure to that antigen. Memory cells respond more rapidly to antigen than naive cells.

Mesenchymal stem cells (MSCs) are self-renewing and multipotent progenitors

Messenger RNA (mRNA) is the intermediate that represents one strand of a gene coding for protein. Its coding region is related to the protein sequence by the triplet genetic code.

Metabolic fingerprinting Unbiased, global screening approach to classify samples based on metabolite patterns or 'fingerprints' that change in response to disease, environmental or

Metabolic footprinting Analysis of extracellular metabolites in cell culture medium as a reflection of metabolite excretion or uptake by cells.

Metabolic profiling Quantitative analysis of set of metabolites in a selected biochemical pathway or a specific class of compounds.

Metabolite A product of biochemical activity.

Metabolomics Technology is the "systematic study of the unique chemical fingerprints that specific cellular processes leave behind"- specifically, the study of their small molecular metabolite profiles.

Metagenomics technology uses a culture independent approach to collect, sort, categorize and identify sequences of microbes retrieved from environmental samples such as soil or water.

Metastasis describes the ability of tumor cells to leave their site of origin and migrate to other locations in the body, where a new colony is established.

Methyltransferase (methylase) is an enzyme that adds a methyl group to a substrate, which can be a small molecule, a protein, or a nucleic acid.

Microarray Technology Microarray is an advanced and high throughput method based on DNA chips, which consists of very high density arrays of short oligonucleotide synthesized on a silicon wafer by a combination of conventional oligonucleotide synthesis chemistry and photolithography.

Microencapsulation Technology is an interesting method of large-scale production of monoclonal antibodies

Micropropagation The use of small pieces of tissue, such as meristem, grown in culture to produce large numbers of plants.

MicroRNAs are very short RNAs that may regulate gene expression.

Microsatellite DNAs consist of repetitions of extremely short (typically <10 bp) units.

Minisatellite DNAs consist of ~10 copies of a short repeating sequence, the length of the repeating unit is measured in 10s of base pairs. The number of repeats varies between individual genomes.

miRNA are the most imported class of endogenous non-coding small RNAs.

Mispairing the occurrence of a base in one polynucleotide strand of duplex DNA that is not complementary to the corresponding base in the second polynucleotide strand.

Missense mutations change a single codon and so may cause the replacement of one amino acid by another in a protein sequence.

Modifier gene *or* modifying gene any gene that affects the phenotypic expression of a gene or genes at other loci.

Molecular Diagnostics Technology Molecular Technology that has been implemented into diagnostic testing is called molecular diagnostics technologies.

Molecular farming is the production of pharmaceutical proteins in transgenic plants.

Molecular Marker Technology has opens exciting now windows through which to view the natural biological world.

Monoclonal antibody An antibody derived from a single source or cone of cells which recognizes only one kind of antigen.

Multiple interval mapping (MIM) It is a multiple-QTL oriented method combining QTL mapping analysis with the analysis of genetic architecture of quantitative traits through a search algorithm to search for number, positions, effects, and interaction of significant QTL.

Multiple Sequence Alignment (MSA) In order to identify the conserved residues, or motifs within many nucleotide/protein sequences, multiple sequence alignment is performed.

Multiplex PCR In multiplex PCR (mPCR), two and more primer pairs specific for different targets are included in the same amplification reaction.

Multipotent cells can give rise to several other cell types, but those types are limited to mostly cells of the blood, heart, muscle and nerves

Muscular Dystrophy (MD) is a collection of disorders caused by genetic defects that lead to increasing muscle weakness over time

Mutagens increase the rate of mutation by inducing changes in DNA sequence, directly or indirectly.

Nano-biotechnology is bridging the gap between inanimate and animate nature and aims at understanding the basic principles of biological functional units as well as creating extremely small components at "nano-scale" in a controlled way with technical materials.

Nested PCR In nested PCR (nPCR), two separate amplifications are used. The first uses a set of primers that yields a larger product, which is then used as a template for the second amplification.

Nick translation a procedure for preparing radioactively labelled DNA, especially for use as probes in hybridization experiments.

Non allelic genes are two (or more) copies of the same gene that are present at *different* locations in the genome (contrasted with alleles which are copies of the same gene derived from different parents and present at the same location on the homologous chromosomes).

Nonsense mutation is any change in DNA that causes a (termination) codon to replace a codon representing an amino acid. A nonsense suppressor is a gene coding for a mutant tRNA able to respond to one or more of the termination codons.

Nopaline plasmids are Ti plasmids of *Agrobacterium tumefaciens* that carry genes for synthesizing the opine, nopaline. They retain the ability to differentiate into early embryonic structures.

Nuclear magnetic resonance (NMR) methods provide metabolite fingerprints with good chemical specificity for compounds containing elements with non zero magnetic moments, such as ^{1}H, ^{13}C, ^{15}N and ^{32}P which are commonly found in most biological metabolites at different levels of low abundance.

Nucleic acid probes technology has been developed that relies on the use of DNA or RNA probes to detect particular gene sequences.

Null mutation completely eliminates the function of a gene, usually because it has been physically deleted.

Oncogenes are genes whose products have the ability to transform eukaryotic cells so that they grow in a manner analogous to tumor cells. Oncogenes carried by retroviruses have names of the form *v-onc.*

Open reading frame (ORF) is a sequence of DNA consisting of triplets that can be translated into amino acids starting with an initiation codon and ending with a termination codon.

Operator is the site on DNA at which a repressor protein binds to prevent transcription from initiating at the adjacent promoter.

Operon is a unit of bacterial gene expression and regulation, including structural genes and control elements in DNA recognized by regulator gene product(s).

Optical-detection Biosensors The output-transduced signal that is measured is light for this type of biosensor.

Orthologs are corresponding proteins in two species as defined by sequence homologies.

Packed bed reactor (PBR) also called plug -flow reactor (PFR), containing a settled bed of immobilized enzyme particles.

Particle gun bombardment A method of introducing DNA into a host plant cell. It involves precipitating DNA onto microscopic particles or projectiles. The particles are then accelerated and penetrate the plant cells, depositing DNA.

PCR Walking allows amplification of DNA with unknown sequences that are present adjoining a known sequence within a DNA fragment.

Phage Display is another technique contributing to proteomics. It involves the creation of peptide or protein libraries on viral surfaces that are screened for activity as a group.

Phasmid a gene-cloning vector consisting of an artificial combination of a plasmid with a phage such that its genome contains functional origins of replication of both; it may thus be propagated either as a plasmid or as a phage in appropriate host strains.

Phosphostaining can also directly be visualized in the gel by using commercially available phosphospecific stains. Phosphostaining is less sensitive method of phosphostains in more convenient than radioactive reagents.

Phylogenetic analysis A phylogenetic or evolutionary tree is composed of branches (edges), nodes and leaves with each leaf representing a protein or gene.

The use of plants for environmental restoration is an emerging cleanup technology to exploit plant potential to remediate soil and water contaminated with a variety of compounds.

Plant transgenic Technology the genetic engineering of plants by inserting a foreign DNA-segregate into the plant genome is called transgenesis and the developed plant a transgenic plant.

Plaque is an area of clearing in a bacterial lawn. It is created by a single phage particle that has undergone multiple rounds of lytic growth.

Plasmid is a circular, extra chromosomal DNA. It is autonomous and can replicate itself.

Pluripotent cells This type of stem cell has the ability to become almost any kind of cells in the body-except the cells of the placenta or other supporting tissues of the uterus. Pluripotent stem cells results after totipotent stem cells undergo the first few divisions.

Point mutation is a change in the sequence of DNA involving a single base pair.

Polonator This system is similar to AB SoLid system in that emulsion PCR is used for clonal amplification of DNA fragments and sequencing is done with the help of DNA ligase.

Polyacrylamide gel electrophoresis is a technique of zone electrophoresis that uses polyacrylamide gel as supporting medium.

Polycation-mediated DNA uptake Direct DNA uptake by protoplasts can be stimulated by using extremely hydrophilic, high molecular weight, long chain polycations such as PEG with or without metal ions such as Zn^{2+}, Li^{+}, Cs^{+}, Rb^{+}, K^{+}, Na^{+}, Ca^{2+} or Mg^{2+}.

Polyclonal antibody an antibody that arises from the immune response to an immunogen. Each epitope on the immunogen has the potential for causing the formation of a clone of B lymphocytes each capable of synthesizing an antibody specific to the particular epitope.

Polymerase chain reaction (PCR) The action of an enzyme (polymerase) in producing many copies of a polynucleotide sequence of DNA.

Polymorphism (more fully genetic polymorphism) refers to the simultaneous occurrence in the population of genomes showing variations at a given position. The original definition applied to alleles producing different phenotypes. Now it is also used to describe changes in DNA affecting the restriction pattern or even the sequence. For practical purposes, to be considered as an example of a polymorphism, an allele should be found at a frequency > 1 % in the population.

Position effect variegation (PEV) is silencing of gene expression that occurs as the result of proximity to heterochromatin.

Potentiometric In this type of sensor the measured parameter is oxidation or reduction potential of an electrochemical reaction.

Primary immune response is an organism's immune response upon first exposure to a given antigen. It is characterized by a relatively shorter duration and lower affinity antibodies than in the secondary immune response.

Primer is a short sequence (often of RNA) that is paired with one strand of DNA and provides a free 3'-OH end at which a DNA polymerase starts synthesis of a deoxyribonucleotide chain.
Prion is a proteinaceous infectious agent, which behaves as an inheritable trait, although it contains no nucleic acid. Examples are PrPSc, the agent of scrapie in sheep and bovine spongiform encephalopathy, and Psi, which confers an inherited state in yeast.
Promoter is a region of DNA where RNA polymerase binds to initiate transcription.
Proofreading refers to any mechanism for correcting errors in protein or nucleic acid synthesis that involves scrutiny of individual units *after* they have been added to the chain.
Protein Engineering is the process of developing useful or valuable proteins.
Protein sorting (targeting) is the direction of different types of proteins for transport into or between specific organelles.
Proteome The collective body of proteins made within an organism's cells and tissues.
Proteomics Technology is an interdisciplinary science that includes biology and protein chemistry.
Protoplast A microbial or plant cell whose wall has been removed so that the cell assumes a spherical shape..
Provirus is a duplex sequence of DNA integrated into a eukaryotic genome that represents the sequence of the RNA genome of a retrovirus.
Pseudogenes are inactive but stable components of the genome derived by mutation of an ancestral active gene. Usually they are inactive because of mutations that block transcription or translation or both.
Pyrimidine dimer is formed when ultraviolet irradiation generates a covalent link directly between two adjacent pyrimidine bases in DNA. It blocks DNA replication.
Pyrosequencing is an alternative to the traditional Sanger method for *de novo* DNA sequencing that allow sequencing of up to hundred bases.

QTL Mapping is defined as 'a region of the genome that is associated with an effect on a quantitative trait.
Quantitative PCR involves co-amplification of two templates: a constant amount of a preparation containing the desired target sequence and serial dilutions of a reference template that is added in known amount to a series of amplification reactions.
Quantum Dots (QDs) represent a class of most used and promising nanostructures available for diagnostic applications.

RACE *abbr. for* rapid amplification of cDNA ends; a variation on the polymerase chain reaction designed for amplification of cDNA corresponding to low-abundance mRNA.
Radioactive isotope any isotope of a chemical element whose nucleus is unstable and emits alpha, beta, or gamma rays.

Radioimmunoassay is an alternative for cancer-therapy. In this, the monoclonal antibody is coupled to a radioisotope such that the cancer cell is killed by irradiation.

RAPD PCR *abbr. for* random polymorphic DNA PCR; a variation of the polymerase chain reaction in which many short (=40 nucleotide) primers are used. The products of the reaction from different sources can lead to recognition of polymorphisms and physical maps.

Reading frame is one of the three possible ways of reading a nucleotide sequence. Each reading frame divides the sequence into a series of successive triplets. There are three possible reading frames in any sequence, depending on the starting point. If the first frame starts at position 1, the second frame starts at position 2, and the third frame starts at position 3.

Real-time PCR (qRT-PCR) is used for the quantification of nucleic acid.

Recombinant clone a population of bacteria or other host derived from a single cell into which a vector containing recombinant DNA has been introduced.

Recombinant DNA The hybrid DNA produced by joining pieces of DNA from different organisms. Recombinant DNA Technologies is a set of molecular techniques for locating, isolating, altering and studying DNA segments.

Red Biotechnology is applied to medical processes.

Redundancy describes the concept that two or more genes may fulfill the same function, so that no single one of them is essential.

Regulator gene codes for a product (typically protein) that controls the expression of other genes (usually at the level of transcription).

Repetitive DNA behaves in a reassociation reaction as though many (related or identical) sequences are present in a component, allowing any pair of complementary sequences to reassociate.

Reporter gene a gene used to disclose the function of potential regulatory sequences. The sequences are placed in plasmids, upstream of the reporter gene; these chimeric plasmids are then introduced into cells and the expression of the reporter gene is measured as an index of the function of the regulatory sequences under the conditions being investigated.

Repression the act of inhibiting gene expression. An example is catabolite repression of the *lac* operon by glucose, mediated through binding of cyclic AMP to catabolite (gene) activator protein (CAP).

Resonance Light Scattering (RLS) technique is utilized in generating strong visual signals when incident light is scattered by metallic nanoparticles of uniform size like gold or silver.

Resonant Biosensors (Acoustic/Mechanical Sensors) In this type of biosensor, an acoustic wave transducer is coupled with an antibody (bio-element).

Restriction enzyme An enzyme used by molecular biologists to cut through DNA at specific points.

Restriction fragment length polymorphism (RFLP) Fragments of differing lengths of DNA that are produced by cutting DNA with restriction enzymes.

Restriction mapping It locates the relative positions of restriction sites for various restriction endonucleases on a DNA fragment.

Reverse mutation a heritable change in a mutant gene that restores a nucleotide sequence to that which obtained prior to mutation.

Reverse transcription is synthesis of DNA on a template of RNA; accomplished by reverse transcriptase enzyme.

Ri plasmids are found in *Agrobacterium tumefaciens.* Like Ti plasmids, they carry genes that cause disease in infected plants. The disease may take the form of either hairy root disease or crown gall disease.

Ribonucleases (RNAases) are enzymes that cleave RNA. They may be specific for single-stranded or for double-stranded RNA, and may be either endonucleases or exonucleases.

Ribozyme an RNA molecule with catalytic activity. Such activity was first discovered by Sidney Altman in 1981 for RNase P. Thomas R. Cech in 1982 discovered the catalysis by RNA of the reactions involved in the splicing of ribosomal RNA from *Tetrahymena.*

RNA editing describes a change of sequence at the level of RNA following transcription.

RNA Induced Silencing Complex The sRNAs provide specificity of the targets in a sequence-dependent manner while the enzymatic machinery called RISC (RNA Induced Silencing Complex) is responsible for the degradation or translation repression of the target mRNA.

RNA interference Some alternate names of RNA interference are PTGS (Post Transcriptional Gene Silencing), VIGS (Virus Induced Gene Silencing) and co suppression in plants, Quelling in fungi, and RNAi in animals.

RNA ligase is an enzyme that functions in tRNA splicing to make a phosphodiester bond between the two exon sequences that are generated by cleavage of the intron.

RNA polymerases are enzymes that synthesize RNA using a DNA template (formally described as DNA-dependent RNA polymerases).

RNA splicing is the process of excising the sequences in RNA that correspond to introns, so that the sequences corresponding to exons are connected into a continuous mRNA.

RNAi pathway The RNAi pathway is initiated by the enzyme dicer, which cleaves long, dsRNA molecules into short double stranded fragments of ranging from 21–24 bp (or even higher) in length.

S

S1 mapping *or* St **nuclease mapping** a commonly used technique depending on the property of S1 nuclease to remove single-stranded DNA or RNA from double-stranded hybrids of DNA and RNA.

Satellite DNA (simple-sequence DNA) consists of many tandem repeats (identical or related) of a short basic repeating unit.

Scale-up The expansion of laboratory experiments to full-sized industrial processes.

Secondary immune response is an organism's immune response upon a second exposure to a given antigen. This second exposure is also referred to as a "booster". The secondary immune response is characterized by a more rapid induction, greater magnitude, and higher affinity antibodies than the primary immune response.

Secondary messenger is a small molecule that is generated when a signal transduction pathway is activated. The classic second messenger is cyclic AMP, which is generated when adenylate cyclase is activated by a G protein (when the G protein itself was activated by a transmembrane receptor).

Selfish DNA describes sequences that do not contribute to the genotype of the organism but have self-perpetuation within the genome as their sole function.

Senescent cells show visible changes in the appearance of a culture as the result of limitations posed by telomere shortening on the number of chromosomal replications that can occur.

Sequence-Tagged Sites (STS) RFLP markers linked to a desired trait can be converted into PCR-based STS markers based on nucleotide sequence of the probe giving polymorphic band pattern, or amplicons specific to different genotypes.

Serial analysis of gene expression (SAGE) technology is based on the principle that a 10-bp cDNA fragment, the tag, contains sufficient information to unambiguously identify a transcript, provided that the tag has been isolated from a defined position within transcript.

Shotgun approach Whole genome shotgun is another widely used strategy for genome sequencing.

Shotgunning Theoretically it is possible to clone any desired gene in one organism from another organism by the technique known as shotgunning.

Shuttle vector a DNA molecule, e.g. a plasmid, that is able to replicate in two different host organisms and can therefore be used to 'shuttle' or convey genes from one to the other.

Signal transduction describes the process by which a receptor interacts with a ligand at the surface of the cell and then transmits a signal to trigger a pathway within the cell.

Signalomics Technology the goal of signalomics technology is to track down faculty cellular signal proteins and to develop custom-made therapeutics and diagnostics for complex illness that result from errors in cellular signal transduction.

Signature *an alternative term for* motif (in protein sequences); the word is used in the PRINTS database.

Silencing describes the repression of gene expression in a localized region, usually as the result of a structural change in chromatin.

Single cell protein Cells or protein extracts of microorganisms grown in large quantities for use as human or animal protein supplements.

Single Nucleotide Polymorphism (SNP) is the ultimate DNA markers consisting of a single base substitution within a given segment of DNA between two individuals.

Single-strand conformation polymorphism analysis *abbr.:* SSCP analysis; a method for comparing mutations by the rate at which DNA migrates on denaturing gels, under conditions in which the conformation adopted by the DNA is critical.

siRNAs are 21-24 nt long sequences that are generally produced from cleavage of exogenous long dsRNA precursors by the RNase III endonuclease, Dicer or DCL.

Somatic cell hybrid a hybrid cell formed from the fusion of different cells, usually from different species. Somatic cell hybrids obtained by the fusion of human and rodent cells are frequently used for gene mapping.

Somatic cell hybrid technology This has been utilized for selecting the specific human chromosome. A specific human chromosome can be selected by fusing the human cell with the rodent cell.

Southern blotting a procedure for transferring denatured DNA from an agarose gel to a solid support membrane such as nitrocellulose or nylon.

Southwestern Blotting is an interesting technique used to study DNA-protein interaction through which the molecular weight of an unknown DNA binding factor can be inferred and hence has an advantage over EMSA, foot priming and other related techniques.

Stem cell technology deals with stem cells that are characterized by the ability to renew themselves through mitotic cell division an able to differentiate into a diverse range of specialized cell types.

Sterility the inability to produce functional gametes, either egg cells, or sperm cells in pollen grains. Male sterility can be cytoplasmic or nuclear in origin; cytoplasmic male sterility involves a factor coded in the mitochondrial genome.

Stirred tank batch reactor (STR) It contains all of the enzyme and substrates) until the conversion is complete.

Stop codon (termination codon) is one of three triplets (UAG, UAA, UGA) that cause protein synthesis to terminate. They are also known historically as *nonsense codons.* The UAA codon is called ochre, and the UAA codon as called amber, after the names of the nonsense mutations by which they were originally identified.

A database of known and predicted protein-protein interactions.

Structural genomics includes construction of high resolution genetic and physical map, determination of complete genome sequence and determination of structures of protein encoded by the genes.

Super family is a set of genes a related by presumed descent from a common ancestor, but now showing considerable variation.

Superbug Ananda Chakrabarty (1979) an India born American scientist, created a single such strain of Pseudomonas that would be able to contain all the genes responsible for oil consumption and thus mop up all the types of hydrocarbon in the oil. This unique bacterial strain, the product of genetic engineering, is called a "superbug".

Suppression describes the occurrence of changes that eliminate the effects of a mutation without reversing the original change in DNA.

Surface plasmon resonance is a phenomenon in which intensity of reflected light decreases when an incident light beam falls on metal surface (gold or silver) at a particular angle.

Surface-enhanced laser desorption ionization (SELDI) mass spectrometry is an ultra high throughput screening system for protein purification, expression profiling or protein interaction profiling.

Symbiosis a relationship between two contrasting organisms showing interdependence rather than exploitation, such as insects taking nectar and/or pollen from flowers, but bringing about pollination; or nitrogen-fixing bacteria living in the security of nodules on roots, exchanging ammonium ions for metabolites and shelter.

Synthetic Biological technology deals with the design and construction of new biological entities, such as enzymes, genetic circuits and cells or the redesign of existing biological systems.

Synthetic Gene cloning An alternative way of avoiding the problem of introns is to synthesize an artificial gene in the test tube starting with deoxyribonucleotides.

Synzymes A number of possibilities now exists for the construction of artificial enzymes. These are generally synthetic polymers or oligomers with enzyme-like activities, often called synzymes that can be immobilized on solid support.

System Biology Technology aims at understanding biological systems at system level.

T cells are lymphocytes of the T (thymic) lineage; may be subdivided into several functional types. They carry TcR (T-cell receptor) and are involved in the cell-mediated immune response.

Tag DNA polymerase a heat-stable DNA polymerase from *Thermus aquaticus,* a thermophilic bacterium. It is used in the polymerase chain reaction.

Tandem Mass Spectrometry (MS/MS) is basically the connection of two MS in series. It provides amino acid sequence information on peptide fragments of the parent protein.

T-DNA is the segment of the Ti plasmid of *Agrobacterium tumefaciens* that is transferred to the plant cell nucleus during infection. It carries genes that transform the plant cell.

Thermal-detection Biosensors (Calorimetric Sensors) This type of biosensor is exploiting one of the fundamental properties of biological reactions, namely absorption or production of heat, which in turn changes the temperature of the medium in which the reaction takes place.

Ti plasmid is an episome of the bacterium *Agrobacterium tumefaciens* that carries the genes responsible for the induction of crown gall disease in infected plants.

Tissue culture A process whereby individual cells, or clumps of plant or animal tissue, are grown artificially.

Totipotent cell These stem cells have the potential to become any kind of cell in the body.

Touchdown PCR is a method used to increase specificity without compromising yield.

Toxicogenomics The goal of toxicogenomics is to find correlations between toxic responses to toxicants and changes in the genetic profiles of the objects exposed to such toxicants.
Toxicological research The goal of toxicogenomics is to find correlations between toxic responses to toxicants and changes in the genetic profiles of the objects exposed to such toxicants.
Transcription describes synthesis of RNA on a DNA template. A transcription factor is required for RNA polymerase to initiate transcription at specific promoter(s), but is not itself part of the enzyme.
Transcriptome is the complete set of RNAs present in a cell, tissue, or organism. Its complexity is due mostly to mRNAs, but it also includes non-coding RNAs.
Transduction The transfer of bacterial genes from one bacterium to another by a virus (bacteriophage).
TRANSFAC A database on transcriptional regulation in eukaryotes, with documentation of transcription factor properties, their genomic and artificial binding sequences, and DNA binding profiles.
Transfer RNA (tRNA) is the intermediate in protein synthesis that interprets the genetic code. Each tRNA can be linked to an amino acid. The tRNA has an anticodon sequence that complementary to a triplet codon representing the amino acid.
Transformation of bacteria describes the acquisition of new genetic markers by incorporation of added DNA.
Transgene is a gene that is introduced into a cell or animal from an external source.**Transgenic** plant a plant that has been transformed by incorporation of a construct that includes a gene or genes from another species of plant, or any other kind of living organism, or a virus.
Translation the process by which a particular sequence of bases in messenger RNA (mRNA) determines a sequence of amino acids in the polypeptide chain being assembled during protein and peptide biosynthesis.
TRANSPATH A database on regulatory network information, mostly in human, mouse and rat cells, originally focusing on signal transduction pathways that aim at gene regulatory molecules (transcription factors), but increasingly expanding to metabolic enzymes and structural proteins as targets.
Transposon (transposable element) is a DNA sequence able to insert itself at a new location in the genome, without having any sequence relationship with the target locus.
Two-dimensional polyacrylamide gel electrophoresis (2-DE) separates proteins based on two parameters, isoelectric point (pI) in the first dimension and molecular size in the second dimension.

Ultrasonication The latest method developed for plant transformation uses ultrasound to facilitate the uptake of nucleic acids into plant cells.
Unipotent A unipotent stem cell refers to a cell that can differentiate along only one lineage.

Untranslated region (UTR) any part of an mRNA molecule not coding for a protein; e.g. in eukaryotes the poly (A) tail.

Upstream identifies sequences proceeding in the opposite direction from expression; for example, the bacterial promoter is upstream of the transcription unit, the initiation codon is upstream of the coding region.

Vaccine is a preparation containing a pathogen (disease-producing organism) either in attenuated or inactivated state.

Vaccine technology deals with the vaccines that are designed for human or veterinary use to prime the immune systems to produce antibodies or cellular responses that ward off future challenge by pathogenic organisms or their toxins.

Variable number tandem repeats *abbr.*: VNTR; a multiallelic DNA polymorphism that results from insertions or deletions of DNA between two restriction sites. The existence of these repeats is exploited in genetic profiling.

Variable region (V region) of an immunoglobulin chain is coded by the V gene and varies extensively when different chains are compared, as the result of multiple (different) genomic copies and changes introduced during construction of an active immunogl obulin.

Variety a distinct type within a species, equivalent to cultivar for cultivated plants.

Vector A vehicle for transferring DNA from one cell to another.

Vermiculture is the process of using worms to decompose organic waste into a material capable of supplying necessary nutrients to help sustain plant growth.

Vesicular Arbuscular Mycorrhiza (VAM) is the most abundant kind of mycorrhiza described as a universal plant symbiosis.

Virion is the physical virus particle (irrespective of its ability to infect cells and reproduce).

Viroid is a small infectious nucleic acid that does not have a protein coat.

Vitrification is a physical process by which a solution is transformed into a stable amorphous glass by rapid cooling, bypassing ice crystal formation while maintaining the properties of liquid in a solidified form.

Western blotting a technique for blotting proteins onto nitrocellulose, nylon, or other transfer membrane after they have been resolved by gel electrophoresis.

White Biotechnology (industrial biotechnology) is biotechnology that applied to industrial processes.

Winding number the number of double-helical turns in a closed-circular DNA measured relative to a surface on which the DNA helix lies.

Wobble hypothesis accounts for the ability of a tRNA to recognize more than one codon by unusual (non-G-C, non-A-T) pairing with the third base of a codon.

Xenobiotic is applied to synthetic chemical compounds, those that are so alien and novel that living organisms may have no previous exposure to anything like them in the course of their evolution, or if such exposure occurred, it was so long ago that the enzymatic capacity to modify such compounds has been lost. They often successfully challenge and overcome our detoxifying enzyme systems and immunological defences, so causing cancers.

Xenobiotics are such synthetic (man-made) organic compounds that are foreign to existing biological system.

X-gal *abbr. for* 5-bromo-4-chloro-3-indolyl-B-D-galactoside, a colourless substrate that is hydrolysed by ?- galactosidase to a blue product. It is used with cloning vectors containing part of the *lacZ* gene to select recombinants in molecular cloning: the peptide produced by the *lacZ* fragment complements the defective ? -galactosidase enzyme in host cells. Insertion of foreign DNA into the vector inactivates the *lacZ* gene, so host cells containing recombinant plasmids will grow as white colonies on medium containing X-gal, whereas host cells containing 'empty' vectors will have a functional ?-galactosidase and thus produce blue colonies.

Yeast artificial chromosome *abbr.:* YAC; a specialized cloning vector that contains a centromere, an autonomously replicating sequence (ARS), a pair of telomeres, selectable marker genes, and the fragment of DNA to be cloned.

Yeast one hybrid system has been developed to trap specific DNA binding protein and is a modification of yeast two hybrid system which is generally used to study the protein-protein interaction.

Yeast two hybrid system In Yeast two hybrid systems, the transcriptional activation of a reporter gene is used as a principle to screen the interacting proteins.

Zinc finger a polypeptide motif present in many DNA-binding proteins and having the consensus sequence.

INDEX

Q

R

S